Women's Health Care

Women's Health Care

A COMPREHENSIVE HANDBOOK

Edited by

CATHERINE INGRAM FOGEL
NANCY FUGATE WOODS

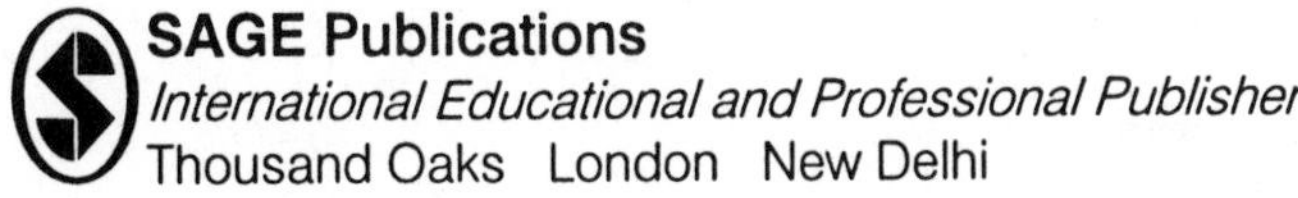
SAGE Publications
International Educational and Professional Publisher
Thousand Oaks London New Delhi

For information address:

SAGE Publications, Inc.
2455 Teller Road
Thousand Oaks, California 91320

SAGE Publications Ltd.
6 Bonhill Street
London EC2A 4PU
United Kingdom

SAGE Publications India Pvt. Ltd.
M-32 Market
Greater Kailash I
New Delhi 110 048 India

Printed in the United States of America

Library of Congress Cataloging-in-Publication Data

Main entry under title:

Women's health care: A comprehensive handbook / edited by Catherine
Ingram Fogel, Nancy Fugate Woods.
p. cm.
Includes bibliographical references and index.
ISBN 0-8039-7022-6.—ISBN 0-8039-7023-4 (pbk.: alk. paper)
1. Women—Health and hygiene. 2. Women's health services—Social aspects. 3. Women—Health and hygiene—Sociological aspects.
I. Fogel, Catherine Ingram, 1941- . II. Woods, Nancy Fugate.
RA564.85.W66684 1995
613′.04244—dc20 94-36836

This book is printed on acid-free paper.

95 96 97 98 99 10 9 8 7 6 5 4 3 2 1

Sage Production Editor: Diane S. Foster

Contents

Part II

Part III

Part IV

Preface

The health of women is inextricably linked to the nature of their lives. Only recently, however, have health scientists and practitioners acknowledged the importance of women's lived experiences for their well-being. The feminist movement and the women's health movement of the 1960s and 1970s prompted critical analysis of women's health and its relationship to the society and women's health care options. Together these social movements gave voice to women's increasing dissatisfaction with health services and prompted the creation of alternative services that reflected new values about women and allowed them to reclaim control over their bodies and assume responsibility for their health. During this same period, the nursing profession, largely composed of women, began to recognize that many assumptions that had limited women's opportunities had also limited those of the nursing profession. As a result of the women's health movement, nurses began to address problems of sexism as they affected the nursing profession and women who sought health care.

The 1980s saw a rapid development of nursing literature focusing on women's health problems, with some works examining women's health from a feminist perspective. The purpose of this text is to inform health professionals, especially practitioners of nursing, about the complex nature of women's health. The book contains an overview of topics and issues that influence women's health in contemporary society. Women's health can no longer be described as synonymous with reproductive health care, yet reproduction and reproductive health problems are central to many women's lives. Therefore this book incorporates several dimensions of women's health in an effort to support the practices of students and practitioners in a wide range of clinical settings, spanning community- and hospital-based practices, health maintenance organizations, and alternative health centers.

Part I focuses on the connections between women's lives and women's health. This section begins with an examination of the paradoxical relationship between gender and health and use of health services. Although women report more sickness and use health services more frequently than men, they experience a significant advantage: a longer life span. Several explanations for this paradox are explored, including biological and social differences between women and men. Women have been engaged in providing health care for themselves and their families since the beginning of recorded history, yet only certain aspects of health care have come to be viewed as women's work. Stratification by gender, ethnicity, and social class will be examined in relation to the health professions.

Women's bodies possess unique strengths and capabilities related to their sexuality and reproduction; these unique characteristics commonly become the target for discrimination and the basis for sexist interpretations affecting women's lives. Only recently has women's development throughout the life cycle attracted the attention of behavioral and social scientists. Revisionist theories about women's moral development, intellectual development, and social role development have illuminated the lives of women in new ways. Midlife and older women have been ignored or subjected to the doubly damaging effects of sexism and ageism, both of which severely limit women's chances for health.

Part II of the book addresses nursing practice with women. This section begins with an examination of women's experiences as recipients of health care. Sexism in the delivery of health services is examined, as are women's health care worlds. Conceptual frameworks for nursing practice that address the complexity of women's health and reflect contemporary views of nursing practice are proposed. Health assessment for well women provides a basis for considering health promotion, prevention, and maintenance strategies for women. Lesbians frequently encounter lack of understanding of their sexual orientation and lifestyle in their encounters with health professionals. The health problems and concerns of lesbians are examined.

Part III focuses on health promotion for women. Current theory and research on health promotion for women are summarized in a series of chapters addressing nutrition, exercise, fertility control, mental health, health in the workplace, and childbearing choices.

Part IV examines common health problems women experience. Violence against women results in rape and sexual assault, including spousal and date assault. In addition, women commonly are the victims of incest and pornography. Women's sexual behavior may also result in unplanned pregnancy and the challenge of deciding whether to carry the pregnancy or terminate it. Women's sexual experiences may be sources of pleasure as well as pain. Sexual concerns and dysfunctions related to sexual desire, arousal, and orgasm and their causes and therapies are discussed. Substance abuse creates significant challenges to women's health, and their unique needs for programs that aid their recovery merit special attention. Although childbirth is commonly regarded as a normal part of women's lives, infertility and high-risk pregnancy represent special challenges to women's health. Symptoms such as pain, vaginal discharge, and bleeding occur commonly, cause women great concern, and prompt them to seek health care. Both their significance to women and their clinical significance and treatment are explored. Common infections, including sexually transmitted diseases and AIDS are also explored. Reproductive surgery represents a major cause of hospitalization for women. Assuming she controls her fertility, the woman who experiences either infertility or unintended pregnancy has her assumptive world and well-being challenged. Special emphasis is given to tubal ligation and hysterectomy and their significance to women's lives. Chronic illnesses such as heart disease, cancer, diabetes, and arthritis challenge the quality of women's lives. Living with these and other chronic health problems and being differently abled will be addressed. Problems related to breast health are examined with a focus on early detection of malignancies and selecting treatment options. While advancements in reproductive technology offer women expanded options for becoming parents, they also present significant challenges, including complicated decisions for women and their partners.

In conclusion, this volume addresses many significant topics for contemporary women and their health care providers. We believe it will be a useful text and reference for students in undergraduate and graduate programs in nursing and for nurses, clinical specialists, and nurse practitioners who care for women.

We thank the many women in our lives who helped to bring this project to fruition, and we dedicate our work to them.

Catherine Ingram Fogel
Nancy Fugate Woods

PART I

1

Women and Their Health

NANCY FUGATE WOODS

The Paradox

One of the most fascinating observations recorded in the annals of health and disease is the paradoxical relationship between morbidity (sickness) and mortality (death) for women and men. Although mortality rates for most causes of death are lower for women than for men, and women in the Western world live longer than men, women report more morbidity and use health services at higher rates than men do.

The purposes of this chapter are to (a) explore sex differences in mortality, morbidity, and the use of health services as well as the factors responsible for these differences; (b) examine patterns of health and illness for women with special consideration of the intersection of gender, race, and class; and (c) consider future prospects for women's health.

Mortality: Comparison of Death Rates for Women and Men

Life Expectancy and Mortality Patterns

In the United States, life expectancy for white women is now approximately 79 years, and for black women it is 73.4 years (National Center for Health Statistics [NCHS], 1993b). Although this may be seen as a reflection of advanced health care technology, life expectancy for women is lower in the United States than in 15 other developed countries (see Table 1.1). In general, women in developed countries live longer than men.

During this century, life expectancy increased significantly for all Americans, regardless of race or gender. During the first half of the century, increases in life expectancy were attributable to reduction in infant and childhood mortality, and in the second half, increases in longevity are attributable to decreasing mortality from chronic disease among middle-aged and elderly persons. White women have the longest life expectancy,

Table 1.1 Life Expectancy at Birth, According to Sex: Selected Countries, 1989 (in years)

Country	*Women*	*Men*
Japan	82.5	76.2
France	81.5	73.1
Switzerland	81.3	74.1
Netherlands	81.1	73.7
Canada	80.6	73.7
Spain	80.3	73.6
Sweden	80.1	74.2
Hong Kong	80.1	74.3
Norway	80.0	73.3
Italy	79.9	73.3
Australia	79.6	73.3
Greece	79.4	74.3
Federal Republic of Germany	79.2	72.6
Finland	79.0	70.9
Austria	78.9	72.1
United States	78.6	71.8
England and Wales	78.4	72.9
Portugal	78.2	71.1
Belgium	78.2	71.4
Denmark	77.9	72.2

SOURCE: National Center for Health Statistics (1993b, tab. 26, pp. 42-43).

and black women began surpassing white men in life expectancy around 1970. Racial differences in life expectancy have narrowed. Now white women live about 5 years longer than black women, and white men live about 6 years longer than black men.

Although more male than female infants are born alive (in a ratio of 106:100) death rates for males exceed those for females at all ages. Moreover, death rates for women and men became more divergent from the 1950s until the 1970s, when the divergence in death rates slowed. The steady increase in the sex differential favoring women between 1900 and 1970 can be attributed to decreasing mortality rates for diseases affecting only women, such as maternal mortality, and increasing mortality rates for diseases affecting mostly men, such as cancer of the lung and heart disease (Wingard, 1982). The sex differences in mortality have stabilized because of increases in some rates for women and decreases in others. For example, lung cancer mortality increased more rapidly for women than for men, thus decreasing the sex differential in lung cancer mortality (Verbrugge, 1980).

Causes of Death

Leading causes of death in the United States have changed since 1900, when infectious disease, such as tuberculosis, claimed the greatest number of lives. In 1985, the leading cause of death was heart disease, with cancer and cerebrovascular disease the second and third leading causes of death. People now survive infectious disease to live to middle and old age, in which they develop chronic diseases.

Table 1.2 displays the most prevalent causes of death for women throughout the adult years. Death rates increase for most causes with increasing age of the population groups. In nearly every case, death rates for men exceed those for women.

Explanations for Sex Differences in Mortality

A number of explanations have been proposed to account for sex differentials in mortality patterns observed both in the United States and in other countries. These include differences in biology, technological advances in health care, stress exposures and responses, and lifestyle.

Table 1.2 Leading Causes of Death for Women (per 100,000) Across the Life Span, 1986

Age Groups							
15-24	*25-34*	*35-44*	*45-54*	*55-64*	*65-74*	*75-84*	*85 and Older*
Accidents	Accidents	Malignant neoplasms	Malignant neoplasms	Malignant neoplasms	Heart disease	Heart disease	Heart disease
23.3	15.9	49.7	160.7	373.6	724.2	2,196.9	6,889
Homicide	Malignant neoplasms	Heart disease	Heart disease	Heart disease	Malignant neoplasms	Malignant neoplasms	Cerebro-vascular disease
6.1	12.8	17.7	72.1	244.1	657.6	954.2	1,804.6
Suicide	Homicide	Accidents	Cerebro-vascular disease	Cerebro-vascular disease	Cerebro-vascular disease	Cerebro-vascular disease	Malignant neoplasms
4.4	6.7	14.1	19.1	46.8	147.6	540.7	1,277.2
Malignant neoplasms	Suicide	Suicide	Accidents	Chronic obstructive pulmonary disease	Chronic obstructive pulmonary disease	Pneumonia	Pneumonia
4.2	5.9	7.6	15.1	36.4	100.5	183.4	902.3
Heart disease	Heart disease	Cerebro-vascular disease	Liver disease	Pneumonia	Pneumonia	Chronic obstructive pulmonary disease	Chronic obstructive pulmonary disease
2.1	5.5	6.5	12.2	12.6	40.3	171.2	211.9
Cerebro-vascular disease	Cerebro-vascular disease	Liver disease	Suicide	Diabetes	Diabetes	Diabetes	Diabetes
0.6	2.2	5.4	8.8	25.5	58.9	122.0	216
Pneumonia	Liver disease	Homicide	Chronic obstructive pulmonary disease	Liver disease	Accidents	Accidents	Accidents
0.6	1.8	4.8	8.7	20.7	35.2	83.3	211.9
Chronic obstructive pulmonary disease	Pneumonia	Diabetes	Diabetes	Accidents	Liver disease	Liver disease	Liver disease
0.4	1.3	2.9	8.7	20.7	25.6	23.9	15.8
Diabetes	Diabetes	Pneumonia	Pneumonia	Suicide	Suicide	Suicide	Suicide
0.4	1.3	2.5	5.0	8.4	7.2	7.5	4.7
Liver disease	Chronic obstructive pulmonary disease	Chronic obstructive pulmonary disease	Homicide	Homicide	Homicide	Homicide	Homicide
0.1	0.6	1.5	3.5	2.4	2.8	3.5	4.0

SOURCE: National Center for Health Statistics (1988b).

Biology. Because the inferior longevity of men is nearly universal in humans, sex differences in mortality have been linked to biological differences between women and men. These differences include genetic makeup, sex hormone elaboration, neuroendocrine effects, and immune system function.

At conception, the ratio of males to females has been estimated at 115 to 100, whereas the sex ratio at birth is usually between 103 to 106.

The mortality difference seems to be accounted for only in part by genetic determinants, and the in utero mortality and postnatal mortality for males may be from different causes (Neel, 1990).

Possible relationships between genes on the sex chromosomes and longevity have prompted studies of the genes on the *X* and *Y* chromosomes that may be critical to longevity. Any essential function mapped on the *X* chromosome, not duplicated elsewhere, could confer greater longevity to women. This would place men at a disadvantage because they have only one *X* chromosome. During most of their lives, women do not express the genes on both of their *X* chromosomes due to *X*-inactivation. Inactivation of one *X* chromosome in each cell occurs early in female development to achieve balanced gene dosage. This process may negate some of the female longevity based on the female genotype. Because biosynthetic defects in some cells can be compensated by neighboring cells with the other *X* chromosome active, however, the fact that women have a mosaic of cells influenced randomly by both *X* chromosomes may provide a survival advantage. Mosaicism means that cell selection is possible, and this selection process could be adaptive, thus contributing to the gender longevity difference (Gartler, 1990). Steroid hormones, particularly estrogen, play a role in the sex differential in human longevity. The presence of estrogen in premenopausal years appears to reduce risk from cardiovascular disease associated with high low-density lipoprotein (LDL) cholesterol levels and low high-density lipoprotein (HDL) levels, whereas androgen has the opposite effect (Hazzard, 1990). Animal studies reveal that young females produce more autoantibodies, monoclonal immunoglobulins, and more specific antibody after immunization with foreign antigens. Moreover, they reject skin grafts more actively and have greater T lymphocyte proliferative responses than do T cells from young male animals. There is speculation that heightened immune activity of females may be related to longer survival of women because of their greater immune function (Weksler, 1990). Questions that remain are what genes on the *X* and *Y* chromosomes may contribute directly to longevity, how the expression of these genes is related, whether there are age-related differences in expression, what biological functions other than sex determination are influenced by sex hormones, and what role immune responsiveness plays in health in later life (Smith & Warner, 1990).

Despite lack of understanding of the mechanisms by which genetic differences influence mortality differentials, it is most likely that genetic, hormonal, neuroendocrine, and immune functional differences act together in complex ways. Waldron (1983) estimated that deaths from these genetically linked conditions account for less than 2% of the excess deaths experienced by men during their adult years. However, genetic differences may account for a greater proportion of the sex differences in infant mortality (Naeye, Burt, Wright, & Associates, 1971) and for the greater susceptibility of male infants and children to infectious diseases (Michaels & Rogers, 1971). Greater resistance to infection for female infants and children may be linked to the *X* chromosome, which carries genes for the production of immunoglobulin M, resulting in higher serum levels for female infants and children (Goble & Konapka, 1973). Also, the *X* chromosome is thought to permit greater options for variability in women than in men because one of women's *X* chromosomes may be active in some cells and the other in different cells, thus permitting more variation (Naeye et al., 1971). Hormonal differences may also account for some of the sex differences in mortality. Stimulation of phagocytosis by macrophages is enhanced by estrogen and progesterone, thus affording women an advantageous response to infectious organisms (Vernon-Roberts, 1969).

In past years, reproduction accounted for high mortality among women of childbearing age. Because this is no longer the case in developed countries, reproductive mortality does not play a major role in explaining sex differences in mortality.

The increases in mortality advantage for women observed over this century cannot be accounted for solely by biology, because genetic variation occurs too slowly for biological differences to have occurred within this time period (Retherford, 1975). Variability in mortality rates for women and men during the adult years suggests that other factors, such as changes in the environment, are most likely responsible.

Technological Improvements in Health Care. No doubt technological advancements have changed mortality patterns. Biomedical technology has aided in decreasing the maternal mortality rate. Improved detection and treatment of women's reproductive cancers have also contributed to the decreased mortality rate for women (Retherford, 1975).

Stress Exposures and Stress Responses. Stress produced by exposure of individuals to conflicting or ambiguous expectations regarding their behavior may account for mortality differences between women and men. However, there is little consensus about whether women or men experience the most stress (Nathanson, 1977a). Some link occupational or economic sources of stress to male mortality patterns (Retherford, 1975), but others suggest that the traditional role of married women is a source of stress (Gove, 1973). What is becoming clear is the difference in the effects of stressors on women and men. Indeed, some suggest that biological effects of reproductive hormones, in interaction with behavioral characteristics, influence the sex differences in coronary heart disease mortality. It is unlikely that only biological or behavioral differences will account for mortality differences and more likely that their joint effects on health will provide important clues to solving the puzzle of sex differences in mortality (Matthews, 1989).

Lifestyle. Many aspects of how women and men live their lives can influence how and when they die (Gove, 1973). Social norms regulating behavior for women and men may encourage higher risk-taking behaviors and in turn higher mortality among men. For example, it is considered more appropriate for men than women to use alcohol and to smoke. Type A, coronary-prone behavior, also believed to be a risk factor for coronary heart disease, reflects typical social expectations for men, whereas aggressive competitiveness is not encouraged for women (Waldron, 1976). Personality differences may also be involved. In concert with Western social norms, the modal male personality is more likely to be aggressive and to take risks than the modal female personality, thus accounting for increasing mortality risks for men.

Lifestyle differences expose women and men to different health-promoting and health-damaging behaviors. Differential exposure to smoking, diets high in saturated fats, excess food intake and use of alcohol, employment hazards, violence, and automobile accidents contribute to higher mortality rates for men from lung cancer and other lung diseases, cardiovascular disease, cirrhosis, fatalities from occupational accidents, homicide, and automobile fatalities (Waldron, 1976).

Some elements of women's lifestyles may have become more protective during the first part of the century. Use of labor-saving devices in the home, such as machines to help with heavy housework, may be responsible for women's improved mortality rates (Spiegelman & Ehrhardt, 1974). Trends toward limiting obesity may also have contributed to reduced mortality for women (Retherford, 1975). In addition, women's learned ability to adapt to role changes during their life spans may account for their relatively greater resilience during old age (Kline, 1975). The ability to tolerate variations in sex roles may indicate flexibility associated with a longer life span and more successful aging (Sinnott, 1977).

A life partner may also influence longevity, but being partnered has different effects for women and men. Single, widowed, and divorced persons have higher mortality rates than do married persons. Men seem to benefit more from marriage than do women (Gove, 1973). The benefit to men is particularly noteworthy for suicide rates, with the protective effects of being married being much greater for men than for women (Gove, 1972a, 1972b).

Future Mortality Patterns

Some suggest that sex differences in mortality may become less dramatic as women's roles in society change. Occupational hazards previously applicable only to men will apply to women's health as women become more integrated into the labor force. In addition, as women's roles change, the norms influencing their behavior may also change, encouraging them to engage in more risk-taking behavior with their health. If women respond to social pressures to behave in ways similar to those of men, they may respond to their environment more like men. Women who combine employment and family roles may be exposed to work overload and may not have access to the same socioemotional supports available to men from their spouses. Whether the positive effects of changing social roles for women and men will outweigh the negative health effects is being explored by many investigators. For example, some find that employment for women buffers the demands of caretaking roles on their health (McKinlay & McKinlay, 1989).

Table 1.3 Number of Acute Conditions per 100 Persons per Year, by Gender, Age, and Type of Condition: United States, 1992

Type of Acute Condition	*Women*		*Men*	
	18-44	*45+*	*18-44*	*45+*
All acute conditions	190.1	135.9	143.3	93.9
Infective and parasitic diseases	21.6	9.0	12.8	3.8
Respiratory conditions	93.2	60.0	70.0	44.1
Common cold	26.6	15.0	19.4	11.7
Other acute upper respiratory infections	9.1	7.2	7.7	3.5
Influenza	50.8	30.5	38.6	22.1
Digestive system conditions	5.8	6.2	5.5	5.7
Injuries	20.6	19.4	32.1	14.5
Selected other acute conditions	35.1	24.4	12.7	13.2
All other acute conditions	13.8	16.9	10.3	12.5

SOURCE: National Center for Health Statistics (1993a, Table 2, p. 15).

The extent to which biology, technological advancements, stressor exposures and stress responses, and lifestyles can explain the narrowing of the mortality differences between women and men remains to be evaluated. The slowing of the more favorable trend for women's longevity may be attributable to changes in lifestyle. Women's longevity may be improving at a slower rate because of exposure to job stressors and risks such as smoking. Alternatively, men's longevity may be improving at a faster rate than previously because they are exercising more, smoking less, and following more healthful diets (Verbrugge & Wingard, 1987).

Morbidity: Comparison of Rates for Women and Men

Although mortality data provide one index of the ill health of a population, these data alone provide an incomplete picture. In developed countries, ill health frequently results from significant but nonfatal conditions, such as mental illness or orthopedic and sensory impairments. Morbidity is a departure from physical or mental well-being that results from disease or injury and that has an effect on the individual's life inasmuch as she or he is aware of both the departure from health and the restrictions or disabilities resulting from the condition (Cole, 1974). Current estimates from the National Health Interview Survey (NCHS, 1993a) data for 1993 show that in the United States women reported more illness than did men, responded to illness differently, and used health services at higher rates than did men. These estimates were based on data from a stratified random sample of households drawn from the civilian noninstitutionalized populations of the United States.

Acute Conditions

Acute conditions are those illnesses and injuries that last less than 3 months and involve 1 day or more of restricted activity or medical attention. The annual incidence of acute conditions is estimated by including only those conditions that began during the 2 weeks before the interview conducted as part of the National Health Interview Survey. Table 1.3 shows the incidence of acute conditions for women and men. Acute conditions for women exceeded those for men for nearly every condition except injuries. For women over 45 years, acute conditions were less prevalent than for those 18 to 44 years. Similar patterns occur for men for most conditions. Rates for whites exceed those for blacks for most conditions.

Chronic Conditions

A chronic condition is one that was noticed at least 3 months or more before the interview or that belongs to a group of conditions (including heart disease, diabetes, and others) that persist for a long period of time, regardless of when the condition began. As seen in Table 1.4, women experienced higher rates of arthritis, cataracts, orthopedic impairments, diabetes, hemorrhoids, hypertension, chronic bronchitis, asthma, and

Table 1.4 Number of Selected Reported Chronic Conditions per 1,000 Persons, by Gender and Age: United States, 1992

Type of Chronic Condition	*Women*				*Men*			
	Under 45	*45-64*	*65-74*	*75+*	*Under 45*	*45-64*	*65-74*	*75+*
Arthritis	42.2	315.9	508.7	611.2	26.1	199.2	364.8	417.2
Visual impairment	14.5	33.1	49.6	99.4	31.1	66.0	96.6	131.9
Cataracts	1.7	32.3	137.1	245.2	2.5	18.7	112.5	193.2
Hearing impairment	30.4	96.9	204.3	392.9	44.3	216.2	322.3	452.7
Deformity or orthopedic impairment	100.5	167.4	167.1	243.0	102.1	181.8	154.9	185.8
Ulcer	13.4	29.5	34.0	26.9	111.1	23.2	38.4	31.8
Hernia of abdominal cavity	6.5	34.1	57.4	67.5	11.5	39.0	61.5	64.8
Diabetes	9.0	59.2	109.2	110.2	6.1	52.5	119.6	96.8
Heart disease	32.9	120.3	220.6	401.2	25.7	150.8	334.7	408.5
Hypertension	30.2	222.1	377.7	374.3	37.5	231.0	341.4	314.7
Hemorrhoids	30.5	65.6	51.6	68.9	19.0	77.3	63.9	56.7
Chronic bronchitis	58.0	71.9	80.0	65.9	41.0	43.6	76.6	40.1
Asthma	53.5	56.6	55.9	32.8	50.7	32.4	28.9	35.7
Chronic sinusitis	155.0	219.3	185.4	183.6	108.5	152.7	123.9	120.2
Emphysema	0.6	10.6	16.4	34.8	0.8	19.7	47.7	51.1

SOURCE: National Center for Health Statistics (1993a, tab. 58, pp. 85-86).

chronic sinusitis than did men in 1992. Men experienced higher rates of visual impairment, hearing impairment, ulcer and abdominal hernia, heart disease, and emphysema than did women. Blacks experienced higher rates of arthritis, diabetes, and hypertension than did whites, who had higher rates of hearing impairment, orthopedic impairment, abdominal hernia, heart disease, hemorrhoids, chronic bronchitis, and asthma than did blacks, particularly during the latter decades of life. Rates of some chronic conditions differed across income categories, with people in lower income categories being at greater risk for diabetes, heart disease, hypertension, emphysema, arthritis, visual impairment, cataracts, and hearing impairment.

Mental Illness

The National Institute of Mental Health sponsored the Epidemiological Catchment Area (ECA) Program, which sampled noninstitutionalized people. For 15 diagnoses studied, there were gender differences in the prevalence rates of lifetime diagnoses. Women more often had a diagnosis of major depressive episodes, agoraphobia, and simple phobia, and men more frequently had diagnoses of antisocial personality disorder and alcohol abuse/dependence. Women were more likely than men to be diagnosed with dysthymia, obsessive-compulsive disorder, schizophrenia, somatization disorder, and panic disorder. There were no gender differences in manic episodes or cognitive impairment (Robins et al., 1984).

Responses to Illness

In response to illness, people may treat themselves, perhaps spending a day away from work or in bed. In the National Health Interview Survey, four types of disability days are reported: restricted activity days, bed-disability days, work-loss days, and school-loss days. A restricted activity day is one on which an individual reduces his or her normal activity for the entire day because of an illness or injury. By definition, bed-disability days are ones in which the person spends all or most of the day in bed; these are counted as days of restricted activity. Each day lost from work or school is also counted as a day of restricted activity. Table 1.5 shows that all types of restriction for acute and chronic conditions increase with age. Moreover, men have higher rates of bed-disability days, but women have higher rates of work- or school-loss days. Blacks have higher rates of bed-disability or work- or school-loss days than do

Table 1.5 Number of Days of Activity Restriction Resulting From Acute and Chronic Conditions per Person per Year, by Type of Restriction and Gender: United States, 1992

	Types of Restrictions		
Age and Gender	*All Types*	*Bed Disability*	*Work or School Loss*
Women			
All ages	18.2	7.3	5.6
5-17	9.2	4.1	5.0
18-24	12.2	4.6	5.1
25-44	15.7	6.0	5.7
45-64	23.7	9.0	6.5
65 and older	36.5	15.2	5.2
Men			
All ages	14.2	5.3	4.3
5-17	7.9	3.3	4.2
18-24	9.1	2.5	4.5
25-44	11.8	4.0	4.1
45-64	18.3	6.4	4.7
65 and older	34.0	14.1	6.1

SOURCE: National Center for Health Statistics (1993a, tab. 69, p. 111).

whites, and people in low-income categories have higher rates of restriction than do those who have a higher income during middle and later years of life.

Use of Health Services

Another response to illness is using health services. People usually contact physicians, nurses, and other health care providers by telephone, by visiting their offices, or by going to the hospital. The use of telephone calls and office visits tends to increase with age. Men make more hospital visits than do women, and women make more telephone calls and office visits than do men (see Table 1.6). Women are hospitalized more frequently than men, but the frequency of hospitalization of women and men is similar when hospitalization for childbirth is excluded (Table 1.7 lists reasons for hospitalization of women in 1991). Whites tend to make more telephone calls and office visits than do blacks, whereas blacks make more hospital visits than do whites. People in low-income categories tend to make more hospital contacts than their socially advantaged counterparts.

Patterns of service use for mental illness differ for men and women. For inpatient facilities, women account for a greater proportion of admissions than men in nonfederal general hospitals and private mental hospitals. Men account for a greater proportion of admissions to state and county mental hospitals and Veterans Administration hospitals. Women account for more admissions to outpatient facilities (Russo, Amaro, & Winter, 1987).

Health Perceptions

As part of the National Health Interview Survey, people rate their own health or that of family members living in the same household as excellent, very good, good, fair, or poor. Only about 3% of the population rated their health as poor, with 42% of men and 36% of women rating their health as excellent. Table 1.8 shows that in general, men are somewhat more likely than women to rate their health as excellent, older adults are more likely than younger adults to rate their health as poor, and older men are more likely than older women to rate their health as poor. Older blacks are more likely than older whites to rate their health as poor, and people with low incomes are more likely than people who are wealthier to rate their health as poor (NCHS, 1993a).

Explanation of Sex Differences in Morbidity Patterns

The data collected in the United States show that women have more acute conditions than do men. Although the rates of chronic conditions do not reflect a clear pattern of sex differences, some have suggested that men have more serious

Table 1.6 Number of Physician Contacts per Person per Year, by Place of Contact, Gender, and Age: United States, 1992

Gender and Age	*Telephone*	*Office*	*Hospital*
Women			
All ages	0.9	3.8	0.9
18-44	0.9	3.6	0.9
45-64	1.1	4.5	1.1
65 and older	0.9	5.8	1.1
Men			
All ages	0.5	2.8	0.9
18-44	0.3	2.0	0.6
45-64	0.6	3.3	1.2
65 and older	0.9	5.3	1.8

SOURCE: National Center for Health Statistics (1993a, tab. 71, p. 115).

chronic conditions (Verbrugge & Wingard, 1987). Women miss work and school more frequently than do men for reasons of illness, but men spend more days in bed. Although women use health services more frequently than do men, men have more hospital visits. Despite these patterns, men are more likely than women to rate themselves as in excellent health, but this sex difference reverses itself after age 60. Taken together, this evidence suggests that women have more episodes of sickness, but men suffer from more fatal conditions. Women seek care for their problems in a variety of ways, while men use hospitalization more than primary care.

Some of the same factors used to explain sex differences in mortality patterns may be invoked to explain sex differences in morbidity and the use of health services: differences in biology, stress exposures and stress responses, and lifestyle. Some sex differences may be linked to biology. For example, some of the restrictions in activity that women experience are attributable to childbearing and problems associated with pregnancy. Others suggest that physiological differences linked to genetic and hormonal differences between men and women contribute to women having milder forms of illness than men, citing women's greater resistance to infection and to degenerative illness (Cole, 1974; Moriyama, Krueger, & Stamler, 1971; Nathanson, 1977a; Verbrugge, 1976).

Stress exposures and stress responses may also help account for sex differences in illness and responses to illness. Some suggest that women's roles are more stressful than men's, thus accounting for the greater frequency of morbidity among women (Gove & Tudor, 1973; Nathanson, 1975). Yet others argue that men's roles are more stressful.

Women and men are exposed to different physical risks of disease and injury as a result of their lifestyles, and these may also help account for sex differences in illness and illness responses. Some have suggested that in the past women tended to engage in less risky behavior than did men and may have been exposed to fewer occupational hazards (Verbrugge, 1976). Whether these protective behaviors will persist remains unknown.

In addition, differences in socialization patterns of health and illness may be responsible for differences in morbidity and responses to illness. Many suggest that women are socialized to be sensitive to bodily discomforts and to report them, whereas men are socialized to ignore symptoms (e.g., Cole, 1974; Mechanic, 1976; Nathanson, 1977b; Verbrugge, 1976; Verbrugge & Wingard, 1987). Likewise, women and men differ in socialization about evaluation of their symptoms, and women may learn to respond to less serious symptoms (Cole, 1974). Women may also learn to reduce their usual activities in response to symptoms, thus receiving earlier diagnosis and treatment than do men (Cole, 1974; Verbrugge, 1976). In addition, women seem more oriented than do men to using preventive services, probably reducing the seriousness of their illnesses and limiting their disabling consequences (Verbrugge & Wingard, 1987).

Differences in the ways in which men and women respond to studies of health and illness may also be responsible for sex differences in health-related statistics. Most interviews are conducted with women who often report as proxy

Table 1.7 Days of Care in Nonfederal Short-Stay Hospitals, by First-Listed Diagnosis and Operations Performed, by Type and by Age: United States, 1991

Age Group and Diagnosis	*Number of Days of Care per 1,000 Persons*
15 to 44 years	
Delivery	186.5
Psychoses	54.0
Pregnancy with abortive outcome	7.3
Cholelithiasis	13.0
Benign neoplasms	11.0
Inflammatory disease of female pelvic organs	7.8
Disorders of menstruation	4.3
45 to 64 years	
Diseases of heart	98.3
Malignant neoplasms	85.4
Cholelithiasis	20.5
Benign neoplasms	18.9
Psychoses	62.9
Diabetes	22.6
65 years and over	
Diseases of heart	480.0
Malignant neoplasms	221.8
Cerebrovascular diseases	196.0
Fracture, all sites	208.5
Pneumonia, all forms	171.3
Eye diseases and conditions	7.2
Age Group and Type of Procedure	
15 to 44 years	
Procedures to assist delivery	43.2
Cesarean section	15.8
Repair of current obstetric laceration	13.4
Bilateral destruction or occlusion of fallopian tube	6.8
Hysterectomy	5.5
Diagnostic dilation and curettage of uterus	1.1
45 to 64 years	
Hysterectomy	6.6
Oophorectomy and salpingo-oophorectomy	6.2
Cardiac catheterization	6.2
Cholecystectomy	5.5
Excision or destruction of intervertebral disc and spinal fusion	2.7
Diagnostic dilation and curettage of uterus	0.9
Biopsies on the integumentary system	0.7
65 years and over	
Cardiac catheterization	11.1
Reduction of fracture	9.2
Arthroplasty and replacement of hip	6.5
Biopsies on the digestive system	5.6
Pacemaker insertion or replacement	6.7
Cholecystectomy	6.1
Extraction of lens	2.5
Insertion of prosthetic lens	2.4

SOURCE: National Center for Health Statistics (1993b, tab. 86, pp. 125-126; tab. 88, pp. 129-130).

respondents for their spouses (Cole, 1974). Because women are socialized differently than men about their health, they may be better able to recall their symptoms and their health activities and may be better prepared to discuss their health than are men (Verbrugge, 1976). Moreover, the types of health problems studied may be biased to include more of the expressions of

Table 1.8 Distribution of Respondent-Assessed Health Status, According to Gender and Age: United States, 1992 (in percentages)

	Health Status—Self-Assessed				
Gender and Age	*Excellent*	*Very Good*	*Good*	*Fair*	*Poor*
Women					
All ages	35.1	29.0	24.7	8.4	2.9
18-24	36.3	32.1	23.8	5.4	0.6
25-44	36.3	32.1	23.8	6.3	1.6
45-64	25.7	27.3	29.2	12.5	5.2
65 and older	15.1	22.7	34.0	19.8	8.5
Men					
All ages	40.9	28.2	21.3	6.8	2.8
18-24	47.5	30.2	18.3	3.4	0.6
25-44	42.9	31.1	19.6	4.9	1.6
45-64	30.8	27.2	25.5	10.8	5.7
65 and older	16.4	22.4	32.0	19.4	9.8

SOURCE: National Center for Health Statistics (1993a, tab. 70, p. 113).

distress common to women (Mechanic, 1976). All self-reports of acute and chronic illness will reflect the different socialization patterns of women and men with respect to the perception, evaluation, and action in response to symptoms (Nathanson, 1977b). Finally, differences in rates of use of health services may reflect variations in (a) the actual prevalence of the symptoms, (b) willingness to seek help from a particular service, (c) attitudes toward the service, (d) expectations regarding the appropriate use of the service, (e) social accessibility of the service, (f) alternative services available, (g) self- versus practitioner-initiated nature of the service, (h) differences in practitioners' attitudes toward men and women, and (i) the process of health care for men and women who report the same complaints (Mechanic, 1976).

In short, there are many explanations for the sex differences in morbidity and responses to illness. What seems most likely is that a combination of these help account for differences in women's and men's experiences.

Patterns of Health and Illness for Women

Mortality Patterns Across the Life Span for Women

In addition to striking sex differences in patterns of mortality, differences in the most prevalent causes of death occur across the life span, as reflected in the U.S. vital and health statistics. Major causes of death for women 15 to 24 years of age include accidents, homicide, and suicide (see Table 1.2). During the adolescent and early adult years, automobiles are responsible for the majority of accidental deaths, some of which could have been prevented by using seat belts and by reduced use of alcohol and drugs. Homicide is a preventable cause of death that occurs in a cultural context that condones use of violence as a means of conflict resolution and in which handguns are readily available. As young women struggle with issues of independence, suicide is a major cause of death for this age group over major cardiovascular disease, cerebrovascular disease, influenza and pneumonia, and other causes. Early identification and treatment of depression could prevent some of these deaths. In young adult women, malignancies, especially leukemias and lymphomas, contribute heavily to deaths. Many cardiovascular disease deaths in this age group are attributable to congenital anomalies and valvular heart disease. Appropriate use of antibiotics could reduce risk of death from chronic rheumatic heart disease, and reduction in smoking and alcohol could lessen the risk of death from pneumonia.

Accidents, especially those caused by motor vehicle injuries, remain the leading cause of death for women aged 25 to 34. During the childbearing years, malignant neoplasms emerge as the second major cause: cancer of the breast, uterus, brain, and nervous system; leukemia; and Hodgkin's disease account for most deaths. Homicide and suicide continue to be major causes of death. The major cardiovascular diseases also claim the lives of many women during this period, with active rheumatic fever and chronic rheumatic heart disease, ischemic heart disease, acute myocardial infarction, and cerebrovascular disease being responsible for most of the deaths. Factors that increase the risk of the major cardiovascular diseases include untreated elevated blood pressure and cholesterol, uncontrolled diabetes, smoking, and untreated rheumatic fever. Sedentary lifestyles and obesity also contribute to cardiovascular disease mortality. Cirrhosis of the liver emerges as an important cause of death for this age group. Alcohol abuse is the primary factor associated with cirrhosis. Influenza and pneumonia remain major causes of death, with alcohol use, smoking, and previous lung diseases, such as bacterial pneumonia and emphysema, increasing the mortality risk for women aged 25 to 34 years (see Table 1.2).

Maternal mortality does not account for a large proportion of deaths during the childbearing years. Most women now survive childbirth. For white women 20 to 24 years old, maternal mortality dropped from 102 deaths per 100,000 live births for women born between 1921 and 1925 to 3 deaths per 100,000 live births for the cohort born between 1961 and 1965. For black women, however, the maternal mortality rate dropped from 300 deaths per 100,000 live births for the 1921 to 1925 birth cohort to 17 deaths per 100,000 live births for the 1961 to 1965 birth cohort. The maternal mortality rate for black women is about five times that for white women (NCHS, 1993b). Maternal mortality rates for complications of pregnancy, childbirth, and the puerperium for white women were 4.9 per 100,000 live births in 1987, but the maternal mortality rate for black women was 14.3 per 100,000 live births. The differences for women are particularly noteworthy for ages 20 and up (NCHS, 1993b; see Table 1.9). Most deaths are attributable to complications of childbirth. Ectopic pregnancy, toxemia, hemorrhage, and sepsis are disproportionately high among non-white women.

The major causes of death for women aged 35 to 44 are similar to those in the previous decade. Malignant neoplasms, including cancer of the breast, lung, uterus, ovary, colon, and rectum, are major causes. In addition, the leukemias and the lymphatic and hematopoietic neoplasms are also major causes of death. Regular breast examination can aid the early detection of breast cancer, and regular Pap smears aid the early detection of cervical cancer. Cardiovascular diseases are the second major cause of death for this group, with injuries from accidents, suicide, cerebrovascular disease, homicide, diabetes, pneumonia and influenza, and chronic obstructive pulmonary disease among the 10 major causes of death. Obesity, a serious health risk for women, has been linked to adult onset diabetes, and diabetes mellitus emerges as a major cause of death for this age group (see Table 1.2).

For women 45 to 54, cancer is the major cause of death, followed by heart disease, cerebrovascular disease, accidental injuries, liver disease, suicide, chronic obstructive pulmonary disease, diabetes, pneumonia and influenza, and homicide. The cardiovascular diseases that affect women in this age group are the ischemic heart diseases. During this decade, most women experience the biological changes of menopause as well as social changes in family and work roles (see Table 1.2).

Women who die between the ages of 55 and 64 years are victims of cancer and heart disease. These two disease groups persist as leading causes of death, followed by cerebrovascular diseases, throughout the remainder of the life span. Accidental injuries, liver disease, suicide, chronic obstructive pulmonary disease, diabetes, pneumonia and influenza, and homicide remain leading causes of death during this decade (see Table 1.2).

Causes of death for women between the ages of 65 and 74 include cardiovascular disease, malignant neoplasms, cerebrovascular disease, chronic obstructive pulmonary diseases, and pneumonia. These five causes remain the principal causes of death throughout the remainder of the life span. In women over 75, cardiovascular deaths are attributable to ischemic heart disease and hypertension. The cancers affecting women over the age of 75 are those of the colon, breast, lung, pancreas, and uterus. Cerebrovascular disease, especially cerebral thrombosis and hemorrhage and arteriosclerosis, also claim many lives (see Table 1.2).

AIDS accounts for recent changes in causes of death for women. The percentage of AIDS cases who are women increased from 6% to 10% from 1984 to 1988, and 5,500 deaths were attributable to AIDS for women aged 13 and over. Among adult and adolescent women, intravenous drug use as an HIV transmission source dropped from 62% to 53%, but HIV transmission from heterosexual contact rose from 17% to 26% (NCHS, 1993b).

Table 1.9 Maternal Mortality Rates[a] for Complications of Pregnancy, Childbirth, and the Puerperium, According to Race and Age: United States, Selected Years

Race and Age	*1950*	*1960*	*1970*	*1980*	*1990*
White					
Under 20	44.9	14.8	13.8	5.8	5.3
20-24	35.7	15.3	8.4	4.2	3.9
25-29	45.0	20.3	11.1	5.4	4.8
30-34	75.9	34.3	18.7	9.3	5.0
35+	174.1	73.9	59.3	25.5	12.6
Black					
Under 20	—	54.8	32.3	13.1	12.0
20-24	—	56.9	41.9	13.9	14.7
25-29	—	92.8	65.2	22.4	14.9
30-34	—	150.6	117.8	44.0	44.2
35+	—	299.5	207.5	100.6	79.7

SOURCE: National Center for Health Statistics (1993b, tab. 41, p. 73).
a. Deaths per 100,000 live births.

Morbidity

During the early adult years, respiratory conditions and injuries account for most of the acute conditions that women experience, with young women experiencing two to three conditions per year. On the average, young adult women restrict their activity about 12 days per year, spend about 4.5 days in bed, and miss about 5 days of work due to acute conditions. For these women, the greatest proportion of accidental injuries occur in the home, and these account for about 3 days of restricted activity per year (NCHS, 1993a).

Morbidity experiences for women over 45 years of age include a lower incidence of acute conditions, with only about 1 per year. Respiratory conditions and injuries account for most, resulting in about 20 days of restricted activity, 9 days of bed rest, and 6.5 days away from work each year (NCHS, 1993a).

Chronic conditions affect many thousands of women. The most prevalent chronic conditions affecting women include arthritis, cataracts, hearing impairment, orthopedic impairment, heart disease, hypertension, varicose veins, and chronic sinusitis (NCHS, 1993a).

Mental Health

Mental health can be assessed in many ways. The Health and Nutrition Examination Survey measures a construct labeled *psychological well-being.* On this index, 77% of women describe themselves at a positive level of well-being, with 27% ranking high on levels of tension, stress, and anxiety (NCHS, 1993a). As indicated earlier, the diagnoses of mental illness for women most commonly include phobias, major depression, dysthymia, and obsessive-compulsive disorders. When women are admitted to mental hospitals, it is most likely to be for depression (Marieskind, 1980; Russo, 1990).

The access to and appropriateness of mental health services for women has been examined also. General practice physicians prescribe psychoactive drugs, such as major tranquilizers, sedatives, and stimulants, for women more frequently than for men (Cooperstock, 1981; Fidell, 1981). In addition, women account for 43% of the drug-related deaths in the United States (Marieskind, 1980).

Use of Health Services

Fewer than half of American women in the National Health Interview Survey had had a Pap smear within the previous year, with younger women more likely than older women to have done so. Women with more education and black women were more likely to have had a Pap smear within the previous year than those with less education and white women. Half of American women had a breast exam by a health professional in the previous year, with younger women more likely to have done so than older women. About 60% of women 18 to 29 years old had a breast exam, but only 39% of those 65 years and older had done so. Women with more education and black women were more likely to have done so than women with less education and white women (NCHS, 1993b).

Young women make about four physician visits and two dental visits per year. Midlife and elderly women make more frequent physician and dental visits (see Table 1.6). When women visit physicians, it is frequently for health maintenance examinations. Most have had both a breast exam and a Pap smear, except for women older than 65 years of age. Most women receive their health care from a general practitioner or a family practice physician.

For all women, the most frequent discharge diagnoses in 1992 were deliveries, heart disease, and malignant neoplasms (NCHS, 1993b). Women 15 to 44 are hospitalized most frequently for delivery, psychoses, abortion, cholelithiasis, inflammatory disease of the pelvic organs, benign neoplasms, and disorders of menstruation. Women between 45 and 64 years are hospitalized for heart disease, malignant neoplasms, benign neoplasms, cholelithiasis, psychoses, and diabetes. For women 65 years and older, hospitalizations are for heart disease, malignant neoplasms, cerebrovascular diseases, fracture, pneumonia, and eye diseases and conditions (NCHS, 1993b) (see Table 1.7).

The high incidence of hospitalization for women during the reproductive years reflects childbearing, and most stays are short. Women's hospitalization rates decrease in midlife, reflecting the effects of childbearing on younger women's patterns of hospitalization and the decreased incidence of childbearing during the middle years. Hospital stays for women in their middle and older years are longer than those for younger women, reflecting the differences in their health problems. Hospital stays exceeding 7 days in 1992 were for heart disease, malignancy, pneumonia, and fractures (NCHS, 1993b).

Women are nearly four times more likely than men to have surgery from the ages of 15 to 44 years, but women's and men's experiences of surgery become more similar from the ages of 45 to 64, and men have 25% more surgeries from age 65 onward (NCHS, 1993b). Gynecologic surgery and obstetric procedures account for the dramatic differences during the reproductive years (NCHS, 1993b).

The most common surgical procedures for girls under 15 years of age were tonsillectomy; myringotomy; appendectomy; reduction of fracture; operations on muscles, tendons, fascia, and bursa; and adenoidectomy without tonsillectomy. Surgeries were performed most commonly for women 15 to 44 years included procedures to assist delivery, cesarean section, repair of current obstetric laceration, bilateral destruction or occlusion of fallopian tubes, hysterectomy, and diagnostic dilation and curettage of the uterus. Surgical procedures for women 45 to 65 years included hysterectomy, oophorectomy and salpingo-oophorectomy, cardiac catheterization, cholecystectomy, excision or destruction of intravertebral disc and spinal fusion, diagnostic dilation and curettage, and biopsies of the integumentary system. For women 65 years and older, surgeries included cardiac catheterization, reduction of fracture, arthroplasty and replacement of the hip, biopsies on the digestive system, pacemaker insertion or replacement, cholecystectomy, arthroplasty and replacement of the hip, and extraction of the lens and insertion of prosthetic lens (NCHS, 1993b).

Women's rates of admission to selected inpatient psychiatric organizations are lower than men's for state and county mental hospitals and private psychiatric hospitals and similar to rates for nonfederal general hospitals. When women are mentally ill, they are most likely to be cared for in nonfederal general hospitals, with about half of admissions to state and county mental hospitals and nearly two thirds of admissions to private psychiatric hospitals (NCHS, 1993b).

Nursing and personal-care home residents who are 65 years of age and over are mostly women. Compared to 334,400 men, 983,000 women were cared for in these institutions in 1985. The rate of admission for women was 57.9 per 1,000 versus 29.0 per 1,000 men (NCHS, 1993b).

Self-Care Activities

Women make a significant contribution to their own health care through self-care, the practice of activities that they initiate and perform on their own behalf in maintaining life, health, and well-being (Orem, 1971). Self-care may be related to universal needs, such as participation in activities of daily living, or to specific illness experiences.

National statistics describing self-care practices are not available. Nonetheless, several studies of women's self-care practices underscore the prevalence and diversity of women's activities. For example, young adult women enrolled in a family practice plan recorded a wide range of universal self-care behaviors. The most frequent was use of vitamins, followed by contraceptive use, prescription medications, and dietary and activity alterations. Over-the-counter medications, except for vitamins, were used infrequently. The most commonly used illness-related self-care measures were over-the-counter medications, alteration of activity, use of prescription medications, and home remedies. Only 3% of activities in response to symptoms involved consulting a health professional, and only 1% involved actually visiting a health professional. The illness-related self-care activities reflected the nature of the women's symptoms (Maunz & Woods, 1988; Woods, 1985b).

Healthy Lifestyles

Lifestyle influences women's health in significant ways. Smoking, alcohol use, nutritional intake, exercise, self-protective practices, exposure to stress, and occupational hazards have all been linked to health. Despite the evidence on the hazards of smoking, nearly 27% of women over the age of 18 years smoke. This compares to 31% of men. Of concern is the increased rate of smoking among women, especially young women. Despite the fact that 90% of women are aware of the risks of smoking, 31% of black women, 28% of white women, and 21% of Hispanic women smoke. Black women between 25 and 44 years of age are slightly more likely to smoke than are white women, but white women 18 to 24 years and those 45 years and older are slightly more likely to smoke than are black women. Smoking is most prevalent among low-income women with the least education; it has declined most among well-educated women and least among the poorly educated. Of women smokers, 21% quit when they became pregnant and 36% decreased the number of cigarettes they smoked (NCHS, 1988b, 1993a).

Young women 12 to 17 years of age are less likely to use alcohol than are young men of the same ages and also less likely to use marijuana and cocaine. Nonetheless, use patterns are much more similar for the ages of 12 to 17 years (NCHS, 1993a).

Although only 3% of women consider themselves heavy drinkers, using over an ounce of alcohol per day, 13% of men consider themselves heavy drinkers. Only 10% of women admit to driving after having had too much to drink compared to 22% of men (NCHS, 1988a, 1993a).

Women are only slightly more likely to eat breakfast (56%) than men (54%), and both groups snack between meals at the same rate (28% women, 29% men). Overweight is more prevalent among women at all ages, with the overall rate being 27.5% for men from 20 to 74 years of age and 46.1% for women of the same ages. Of black women, 36% are overweight, as are 21% of white women, and these percentages increase to 55% and 28%, respectively, during midlife (NCHS, 1988a, 1993a).

Although fewer women than men exercise regularly (38% of women compared to 43% of men), 46% of women report walking and 38% of men do so. Half of women aged 18 to 29 years report walking regularly for exercise (NCHS, 1988a).

Women are more likely than men to observe self-protective practices. For example, they are more likely than men to use seat belts (38% vs. 34%) in a car. Women are more likely than men (89% vs. 81%) to have had their blood pressure checked within the past year. In 1985, 87% of women knew how to do breast self-examination (BSE), but only 37% of those who knew how to do BSE actually did it 12 or more times per year. Although women with more education were more aware of how to perform BSE, education had no effect on actually performing BSE. For women 65 years and older, 60% of blacks and 80% of whites knew how to perform BSE, but three quarters of blacks who knew the procedure practiced it, compared with only a little more than half of whites. Hispanic women were aware of the procedure (75%), but there was no difference in the proportion of Hispanic and non-Hispanic women practicing BSE (NCHS, 1988a).

In 1985, women were somewhat more likely than men to report experiencing moderate stress levels during the previous two weeks. Women with more education and higher incomes were most likely to experience a moderate level of stress. White women were more likely to report this level of stress than black women, with those currently employed more likely than those not employed or looking for work. Of women, 50% believed that stress had affected their health, but the proportion dropped in those over 65 years of age. Women were twice as likely as men to have sought help for a personal problem (14% vs. 8%; NCHS, 1988a).

Occupational exposure to one or more health hazards differentiated men and women, with 72% of men and 48% of women reporting such exposure. However, exposure to mental stress was similar: 17% of men and 16% of women reported exposure to mental stress on the job (NCHS, 1988a).

Women's Chances for Health

Many characteristics of contemporary Western societies influence women's chances for health. Those of particular significance include recent dramatic changes in women's labor force participation, poverty, longevity, racism, and sexism.

The most dramatic change in women's lives during the past few decades is that a majority of women remain employed throughout their lives regardless of marital status or the ages of their children (McLaughlin & Melber, 1986). In addition, contemporary women live alone more of their adult lives than in the past. The number of women-headed households has increased dramatically, reflecting the difference in marriage and divorce rates. As a result, women are married for a smaller proportion of their lifetimes than were their mothers. Contemporary women are better educated than in the past. They have lower fertility rates, with fewer having their first child by the age of 23.

Women's Labor Force Participation

Since the mid 1970s, researchers have focused on the effects of employment on women's health (Nathanson, 1975). Some worried that changes in employment patterns would have negative effects on women's health. They argued that women would experience more morbidity than men because their lives would be more stressful as they combined employment and parenting (Woods & Hulka, 1979). Others argued that women's traditional roles were more compatible with illness than were men's and that as women enter the labor force they would have less opportunity to be ill and to use health services. Some believed that women would continue to report more illness than men simply because they are socialized to express symptoms more readily and are more aware of their health than are men. Others argued that as women enter the traditionally male domains, they would take on risks associated with changes in behavior patterns, such as smoking and use of alcohol, thus compromising their health.

Since the early studies examining the positive and negative health effects of women's labor force participation, investigators have focused on the constellation of a woman's roles, such as parenting and employment (McBride, 1990). Verbrugge (1986) found that women who were employed and married, regardless of whether they had children, were in the best health (reflected in a number of indicators). The relationships between roles and health for black women were less clear-cut than were the patterns for white women (Verbrugge, 1986).

Some have focused on the type of women's employment. For example, Stellman (1987) examined exposure to toxic substances in the workplace, calling attention to physical, chemical, and biological hazards of the workplace and occupational stress (see Chapter 16). Haynes and Feinleib (1980) examined data from the Framingham study of heart disease, finding that clerical workers, especially those who had unsupportive bosses and were unable to express anger were at greatest risk of developing heart disease, especially if they had several children and were married to blue-collar husbands.

Others have examined the subjective appraisals women make of their roles, linking them to their health effects. For example, Nathanson (1980) and Hibbard and Pope (1985) stressed the importance of social support and integration as dimensions of the employment experience. Muller (1986) explored the health effects of desired positive roles, such as marriage and married parenthood, in contrast with unwelcome role expansions, such as single parenthood, child illness, illness in a spouse, or dissolution of a marriage. She concluded that inability to choose one's roles and organize one's resources to meet their demands may explain health effects. Muller also found that more complex, challenging jobs and those offering more autonomy were associated with better health.

Verbrugge (1986) suggested that role burden, subjective feelings of oppression rather than objective characteristics of women's roles, accounted for their health effects. She found that dissatisfaction with roles in life and very great or very little time pressure on the job were associated with poor health. Time constraints, irregular and short job schedules, little or high family dependency, and a low or high responsibility for family income were also associated with poor health. Waldron and Herold (1986) confirmed that subjective appraisals of roles were important. Women whose labor force status was compatible with their attitudes toward employment experienced better health than did those with negative attitudes. Although being a homemaker was detrimental to health for women with favorable attitudes toward employment, there were no health effects of employment on women with unfavorable attitudes toward employment. Waldron and her colleagues also have demonstrated that healthy women get selected into the labor force. Probably these healthy women have positive attitudes toward employment (Waldron, Herold, Dunn, & Straum, 1982).

Support for women's roles is also important. Married women in certain constellations of roles exhibited better mental health when their spouses provided specific types of support. For married employed women without children, sharing household tasks was important. For employed married women with children, both task sharing and emotional support were important, and for married women not employed with children, emotional support from a spouse was most important (Woods, 1985a).

What is missing from the literature about women and work is a picture of how low-income women always have struggled to balance child care and employment. Nonetheless, the bulk of contemporary research has focused on middle-class women choosing to combine career and parenting.

Poverty

Despite women's growing representation in the labor force, women are still overrepresented in low paying jobs. Not surprisingly, poverty is one of the major social issues affecting women's lives and their health (Belle, 1990).

In general, there are more women than men living in poverty, and women remain poor for longer periods than do men. Indeed, women who are heads of households are five times more likely than men to be poor. Over the past 25 years, the number of poor people living in American woman-headed households (WHHs) has risen from 18% to 35%, and the poverty rates for WHHs are much higher among blacks and Hispanics (Willson, 1987). Poverty among women persists despite the decreased number of elderly WHHs below the poverty level over the last 15 years and despite the decreased size of families of WHHs (from 3.85 to 3.39). Indeed, there are as many poor married women as there are poor women who head households. Of poor WHHs, over one third are in the labor force, and nearly one of two have at least one wage earner present (working poor). Only 4 of 10 women who head households have completed high school, and only 1 of 5 receives financial support from the father of her children; 6 of 10 receive public assistance of some form.

At special risk are teen mothers. Although fertility rates have dropped for teens, teens still have more children than do their peers who delay childbearing. Teen mothers are less likely to be in the labor force, less well educated, and more likely to be receiving public assistance than are their peers without children. Teen mothers are less likely to marry, and when they do, they are more likely to divorce. Moreover, when they marry, spouses of teen mothers have lower earnings (Willson, 1987).

Rural poverty also affects women disproportionately. Although rural women enter the labor force, many are working in low-skilled, low-wage jobs. Of rural families, 17% are WHHs with incomes of less than $10,000 per year. Conservative rural governments and lower tax bases contribute fewer dollars for services. Many rural women are uninsured, lack transportation, and have fewer services available in their communities. They also suffer from many chronic conditions, including arthritis, bursitis, back disorders, hearing or vision problems, ulcers, and hernias (Richardson, 1987).

It is important to recognize the diversity of poor women and the multiple reasons for their lives of poverty. Some of these include divorce, chronic illness, job-related injuries, involvement in low-wage occupations, single parenting, retirement, and loss of income with death of a spouse.

Consequences of poverty for women's health are complex. Poor women suffer from lack of access to reproductive health care. In 1985 in the United States, 4 of 10 obstetrics/gynecology (OB/GYN) physicians did not accept Medicaid clients (McBarnette, 1987). In the United States, although sterilizations are federally financed (200,000 in 1970 to 700,000 in 1980), abortions are restricted in many states.

There is a greater incidence of sexually transmitted diseases (STDs) among women with low versus high incomes. Chlamydia produces pelvic inflammatory disease (PID) disproportionately in many poor women. In the United States, 6.6%

of AIDS cases are women (compared with Africa, where 50% of AIDS cases are women). However, in New York City, AIDS is the leading cause of death for women 25 to 29 years of age and is particularly prevalent among black and some Hispanic women. Ectopic pregnancy is the leading cause of death in the first trimester of pregnancy. It is the leading cause of maternal death among black women (17,000 in 1970 and 52,000 in 1980). Black women in the United States are three times more likely to die in childbirth than are white women. Moreover, cervical cancer incidence is greatest among lower socioeconomic status women (McBarnette, 1987).

Ethnic minority women experience more poverty and more reproductive health problems than do white women in the United States. In addition, they have lower life expectancy—5 to 7 years less—than do white women and more have diabetes, cardiovascular disease, and certain cancers (Zambrana, 1987).

Racism

Although ethnicity is linked to health, the ways in which ethnicity influences health remain poorly understood (U.S. Department of Health and Human Services, 1985). Recently, attention has turned from examining race as a marker for biology to ethnicity and race as social experiences. This line of inquiry has raised questions about the consequences of racism for health. Racism places women from certain ethnic groups at a social disadvantage and reduces significantly their chances for health. Audre Lorde (1988) proposed that "institutionalized rejection of difference" is necessary in an economy that requires "surplus people." She cautions that members of such an economy have all been programmed to respond to human differences with fear and loathing. As a result, we have been programmed to ignore difference, imitate it if the difference is dominant, or destroy the difference if it is subordinate. These operations allow some to feel personally adequate and secure at the expense of others. The predominant form of racism in the United States is based on the premise that white skin color is superior to the skin color of others (Gordon-Bradshaw, 1987).

Racism severely limits the chances for education, and the gap between white students and blacks and Hispanics who complete college has widened since the 1970s. Living environments include housing, nutrition, and access to health services as well as to education. Poor women from American ethnic groups termed *minorities* are concentrated in inner cities in the United States, where they are exposed to hazards to their health and poor housing or homelessness. Employment opportunities are limited and carry exposure to occupational hazards and little opportunity for advancement. Fewer blacks, Asians, Native Americans, and Hispanic women are represented in white-collar occupations. Little opportunity to access pension funds exists, and many elderly women from minority groups rely on only their social security in their old age. Stagnation of the minimum wage has kept poor minority women and their families in poverty even when they are employed.

Violence against women of color is reflected in their death rates. A black woman has more than four times the likelihood of being murdered than does a white woman, twice the chance of dying from cirrhosis, three times the chance of dying from diabetes, and is four times more likely to die in childbirth (NCHS, 1993b). Infant mortality rates for black women are more than double those for whites.

Longevity

By 2050, there will be a 9-year difference in the life expectancy for women and men, with an average life expectancy for women of 81 years versus 72 years for men. The number of white women older than the age of 85 will increase 150% in the next 30 years, with the number of black women in this older age group increasing by 300%. These dramatic differences in life span may seem advantageous for women, but our society has not adapted well to caring for older women, and as a result, women's last years are often spent in poverty. Although women compose 60% of the elderly, they account for 72% of the aged poor in the United States. Only 20% of American women have access to pensions, and fewer than 7% of women work after the age of 65, with 17% of men doing so. Poverty is especially acute among unmarried and minority elderly women (Grau, 1987). Moreover, the median annual income level for many elderly women is about $800 over the poverty level. Fifty percent of blacks, 25% of Hispanics, and 15% of white elderly women live in poverty (Grau, 1987).

In the United States, older women's lives are likely to end in poverty as they spend down their income and savings, exhaust their Medicare benefits, and qualify for Medicaid, usually as a result of expenses associated with their husband's dying (Lewis, 1986). Because health policy has been based on "men as the norm," women's needs are not well served. Older men are more likely to die when ill and spend more days in a hospital, whereas older women are more likely than men to spend time in a nursing home (Lewis, 1986). Medicare supports care for acute illness, such as hospitalization, but provides limited support for nursing home and home care. Many American women have no source of private insurance, and most carriers do not pay for nursing home care. As a result, "Medi-gap," the gap between Medicare coverage and the cost of services women really need, is responsible for some women's poverty as they age (Rathbone-McCuan, 1985).

Of nursing home residents, 75% are women, reflecting that women live longer than men, outlive their spouses, accumulate disabilities over the life span, and develop organic brain syndrome as they age, which increases their requirements for care; 50% are childless or have outlived their children due to the low fertility of the depression years. Although women usually care for their elderly husbands, there frequently is no one available to care for older women. Now female caregivers are in the labor force, and as many as five or six generations in one family require support: An 80-year-old mother may be cared for by her 60-year-old daughter, who has a 40-year-old daughter, a 20-year-old granddaughter, and an infant great-granddaughter requiring care. Women who once cared for their elderly relatives at home now care for them in nursing homes for pay (Miller, 1985).

The typical nursing home resident is over 80 years of age, chronically ill with multiple-organ pathology, white, and has an income below the poverty level and less than 8 years of schooling. Fewer than 10% have a living spouse, and over 50% have no living relatives. For about 91%, the stay is about 2.5 years. Only 10% improve and are discharged; most die in 18 to 20 months. Although some nursing home admissions are attributable to major illness, 70% to 80% are a result of mental disturbances such as organic brain syndrome as a consequence of strokes or Alzheimer's disease.

In addition to nursing home care, women have needs for noninstitutional long-term care. Some communities provide home health care, as in the nursing home without walls model. This care is not available to everyone because it is reimbursed for less than 75% of costs for nursing home care and requires family involvement. Another type of care necessary for elderly women is respite care to provide an interval of rest or relief for the family caring for a member at home. The goal is to deter nursing home admission by providing the family with an opportunity for relief of their caregiving. Community-based services, including home care, day care, enriched housing, and hospice care are needed to augment nursing home care (Miller, 1985).

Bader (1985) points out that there are typically multiple women involved in providing care to the elderly: the very old patient, the caregivers who are usually women, and the respite care providers who are likely to be women receiving low pay, poor benefits, and little opportunity for advancement. Caregivers, who are usually the young old, incur costs and risks to their health as their social circles contract and they lose wages from better-paying employment. Moreover, deterioration in affectional bonds between the family caregiver and the patient may occur, with some families being incapable of assuming caregiving responsibilities.

Older women's experiences with the health care system often mirror the disrespect and neglect of the larger society for the poor and elderly, the difficulty of treating chronic illness, and the paucity of emphasis on self-care and wellness for the old (Lewis, 1986). Moreover, women are likely to be victimized by the double standard applied to aging men and women, with older women being less valued than older men. Sexuality for elderly women is largely ignored by health professionals, with women's experiences often characterized by loss of a partner and society's view of the elderly woman as sexless. Widowhood, divorce, and loneliness are likely to be part of women's experience. Alcoholism and drug dependency, particularly with legally prescribed medications, have become more common among older women. Although valuing oneself may be difficult for older women given Western societies' images of aging, the women's movement has deterred the loss of self-esteem for some women.

Sexism

Sexism pervades Western societies in subtle as well as overt ways (Faludi, 1991). Sexual harassment of women in the workplace, sexual discrimination in hiring and promotion practices, and differential access to education persist despite changes in the law. Incest and sexual abuse has become more prevalent and more recognized. Unwanted sex or "date rape," homicide, and violent acts against women, such as rape and battering, continue. Indeed, homicide is the second most common cause of death for American women 15 to 24 years of age and among the 10 leading causes of death for women 25 to 54 years of age.

Sexism creates differential chances for wellness for women and men by restricting their human development and access to resources. Control of women and views of women as sexual objects remain pervasive and dehumanizing among the health services. The dehumanizing consequences of sexism for women's health care are discussed in greater detail in Chapter 7.

Women's Health: Future Prospects

Women's future prospects for health depend on multiple factors (Rodin & Ickovics, 1990). Among the most important factors are changing health care technologies, women's changing lifestyles, institutionalized sex role expectations, health care delivery, and changing biology.

Two possible outcomes linked to changing health technology are improved detection and treatment methods and development of iatrogenic mortality and morbidity. Improved early detection and treatment methods for diseases affecting women, such as breast cancer, may contribute to a longer life span and improved quality of life. Iatrogenic problems such as vaginal cancer in DES (diethylstilbestrol) daughters, endometrial cancer in estrogen replacement therapy users, and thrombophlebitis and increased risk of death from vascular diseases among women using birth control pills, may shorten women's lives or contribute to their morbidity. Careful analysis of the merits and risks of each new technological advance will be essential to safeguard women's health in the future.

Lifestyles that women will adopt may improve or harm their health. As social norms promote more opportunity for women in the labor force, women may be exposed to toxic substances and other hazards that currently account for work-connected disability and mortality among men. If women adopt health behavior, illness behavior, and sick role behavior patterns that are more like those that men observe, then it is possible that the protection once afforded women by their self-care and use of health services may become a lost advantage. On the other hand, if women maintain their previous patterns of self-care as well as health services use, they may be affected to a lesser extent by hazards of the workplace. If sex discrimination in employment is abolished and women truly have equal opportunity to achieve their goals in their place of employment, their health may improve. On the other hand, if more women adopt characteristics such as aggressive competitiveness, the advantages accrued through improved opportunities may be erased.

As the current institutionalized sex role expectations among clinicians are changed, the reported "excess" of mental illness among women may decrease. However, symptoms of mental illness reported by women and men may become more similar as sex role expectations converge. As women's roles more closely approximate those of men, assumptions about appropriate therapies may be revised. For example, prescription of psychotropic drugs might be weighed differently than in the past as their effects on women's work functions become more visible.

Women's adoption of self-care may make certain contacts with formal health services unnecessary. For example, women may choose to perform their own pregnancy tests. This trend may have positive outcomes linked to women's increased knowledge about their health or negative effects if self-care replaces services that require professional expertise, such as diagnoses and treatment of certain conditions. As clinicians realize that women are knowledgeable about their health, social stratification between clinician and client is less likely to influence the process of health care. The demystification of health that brought about the dissemination of health information to women is likely to result in consumers of services who are increasingly able to question decisions about treatment, explore alternative methods of healing, and carefully examine the ramifications of procedures such as surgery, drug therapy, and sterilization.

Changes in women's own biology are least likely to influence their health in the coming decades, aside from the aging of the population. However, changes in biology brought about by current research in genetics and technologies developed as a result of this research may provide hope for women with genetically determined diseases. Although it is important to remain hopeful about these future technologies, it is equally important to remain vigilant about their potentially health-damaging consequences.

References

Bader, J. (1985). Respite care: Temporary relief for caregivers. *Women and Health, 10*(2/3), 39-52.

Belle, D. (1990). Poverty and women's mental health. *American Psychologist, 45,* 385-389.

Cole, P. (1974). Morbidity in the United States. In C. Erhardt & J. Berlin (Eds.), *Mortality and morbidity in the United States* (pp. 65-104). Cambridge, MA: Harvard University Press.

Cooperstock, R. (1981). A review of women's psychotropic drug use. In E. Howell & M. Ayes (Eds.), *Women and mental health* (pp. 131-140). New York: Basic Books.

Faludi, S. (1991). *Backlash.* New York: Crown.

Fidell, L. (1981). Sex differences in psychotropic drug use. *Professional Psychologist, 12*(1), 156-162.

Gartler, S. (1990). The relevance of X chromosome inactivation to gender differentials in longevity. In M. Ory & H. Warner (Eds.), *Gender, health, and longevity: Multidisciplinary perspectives* (pp. 73-85). New York: Springer.

Goble, F., & Konapka, E. (1973). Sex as a factor in infectious disease. *Transactions of the New York Academy of Sciences, 2,* 325-346.

Gordon-Bradshaw, R. (1987). A social essay on special issues facing poor women of color. *Women and Health, 12*(3/4), 243-259.

Gove, W. (1972a). The relationship between sex roles, mental illness, and marital status. *Social Forces, 51*(1), 34-44.

Gove, W. (1972b). Sex, marital status, and suicide. *Journal of Health and Social Behavior, 13,* 304-313.

Gove, W. (1973). Sex, marital status, and mortality. *American Journal of Sociology, 79,* 45-67.

Gove, W., & Tudor, J. (1973). Adult sex roles and mental illness. *American Journal of Sociology, 78,* 812-835.

Grau, L. (1987). Illness-engendered poverty among the elderly. *Women and Health, 12*(3/4), 103-118.

Haynes, S., & Feinleib, M. (1980). Women, work, and coronary heart disease: Prospective findings from the Framingham Heart Study. *American Journal of Public Health, 70*(2), 133-141.

Hazzard, W. (1990). A central role of sex hormones in the sex differential in lipoprotein metabolism, atherosclerosis, and longevity. In M. Ory & H. Warner (Eds.), *Gender, health, and longevity: Multidisciplinary perspectives* (pp. 87-108). New York: Springer.

Hibbard, J., & Pope, C. (1985). Employment status, employment characteristics, and women's health. *Women and Health, 10*(1), 59-78.

Kline, C. (1975). The socialization process of women. *The Gerontologist, 15,* 486-492.

Lewis, M. (1986). Older women and health: An overview. *Women and Health, 11*(1), 1-16.

Lorde, A. (1988). Age, race, class, and sex: Women redefining difference. In C. McWeven & S. O'Sullivan (Eds.), *Out the other side* (pp. 269-276). London: Virgo.

Marieskind, H. (1980). *Women's health.* St. Louis: C. V. Mosby.

Matthews, K. (1989). Interactive effects of behavior and reproductive hormones on sex differences in risk for coronary heart disease. *Health Psychology, 8*(4), 373-387.

Maunz, E., & Woods, N. (1988). Self care practices among young adult women: Influence of symptoms, employment, and sex role orientation. *Health Care for Women International, 9,* 29-41.

McBarnette, L. (1987). Women and poverty: Effects on reproductive status. *Women and Health, 12*(3/4), 55-82.

McBride, A. (1990). Multiple roles. *American Psychologist, 45,* 381-384.

McKinlay, S., & McKinlay, J. (1989). The impact of menopause and social factors on health. In C. Hammond, F. Haseltine, & I. Schiff (Eds.), *Menopause: Evaluation, treatment and health concerns* (pp. 137-161). New York: Alan Liss.

McLaughlin, S., & Melber, B. (1986). *The changing lifecourse of American women: Life-style and attitude changes.* Unpublished manuscript, Battelle Human Affairs Research Centers, Seattle, WA.

Mechanic, D. (1976). Sex, illness, illness behavior, and the use of health services. *Journal of Human Stress, 2*(2), 29-40.

Michaels, R., & Rogers, K. (1971). A sex difference in immunologic responsiveness. *Pediatrics, 47,* 120-123.

Miller, D. (1985). Women and long-term nursing care. *Women and Health, 10*(2/3), 29-38.

Moriyama, I., Krueger, D., & Stamler, J. (1971). *Cardiovascular diseases in the United States.* Cambridge, MA: Harvard University Press.

Muller, C. (1986). Health and health care of employed women and homemakers: Family factors. *Women and Health, 11*(1), 7-26.

Naeye, R., Burt, L., Wright, D., & Associates. (1971). Neonatal mortality, the male disadvantage. *Pediatrics, 48*(6), 902-906.

Nathanson, C. (1975). Illness and the feminine role: A theoretical review. *Social Science and Medicine, 9*(2), 57-62.

Nathanson, C. (1977a). Sex, illness, and medical care: A review of data, theory, and method. *Social Science and Medicine, 2*(1), 13-25.

Nathanson, C. (1977b). Sex roles as variables in preventive health behavior. *Journal of Community Health, 3*(2), 142-155.

Nathanson, C. (1980). Social roles and health status among women: The significance of employment. *Social Science and Medicine, 14a,* 463-471.

National Center for Health Statistics. (1988a). *Health promotion and disease prevention: United States, 1985* (Series 10, No. 163, DHHS Publication No. 88-1591). Hyattsville, MD: U.S. Department of Health and Human Services.

National Center for Health Statistics. (1988b). *Vital statistics of the United States, 1986* (Vol 2., Part A). Washington, DC: Government Printing Office.

National Center for Health Statistics. (1993a). *Current estimates from the National Health Interview Survey, 1992* (Series 10). Hyattsville, MD: U.S. Department of Health and Human Services.

National Center for Health Statistics. (1993b). *Health in the United States and prevention profile, 1992.* Hyattsville, MD: U.S. Department of Health and Human Services.

Neel, J. (1990). Toward an explanation of the human sex ratio. In M. Ory & H. Warner (Eds.), *Gender, health, and longevity. Multidisciplinary perspectives* (pp. 57-72). New York: Springer.

Orem, D. (1971). *Nursing: Concepts of practice.* New York: McGraw-Hill.

Rathbone-McCuan, E. (1985). Health needs and social policy. *Women and Health, 10*(2/3), 17-28.

Retherford, R. (1975). *The changing sex differential in mortality.* Westport, CT: Greenwood.

Richardson, H. (1987). The health plight of rural women. *Women and Health, 12*(3/4), 41-54.

Robins, L., Helzer, J., Weissman, M., Orvaschel, H., Gruenberg, E., Burke, J., & Regier, D. (1984). Lifetime prevalence of specific psychiatric disorders in three sites. *Archives of General Psychiatry, 41,* 949-958.

Rodin, J., & Ickovics, J. (1990). Women's health: Review and research agenda as we approach the 21st century. *American Psychologist, 45*(9), 1018-1034.

Russo, N. (1990). Overview: Forging research priorities for women's mental health. *American Psychologist, 45*(3), 368-373.

Russo, N., Amaro, J., & Winter, M. (1987). The use of inpatient mental health services by Hispanic women. *Psychology of Women Quarterly, 11,* 427-442.

Sinnott, J. (1977). Sex role inconsistency, biology, and successful aging: A dialectical model. *The Gerontologist, 17*(5), 459-463.

Smith, D., & Warner, H. (1990). Overview of biomedical perspectives: Possible relationships between genes on the sex chromosomes and longevity. In M. Ory & H. Warner (Eds.), *Gender, health, and longevity: Multidisciplinary perspectives* (pp. 41-55). New York: Springer.

Spiegelman, M., & Ehrhardt, C. (1974). International comparisons of mortality and longevity. In C. I. Ehrhardt & J. E. Berlin (Eds.), *Mortality and morbidity in the United States.* Cambridge, MA: Harvard University Press.

Stellman, J. (1987). The working environment of the working poor: An analysis based on worker's compensation claims, census data and known risk factors. *Women and Health, 12*(3/4), 83-102.

U.S. Department of Health and Human Services. (1985). *Report of the Secretary's Task Force on Black and Minority Health.* Washington, DC: Author.

Verbrugge, L. (1976). Females and illness: Recent trends in sex differences in the United States. *Journal of Health and Social Behavior, 17,* 387-403.

Verbrugge, L. (1980). Sex differences in complaints and diagnoses. *Journal of Behavioral Medicine, 3,* 327-355.

Verbrugge, L. (1986). Role burdens and physical health of women and men. *Women and Health, 11*(1), 47-77.

Verbrugge, L., & Wingard, D. (1987). Sex differentials in health and mortality. *Women and Health, 12*(2), 103-145.

Vernon-Roberts, B. (1969). The effects of steroid hormones on macrophage activity. *International Review Cytology, 25,* 131-159.

Waldron, I. (1976). Why do women live longer than men? *Social Science and Medicine, 10,* 349-362.

Waldron, I. (1983). Sex differences in human mortality: The role of genetic factors. *Social Science and Medicine, 17,* 321-333.

Waldron, I., & Herold, J. (1986). Employment, attitudes toward employment and women's health. *Women and Health, 11*(1), 79-98.

Waldron, I., Herold, J., Dunn, D., & Straum, R. (1982). Reciprocal effects of health and labor force participation among women: Evidence from two longitudinal studies. *Journal of Occupational Medicine, 24*(1), 126-132.

Weksler, M. (1990). A possible role for the immune system in the gender-longevity differential. In M. Ory & H. Warner (Eds.), *Gender, health, and longevity: Multidisciplinary perspectives* (pp. 109-115). New York: Springer.

Willson, J. (1987). Women and poverty: A demographic overview. *Women and Health, 12*(3/4), 21-40.

Wingard, D. (1982). The sex differential in mortality rates: Demographic and behavioral factors. *American Journal of Epidemiology, 115*(2), 205-216.

Woods, N. (1985a). Employment, family roles, and mental ill health in young adult married women. *Nursing Research, 34*(1), 4-9.

Woods, N. (1985b). Self care practices among young adult married women. *Research in Nursing and Health, 8,* 227-234.

Woods, N., & Hulka, B. (1979). Symptom reports and illness behavior among employed women and homemakers. *Journal of Community Health, 5*(1), 36-45.

Zambrana, R. (1987). A research agenda in issues affecting poor and minority women: A model for understanding their health needs. *Women and Health, 12*(3/4), 137-160.

2

Women as Health Care Providers

CAROL J. LEPPA

Health care is women's work. This is true for both the highly visible, paid public health care provider roles and the nearly invisible, unpaid family health care provider roles that women occupy. This chapter explores both of these realms of health care and provides an overview of how women provide the vast majority of health care work in the world.

Women as Paid Health Care Providers

Women provide the majority of paid health care. Women health care providers outnumber men by 3 to 1, yet women are clustered in those professions and occupations that are lower paying, less prestigious, and less autonomous than those that are predominantly occupied by men (Butter, Carpenter, Kay, & Simmons, 1985, 1987). This is not new. Bullough and Bullough described the phenomenon in 1975 and Butter and colleagues elaborated on it in the 1980s. As we move toward the 21st century there is little indication of change. Although women are making significant advances in the traditionally male occupations of medicine, dentistry, and pharmacy, they continue to far outnumber men in the traditionally female occupations: nurse, occupational and physical therapist, dietition, dental assistant/dental hygienist, nursing assistant, and health technician.

The statistics presented in Figure 2.1 illustrate the state and status of women in the paid health care occupations. Overall, Figure 2.1 is, again, not new information. Many authors have compared the percentage of women in the varied health occupations and explored the gender hierarchies in the health labor force (Brown, 1982; Butter et al., 1985, 1987; Marieskind, 1980). The statistics are followed and updated annually by the federal government and reported in various government reports available to the public—for example, reports from the U.S. Bureau of the Census and the U.S. Public Health Service. The occupations listed in Figure 2.1 are not all of those on which information is available, but they provide a good representation and clear picture of the continued disparity between women's and men's paid health care roles. The

Health Occupation	Percentage of Women of Total	Total Workers (1,000s)	Average Earnings (in dollars)
MDs	17.9	548	132,300
Dentists	8.6	170	70,000
Pharmacists	32.3	174	37,336
RNs	94.2	1,599	32,100
Dietitians	90.8	83	25,650
Therapists	76.3	324	24,566
Dental assistants	98.9	210	15,000
Health aides	84.5	416	12,480
Nurses' aides/orderlies	90.4	1,439	11,500

Figure 2.1. Women Workers in Selected Health Occupations, 1990
SOURCE: Figures for the percentage of women of total and number of total workers are from the U.S. Bureau of the Census (1991). Figures for average earnings are from the U.S. Department of Labor, Bureau of Labor Statistics (1990-1991).

occupations were listed in order of median reported income (Butter et al., 1985) and in a relatively comparable order of percentage of women in each occupation. It is also important to look at the numbers of people employed in each occupation. In particular, the large numbers of nurses and nurses' aides/orderlies, of which over 90% are women, account for the majority of women in all health care occupations. Women are indeed clustered in jobs and occupations that are lower in pay, less prestigious, and less autonomous than jobs of men in the health care field (Butter et al., 1987).

In 1975 Navarro wrote that the occupational, class, and sex structure in the U.S. health labor force reflects that structure seen in the competitive sector of the economy. He compared the distribution of health workers by class and sex with the distribution of workers in other sectors of the labor force. Ehrenreich (1975) commented that "the stratification within the U.S. health industry has been documented again and again—in tones ranging from academic resignation to feminist outrage" (p. 7). The stratification of the health labor force in general is further explored in Table 2.1.

Table 2.1 compares four traditionally male health care occupations and nursing and makes projections for the future composition in terms of numbers and gender. The occupations of medicine, dentistry, and pharmacy were chosen not only because they have the highest visibility and occupy the three top spots in terms of income in Figure 2.1 but also because the data exist in current federal reports. Nursing is included for comparison in the years 1970 and 1990. No projections have been made for the percentage of nurses who will be female in the future. Evidently, no one expects a great deal of change. Although it is true that for male nurses a change from 2.7% in 1970 to 5.8% in 1990 represents a greater than 100% increase and that in 1990 some 93,000 nurses were men, the effect on the profession as a whole is minimal. Nursing remains a profession dominated by women. The importance of Table 2.1 is the illustration of how the health labor force is changing. According to U.S. government reports and projections, all of the traditionally male health care occupations have experienced and will continue to experience dramatic increases in the percentage of women in their ranks. The 21st century will see the health care occupations more solidly female than they are today in terms of the number and percentage of women occupying jobs in the

Table 2.1 Percentage of Women in Selected Health Care Occupations

Occupation	*1970*	*1990*	*2000*	*2020*	*Number of Women in 2020*
RNs	97.3	94.2	NA	NA	1,642,900
MDs	9.2	17.9	22.7	29.8	252,790
Dentists	3.4	8.6	16.0	30.2	42,400
Pharmacists	11.9	32.3	38.3	49.5	105,900

SOURCES: Adapted from Fogel and Woods (1981); U.S. Bureau of the Census (1991); and U.S. Public Health Service (1990).

health labor force. Other implications of the changes in the traditionally male and female health occupations will be explored further.

Traditional Women's Occupations in Health Care

The idea of formal education for women in the 19th century was not well accepted, let alone an occupation for women outside the home. Women in the 1800s were struggling to define a role for themselves in society through the women's suffrage movement of the 1840s as well as through the early women's health organizations of the time (Ehrenreich & English, 1973). Tremendous resistance was presented with "scientific reasons" for women to stay in what were their supposed physically and intellectually inferior positions in society. Hamilton (1885) wrote that "the best education for girls, then, is that which best prepares them for the legitimate duties of womanhood" (p. 319; e.g., wife, motherhood, homemaking). He further asserted that attainment of high intellectual culture exacts too great a price and results in a "ruined or physically damaged constitution." Hamilton based his theory about education for women on a set of assumptions about physical and intellectual differences between the sexes. With respect to women, he described how "brain work" competes with the "vital forces of the body," and that such a diversion of "nerve power" to the mental labor involved in education could only lead to "greatly impaired or permanently ruined health, a life of sterility, general unhappiness, and uselessness" (p. 320). In the face of such heated (if erroneous) opposition as this, nursing was seen as at least a marginally respectable occupation for women given the close approximation of nursing work with the "legitimate duties of womanhood."

Nursing is the largest single health care occupation and, as illustrated earlier, it continues to be a women's work world. Nursing will be the first focus of this discussion of the traditionally women's health occupations.

Historical Perspective

The history of nursing has been explored extensively from multiple perspectives. Modern nursing is traditionally associated with its beginnings with Florence Nightingale, who asserted that "every woman is a nurse" (Nightingale, 1860/1969). The 19th century saw the organization of hospitals as centers for care for the sick as well as the organization of the nursing profession. England's Crimean War and the United States' Civil War during the 19th century helped create a demand for nurses and an opportunity for women to provide a socially acceptable contribution outside the home. While carving out a respectable occupation for women in the 19th century, Nightingale set in motion many of the norms and traditions that structure nursing today. The Nightingale model for nursing education (e.g., practical experiential training in the hospital setting) was the gold standard for early nursing education both in England and in the United States.

The 19th-century profession of nursing was created for women and by women—primarily middle- and upper-class women—and was molded by the restraints on women at that time (Ehrenreich & English, 1973). Historians have chronicled the developments of the nursing profession, nursing schools, nursing work in private duty and hospital environments, public health nursing, and war work; the recurrent cycles of nursing shortage; and the expanded roles of nurses. The close association between the status of women and the status of nursing and how this has affected the development of nurses and nursing has not been attended to well. Beyond the work of Ehrenreich and English there are a few classic works that explore how gender has affected nursing and nurses.

Jo Ann Ashley (1976) was one of the first to explore in-depth the influence of gender on nursing and nurses. Her book, *Hospitals, Paternalism, and the Role of the Nurse,* is the first history of American nursing from a feminist point of view. Ashley describes the discriminatory attitudes toward women that institutionalized their servitude in hospitals. By exploring and exposing the sexism of the "hospital family" with its systematic oppression of the nursing profession, Ashley points out the far-reaching effects on the quality and delivery of health care in American hospitals.

How sexism has affected nurses and nursing has been explored by others (Cleland, 1971; Darbyshire, 1987; Levitt, 1977; Weaver & Garrett, 1983). Of these, Cleland (1971) was the first to discuss how sexism is nursing's most pervasive problem. Roberts (1983) explored oppression and oppressed group behavior in nursing, discussing how oppression has fostered the horizontal violence of nurse against nurse. Muff (1988) and her colleagues identify the problems of nurses as the problems of women in the collection *Socialization, Sexism, and Stereotyping: Women's Issues in Nursing.* These authors explore the problems of rigid sex role socialization and the distortions (stereotypes) that reflect societal values and prejudices. Feminism has brought both positives and negatives to nursing. On the positive side, feminists have encouraged women's participation and recognition in all work environments. On the negative side, some feminists have identified nursing as one of the female ghettos that should be avoided by career-minded women.

The historical development of the nursing work culture has also been explored by Barbara Melosh (1982) in her book *The Physician's Hand.* Complementing the history of nursing portrayed in professional nursing journals and texts (which promotes the ideal of professionalism), Melosh presents the history from the perspective of working nurses and the active and passive resistance that many nurses displayed toward professionalism in nursing. Melosh describes the nursing work culture as the distinctive language, lore, and social rules that nurses create on the job that suggest the coherence and structure of work activities. This is in contrast to the culture of professionalism created by academics and nursing leaders. Melosh explores the culture of nursing and "recasts nursing history from the viewpoint of nurses on the job and places it in the context of women's history, labor history, and medical history and sociology"(p. 6). In so doing, she illuminates the origins of some of the divisive issues within nursing that exist today—for example, the continued controversy over the required level of education for entry to practice. Melosh views this topic through the lens of history in describing the different methods of nursing training that developed for licensed practical nurses (LPNs) and registered nurses (RNs). She traces the labor history and the professional organizations that grew out of and supported both the LPN and RN educational methods. In addition, she describes the class differences between the educational elite (RNs) and the labor class workers (LPNs). The title of her work reflects the establishment and development of nursing as an extension of the physician—an image of handmaiden that nurses have long fought to eliminate.

The central work of nursing, caring, is the focus of Reverby's (1987a, 1987b) historical study of nursing. The history of nursing is inextricably intertwined with the development of medicine and the political economy of the hospital as an institution. The "dilemma of caring" involves nurses being ordered to care (and to provide care) in a society that does not value caring. Taking the struggle that Nightingale faced in developing a respectable occupation for women one step further, Reverby examines how society has failed to value caring and caring activities. The profession of nursing has been demanding the right to care as opposed to obeying the order to care. This challenges the deeply held beliefs about the gender relations in and the structure of the health care hierarchy in that it opposes the traditional physician-male ordering the nurse-female to care for the patient-child. The nurse and physician decide collaboratively on, in consultation with the patient, the methods and modes of care, enacting the ideal of having the "right to care." The difficulty of finding a way to "care with autonomy" and the inability to separate caring from its societal (lack of) value leads many nurses to abandon the effort to care or to abandon nursing altogether. Reverby makes a strong argument to support the close connection between the social status of women and nurses and the problems that both face.

Expanded Roles for Nurses

It might be argued that the struggles of nurses reviewed earlier hold only for those nurses working in hospitals. Although this may be true to some extent, it must be remembered that the majority (68%) of nurses continue to be employed by hospitals (U.S. Public Health Service, 1990) with this majority decreasing only slightly (61%) in projections for 2020. Nevertheless, there are other areas in which nurses provide health care.

As well as the areas of home health care, nursing homes, and physician's offices, there are the more autonomous expanded nursing roles of clinical nurse specialist, nurse practitioner, nurse-midwife, and nurse anesthetist. These expanded roles require advanced educational preparation and have relatively small but active populations of nurses in their ranks. The expansion of the nursing role by these advanced practitioners has met with opposition from the medical practitioners who occupy the respective markets. Nurse-midwives have had to fight obstetricians and gynecologists for practice privileges and reasonable insurance rates (Kendellen, 1987; Lubic, 1987). In addition, nurse-midwives have struggled with the dilemma of lay midwives (whether or how to officially recognize/identify with these less formally educated practitioners), who have been making a comeback in the past 10 years (Kay, Butter, Chang, & Houlihan, 1988). The role of nurse practitioner requires a close collaboration with a physician because the authority to prescribe medications is limited for these nurses (Bezjak, 1987; Jacox, 1987). Direct reimbursement for nurse practitioner services by insurance and government programs is also an issue. Nurse practitioners have had to bill their services under the name of a physician to receive payment from these third-party payers. Nurse practitioners (just like physicians) can bill patients directly, but this has become the exception rather than the rule in patient care reimbursement.

Although the practice of anesthesia began as a nursing practice in 1919, it was recognized as a medical specialty after World War II (Gunn, Nicosia, & Tobin, 1987). Consequently, nurse anesthetists must fight for their legal practice position with anesthesiologists, and because nurse anesthetists cannot prescribe the anesthetic agents they use and must work in close association with surgeons, they are at a decided disadvantage. It is important to note that nurse anesthetists have been accorded a high status and correspondingly high salaries in nursing. It is also interesting that whereas men make up only 5.8% of all nurses, 40% of nurse anesthetists are male (Bernhardt & Pardue, 1987).

This discussion of women's health occupations has focused on nursing. Referring back to Figure 2.1, it is clear that nursing is not the only health job occupied primarily by women—it is only the largest. It is also the most organized and vocal about the issues the profession faces. The issues for dietitians, therapists, dental hygienists, and the health service occupations of nurse aide, orderly, and nonnursing health aide will not necessarily be the same as those described for nursing. What can be assumed is that working in a health care field that continues to be segregated by sex and class affects all workers in terms of working conditions and wages (Butter et al., 1987).

Traditional Men's Occupations in Health Care

Three health care occupations—medicine, dentistry, and pharmacy—are identified as traditionally male in Figure 2.1, which also identifies them as the highest paid health occupations. There is a considerable literature on women in medicine, less on women in dentistry, and very little on women in pharmacy. This discussion will focus on women in medicine as representative of the challenges facing women in these male-identified occupations.

As described earlier in the history of the development of nursing, the history of women in medicine is inextricably entwined with women's social and political history. It is not surprising that women faced resistance in seeking entrance into the medical profession. In the 19th century, when women were organizing and fighting for their political (right to vote) and social (right to work outside the home and own property) rights and some women were fighting to establish nursing as a respectable career for women, others were arguing that women ought to be physicians "by virtue of their natural gifts as healers and nurturers" (Morantz-Sanchez, 1985). Although the feminist movement of the 19th century helped women gain access to medical education and careers, at the same time the feminist movement also incited a strong resistance to women in medicine (Shryock, 1966).

The early relative success in the 1850s in opening medicine to women was minimized or reversed in the late 19th and early 20th centuries. During this time the Flexner Report was contracted by the Carnegie Corporation and published in 1910. The wealth of the industrial revolution had allowed the development of organized philanthropy, and medical reform was a high priority for these new foundations. In the name of standardizing (in accordance with the Johns Hopkins medical education model) and ensuring the quality of medical education, the majority of smaller, less well endowed and supported medical schools that trained women and minority physicians were effectively closed. Although this process did eliminate those ineffective and dangerous small schools, it also eliminated those that were effective and successful but unable to finance the newly "required" facilities. Without access to training opportunities, the number of women physicians decreased markedly. Not until the 20th century women's movement, which gained momentum in the 1960s, did women begin to increase significantly in numbers and percentage of medical school applicants, admissions, and graduates (Walsch, 1977).

As indicated in Table 2.1, the percentage of physicians who are women has been increasing significantly and is projected to continue to increase to nearly 30% of physicians in 2020. These women have made it into a traditionally male work world, and although they are a part of the top of the health care occupations hierarchy, they face problems similar to those faced by women in other occupations and in society as a whole.

First, making it into the world of medicine does not mean making it within the world of medicine—if "making it" means status and monetary success in our society. Women in medicine are disproportionately concentrated in the relatively lower paying and lower status medical specialties of family practice (10%), internal medicine (22%), pediatrics (14%), psychiatry (9%), and obstetrics/gynecology (9.3%) (Adams & Bazzoli, 1986; Cohen, Ferrier, Woodward, & Goldsmith, 1991; Lorber, 1987; Shye, 1991). The higher paying (and therefore higher status) specialties of diagnostic radiology (4%) and surgery (4.4%) (in particular cardiothoracic surgery [less than 0.1%]) have the lowest percentage of women (Council of Medical Specialty Society, 1990; Heins, 1985; Martin & Woodring, 1986). Whether these specialty choices reflect women's preferences for practice type and environment or reflect a subtle pressure to choose "appropriate" specialties, it remains interesting that those specialties with a higher percentage of women are at the bottom of the medical hierarchy. Also, those women in the highest paid/highest status specialties are at the bottom of their particular specialty hierarchy (Janus & Janus, 1987).

The discrimination and problems that women physicians have faced within medicine have been well documented (Lorber, 1984, 1986, 1987; Morantz-Sanchez, 1985; Walsch, 1977). The problems of combining a family with a demanding medical career have been explored with the not surprising finding that women physicians will feel the most strain on their personal lives, some strain in their family role, and minimal, if any, strain in their professional role (Ducker, 1986). Women physicians, like women in general, sacrifice their own health and well-being for the sake of others. Women physicians struggle to combine a family life and a career (Mikell, 1987; Shye, 1991; Sinal, Weavil, & Camp, 1989; Woodward, Cohen, & Ferrier, 1990). The female surgery resident who is married starts out "with a strike against her" because her attention is assumed to be divided between her career and her marriage/family responsibilities (Burnley & Burkett, 1986). The struggles that men physicians face in combining a family and career are not documented in the literature on physicians; therefore, comparisons are not currently possible. Finally, echoes of Hamilton's 19th-century admonition that women are at best ill suited for education and risk sterility when they use their minds are found in a study on how menstrual cycles and pregnancy negatively affect the practice of female family practitioners via the decreased time in practice and the increased "emotionality" found by these researchers (Tucker & Margo, 1987).

The prediction that women will make up a growing proportion of physicians is not taken lightly by those who are keeping track of these statistics. The American College of Obstetricians and Gynecologists (1987) conducted a study of what the increasing percentages of women and the women's movement in general mean for the future of the practice of obstetrics and gynecology. One particular effect of note is that, the women's movement has changed the conventional practice of obstetrics with the demand for alternative birthing methods and the resultant major change toward birthing rooms and partner participation in delivery in obstetric practice. Women patients also prefer women physicians (1.5 to 3 times more often) in the areas of obstetrics and gynecology, family practice, internal medicine, and psychiatry according to one study (Fenton, Robinowitz, & Leaf, 1987).

Lorber (1987) and Wilson (1987) sum up the issues of women physicians by stating that women physicians face a choice—either they can align themselves with male physicians and perpetuate physician dominance of the health care system or they can align themselves with other women and work toward change of the health care system. Whether the higher percentage of women physicians will result in women influencing the practice of medicine or if the established medical profession will influence women physicians—or a combination of the two—the status of women physicians will continue to be linked with the status of women in society.

Women as Unpaid Health Care Providers

As mentioned earlier in this chapter, health care is women's work, with the majority of health care providers being women. Turning the phrase around presents another truth—women's work is health care. Much of the work that women do in their unpaid, private lives is health care for themselves and their families. The arguments that were used to gain women's access into the paid fields of health care were based on women's natural talents and interests in caring for their families. Chodorow (1978) argued that women's greater interest in and ability to care for family members is a socially constructed gender difference, not a biologically determined difference. The ancient socially proscribed roles of food gathering, cultivation, and preparation; keeping the home environment clean and safe; and the biological role of bearing and caring for children had singularly prepared women to care for the health and welfare of society.

Today, women do the majority of the housework, shopping, and cooking and are the primary caregivers in the family, whether they are employed outside of the home or not (Brody, Kleban, Johnson, Hoffman, & Schoonover, 1987). The fact that more women are in the labor force and that the two-income family is fast becoming a necessity rather than a luxury has not altered women's socially proscribed roles and rarely challenged responsibility for the care of the family.

One way of evaluating the socially recognized importance of women as health care providers for the family is an exploration of the marketing aimed at women as the health care decision maker for the family (e.g., the "ask Doctor Mom" commercial for cough medicine). Women provide health care and also decide from whom and where they will seek help for themselves and their families. To guide women consumers toward healthy choices in providing family health care, women are also targeted by food product advertisements that promote healthy children, heart health, low fat, low sugar, and smart buying as healthy buying, including all types of food products from soup to peanut butter. The importance of a clean house, clean clothes, healthy exercise—not to mention a beautiful body, preferably looking like a model—are primarily advertised using women models and targeted to women who are responsible for the health and welfare of their families (Graham, 1985).

Beyond the standard of daily health care provided by women in families is the role of health care provider for the ill and infirm in the family (Finch & Groves, 1983). Women as mothers and daughters have traditionally been the caregivers for family members in need (O'Neill & Ross, 1991; Pasquali, 1991), with one study finding that 75% of the caregivers of ill elders are women (Travelers Insurance Companies, 1988). Elaine Brody (1981) was the first to define the role of "women in the middle" as those women who have primary responsibility for dependent children as well as assuming care for their elderly parents and in-laws as the advances of modern medicine have resulted in an extended life span. In addition, the U.S. demographics are not encouraging for this group of women in the middle. Only 4% of the U.S. population was aged 65 or older in 1900. In 1990, 12% of the population was 65 or older, which is projected to be 14% by the year 2010 (Bowers & Liegel, 1990). Not all people over the age of 65 are infirm; in fact, the majority are in good health. However, the increasing disability and episodic health needs of this age group rely primarily on daughters or daughters-in-law for assistance. The aging of the population has combined with a decrease in the birthrate (4 per family in 1900 to 1.8 per family in 1990). This means that there will be an increase in the number of needy elderly in the population corresponding to a decrease in the number of women (or men) available to provide health care assistance. These caretakers, these women in the middle, will likely attend to the needs of their aging and young dependent family members to the detriment of their own health needs (Bull, 1990; Lindgren, 1990).

It is not only the increase in the numbers of elderly in the population that has placed additional burden on women as family health care providers. The changes resulting from the implementation of diagnostic related groupings (DRGs)—which effectively limits the amount of time any particular patient stays in the hospital—have resulted in patients who are discharged sooner and sicker than in the past. The majority of these patients are discharged home with the assumption that home care is cheaper than hospital care and just as safe, if not beneficial, after a certain stabilized point in recovery (Bull, 1990; Cawley & Gerdts, 1988; Dewis & Chekryn, 1990). The majority of this at-home care—from assistance with daily living activities to complex cancer pain and treatment management to managing with the ever changing demands of the Alzheimer's patient—is provided by women, either an unpaid family member (80% to 90%) or a home health aid (Brody, 1985).

Beyond the family health care needs that women attend to, women are community activists in promoting health care. Whether it is campaigning for safe living environments in the inner city, combating toxic waste hazards, or working for clean water and proper sanitation in the developing countries, women are leaders in identifying the problems and organizing the solutions (Pizurki, Mejia, Butter, & Ewart, 1987). The World Health Organization has recognized the importance of women as health care providers in its emphasis on Women, Health and Development in the push for Health for All by the Year 2000 through the mechanisms of primary, preventive health care (Pizurki et al., 1987).

Summary

Health care is women's work. Those women who work in the traditionally defined male health care roles receive a lot of attention and praise for "making it in a man's world." But health care is not a man's world, although it is still controlled primarily by men. The world of health care is a woman's work world, in both the paid/public and unpaid/private realms.

References

Adams, K. E., & Bazzoli, G. J. (1986). Career plans of women and minority physicians: Implications for health manpower policy. *Journal of the American Medical Women's Association, 41*(1), 17-20.

American College of Obstetricians and Gynecologists and American Medical Association Council on Long Range Planning and Development. (1987). The future of obstetrics and gynecology. *JAMA, 258*(24), 3547-3553.

Ashley, J. (1976). *Hospitals, paternalism, and the role of the nurse.* New York: Teachers College Press.

Bernhardt, M. L., & Pardue, N. (1987). Career trends in nursing. *Imprint, 34*(5), 36-37.

Bezjak, J. E. (1987). Physician-perceived incentives for association with nurse practitioners. *Nurse Practitioner, 12*(3), 66-74.

Bowers, B., & Liegel, B. (1990). Women as health care providers: Family caregivers of the elderly. In C. J. Leppa (Ed.), *Women's health perspectives: An annual review* (Vol. 3, pp. 261-292). Phoenix, AZ: Oryx.

Brody, E. M. (1981). "Women in the middle" and family help to older people. *The Gerontologist, 21*(5), 471-480.

Brody, E. M. (1985). Parent care as a normative stress. *The Gerontologist, 25*(1), 19-29.

Brody, E. M., Kleban, M. H., Johnson, P. T., Hoffman, C., & Schoonover, C. B. (1987). Work status and parent care: A comparison of four groups of women. *The Gerontologist, 27*(2), 201-208.

Brown, C. A. (1982). Women workers in the health service industry. In E. Fee (Ed.), *Women and health: The politics of sex in medicine* (pp. 105-116). New York: Baywood.

Bull, M. J. (1990). Factors influencing family caregiver burden and health. *Western Journal of Nursing Research, 12*(6), 758-770.

Bullough, B., & Bullough, V. (1975). Sex discrimination in health care. *Nursing Outlook, 23*(1), 40-45.

Burnley, C. S., & Burkett, G. L. (1986). Specialization: Are women in surgery different? *Journal of the American Medical Women's Association, 41*(5), 144-147.

Butter, I., Carpenter, E., Kay, B., & Simmons, R. (1985). *Sex and status: Hierarchies in the health workforce.* Ann Arbor, MI: American Public Health Association.

Butter, I., Carpenter, E., Kay, B., & Simmons, R. S. (1987). Gender hierarchies in the health labor force. *International Journal of Health Services, 17*(1), 133-149.

Cawley, M. M., & Gerdts, E. K. (1988). Establishing a cancer caregivers program: An interdisciplinary approach. *Cancer Nursing, 11*(5), 267-273.

Chodorow, N. (1978). *The reproduction of mothering: Psychoanalysis and the sociology of gender.* Berkeley: University of California Press.

Cleland, V. (1971). Sex discrimination: Nursing's most pervasive problem. *American Journal of Nursing, 71*(8), 1542-1547.

Cohen, M., Ferrier, B. M., Woodward, C. A., & Goldsmith, C. H. (1991). Gender differences in practice patterns of Ontario family physicians. *Journal of the American Medical Women's Association, 46*(2), 49-54.

Council of Medical Specialty Society. (1990). *Choosing a medical specialty.* Lake Forest, IL: Author.

Darbyshire, P. (1987). Nurses and doctors: The burden of history. *Nursing Times, 83*(4), 32-34.

Dewis, M. E., & Chekryn, J. (1990). The older dyadic family unit and chronic illness. *Home Health Care Nurse, 8*(2), 42-48.

Ducker, D. G. (1986). Role conflict in women physicians: A longitudinal study. *Journal of the American Medical Women's Association, 41*(1), 14-16.

Ehrenreich, B. (1975). The status of women as health providers in the United States. In *Proceedings of the International Conference on Women in Health, June 16-18* (DHEW Publication No. HRA 76-51, pp. 7-13). Washington, DC: Department of Health, Education and Welfare.

Ehrenreich, B., & English, D. (1973). *Witches, midwives, and nurses: A history of women healers.* New York: Feminist Press. [An article condensing the information in this pamphlet is found as the following: Witches, midwives, and nurses. *Monthly Review, 25*(5), 25-40.]

Fenton, W. S., Robinowitz, C. B., & Leaf, P. J. (1987). Male and female psychiatrists and their patients. *American Journal of Psychiatry, 144*(3), 358-361.

Finch, J., & Groves, D. (Eds.). (1983). *A labour of love: Women, work and caring.* Boston: Routledge & Kegan Paul.

Fogel, C. I., & Woods, N. F. (1981). *Health care of women: A nursing perspective.* St. Louis, MO: C. V. Mosby.

Graham, H. (1985). Providers, negotiators, and mediators: Women as the hidden carers. In E. Lewin & V. Olesen (Eds.), *Women, health, and healing: Toward a new perspective* (pp. 25-52). New York: Tavistock.

Gunn, I. P., Nicosia, J., & Tobin, M. (1987). Guest editorial—Anesthesia: A practice of nursing. *Journal of the American Association of Nurse Anesthetists, 55*(2), 97-100.

Hamilton, S. H. (1885, September 19). Female education from a medical standpoint. *JAMA,* pp. 318-320.

Heins, M. (1985). Update: Women in medicine. *Journal of the American Medical Women's Association, 40*(2), 43-50.

Jacox, A. (1987). The OTA report: A policy analysis. *Nursing Outlook, 35*(6), 262-267.

Janus, C. L., & Janus, S. S. (1987). Career adjustment of women radiologists. *Journal of the American Medical Women's Association, 42*(2), 54-56.

Kay, B. J., Butter, I. H., Chang, D., & Houlihan, K. (1988). Women's health and social change: The case of lay midwives. *International Journal of the Health Services, 18*(2), 223-236.

Kendellen, R. (1987). The medical malpractice insurance choice: An overview of the issues. *Journal of Nurse-Midwifery, 32*(1), 4-10.

Levitt, J. (1977). Men and women as providers of health care. *Social Science and Medicine, 14,* 395-398.

Lindgren, C. L. (1990). Burnout and social support in family caregivers. *Western Journal of Nursing Research, 12*(4), 469-482.

Lorber, J. (1984). *Women physicians: Careers, status, and power.* New York: Tavistock.

Lorber, J. (1986). Sisterhood is synergistic. *Journal of the American Medical Women's Association, 41*(4), 116-119.

Lorber, J. (1987). A welcome to a crowded field: Where will the new women physicians fit in? *Journal of the American Medical Women's Association, 42*(5), 149-152.

Lubic, R. W. (1987). Nurse midwives and liability insurance. *Nursing Outlook, 35*(4), 174-177.

Marieskind, H. I. (1980). *Women in the health system: Patients, providers, and programs.* St. Louis: C. V. Mosby.

Martin, C. A., & Woodring, J. H. (1986). Attitudes toward women in radiology. *Journal of the American Women's Medical Association, 41*(2), 50-53.

Melosh, B. (1982). *The physician's hand: Work culture and conflict in American nursing.* Philadelphia: Temple University Press.

Mikell, J. L. (1987). To the editor: Dr. Mom [Letter to the editor]. *JAMA, 257*(19), 2594-2595.

Morantz-Sanchez, R. M. (1985). *Sympathy and science.* New York: Oxford University Press.

Muff, J. (Ed.). (1988). *Socialization, sexism, and stereotyping: Women's issues in nursing.* Prospect Heights, IL: Waveland.

Navarro, V. (1975). Women in health care. *New England Journal of Medicine, 292*(8), 398-402.

Nightingale, F. (1969). *Notes on nursing. What it is and what it is not.* New York: Dover. (Original work published 1860)

O'Neill, G., & Ross, M. M. (1991). Burden of care: An important concept for nurses. *Health Care for Women International, 12*(1), 111-121.

Pasquali, E. A. (1991). Humor: Preventive therapy for family caregivers. *Home Health Care Nurse, 9*(3), 13-17.

Pizurki, H., Mejia, A., Butter, I., & Ewart, L. (1987). *Women as providers of health care.* Geneva: World Health Organization.

Reverby, S. (1987a). A caring dilemma: Womanhood and nursing in historical perspective. *Nursing Research, 36*(1), 5-11.

Reverby, S. (1987b). *Ordered to care: The dilemma of American nursing, 1850-1945.* New York: Cambridge University Press.

Roberts, S. J. (1983). Oppressed group behavior: Implications for nursing. *Advances in Nursing Science, 5*(4), 21-30.

Shryock, R. H. (1966). *Medicine in America: Historical essays.* Baltimore: Johns Hopkins Press.

Shye, D. (1991). Gender differences in Israeli physicians' career patterns, productivity and family structure. *Social Science and Medicine, 32*(10), 1169-1181.

Sinal, S., Weavil, P., & Camp, M. G. (1989). Child care choices of women physicians. *Journal of the American Medical Women's Association, 44*(6), 183-184.

Travelers Insurance Companies and the American Association of Retired Persons. (1988). *National survey of caregivers: Summary of findings.* Hartford, CT: Author.

Tucker, J. B., & Margo, K. L. (1987). Profile of women family practice residents. *Family Medicine, 19*(4), 269-271.

U.S. Bureau of the Census. (1991). *Statistical abstracts of the United States: 1991* (11th ed.). Washington, DC: Author.

U.S. Department of Labor, Bureau of Labor Statistics. (1990-1991). *Occupational outlook handbook.* Washington, DC: Author.

U.S. Public Health Service. (1990). *Seventh report to the President and Congress on the status of health personnel in the United States* (DHHS Publication No. HRS-P-OD-90-1). Washington, DC: U.S. Department of Health and Human Services.

Walsch, M. R. (1977). *"Doctors wanted: No women need apply": Sexual barriers in the medical profession, 1835-1975.* New Haven, CT: Yale University Press.

Weaver, J. L., & Garrett, S. D. (1983). Sexism and racism in the American health care industry: A comparative analysis. In E. Fee (Ed.), *Women and health: The politics of sex in medicine* (pp. 79-104). New York: Baywood.

Wilson, M. P. (1987). Making a difference: Women, medicine, and the twenty-first century. *Yale Journal of Biology and Medicine, 60*(3), 273-288.

Woodward, C. A., Cohen, M. L., & Ferrier, B. M. (1990). Career interruptions and hours practiced: Comparison between young men and women physicians. *Canadian Journal of Public Health, 81*(2), 16-20.

3

Women's Bodies

NANCY FUGATE WOODS

The women's health movement has encouraged women to feel ownership of their bodies, appreciate their uniqueness as women, increase their awareness of their physical bodies and the feelings associated with them, and use their bodies in ways that they choose to give them positive feelings. These goals are being fostered by women providing other women with information about their bodies and encouraging them to appreciate their uniqueness (Boston Women's Health Book Collective, 1976, 1990, 1992; Federation of Feminist Women's Health Centers, 1981; Martin, 1991; Scheper-Hughes & Lock, 1987).

The purpose of this chapter is to provide nursing practitioners with knowledge about women's bodies that can be shared with women who seek nursing services, consultation, and information. The chapter begins with an overview of the structural and functional aspects of a woman's body. The procreative and recreative functions of women's anatomy will be compared and contrasted. Women's bodies develop across the life span. The chapter includes a description of sexual differentiation and development, pubertal development, changes occurring during pregnancy, and menopause. Two important cyclic phenomena are women's menstrual cycles and sexual response cycles. The chapter describes how women's bodies participate in these cycles.

Women's Anatomy

Breasts

Although some Western societies socialize women to regard their breasts as symbols of their feminine attractiveness and nurturance and socialize men to regard women's breasts as sexual objects, women's breasts serve both procreative powers and recreative pleasures. Indeed, the mammary gland is the distinguishing feature of an entire zoological class—mammals! These structures have a unique and complex anatomy.

Location. The breasts are paired, highly specialized variants of sebaceous glands, located between the second and sixth ribs and between the sternal and midaxillary line. About two thirds of the breast lies superficial to the pectoralis major, the remainder to the serratus anterior.

Appearance. The breasts of healthy women are usually symmetrical in size and shape, although they are often not absolutely equal in size. The skin covering the breasts is similar to that of the abdomen, and, often, hair follicles are noted around the pigmented area surrounding the nipple, called the *areola.* Often, women with fair complexions can note a vascular pattern in a horizontal or vertical dimension. When present, this pattern is usually symmetrical.

The areolar pigment varies from pink to brown, and the size is also highly variable from woman to woman. The nipple is located in the center of each breast, surrounded by the areola. Several sebaceous glands are seen on the areola as small elevations. The nipples are pigmented and usually protuberant, although some are inverted. Nipple size and shape are highly variable from woman to woman, and the same woman may notice a great deal of variation in the size and shape of her nipples depending on the extent to which they are contracted. Some women have inverted nipples, a condition in which the nipple is invaginated or its central portion depressed. Some women have supernumerary nipples, nipples and breasts, or breast tissue. This supernumerary tissue develops along the longitudinal ridges extending from the axilla to the groin, which existed during early embryonic development.

Visible changes in the woman's breast occur in conjunction with her development. Prior to the age of 10, there is little visible distinction between boys' and girls' breasts. At approximately the age of 10 the mammary buds appear in girls' breasts. The subareolar mammary tissue is not prominent at this point. The adult breast develops under the influence of estrogen and progesterone. During the transition to adulthood, the prominent subareolar tissue of adolescence recedes into the contour of the remainder of the breast and the nipple protrudes. (See p. 47 for a more complete description of breast changes with puberty.)

Breast size is influenced by nutrition, heredity, and the woman's individual sensitivity to hormones. Nodularity, tenderness, and size of the breasts may fluctuate with the menstrual cycle. Usually, women's breasts are smallest during days 4 to 7 of the menstrual cycle, shortly after menstruation. An increase in breast volume, tenderness, heaviness, fullness, and general or nipple tenderness may be experienced before menstruation.

Short-lived changes of appearance are observed in many women during sexual response, including protuberance of the nipple, increase in breast size, and so forth. The breasts are highly erogenous organs for many women. They do not merely vary in shape and size with sexual excitement, but there is also a great deal of variation from woman to woman in those parts of the breasts perceived as erotic. For example, some women perceive erotic sensations in the areolae, others in the nipple, and still others in the breast tissue near the axilla.

A woman's breasts may also double or triple in size during pregnancy. Striae, engorgement of veins, and increased prominence and pigmentation of nipple and areolae are common during pregnancy. The glandular tissue of the breast gradually involutes after menopause and fat is deposited in the breasts. The breasts of postmenopausal women, therefore, take on a flattened contour and appear less firm than prior to menopause.

A convention useful in describing the appearance of women's breasts is division into four quadrants by vertical and horizontal lines crossing at the nipple. The axillary tail, a portion of breast tissue that extends into the axilla, is another important landmark. A more precise description of breast landmarks is one that incorporates an analogy to the face of a clock: A lump could be described at 2 o'clock and the appropriate number of centimeters from the nipple.

Although women are encouraged to wear brassieres to prevent a drooping of Cooper's ligaments, which makes breasts appear pendulous, there is no compelling evidence for the efficacy of the practice. Aside from fatigue or pain that some women with large breasts experience, there are no health consequences associated with not wearing a brassiere.

Components of Breast Tissue. There are three main components of tissue in women's breasts: glandular, fibrous, and fatty tissue. Most of the breast is composed of subcutaneous and retromammary (behind the breast) fat. Breast tissue is supported by fibrous tissue, including suspensory ligaments, extending from the subcutaneous connective tissue to the muscle fascia (see Figure 3.1).

An important functional component of the breast is the glandular tissue, which consists of 12 to 25 lobes that terminate in ducts that open

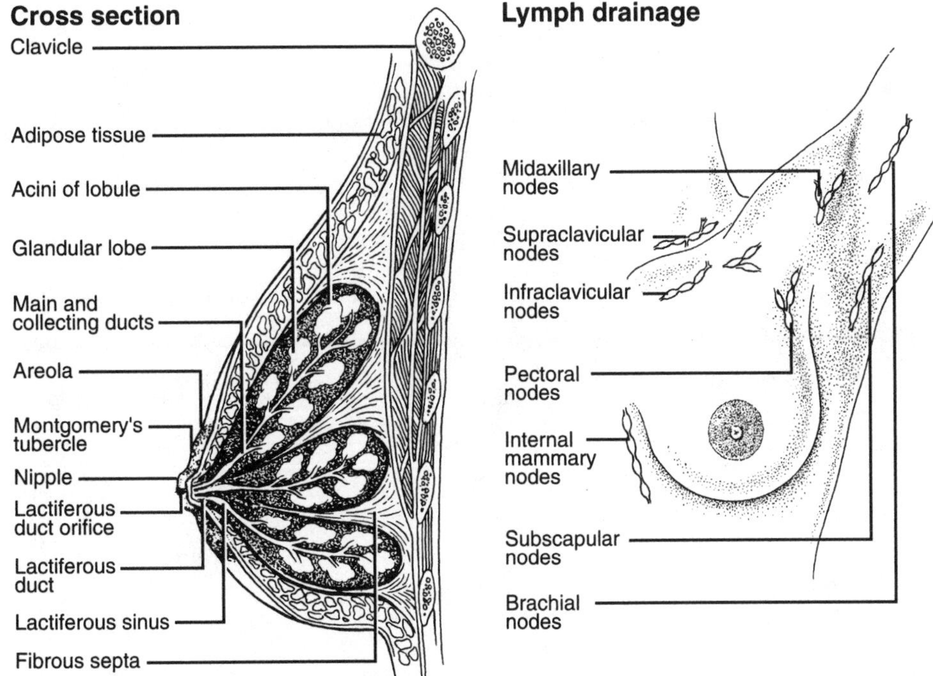

Figure 3.1. Components of breast tissue and lymph drainage. Breast tissue is composed of glandular, fibrous, and fatty tissue. Lymph from the skin of the breast flows to the axillary nodes and lymph from the medial cutaneous area of the breast flows to the opposite breast. Lymph from the areolae and the nipple flows into the mammary nodes.

on the surface of the nipple. Each lobe is composed of 20 to 40 lobules, each of which contains 10 to 100 alveoli (sometimes called *acini*).

The alveolus is the basic component of the breast lobule. The hollow alveolus is lined by a single layer of milk-secreting columnar epithelial cells, which are derived prenatally from an ingrowth of epidermis into the mesenchyme between 10 and 12 weeks of gestation. These cells enlarge greatly and discharge their contents during lactation. The individual alveolus is encased in a network of myoepithelial strands and is surrounded by a rich capillary network. The lumen of the alveolus opens into a collecting intralobar (within the lobe) duct through a thin, nonmuscular duct. The intralobar ducts eventually end in the openings in the nipple, and these ducts are surrounded by muscle cells.

Supporting Structures. The third and fourth branches of the cervical plexus provide the cutaneous nerve supply to the upper breast and the thoracic intercostal nerves to the lower breast. The perforating branches of the internal mammary artery constitute the chief external blood supply, although additional arterial blood supply emanates from several branches of the axillary artery. Superficial veins of the breast drain into the internal mammary veins and the superficial veins of the lower portion of the neck and from the latter into the jugular vein. Veins emptying into the internal mammary, axillary, and intercostal veins serve deep breast tissue.

The lymphatic drainage of the breast is of special interest and importance to women because of its role in dissemination of tumor cells as well as its ability to respond to infection. The lymphatic system of the breast is both abundant and complex. In general, the lymphatics drain both the axillary and internal mammary areas. Lymph from the skin of the breast, with the exception of areolar and nipple areas, flows into the axillary nodes on the same side of the body, whereas the lymph from the medial cutaneous breast area may flow into the opposite breast. The lymph from the areolar and nipple areas flows into the anterior axillary (mammary) nodes. Lymph from deep within the mammary tissues flows into the anterior axillary nodes but may also flow into the apical, subclavian, infraclavicu-

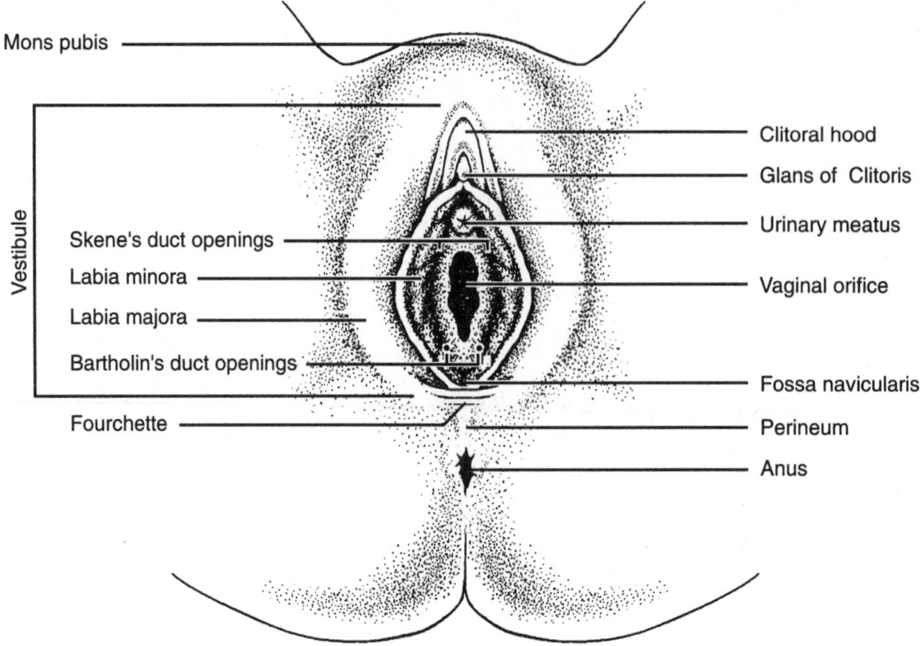

Figure 3.2. External Genitalia

lar, and supraclavicular nodes. Lymph from areas behind the areolae and the medial and lower glandular areas of breast tissue communicates with the lymphatic systems draining into the thorax and abdomen (see Figure 3.1).

Pelvic Organs

Like her breasts, many of a woman's pelvic structures serve both procreational powers and sexual pleasures. Despite the unique functions served by their pelvic structures, women may be unaware of their appearance because they have not had an opportunity to visualize them or because they have been discouraged from examining themselves.

Many of a woman's genital structures can be visualized easily with a mirror (see Figure 3.2). The configuration of the genitals is strikingly unique to each woman and highly variable from woman to woman. For example, many paired structures, such as the labia, are not perfectly symmetrical.

Vulva. The external female genitalia are commonly referred to as the *vulva.* The older term for the vulva, the *pudendum,* derives from the Latin word meaning "to be ashamed." For this reason, the term *vulva* is preferable.

The most obvious feature on an adult woman is the pubic hair, which is rather coarse and curly and not only covers parts of the vulvar area (mons, labia majora) but extends upward toward the abdomen. The flattened area of pubic hair over the abdomen forms the base of an inverted triangle. The triangle is sometimes referred to as the *female escutcheon.* Although this is a somewhat typical pattern, it is not uncommon for healthy women to exhibit variation in this pattern. For example, hair growth may extend up toward the umbilicus, to the anus, and toward the inner portion of the thighs.

The mons veneris or mons pubis is composed of fat and lies over the symphysis pubis. The labia majora consist of two raised folds of adipose tissue. They are heavily pigmented, and in postpubertal women their outer surfaces are covered with hair, whereas the inner surfaces are smooth and hairless. In postmenopausal women the hair on the labia becomes thinner and the labia and mons appear less full as a result of the loss of fatty tissue. The labia minora are two folds of skin heavily endowed with blood vessels that lie within the labia majora and extend from the clitoris to the fourchette (vaginal outlet).

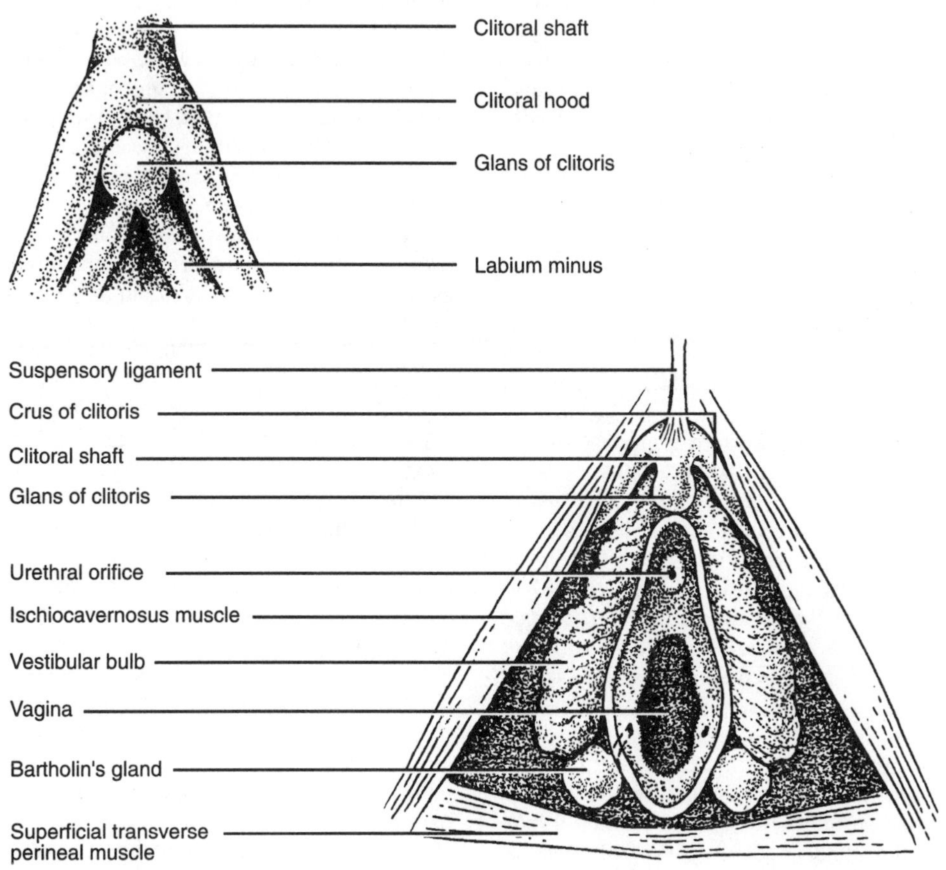

Figure 3.3. The clitoris. The sole purpose of the clitoris is reception and transformation of sexual stimuli.

Each of the labia minora divides into a medial and lateral part. The medial parts join anteriorly to the clitoris to form the clitoral hood and the lateral parts join posterior to the clitoris. In some women, the labia minora are completely hidden from view by the labia majora, but in other women the labia minora protrude between the labia majora. The color and texture of the labia minora are highly individual, varying from pink to brown. The clitoral hood covers the clitoris and is believed to protect this extremely sensitive organ from irritation. In some women the clitoral hood will adhere to the clitoris so that the hood cannot be pulled back very far to reveal the clitoris (see Figure 3.3).

The area between the labia minora is called the *vestibule*. It contains both the urethral and vaginal orifices. The hymen, a membranous fold at the vaginal opening, may be intact, but more commonly is seen as small, rounded fragments attached to the margins of the vaginal opening. Skene's glands are tiny, multiple paraurethral organs, the ducts of which open laterally and posteriorly to the urethral orifice. Bartholin's glands, located lateral and slightly posterior to the vaginal introitus, open into the groove between the labia minora and the hymen at the 5 and 7 o'clock positions in relation to the vaginal orifice. Both Skene's and Bartholin's glands are usually not visible, although they are located in tissues that can be visualized, and their openings on the vulva can be seen in some women. The perineum consists of the tissues between the vaginal orifice and the anus. Beneath the vestibule are two bundles of vascular tissue referred to as the bulbs of the vestibule. These tissues become congested during sexual response.

Clitoris. A woman's clitoris is an organ unique to all of human anatomy. Its sole purpose is to serve as a receptor and transformer of sensual stimuli. This unique structure exists to initiate or elevate levels of sexual tension for women (Masters & Johnson, 1966).

The clitoris consists of two corpora cavernosa (cavernous bodies) enclosed in a dense fibrous membrane that is made up of elastic fibers and smooth muscle bundles. Each corpus is connected to the pubic ramus and the ischium. The tip of the clitoris is called the *glans* and is exquisitely sensitive. The clitoris is held in place by a suspensory ligament and two small ischiocavernosus muscles that insert into the crurae of the clitoris (Masters & Johnson, 1966).

Blood supply to the clitoris emanates from the deep and dorsal clitoral arteries that branch from the internal pudendal artery. The vasculature of the clitoris plays an important role in increasing size during sexual response.

The length of the clitoral body (consisting of glans and shaft) varies markedly. The size of the clitoral glans may vary from 2 mm to 1 cm in healthy women and is usually estimated at 4 to 5 mm in both the transverse and longitudinal planes. There is also variation in the position of the clitoris, a function of variation in the points of origin of the suspensory and crural ligaments. The glans is capable of increasing in size with sexual stimulation, and marked vasocongestive increases in the diameter of the clitoral shaft have also been noted (Masters & Johnson, 1966).

The dorsal nerve of the clitoris is the deepest division of the pudendal nerve, and it terminates in the nerve endings of the glans and corpora cavernosa. Pacinian corpuscles, which respond to deep pressure, are distributed in both the glans and the corpora but have greater concentration in the glans. Their distribution is highly variable from woman to woman, which probably accounts for the rich variation in women's self-pleasuring techniques. For example, some women prefer very light touch whereas others prefer deep pressure. In some women, the anatomic arrangement of the labia minora that forms the clitoral hood makes it possible for mechanical traction on the labia to stimulate the clitoris indirectly. The clitoris is endowed with sensory nerve endings that respond to tactile stimuli as well as pressure. Although afferent stimuli can be received through afferent nerve endings in the clitoral glans and shaft, it is also possible that the clitoris serves as the subjective end point or transformer for efferent stimuli from higher neurogenic pathways (Masters & Johnson, 1966).

Vagina. Although the vagina can be considered an internal structure, it can be easily visualized with assistance of a speculum, a light source, and a mirror. The vagina is a musculomembranous canal connecting the vulva with the uterus. It is lined with a reddish pink mucous membrane that is transversely rugated. Under the stratified squamous epithelial lining is a muscular coat that has an inner circular layer and an outer fibrous layer (see Figure 3.4).

The vagina is a potential rather than a real space. Although highly distensible, its unstimulated length is approximately 6 to 7 cm anteriorly and about 9 cm posteriorly. The vaginal canal inclines posteriorly at about a 45° angle. The cervix is inserted into the vagina anteriorly and superiorly. There is a recessed portion of the vagina adjacent to the cervix, which, together with the cervix, is called the vaginal fornix. The fornix has anterior, posterior, and lateral portions.

Unlike the clitoris, the vagina has procreative as well as recreative functions. One of the important physiological functions of the vagina during sexual response is its ability to produce lubrication by means of transudation of mucoid material across its rugal folds. In addition, vaginal lubrication occurs in a rhythmic 90-minute cycle throughout the day and night. The venous plexus (including the bulbus vestibuli, plexus pudendalis, plexus uterovaginalis, and possibly the plexus vesicalis and plexus rectalis) encircling the vaginal barrel probably provides the circulatory support for vaginal lubrication. In addition to producing lubrication, the vagina demonstrates a fascinating distensive ability during both sexual response and childbirth. Both a lengthening of the vagina and a ballooning out of its inner portions have been observed during sexual response. The vascular changes occurring in conjunction with sexual response are profound. The reddish pink hue of the premenopausal woman's vagina changes to a darker purplish vasocongested appearance. In postmenopausal women the color changes in the vagina and its expansion during sexual response are less pronounced. As the vagina distends, the rugae become flattened as a result of the thinning or stretching of the vaginal mucosa. The vagina, unlike the clitoris, is not well endowed with nerve endings; although there are deep pressure receptors in the innermost portion of the vagina, it is primarily in the outer third of the vagina that women report pleasurable sexual sensations (Masters & Johnson, 1966).

Cervix. Although the cervix might be regarded as an internal structure because it is a part of the

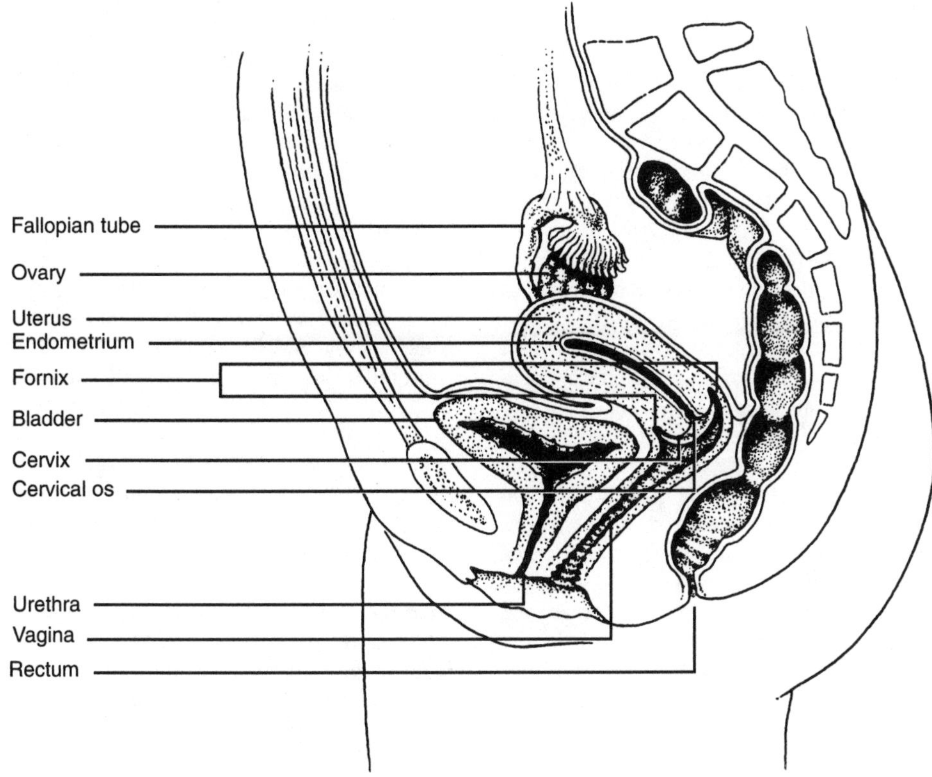

Figure 3.4. The internal genitalia. The vaginal canal is a potential rather than a real space and inclines posteriorly at a 45 degree angle. The cervix pierces the anterior superior wall of the vagina.

uterus, it can be readily visualized for a clinician's exam with the aid of a speculum and a light source. The cervix extends from the isthmus of the uterus into the vagina and it is through the small cervical opening (os) that the uterus and vagina communicate. The cervical os appears as a small closed circle in nonparous women and may be enlarged or of an irregular shape in parous women. The cervix appears as an oval-shaped organ and is usually shiny and pink. In postmenopausal women it may be smaller and less colorful than in premenopausal women. The stroma (connective tissue forming the framework) of the cervix consists of connective tissue with unstriated muscle fibers as well as elastic tissue.

The stratified squamous epithelium of the outer cervix (portio) is made up of several layers. The basal layer is a single row of cells resting on a thin basement membrane and is the layer where active mitosis (cell division) is seen. The parabasal and intermediate layers are next. In the intermediate layer are vacuoles containing glycogen. The superficial layer varies in thickness in response to estrogen stimulation. The desquamation of this surface layer occurs constantly. The superficial layer contains a large amount of glycogen, as does the intermediate layer. It appears that glycogen plays an important role in maintaining the acid pH of the vagina. Glycogen released by cytolysis of the desquamated cells is acted on by the glycolytic bacterial flora in the vagina, forming lactic acid.

Just as the endometrium is influenced by the hormonal fluctuations of the menstrual cycle, so is the mucus produced by the secretory cells of the endocervical (within the cervix) glands. This is especially noticeable in premenopausal women. The fluctuations of the cervical mucus over the menstrual cycle will be discussed later in this chapter. The endocervical canal shows an abrupt transition from the stratified squamous epithelium covering the vagina and the outer surface of the cervix to a tall, columnar epithelium rich in mucin (proteinaceous substance in mucus).

Uterus. The uterus is a hollow, pear-shaped organ that is from 5.5 to 9 cm long, 3.5 to 6 cm wide, and 2 to 4 cm thick in nonparous women. The uterus of a parous woman may be 2 to 3 cm larger in any of these three dimensions. The uterus is usually inclined forward at a 45° angle from the longitudinal plane of the body. Usually, the uterus is anteverted and slightly anteflexed in positions. However, it may also be retroflexed, retroverted, or in midposition.

The portion of the uterus above the cervix is termed the *corpus* (body) and is constructed of a thick-walled musculature. It is covered with peritoneum on the exterior and lined with a mucous surface called the *endometrium.* The body of the uterus is divided into three portions: the fundus, the corpus, and the isthmus. The fundus is the prominence above the insertion of the fallopian tubes, the corpus is the main portion, and the isthmus is the narrow lower portion of the uterus adjacent to the cervix. The uterus is not a fixed organ but can be moved about; for example, during the sexual response cycle, the entire uterus elevates from the true pelvis into the false pelvis.

Uterine Tubes. Two uterine (fallopian) tubes function as oviducts for the transport of ova from the ovary to the uterus. They are inserted into the upper part of the uterus and run laterally to the ovaries. Each tube is approximately 10 to 12 cm long. The distal portions of the tube are fimbriated (fringed); the middle portion (ampulla) and the portion of the tube closest to its insertion in the uterus (isthmus) are extremely narrow. The wider fimbriated end of the tube is not actually attached to the ovary but is partly wrapped around the ovary. The outer, serous coat of the tubes covers a muscular portion consisting of an inner circular and outer longitudinal layer. The mucosal layer, composed of a number of rugae that become more numerous approaching the fimbriated portions, lines the tubes. The tubes are lined with cilia.

Ovaries. The ovaries are paired oval organs approximately 3 to 4 cm long, 2 cm wide, and 1 to 2 cm thick. They are located near the pelvic wall at the level of the anterior superior iliac spine. The ovaries float freely in the pelvis except for their attachment to the broad ligaments. The external ovarian surface has a dull, whitish, opaque appearance. The ovary is composed of an outer cortex lined by a single layer of cuboidal (cube-shaped) epithelium. Through this layer, blood vessels and nerves enter and leave the ovary. Beneath the outer layer is the stroma, which consists of spindle-shaped cells. The stroma of the ovary contains the primordial follicles. Not only do the ovaries release gametes, but they also produce steroid hormones, including estrogen and progesterone. The medullary portion of the ovary is composed of loose connective tissue, lymphatics, and blood vessels. The ovary has a rich lymphatic drainage, and an abundant supply of unmyelinated nerve fibers also enters the medulla.

At birth, the ovary contains about one million germ cells. The follicle is the functional unit of the ovary, the source of both the gametes and the ovarian hormones. Each follicle is surrounded by a theca folliculi. The theca contains an inner rim of secretory cells, the theca interna, and an outer rim of connective tissue, the theca externa. Within the theca, but separated from it by a layer of thin basement membrane, are the granulosa cells, which in turn surround the ovum. An acellular layer of protein and polysaccharide, the zona pellucida, separates the ovum from the granulosa cells. The theca interna is richly vascularized although neither the ovum nor the granulosa cells are in contact with any capillaries. Development and maturation of the follicle consists of proliferation of the granulosa cells and the gradual elaboration of fluid within the follicle. Accumulation of the fluid increases rapidly with follicular maturation and causes the follicle to bulge into the peritoneal cavity. As the follicle swells, the ovum remains embedded in granulosa cells (cumulus oophorus), which remain in contact with the theca. As fluid accumulates, the cumulus thins out until only a narrow thread of cells connects the ovum with the rim of the follicle. At ovulation the ovum, surrounded by the corona of granulosa cells (sometimes called the corona radiata) and floating in the follicular fluid, ruptures. The ovum and its corona extrude into the peritoneal cavity in a bolus of follicular fluid. After ovulation, ingrowth and differentiation of the remaining granulosa cells fill the collapsed follicle to form a new endocrine structure called the *corpus luteum.* The corpus luteum continues to develop when a pregnancy occurs. When the ovum is not fertilized and dies, the corpus luteum no longer develops and leaves a remnant on the surface of the ovary called a *corpus albicans* (see Figure 3.5).

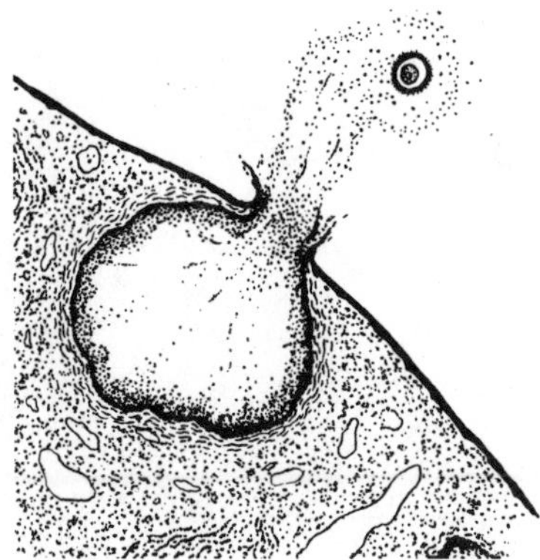

Figure 3.5. Ovulation. At ovulation the ovum, surrounded by the corona radiata and floating in the follicular fluid, ruptures into the peritoneal cavity.

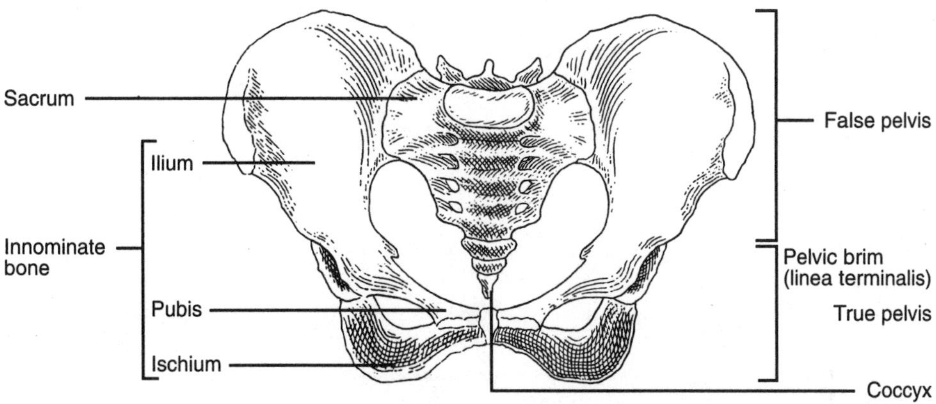

Figure 3.6. The bony pelvis. The pelvis is composed of two innominate bones, the sacrum and the coccyx. The innominates are composed of the ilium, the ischium, and the pubis.

Pelvic Supporting Structures

Bones, muscles, ligaments, blood vessels, and nerves form supporting structures of the pelvic organs.

Bony Pelvis. The pelvis is composed of two innominate bones, the sacrum and coccyx. The innominate bones, in turn, are composed of the ilium, ischium, and pubis. The pubic bones join at the symphysis pubis. The pubic arch is formed by the inferior borders of the pubic bones and symphysis. The ilium joins with the sacrum posteriorly to form the sacroiliac joint. A woman's pelvis is wider and more shallow than a man's because of the flaring of the woman's iliac bones (see Figure 3.6).

Muscle. Several sets of muscles attach to the bony pelvis to constitute the pelvic floor. These muscles actively and passively support the pelvis and are involved in the voluntary contraction of the vagina and the anus. The pubococcygeus muscle, part of the levator ani group, has particular significance in women because it is important not only in sexual sensory function but also in bladder control and birthing for controlling relaxation of the perineum and expulsion of the infant. Also of importance for sexual pleasure is the bulbocavernosus (see Figure 3.7).

Ligaments. Four pairs of ligaments, the cardinal, uterosacral, round, and broad ligaments, provide primary support for the uterus, and the ovarian ligaments and infundibulopelvic ligaments

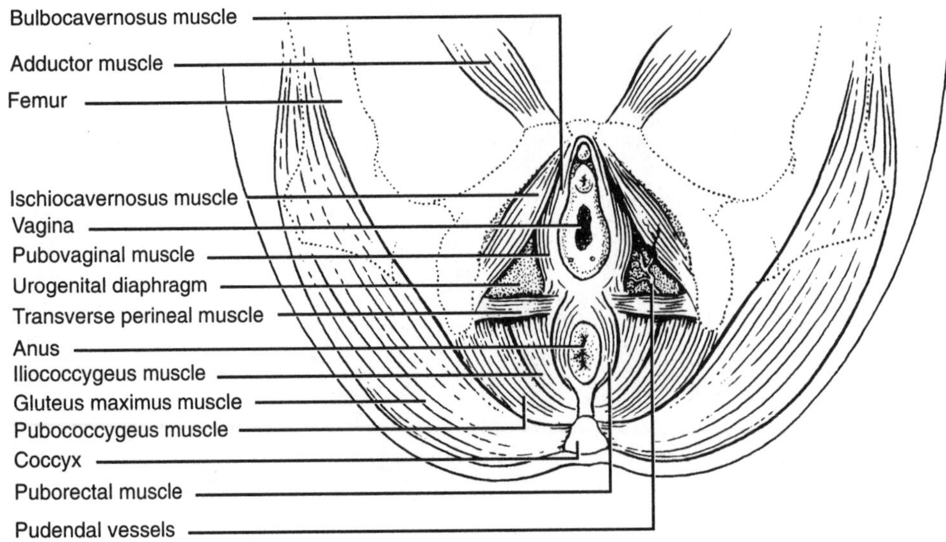

Figure 3.7. Pelvic muscles. Several sets of muscles support the pelvic floor. The bulbocavernosus and the pubococcygeus have special significance for sexual function.

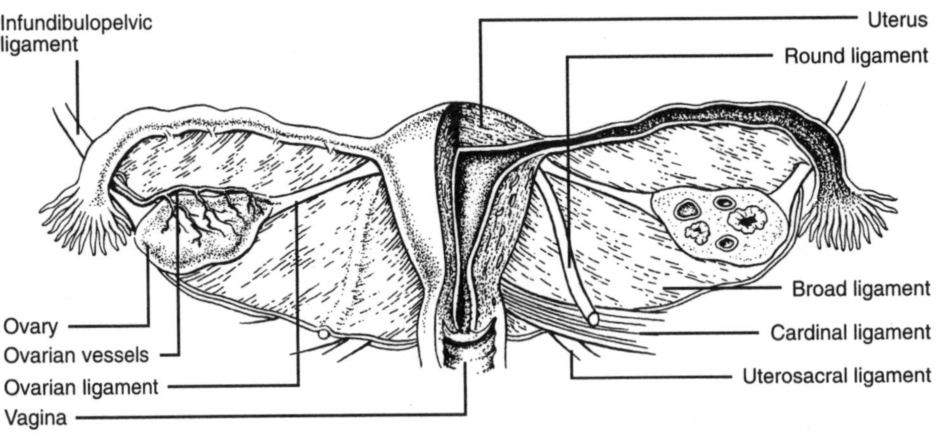

Figure 3.8. Ligaments. Four pairs of ligaments support the uterus, tubes, and ovaries. These are the cardinal, uterosacral, round, and broad ligaments.

provide ancillary support (see Figure 3.8). Stretching of the ligaments is sometimes associated with minor discomfort during strenuous exercise or during pregnancy.

Vasculature. The ovarian arteries arise from the abdominal aorta, supply the tube and ovary, and ultimately anastamose with the uterine artery. The uterine artery arises from the anterior branch of the hypogastric artery and supplies the cervix and uterus. The vaginal artery arises similarly from the anterior branch of the hypogastric artery. The uterine veins run along the same channels as the uterine artery. The ovarian veins from the vena cava pass through the broad ligament en route to the ovarian hilus. On the right, the ovarian vein empties into the inferior vena cava; on the left it empties into the renal vein.

Innervation. The internal genitalia are supplied by autonomic as well as spinal nerve pathways. The main autonomic supply to the uterus appears to consist of both sympathetic and parasympathetic fibers of the superior hypogastric plexus. The pudendal nerve is the main spinal nerve, providing the source of motor and sensory activation of the lower genital tract.

Sexual Differentiation and Development

Sexual differentiation and development involves a complex series of events that ultimately transform an undifferentiated embryo into a human with a gender identity of female or male. As a result of the complexity of differentiation, one can be born with genotypic sex that is inconsistent with phenotypic sex. The developmental process of sexual differentiation begins at fertilization with establishment of genetic sex. Genetic sex refers to the chromosomal combination from the ovum and sperm, resulting in an XX (female), XY (male), or other combination. Gonadal sex refers to the structure and function of the gonads, whereas somatic sex involves the genital organs other than the gonads. Neuroendocrine sex refers to the cyclic or continuous production of gonadotropin releasing hormones. Although gonadal, somatic, and neuroendocrine sexual differentiation begin prior to birth, sexual differentiation continues after birth. Development of social, psychological, and cultural dimensions of sexuality as well as secondary sex characteristics occur after birth (Blackburn & Loper, 1992; George & Wilson, 1988).

Genetic Sex

Genetic sex is determined at the time of fertilization and is defined by the contribution of an X or Y chromosome from the father. Of interest is that despite the genotype, sexual differentiation will produce a basic female phenotype unless testosterone is present and can be used by the cells of the developing human.

Gonadal Sex

At about 4 to 6 weeks of gestation, germ cells migrate to the site of the fetal gonad. At the 6th week, the gonads are sexually indistinguishable, containing a cortex and medulla layer. If the chromosomal sex is XX, the cortex will differentiate into the ovary, and the medulla will regress; if the chromosomal sex is XY, the medulla will differentiate into a testis and the cortex will regress under the influence of SRY, a gene from the sex-determining region of the Y chromosome.

Differentiation of the gonad occurs slightly earlier in males than in female fetuses. At seven weeks testicular differentiation begins under the influence of testosterone, which is stimulated by human chorionic gonadotropin (HCG). The ovary differentiates about 2 weeks after testicular differentiation and is identifiable by 10 weeks. By 16 weeks, the oogonia become surrounded by follicular cells, composing the primordial follicle. At 20 weeks gestation, the fetal ovary contains mature compartmentalization with primordial follicles and oocytes. At 20 weeks gestation, there are 5 to 7 million germ cells present. Follicular maturation and atresia is already progressing. Approximately 1 million germ cells remain in the ovary at birth. The oocytes are surrounded by primordial follicles and are arrested in the prophase of the first meiotic (cellular division in which the diploid number of chromosomes is reduced to the haploid) division until the follicle is reactivated at the time of puberty.

Female differentiation is probably linked to a gene on the X chromosome that acts in the absence of androgen. Only one X chromosome is needed for primary ovarian differentiation, explaining why female differentiation may occur in fetuses with XY chromosomes who lack testosterone elaboration at a critical point in development or are unable to use testosterone.

Somatic Sex

The mesonephric (Wolffian duct) and the paramesonephric (Mullerian duct) coexist in all embryos regardless of chromosomal sex. During the third fetal month, one persists and the other disappears. The intrinsic tendency toward feminization produces differentiation of the paramesonephric (Mullerian) system. In the absence of Mullerian inhibiting factor, which inhibits the further development of the Mullerian ducts in male embryos, the paramesonephric system differentiates into the uterine tubes, uterus, and upper vagina.

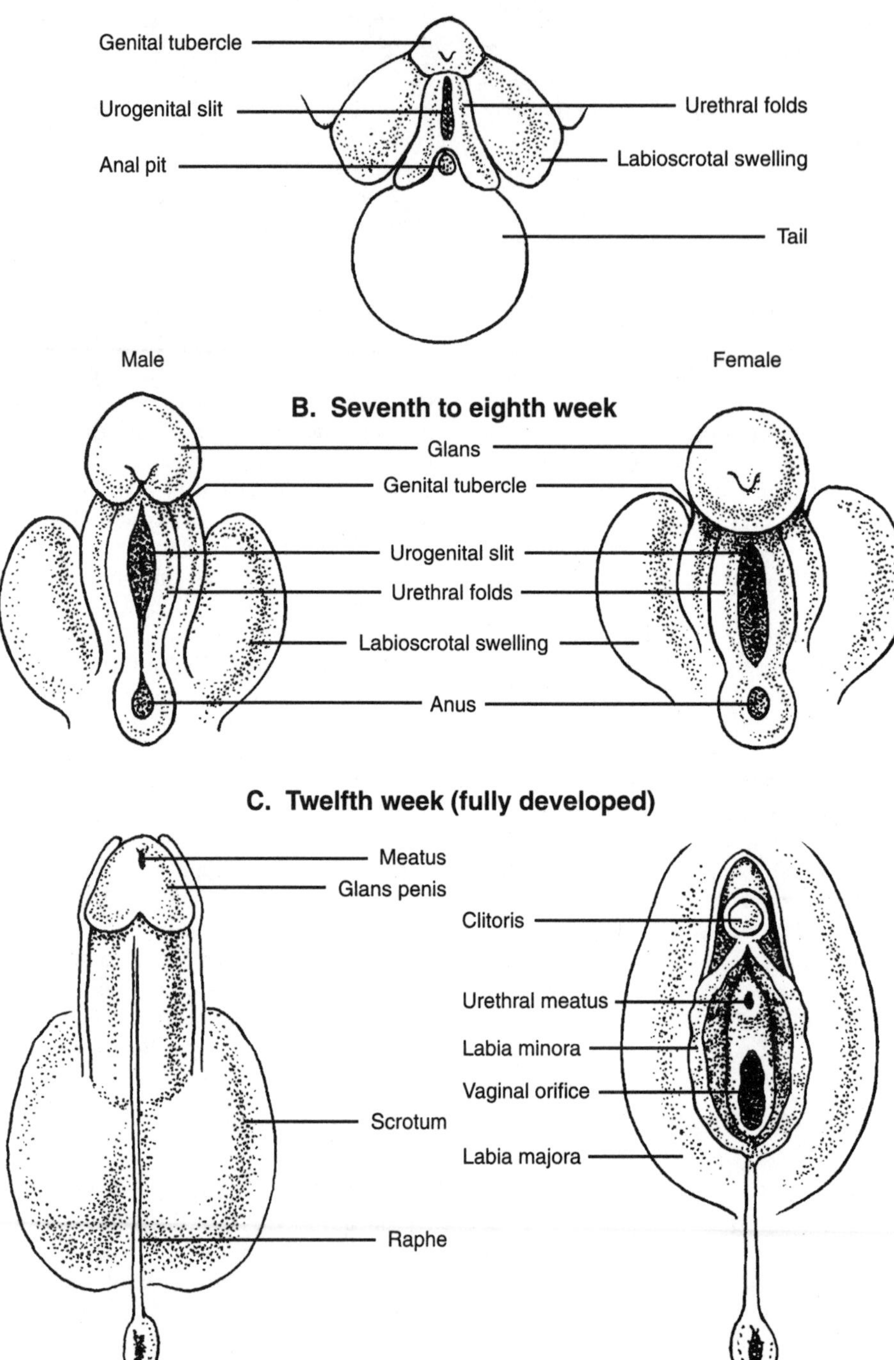

Figure 3.9a. Sexual differentiation of the external genitalia. As early as the 7th to 8th weeks of fetal life, gender differentiation has begun. Before the 6th week, the embryo appears undifferentiated. By the 12th week, the external genitalia assume the differentiated appearance.

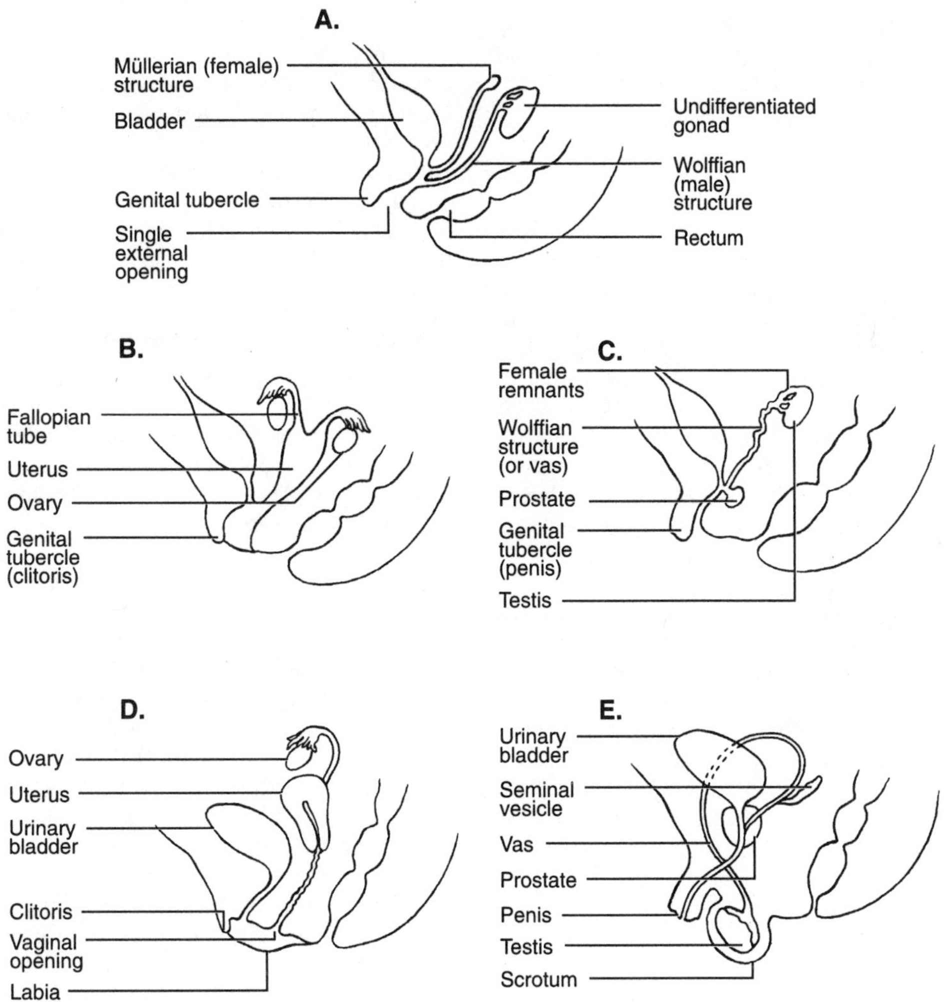

Figure 3.9b. Sexual Differentiation of the Internal Genitalia

NOTES: A. Undifferentiated structures; B. Female structure at the 3rd month; C. Male structure at the 3rd month; D. Female mature form; E. Male mature form.

At the 8th week of gestation, the embryo is bipotential, that is, it can differentiate into either a female or a male. Between 9 to 12 weeks of gestation, differentiation of external genitalia becomes evident. The urogenital sinus, labioscrotal swellings, and genital tubercle will differentiate into a female pattern in the absence of androgen stimulation and without a Y chromosome. In females, the urogenital folds remain open, developing into the labia minora. The labioscrotal folds differentiate into the labia majora, and the genital tubercle differentiates into the clitoris. The urogenital sinus becomes the vagina and the urethra. The lower vagina is formed as part of the external genitalia. The differentiation of these structures is illustrated in Figures 3.9a and 3.9b.

Fetal endocrines are supported by the placenta as well as the fetal gonads. By the 10th week of gestation, most of the pituitary hormones are apparent. They rise during the first 20 weeks of pregnancy, and then negative feedback mechanisms begin to limit their levels. Luteinizing hormone (LH) and follicle-stimulating hormone (FSH) are apparent at 9 to 10 weeks and peak at about 20 to 22 weeks gestation. FSH stimulates follicular development in females and LH stimulates steroid synthesis in the ovary and will later induce ovulation in FSH-primed follicles. Hypothalamic-releasing hormones stimulate adrenocorticotropin hormone (ACTH) production by about 8 weeks gestation.

Puberty

Puberty refers to the period of becoming capable of reproducing sexually and is indicated by the maturation of the genital organs, the development of secondary sex characteristics and by the first occurrence of menstruation in young women. Puberty and the climacteric share the characteristic of a transitional period during which a biological series of events culminating in a change in fertility occurs. During puberty, menarche occurs in girls; during the climacteric, menopause occurs in women (Cacciari & Prader, 1980).

A time interval of a decade or more separates birth and puberty. Puberty occurs during the later phases of human growth, long after the initial sexual differentiation. Both growth and differentiation continue during puberty, making it a distinctive part of the life span and requiring complex physiological mechanisms to initiate its occurrence (Plant, 1988; Venturoli, Flamigni, & Givens, 1985).

Initiation of Puberty

Initiation of puberty remains poorly understood. Currently, two theories account for pubertal initiation. The first implicates a central neural timekeeping mechanism that measures age and gates (controls) the gonadotropin-releasing hormone (GnRH) pulse generator. The second involves a central neural mechanism that tracks one or more parameters of growth, a type of somatometer. Regardless of whether either or both mechanisms are responsible for pubertal onset, neuroendocrine control systems play an important role in orchestrating pubertal events. The GnRH pulse generator, a mechanism within the hypothalamus, plays an important role in stimulating the pulsatile gonadotropin release that is responsible for certain pubertal changes. What increases the responsiveness of the anterior pituitary to GnRH remains uncertain (Plant, 1988; Turek & Van Cauter, 1988).

Physiological Development and Puberty

Shortly after birth, FSH and LH levels are elevated due to the release of negative feedback provided by maternal ovarian hormones during pregnancy. The gonadotropins remain high for approximately 3 months with resulting transient elevations of estradiol. Low levels of estradiol provide negative feedback, depressing gonadotropins until about 8 years of age. Gonadotropin control of the pituitary-ovarian axis is sensitive to low levels of estradiol feedback, which in turn, limit the secretions of gonadotropins. LH pulses appear during infancy. Thus it appears that immaturity of the endocrine systems is not the factor limiting onset of puberty. Indeed, all components of the hypothalamic-pituitary-ovarian axis below the level of the hypothalamus can respond to GnRH from birth.

Prepubertal Phases. During the prepubertal years, three phases are evident: adrenarche, decreasing repression of the "gonadostat," and amplification of interactions leading to gonadarche. Adrenarche refers to the development of pubic and axillary hair and is a function of increased adrenal androgen production. Elevations in dehydroepiandrosterone (DHA), dehydroepiandrosterone sulfate (DHAS), and androstenedione occur from about 6 to 15 years of age. An increase in the size of the inner zone of the adrenal cortex precedes the growth spurt by about 2 years. In addition, it precedes elevation of estrogens and gonadotropins seen during early puberty and menarche in midpuberty. However, the mechanisms governing adrenarche probably are not the same as those influencing GnRH-pituitary-ovarian axis maturation and gonadarche. Early adrenarche, occurring before 8 years, is not associated with early gonadarche. The mechanisms producing adrenarche remain obscure.

Derepression of the gonadostat refers to the increased responsiveness of the anterior pituitary to GnRH and follicular activity to FSH and LH. LH and FSH are suppressed to very low levels until about 8 years of age due to two factors. First, during early childhood, there is a very sensitive negative feedback effect of low levels of gonadal estrogens on the hypothalamus and pituitary sites. Second, during midchildhood, there is an intrinsic central inhibitory influence on GnRH that reduces gonadotropin concentrations. Factors that are responsible for derepressing the gonadostat, allowing the hypothalamus and pituitary to become less sensitive to the negative feedback of low levels of estrogens and permitting gonadotropin concentrations to rise, remain uncertain. Sustained elevation of growth hormone levels may play a role as the factor responsible for derepressing the gonadostat.

Endogenous GnRH is important in establishing and maintaining puberty. An increasing amplitude and frequency of pulsatile GnRH probably enhances the responses of FSH and LH secretion. GnRH appears to induce cell surface receptors specific for itself and necessary for its action on the surface of gonadotrope cells of the anterior pituitary. Sleep-related pulsations of LH are seen during early puberty. By midpuberty, estrogen enhances LH secretory responses to GnRH (creating positive feedback) and maintains its negative feedback of FSH responses.

Puberty. A cascade of endocrine events initiated by release of pulsatile GnRH results in elevated gonadotropin levels and gonadal steroids, with subsequent appearance of secondary sexual characteristics and, later, menarche and ovulation. Between the ages of 10 and 16, the usual sequence includes the appearance of a pulsatile pattern of LH during sleep, followed by pulses of lesser amplitude throughout the entire day. Increasing levels of estradiol result in menarche, and by the latter part of puberty, the positive feedback relationship exists between estradiol and LH that is necessary to stimulate ovulation.

Progression of puberty through a sequence of increased rate of growth, breast development, pubarche (onset of pubic hair growth), and menarche occurs over a period of approximately 4.5 years. Usually the first sign of puberty is acceleration of growth, which is followed by breast budding (thelarche). The growth peak (about 2 to 4 inches within 1 year) usually occurs about 2 years after breast budding. Pubarche usually appears following the appearance of breast budding, and axillary hair growth occurs approximately 2 years later. In some girls, pubic hair growth is the first sign of puberty. The growth peak in height occurs about 1 year prior to menarche. Menarche occurs late in this sequence with a median age of about 12.8, after the growth peak has occurred. Growth hormone and gonadal estrogen are important factors in the increased growth velocity. In addition, increasing estrogen levels produce breast development, female fat distribution, vaginal and uterine growth, and skeletal growth.

Menarche. Menarche is a function of genetic and environmental influences and occurs between 9.1 and 17.7 years of age, with a mean age of 12.8 years. Improvements in the standard of living and nutrition have produced children who mature earlier than in the past. In cultures that are affluent, menarcheal age has become lower. After menarche, growth slows, with approximately 2.5 inches in height gained after menarche. Age of menarche is correlated for mothers and daughters and between sisters. Although there has been discussion of a critical weight for menarche to occur (47.8 kg), it is likely that the shift in body composition from 16% to 23.5% fat is a more important factor. Whether there is a central mechanism responsible for production of a critical weight, proportion of body fat, and onset of menarche is unclear. What is clear is that estrogen secretion, which produces endometrial proliferation, is essential for menarche to occur.

Fertility. Development of positive feedback effects of estrogen on the pituitary and hypothalamus that stimulates the midcycle LH surge necessary for ovulation is a late event in puberty. For this reason, menstrual cycles are often anovulatory for about 12 to 18 months after menarche. The frequency of ovulation becomes more regular with each menstruation and as girls progress through pubertal changes.

Development During Puberty. The Tanner (1981) stages are a commonly used indicator of the stage of pubertal development. On the basis assessment of breast and pubic hair growth, it is possible to assess progression through puberty (see Figure 3.10a & b).

In Stage 1, a prepubertal stage, there is elevation of the papilla of the breast only. Although the feminine pelvic contour is evident, the breasts are flat. The labia majora are smooth and the labia minora are poorly developed. The hymenal opening is small, the mucous membranes are dry and red, and the vaginal cells lack glycogen.

In Stage 2, there is elevation of the nipple, with a small mound beneath the areola, which is enlarging and beginning to become pigmented. The labia majora become thickened, more prominent, and wrinkled. The labia minora are easily identified due to their increased size along with the enlarging clitoris. The urethral opening is more prominent, mucous membranes are moist and pink, and some glycogen is present in vaginal cells. Pubic hair first appears on the mons

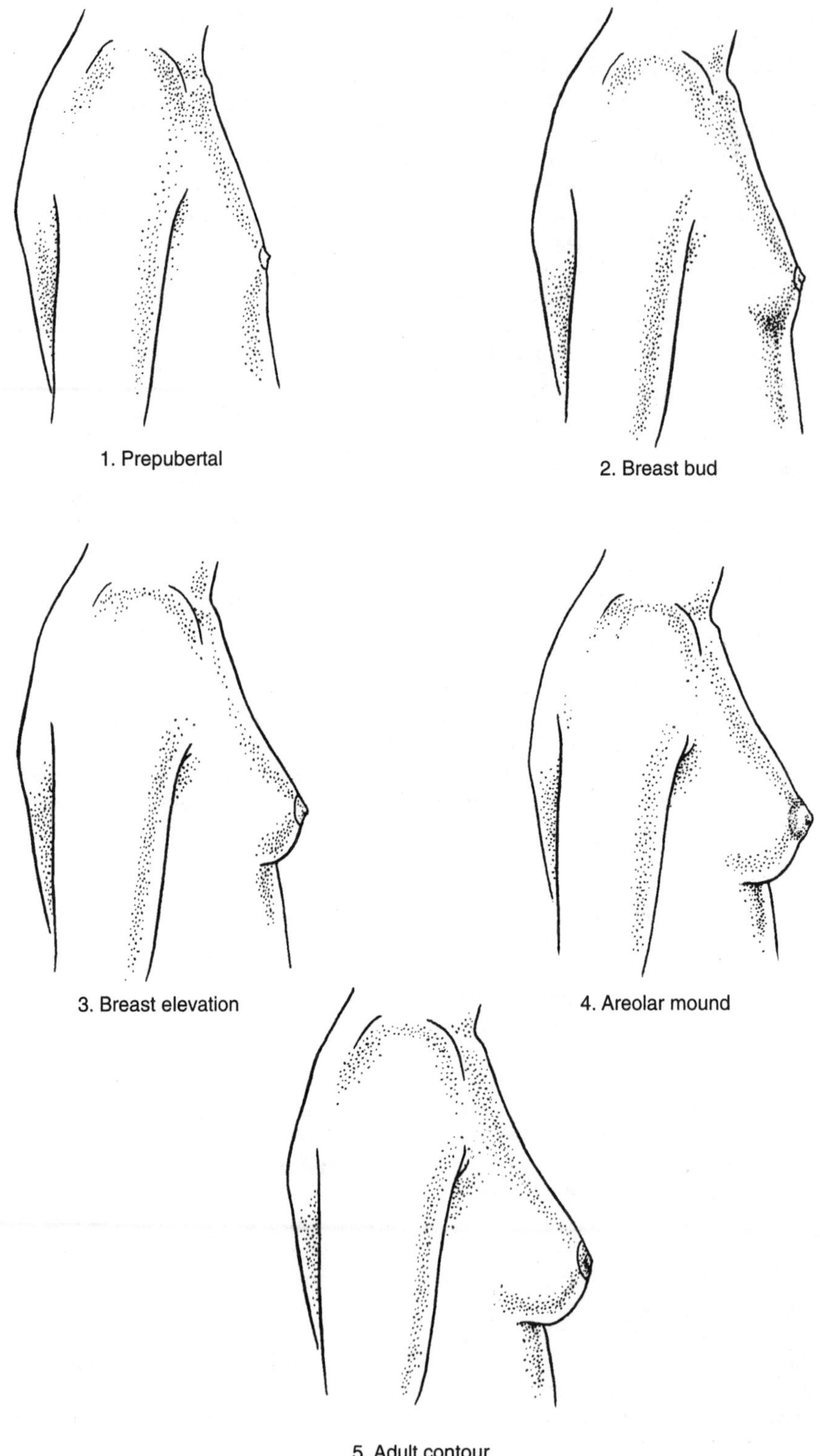

Figure 3.10a. Tanner Stages for Breast Development

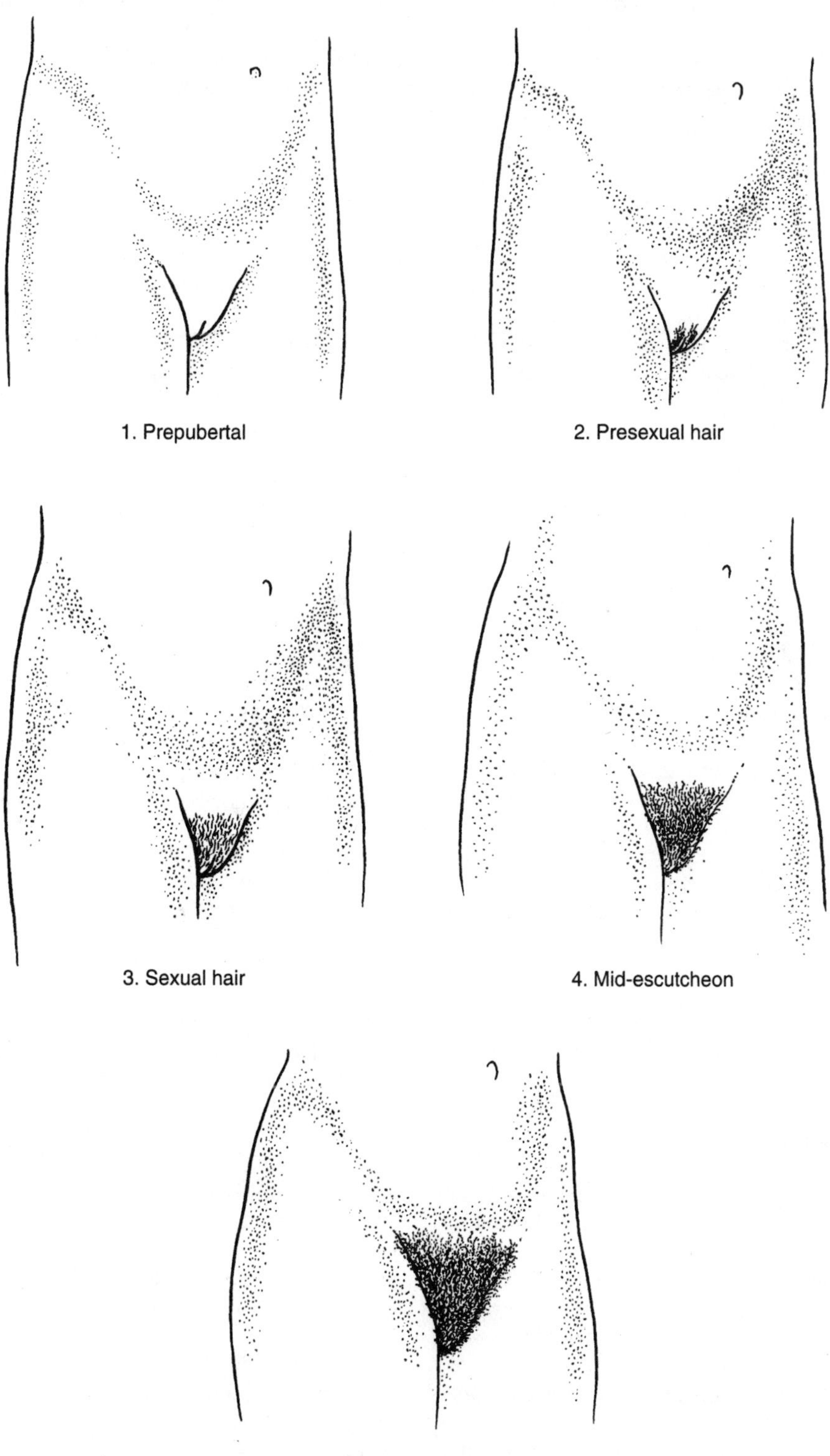

Figure 3.10b. Tanner Stages for Pubic Hair Development

and then on the labia about the time of menarche. The pubic hair is scanty, soft, and straight. There is increased activity of the sebaceous and merocrine sweat glands and the initial functions of the apocrine glands in the axilla and vulva.

In Stage 3, the rapid growth peak has occurred, and menarche occurs most frequently during this stage following the acceleration of the growth peak. The areola and nipple enlarge and pigmentation is more evident along with increased glandular size. The labia minora are well developed and the vaginal cells have increased glycogen content. The mucous membranes are increasingly more pale. The pubic hair is thicker, coarser, often curly at this time. There is increased activity of the sebaceous and sweat glands with the beginning of acne in some girls along with adult body odor.

In Stage 4, the areola project above the plane of the breast and the areolar glands are apparent. Glandular tissue is easily palpable. Both the labia major and minora assume the adult structure, and the glycogen content of the vaginal cells begins its cyclic pattern. Pubic hair is more abundant and axillary hair is present.

In Stage 5, the breasts are more mature, with the nipples enlarged and protuberant and the areolar glands well developed. Pubic hair is more abundant and spreads to thighs in some women or may extend to the umbilicus. Facial hair may increase. Increased sebaceous gland activity of the skin and increased severity of acne may appear.

The Menstrual Cycle

Coordination of the Menstrual Cycle

The menstrual cycle requires a complex sequence of physiological events coordinated by the hypothalamus in conjunction with the pituitary, ovary, and uterus, and that adapts to environmental phenomena. Major components of the system coordinating the menstrual cycle include the GnRH pulse generator, GnRH released by the hypothalamus, the gonadotropins (FSH and LH) secreted by the pituitary, and estrogen and progesterone produced by the ovary and corpus luteum, respectively. GnRH is released from the hypothalamus in a pulsatile fashion into the pituitary portal circulation. The pituitary gonadotropins respond to the stimulus from GnRH with pulses of LH and FSH released into the peripheral circulation. In response to GnRH and the gonadotropic hormones, the follicles produce estradiol and the corpus luteum produces progesterone in response to LH.

This coordinating system can be modulated by many inputs from higher neural centers and peripheral factors influencing the GnRH pulse generator as well as other hormones. Norepinephrine seems to amplify GnRH secretion, whereas dopamine dampens GnRH secretion. Increased endorphin release inhibits gonadotropin secretion through suppression of the release of GnRH (Knobil & Hotchkiss, 1988; Turek & Van Cauter, 1988; Vollman, 1977).

Ovarian Cycle: The Follicular Phase

The menstrual cycle consists of an ovarian and an endometrial component. The ovarian component is customarily divided into three phases to facilitate discussion: the follicular, ovulatory, and luteal phase (see Figure 3.11). The follicular phase consists of 10 to 14 days of hormonal influence that support the growth of the primordial follicle through the preantral, antral, and preovulatory phases. The primordial follicle consists of the oocyte arrested in the diploid stage of development in which it still has 46 chromosomes. The initiation of follicular growth does not appear to be dependent on gonadotropins or estrogen. In fact, follicular growth may have begun during the days of the previous luteal phase when the regressing corpus luteum secretes decreasing amounts of steroids. Indeed, follicles grow continuously, even during pregnancy, ovulation, and anovulation.

Within the first few days of the cycle, the follicle that will ovulate is identified. The mechanism for determining which follicles or how many will grow is unknown. The granulosa cells around the ovum become cuboidal and gap junctions develop, probably as a pathway for nutrients and metabolic interchange (Speroff, Glass, & Kase, 1994; Yen & Jaffee, 1989).

Preantral Follicle. A rise in FSH stimulates a group of follicles to grow to the preantral phase (the phase before the antrum is identifiable). During this phase, the zona pellucida appears around the ovum and the thecal layer begins to organize. The granulosa cells synthesize steroids, producing more estradiol than pro-

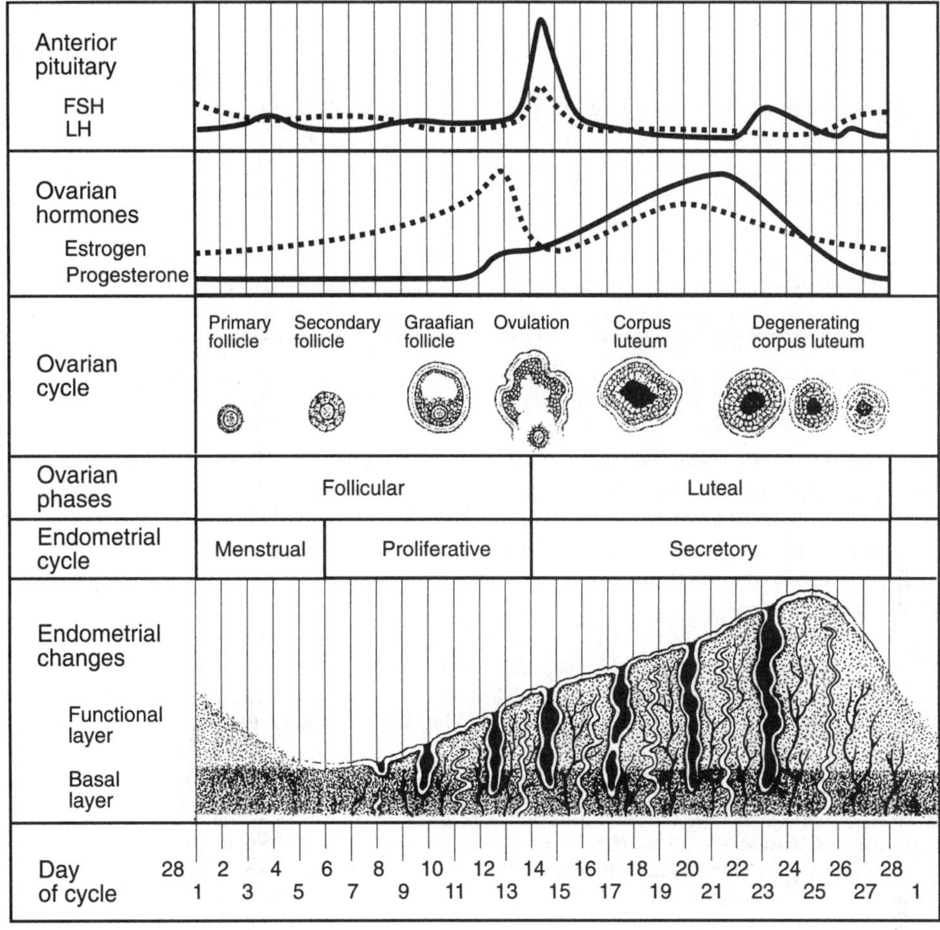

Figure 3.11. Coordination of the Menstrual Cycle

gestins or androgens. The follicle can also convert androgens to estrogens. Activated by FSH, the preantral follicle can generate its own estrogenic microenvironment. FSH can increase the concentration of its own receptors on the granulosa cells, thus inducing the production of estradiol. Moreover, at low concentrations, androgen enhances its transformation to estradiol. At higher levels, androgens cause the follicle to produce a more androgenic environment leading to atresia of the follicle. The follicle's development depends on its ability to convert androgen to estrogen.

Antral Follicle. Accumulation of follicular fluid in the antral follicle provides nurturance in an endocrine microenvironment. Influenced by FSH, estradiol becomes the dominant substance in follicular fluid. During the follicular phase, estrogen production occurs by a two-cell, two-gonadotropin mechanism. LH stimulates the theca cells to liberate androgens that are converted to estrogen, and FSH stimulates the granulosa cells to produce estradiol. Sensitivity to FSH determines the capacity for conversion of androgenic to an estrogenic environment in the follicle.

Selection of the follicle that will ovulate (often called dominant follicle) occurs during cycle days 5 through 7 and requires estrogenic action. By day 7, peripheral estradiol levels begin to rise significantly. Estradiol produces negative feedback that decreases gonadotropin support to other follicles. To survive, the selected follicle must increase its own FSH production. Because the dominant follicle has FSH receptors in the granulosa cells, it can enhance FSH action. These actions effectively allow the selected follicle to increase its own estradiol levels and suppress FSH release to other follicles. The theca doubles in vascularity by day 9, producing a siphon for gonadotropins for the selected follicle.

Although the midfollicular increase in estradiol levels produces negative feedback to suppress FSH, it exerts a positive feedback on LH. When estradiol levels reach a concentration necessary for positive feedback (more than 150-200 pg/ml for at least 36-50 hours), the LH surge occurs (Knobil & Hotchkiss, 1988; Speroff, 1994).

Feedback systems involving the pituitary and hypothalamus also enable the selected follicle to control its own development. Estradiol exerts negative feedback effects at the hypothalamus and anterior pituitary. Progesterone exerts inhibitory feedback at the level of the hypothalamus and positive feedback at the level of the pituitary. FSH is particularly sensitive to estradiol, whereas LH is sensitive to negative feedback of estradiol at low levels and to positive feedback by estradiol at higher levels. Progesterone slows LH pulses.

GnRH is secreted in the hypothalamus in a pulsatile fashion that changes in amplitude and duration across the menstrual cycle. During the early follicular phase, GnRH is secreted at approximately 94-minute intervals; in the late luteal phase it is secreted at 216-minute intervals with a decreased amplitude. In turn, the pituitary releases gonadotropic hormones in a pulsatile fashion.

Preovulatory Follicles. Initiated by the LH surge, the oocyte resumes meiosis, approaching completion of reduction division. Estradiol concentrations rise to maintain the peripheral threshold necessary for ovulation to occur. LH initiates luteinization of the granulosa cells and the production of progesterone in the granulosa. The preovulatory increase in progesterone facilitates positive feedback of estradiol and may be necessary for induction of the midcycle FSH peak. The midcycle increase in local and peripheral androgens deriving from the theca of the nonselected follicles may account for the increased libido some women report at midcycle.

Ovulation. Ovulation occurs about 10 to 12 hours after the LH peak, 24 to 36 hours after the estradiol peak. The onset of the LH surge is estimated to occur approximately 34 to 46 hours before the follicle ruptures. LH stimulates the completion of the reduction division in the oocyte (to 23 chromosomes), luteinization of granulosa cells, and synthesis of progesterone and prostaglandins. The continuing rise in progesterone in the follicle up to the time of ovulation may act to end the LH surge. Progesterone also enhances proteolytic enzymes and prostaglandins needed for digestion and rupture of the follicle. Progesterone influences the midcycle rise in FSH, which in turn frees the oocyte from the follicular attachments, converts plasminogen to plasmin (a proteolytic enzyme involved in follicular rupture), and ensures sufficient LH receptors for a normal luteal phase.

Ovarian Cycle: Luteal Phase

The luteal phase is named for the process of luteinization, which occurs following rupture of the follicle and release of the ovum. The granulosa cells increase in size and take on a yellowish pigment, lutein, from which they were named the corpus luteum or yellow body. Luteinization involves synthesis of androgens, estrogens, and progestins. The process of luteinization requires the accumulation of LH receptors during the follicular phase of the cycle and continuing levels of LH secretion. Progesterone acts during this phase to suppress new follicular growth, rising sharply after ovulation with a peak at about 8 days after the LH surge. Luteal phases ranging from 12 to 17 days are considered to be within normal limits. The corpus lutuem begins a rapid cessation of activity at about 9 to 11 days after ovulation, and the mechanism triggering this remains unknown. Some speculate that estrogen production and alteration in prostaglandin concentrations within the ovary are responsible. When pregnancy occurs, the corpus lutuem continues to function with the stimulus of HCG, which appears at the peak of corpus luteum function, 9 to 13 days after ovulation. HCG maintains corpus luteum function until approximately the 9th or 10th week of gestation.

The Endometrial Cycle

The first portion of the menstrual cycle is dominated by follicular development and follicular secretion and causes proliferation of the endometrium. The first portion of the menstrual cycle is named the *follicular phase* with respect to the ovary and the *proliferative phase* with respect to the endometrium. The second portion of the cycle is influenced by the corpus luteum, and the increasing levels of progesterone evoke secretory changes in the endometrium. The second portion of the menstrual cycle is named the *luteal phase* with respect to the ovary and the *secretory phase* with respect to the endometrium.

Immediately following menstruation, the endometrium is thin, only about 1 to 2 mm thick. Its surface endometrium is composed of low cuboidal cells, the stroma is dense and compact, and the glands appear straight and tubular.

Proliferative Phase. Under the influence of estrogen, the endometrium proliferates and increases in thickness. The endometrium becomes somewhat taller and the surface epithelium becomes columnar. The epithelial lining becomes continuous with the stromal component containing spiral vessels immediately below the epithelial-binding membrane that form a loose capillary network. Although the stroma is still quite compact, the endometrial glands have become more tortuous. Mitotic activity is evident in both the surface epithelium and the basal nuclei of the epithelial cells lining the endometrial glands. Estrogenic effects are also seen in the secretions of the cervical glands and in the vaginal lining. The variability in length of this phase of the menstrual cycle is greater than that for the luteal phase. Indeed, the varying number of proliferative or follicular phase days accounts for the variation in total cycle length.

Secretory Phase. As a result of the developing corpus luteum, progesterone evokes and increases the secretory changes in the endometrium. The surface epithelium is now tall and columnar; the stroma is less compact than earlier in the cycle and somewhat edematous and vascular. The endometrial glands become increasingly tortuous and convoluted. In addition, by 7 days after ovulation, the spiral vessels are densely coiled. The confinement of the growing endometrium to a fixed structure produces the tortuosity of the glands and spiral vessels.

Implantation usually occurs within 7 to 13 days after ovulation. At this point, the midportion of the endometrium appears lacelike, a stratum spongiosum. The stratum compactum overlies the inner layers of the endometrium and is a sturdy structure.

Premenstrually, the surface epithelium is quite tall, about 8 to 9 mm. The stroma consists of large polyhedral cells. The endometrial glands are very convoluted and serrated, resembling a corkscrew. The lining epithelium of endometrial glands is less well demarcated and smaller because of loss of glycogen into the gland lumen. A large number of lymphocytes and leukocytes are seen, probably as a result of the beginning necrosis of the endometrium.

Menstruation. In the absence of fertilization, implantation, and sustaining HCG, estradiol and progesterone levels wane as the corpus luteum ceases to function.

Endometrial growth regresses a few days before the onset of menstruation; at the same time, there is stasis of blood flow to the coiled arteries, with intermittent vasoconstriction. Between 4 and 24 hours prior to the onset of menstrual bleeding, intense vasoconstriction occurs. The menstrual blood flows from coiled arteries that have been constricted for several hours. Prostaglandins, synthesized in the endometrium as a result of progesterone stimulation, are released and produce more intense vasoconstriction. Dissolving of the endometrium liberates acid hydrolases from the cell lysosomes. The acid hydrolases further disrupt the endometrial-cell membranes, completing the process of menstruation. White cells migrate through capillary walls and red blood cells escape into the interstitial space along with thrombin-platelet plugs that appear in the superficial vessels. Leakage and interstitial hemorrhage occur. With increased ischemia, the continuous-binding membrane becomes fragmented and intercellular blood is extruded into the endometrial cavity. The loose, vascular stroma of the spongiosum desquamates. Menstrual flow stops due to prolonged vasoconstriction, desquamation of the spongy layer of the endometrium, vascular stasis, and estrogen-induced rebuilding. The lower layer of the endometrium (basalis) is retained and the stumps of the basal glands and stroma for the ensuing cycle continue to grow from them. The surface epithelium regenerates rapidly and may begin even while other areas are being desquamated.

With menstruation, as much as two thirds of the endometrium is lost. The menstrual flow may last from 2 to 8 days. Menstruation fluid consists of cervical and vaginal mucus as well as degenerated endometrial particles and blood. Sometimes clots may appear in the menstrual fluid. Usually from 2 to 3 ounces of fluid is lost with menses, but the amount of flow is highly variable. Women with more rapid loss experience a shorter duration of flow. Heavier flow and greater blood loss may indicate delayed or incomplete shedding of the endometrium.

Cyclic Changes in Other Organs

In addition to the uterus and ovary, other organs experience cyclic changes. The cervical canal contains about 100 crypts referred to as glands; the secretory cells of these crypts secrete mucus into the endocervical canal. The mucus undergoes qualitative and quantitative changes during the menstrual cycle depending on the hormonal environment. Immediately after menstruation, the mucus is sparse, viscid, and sticky. When examined under a microscope, an abundance of vaginal and cervical cells and lymphocytes can be seen. From about the 8th day of the cycle until ovulation, the quantity and viscosity of the mucus increase. Sometimes an obvious plug of yellow, white, or cloudy mucus of a tacky consistency is present. At midcycle the mucus is a thin hydrogel containing only 2% solids and 98% water. The mucus resembles raw egg white, being clear, stretchy, and slippery. It will stretch without breaking or spin a thread (spinnbarkheit). Ability of the mucus to stretch at least 5 to 6 cm has been established as a guideline for determining adequacy of the cervical mucus to support sperm transport. When the midcycle mucus is allowed to dry on a slide, it gives a fern or palm-leaf pattern. This pattern is absent after ovulation, during pregnancy, and after menopause. After ovulation, the mucus may again become cloudy, white, or yellow and tacky and may disappear altogether. Women can use the changes in cervical mucus as an indirect index of ovulation.

The cervix itself changes with the menstrual cycle. During the proliferative phase, the os progressively widens, reaching its maximum width just prior to or at ovulation. At the point of maximal widening, mucus can be seen extruding from the external os. After ovulation, the os returns to a smaller diameter, with the profuse and watery mucus becoming scanty and viscid. These changes are believed to be estrogen induced and are not seen in prepubertal or postmenopausal women or in those whose ovaries have been removed.

The motility of the uterine tubes is greatest during the estrogen-dominant portion of the menstrual cycle. They demonstrate a decreased motility during the progesterone-dominant phase.

Estrogen stimulation leads to cornification of the vagina. Following progesterone stimulation the vaginal epithelium shows an increase in the number of precornified cells, mucus shreds, and aggregates of cells.

Menopause

At between 38 and 42 years of age, ovulation becomes less frequent. Residual follicles have decreased in number from about 300,000 at puberty to a few thousand and are less sensitive to gonadotropin stimulation than earlier in life, are less likely to mature, and produce less estrogen. Menopause occurs when estrogen is insufficient to stimulate endometrial growth so that a woman no longer menstruates (Vom Saal & Finch, 1988; Wise, 1989; Wise, Weiland, Scarbrough, Larson, & Lloyd, 1990).

Menopause is said to have occurred when a woman has not menstruated for a period of 1 year. The climacteric, on the other hand, is analogous to puberty: It is a period of transition punctuated by a biological event, in this case menopause. Prior to menopause, women notice changes in their menstrual cycles, most likely due to a shortening of the follicular phase as a result of lower estradiol secretion. As a woman's cycles become more irregular, vaginal bleeding may occur at the end of a short luteal phase or after an estradiol peak without ovulation or corpus luteum formation.

Elevated FSH levels reflect an attempt to stimulate a follicle to produce estrogen. FSH levels of over 40 IU/L are used as an indicator that menopause is approaching, although women may still be bleeding. Elevated FSH levels probably reflect the decreased regulation by the negative feedback of inhibin produced by the granulosa cells. Although FSH rises to 10 to 20 times its premenopausal level and LH rises to 3 times its premenopausal level within 1 to 3 years after menopause, there is a subsequent decrease in both gonadotropins to a new steady state. In postmenopausal women, the ovary continues to secrete testosterone from the stromal tissue, and androstenedione secretion decreases to approximately one half the level seen premenopausally. As the follicles disappear and less estrogen is produced, the gonadotropins may stimulate secretion of testosterone. However, the total amount of testosterone produced is lower than premenopausally because peripheral conversion of androstenedione is reduced.

Circulating estradiol levels after menopause range from approximately 10 to 20 pg/ml. Most of this is derived from the conversion of estrone to estradiol in adipose tissue. Circulating levels of estrone are higher than estradiol with the mean levels approximately 30 to 70 pg/ml. As women age, there are lower levels of DHA and DHAS, but estrone, testosterone, and androstenedione remain relatively constant. Although estrogen production by the ovaries does not persist beyond menopause, estrogen levels in postmenopausal women may be significant due to the conversion of androstenedione and testosterone to estrone. Consequently, estrone levels will vary with the individual characteristics of women. Because fat aromatizes androgen, women with more body fat have higher estrone levels than do those with less body fat. An increase in substrate for estrogen production, as occurs in stressful situations that increase adrenal androstenedione, may induce a menstrual flow in a woman who is postmenopausal. Estrogens from nonovarian sources sustain the breasts and other estrogen-stimulated surfaces such as the urethra. Thin women are more likely to experience more symptoms related to lower estrogen levels, such as vaginal dryness, whereas obese women are more likely to experience dysfunctional uterine bleeding, endometrial hyperplasia, and endometrial neoplasms.

Occasionally, ovulation occurs and may result in an unplanned pregnancy during the menopausal transition. Elevation of both FSH and LH are thought to indicate that pregnancy cannot occur. Nonetheless, to prevent unwanted conception, women who are experiencing the menopausal transition need to be aware of their fertility status.

Physiological Aspects of Sexual Response

Masters and Johnson (1966) characterized physical phenomena that occur as humans responded to sexual stimulation as well as the psychosocial factors that influenced how people responded. Their observations during sexual response in 382 women and 312 men ranging from 18 to 89 years of age and representing a wide range of educational levels and ethnic groups contributed significantly to understanding sexual physiology.

There are two principal physiological changes responsible for events during the human sexual response cycle: vasocongestion and myotonia. Vasocongestion is congestion of blood vessels, usually venous vessels, and is the primary physiological response to sexual stimulation. Myotonia, increased muscular tension, is a secondary physiological response to sexual stimulation. These two changes are responsible for the phenomena observed during the sexual response cycle. Human sexual response is a total body response, not merely a pelvic phenomenon. Changes in cardiovascular and respiratory function as well as reactions involving skin, muscle, breasts, and the rectal sphincter occur during sexual response. The sexual response cycle includes four phases: excitement, plateau, orgasm, and resolution (Masters & Johnson, 1966).

Excitement Phase

Excitement phase develops from any source of bodily or psychic stimuli, and if adequate stimulation occurs, the intensity of excitement increases rapidly. This phase may be interrupted, prolonged, or ended by other competing stimuli. During the excitement phase, the clitoral glans becomes tumescent or enlarged, and the clitoral shaft increases in diameter and length. The appearance of vaginal lubrication, caused by vasocongestion and transudation of fluid across the vaginal membrane, occurs within 10 to 30 seconds after initiation of sexual stimulation. The vaginal barrel expands about 3.75 to 4.25 cm in transcervical width and lengthens 2.5 to 3.5 cm. In addition, the vaginal wall develops a purplish hue due to vasocongestion. Partial elevation of the uterus may occur if it lies in the anterior position.

In nulliparous women, flattening and separating of the labia majora occur. In multiparous women the labia majora move slightly away from the introitus due to a vasocongestive increase in their diameter. The vaginal barrel is lengthened approximately 1 cm as a result of the thickening of the labia minora.

During the excitement phase, changes also occur in women's extragenital organs. Nipples may protrude, breast size increases, the areolae become engorged, and the venous pattern on the breast becomes more obvious. The "sex flush," a maculopapular rash, may appear over the epigastric area, spreading quickly over the breasts. Some involuntary muscle tensing may be evident, as in the tensing of intercostal and abdominal muscles. The heart rate and blood pressure

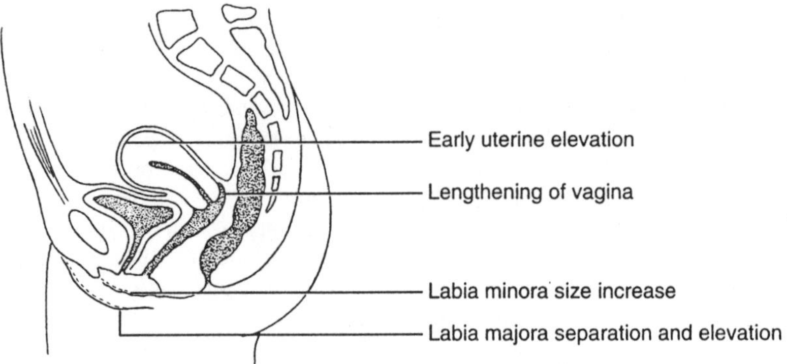

Figure 3.12a. Excitement Phase

also increase as sexual tension increases (see Figure 3.12a).

Plateau Phase

The plateau phase is a consolidation period following excitement when adequate stimulation is maintained. Sexual tension becomes intensified to the level at which a person may experience orgasm. Like excitement, this phase also may be affected by competing stimuli. During the plateau phase, the clitoris retracts against the anterior body of the symphysis pubis, underneath the clitoral hood. Vasocongestion of the tissues of the outer third of the vagina and the labia minora causes an increase in size of this highly sensitive tissue, referred to as the orgasmic platform. Further increase in the depth and width of the vaginal barrel occurs. The uterus becomes fully elevated, and as the cervix rises, it produces a tenting effect in the inner part of the vagina. Irritability of the corpus uteri continues to intensify.

In both nulliparous and multiparous women, the labia majora continue to become engorged, with the phenomenon being more pronounced in nulliparous women. The labia minora undergo a vivid color change from bright red to a deep wine-colored hue, considered a sign of impending orgasm. During the plateau phase, a drop or two of mucoid material is secreted from Bartholin's glands; this secretion probably assists slightly in vaginal lubrication.

Several extragenital responses occur in women during the plateau phase. Nipple stiffness continues to develop along with an increase in breast size and marked engorgement of the areolae. The sex flush, which began during excitement, may spread over the body. Facial, abdominal, and intercostal muscles contract; muscle tension is increased both voluntarily and involuntarily. Some women use voluntary rectal contractions to enhance stimulation during this phase. Hyperventilation occurs along with a heart rate of 120 to 175 beats per minute, elevation of the systolic blood pressure of 20 to 60 mm Hg, and diastolic elevation of 10 to 20 mm Hg (see Figure 3.12b).

Orgasmic Phase

Orgasm, the involuntary climax of sexual tension increment, involves only a few seconds of the cycle during which vasocongestion and muscle tension are released. During the orgasmic phase, the primary response occurs in women's orgasmic platform, as illustrated in Figure 3.12c. Approximately 5 to 12 contractions occur in the orgasmic platform at 0.8-second intervals. After the first three to six contractions, the interval between contractions increases and the intensity diminishes. The pelvic floor muscles that surround the lower third of the vagina contract against the engorged vessels, thus forcing out the blood trapped in them. Contractions of the uterus begin at the fundus and progress to the lower segment of the uterus. The contractile excursion of the uterus parallels women's ratings of the intensity of the orgasmic experience.

Extragenital responses involve several organ systems during orgasm. The sex flush parallels the intensity of orgasmic experience and is present in about 75% of women. Involuntary contraction and spasm of muscle groups may be

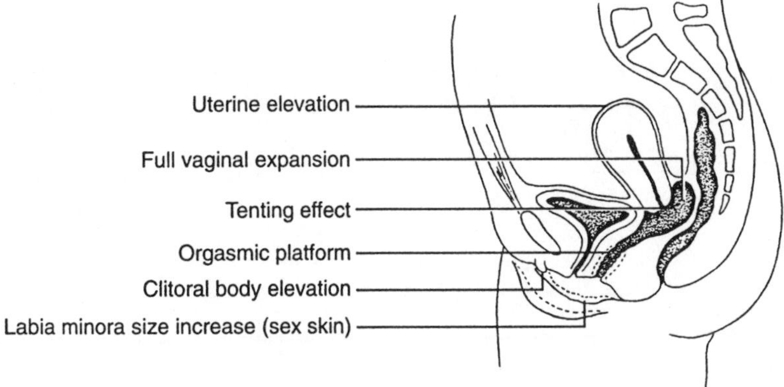

Figure 3.12b. Plateau Phase

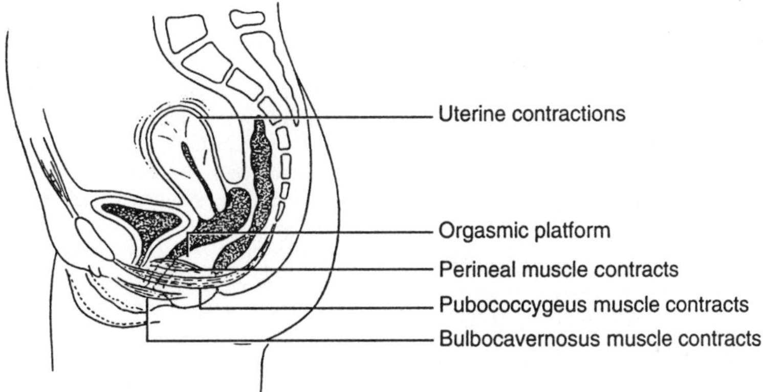

Figure 3.12c. Orgasmic Phase

seen, including contractions of the rectal sphincter, which occur at the same intervals as those of the orgasmic platform. Respiratory rates as high as 40 breaths per minute have been recorded, along with pulse rates from 110 to 180 beats per minute. Fluctuations in the pulse and respiratory rate tend to parallel the level of sexual tension. The systolic blood pressure may be elevated 30 to 80 mm Hg and the diastolic 20 to 40 mm Hg.

Resolution Phase

During the resolution phase, involutional changes restore the preexcitement state. With adequate stimulation, women may begin another sexual response cycle immediately before sexual excitement totally resolves. Usually the length of the resolution period parallels the length of the excitement phase. During the resolution phase, the clitoris returns to its usual position within 5 to 10 seconds after the contractions of the orgasmic platform cease. Vasocongestion and tumescence of the clitoris dissipate more slowly. There is rapid detumescence (loss of vasocongestion) of the orgasmic platform and relaxation of the walls of the vagina. The vaginal wall returns to its normal coloring in about 10 to 15 minutes. Gaping of the cervical os continues for 20 to 30 minutes. The uterus returns to its unstimulated position in the true pelvis, and the cervix descends into the dorsal area of the vagina. The nulliparous labia majora return to their preexcitement position, but in multiparas, the labial vasocongestion dissipates

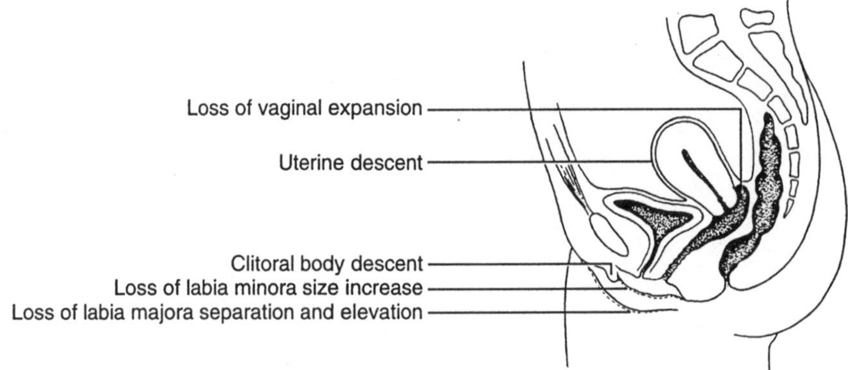

Figure 3.12d. Resolution Phase

more slowly. The labia minora change from deep red to light pink, and they decrease in size as vasocongestion is lost.

Involution of nipple stiffness, a slow decrease in breast size, and rapid reversal of the sex flush are seen. Some myotonia may still be seen during resolution. The respiratory rate, pulse rate, and blood pressure return to usual levels. An involuntary widespread film of perspiration may appear.

Although these physiological changes are common in women's sexual response, not every woman experiences each response. Indeed, the same woman may experience different aspects from cycle to cycle. Regardless of the difference in stimuli, some women will experience the same sexual responses whether the stimulus is self-pleasuring, pleasuring from another woman or from a man, or intercourse (Sherfey, 1972; Figure 3.12d).

Summary

From this discussion, it is evident that certain structures and functions are unique to a woman's body. These are involved in the menstrual cycle and women's sexual response cycles. Several of the structures of a woman's body serve her procreative powers as well as her pleasures, with the exception of the clitoris, an organ whose sole raison d'être is to receive and transduce sexual pleasure. Women's bodies develop uniquely from the time of conception and early differentiation through pubertal and menopausal transitions.

References

Bates, B. (1990). *A guide to the physical examination.* Philadelphia: J. B. Lippincott.

Blackburn, S., & Loper, D. (1992). *Maternal, fetal, and neonatal physiology: A clinical perspective.* Philadelphia: W. B. Saunders.

Boston Women's Health Book Collective. (1976). *Our bodies, ourselves.* New York: Simon & Schuster.

Boston Women's Health Book Collective. (1990). *Ourselves, growing older.* New York: Simon & Schuster.

Boston Women's Health Book Collective. (1992). *The new our bodies, ourselves.* New York: Simon & Schuster.

Cacciari, E., & Prader, A. (Eds.). (1980). *Pathophysiology of puberty.* New York: Academic Press.

Federation of Feminist Women's Health Centers. (1981). *A new view of a woman's body.* New York: Simon & Schuster.

George, F., & Wilson, J. (1988). Sex determination and differentiation. In E. Knobil, J. Neill, & Associates (Eds.), *The physiology of reproduction* (pp. 3-25). New York: Raven.

Knobil, E., & Hotchkiss, J. (1988). The menstrual cycle and its neuroendocrine control. In E. Knobil, J. Neill, & Associates (Eds.), *The physiology of reproduction* (pp. 1971-1994). New York: Raven.

Martin, E. (1991). The egg and the sperm: How science has constructed a romance based on stereotypical male-female roles. *Signs: Journal of Women in Culture and Society, 16,* 485-501.

Masters, W., & Johnson, V. (1966). *Human sexual response.* Boston: Little Brown.

Plant, T. (1988). Puberty in primates. In E. Knobil, J. Neill, & Associates (Eds.), *The physiology of reproduction* (pp. 1763-1788). New York: Raven.

Scheper-Hughes, N., & Lock, M. (1987). The mindful body: A prolegomenon to future work in medical anthropology. *Medical Anthropology Quarterly, 1*(1), 6-39.

Sherfey, M. (1972). *The nature and evolution of female sexuality.* New York: Random House.

Speroff, L., Glass, R., & Kase, N. (1994). *Clinical gynecologic endocrinology and infertility.* New York: Williams & Wilkins.

Tanner, J. (1981). Growth and maturation during adolescence. *Nutrition Reviews, 39*(2), 43-55.

Turek, F., & Van Cauter, E. (1988). Rhythms in reproduction. In E. Knobil, J. Neill, & Associates (Eds.), *The physiology of reproduction* (pp. 1789-1830). New York: Raven.

Venturoli, S., Flamigni, C., & Givens, J. (Eds.). (1985). *Adolescence in females.* Chicago: Medical Year Book Publishers.

Vollman, R. (1977). *The menstrual cycle.* Philadelphia: Saunders.

Vom Saal, F., & Finch, C. (1988). Reproductive senescence: Phenomena and mechanisms in mammals and selected vertebrates. In E. Knobil, J. Neill, & Associates (Eds.), *The physiology of reproduction* (pp. 2351-2413). New York: Raven.

Wise, P. (1989). Influence of estrogen on aging of the central nervous system: Its role in declining female reproductive function. In C. Hammond, F. Haseltine, & I. Schiff (Eds.), *Menopause: Evaluation, treatment, and health concerns* (pp. 53-70). New York: Alan Liss.

Wise, P., Weiland, N., Scarbrough, K., Larson, G., & Lloyd, J. (1990). Contribution of changing rhythmicity of hypothalamic neurotransmitter function to female reproductive aging. In M. Flint, F. Kronenberg, & W. Utian (Eds.), *Multidisciplinary perspectives on menopause* (pp. 31-43). New York: New York Academy of Sciences.

Yen, S., & Jaffee, R. (1989). *Reproductive endocrinology, physiology, pathophysiology, and clinical management.* Philadelphia: W. B. Saunders.

4

Young Women's Health

NANCY FUGATE WOODS

The health of young women, beginning with adolescence and extending through the young adult years, has profound effects on the health of women during their middle and older years. Despite this realization, only recently have clinicians and researchers accorded the health of young women—and not merely their reproductive health—the serious attention it deserves.

The purposes of this chapter are to examine the biological, personal, and social aspects of young women's healthy development. In addition, the chapter includes an overview of health concerns common during young women's adolescent and young adult years.

Central to the discussion in this chapter and in the chapters following is the notion that women are simultaneously embodied selves and relational selves. The embodied self refers to the simultaneity of physical experiences with the self. The body is inseparable from the self, and yet a woman can contemplate her body (Gadow, 1980). Although women's lives have sometimes been limited by other's assumptions that they are reducible to their bodily functions (for example, as reproductive machines), women also have unique bodily experiences, such as menstruation, that influence their life experiences and how they experience their bodies. Understanding embodiment means just embracing the bodily being, not accepting the dualistic notions about the separateness of body and self.

The relational self refers to the self as one in which relationships are a central, positive aspect of development throughout the life span. Self-in-relation theory, a product of thinkers such as Jean Baker Miller and Carol Gilligan, defines a woman's orientation as it is influenced by socialization. Whereas young men are socialized to achieve intimacy only after they have pursued individuation, girls develop a sense of self in the context of relationships (Miller, 1991b). Consequently, a woman's concept of her self is a relational self, one that exists in a web of relationships with others. Social intimacy, rather than individuation and separation, organizes her experiences. Women's self-esteem develops in a basis of feeling part of relationships and taking care of relationships. Growth occurs in emotional connections. For women, then, seeking an identity as a being-in-relation means developing all aspects of oneself in increasingly complex ways in the context of increasingly complex relationships (Jordan, Kaplan, Miller, Stiver, & Surrey, 1991).

Changing Bodies, Changing Selves

Experiencing Puberty

Women's relationships to their bodies evolve over the life span, and adolescence appears to be a critical period for changes in young women's self-concept and body image (Martin, 1987; Petersen, 1980). Prior to menarche, young women experience dramatic changes in their bodies during a relatively short period, including a deposition of fatty tissue, sometimes called the *fat spurt* (up to 11 kg of body fat), as well as an increase in height (up to 25 cm), called the *growth spurt* (Frisch, 1983). In addition, premenarcheal girls experience adrenarche (growth of pubic hair, stimulated by androgens), thelarche (breast development stimulated by estradiol), and late in puberty, menarche. Nearly two thirds of girls experience menarche during Tanner's (1981) Stage 4 (Brooks-Gunn & Warren, 1985b; Brooks-Gunn, Warren, Rosso, & Gargiulo, 1987). (The physiological basis of puberty and menarche is discussed more fully in Chapter 3, "Women's Bodies.")

Although the physical changes of puberty are likely to stimulate concern about one's body, the self-concept and body image changes do not occur in isolation from the dominant culture. Moreover, the timing of developmental events appears to be very important (Brooks-Gunn, 1984; Brooks-Gunn & Petersen, 1983; Brooks-Gunn & Ruble, 1983).

For girls, being in the middle of puberty and perceiving oneself to be on-time rather than early or late is related to a more positive body image and greater feelings of attractiveness. Girls who perceive themselves as late developers feel better about themselves than do those who are early (Brooks-Gunn, Petersen, & Eichorn, 1985; Brooks-Gunn & Warren, 1985a). Both perceptions of and satisfaction with weight affect a girl's body image and to a greater extent than that seen in boys. Being average in weight is most valued, but being thin is next. Being overweight is least valued. In general, physical maturation does not stimulate the positive response for girls that it does for boys. Of concern is that for postpubertal girls, a lower sense of self-esteem occurs. This finding elicits concern about the physical maturation in girls eliciting a more sexualized response from others, perhaps reinforcing their less-valued status in the overall society (Tobin-Richards, Boxer, & Petersen, 1983).

Meanings of Menarche

Early work from the 1970s shows that premenarcheal girls and young boys had negative attitudes and expectations about menstruation. Most thought menstruation would be accompanied by physical discomfort, emotionality, and a disruption of activities and interactions. Moreover, the postmenarcheal girls had more negative evaluations of menstruation than did the premenarcheal girls. Physiological aspects of menstrual distress may have been overemphasized in menstrual socialization, creating a negative frame of reference for construction of menstrual meanings (Clarke & Ruble, 1978).

In contrast, Whisnant and Zegans (1975) found that premenarcheal girls believed that menses would signal "being really grown up" and expectations that they should act differently but also denial that anyone but their mothers would view them or treat them differently. Postmenarcheal girls emphasized that they were still "the same person" after menarche. Nevertheless, some reported feeling closer to their mothers and becoming more private, introspective, and concerned with their relationships to other people. Some thought their fathers felt differently about them. Most of the postmenarcheal girls felt that a menstrual period should be "no great thing," emphasizing a need to be casual about the experience (Whisnant & Zegans, 1975).

Body Image and Sexual Identity

Menarche seems to be a pivotal event for reorganization of the adolescent girl's body image and sexual identity (Doan & Morse, 1985; Golub, 1983; Grief & Ullman, 1982; Koff, 1983). For example, Koff, Rierdan, and Silverstone (1978) found that postmenarcheal girls produced more sexually differentiated human drawings, were more likely to draw a female figure when asked to draw a person, and indicated greater satisfaction with female body parts on a body-cathexis scale than did premenarcheal girls. There is also evidence that the effect of menarche is primarily integrative rather than disruptive and can be viewed as a normal developmental crisis; postmenarcheal girls demonstrated clearer sexual differentiation and sexual identification than did premenarcheal girls of the same age but no more anxiety than the premenarcheal girls (Rierdan & Koff, 1980).

Responses to Menarche

Menarche may have a positive personal significance because it is associated with greater maturity, but this positive effect may be overshadowed by its negative interpersonal significance as girls become more self-conscious, embarrassed, and secretive regarding their experiences. Girls emphasized the central role of their mothers in menarche, with little mention of fathers (Koff, Rierdan, & Jacobson, 1981), and reports on relationships with mothers changed after menarche with respect to limits, closeness, distance, conflict, and daughters' roles in the family (Danza, 1983). Disclosure about menarche to friends was more likely to occur between close friends with high reciprocity and less likely among girls who were postmenarcheal and who had advanced breast development but was unrelated to pubic hair growth (Brooks-Gunn, Warren, Samelson, & Fox, 1986). Although adolescent girls can describe pubertal changes, discussing feelings was more difficult for them (Petersen, Tobin-Richards, & Boxer, 1983). Girls' secretiveness about their menarche seems limited to the first two or three cycles (Ruble & Brooks-Gunn, 1982b).

Significance of Menarche Versus Other Pubertal Changes

Different pubertal events seem to play different roles in self-definitions of adolescents, making it imperative to differentiate responses to menarche from responses to other pubertal events. Moreover, it is important to consider the influences of peers and others on the meanings ascribed to the events. Both breast development and height are public events and more likely to elicit responses from others than is development of pubic hair, which is not apparent to others (Brooks-Gunn & Warren, 1988).

Attitudes Toward Menarche

Menstrual attitudes are multidimensional and reflect attitudes toward menstruation as debilitating, bothersome, positive, or predictable. Some deny any effects of menstruation. Moreover, attitudes are linked to symptoms so that women who experience more symptoms view menstruation as more debilitating and predictable and are less likely to deny effects of menstruation than are women without symptoms (Brooks, Ruble, & Clarke, 1977). Adolescent girls resemble their peers more than they do their mothers with respect to both attitudes and symptoms. Adolescents are more likely to view menstruation as debilitating, bothersome, and unsanitary than are their mothers and are also more likely to report several types of symptoms than are their mothers (Menke, 1983; Stoltzman, 1986).

Symptoms

Ruble and Brooks-Gunn (1982a) found that shortly after menarche, often within the first year, young women reported symptoms of menstrual distress. Symptoms appeared to increase with age after menarche, but anticipated symptoms decreased with age in premenarcheal girls. Ruble and Brooks-Gunn suggested that the type of information that premenarcheal girls receive may change with their ages and that socialization processes rather than biology may be responsible for their expectations about symptoms. Moreover, as young women get older, they discuss their menstrual experiences with an increasingly large group of friends, and the nature of their information about menarche changes.

Longitudinal studies conducted in Finland (Kantero & Widholm, 1971; Widholm, 1979; Widholm & Kantero, 1971) revealed that girls experienced increasing incidence of dysmenorrhea with chronological and gynecologic age, with 75% of those experiencing dysmenorrhea reporting onset by the end of the first year after menarche. Widholm (1979) found that 36% of 13- to 14-year-olds and 56% of 17- to 20-year-olds experienced menstrual pain, with the pain lasting 1 to 2 days. In the United States, 60% of 12- to 17-year-olds experienced dysmenorrhea, with 14% reporting severe symptoms. The prevalence of dysmenorrhea increased with the progression through the Tanner (1981) stages of puberty, age, and gynecologic age (Klein & Litt,

1983). Brooks-Gunn and Ruble (1980) found that more than 75% of college women and late adolescents in New Jersey experienced dysmenorrhea. The role of ovulation is uncertain; 60% of those with dysmenorrhea were anovulatory according to vaginal smears (Widholm, 1979). Of interest was that very few girls remembered experiencing any symptoms with their first period (Brooks-Gunn & Ruble, 1980).

Another set of symptoms commonly experienced by adult women is premenstrual tension. Approximately 30% of the Finnish girls reported premenstrual tension, and about 60% reported fatigue and irritability premenses (Widholm & Kantero, 1971). Girls in the New Jersey studies reported expecting cycle phase differences in water retention and negative affect symptoms. Beliefs about symptoms were acquired early with more premenarcheal fifth to sixth graders expecting to experience more water retention and negative affect than did premenarcheal seventh to eighth graders. Similar to their experiences with pain symptoms, 79% of the girls recalled no premenstrual symptoms associated with their first menses (Ruble & Brooks-Gunn, 1982a).

Hygiene Behaviors

One important set of behaviors related to menarche is the hygienic management of menses. Napkin use decreased and tampon use increased from the elementary grades to high school, with 75% of 12th graders using tampons. Most girls learned tampon use from their mothers. Tampon users were less self-conscious and more comfortable with menstruation and reported a positive family atmosphere (Brooks-Gunn & Ruble, 1982b).

Menarcheal Age and Menarcheal Experience

Menarcheal age influences girls' experiences of menarche and puberty in several ways. Timing of menarche has been used as an indicator of pubertal maturation. Timing of menarche seemed to influence middle school girls' ratings of how grown-up a girl was and to her having older friends (Faust, 1983). Timing of menarche also influenced girls' level of preparation for menarche. Koff, Rierdan, and Sheingold (1982) found that girls who had a later menarche were better prepared for the experience. Girls experiencing later menarche had more opportunity for exposure to information about menstruation and greater maturity when they experienced their first menses.

Timing and Context for Menarche. Evidence from studies of menarche suggests that consideration of context is important in understanding the effects of timing of developmental events. First, subjective, not objective, timing of menarche seemed most important. Girls who perceived that they were early versus on-time or late had more negative menarcheal experiences. Girls who were early, late, or on-time according to objective criteria, did not differ in their experiences. These results underscore the importance of social clocks as well as biological clocks for adolescents (Rierdan & Koff, 1985). The importance of the context for maturation was illustrated in studies of menarcheal timing among dancers and nondancers. Dancers enrolled in national ballet company schools experienced more psychopathology when they began menarche on-time, whereas nondancers did not differ on any of the measures when timing of menarche was taken into account. Because of their low body fat, more of the dancers than nondancers were late in experiencing their menarche.

Timing and Social Relationships. Timing of menarche has been related to social relationships with family and peers. Adolescents' and parents' transactions differed according to their maturational status, with the earlier maturing adolescents engaging in more mutual explaining than did other parent-adolescent pairs (Hauser et al., 1985). In addition, mothers were more constraining and less explaining with on-time adolescents, although the mother-adolescent pairs were more mutually enabling in transactions in the on-time adolescents' families. Hill, Holmbeck, Marlow, Green, and Lynch (1985) assessed the relationship between menarcheal status and parent-child relations in families of seventh-grade girls. They found that most of the significant relationships occurred within the mother-daughter dyad and that most were curvilinear. Girls with early menarcheal status had less involvement in family activities, less parental influence, and less acceptance. The authors concluded that when menarche occurred around the modal time, the changes in the parent-child relationship were probably temporary perturbations, but when menarche occurred early, effects may persist in family relationships.

Preparation for Menarche

Types of Preparation. Most girls studied in the 1970s had received information through commercial educational materials that emphasized hygiene measures to deal with menstruation rather than with the emotional needs and anxieties that young girls might be experiencing (Whisnant, Brett, & Zegans, 1975). Most of the audiovisual and printed materials were produced by industry and included a technical, medical presentation of anatomy and physiology of menstruation, much as that seen in an anatomy text. Little material about the physiological changes of puberty was included. Although there was emphasis on the significance of menarche, womanhood and motherhood were emphasized rather than the significance of menstruation itself. Most materials encouraged girls not to acknowledge their menstruation and emphasized concealment of menses. Indeed, girls were encouraged to compensate for menstruation by following regimens to make themselves more attractive and to pamper themselves. Managing their emotions and learning to select and use menstrual hygiene products constituted the major emphasis of the materials, with little description of the experience of menstruation itself. Only the materials prepared for retarded girls' mothers were explicit about what menstruation would be like. Some materials prepared for mother-daughter interaction about menstruation provided scripts for the mothers, but others emphasized the girls' independence of their mothers. Generally, the materials dictated what a girl should feel rather than emphasizing her personal exploration of her unique responses to menarche. A more recent review of ads for sanitary products and products for relief of menstrual symptoms from *Seventeen* magazine for the years 1976 to 1986 revealed themes of menstruation as a hygienic crisis that required an effective security system to protect from soiling, staining, embarrassment, and odor and promote peace of mind. Menstruating women were portrayed as dynamic, energetic, and always functioning at their optimal level (Havens & Swenson, 1988; Swenson & Havens, 1987).

Menarcheal Preparation and Menarcheal Experiences. Although girls learned about their bodies and menstruation from commercial booklets, school, and parents, their friends were an important source. Most had seen commercially prepared films or attended health lectures augmented with printed materials. Both premenarcheal and postmenarcheal girls perceived themselves as knowledgeable about menstruation and were able to give superficial explanations of the anatomy and physiology of menstruation. Nonetheless, they had many misconceptions about their genitalia and about why menstruation occurs. Their concerns were not centered on the emotional response or meaning of menstruation but on the hygiene measures for dealing with menstruation, about which they were well informed. Premenarcheal girls anticipated announcing their menarche to their families and friends, but the postmenarcheal girls were quite secretive. Few told anyone except their mothers about their menarche. These findings support the cultural orientation toward menarche as a hygienic crisis to be concealed (Whisnant & Zegans, 1975).

Women from 23 countries reported that although their mothers were the main source of information about menstruation, nearly one third received no maternal preparation prior to menarche. The most common reaction was centered on getting help with the hygienic management issues. For some, needing reassurance of the normality was often reported. Emotional reactions differed, with Asians most often reporting feeling embarrassed and surprised and Iranian women feeling more grown up (Logan, 1980).

In the United States, as early as fifth grade, premenarcheal girls had expectations regarding menstrual symptoms. They anticipated experiencing cyclic symptoms much like those of older adolescents and adult women. Those who had begun menstruating experienced less severe menstrual distress (pain, water retention, negative affect, and behavioral changes) than the premenarcheal girls expected to experience. Among girls who experienced menarche during the course of the study, those who expected symptoms were more likely to experience them after they began menstruation. There were few changes in the amount of information girls learned from various sources as they experienced menarche. Of interest was that those who learned more information from males about menstruation rated menstruation as more debilitating and negative than did those who learned less from males (Brooks-Gunn & Ruble, 1982a).

Midwestern grade school girls demonstrated relatively poor knowledge of reproductive anatomy and menstrual physiology. Moreover, they had a wide variety of beliefs about menstruation, including the belief that menstrual blood had a bad odor. They ascribed to three menstrual taboos: the restriction of communication about menstruation with boys and in public; concealment of menstruation; and restriction of activity, such as swimming, during menstruation. They also attributed changes in emotion to menstruation, such as being more nervous and upset during menstruation (Williams, 1983).

Emotional and cognitive limitations of preadolescence may lead well-informed girls to have misconceptions about menstruation. For example, 40% assumed bleeding would be painful and associated it with injury. More than 50% expected to experience cramps. Nearly 80% had correct information about the frequency and duration of menstruation, and 86% had been informed about sanitary products. Many were convinced that their menstruation was obvious to others. It is likely that premenarcheal girls lacked a framework in which to integrate much menstrual information, especially information that was subjective and abstract, such as what it feels like to menstruate (Rierdan, Koff, & Flaherty, 1985-1986).

Preparation for Menarche and Adult Menstrual Experiences. Inadequate emotional preparation for menstruation was associated with more negative feelings at menarche, but menarcheal circumstances were not predictive of adult menstrual distress (Pillemer, Koff, Rhinehart, & Rierdan, 1987). The incidence of menstrual symptoms in adult college women and adults 30 to 45 years of age was not related to either preparation for menstruation or to whether menarche was a positive event (Golub & Catalano, 1983; Golub & Harrington, 1981; Woods, Dery, & Most, 1982).

Personal and Social Dimensions of Young Women's Lives

Women's lives have been examined from many perspectives, yet we know remarkably little about unique aspects of women's development because much of our knowledge about human development has been based on studies of men. Life stage models for understanding human development have been grounded in works in which men provided the information about the life span and women constituted a residual category—the complement to a man's life. Taking male development as the norm has produced a distorted view of women, recently replaced by a careful reexamination of women's development across the life span. This work, much of it still in progress, is revolutionizing how we think about women and our development. These new frames of reference provide a rich background for clinical practice with women.

Self-in-Relation

Infants can appreciate their ability to be in relationships, learning quickly to influence their caretakers. They learn about a self as inseparable from a dynamic interaction with a caretaker. Yet the literature on human development has ignored the complexity of mother-child interaction and the character of that interaction that involves attending to and responding in caretaking relationships. Young girls, socialized differently than young boys, learn to be caretakers. Their self-esteem is based on feeling a part of relationships and taking care of relationships. Thus growth occurs within emotional connections. Young boys, socialized to separation, may not develop a sense of self as interactive. They may envision themselves as doing rather than doing for or doing with.

Doing for others within the context of relationships involves using increased power and assertion and results in a change in internal configurations of self and others. Actions and feelings in relationships allow children to move to a larger and more articulated sense of self (Miller, 1991c).

During childhood, the social context plays an important role in how children view their parents. Devaluation of women undermines the influence of the mother-child relationship at the same time that it reinforces the importance and power of men. How children are socialized also affects their activities within relationships with one another. Girls' friendships with other girls often involve a focus on relational issues.

Adolescence brings the development of enhanced capacities in many arenas, including sexual, agentic, and cognitive arenas. With development of formal thought processes, girls explore fulfillment of their cognitive capacities. During adolescence, however, they are encouraged often to defer to the thoughts of others rather than to use their own cognitive capacities. Sexual development provides a conflictual situation for girls. Although desiring to integrate their sexuality into relationships, girls have been taught that their bodily and sexual feelings are unacceptable to bring into the context of relationships. Moreover, girls acting on the basis of their own sexuality often experience conflict with their male partners. As a result, they are encouraged to be passive or submissive in sexual relationships.

Agency refers to the capacity to perceive and use powers. Although girls have learned to do many things within relationships, they often discover that to act with a sense of self as agent is discouraged. Instead, adolescent girls often receive strong pressures not to do so.

Seeking an identity as a being-in-relation means developing all aspects of oneself in increasingly complex ways in the context of increasingly complex relationships. When the nature of those relationships is suppressive or oppressive, as often is the case for girls in many cultures, their development is thwarted (Miller, 1991c).

Empathy

Basic to human development is the concept of empathy, a complex process relying on a high level of psychological development and ego strength (Jordan, 1991a). Jordan points out that empathy involves affective and cognitive function that requires a well-differentiated sense of self and an appreciation of and sensitivity to the differences as well as the similarities of other persons. Empathy begins with motivation for human relatedness that allows one to perceive affective cues. Affective arousal in oneself follows, producing a temporary identification with the other's emotions. Finally, one regains a separate sense of self in which one can understand the emotional experience.

Mothering relies on empathic involvement with the infant, and young girls are encouraged to attend to others' emotional states. Young boys are socialized to contain their emotions, focusing on self-reliance and autonomy.

The mother-daughter relationship fosters development of empathy in young girls. Because of cultural norms and social practices that encourage young boys not to identify with their mothers, girls have greater opportunity to learn about empathy. This, in turn, may strengthen girls' sense of connection and being emotionally understood. The advantage that girls have in learning empathy may help make women in Western cultures the "carriers" of some aspects of human experience, including emotionality, vulnerability, and growth fostering.

Relationship Differentiation

Instead of emphasizing separation-individuation, the self-in-relation theorists have proposed that relationship-differentiation is central to women's development. Relationship-differentiation is a dynamic process encompassing increasing levels of complexity, structure, and articulation within the context of human attachments (Surrey, 1991a).

The mutual identification between mothers and daughters may create an advantageous situation for girls, who have opportunities to learn to take the role of other. Thus more accurate empathy, mutual identification, and mirroring of one another may strengthen girls' sense of being emotionally understood (Jordan, 1991a).

The developmental precursors of women's relational self-structure are further elaborated in adult women. In the context of relationship, women experience a heightened sense of their personal identity and powers. Early emotional sensitivity develops into complex cognitive and affective interactions later identified as empathy. Connectedness and the capacity for identification provide a basis for later feelings that to understand and to be understood are essential for self-acceptance and fundamental to feeling part of a larger network. Relationship differentiation, then, implies that (a) critical relationships such as that between mother and daughter continue to evolve throughout the life cycle; (b) the capacity to maintain relationships with tolerance, consideration, and mutual adaptation to the growth of each person requires developmental movement in many directions; (c) the ability to move closer to and further away from people depends on needs of the individuals and situational context; and (d) the capacity for developing additional relationships that are based on broader, more diverse identifications and corresponding patterns of relational networks can be understood through tracing development of one's identity through relational networks. Potential problems in the development of relational capacities can be understood from this perspective. For example, women experience difficulty attending to themselves and problems in separating from their families (Surrey, 1991a).

The mother-daughter relationship is a model for relationships with three crucial aspects: (a) the girl's ongoing interest in and desire for connection to her mother, (b) the girl's increasing capacity for mutual empathy developed in emotional connectedness, and (c) mutual empowerment that involves taking care of her relationship with her mother (Surrey, 1991a). Mothers empower their daughters by allowing them to feel successful in their abilities to understand and give support. Being able to perceive, respond, and relate to the needs and feelings of the other person contributes to a sense of empowerment that, in turn, creates a sense of effectiveness and motivates response to one another (Surrey, 1991a).

Reciprocity contributes to a mutual sense of self-esteem. Emotional sharing, openness, shared understanding, and regard contribute to self-esteem. Accurate empathy requires interactive validation of the differences between self and other. Oscillating between the capacity to see the other and to make oneself known to the other fosters growth in the other person as well as in oneself. Both reciprocity and flexibility are essential for the processes of growth.

Basic elements of women's core self, then, are (a) interest in and attention to the other person, forming the base for emotional connection and empathy; (b) expectation of a mutual empathic process in which sharing of experience enhances development of oneself and another; and (c) expectation of interaction and relationships as a process of mutual sensitivity and responsibility that stimulates growth of empowerment and self-knowledge (Surrey, 1991b, p. 59). This perspective of a core self-in-relation has important consequences for viewing development during adolescence. Adolescent girls may not want to separate from their parents but may want to change the nature of their relationships, to affirm their own development and allow the development of new relationships.

Relationship

In the context of self-in-relation theory, relationship has a specific meaning. *Relationship* means the "experience of emotional and cognitive intersubjectivity." It is being aware of and responsive to the other or others and the expectation that this awareness/responsiveness will be mutual (Surrey, 1991b). One comes to know oneself and others in the context of mutual relational interaction and in the continuity of emotional-cognitive dialogue. Communication is interaction rather than debate.

Relationships and identity develop in synchrony. Growing children move from emotional responsivity to conscious adult responsibility. Women's development moves from a caretaking relationship to one involving consideration, caring, and empowering.

Mutuality refers to reciprocity. In a mutual exchange, one affects the other and is affected by the other. In mutuality, both are open to influence, emotionally available, and engaged in a constantly changing pattern of responding to and affecting the other's state. Central to mutuality is having an influence on the other. The influence is conveyed through emotional reaction or change in behavior. Women often are more attuned to shifts in feelings, whereas men are more alert to behavioral change or action. As a result, heterosexual couples may struggle to "be with the other," with each responding to different cues (Jordan, 1991b; Surrey, 1991b).

Imbalances in mutuality arise from many sources. In some relationships, one person may be inaccessible or disconnected. In others, one person may use the other to shore up herself or himself. With depression, withdrawal into oneself may produce pain in one's inability to transcend self-interest. Mutuality suffers when one person does most of the giving and expects less in return. Often women get involved in one-sided nurturing. Power dynamics may create a dominance that interferes with mutuality. Problems can occur not only in couple relationships but in workplace relationships. Most workplaces are not structured to foster mutuality. Instead, productivity is emphasized through competition and individualism.

Through empathy, one develops the capacity to allow the other person's differentness and ultimately value and encourage the qualities that make that person unique. In an empathic relationship, one paradoxically experiences affirmation of the self and a transcendence of the self as part of a larger relationship (Jordan, 1991b; Jordan, Surrey, & Kaplan, 1991). Intersubjectivity implies the motivation to understand another's meaning system from his or her frame of reference, a type of relational frame of reference in which empathy is most likely to occur. A model of mutual intersubjectivity suggests that each person in a relationship (a) has interest in and cognitive-emotional awareness of and responsiveness to the other through empathy; (b) is willing to reveal one's inner states to the other person, giving the other access to one's subjective world; (c) has the capacity to acknowledge one's needs without manipulating the other to gain gratification while overlooking the other's experience; (d) values processes of knowing, respecting and enhancing the growth of the other; and (e) establishes an interactive pattern in which both are open to change in the interaction—for example, matching intensity of interest and involvement in exchange for both self and other (Surrey, 1991b).

Mother-Daughter Relationships

Self-in-relation theory provides an alternative explanation for the conflict in mother-daughter relationships that Freudians attribute to the Oedipal complex. In the context of self-in-relation theory, context is emphasized. Small children see their valued mothers devalued by the society. They are constantly exposed to situations demonstrating that women are accorded less power and authority than men. Girls come to idealize their fathers as a result of the respect the society accords them. In addition, girls develop different relationships with their fathers as a result of their differential exposure to their parents. The fathers are often less present in girls' lives than are mothers, so the father-daughter relationship is less real to the daughters. Indeed, mothers' relationships with daughters may facilitate their empathic development and ability to identify and respond to emotions, whereas fathers' relationships with daughters may help them to feel competent.

Evidence from studies by Kaplan and Klein (Kaplan, Klein, & Gleason, 1991) suggest that girls' conflicts with their mothers get resolved by late adolescence. The authors suggest that conflict is one way of elaborating connection, as one aspect of development. Disconnection, characterized by withdrawal or indifference, does not include the possibility for conflict. Indeed, conflict in relationships is a necessary part of development. Conflict may test relationships, such as occurs when adolescents want the nature of the relationship with their mothers to change. Connection and mutuality of concern, however, are possible even in the face of conflict.

Adolescents face dual relationship tasks of developing new networks while maintaining their continuing relationships. Tasks for college women include building on their parental and peer relationships so as to enhance their sense of self as a competent and able person (Kaplan et al., 1991). Late adolescence involves critical aspects of development of a core relational self-structure. Among the aspects of growth are (a) an increased potential for entering into mutually empathic relationships; (b) relational flexibility, the capacity to permit relationships to evolve; (c) ability and willingness to work through relational conflict; and (d) capacity to feel more empowered resulting from one's sense of relational connection to others, particularly to mothers. Of interest is that college women tend to look for changes in the mother-daughter relationship to accommodate changing maturity, not decreased closeness (Kaplan et al., 1991).

Dependency

Dependency is expecting other people to provide help as we cope physically and emotionally with those experiences and tasks for which we do not have "sufficient skill, confidence, energy, and/or time" (Stiver, 1991b). Conflicts around dependency arise in many types of relationships but are particularly noted in heterosexual relationships. Often, women are characterized as being more dependent than men. Adult development for men is often described in terms of achievement in work, with relationships with women subordinate to their occupational growth. Men tend to segregate work and family, whereas women tend to maintain interpersonal connections in and out of the workplace. For men, moving from attachment to separation is emphasized, whereas for women, moving from attachment to continued connection in the context of a relationship is emphasized. In the context of relationships, gender differences in styles of relating become apparent and often are responsible for miscommunication. Women's skills at empathizing permit them to respond to emotional needs and feelings, but women often feel that their needs are not met because men have been socialized to help through acting in concrete ways rather than listening. One can be enhanced and empowered through the process of depending on others for help. Dependency can promote growth and development of a sense of self (Stiver, 1991b).

Relationship and Empowerment

Power is the capacity to move or produce changes. Power, in the context of self-in-relation theory, is the capacity to move or produce changes.

This definition is in contrast to power as dominion, control, or mastery. Power is not seen as "power over" but "power with" (Surrey, 1991a). In contrast to empowerment is disempowerment, which is difficulty in creating or sustaining a healthy relational context.

As one develops power with others, one has a sense of being part of the growth and empowerment of others. One develops while seeing another become more of who he or she is as one does the same. The power-over model limits growth because it limits the relational context (Surrey, 1991a).

Anger in relationships is especially problematic for women. Although women suffer from many constraints against expressing anger, they live in a social milieu that engenders anger. Moreover, the conditions producing anger for women may grow from a reality that expressing anger is encouraged only for men. Because women are treated as a subordinate group, they learn to suppress anger, and that learning is encouraged by the threat of social or physical force against subordinates. However, the belief that subordinates shouldn't be angry discourages women from expressing their distress. Anger not expressed often manifests as depression (Miller, 1991a). An alternative to expressing anger is using one's power. Yet when some women use their power, they may feel selfish or destructive. Some are unable to reconcile their use of power with their feminine identity. Finally, when some women use their power they may precipitate abandonment.

Women's Networks

Women have overlapping relational networks that span many domains, such as relational structures for their personal, educational, work, social, and political development. Women have been involved in conscious-raising groups and support groups for a variety of purposes. Moreover, women's networks tend to overlap so that their personal friends are often their coworkers or their student friends (Surrey, 1991a).

Women's friendships evolve within a relational network seemingly designed to support and sustain it. Yet, in the broader social context, there exist many obstacles to female friendship. Raymond (1986) proposed the concept "gyn-affection," a unique feature of female friendship, in which vision is a central feature. Vision refers to the use of ordinary sight to see what exists as well as the ability to see beyond the ordinary to what can be. In a patriarchal society, men have established patterns of language and meaning to define what is "realistic." Some men regard feminism as utopian rather than realistic. Raymond emphasizes the importance of women seeing the material conditions of women's lives, their illiteracy, poverty, underemployment, victimization by rape, and other types of abuse. She points out the need for two perspectives, one focusing on what is and another focusing on what is possible.

Raymond (1986) asserts that the process of women's friendship moves between the ideal and the real. Women friends can help one another transcend the limits of what is to see new possibilities. Female friendship requires both thoughtfulness and passion. Thoughtfulness means a thinking participation in the world. Passion is evident in a friend manifesting a thinking heart. Friendship needs to be sustained and nurtured, yet gyn-affection in a patriarchal context is carefully contained and not allowed to expand in political or passionate senses.

Gyn-affection creates a context in which women can live as women, among women, among men. Living as a woman, among women, among men, implies simultaneously questioning the man-made world without dissociating from it, assimilating into it, or allowing it to define oneself as a victim in it. Raymond (1986) uses the term *inside outsider* to describe the dual tension of women who can see a man-made world for what it is and who can exist in it with integrity but simultaneously see beyond it to something different. Also the term highlights the importance of women recognizing that they can never truly be insiders but still recognizing the problems associated with becoming a dissociated outsider. Women's friendships, gyn-affection, can support women in living in a world fabricated by men while working for a world that women imagine.

Female friendship provides a context in which women can experience happiness, the feeling of gladness about life, as well as the experience of living life with a purposeful energy. In this context, women's happiness is defined not in relation to the lives of men but in relation to the lives of women.

Finally, female friendship makes women visible to one another. The dual vision of what is and what can be includes making women visible to themselves and to one another in a world that frequently keeps women and women's doings invisible by design (Raymond, 1986).

Cognitive Development and Moral Reasoning

The new accounts of women's development have also examined women's cognitive development and women's moral reasoning. Belenky, Clinchy, Goldberger, and Tarule (1986) studied women's ways of knowing by interviewing women from widely different ages, life circumstances, and backgrounds. They heard women describe a variety of epistemological perspectives from which they knew and viewed the world. In brief, the investigators found that some women were locked in a world of silence in which they obeyed external authority and remained voiceless. Others experienced received knowledge, that is, information they had learned from others and were able to reproduce. Still others experienced subjective knowledge and were able to hear their own inner voices and perceive truth as personal, private, and intuitive. Some had procedural knowledge that they derived from listening to the voice of reason and learning to incorporate others' ideas as something of value. Procedural knowledge includes two forms: separate procedures to support one's point of view, and connected knowing that involves understanding through relating to others and using empathy to gain knowledge about others. Some women experienced constructed knowledge, an integration of many voices. They recognized that truth is constructed in relation to context, that objective and subjective knowledge can be integrated. They appreciated the uniqueness of self and its contribution to constructed knowledge.

Some have suggested that relational experiences contribute to a special style of knowing for women. Belenky and colleagues (1986) have proposed that connected learning, taking the views of others and connecting them to one's own knowledge, contributes to a larger understanding of human experience. This approach discourages a split between thinking and feeling. In addition, their work illustrates how differential access to social resources and definitions of self have kept some women silent rather than promoted their ability to construct knowledge.

Carol Gilligan's works demonstrate that women's ethical development differs from men's and evolves around an ethic of caring versus a rights orientation. Gilligan found that women live in networks or webs of attraction, a fact that influences our development of an ethic of care. Women make decisions about moral acts using the criterion of caring or responsibility versus a rights orientation. Illustrating this distinction are the results of Gilligan's testing of a group of young women using a story about a man named Heinz who stole an expensive drug to save his wife's life. Heinz was judged by men to have been wrong—he took another's property. Women, on the other hand, tended to see this story from the perspective of relationships: Heinz's relationship to his wife and his relationship to the druggist. This pattern of the ethic of caring as distinct from an ethic of rights has permeated many other studies conducted by Gilligan and her colleagues (Brown & Gilligan, 1992; Gilligan, 1982). For example, stories of intimacy elicit fears of entrapment or betrayal from men, whereas they elicit fears of isolation from women.

Health and Health Risks During Adolescence and the Young Adult Years

In general, the adolescent and young adult years are healthy ones (Graham & Uphold, 1992). Although death rates are relatively low, deaths related to injury are the most prevalent cause of death for women 15 to 34 years of age. Nearly 75% of unintentional injury deaths are due to motor vehicle accidents (National Center for Health Statistics [NCHS], 1992). For young women 15 to 24 years of age, homicide ranks second in frequency, with suicide third. Both homicide and suicide remain among the first four causes of death for women 25 to 34 years of age. Punctuated by acute illnesses, such as colds and influenza, and hospitalizations primarily due to childbirth, the young women's use of health services is relatively infrequent when compared with women in midlife and older women. In addition, most young women assess their health as very good or excellent (NCHS, 1992).

Despite young women's good health, there are several serious health risks during this period. Risky behavior, including use of drugs and alcohol and lack of use of safety restraints, increases the risk of motor vehicle injuries, which account for the greatest proportion of accidental deaths for women. Exposure to violence (see Chapter 18) accounts for many of the homicides and injuries among young women. In addition, suicides are linked to young women's depression, exposure to drugs and alcohol, and abusive lifestyles (Strasburger & Greydanus, 1992).

Sexual Behavior, Sexually Transmitted Diseases, and Pregnancy

Among the most serious risks for young women are unsafe sexual practices and injectable drug use. Both may expose women to HIV and subsequent AIDS. During 1991, there were 75 cases of AIDs among women 13 to 19 years of age, with 5,061 among those 20 to 29, and 13,368 among those 30 to 39 years of age. The incidence drops to 7,341 among women 40 to 49 years (NCHS, 1992, p. 188). That AIDS occurs at all in adolescent females may reflect a greater vulnerability than that of adult women to sexually transmitted diseases (STDs). The heterosexual transmission of HIV has been forecast as a coming epidemic unless safe sexual practices become institutionalized (Bowler, Sheon, D'Angelo, & Vermund, 1992).

Young women become sexually active during their teen years (Brooks-Gunn & Furstenberg, 1989). Nearly 20% of white girls have had intercourse by 15 years of age, about 30% by 16 years of age, and about 40% by 17 years of age. For black girls, about 40% have had intercourse by age 16 and about 60% by age 17 (Newcomer & Baldwin, 1992).

During 1989, there were approximately 11,500 births to girls 14 years of age and younger (NCHS, 1992). The percentage of abortions for young women is significant and age related (NCHS, 1992, tab. 13, p. 28):

Age	*Abortions/100 Live Births*
<15 years	83.5
15-19	54.8
20-24	36.1
25-29	20.9
30-34	18.4
35-39	26.8
>40	49.4

Contraceptive methods vary greatly with young women's age. As seen below, the percentage of ever-married women using each type of contraceptive varies with the woman's age, with sterilization becoming increasingly prevalent with age, and oral contraceptives and condoms being the most common among very young women (NCHS, 1992, p. 138):

Age	*Any Method*	*Sterilization*	*Oral Contraceptives*
15-24	69.6	8.4	61.4
25-34	70.6	27.6	28.6
35-44	71.4	48.5	3.8

Age	*IUD*	*Diaphragm*	*Condom*	*Male Sterilization*
15-24	0.4	3.1	16.3	2.8
25-34	2.1	6.7	13.9	11.8
35-44	2.8	5.9	11.0	21.3

Smoking, Alcohol, and Other Drugs

Statistics for 1990 reveal a higher incidence of cigarette and alcohol use among teens than older women, with a similar pattern for marijuana and cocaine use.

The percentage of young women using cigarettes, alcohol, marijuana, and cocaine by age is as follows (NCHS, 1992, p. 205):

Age	*Cigarettes*	*Alcohol*	*Marijuana*	*Cocaine*
12-17	10	18	4	0.3
18-25	32	58	11	1.3

Weight Concerns and Eating Problems

Weight concerns and eating problems are among the most commonly reported concerns for young women. Recent data from adolescents enrolled in school revealed that 25% thought they were too fat, with 68% of those trying to lose weight. Young women accounted for 75% of those who believed they were too fat and were trying to lose weight. More white than black adolescent girls believed they were too fat and were trying to lose weight. Those who believed they were too fat engaged in less strenuous activity and watched more television on school days (Felts, Tavasso, Chenier, & Dunn, 1992). Girls tend to report more weight and eating concerns than do boys of the same age (Richards, Casper, & Larson, 1990). Indeed, some find that feeling fat and wishing to lose weight are becoming normative for young adolescent girls. Most weight concerns emerged between the ages of 9 and 11 (Koff & Rierdan, 1991). (For more information about nutrition and eating disorders see Chapter 12 and Nussbaum and Dwyer, 1992.)

Dysphoric Mood

Hormone levels account for little variation of mood among adolescent girls. Instead, negative life events and hormonal changes seem to have important joint influences on mood (Brooks-Gunn & Warren, 1989). (Warren & Brooks-Gunn, 1989). (For a full discussion of depression and dysphoric mood, see Chapter 15.)

The role of abuse, particularly sexual abuse, is not yet completely understood in the generation of adolescent health problems, including depression. Nonetheless, the victimization of young girls continues and is likely to have long-term consequences for their health throughout the life span. (For an extensive discussion of psychosocial issues, see Brown and Cromer, 1992.) Young women's constant exposure to sexual harassment, including verbal and physical harassment in their school settings, has recently received public attention. Moreover, court cases that are pending could influence the quality of the environments to which girls are exposed on an everyday basis.

Social Concern About Health and Health Promotion for Adolescents and Young Adults

Significant concern about the health of American adolescents has prompted an Office of Technology Assessment Report on Adolescent Health, with recent publication of results in the *Journal of Adolescent Health* ("Introduction," 1992). In addition, special concern about the growing problems of homeless and runaway youths and their associated health problems has received recent attention (Farrow, Deisher, Brown, Kulig, & Kipke, 1992). Besides work with youths and their families, both school-based health programs and communitywide efforts have been coupled with traditional health services to reach young women.

School-Based Health Programs

School-based health promotion programs, along with school-based clinics, have become increasingly common during the past decade. A recent review of reports about school-based health promotion program reveals consensus about five program elements:

1. Education and health are interrelated, each affecting the other.
2. The biggest threats to health are social morbidities.
3. A more comprehensive, integrated approach is needed.
4. Health promotion and education efforts should be centered in and around school.
5. Prevention efforts are cost-effective, with the costs of inaction too high and escalating (Lavin, Shapiro, & Weil, 1992).

Exercise and Fitness

Community-based interventions to increase exercise have had significant effects, especially in young women. A program begun in sixth grade had positive effects on children and adolescents of both genders, with increased exercise and activity observed among girls (Kelder, Perry, & Klepp, 1993).

Sex Education

Results of the Youth Risk Behavior Survey from 1991 indicated that 80% of adolescents received HIV instruction in school and 60% from their parents. In addition, risky behaviors were decreasing, with those having ever had intercourse fewer than 60% and those with two or more partners having dropped to fewer than 40%. Condom use was increasing, especially among those 14 years of age and younger ("HIV Instruction," 1991). Little is known about programmatic efforts to help adolescents address sexual orientation. As greater understanding of lesbian experiences becomes available, more supportive efforts for young women can be integrated into sexuality education programs (see Chapter 10). For an extensive review of sexuality programs, see Coupey and Klerman, 1992.

Prevention of Drug Use

A youth drug prevention program was tested through Boys and Girls Clubs of America, using their Stay SMART program, which was adapted from a school-based personal and social competence drug prevention program. Both the Stay SMART program and the Stay SMART program with a 2-year booster program had positive effects on marijuana-related, cigarette-related, alcohol-related, and overall drug-related behavior and knowledge about drug use. Booster programs produced added effects for alcohol attitudes and marijuana attitudes after each year of the booster programs (St. Pierre, Kaltreider, Mark, & Aikin, 1992).

Nutrition Programs

Although there have been many attempts to promote healthy nutritional patterns among adolescents, there have been few long-term controlled studies evaluating curriculum about eating attitudes and unhealthful weight regulation practices of young adolescent girls. A prevention intervention developed around instruction on harmful effects of unhealthful weight regulation, promotion of healthful weight regulations through nutrition and dietary principles and regular aerobic physical activity, and development of coping skills for resisting influences linking popular obsessions with thinness and dieting was tested with sixth- and seventh-grade girls. Although there was a significant increase in knowledge, there was only a small effect on body mass index. Targeting those at greatest risk, rather than the general population of young adolescent girls, may be more appropriate and effective (Killen et al., 1993).

Perimenstrual Symptoms and Dysmenorrhea

As discussed earlier, adolescents experience dysmenorrhea and perimenstrual symptoms similar to those experienced by older women. (See Chapter 23 for a discussion of these symptoms and their management.)

Screening Recommended for the General Population of Adolescents

For adolescents, in general, an annual screening for growth, vision, iron status, dental status, scoliosis, blood pressure, thyroid disease, behavior (including school performance and attendance, substance use, affective state, sexual activity and abuse, and somatic symptoms) is recommended. In addition, immunity to measles, mumps, rubella, and poliovirus infection and tetanus should be ensured at least once during adolescence. Special populations in which tuberculosis, sickle cell trait, and thalassemia conditions are prevalent should be screened for these conditions (Cromer, McLean, & Heald, 1992).

The first pelvic exam often occurs during adolescence or the early adult years (see Chapter 9). Although high school girls are beginning to have pelvic exams and Pap smear testing for cervical cancer, they may not comprehend the significance of early detection of cancer (Sharp, Dignan, Dammers, Michielutte, & Jackson, 1990). Young girls' exposure to information about the value of cancer screening, in particular learning about breast self-examination and Pap smears, provides an important foundation for future health protection practices.

Menarcheal Preparation

The dominant emphasis of materials designed for preparing young girls for menarche is coping with a hygienic crisis rather than a developmental event. In addition, most materials have emphasized provision of technical information rather than addressing the psychosocial impact of menarche. College women recommended inclusion of knowledge, providing emotional support, and addressing the psychosocial significance of menstruation in preparing young girls for menstruation. In particular, they mentioned that prior knowledge about menstruation would make the experience of the first period easier. Most thought that the biology behind menstruation was important to include, and many thought it important to discuss the sexual implications of menstruation. The majority acknowledged the need for information about the experiential aspects of menstruation: how menstruation feels. In addition, emphasizing variability in the experience was important. Knowledge about hygiene, including demonstrations of how to use a pad or tampon, was seen as important. Emotional support was particularly helpful, and the women emphasized the importance of mothers offering to be available to talk to them about their concerns and answer their questions. Many emphasized reassurance about the normalcy of menstruation and the importance of differentiating it from a disease. There were mixed opinions about the psychosocial significance of menstruation, with many emphasizing minimizing the significance of the event. Others recommended presenting menstruation as a positive thing in which one could take pride. Still others emphasized the menstrual experience as unique to women (Rierdan, 1983). Rierdan, Koff, and Flaherty (1983, p. 14) recommend that "preparation for menarche should be construed as a continuous learning process, taking place before and after menarche, with the content of what is to be learned varying with the girl's ability to assimilate such material." The task of preparing girls intellectually and, insofar as possible, emotionally before menarche needs to be coordinated with the task after menarche of helping the girl interrelate her abstract knowledge with her personal experience to provide a more positive, integrated type of knowing. In addition, they recommend acknowledging the wide range of meaning that menstruation has for girls, the significance of the affective response to menarche indicated by the richness of women's memories of their own menarche, and the importance of a supportive, emotionally available mother as an important aspect of preparation for menarche.

McKeever (1984) recommended acknowledging the cyclicity that is part of women's lives, enhancing awareness of the young woman's uterus and vagina through use of concrete models and experiences with tampons and cramps, and emphasizing the normal variation of menstruation. In addition, she stressed the need to help mothers prepare for and support their daughters during their menarcheal experiences.

Adolescent girls want simple acknowledgment of their menarche, indicating that something special has happened to them. They do not want emphasis on becoming a woman or their ability to become pregnant. They want to safeguard their privacy and prefer a simple hug or toast to mark the event (Logan, Calder, & Cohen, 1980).

Relationships, Parental, and Peer Support

Although relationships with peers are significant for adolescents, there is evidence that relationships with parents, especially one's mother, can be significant for adolescent girls. Among a community population of girls between the ages of 15 and 20, a clear preference was seen for using other girls and women as problem solvers and intimate confidants. Mothers were the most frequently named problem solvers, but confiding was affected by quality of the mother-daughter relationship. Girlfriends were the most commonly named intimate confidant (Monck, 1991).

References

Belenky, M., Clinchy, B., Goldberger, N., & Tarule, J. (1986). *Women's ways of knowing: The development of self, voice, and mind.* New York: Basic Books.

Bowler, S., Sheon, A., D'Angelo, M., & Vermund, S. (1992). HIV and AIDS among adolescents in the U.S.: Increasing risk in the 1990s. *Journal of Adolescence, 15,* 345-371.

Brooks-Gunn, J. (1984). The psychological significance of different pubertal events to young girls. *Journal of Early Adolescence, 4*(4), 315-327.

Brooks-Gunn, J., & Furstenberg, F. (1989). Adolescent sexual behavior. *American Psychologist, 44*(2), 249-257.

Brooks-Gunn, J. & Petersen, A. (1983). *Girls at puberty: Biological and psychosocial perspectives.* New York: Plenum.

Brooks-Gunn, J., Petersen, A., & Eichorn, D. (1985). The study of maturational timing effects in adolescence. *Journal of Youth and Adolescence, 14*(1), 149-161.

Brooks-Gunn, J., & Ruble, D. (1980). Menarche: The interaction of physiological, cultural, and social factors. In A. Dan, E. Graham, & C. Beecher (Eds.), *The menstrual cycle: Vol. 1. A synthesis of interdisciplinary research* (pp. 141-159). New York: Springer.

Brooks-Gunn, J., & Ruble, D. (1982a). The development of menstrual-related beliefs and behaviors during early adolescence. *Child Development, 53,* 1567-1577.

Brooks-Gunn, J., & Ruble, D. (1982b). Psychological correlates of tampon use in adolescents. *Annals of Internal Medicine, 96*(part 2), 962-965.

Brooks-Gunn, J., & Ruble, D. (1983). The experience of menarche from a developmental perspective. In J. Brooks-Gunn & A. Petersen (Eds.), Girls at puberty (pp. 155-177). New York: Plenum.

Brooks, J., Ruble, D., & Clarke, A. (1977). College women's attitudes and expectations concerning menstrual related changes. *Psychosomatic Medicine, 39,* 288-298.

Brooks-Gunn, J., & Warren, M. (1985a). The effects of delayed menarche in different contexts: Dance and nondance students. *Journal of Youth and Adolescence, 14*(4), 285-300.

Brooks-Gunn, J., & Warren, M. (1985b). Measuring physical status and timing in early adolescence: A developmental perspective. *Journal of Youth and Adolescence, 14*(3), 163-189.

Brooks-Gunn, J., & Warren, M. (1988). The psychological significance of secondary sexual characteristics in nine to eleven year old girls. *Child Development, 59,* 1061-1069.

Brooks-Gunn, J., & Warren, M. (1989). Biological and social contributions to negative affect in young adolescent girls. *Child Development, 60*(1), 40-55.

Brooks-Gunn, J., Warren, M., Rosso, J., & Gargiulo, J. (1987). Validity of self report measures of girls' pubertal status. *Child Development, 58,* 829-841.

Brooks-Gunn, J., Warren, M., Samelson, M., & Fox, R. (1986). Physical similarity of and disclosure of menarcheal status to friends: Effects of grade and pubertal status. *Journal of Early Adolescence, 6*(1), 3-14.

Brown, L. M., & Gilligan, C. (1992). *Meeting at the crossroads.* Cambridge, MA: Harvard University Press.

Brown, R., & Cromer, B. (Eds.). (1992). *Psychosocial issues in adolescents.* Philadelphia: Hanley & Belfus.

Clarke, A., & Ruble, D. (1978). Young adolescents' beliefs concerning menstruation. *Child Development, 49,* 231-234.

Coupey, S., & Klerman, L. (Eds.). (1992). *Adolescent sexuality: Preventing unhealthy consequences.* Philadelphia: Hanley & Belfus.

Cromer, B. A., McLean, C. S., & Heald, F. P. (1992). A critical review of comprehensive health screening in adolescents. *Journal of Adolescent Health, 13* (Suppl. 2), 1S-65S.

Danza, R. (1983). Menarche: Its effects on mother-daughter and father-daughter interactions. In S. Golub (Ed.), *Menarche* (pp. 99-105). Lexington, KY: Lexington Books.

Doan, H., & Morse, J. (1985). The last taboo: Roadblocks to researching menarche. *Health Care for Women International, 6*(5-6), 277-283.

Farrow, J., Deisher, R., Brown, R., Kulig, J., & Kipke, M. (1992). Health and health needs of homeless and runaway youth. *Journal of Adolescent Health, 13,* 717-726.

Faust, M. (1983). Alternative constructions of adolescent growth. In J. Brooks-Gunn & A. Petersen (Eds.), *Girls at puberty* (pp. 105-125). New York: Plenum.

Felts, M., Tavasso, D., Chenier, T., & Dunn, P. (1992). Adolescent's perceptions of relative weight and self reported weight loss activities. *Journal of School Health, 62*(8), 372-376.

Frisch, R. (1983). Fatness, puberty, and fertility: The effects of nutrition and physical training on menarche and ovulation. In J. Brooks-Gunn & A. Petersen (Eds.), *Girls at puberty* (pp. 29-49). New York: Plenum.

Gadow, S. (1980). Body and self: A dialectic. *Journal of Medicine & Philosophy, 5*(3), 172-185.

Gilligan, C. (1982). *In a different voice: Psychological theory and women's development.* Cambridge, MA: Harvard University Press.

Golub, S. (Ed.). (1983). *Menarche: The transition from girl to woman.* Lexington, MA: D. C. Heath.

Golub, S., & Catalano, J. (1983). Recollections of menarche and women's subsequent experience with menstruation. *Women and Health, 8*(1), 49-61.

Golub, S., & Harrington, D. (1981). Premenstrual and menstrual mood changes in adolescent women. *Journal of Personality and Social Psychology, 41*(5), 961-965.

Graham, M., & Uphold, C. (1992). Health perceptions and behaviors of school-age boys and girls. *Journal of Community Health Nursing, 9*(2), 77-86.

Grief, E., & Ullman, K. (1982). The psychological impact of menarche on early adolescent females: A review of the literature. *Child Development, 53,* 1413-1430.

Hauser, S., Liebman, W., Houlihan, J., Powers, S., Jacobson, A., Noam, G., Weiss, B., & Follansbee, D. (1985). Family contexts of pubertal timing. *Journal of Youth and Adolescence, 14*(4), 317-337.

Havens, B., & Swenson, I. (1988). Imagery associated with menstruation in advertising targeted to adolescent females. *Adolescence, 23*(89), 89-97.

Hill, J., Holmbeck, G., Marlow, L., Green, T., & Lynch, M. (1985). Menarcheal status and parent-child relations in families of seventh-grade girls. *Journal of Youth and Adolescence, 14*(4), 301-316.

HIV instruction and selected HIV risk behaviors among high school students. (1991). *Journal of School Health, 62*(10), 481-482.

Introduction. (1992). *Journal of Adolescent Health, 13*(2S), 3S-6S.

Jordan, J. (1991a). Empathy and self boundaries. In J. Jordan, A. Kaplan, J. Miller, I. Stiver, & J. Surrey (Eds.), *Women's growth in connection: Writings from the Stone Center* (pp. 67-80). New York: Guilford.

Jordan, J. (1991b). The meaning of mutuality. In J. Jordan, A. Kaplan, J. Miller, I. Stiver, & J. Surrey (Eds.), *Women's growth in connection: Writings from the Stone Center* (pp. 81-96). New York: Guilford.

Jordan, J., Kaplan, A., Miller, J., Stiver, I., & Surrey, J. (Eds.). (1991). *Women's growth in connection: Writings from the Stone Center.* New York: Guilford.

Jordan, J., Surrey, J., & Kaplan, A. (1991). Women and empathy: Implications for psychological development and psychotherapy. In J. Jordan, A. Kaplan, J. Miller, I. Stiver, & J. Surrey (Eds.), *Women's growth in connection: Writings from the Stone Center* (pp. 27-50). New York: Guilford.

Kantero, R., & Widholm, O. (1971). The age of menarche in Finnish girls in 1969 (Series II). *Acta Obstetrica Gynecologica Scandinavica, 14*(Suppl.), 7-18.

Kaplan, A., Klein, R., & Gleason, N. (1991). Women's self development in late adolescence. In J. Jordan, A. Kaplan, J. Miller, I. Stiver, & J. Surrey (Eds.), *Women's growth in connection: Writings from the Stone Center* (pp. 122-142). New York: Guilford.

Kelder, S., Perry, C., & Klepp, K. (1993). Community based youth exercise program: Long-term outcomes of the Minnesota Heart Health Program and Class of 1989 Study. *Journal of School Health, 64*(5), 218-223.

Killen, J., Taylor, C., Hammer, L., Litt, I., Wilson, D., Rich, T., Hayward, C., Simonds, B., Kraemer, H., & Varady, A. (1993). An attempt to modify unhealthful eating attitudes and weight regulation practices of young adolescent girls. *International Journal of Eating Disorders, 13*(4), 369-384.

Klein, J., & Litt, I. (1983). Menarche and dysmenorrhea. In J. Brooks-Gunn & A. Petersen (Eds.), *Girls at puberty* (pp. 73-88). New York: Plenum.

Koff, E. (1983). Through the looking glass of menarche: What the adolescent girl sees. In S. Golub (Ed.),

Menarche (pp. 77-86). Lexington, MA: Lexington Books.

Koff, E., & Rierdan, J. (1991). Perceptions of weight and attitudes toward eating in early adolescent girls. *Journal of Adolescent Health, 12*(5), 307-312.

Koff, E., Rierdan, J., & Jacobson, S. (1981). The personal and interpersonal significance of menarche. *Journal of the American Academy of Child Psychiatry, 20*(6), 148-158.

Koff, E., Rierdan, J., & Sheingold, K. (1982). Memories of menarche: Age, preparation, and prior knowledge as determinants of initial menstrual experience. *Journal of Youth and Adolescence, 11*(1), 1-9.

Koff, E., Rierdan, J., & Silverstone, E. (1978). Changes in representation of body image as a function of menarcheal status. *Developmental Psychology, 14,* 635-642.

Lavin, A., Shapiro, G., & Weil, K. (1992). Creating an agenda for school based health promotion: A review of 25 selected reports. *Journal of School Health, 62,* 212-228.

Logan, D. (1980). The menarche experience in twenty-three foreign countries. *Adolescence, 15*(58), 247-256.

Logan, D., Calder, J., & Cohen, B. (1980). Toward a contemporary tradition for menarche. *Journal of Youth and Adolescence, 9*(3), 263-269.

Martin, E. (1987). *The woman in the body: A cultural analysis of reproduction.* Boston: Beacon.

McKeever, P. (1984). The perpetuation of menstrual shame: Implications and directions. *Women and Health, 9*(4), 33-47.

Menke, E. (1983). Menstrual beliefs and experiences of mother-daughter dyads. In S. Golub (Ed.), *Menarche* (pp. 133-137). Lexington, MA: Lexington Books.

Miller, J. (1991a). The construction of anger in women and men. In J. Jordan, A. Kaplan, J. Miller, I. Stiver, & J. Surrey (Eds.), *Women's growth in connection: Writings from the Stone Center* (pp. 181-196). New York: Guilford.

Miller, J. (1991b). The development of women's sense of self. In J. Jordan, A. Kaplan, J. Miller, I. Stiver, & J. Surrey (Eds.), *Women's growth in connection: Writings from the Stone Center* (pp. 11-26). New York: Guilford.

Miller, J. (1991c). Women and power. In J. Jordan, A. Kaplan, J. Miller, I. Stiver, & J. Surrey (Eds.), *Women's growth in connection: Writings from the Stone Center* (pp. 197-205). New York: Guilford.

Monck, E. (1991). Patterns of confiding relationships among adolescent girls. *Journal of Child Psychology and Psychiatry, 32*(2), 333-345.

National Center for Health Statistics. (1992). *Health, United States.* Hyattsville, MD: Public Health Service.

Newcomer, S., & Baldwin, W. (1992). Demographics of adolescent sexual behavior, contraception, pregnancy, and sexually transmitted diseases. *Journal of School Health, 62,* 265-270.

Nussbaum, M., & Dwyer, J. (Eds.). (1992). *Adolescent nutrition and eating disorders.* Philadelphia: Hanley & Belfus.

Office of Technology Assessment. (1993). The role of federal agencies in adolescent health. *Journal of Adolescent Health, 13*(3), 183-235.

Petersen, A. (1980). Puberty and its psychological significance in girls. In A. Dan, E. Graham, & C. Beecher (Eds.), *The menstrual cycle: Vol. I. A synthesis of interdisciplinary research* (pp. 45-55). New York: Springer.

Petersen, A., Tobin-Richards, M., & Boxer, A. (1983). Puberty: Its measurement and its meaning. *Journal of Early Adolescence, 3*(1-2), 47-62.

Pillemer, D., Koff, E., Rhinehart, E., & Rierdan, J. (1987). Flashbulb memories of menarche and adult menstrual distress. *Journal of Adolescence, 10*(2), 187-199.

Raymond, J. (1986). *A passion for friends: Toward a philosophy of female affection.* Boston: Beacon.

Richards, M. H., Casper, R. C., & Larson, R. (1990). Weight and eating concerns among pre- and young adolescent boys and girls. *Journal of Adolescent Health Care, 11*(3), 203-209.

Rierdan, J. (1983). Variations in the experience of menarche as a function of preparedness. In S. Golub (Ed.), *Menarche* (pp. 119-125). Lexington, MA: Lexington Books.

Rierdan, J., & Koff, E. (1980). The psychological impact of menarche: Integrative versus disruptive changes. *Journal of Youth and Adolescence, 9*(1), 49-58.

Rierdan, J., & Koff, E. (1985). Timing of menarche and initial menstrual experience. *Journal of Youth and Adolescence, 14*(3), 237-244.

Rierdan, J., Koff, E., & Flaherty, E. (1983). Guidelines for preparing girls for menstruation. *Journal of the American Academy of Child Psychiatry, 22,* 480-486.

Rierdan, J., Koff, E., & Flaherty, J. (1985-1986). Conceptions and misconceptions of menstruation. *Women and Health, 10*(4), 33-45.

Ruble, D., & Brooks-Gunn, J. (1982a). A developmental analysis of menstrual distress in adolescence. In R. Friedman (Ed.), *Behavior and the menstrual cycle* (pp. 177-197). New York: Marcel Dekker.

Ruble, D., & Brooks-Gunn, J. (1982b). The experience of menarche. *Child Development, 53,* 1557-1566.

Sharp, P., Dignan, M., Dammers, P., Michielutte, R., & Jackson, D. (1990). Knowledge and attitudes about cervical cancer and the Pap smear among 10th grade girls. *Southern Medical Journal, 83*(9), 1016-1018.

St. Pierre, T., Kaltreider, D., Mark, M., & Aikin, K. (1992). Drug prevention in a community setting: A longitudinal study of the relative effectiveness of a three-year primary prevention program in boys and girls clubs across the nation. *American Journal of Community Psychology, 20*(6), 673-706.

Stiver, I. (1991a). Beyond the Oedipus complex: Mothers and daughters. In J. Jordan, A. Kaplan, J. Miller, I. Stiver, & J. Surrey (Eds.), *Women's growth in connection: Writings from the Stone Center* (pp. 97-121). New York: Guilford.

Stiver, I. (1991b). The meanings of "dependency" in female-male relationships. In J. Jordan, A. Kaplan,

J. Miller, I. Stiver, & J. Surrey (Eds.), *Women's growth in connection: Writings from the Stone Center* (pp. 143-161). New York: Guilford.

Stoltzman, S. (1986). Menstrual attitudes, beliefs, and symptom experiences of adolescent females, their peers, and their mothers. *Health Care for Women International, 7*(1/2), 97-114.

Strasburger, V., & Greydanus, D. (Eds.). (1992). *The at-risk adolescent.* Philadelphia: Hanley & Belfus.

Surrey, J. (1991a). Relationship and empowerment. In J. Jordan, A. Kaplan, J. Miller, I. Stiver, & J. Surrey (Eds.), *Women's growth in connection: Writings from the Stone Center* (pp. 162-180). New York: Guilford.

Surrey, J. (1991b). The "self-in-relation": A theory of women's development. In J. Jordan, A. Kaplan, J. Miller, I. Stiver, & J. Surrey (Eds.), *Women's growth in connection: Writings from the Stone Center* (pp. 51-66). New York: Guilford.

Swenson, I., & Havens, B. (1987). Menarche and menstruation: A review of the literature. *Journal of Community Health Nursing, 4*(4), 199-210.

Tanner, J. (1981). Growth and maturation during adolescence. *Nutrition Reviews, 39*(2), 43-55.

Tobin-Richards, M., Boxer, A., & Petersen, A. (1983). The psychological significance of pubertal change: Sex differences in perceptions of self during early adolescence. In J. Brooks-Gunn & A. Petersen (Eds.), *Girls at puberty* (pp. 127-154). New York: Plenum.

Warren, M., & Brooks-Gunn, J. (1989). Mood and behavior at adolescence. Evidence for hormonal factors. *Journal of Clinical Endocrinology and Metabolism, 69*(1), 77-83.

Whisnant, L., Brett, E., & Zegans, L. (1975). Implicit messages concerning menstruation in commercial educational material prepared for young adolescent girls. *American Journal of Psychiatry, 132,* 815-820.

Whisnant, L., & Zegans, L. (1975). A study of attitudes toward menarche in white middle-class American adolescent girls. *American Journal of Psychiatry, 132,* 809-820.

Widholm, O. (1979). Dysmenorrhea during adolescence. *Acta Obstetrica Gynecologica Scandinavica, 87,* 61-66.

Widholm, O., & Kantero, R. (1971). Menstrual pattern of adolescent girls according to chronological and gynecological ages (Series III). *Acta Obstetrica Gynecologica Scandinavica, 14*(Suppl.), 19-29.

Williams, L. (1983). Beliefs and attitudes of young girls regarding menstruation. In S. Golub (Ed.), *Menarche* (pp. 139-148). Lexington, MA: Lexington Books.

Woods, N., Dery, G., & Most. A. (1982). Recollections of menarche, current menstrual attitudes, and perimenstrual symptoms. *Psychosomatic Medicine, 44,* 285-293.

5

Midlife Women's Health

CATHERINE INGRAM FOGEL
NANCY FUGATE WOODS

Midlife women account for a growing proportion of the U.S. population. Despite their numbers, however, midlife women's health concerns have received little attention from health researchers and clinicians. Aside from studies of menopause, little existing research focuses on middle-aged women's health. The purpose of this chapter is to summarize knowledge about midlife women's health, emphasizing findings from contemporary work. The chapter begins with definitions of midlife; next, biological, personal, and social changes accompanying midlife are addressed. Health status and assessment of midlife women is described next, and preventive and therapeutic management of midlife health concerns and problems are discussed.

Definitions of Midlife

Midlife has been defined in a variety of ways. Some use age boundaries, such as 35 to 65 years, to differentiate midlife from young adulthood and old age. Others base their definitions on women's reproductive capacity, using menopause or hormonal changes consistent with menopause as markers. Still others base their definitions on women's role patterns, using indicators such as a child leaving home or a woman's return to the workplace to designate the beginning of midlife. Another option is using women's own perceptions about whether they are in the middle of their lives (Brooks-Gunn & Kirsh, 1984).

Midlife has been characterized as a transition rather than a distinct life cycle phase. But midlife is more than preparation for old age and death; it can be a period of generativity, satisfaction, and competence. Brooks-Gunn and Kirsh (1984) stress the multidimensional and multidirectional nature of change in midlife, describing the boundaries as fluid and constructed by the society and the individual rather than being determined by chronological age.

Whatever the markers might be, understanding the context for the experience of midlife for any woman under consideration is extremely important. Anticipation of midlife by each woman's age cohort—those women born at the same time—as well as socialization during midlife by these same women and others will influence how women interpret the events of midlife. For example, socialization may occur in observation of role models, seeking of new referent groups, asking friends for information, and being offered information. As a result of their combined early and later socialization, some cohorts of women may anticipate one pattern for midlife yet encounter another. Both anticipated and actual midlife experiences can influence women's health.

Perimenopause is the term often used to describe the years during which women are making this transition; it encompasses the period of changing ovarian activity prior to menopause and the first few years of amenorrhea. The climacteric is the transitional period of lessening ovarian activity. Menopause itself refers to the complete cessation of menses and is a single physiological event said to occur when women have not experienced menstrual flow or spotting for 1 year (Voda, 1984). Postmenopause is the time after actual menopause.

The perimenopause spans a 25-year period, from approximately age 35 to age 60. In the United States most women experience menopause during their late 40s and early 50s, with the median age being approximately 51 years. The popular belief that an early menarche predisposes to a late menopause is not substantiated. Unlike the average age at menarche, the average age at menopause has remained about the same since the Middle Ages. As the life span of American women has increased in recent decades, the potential for spending more than a third of one's life in the postmenopausal years has increased.

Women may define themselves as menopausal as they notice changes in bleeding patterns or cyclicity prior to noticing the absence of menstrual periods. As a result, they may define menopause differently than do clinicians or researchers (Kaufert, 1986). Clinicians may define women who have regular periods, regardless of their age, as premenopausal. Yet this definition becomes less clear as more women use hormone replacement therapy that causes them to continue to menstruate. In the latter case, clinicians and researchers may use follicle-stimulating hormone (FSH) as a marker for menopause, inferring that women with elevated FSH levels are postmenopausal. In addition, clinicians consider women who have not menstruated within the past 3 months but have menstruated during the past year to be perimenopausal. Those who have menstruated during the past 3 months but who have noted a change in regularity or flow during the last year may be considered to be in transition to menopause or to be perimenopausal (Kaufert, 1986).

Physiological Alterations During the Perimenopausal Period

Menopause is a nearly universal experience during midlife, with every woman experiencing the biological transition as a natural event or as a medical or surgical event during midlife or earlier. Natural menopause is a gradual process with progressive increases in anovulatory cycles and eventual cessation of menses. In the 8 to 10 years preceding menopause, subtle hormonal changes occur, which eventually lead to altered menstrual function and later to amenorrhea. (See Chapter 3, "Women's Bodies," for a full discussion of these changes.)

Physical Changes During the Perimenopausal Period

Menopausal/Postmenopausal Bleeding

During the perimenopausal years (ages 40 to 50), women may experience longer menstrual periods that differ in type of bleeding. They may experience 2 to 3 days of spotting, followed by 1 to 2 days of heavy bleeding, or they may have regular menses followed by 2 to 3 days of spotting. Such symptoms are characteristic of degenerating corpus luteum function.

During the past three decades, investigators have devoted significant attention to identifying ovarian, hypothalamic, and pituitary hormonal mechanisms producing symptoms related to menopause. Nonetheless, only two symptoms appear to increase in incidence as women progress through menopause: hot flashes and hot flushes (Kaufert, Gilbert, & Hassard, 1988; Kaufert & Syrotiuk, 1981; McKinlay, McKinlay, & Brambilla, 1987). Table 5.1 lists physical changes associated with changing estrogen levels. Many of the other changes commonly associated with meno-

Table 5.1 Physical Changes Associated With Decreased Estrogen Production During the Perimenopausal Years

Menstrual cycle	Cycle pattern alters with decrease in cycle length followed by increasing cycle irregularity. Flow may be lighter or heavier. Cessation of menses.
Fertility	Decrease in fecundity (ability to conceive per month of exposure). Increased spontaneous abortion rate.
Vasomotor	Hot flash (sudden warm sensation in neck). Hot flush (visible red flush of skin) and perspiration.
Genital	Vaginal membrane thins.

pause, such as decrease in size of genital structures, skin changes, and changes in breast size, are more correctly attributed to aging. The reader is referred to Chapter 3 for a discussion of physiology of menopause and to Chapter 6, "Older Women," for a discussion of the physical effects of aging.

Mood and Behavioral Responses. The tendency to associate hormonal changes with psychological symptoms in midlife began early in the medical literature, was fueled by the attitude that postmenopausal women suffer from "estrogen deficiency," and continues today. The well-documented preponderance of female depression and anxiety seen in midlife women has often been attributed to events relating to loss of reproductive capability and menopause. More recently, however, authorities have criticized this body of research, asserting that it is primarily based on clinical observations and case studies and uses biased samples of women—namely those who seek medical help for menopausal symptoms and complaints (Koeske, 1982; McKinlay & McKinlay, 1986). There is growing evidence that psychosocial factors, including stressful life events and socioeconomic status, have more influence on mood than does menopause itself (Cooke & Greene, 1981; Greene & Cooke, 1980; Hunter, 1988, 1990).

The effect of hormonal alterations during menopause on mood is not yet explicit. In fact, the interaction of biological, psychological, and sociocultural variables is so complex that it is difficult to determine if the mood changes reported by some menopausal women (a) are the result of hormonal changes associated with menopause, (b) are phenomena resulting from normal aging processes, (c) are related to psychological transitions that may occur in the midlife decades, or (d) arise from cultural beliefs and expectations and from dietary and lifestyle habits.

Midlife Experiences: Personal Continuity and Change

Women continue to grow and develop through the life span, and midlife is no exception. Indeed, midlife is a dynamic period of development, noteworthy for the number and complexity of changes that occur.

Self

Contrary to popular belief, women are not devastated by the "empty nest," the time when their children leave home. Gilligan (1982a, 1982b) proposed that the middle years of a woman's life are not simply a time of return to the unfinished business of adolescence. Instead, women's embeddedness in relationships, their orientation to interdependence, their ability to subordinate achievement to care, and their conflicts over competitive success place them at risk in midlife. Such a dilemma is a commentary on the society more than a problem in women's development. Gilligan argues that the events of midlife can alter a woman's activities of care in ways that affect her sense of herself. For example, if midlife brings an end to relationships, and with that the sense of connection on which she relies and the activities of care through which she judges her worth, the life transition can lead to despair. The meaning of midlife events for a woman is contextual, arising from the interaction between the structures of her thought and the realities of her life. Women face midlife with a psychological history different from that of men and make sense out of experiences on the basis of their knowledge of human relationships. Rubin (1979) interviewed 160 women between 35 and 54 years of age. She asked women if they could briefly describe themselves in some way that would give her a good sense of who and what they were. Nearly 25% could not answer the question. Those who could described themselves as physical beings; others used words such as *warm, sensitive, kind, outgoing, considerate, caring, concerned,* and *responsible* to describe themselves. Most mentioned that they were wives and mothers. Although half the women held paid jobs outside their homes, not one described herself in relation to her work. Many were surprised when this was pointed out to them. A fundamental theme found in these women's identity was the distinction they experienced between being (internal, identity) and doing (external, work). In short, their work was what they did, not what they were. These findings reflect the complexity of women's views of themselves.

Ageism and Aging

Ageism permeates Western society, and the meanings of aging for women reflect this. Rossi (1980) explored the meanings of age and aging for women 33 to 55 years of age. Although none wanted to be older than they were, only half wanted to be under 30. Most expressed a desire to live to be at least 75 years. Those who wanted to be younger than they were and those who had very short longevity preferences were those with very high levels of stress in their current lives, having marital tension, difficulty with children, large family size, economic strain, or sharp increases in symptoms of aging.

Berkum (1983) interviewed 60 physically and mentally healthy white suburban women between 40 and 55 years of age. Most were married or had been married and said they had been married largely because it was the only desirable option available to them. Most had internalized the social ideology about women's appearance. For example, 68% felt different without makeup, 57% thought they looked older without makeup, and 85% thought they were less attractive without makeup. For all but 3 women, cosmetic surgery was only a fantasy but not to be realized because of the expense and risk. Some thought middle age was frightening, but others perceived that they had more self-confidence, social ease, and a better perspective on life than they had held earlier. Others pointed out the negative aspects of aging on their appearance, especially those facing a harsh social reality—trying to attract men or needing to find work. For many women, changing appearance was not problematic. Only 23% expressed a great desire to look younger; 21% felt they had lost attractiveness as they aged; but 58% felt positive about their appearance. Berkum recommends the following considerations: Feminine stereotypes may be dysfunctional for middle-aged women, and midlife women may benefit from an educational process that involves learning new ways of thinking about themselves and their behavior and understanding that there may be no social reinforcements for these new ways of thinking. Women who have discarded old patterns of thought and behavior may experience difficulty with others whose beliefs reflect agist assumptions.

Sexuality

Cutler (1987) interviewed 124 women during the perimenopause about their sexual responses and correlated the results of 52 of these women's prospective coital records over 3 months with concomitant ovarian hormones. She found that women around 49 years do not suffer from a particular deficit in sexual desire, response, or satisfaction. A subset of women with especially low estradiol levels (less than 35 pg/ml) tended to have reduced coital activity.

One difficulty with much of the research on midlife women's sexuality is that it is based on defining sex as sexual acts—for example, masturbation or sexual intercourse. Women experience coitus as relational, whereas they experience masturbation as a solitary act. Thus the meanings ascribed to different sexual behaviors for women are likely to be different from those ascribed by men. Luria and Meade (1984) predict that as the baby boom generation becomes older, middle-aged women will be seen as sexual rather than asexual, a function of greater acceptance of sexuality across the life span. In addition, they predict a growing absence of stable male sexual partners for many women because of divorce rates and shorter life spans for men. Finally, they anticipate that labor force participation for women could have variable effects on sexual activity, interfering with sexual frequency because of increased responsibilities or enhancing it because of increased social skills development for women. Anticipated consequences also may include more "safe" sexual behaviors, with many women considering sex risky and weighing the benefits and risks.

Toward a New View of Midlife: Prime Time for Women

Contrary to the belief that midlife is a negative period for women, Mitchell and Helson (1990) tested the hypothesis that the early 50s is women's prime of life, a time of good health combined with autonomy and relational security. College graduates in their early 50s mostly described their lives as very satisfying. Women in their early 50s rated their quality of life as high. The conditions distinguishing the early 50s from earlier and later periods of the middle years included more "empty nests," better health, higher income, and more concern for parents. The first three of these factors accounted for the quality of life of women in their early 50s. The investigators offer prime of life as a useful concept in women's adult development.

Women's adult development as chronicled in textbooks focuses on the woman as a biological creature, especially a mother; the proposed life cycle trajectory is one of decline for women after 40; little attention is paid to the character of women's life stories (Gergen, 1990). These approaches to understanding adult womanhood reinforce patriarchal systems of power. Gergen (1990) recommends a social constructionist approach to create theories that liberate interpretations of women from an exclusive focus on their reproductive roles, support feminist methodologies, emphasize relational networks over autonomous individualism, create new narrative life forms for women that are multiple and nonlinear, and support a critical function with psychology and society. Emphasis on the value of relational theory rather than on developing another theory about the single self changing over time could stimulate studies of relational networks that might encompass intergenerational activities, family relations, collegial interactions, and social group performances and might provide a fuller account of women's lives than do theories focusing only on individual development.

Social Changes in Midlife

Several social changes occur during the course of midlife for women. These may include returning to or changing employment, watching and helping children as they leave home or move back in with parents, changing the nature of marital relationships, and caring for aging parents whose care needs are often met by midlife women.

Roles

To understand the effects of roles for women in midlife, it is important to consider work rewards, success, satisfaction, and economic security. In addition, one needs to distinguish between women's experiences in occupations as opposed to careers. The usual mechanisms for reducing role conflict, such as compartmentalization of roles, delegation of role performance, elimination of roles, and role accumulation, have been based on studies of male roles, and their application to women's lives is often inappropriate. Women's role partners can be sources of role conflict, particularly spouses and coworkers. In addition, the economic consequences of women's discontinuous work life experiences make their situations different from those of men.

Lopata and Barnewolt (1984) studied role conflict and role strain as they may be relevant to women in midlife. Nearly 1,000 Chicago-area women were asked to respond to the question, "What are the most important roles of a woman?" Few women considered a role in which they were not involved currently as the most important. In all, the role of mother outweighed any other role, including wife, as most important for the Chicago women. Blue-collar women were most apt to list the role of employee first in the absence of wife and mother roles. Work-oriented women saw themselves as leaders and successful people and were less likely to see themselves as emotional than were women who gave first importance to other roles. The age of her children rather than the age of the woman was the crucial variable. Presence of small children, especially under the age of six, decreased the choice of employee as the most important role. Women who chose the wife role as most important were married to men with more education, prestigious occupations, and higher incomes. Women who chose mother as the most important role were most likely to have a child under the age of 3 at home. Also, those who had their first child at the age of 27 or later were more likely to list the role of mother first. Generally, child-oriented women were of lower socioeconomic background than others because they lived alone or shared a household with someone other than a husband. Women tended to see their involvement in social roles in life course terms, with those currently involved as a mother expecting to shift from the role of mother to the role of wife more as they grew older. Those nearing 55 did not anticipate major changes in the near future with the exception of an increased involvement in roles outside the complex of wife and mother. Over the past two decades, the major shift has been in the devaluation of the role of housewife. The importance that women assign to their roles may influence their sense of well-being in midlife.

Jennings, Mazaik, and McKinlay (1984) analyzed the results of the first large U.S. epidemiological study of 8,114 women aged 45 to 54 randomly selected from Massachusetts. Women employed for pay (69%), full-time homemakers (24%), and women unemployed (5%) or living with an unemployed spouse (2%) were included in the analyses. Employed women had the fewest health problems and reported the fewest illness behaviors, whereas unemployed women reported the most health problems and the most illness behaviors. Homemakers reported intermediary levels.

Ackerman (1990) studied job transition behaviors in 71 midlife women with professional careers who had changed jobs in the past 3 years. All were employed in a utility company in a midwestern city where 11% of jobs were eliminated. She classified women according to their job transition attitudes and behaviors into groups who wanted and did not want change and those who planned for and those who did not plan for the change. She found that personal characteristics (including demographic, personality, and attitude factors), situational characteristics (intrafamily life events and outside-of-family life events), and person-by-situation characteristics (coping behaviors, job-changing strategies, and job and life satisfaction) significantly discriminated between the four groups of women. Creators, those who wanted and planned for change, were positively attuned to their change and used family, professional, and community supports. Reactors, who did not want change and did not plan for it, experienced the highest levels of stress, physical illness, hostile behavior, and legal problems; these women did not have support from the family or community, had the lowest incomes, and did not readily adapt to incorporate new skills in their job transitions. Most were single or single parents, and family needs ranked as a high priority in their lives. Maintainers (wanted change but did not plan for it) and conventionalists (who did not want change but planned for it) had intermediate levels of stress. For all groups, family priorities created tensions about changing work roles.

Relationships With Parents

Relationships with parents, especially mothers, have important health effects for midlife women. Rapport with one's mother is related to a woman's sense of mastery and happiness and is contingent on the entire constellation of a woman's roles (Baruch & Barnett, 1983). Baruch and Barnett (1983) used a three-item index of "maternal rapport" to examine perceived relationships between mothers of 171 women aged 35 to 55 years. They found that, overall, the relationships were seen as rewarding, especially by women who were not currently mothers. Although the age of the daughter and the mother's marital status (widowed or currently married) were not significantly related to maternal rapport scores, the mother's health was significantly related to such scores. In addition, psychological well-being, as measured by sense of mastery and pleasure, was significantly correlated with maternal rapport, with relationships being stronger for the women who were not mothers themselves. The gratifications of adult women in the role of daughter seem contingent on their entire constellation of roles.

Caretaking responsibilities for one's parents depend on the parents' health status, and the extent of responsibility that women assume seems to be a function of the woman's social class and the nature of her own family timing patterns and employment responsibilities (Stueve & O'Donnell, 1984). Stueve and O'Donnell (1984) studied adult daughters, including 81 working women 30 to 60 years of age who had one living parent more than 70 years of age. They found that variation among family timing patterns shaped how the daughters dealt with issues and considerations of their aging parents, for example, some framed their parent's death as their own loss or as being inevitable. Parents' needs depended on health and life circumstances. Most instrumental support (e.g., cleaning house) was provided by working-class daughters who assumed interdependence and the necessity of helping out. Middle-class, college-educated daughters had tighter boundaries around their nuclear families and were less likely to integrate their aging parents. Middle-class children were more likely to buy care from others outside the family. Daughters were more likely than sons to provide care to their parents. The authors concluded that the "caught in the middle" label assigned to midlife women was inaccurate for all women. Although employment, per se, made little difference in caregiving, features of employment, such as freedom to negotiate schedules and the number of hours worked, did affect caregiving to parents. The authors point out the need to consider the birth cohort of midlife women when considering the effects of employment on patterns of caregiving for elderly relatives: Employment had different meanings for different birth cohorts. In addition, those concerned about midlife women's health should consider women's involvements with other elderly kin, not just their parents but also their in-laws. Whether women with elderly kin feel caught in the middle and feel competing demands of their roles can be determined only by exploring each woman's situation. Finally, consideration needs to be given to caregiving for the midlife women who are currently providing care to their elderly relatives.

Current literature on parent care asserts that modern women at some time in their lives may expect to be sandwiched between responsibilities to old parents and their other commitments. Rosenthal, Matthews, and Marshall (1989) studied a random sample of 163 women between 40 and 69 years of age to determine their commitments. They found that considering the multiple commitments of children in the household, husbands, and employment, women younger than 55 are most likely to be affected by competing commitments. Although these women are most likely to have living parents, many of their parents are younger and relatively healthy. Older respondents are less likely to have living parents, but when they do, their parents are less healthy than those of younger women. The risk to midlife women of actually providing extensive parent care was estimated as less than that which current studies are based on, rather than what a cross section of the population would suggest.

Much worry about women's multiple roles as a source of poor health seems to have been misdirected. Uphold and Sussman (1981) examined the influence of role and child rearing, marital, recreational, and work role integration in 185 healthy midlife women. Women involved in more roles complained of fewer symptoms commonly attributed to the climacteric (e.g., depression). Women who participated in recreation and had good marital adjustment were less likely to have symptoms. Child rearing and work roles were unrelated to symptoms.

Baruch (1984) examined the psychological well-being of midlife women and its relation to women's roles. Well-being is a good or satisfactory condition of existence. In earlier studies, Baruch had found that for women 35 to 55 years, eight measures of well-being—happiness, satisfaction, optimism, anxiety, depression, mastery, self-esteem, and the balance of rewards and concerns—factored into two primary dimensions: mastery and pleasure. In studies with Barnett and others, Baruch provided evidence of little change in well-being between the years of 35 and 55. Being employed was not associated with pleasure; instead, being married was associated with higher pleasure scores. Employed women had a greater sense of mastery regardless of their marital or parental status. A subset of 72 women was interviewed intensively about the rewarding and distressing aspects of their various roles, and later 238 women indicated to what extent each aspect of their roles was rewarding or distressing. For employment, major reward factors were challenge and social relationships, whereas factors of major concern were the dullness of the job and whether it was perceived as a dead end. Both rewards and concerns were significantly related to mastery and pleasures, with the exception of social relationships, which had no effect on mastery. In addition, women asked about homemaker's rewards indicated the satisfaction of being available to one's family, freedom from supervision, and opportunity to do tasks fitting one's skills. Concerns were related to boredom and isolation and not earning money. The balance between rewards and concerns was related to both mastery and pleasure. Like employment and homemaking, marriage and child rearing had associated rewards and concerns. Feeling emotionally supported and appreciated was the major reward of marriage, with the major concern being marital conflict. Both affected mastery and pleasure. The central concern about not being married was lack of an intimate relationship. Women who reported distress about the lack of an intimate relationship had lower pleasure scores but not a lower sense of mastery. Marriage enhanced happiness when married women were free to choose their employment status and end an unhappy marriage. However, a good job was the key to self-esteem and protection against anxiety and depression. The balance of rewards and concerns related to motherhood was related to both mastery and pleasure. Conflict with children was the major concern and was related to lower pleasure, but for employed women mastery was also lower. Women's relationships with their mothers were also important. Maternal rapport was positively related to both pleasure and mastery, but for divorced women, maternal rapport and mastery were negatively related. In the Barnett and Baruch study, employed married women who had children were the highest in well-being despite their busy lives.

Stress and Coping

Stressors during midlife have been linked to both psychological and somatic symptoms. Of particular importance are exit stresses or losses from one's social network. Vulnerability to psychological and somatic distress seems related to the vulnerability associated with loss of one's mother early in one's life but also to the number of losses from one's current network—for example, through divorce or death (Cooke, 1985; Cooke & Greene, 1981).

Cooke and Greene (1981) studied life stress, social support, and adjustment using semistructured interviews with 408 women between the ages of 25 to 64 years. They found that psychological symptoms increased between the ages of 35 and 44, when there was also a high rate of exits, including deaths, from the social network. Women who experienced somatic symptoms were exposed to a high level of miscellaneous stress as well as exits.

Cooke (1985) explored the influence of eight social relationship variables on both psychological and somatic distress in a sample of 78 midlife women between 35 and 54 years of age residing in Glasgow. The psychological symptoms included depressed mood, panic attacks, crying spells, and worrying. Somatic symptoms included faintness, dizziness, headaches, and tingling or numbness of the body. The total number of vulnerability factors was calculated on the basis of women's situations. These included loss of or separation from the mother before age 11, number of children under 15 years living at home, lack of full-time employment outside the home, extent of confiding with spouse, and number of confiding relationships available. Number of children under the age of 15 and degree of confiding in the spouse had no effects on psychological or somatic symptoms. Both loss of the mother and being unemployed had important interactive effects on somatic and psychological symptoms. Number of confidants available interacted with total life stress to reduce both psychological and social symptoms. Although degree of involvement with children had no effect on psychological symptoms, it reduced the experience of somatic symptoms.

Investigators have attempted to characterize the stressors to which midlife women are exposed and to describe how they cope with them. Griffith (1983b) studied 579 women 25 to 64 years of age. Women indicated their personal life goals and values and their satisfaction in achieving them. Six major stressors were identified: love relationships, personal success, physical health, parent-child relationships, personal time, and social relationships. Women 35 to 44 years indicated that the major stressors for them were physical health, personal time, love relationships, and personal success. Those 45 to 54 indicated physical health, personal time, love relationships, parent and child issues, and personal success. Those 55 to 65 years listed physical health and personal time. In addition to gender differences, Griffith (1983a) found that women experienced different stressors depending on their age group. Of six major stressor areas, love relationships, personal success, physical health, parent-child relationships, personal time, and social relationships, the major stressors for midlife women included physical health and personal time. Women used a variety of strategies to cope with these stressors. Talking, work, and religion were most commonly used by women between 35 and 64 years of age (Griffith, 1983b). In the same study, the author also analyzed the relationships between women's age groups, their physical and emotional symptoms of stress, and their usual coping patterns. Age-related patterns of symptoms appeared for many types of symptoms. For women aged 35 to 65, feeling fat and frequently nervous and tense were the most prevalent symptoms. In addition, women used a variety of coping styles. Those 35 to 44 years used talking, work, religion, and food consumption. Those 45 to 54 used work, religion, talking, and food consumption, and those 55 to 64 used work, religion, talking, and food consumption.

The importance of women's friendship networks as a means of support during stressful periods has been emphasized (Brooks-Gunn & Kirsh, 1984). Indeed, the number of confidants available to women reduces the health-threatening effects of stressors (Cooke, 1985). Further understanding of how women's support networks enhance their health or prevent illness is needed, however. (See Chapter 4 for a discussion of women's friendships.)

Health Risks in Midlife Women

Until recently, women entering their middle years were thought to be on the threshold of declining health. Today, women recognize that they can offset many of the health risks associated with aging by incorporating health-promoting and protective behaviors into their lifestyle.

During midlife, a woman's risk of developing and dying from cardiovascular disease increases after menopausal age. Known risk factors for coronary heart disease include obesity, cigarette smoking, elevated cholesterol and blood pressure levels, diabetes mellitus, family history of cardiac disease, alcohol abuse, and the effects of aging on the cardiovascular system (Philosophe & Seibel, 1992). (See Chapter 27, "Chronic Illness and Women," for a discussion of hypertension and heart disease in women.)

Obesity has long been known to be a risk factor for heart disease among men; however, until recently, obesity, defined as a weight 20% or more above desired weight, was thought to be a weak risk factor in women. Recent data from the Nurses' Health Study, however, reveal that obesity is a strong risk factor for cardiovascular mortality and morbidity even after controlling for smoking (Manson et al., 1990). The proportion of overweight adult women in the United States has increased steadily over the past several decades. The prevalence of obesity in women increases with age, and more than 35% of all midlife women are overweight. Often, women end their reproductive years overweight, having gained excess weight with each pregnancy and never having lost it.

Whether menopause is a risk factor for heart disease and stroke is not clear. A healthy woman with no underlying risk factors who experiences a natural menopause (as opposed to a surgically induced one) does not appear to be at an increased risk of cardiovascular disease (Philosophe & Seibel, 1992). However, it is not known if menopause alters or modifies other risk factors to promote cardiovascular disease at a later age. It is possible that the increase in cardiovascular disease seen in women in their 70s and 80s is related to estrogen-related changes. Currently, however, there is little statistical evidence for the effect of menopause on heart disease, and it is thought that the known risk factors for heart disease are so strongly predictive that they may overwhelm menopausal status considered alone (Perlman, Wolf, Finucane, & Madans, 1989).

A significant health risk for midlife women is cancer—specifically breast and lung cancer. Lung cancer in women is discussed in Chapter 27, and breast cancer is discussed in Chapter 28.

Osteoporosis

Aging is associated with a progressive decline in bone density in both males and females. Losses in bone density severe enough to result in fractures after minimal trauma define the condition *osteoporosis,* which accounts for more than 1 million fractures in the United States each year (Rowe & Kahn, 1987). Osteoporosis, a debilitating disease found predominantly in aging women, affects 24 million Americans—50% of women and 25% of men over the age of 45—with a cost estimated at $7 billion annually in health care and lost productivity (Bond, 1992). By age 65, one third of women will have vertebral fractures, and by age 81, one third of women will have suffered a hip fracture, often a catastrophic, if not terminal, event. Risk factors of osteoporosis are given in Table 5.2.

Peak bone mass is probably reached between the ages of 25 and 35. Bone loss after 35 is a universal phenomenon in the same way that loss of lean body mass occurs with age. Although all women eventually develop osteoporotic changes to some degree, one in four women over the age of 45 will have progressive loss of bone predisposing them to fractures. The majority of these are hip, vertebral, and distal radial fractures.

Research and clinical evidence suggest a relationship between osteoporosis and menopause. In the first few years after menopause, accelerated bone loss occurs in one in four women (Bond, 1992). The decreased estrogen acts on bone osteoclasts to trigger bone resorption. Low estrogen also increases excretion of calcium in the urine and decreases production of the hormone calcitonin. Calcitonin, produced by the thyroid

Table 5.2 Risk Factors for Developing Osteoporosis[a]

Nonmodifiable	*Modifiable*
Female gender	Diet deficient in calcium
Age 60 and over	Sedentary lifestyle
Small, thin frame	Smoking
European or Asian heritage	Excessive alcohol intake
Early age at menopause	Long-term steroid medication use
	Endocrine disorders (hyperparathyroidism)
	Gastrointestinal disorders that affect digestion and absorption of nutrients

a. Risk factors for developing osteoporosis are classified as nonmodifiable (those risk factors that cannot be changed by a woman's actions) and modifiable (those that can be changed by a woman's actions). Nurses should assist their midlife women clients in identifying modifiable risk factors and planning strategies to change these.

gland, inhibits resorption. Low estrogen levels also reduce parathyroid hormone (PTH), which triggers a decrease in the production of 1.25 dihydroxy vitamin D, the most active metabolite of vitamin D; this metabolite aids in the absorption of dietary calcium from the intestines (Bond, 1992).

There are a number of differences in the factors associated with bone mineral metabolism in perimenopausal and older women. The majority of perimenopausal women have normal serum concentrations of vitamin D and plenty of exposure to the sun and dietary sources of vitamin D. This is often not true for the elderly, particularly women in nursing homes. Cortical bone, and probably trabecular bone, is rapidly lost around menopause, whereas in older women bone loss slows and may even stop.

The relative importance of age and menopause in the development of osteoporosis has not yet been fully established. Richelson, Wahner, Melton, and Riggs (1984), studying women who had had a surgical menopause, women who were perimenopausal, and women who were postmenopausal, concluded that the predominant cause of bone loss during the first two decades of life after natural menopause was decreased estrogen. However, more recent findings from this same group of researchers suggest a more complicated explanation: They have found significant bone loss in women before menopause, probably beginning as early as age 35 (Riggs, 1987). Women with small bones who are underweight for height have less bone to start with and will experience the effects of bone loss to a greater degree than women with larger frames who are heavier. Most of the estrogen production in postmenopausal women results from peripheral conversion of adrenal androgen to estrone that occurs mostly in fat tissue.

Women with osteoporosis are commonly middle-aged women who first had symptoms 5 to 10 years after menopause or oophorectomy. Typically, they complain of acute, nonradiating pain localized in the midline of the lower thoracic lumbar spine. The pain may be severe enough to require bed rest and potent analgesics. The five classic signs or symptoms of osteoporosis are loss of height, thoracic kyphosis, back pain, shortened waist, and fractures—usually of the wrist, hip, rib, or vertebrae.

Assessment

Comprehensive assessment of midlife women includes a complete database with attention to physiological and psychological changes in midlife, identification of risk factors, presence of misinformation and gaps in knowledge, and individual counseling needs. A meticulous history, careful physical examination, and appropriate laboratory studies provide the data necessary to carry out such an assessment. (See Chapter 9, "Well-Woman Assessment," for information necessary to perform assessments of midlife women.)

Midlife women experience menopause within the context of society's stereotypes regarding aging women and the numerous myths and misconceptions about menopause. Thus it is important to assess a woman's knowledge of menopause. What has she heard about menopause? What have the middle years been like for family members, for friends? Napholtz (1985) found that a sample of 67 working women seemed to be knowledgeable about menopause and were able to differentiate between changes associated with menopause and those associated with midlife and aging. Leiblum and Swartzmann (1986) found that 244 general-population American women thought menopause should be viewed as a "medical condition" and treated as one; yet they did not regard it as a particularly serious one and preferred natural treatments to hormonal ones. Also important is an understanding of the client's beliefs and attitudes about menopause and the aging process. What do you think it will be like for you? What do you think when you see women in their 40s, 50s, and 60s on TV or in magazines? Studies conducted in 1963 (Neugarten, Wood, Kraines, & Loomis, 1963) and 1980 (Eisner & Kelly, 1980, cited in Greene, 1990) found that younger women who had no direct personal experience of menopause had more negative attitudes than did those who were currently experiencing or had passed through that phase of their lives. In addition, Eisner and Kelly (1980, cited in Greene, 1990) found that the attitudes of black women were, in general, less positive than those of white women; low income and low levels of education were also found to be associated with a negative attitude. A common theme in the literature is that one of women's main concerns at menopause is loss of reproductive capacity; very little support for this long-held truism emerged from the Neugarten (Neugarten et al., 1963) study, however.

Osteoporosis

Women should be asked about risk factors for osteoporosis (see Table 5.2). Height is obtained on the initial examination and yearly thereafter and compared to previous measurements; diminished height may be an indication of osteoporetic changes. The client should be observed carefully for clinical features of osteoporosis. The first sign may be loss of height with kyphosis of the dorsal spine resulting from compression of the vertebrae. In the past, laboratory assessments for osteoporosis were problematic, and neither X-ray nor blood chemistry studies were useful for early diagnosis. Radiographic evidence indicates serious bone mass loss, and circulating calcium is not necessarily an indication of calcium balance. Bone density measures are expensive, experimental, and insensitive (Kirkpatrick, Edwards, & Finch, 1991). Prevailing medical opinion is that bone loss and bone mass measurements should not be used indiscriminately to screen for osteoporosis—instead, these methods may be used to guide treatment decisions (Bond, 1992). In addition, a single determination of body fat mass, urinary calcium and hydroxyproline, and serum alkaline phosphatase has been shown to correctly identify more than 78% of women who will have bone loss (Christensen, Riis, & Rodbro, 1987). Health care providers may elect to measure bone density in the woman who has major risk factors for osteoporosis or in whom there is other evidence of osteoporosis.

Health Strategies

Nutrition

Table 5.3 shows the recommended daily food allowances for midlife women. These recommendations seek to decrease the risk of chronic disease and maintain health. At present, there is no well-designed and controlled research demonstrating that any particular foods or nutritional supplements are effective in alleviating the discomforts that may accompany aging. As can be seen from this table, women should change their diets as they move out of the childbearing years. Because metabolic rates decrease with age and many women also exercise less, fewer calories are needed for weight maintenance as women grow older. In general, foods chosen by midlife women should be high in nutrients but moderate or low in calories to allow for adequate nutrient intake while maintaining body weight—for example, using skim milk instead of whole milk. Iron needs also decrease with age, whereas calcium requirements increase. An essential component of all adult women's diets should be adequate fluid intake (eight to ten 8-oz glasses of water/day) for body metabolism and temperature regulation. With aging, the gastrointestinal (GI) tract functions less efficiently; adequate fluid and fiber intake are important in helping GI functioning and preventing constipation.

One of the most important aspects of prevention of cardiovascular disease in women is prevention of obesity. Most overweight individuals do not seek treatment for obesity. Of those who do seek help in losing weight, the majority will not follow through, and of those who do lose weight, most do not maintain the weight loss. (See Chapter 12, "Nutrition," for information on obesity and weight management.)

Table 5.3 Nutritional Needs of Midlife and Older Women

	Fat-Soluble Vitamins						
Women (age)	*Weight (lb)*	*Height (in)*	*Energy (kcal)*	*Protein (gm)*	*Vitamin A (g RE)*	*Vitamin D (g)*	*Vitamin E (mg TE)*
25-50 years	138	64	2,200	50	800	5	8
51+ years	143	63	1,900	50	800	5	8
	Water-Soluble Vitamins						
Women (age)	*Ascorbic Acid (mg)*	*Folate (g)*	*Niacin (mg)*	*Riboflavin (mg)*	*Thiamin (mg)*	*Vitamin B6 (mg)*	*Vitamin B^{12} (mg)*
25-50 years	60	180	15	1.3	1.1	1.6	2.0
51+ years	60	180	13	1.2	1.0	1.6	2.0
	Minerals						
Women (age)	*Calcium (mg)*	*Phosphorus (mg)*	*Iodine (gm)*	*Iron (mg)*	*Magnesium (mg)*	*Zinc (mg)*	*Selenium (g)*
25-50 years	800	800	150	15	280	12	55
51+ years	800	800	150	10	280	12	55

SOURCE: From the National Research Council (1989).
NOTE: Weight and height are actual medians for U.S. population of the designated ages. The use of these figures is not meant to imply that the height-to-weight ratios are ideal.

Hypercholesterolemia is another significant risk factor for cardiovascular disease in women. It is important to ensure that a woman's daily diet includes all the essential nutrients while simultaneously reducing the amount of cholesterol and saturated fats consumed. In the typical American diet, almost 40% of calories are from fat; there are approximately 175 to 200 mg of cholesterol in every 1,000 calories. Current dietary recommendations are that total fat in the diet be decreased to approximately 30% of calories and that cholesterol be reduced to about 300 mg per day.

There is a chronic insufficiency of dietary calcium in the majority of American women's diets (Ausenhus, 1988). Dietary surveys of American women indicate that the usual daily intake is 450 to 550 mg of calcium, or less than half the amount needed to maintain bone mass. Furthermore, it appears that milk and dairy products supply 60% to 80% of the calcium in American diets (Sutnick, 1987). Many of these foods are high in calories and are contraindicated for women attempting to lose weight. Many other women drastically reduce their consumption of dairy products in an effort to reduce fat intake, thus omitting a major source of calcium. Still other women are lactose intolerant and are unable to eat dairy products. The propensity for most women to consume less than the minimum recommended daily allowance of calcium takes on added significance in midlife, when women are at greater risk for the development of osteoporosis. The current recommendations for prevention of osteoporosis are a calcium intake of 1,200 mg per day for women aged 19 to 24, 800 mg for women prior to menopause, 1,000 mg for estrogen-treated women of any age, and 1,000 mg for postmenopausal women not taking estrogen (Bond, 1992; National Research Council, 1989). The recommended daily allowances published by the National Research Council (1989) do not reflect the increased calcium supplements of 1,000 mg premenopausally and 1,500 mg postmenopausally recommended by most experts (Bilezikian & Silverberg, 1992). Women should be counseled regarding other dietary factors, such as high protein or caffeine intake, that increase the excretion of calcium by the kidney, inducing a systemic acidosis that stimulates osteoelastic bone resorption (Sutnick, 1987). Women should also be informed that cigarette smoking intensifies acidosis and decreases endogenous estrogen production.

Exercise

All too often, exercise patterns developed in adolescence or young adulthood are dropped by the time a woman reaches midlife and family demands and work constraints increase and energy level deceases. Unfortunately, a sedentary lifestyle predisposes women to weight gain, muscle atrophy, stress, and insomnia. Because exercise has so many positive effects on total health, it should be encouraged for all midlife women. (See Chapter 13, "Exercise," for a thorough discussion of the effect of exercise on health and well-being.)

An exercise program for midlife women should include both aerobic conditioning and muscle training. Regular aerobic exercise may improve cardiorespiratory endurance, reduce the risk of cardiovascular disease, and prevent some age-related increases in body fat. Resistance training is used to improve muscle strength and bone density. Increases in lumbar vertebral and distal radial bone mineral content have been reported in women who participated in a regular exercise program (Simkin, Ayalon, & Leitcher, 1987).

Examples of appropriate aerobic exercises are brisk walking, bicycling, stationary cycling, jogging or running, swimming, and low-impact aerobic programs. All such types of exercises include activities that maintain or improve cardiovascular fitness, muscle strength and endurance, flexibility, and body composition.

Regardless of the form of exercise a woman chooses, it should contain a level of activity that allows her to feel refreshed and relaxed rather than exhausted. It should also consist of activities that are enjoyable. If these two guidelines are not followed, it is unlikely that a woman will continue to exercise on a regular basis. Women beginning an exercise program are counseled to plan to exercise at least four times a week and preferably more. Thus the type of exercise selected should be one that fits into the woman's lifestyle and does not require large expenditures of money or a complete reordering of daily activities. Nurses might suggest that clients ask themselves questions such as these: Do I want to exercise inside or outside? With music or without? Do I want to take a class and be with people at a set time, or do I want to exercise alone on my own schedule? Do I like team sports and competition, or do I want individual exercise with my own thoughts and agenda? Is there anything I did in childhood that would be fun to take up again? Do I need to do different things on different days? Although, ultimately, the woman should exercise vigorously for 30 to 45 minutes at a time, she should be counseled to start slowly with any exercise if she has been inactive.

Exercise can be a significant component of a program to prevent osteoporosis. Muscle mass and bone mass are directly related, and recent research has demonstrated that an increase in physical activity delays bone loss and increases bone mass (Birge & Dalsky, 1989; Sinaki, 1989). However, physical activity is an important determinant of bone mass only when there is a significantly high calcium intake to produce a positive calcium balance.

Sexuality

Sexual activity can continue throughout one's life. The perimenopausal woman and her partner will need information about the normal aging changes in sexual functioning. Nurses should review sexual behaviors that may need modification. Specific suggestions may include increased time for stimulation to allow time for orgasm, use of water-soluble lubricants, more gentle stimulation of vaginal and clitoral tissues, frequent communication between partners about changing needs and desires, and alterations in accustomed sexual positions. Estrogen therapy, either local or systemic, may be warranted. Kegel exercises, which improve perineal muscle tone, relieve hemorrhoids, and help prevent or correct stress urinary incontinence, should be taught to all women (described in Chapter 21, "Sexuality in Women's Lives").

Therapies

Calcium

Calcium is an integral part of any therapeutic regimen for women with osteoporosis and those wishing to prevent osteoporosis. The best source of calcium is food; however, calcium supplements are recommended when dietary intake does not supply the recommended amount. Some authorities suggest that except for women who have a history of kidney stones, kidney failure, or hypercalcemia (absolute contraindications), calcium therapy should be prescribed for all postmenopausal women regardless of their individual risk for osteoporosis (Consensus Development Conference, 1987). Riis, Thomsen, and Christiansen (1987) examined the effects of calcium supplementation on postmenopausal bone levels in 43 women in the early postmenopausal period and found that calcium supplementation

Table 5.4 Calcium Content of Common Supplements

Calcium Salt	*Percentage of Elemental Calcium (by weight)*	*Amount Found in Common Dose*
Calcium gluconate	9.3	500 mg - 45 mg Ca
Calcium lactate	13.0	325 mg - 42.25 mg Ca
Calcium citrate	21.0	950 mg - 200 mg Ca
Tricalcium phosphate	23.3	1565.2 mg - 600 mg Ca
Calcium carbonate	40.0	1250 mg - 500 mg Ca

might have had a minor effect on loss of cortical bone but had no effect on trabecular bone loss. More recently supplementation with vitamin D and calcium (1,200 mg) was found to reduce the risk of hip fractures and other nonvertebral fractures in elderly women (Chapuy et al., 1992). Concern about the possibility of calcium supplements interfering with the absorption of other nutrients has been expressed. Furthermore, there may be cost, convenience, and compliance problems associated with calcium supplementation. Thus perhaps calcium should not be routinely prescribed for all postmenopausal women. Rather women should be encouraged to consume a diet that has 1,000 to 1,200 mg of calcium per day or to add an amount of calcium supplementation that will increase their dietary intake to this level.

When calcium supplementation is indicated, the nurse and client are faced with many products but little information (see Table 5.4). When choosing a calcium supplement several factors should be kept in mind: It should be inexpensive, safe, effective, and well tolerated. When advising women about calcium supplements, it is important to clarify the difference between total calcium and amount of elemental calcium that a tablet contains, because it is the total number of milligrams of elemental calcium, not the total milligrams of calcium, that is important. Clients should also be counseled about possible side effects and overdose reactions, such as nausea, anorexia, constipation, abdominal cramping, and flatulence. Calcium carbonate is generally considered to be the most effective product, but some women report bloating and flatulence when using this preparation. Calcium lactate and calcium gluconate may be better tolerated. Women should be cautioned about "natural" products such as dolomite and bone meals. Both are sold as calcium supplements, and samples of both have been shown to be contaminated with lead and other heavy metals; cases of toxicity have been reported with use (Sutnick, 1987).

Chestnut (1992) suggests that in addition to calcium and exercise, one of two agents approved by the Food and Drug Administration—estrogen or calcitonin—should be offered to women with documented postmenopausal osteoporosis. Calcitonin has been shown to reduce the rate of bone turnover and to stabilize bone mass in women with osteoporosis; in addition, it may have beneficial analgesic effects (Ljunghall et al., 1991). However, as yet, it has not been shown to reduce fractures in osteoporosis. Calcitonin may be an alternative form of therapy when estrogen therapy is contraindicated or not tolerated. The drug is very safe, although anorexia, nausea, and vomiting have been reported. Its usage is limited by prohibitive cost and parenteral administration. A potential therapeutic option being investigated is calcitriol, the principal determinant of intestinal calcium absorption. Clinical trials have had mixed results, with two indicating its usefulness in stabilizing bone mass (Aloia, Vaswani, Yoh, Yasumura, & Cohn, 1988; Gallagher & Goldgar, 1990), one demonstrating significant reductions in vertebral fractures (Tilyard, Spears, Thomas, & Dovey, 1992), and one finding no effect (Ott & Chestnut, 1989).

Menopausal Hormonal Therapy

Menopausal hormonal therapy is the most commonly prescribed therapy for symptoms associated with the perimenopausal years. In this text, the terms *estrogen therapy* and *hormonal therapy* are used to refer to the more commonly used estrogen replacement therapy (ERT) and hormonal replacement therapy (HRT) for several reasons: First the serum levels of estrogen and progesterone achieved with oral use are not true replacement levels; second, there is growing evidence that the benefits and risks of these therapies are due to pharmacological as well as physiological effects; and third, replacement implies deficiency rather than a natural lessening.

The use of menopausal hormonal therapy, for either therapeutic or, more recently, preventive reasons, has remained a highly controversial issue in women's health. On the one hand, some authorities, viewing the perimenopause as a disease or deficiency state, recommend menopausal hormonal therapy for all women. Others insist that the use of hormones is never indicated for menopausal symptoms. A middle ground approach advocates the use of hormonal therapy for women who have specific symptoms and for women in certain high-risk groups.

Symptom Relief. Numerous studies have demonstrated the usefulness of menopausal hormonal therapy, including estrogen, progestin, or both, in alleviating vasomotor and urovaginal symptoms. The first reports of these benefits of hormonal therapy appeared in 1935, and clinical research continues to substantiate these findings today. Whether or not menopausal hormonal therapy is indicated for hot flushes depends on the extent to which the individual woman is disturbed by them. The frequency and severity of the flushes, the extent to which they interrupt her sleep and activities of daily life, will influence her decision. Short-term therapy (up to 5 years) is usually effective for relief of hot flushes. Gradual withdrawal, to prevent return of symptoms by rapid withdrawal of estrogen, is advised (Lichtman, 1991). Once symptoms no longer recur, treatment is stopped.

Although the urogenital changes seen in postmenopausal women are a normal part of aging, they may be quite uncomfortable for individual women and interfere with sexual activity and pleasure. Vaginal symptoms such as dryness, irritation, pruritus, bleeding, and infection have been shown to respond to both vaginal and systemic estrogen (Lichtman, 1991). However, it may take 12 to 18 months after beginning systemic therapy for benefits to be seen. Vaginal estrogens are very well absorbed systemically in very low doses, and symptom relief is more rapid (Deutsch, Ossowski, & Benjamin, 1981). Urinary symptoms also respond to oral estrogen use. If estrogen withdrawal occurs, vaginal and urinary symptoms may recur; thus relief may require long-term, or even lifelong, therapy.

Cardiovascular Disease. The relationship between estrogen and cardiovascular disease has not been studied extensively. Findings from a study of 8,841 women aged 44 to 101 revealed that women who had used estrogen therapy had reduced mortality when compared to women who had never used estrogen; much of this reduced mortality rate was caused by a marked reduction in death rate from acute myocardial infarction (Henderson, Paganini-Hill, & Ross, 1988). In a study of 1,944 white menopausal women, Wolf, Madans, Finucane, Higgins, and Kleinman (1991) found that, after adjusting for known cardiovascular risk factors, the use of postmenopausal hormones was associated with reduced risk of death from cardiovascular disease. Epidemiological evidence for benefit of estrogen therapy is especially strong for secondary prevention in women with prior cardiovascular heart disease (National Cholesterol Education Program [NCEP], 1993). Barrett-Connor (1991), reviewing evidence that endogenous or exogenous estrogen plays a role in heart disease risk in women, concluded that the evidence suggesting that unopposed oral estrogen reduces the risk of cardiovascular heart disease is "strong, reasonably consistent, and biologically plausible." She found that estrogen therapy is especially beneficial in women who have had an oophorectomy and that its effect is most likely attributable to its favorable influence on lipid/lipoprotein profiles. Natural estrogens used in hormonal therapy increase high-density lipoprotein (HDL) levels and decrease low-density lipoprotein (LDL) levels, thus promoting favorable lipid profiles (Haarbo, Hassager, Jensen, Riis, & Christiansen, 1991). On the basis of current evidence, Barrett-Connor (1991) recommend that the prescription of estrogen solely or primarily to prevent heart disease should be considered for women at high risk—particularly those women who have high LDL cholesterol or low HDL cholesterol. The NCEP expert panel has recommended estrogen therapy for postmenopausal women with high serum cholesterol (NCEP, 1993). Because combination (estrogen and progesterone) therapy is recommended for women with a uterus, the effect of progesterone on lipids and lipoprotein is a critical issue. Concern has been expressed that adding progestin may negate the benefit of estrogen in preventing cardiovascular disease (Barrett-Connor, 1986). Furthermore, the type of progestin used may be significant in terms of its effect on HDLs (Lichtman, 1991). Findings from two recent studies (Gambrell & Teran, 1991; Metka, Hanes, & Heymanek, 1992) suggest that progesterones do not adversely affect lipids and lipoproteins in postmenopausal women. These findings need to be supported with additional studies, and there is a need to investigate whether or not the continuous addition of low-dose progesterone affects lipids over longer periods of time.

Osteoporosis. Menopausal hormonal therapy may be prescribed as a preventive agent for women at high risk for osteoporosis. The protective effects of estrogen on the bone have been well documented (Christiansen, 1990). A number of well-designed, tightly controlled studies have shown that estrogen therapy for postmenopausal women significantly slows bone loss for at least as long as the woman continues therapy (Marslew, Overgaard, Riis, & Christiansen, 1992). The value of estrogen therapy in preventing osteoporosis varies according to risk, with women at high risk showing the greatest benefit and heavy, nonsmoking women showing little if any benefit. At this time there is no definite answer as to how long estrogen therapy should be continued for osteoporosis prevention. Lichtman (1991) states 10 years as the minimum, to account for the years of accelerated bone loss following menopause; thus lifetime therapy must be considered. The minimum effective dose seems to be 0.625 milligrams of conjugated estrogens daily (American Medical Women's Association, 1990). When estrogen therapy is stopped, bone mass decreases at a rate similar to that in the immediate postmenopausal period.

Hormonal Therapy and Breast Cancer. Currently, one in eight women will experience breast cancer in her lifetime. Recent studies showing increased risks of breast cancer associated with estrogen or estrogen/progestin use (Bergkvist, Adami, Persson, Hoover, & Schairer, 1989) raise concern as to the risks associated with menopausal hormonal therapy use. Hulka (1990) reviewed 30 epidemiological studies designed to identify an association between hormone therapy and breast cancer and concluded the following: (a) Analysis of use versus nonuse of estrogen therapy shows no association with breast cancer. (b) Duration of estrogen therapy affects risk. On the basis of studies in the United States, a relative risk of about 1.5 may be reached after 15 or more years of use. (c) The increase in risk after long duration hormone use is present for women with either a natural or surgical menopause. (d) The type of estrogen used and the addition of progestins may alter risk of breast cancer. Two studies suggested an adverse effect with the addition of progestins. Steinberg and associates (1991) conducted a meta-analysis of the results of 16 studies on the effects of estrogen therapy on breast cancer risks and found that for women experiencing any type of menopause, risk of breast cancer did not increase until after at least 5 years of estrogen use. After 15 years of estrogen use, they found a 30% increase in the risk of breast cancer. Furthermore, women with a family history of breast cancer or who had ever used estrogen replacement had a significantly higher risk than did those with a family history and who had not used estrogen therapy. A recent meta-analysis by Sillero-Areneas, Delgado-Rodriguez, Rodigues-Canteras, Bueno-Cavanillas, and Galve Vargas (1992) of 37 original studies revealed a small but statistically significant relative risk of 1.06. Women who experienced natural menopause seemed to have a slightly higher (1.13) risk. A nonsignificant increasing trend was found between duration of hormone therapy and breast cancer risk. Although accumulating research results seem to imply that menopausal hormonal therapy could promote breast cancer, the extent to which estrogen therapy increases the risk of breast cancer and what role progestins play in that risk need further assessment.

Risks Associated With Hormonal Therapy. The risk of endometrial cancer is increased with unopposed estrogen therapy; the risk appears to be negated when a progestin is added at an adequate dose and duration for each cycle of use (see Treatment Guidelines, p. 95). The risk of ovarian or cervical cancer is not increased with estrogen therapy. There are contraindications to the use of estrogen therapy, including presence or suspicion of certain cancers, such as breast cancer or endometrial cancer; current problems with blood clots in the arteries or veins; and unexplained vaginal bleeding. In addition, estrogen therapy is not recommended for a woman with a blood relative who has had breast cancer (Peck, 1990). Because a small percentage of noncancerous breast lumps contain precancerous lesions, these conditions should be evaluated before estrogen therapy is begun. Estrogen therapy may worsen myomas of the uterus and porphyria. Pregnancy is a contraindication for estrogen therapy.

In some instances, menopausal hormonal therapy is not recommended but also is not strictly contraindicated. Conjugated estrogens are associated with an increased incidence of gallbladder disease, and women with a known history of gallbladder disease should not use estrogen therapy. It is not a good idea to smoke cigarettes while using estrogen, and smoking decreases its effectiveness (Peck, 1990). If thrombi develop or if surgery is anticipated, estrogen therapy should be discontinued.

Side effects associated with estrogen therapy may include headaches, nausea and vomiting, bloating, ankle and feet swelling, weight gain, breast soreness, brown spots on the skin, eye irritation with contact lenses, and depression. Although unlikely to appear with current levels of estrogen therapy, they disappear with change in estrogen preparation or decrease in prescribed dose.

Decision to Use Menopausal Hormonal Therapy. All midlife and older women considering hormonal therapy need to understand the unresolved issues in this therapy. Lichtman (1991) asserts that to some extent all postmenopausal users are part of an experimental therapy, often without the benefits of the surveillance found in actual research studies. Each woman considering hormonal therapy should be counseled regarding its benefits and risks so that she may make an informed decision about its use. Currently, the only valid treatment reasons for hormonal therapy are relief of moderate to severe hot flashes/flushes and urovaginal symptoms. In high-risk women, prevention of osteoporosis or cardiovascular disease may also be an acceptable reason for instituting HRT. Harper (1990) identified factors on which the decision to use HRT is dependent: (a) the balance between potential risks and benefits, (b) presence of symptoms or risk factors as indicators of need, (c) a woman's decision to choose HRT, and (d) the ability of the provider and woman to follow through on a plan of therapy.

The decision of whether or not to use HRT is complex because it involves weighing gains and losses related to physical risk. There are no clear-cut answers that care providers can give perimenopausal women. Rothert and her colleagues (1990) studied how women make judgments regarding estrogen therapy and found that relief of hot flashes was the most frequent concern; osteoporosis, side effects of estrogen/progestin therapy, and worry about increased cancer risk were also of concern. They suggested that these results indicate that nursing interventions should anticipate differences in women's concerns and tailor counseling appropriately. A community survey of self-reported estrogen and progestin use revealed that 32% of postmenopausal women (n = 954), aged 50 to 65, used hormones. There were significant social network and medical care use differences in these women: HRT users were younger, thinner, lived in smaller households, and were less likely to be widowed (Harris, Laws, Reddy, King, & Haskell, 1990).

Treatment Guidelines. There are many different estrogen preparations, natural and synthetic, which are administered in different ways—oral tablets, topical creams, transdermal preparations, injectables, suppositories, and vaginal implants. Most women today use either tablets or the transdermal patch.

Estrogen is prescribed in combination with progesterone to simulate the normal menstrual cycle. The usual recommended dosage is 0.625 mg of estrogen for 25 days. This dosage is effective in osteoporosis prevention; higher dosages (0.9 mg or 1.25 mg) may be necessary to relieve hot flashes in some women. Estrogen is taken on calendar days 1 to 25. Until recently, progestin (5 mg norethindrone or 5 to 10 mg medroxyprogesterone acetate) also was prescribed for women who had a uterus. Progestin was taken on days 16 to 25 of the cycle. There was a brief rest each month during which no medications were taken and menstrual bleeding occurred. More recently, other cycle regimens in which a continuous low dose of progestins (2.5 mg medroxyprogesterone) is used are being recommended. It is thought that this dose of progestins will have less adverse effects on lipid profiles than do the higher doses. Women usually do not experience cyclical bleeding with this regimen and are less likely to have progestin side effects.

The estrogen patch is applied two times a week to a hairless area of skin. Each patch is designed to last 3.5 days. Any site on the trunk or upper arms provides adequate absorption (Youngkin, 1990). The patches should not be placed on the breasts because of their sensitivity. Some women report minor skin irritation and reddening at the patch site. Generally, transdermal estrogen offers the same relief of menopausal symptoms as the oral preparation. The transdermal method of delivery of estrogen does not have the same adverse effect on the liver that oral estrogen does (Judd, 1987), and other side effects, such as breast tenderness and fluid retention, have been limited (Utian, 1987).

Estrogen is available in cream form for vaginal application. The primary effect is systemic, estrogen being absorbed by the vaginal mucosa. However, in one study, daily administration of

0.3 mg of conjugated estrogens did not reveal systemic absorption after 1 week while relief of vaginal symptoms was achieved (Harper, 1990).

Two federally sponsored, large studies in progress are the Postmenopausal Estrogen and Progestin Intervention (PEPI) trial and the Women's Health Initiative (WHI). The results of PEPI (which are not available at this printing) reveal effects of estrogen therapy or menopausal hormonal therapy on risk factors of cardiovascular disease. The WHI will be ongoing over the next decade to assess benefits and risks of estrogen therapy or menopausal hormonal therapy in regard to heart disease, osteoporosis, and cancer.

Alternative Therapies

Women who do not choose menopausal hormonal therapy may find other modalities useful for relieving hot flashes. *Menopause Me and You* (Voda, 1984) and *The Pause* (Barbach, 1993) are useful references for all menopausal women. Homeopathy, acupuncture, and Chinese herbs have been used successfully for menopausal problems such as heavy bleeding, hot flashes, irritability, and headaches. Homeopathy views menopausal symptoms as the body's efforts to heal itself from the hormonal changes it is experiencing. Examples of remedies commonly prescribed during menopause by homeopaths include the following: sepia, made from the inky juice of the cuttlefish, to relieve symptoms such as dry mouth, eyes, and vagina; nux vomica, derived from the poison nut to relieve backaches, constipation, and frequent awakenings; and pulsatilla, made from the windflower, to relieve severe menstrual symptoms and hot flashes (Barbach, 1993). Acupuncturists also treat hot flashes, but it is important that women evaluate their acupuncturists carefully. The American Association of Acupuncturists and Oriental Medicine will supply a list of acupuncturists in a given state. Write to AAAOM Referrals, 4101 Lake Boone Trail, Suite 201, Raleigh, NC 27607-6518; (919) 787-5181.

Chinese herbal therapy also has been used to treat menopausal discomforts. In addition to resolving physical symptoms, Chinese herbs are also used to combat mood swings and depression. Ginseng has been reported as helpful in alleviating hot flashes, although research studies have not supported this assertion. Women should be advised against prolonged use of ginseng in high doses because it can increase blood pressure (Greenwood, 1989). Oriental herbal teas composed of licorice, ginseng, coptis, and Chinese rhubarb may be of some help in relieving hot flashes (Kahn & Hughey, 1987). Red raspberry leaf tea may ease hot flashes. Nurses who are interested or who have clients who are interested in herbal remedies may write to Feminist Health Works, 487-A Hudson Street, New York, NY 10014. Additional information about herbal therapies may be found in the book *Hygiegia* by Jeannine Parvati (1983).

Layered clothing, ice packs, iced water, or freshen-up tissues and fans may offer symptomatic relief. Women can be counseled to avoid hot curries or spicy foods. Reassurance that hot flushes will not last forever may be of comfort even if duration of the problem cannot be predicted accurately. Most women find that hot flushes disappear within 4 to 6 years after menopause.

Summary

Midlife is a complex time for women, with personal and social changes having health effects that are as important as, if not more important than, the biological changes of menopause. Although there are probably biological changes of aging that progress in a relatively immutable fashion, women's well-being during midlife appears to be inextricably linked to the fabric of their lives.

Assisting women with the transition through midlife and aging is a critical role for nurses involved in the provision of health care for women. It is essential that all remember that midlife can be a time of rewarding, positive change. Although a number of physical, psychosexual, developmental, and, possibly, environmental alterations can occur during this period; it is also a time of potential growth and an opportunity to do those things delayed or deferred. Sheehy (1991) views menopause as the gateway to a second adulthood and proposes four demarcations of this second adulthood for contemporary Western women: perimenopause (start of the transition); menopause (completion of the ovarian transition); coalescence, during which the woman sheds the shell of her reproductive self and begins to tap the vitality that Margaret Mead labeled *postmenopausal zest*; and, lastly, maturescence, the passage to full maturity.

References

Ackerman, R. (1990). Career developments and transitions of middle-aged women. *Psychology of Women Quarterly, 14,* 513-530.

Aloia, J. F., Vaswani, A., Yoh, J. H., Yasumura, S., & Cohn, S. H. (1988). Calcitriol in the treatment of postmenopausal osteoporosis. *American Journal of Medicine, 84*(3), 401-408.

American Medical Women's Association. (1990). AMWA position statement on osteoporosis. *Journal of the American Medical Women's Association, 45*(3), 75-79.

Ausenhus, M. K. (1988). Osteoporosis prevention during adolescent and young adult years. *Nurse Practitioner, 13*(9), 42-48.

Barbach, L. (1993). *The pause.* New York: Dutton.

Barrett-Connor, E. (1986). Postmenopausal estrogen, cancer and other considerations. *Women and Health, 11*(3-4), 179-195.

Barrett-Connor, E. (1991). Estrogen and coronary heart disease in women. *JAMA, 265,* 1861-1867.

Baruch, G. (1984). The psychological well-being of women in the middle years. In G. Baruch & J. Brooks-Gunn (Eds.), *Women in midlife* (pp. 761-780). New York: Plenum.

Baruch, G., & Barnett, R. (1983). Adult daughters' relationships with their mothers. *Journal of Marriage and the Family, 45*(3), 601-606.

Bergkvist, L., Adami, H-O., Persson, I., Hoover, R., & Schairer, C. (1989). The risk of breast cancer after estrogen-progestin replacement. *New England Journal of Medicine, 321,* 293-297.

Berkum, C. (1983). Changing appearance for women in the middle years of life: Trauma. In E. Markson (Ed.), *Older women* (pp. 11-35). Lexington, MA: D. C. Heath.

Bilezikian, J. P., & Silverberg, S. J. (1992). Osteoporosis: A practical approach to the perimenopausal women. *Journal of Women's Health, 1*(1), 21-27.

Birge, S. J., & Dalsky, G. (1989, September/October). The role of exercise in preventing osteoporosis. *Public Health Reports,* pp. 54-58.

Bond, K. (1992). Osteoporosis. *NAACOG'S Clinical Issues in Perinatal and Women's Health Nursing, 3*(2), 497-508.

Brooks-Gunn, J., & Kirsh, B. (1984). Life events and the boundaries of midlife for women. In G. Baruch & J. Brooks-Gunn (Eds.), *Women in Midlife* (pp. 11-30). New York: Plenum.

Chapuy, M. C., Arlot, M. E., Duboeuf, F., Brun, J., Crouzet, B., Arnaud, S., Delmar P. D., & Meanier, P. J. (1992). Vitamin D_3 and calcium to prevent hip fractures in elderly women. *New England Journal of Medicine, 327,* 1637-1642.

Chestnut, C. H. (1992). Osteoporosis and its treatment. *New England Journal of Medicine, 326,* 406-407.

Christiansen, C. (1990). Hormonal prevention and treatment of osteoporosis—State of the art 1990. *Journal of Steroid Biochemistry Molecular Biology, 37,* 447-449.

Christiansen, C., Riis, B. J., & Rodbro, P. (1987). Production of rapid bone loss in postmenopausal women. *Lancet, 1,* 1105-1108.

Consensus Development Conference. (1987). Prophylaxis and treatment of osteoporosis. *British Medical Journal, 295,* 914-915.

Cooke, D. J. (1985). Social support and stressful life events during mid-life. *Maturitas, 7*(4), 303-313.

Cooke, D. J., & Greene, J. G. (1981). Types of life events in relation to symptoms at the climacterium. *Journal of Psychosomatic Research, 25,* 5-11.

Cutler, W. (1987). Perimenopausal sexuality. *Archives of Sexual Behavior, 16,* 225-234.

Deutsch, S., Ossowski, R., & Benjamin, I. (1981). Comparison between degree of systemic absorption of vaginally and orally administered estrogens at different dose levels in postmenopausal women. *American Journal of Obstetrics and Gynecology, 139,* 967-968.

Gallagher, J. C., & Goldgar, D. (1990). Treatment of postmenopausal osteoporosis with high dose of synthetic calcitriol: A random controlled trial. *Annals of Internal Medicine, 113,* 649-655.

Gambrell, R. D., & Teran, A-Z. (1991). Changes in lipids and lipoproteins with long-term estrogen deficiency and hormone replacement therapy. *American Journal of Obstetrics and Gynecology, 165,* 307-317.

Gergen, M. (1990). Finished at 40: Women's development within the patriarchy. *Psychology of Women Quarterly, 14,* 471-493.

Gilligan, C. (1982a). Adult development and women's development: Arrangements for a marriage. In J. Giele (Ed.), *Women in the middle years: Current knowledge and directions for research and policy* (pp. 89-114). New York: John Wiley.

Gilligan, C. (1982b). *In a different voice: Psychological theory and women's development.* Cambridge, MA: Harvard University Press.

Greene, J. G. (1990). Psychosocial influences and life events at the time of menopause. In R. Formanek (Ed.), *The meanings of menopause: Historical, medical and clinical perspectives* (pp. 79-115). Hillsdale, NJ: Analytic Press.

Greene, J. G., & Cooke, D. J. (1980). Life stress and symptoms at the climacterium. *British Journal of Psychiatry, 136,* 486-491.

Greenwood, S. (1989). *Menopause naturally.* San Francisco: Volcano Press.

Griffith, J. (1983a). Women's stress responses and coping patterns according to age groups. *Issues in Health Care of Women, 6,* 327-340.

Griffith, J. (1983b). Women's stressors according to age groups: Part I. *Issues in Health Care of Women, 6,* 311-326.

Haarbo, J., Hassager, C., Jensen, S. B., Riis, B. J., & Christiansen, C. (1991). Serum lipids, lipoproteins, and apolipoproteins during postmenopausal estrogen replacement therapy combined with either 19-nortestosterone derivatives or 17-hydroxyprogesterone derivatives. *American Journal of Medicine, 90,* 584-589.

Harper, D. C. (1990). Perimenopause and aging. In R. Lichtman & S. Papera (Eds.), *Gynecology well-woman care* (pp. 405-424). Norwalk, CT: Appleton & Lange.

Harris, R. B., Laws, A., Reddy, V. M., King, A., & Haskell, W. L. (1990). Are women using postmenopausal estrogens? A community survey. *American Journal of Public Health, 80,* 1266-1268.

Henderson, B. E., Paganini-Hill, A., & Ross, R. K. (1988). Estrogen replacement therapy and protection from acute myocardial infarction. *American Journal of Obstetrics and Gynecology, 159,* 312-317.

Hulka, B. S. (1990). Hormone replacement therapy and the risk of breast cancer. *CA-A Cancer Journal for Clinicians, 40,* 289-296.

Hunter, M. S. (1988). *Psychological and somatic experience of the climacteric and postmenopause: Predicting individual differences and helpseeking behavior.* Unpublished doctoral dissertation, University of London.

Hunter, M. S. (1990). Somatic experience of the menopause: A prospective study. *Psychosomatic Medicine, 52,* 357-367.

Jennings, S., Mazaik, C., & McKinlay, S. (1984). Women and work: An investigation of the association between health and employment status in middle-aged women. *Social Science and Medicine, 19,* 423-421.

Judd, H. (1987). Efficacy of transdermal estradiol. *American Journal of Obstetrics and Gynecology, 156,* 1326-1331.

Kaufert, P. (1986). Menstruation and menstrual change: Women in midlife. *Health Care for Women International, 7*(1-2), 63-76.

Kaufert, P., Gilbert, P., & Hassard, T. (1988). Researching the symptoms of menopause: An exercise in methodology. *Maturitas, 10,* 117-131.

Kaufert, P., & Syrotiuk, J. (1981). Symptom reporting at the menopause. *Social Science and Medicine, 15E,* 173-184.

Kirkpatrick, M. K., Edwards, M. K., & Finch, N. (1991). Assessment and prevention of osteoporosis through use of a client self-reporting tool. *Nurse Practitioner, 16,* 16-17, 20-25.

Koeske, R. (1982). Toward a biosocial paradigm for menopause research: Lessons and contributions from the behavioral sciences. In A. Voda, M. Dinnerstein, & S. O'Donnell (Eds.), *Changing perspectives on menopause* (pp. 3-23). Austin, TX: University of Austin Press.

Leiblum, S. R., & Swartzmann, L. C. (1986). Women's attitudes toward the menopause: An update. *Maturitas, 8*(1), 47-56.

Lichtman, R. (1991). Perimenopausal hormone replacement therapy. *Journal of Nurse-Midwifery, 36*(1), 30-48.

Ljunghall, S., Gardsell, P., Johnell, O., Larsson, K., Lindh, E., Obrant, K., & Sernbo, I. (1991). Synthetic human calcitonin in post menopausal osteoporosis: A placebo-controlled, double-blind study. *Calcified Tissue International, 49*(1), 17-19.

Lopata, H., & Barnewolt, D. (1984). The middle years: Changes and variations in social-role commitments. In G. Baruch & J. Brooks-Gunn (Eds.), *Women in midlife* (pp. 83-108). New York: Plenum.

Luria, Z., & Meade, R. (1984). Sexuality and the middle-aged woman. In G. Baruch & J. Brooks-Gunn (Eds.), *Women in midlife* (pp. 371-398). New York: Plenum.

Manson, J. E., Colditz, G. A., Stampfer, M. J., Willet, W. C., Rosner, B., Monson, R. R., Speizer, F. E., & Hennekens, C. H. (1990). A prospective study of obesity and risk of coronary heart disease in women. *New England Journal of Medicine, 322,* 882-889.

Marslew, U., Overgaard, K., Riis, B. J., & Christiansen, C. (1992). Two combinations of estrogen and progestogen for prevention of postmenopausal bone loss: Long-term effects on bone, calcium and lipid metabolism, climacteric symptoms, and bleeding. *Obstetrics and Gynecology, 79,* 202-210.

McKinlay, S. M., & McKinlay, J. B. (1986). Aging in a "healthy" population. *Social Science and Medicine, 23*(5), 531-535.

McKinlay, J., McKinlay, S., & Brambilla, D. (1987). The relative contributions of endocrine changes and social circumstances to depression in mid-aged women. *Journal of Health and Social Behavior, 28,* 345-363.

Metka, M., Hanes, V., & Heymanek, G. (1992). Hormone replacement therapy: Lipid response to continuous combined oestrogen and progestogen versus oestrogen monotherapy. *Maturitas, 15*(1), 53-59.

Mitchell, V., & Helson, R. (1990). Women's prime of life: Is it the 50's? *Psychology of Women Quarterly, 14,* 451-470.

Napholtz, L. (1985). A descriptive study on working women's knowledge about midlife menopause and health care practices. *Occupational Health Nursing, 33*(10), 510-512.

National Cholesterol Education Program. (1993). Summary of the second report of the National Cholesterol Education Program (NCEP) expert panel on detection, evaluation, and treatment of high blood cholesterol in adults (adult treatment panel II). *JAMA, 269,* 3015-3023.

National Research Council. (1989). *Recommended dietary allowances* (10th ed.). Washington, DC: National Academy Press.

Neugarten, B., Wood, V., Kraines, R., & Loomis, B. (1963). Women's attitudes toward the menopause. *Vita Humana, 6,* 140-151.

Ott, S. M., & Chestnut, C. H. (1989). Calcitriol treatment is not effective in postmenopausal osteoporosis. *Annals of Internal Medicine, 110,* 267-274.

Parvoti, J. (1983). *Hygieia.* Monroe, UT: Freestone.

Pearlman, J., Wolf, P., Finucane, F., & Madans, J. (1989). Menopause and the epidemiology of cardiovascular disease in women. In C. B. Hammond, F. P. Haseltine, & I. Schiff (Eds.), *Menopause evaluation, treatment, and health concerns* (Proceedings of a National Institute of Health Symposium, pp. 313-332). New York: Alan R. Liss.

Peck, W. A. (1990). Estrogen therapy (ET) after menopause. *Journal of American Medical Women's Association, 45*(3), 87-90.

Philosophe, R., & Seibel, M. M. (1992). Menopause and cardiovascular disease. *NAACOG's Perspectives in Perinatal and Women's Health Nursing, 3*(2), 335-342.

Richelson, L. S., Wahner, H. W., Melton, L. J., & Riggs, B. L. (1984). Relative contributions of age and estrogen deficiency to postmenopausal bone loss. *New England Journal of Medicine, 311,* 1273-1275.

Riggs, B. L. (1987). Pathogenesis of osteoporosis. *American Journal of Obstetrics and Gynecology, 156,* 1342-1346.

Riis, B., Thomsen, K., & Christiansen, C. (1987). Does calcium supplementation prevent postmenopausal bone loss? *New England Journal of Medicine, 316,* 173-177.

Rosenthal, C., Matthews, S., & Marshall, V. (1989). Is parent care normative? The experiences of a sample of middle-aged women. *Research on Aging, 11,* 244-260.

Rossi, A. (1980). Life span theories and women's lives. *Signs, 6*(1), 4-32.

Rothert, M., Rovner, D., Holmes, M., Schmitt, N., Talarczyk, G., Kroll, J., & Gogate, J. (1990). Women's use of information regarding hormone replacement therapy. *Research in Nursing & Health, 13,* 355-366.

Rowe, J. W., & Kahn, R. L. (1987). Human aging: Usual and successful. *Science, 237,* 143-149.

Rubin, L. (1979). *Women of a certain age.* New York: Harper.

Sheehy, G. (1992). *Menopause: The silent passage.* New York: Random House.

Sillero-Arenas, M., Delgado-Rodriguez, M., Rodigues-Canteras, R., Bueno-Cavanillas, A., & Galve Vargas, R. (1992). Menopausal hormone replacement therapy and breast cancer: A meta-analysis. *Obstetrics and Gynecology, 79,* 286-294.

Simkin, A., Ayalon, J., & Leitcher, I. (1987). Increased trabecular bone density due to bone-loading exercises in postmenopausal osteoporetic women. *Calcification Tissue International, 40*(2), 59-63.

Sinaki, M. (1989). Exercise and osteoporosis. *Archives of Physical Medicine and Rehabilitation, 70,* 220-229.

Steinberg, K. K., Thacker, S. B., Smith, J., Stroup, D. F., Zack, M. M., Flanders, W. D., & Berelman, R. L. (1991). A meta-analysis of the effect of estrogen replacement therapy on the risk of breast cancer. *JAMA, 265,* 1985-1990.

Stueve, A., & O'Donnell, L. (1984). The daughter of aging parents. In G. Baruch & J. Brooks-Gunn (Eds.), *Women in midlife* (pp. 203-226). New York: Plenum.

Sutnick, M. R. (1987). Nutritional aspects of the menopause. In B. A. Eskin (Ed.), *The menopause: Comprehensive management* (pp. 123-134). New York: Macmillan.

Tilyard, M. W., Spears, G. F. S., Thomson, J., & Dovey, S. (1992). Treatment of postmenopausal osteoporosis with calcitriol or calcium. *New England Journal of Medicine, 326,* 357-362.

Uphold, C., & Sussman, E. (1981). Self-reported climacteric symptoms as a function of the relationships between marital adjustment and childrearing stage. *Nursing Research, 30*(2), 84-88.

Utian, W. H. (1987). Transdermal estradiol overall safety profile. *American Journal of Obstetrics and Gynecology, 156*(5), 1335-1338.

Voda, A. (1984). *Menopause me and you.* Salt Lake City: College of Nursing University of Utah.

Wolf, P. H., Madans, J. H., Finucane, F. F., Higgins, M., & Kleinman, J. C. (1991). Reduction of cardiovascular disease-related mortality among postmenopausal women who use hormones: Evidence from a national cohort. *American Journal of Obstetrics and Gynecology, 164,* 489-494.

Youngkin, E. Q. (1990). Estrogen replacement therapy and the estraderm transdermal system. *Nurse Practitioner, 15*(5), 19-20, 22-25, 31.

Supplemental Reading

Barrett-Connor, E. (1989). Postmenopausal estrogen replacement and breast cancer. *New England Journal of Medicine, 321,* 319-320.

Brown, W. V. (1987). Changing the diet to reduce plasma cholesterol levels. *Cholesterol and Coronary Disease . . . Reducing the Risk, 1,* 1-6.

Bush, T. L. (1992). Feminine forever revisited: Menopausal hormone therapy in the 1990s. *Journal of Women's Health, 1*(1), 1-4.

Carter, L. W. (1987). Calcium intake in young adult women: Implications for osteoporosis risk assessment. *JOGNN, 16,* 301-308.

Cust, M. P., Gangar, K. F., Hillard, T. C., & Whitehead, M. I. (1990). A risk-benefit assessment of estrogen therapy in postmenopausal women. *Drug Safety, 5,* 345-358.

Dan, A., Wilbur, J., Hedricks, C., O'Connor, E., & Homn, K. (1990). Lifelong physical activity in midlife and older women. *Psychology of Women Quarterly, 14,* 531-542.

Ettinger, B. (1987). Overview of the efficacy of hormonal replacement therapy. *American Journal of Obstetrics and Gynecology, 156,* 1298-1303.

Ettinger, B., Genant, H. K., & Cann, C. E. (1987). Postmenopausal bone loss is prevented by treatment with low-dose estrogen with calcium. *Annals of Internal Medicine, 106*(1), 40-45.

Fogel, C. I. (1981). Nutrition. In C. I. Fogel & N. F. Woods (Eds.), *Health care of women* (pp. 450-483). St. Louis, MO: C. V. Mosby.

Gannon, L. (1990). Endocrinology of menopause. In R. Formanek (Ed.), *The meanings of menopause:*

Historical, medical and clinical perspectives (pp. 170-238). Hillsdale, NJ: Analytic Press.

Jenson, J., Riis, B. J., Strom, V., Nilas, L., & Christiansen, C. (1987). Long-term effects of percutaneous estrogens and oral progesterone on serum lipoproteins in postmenopausal women. *American Journal of Obstetrics and Gynecology, 156,* 66-77.

Johnson, J. E. (1989). Prevention of osteoporosis: The calcium controversy. *Journal of the American Academy of Nurse Practitioners, 1*(4), 126-131.

Kaplan, F. S. (1987). Osteoporosis, pathophysiology and prevention. *Clinical Symposium, 39*(1), 4-28.

Kaufert, P. (1980). The perimenopausal woman and her use of health services. *Maturitas, 2*(1), 191-205.

Kaufert, P. (1984). Women and their health in the middle years: A Manitoba project. *Social Science and Medicine, 18,* 279-281.

Krolner, B., Toft, B., Nielson, S. P., & Tondefold, E. (1983). Physical exercise as prophylaxis against involutional vertebral bone loss. A controlled trial. *Clinical Science, 64,* 541-546.

Lebherz, T. B., & French, L. (1969). Nonhormonal treatment of the menopause syndrome. *Obstetrics & Gynecology, 33,* 759-799.

Long, J., & Porter, K. (1984). Multiple roles of midlife women: A case for new directions in theory, research, and policy. In G. Baruch & J. Brooks-Gunn (Eds.), *Women in midlife* (pp. 109-160). New York: Plenum.

Madson, S. (1989). How to reduce the risk of postmenopausal osteoporosis. *Journal of Gerontological Nursing, 15*(2), 20-24.

National Center for Health Statistics. (1986). *Current estimates from the National Health Interview Survey, United States, 1985* (U.S. Public Health Service Publication No. 8601588). Washington, DC: Government Printing Office.

National Institutes of Health Consensus Conference. (1984). Osteoporosis. *JAMA, 252,* 799.

National Institutes of Health Consensus Development Conference Panel on Lowering Blood Cholesterol to Prevent Heart Disease. (1985). [Recommendations]. *JAMA, 252,* 2080-2086.

Prince, R. L. (1991). Prevention of postmenopausal osteoporosis. *New England Journal of Medicine, 325,* 1189-1195.

Riley, M. (1985). Women, men and the lengthening life course. In A. Rossi (Ed.), *Gender and the life course* (pp. 333-347). New York: Aldine.

Rosen, M. (1990). Health maintenance strategies for women of different ages. *Obstetrics and Gynecology Clinics of North America, 17,* 673-694.

Schultheis, A. H. (1990). Hypercholesterolemia: Prevention, detection and management. *Nurse Practitioner, 15*(1), 40-46, 51-56.

Shangold, M. M. (1990). Exercise in the menopausal women. *Obstetrics and Gynecology, 75*(Suppl.), 53S-58S.

Sherwin, B. B., & Gefland, M. M. (1985). Differential symptoms response to parental estrogen and/or androgen administration in the surgical menopause. *Obstetrics and Gynecology, 151*(2), 153-161.

Sutnick, M. R. (1987). Nutrition: Calcium, cholesterol, and calorie. *Medical Clinics of North America,* 128-134.

Ulerner, D. J., & Kannel, W. B. (1986). Patterns of coronary heart disease morbidity and mortality in the sexes. *American Heart Journal, 111,* 383-390.

Viliet, E. L. (1992). The relationship of hormonal changes to defective disorders in the perimenopause. *NAACOG's Perspectives on Perinatal and Women's Health Nursing, 3*(2), 453-472.

Voda, A. (1981). Climacteric hot flash. *Maturitas, 3*(2), 73-90.

Wahl, P., Walden, C., Knopp, R., Hoover, J., Wallace, R., Heiss, G., & Riskind, B. (1983). Effect of estrogen/progestin potency on lipid/lipoprotein cholesterol. *New England Journal of Medicine, 308,* 862-867.

Weinstein, L. (1987). Efficacy of a continuous estrogen-progestin regimen in the menopausal patient. *Obstetrics and Gynecology, 69,* 929-932.

Westcott, P., & Black, L. (1987). *Alternative health care for women.* Rochester, VT: Thorsons.

Willett, W. C., Green, A., Stampfer, M. J., Speizer, F. E., Colditz, G. A., Rosner, B. S., Monson, R. R., Stason, W., & Hennekens, C. H. (1987). Relative and absolute excess risks of coronary heart disease among women who smoke cigarettes. *New England Journal of Medicine, 317,* 1303-1309.

6

Older Women's Health

MARGARET DIMOND

What nurses believe about older women, their capabilities, desires, and interests, influences how we behave toward them. Likewise, our behavior and caring about them affects their image of themselves. The goal of this chapter is to increase our understanding of the multifaceted nature of being an old woman in America and to provide a knowledge base for nursing practice. The term *older women* as it is used in this chapter refers to women who have completed menopause. Topics included are demographics of aging, a review of selected biopsychosocial aspects of aging, and the economic and political forces that affect older women's lives.

Demographic Patterns

The phrase "graying of America" has been coined to represent the increasing proportion of the population that is over the age of 65. Between 1990 and 2050, the population over 65 years of age will increase 117%; the population over 85 will quadruple. The population 65 years and older will increase from 12.6% to about 22.9%, and the population 85 years and older will increase from 1.3% to 5.1% between 1990 and 2050 (U.S. Bureau of the Census, 1989). The fastest growing group in the older population is 85 years and older. Of the total number of older persons, there are more older women than men. In 1900, for every 100 women over the age of 75 there were 96.3 men; in 1979, for every 100 women over the age of 85 there were 45 men. The projected ratios of women over 85 to men in 2000 and 2050 are 39.4 men per 100 women and 38.8 men per 100 women, respectively (Department of Health and Human Services [DHHS], 1980).

It is likely, although unfortunate, that many in this increasing population of older women will live lives of poverty and chronic disease (Dimond, 1989; Lewis, 1985). Women from underrepresented ethnic groups will face the greatest problems with disease and poverty; and it is this segment of the older female population that is growing the fastest. Any consideration of the status of older women of color must be tempered by the fact that accurate information on the demographics of this population has been lacking until recent times. Zambrana (1988) notes that the undercount of black and Hispanic populations in the 1970 census led to a political advocacy movement by these groups to obtain more accurate national data. The 1980 census showed that blacks constitute 8% of the over 65 age group in America; Asian Americans and Pacific Islanders represent 6%; American Indians/Alaskan Natives and Hispanics represent 5% (DHHS, 1990). Given that the population of older adults in America is composed mostly of women, many of whom are poor and have chronic illnesses, it is clear that most of the issues of aging are women's issues, including issues of women's health. Although many of the solutions to the problems facing older women today are gender based, the context within which these issues arise can be more broadly described as a general societal attitude that glorifies all that is youthful and devalues, or considers of limited value, aging persons of either gender.

Ageism

Ageism is a process of systematic stereotyping of and discrimination against people because they are old (Butler & Lewis, 1975). Just as sexism and racism accomplish stereotyping and discrimination because of gender and skin color, ageism results in similar stereotyping and discrimination on the basis of age. *Sociogenic aging*, a much more devastating form of aging than biological aging, has been described by Comfort (1976) as a consequence of societal folklore, prejudices, and misconceptions about aging that are imposed on "the old." Societal attitudes are not easily influenced, but increased knowledge and understanding of aging issues may begin to modify them.

Biology of Aging

Is the end of life built into its beginning? Several theories of aging focus on aging at a cellular level. For example, the free radical theory of aging suggests that aging is due in part to by-products of oxidative metabolism that attack cellular DNA and result in mutations (Martin, 1992); the thesis of genetic instability refers to faulty copying in dividing cells or the accumulation of errors in information-containing molecules (Kane, Ouslander, & Abrass, 1989).

The Baltimore Longitudinal Study of Aging investigators (DHHS, 1984, p. 208) identified six patterns of aging: (a) stability—the absence of any significant change with age in important functions, such as resting heart rate and personality characteristics; (b) declines with age that are due to illnesses associated with age (e.g., arthritis); (c) steady declines in functions, such as creatinine clearance time, in spite of good health; (d) precipitous functional changes with aging often associated with disease, such as dementias; (e) compensatory changes to maintain function with advancing age, such as the Frank-Starling mechanism which maintains cardiac output during exercise; and (f) changes that occur over time but that have nothing to do with aging and reflect cultural or societal changes—for example, a reduced dietary intake of cholesterol that has occurred in all age groups over the past several decades. Findings from this extensive and well-designed study are tempered by the fact that the sample included no women until 1978; consequently, little is known about what patterns of aging may be unique to women.

Immune Function

Immunosenescence is often accompanied by an increased incidence of neoplasia, autoimmune diseases, and infections (Chatta & Dale, 1991, p. 37). Infections are dramatically increased with age. For example, with increasing age there is an increase in bacterial pneumonias and bacteremia, including afebrile bacteremia, which occurs almost exclusively in older adults (Gleckman & Hibert, 1981). The reactivation of the herpes zoster virus in older adults is linked to a decline in the immune system with age (Chatta & Dale, 1991). However, precise mechanisms of the declining efficacy of the immune system, and therefore the specific effects of this process, remain unclear. More gender-related research is necessary to determine gender-related distinctions in the immune system and, subsequently, the implications for the health of both older women and men (National Institute on Aging [NIA], 1991, p. 13).

Cardiovascular Function

Age-related structural and functional changes in the heart are similar for both older men and women. Increasing heart wall thickening and resultant stiffness, which correlates with the onset of hypertension in advancing age, is found in both sexes. Coronary heart disease (CHD) and hypertension are known to develop at a later age in women than men (NIA, 1991). Once diagnosed with CHD, older women are more likely than older men to have angina than myocardial infarcts. These findings suggest significant differences in the development of heart disease and hypertension by gender. Additional research will identify the mechanisms of these findings and their implications for cardiovascular health of women. (See Chapter 5, "Midlife Women's Health," for a discussion of the effect of menopause on heart health.)

Osteoporosis and Bone Loss

Osteoporosis and bone loss dramatically increase the risk of bone fractures in postmenopausal women. Bone loss occurs in women at a faster rate when compared to bone loss in sameage men (NIA, 1991). The precise mechanisms for this phenomena are not well understood. Research to determine both the mechanisms of bone loss and the differences between men and women in rate of bone loss has focused on age-related changes in vitamin D, parathyroid hormone levels, kidney function, and serum calcium among men and women. This research has not yet resulted in unequivocal answers to questions about bone loss, age, and gender. Although some biological distinctions between older women and men are becoming known, the mechanisms for these differences remain unknown. (See Chapter 5 for a discussion of the effects of menopause on bone health.)

Psychology of Aging

Cognitive Abilities

Cognition can be defined as the various thinking processes through which knowledge is gained, stored, manipulated, and expressed (Rabins, 1992, p. 479). Changes in cognition associated with old age involve a range of capacities: motivation, short- and long-term memory, intelligence, learning and retention of tasks, and a host of factors that seem to facilitate or impede cognitive capacities. It is difficult to attribute changes in cognitive functioning to the process of aging because few studies have been done that include repeated measures over time with the same subjects. The NIA (1991, p. 10) report on older women states that older men and women respond in similar ways on most tasks of cognitive function performed in experimental conditions in laboratories, and, overall, only gradual and modest changes in cognitive performance occur in women with aging. There appear to be no differences between men and women on any measures used to identify senile dementia of the Alzheimer's type (SDAT).

Personality and Patterns of Aging

Several theories have been proposed to explain aging from a sociopsychological perspective. *Disengagement theory* (Cumming, 1975; Cumming & Henry, 1961) postulates a mutual withdrawal between the older person and society. Theoretically, when disengagement is complete there is an increased sense of freedom as the individual feels less controlled by norms governing everyday behavior. However, there is no compelling empirical evidence to confirm this theory. In fact, disengagement theory contradicts other theories that are based on the assumption that older people keep active (i.e., resist disengagement) to ward off a sense of failure, diminished self-esteem, and loss of involvement in meaningful activities. The *activity theory* of aging (Havighurst, 1968) advocates successful aging through continuing the interests, activities, and attitudes of middle age. From this perspective, if older people can find substitutes for activities they must give up, adjustment and successful aging will be enhanced. In other words, the older individual who ages optimally is one who stays active and manages to resist the shrinkage of his or her social world. Empirical support for this perspective is mixed (Longino & Kart, 1982). Hooyman and Kiyak (1988) note that socioeconomic status, lifestyle, and other factors may be more important than age as an explanation of social behavior. Older persons with better education and adequate financial resources have more options for remaining active and engaged in life. The current cohort of older women are at risk of having few educational or financial resources for engaging in satisfying life activities. *Continuity theory* (Atchley, 1989; Neugarten, Havighurst, & Tobin, 1968) suggests that the older person makes adjustments in living based on lifelong patterns, societal constraints, particular likes and/or dislikes, and physical abilities (Watson, 1982). This is a reasonable theoretical stance, but it is not adequately substantiated by empirical data.

Sociology of Aging

Family Relations

Even though older women live alone, their connectedness to other family members is substantial (Brody, 1985). The majority of older women (59%) live in family situations or in their own homes. Only 5% of the aged are institutionalized at any one time, although 20% of older adults (again, mostly women) can expect to be institutionalized at some time. Older women have many roles in the lives of their families. One of the most important roles, and until recently overlooked, is that of caregiver. Midlife and older women are the most frequent caregivers of aging parents and spouses. These women can expect to spend up to 18 years caring for aged parents or other aged family members. This fact is quite extraordinary when compared with the 17 years spent, on average, caring for dependent children (Estes, 1991). Informal caregivers in the home are 72% female and 28% male. The average age of women caregivers is 57 years, and some may expect to remain in the caregiver role until well into their seventh decade.

For older women caregivers of spouses, release from caregiving responsibilities comes with the death of the spouse. Death of a spouse is one of the most significant losses for older women, often requiring great changes in lifestyle. Along with the death of friends, family, and other relatives, most aging females will eventually cope with widowhood. By age 75 or older, 67% of women are widows, whereas at the same age only 37% of men are widowed. Given the mean age of widowhood for women at 56 years and life expectancy at 80 years, many women can expect more than 20 years of widowhood (U.S. Senate Special Committee on Aging, 1986). Thus spousal bereavement and widowhood have become almost natural components of aging women's lives.

The death of a spouse in later life has been the focus of several recent large studies. Most do not support major gender distinctions with respect to coping with this event but do support considerable diversity in the adjustment process among older bereaved spouses. Loneliness is the single greatest difficulty experienced by older bereaved spouses, and it persists at least for 2 years and possibly longer. Older bereaved spouses demonstrate an extraordinary degree of resiliency, resourcefulness, and adaptability. The idea that there are defined stages of bereavement adjustment has not been demonstrated in samples of older bereaved spouses. It is more accurate to compare the process to a roller coaster having many ups and downs with gradual improvement over time. Among the internal resources of the bereaved person, high self-esteem and a sense of competence are very important predictors of bereavement adjustment. Strong social relationships with others, good health, and prebereavement marital happiness are also good predictors of adjustment after bereavement. Factors such as age, gender, education or income level, and religious affiliation have not been found to be good predictors of adjustment (Lund, 1989).

Living Arrangements

Older women, because of their increased longevity and fewer available potential mates for remarriage, are more likely than men to live alone after being widowed or divorced. By 2020, women will account for close to 85% of those who live alone, and of these, approximately 50% will be 75 years or older. In every ethnic and racial group, as well as in each age group, women are more likely than men to live alone. However, among Caucasian, African American, and Hispanic women, the latter group is least likely to live alone (Commonwealth Fund Commission, 1988). The reasons for this are not clear, but it may be due in part to cultural variations in beliefs about the care of older relatives or more available extended family members and thus more resources for care. Although relatives are the main source of assistance for older adults who live alone, approximately 20% of those who live alone have no one to help them even for a few days. Many have no living children, and this becomes more critical for African American elders living alone, 37% of whom have no living children. This compares with 26% of older white persons who live alone (Commonwealth Fund Commission, 1988). A variety of new living arrangements for older adults are emerging on the national scene—for example, residential care settings, continuing care retirement communities, life care communities, and adult day care. Although these trends in housing are promising, a negligible amount of research has been done, and little is known about the health and well-being outcomes of older adults who live in these settings. There is considerable concern about the affordability of these living arrangements for the majority of older women. This is particularly true considering the poverty level for many older women, as described next.

Economic Status

The economic status of older women is a significant factor in determining health status. Although, as will be noted, there are various national and state health programs (most notably Medicare and Medicaid) to which older women may turn, significant barriers still exist for the receipt of good health care. In many situations, the criteria for eligibility for medical insurance are more easily met by men than by women. Thus out-of-pocket costs for health care are a considerable worry for many older women and may in fact limit or prevent access to care. Adult women, regardless of race or ethnicity, urban or rural residence, age or labor force participation, are more likely than men to be poor (Perales, 1988). Compared to urban-dwelling older adults, those who live in rural settings (80% of whom are women living alone), have lower incomes (Coward, Lee, Dwyer, & Seccombe, 1993). For all women over the age of 65 in 1987, 12.5% of Caucasian women were below the poverty level, compared with 40.2% of the African American female population and 30.5% of Hispanic women. The rates for men were one half to one third less (U.S. Senate Special Committee on Aging, 1989). Many older women have grown old functioning in the dual role of homemaker and head of household while employed in low- or minimum-wage jobs, and as older females, they are far more likely than older men to be poor on the basis of the Social Security benefits earned in the workplace. In 1987, the median income for Caucasian women 65 years and older was $7,055; for African American women the median income was $4,494 compared to the poverty level of approximately $6,000. The median income for men at the same time was almost double that of women (U.S. Senate Special Committee on Aging, 1989). In 1986, poverty was an issue for more than 2.5 million women and 1 million men. This is a ratio of 255:100 at a time when the ratio of women to men was 160:100 (Lewis, 1985). For all persons 65 years of age and over, being female, a member of a minority group, and living alone constitutes the greatest risk for poverty. For example, 64.3% of all African American women, aged 72 and older and who lived alone in 1987 had incomes below the poverty level (DHHS, 1990, p. 285).

Even though poverty is largely a concern for older women, especially widows, the special concerns of older women and their economic status have been mostly ignored in research on aging. Statistics confirm the increasing percentage of older women in our population, but this differential is not adequately reflected in public policies that influence aging women. Many of the current cohort of older women worked in low-paying jobs, and even today, women are likely to be paid less than men for the same work. Both of these situations have resulted,and will continue to result, in diminished economic well-being for older women.

Social Security and Pensions

Initially planned in 1935 as a compromise between the insurance principle and society's responsibility for the aging, Social Security benefits were designed for dependents at retirement, disability, or death of the wage earner. Under the current regulations, Social Security is biased against some older adults and nearly all older women. Older persons born at the turn of the century have had fewer years of employment under the Social Security Act and thus fewer years on which to base their retirement benefits. Many women are penalized because of a work history interrupted by childbearing and child rearing. Women who chose to be homemakers have no individual eligibility for Social Security, and although they can receive retirement benefits after the death of their spouses, they cannot receive disability supports on their own, despite the economic value of their household labor to their families (Hooyman & Kiyak, 1988, p. 504).

Very few older women have private pensions, in part because of their interrupted work careers and because mandatory laws addressing work-related private pensions were not in effect during the years that the current cohort of older women were employed. In 1982, women composed nearly 75% of the total beneficiary pool of the supplemental security income (SSI) program, which supports persons whose Social Security or private pension income falls below the poverty level. Although this may represent a safety net against outright destitution, it can also be a source of psychological distress because many older women feel ashamed to ask for SSI. For those who feel this way but must request SSI to survive, many experience diminished self-esteem and loss of personal control and independence (Hooyman & Kiyak, 1988, p. 505).

Retirement

The average number of years worked by women increased from 6.3 years in 1900 to 22.9 years in 1970 and to 30 years in 1980. These trends mandate a closer examination of women's adjustment to retirement and the changes in social and personal resources as well as psychological and physical well-being following retirement. To date, retirement research has focused almost exclusively on men, and that which includes both men and women does not provide adequate information on gender differences. One exception is a study on early retirement that concludes that there are different motivations toward early retirement for women and men and for blacks compared with whites (Belgrave, Haug, & G'omez-Belleng'e, 1987). For example, activity limitations were related to early retirement in men but not in women, and although white women who assessed their health as poor were likely to be retired, black women in poor health were apt to still be working.

The few early studies that examined women's retirement suggest that it may be a difficult transitional period. Atchley (1976), who compared men and women retirees, found that women report taking longer to get used to retirement and are more lonely and depressed than men. Additional research is needed to clarify the contemporary relationships between retirement and measures of women's health.

Rural/Urban Inequities

Access to economic security is a significant problem for rural dwelling persons. Rural residents have lower average incomes and higher poverty rates than do urban residents. They are more likely to be without a regular source of health care and to have insufficient or no health insurance (NIA, 1991; Rosenblatt & Moscovice, 1982). Rural-dwelling older persons living alone are more dependent on Medicaid than their urban-dwelling counterparts, are unlikely to have private insurance, and rely heavily on Medicare (Coward et al., 1993). At the same time, rural dwellers are more likely to have higher rates of chronic illness (little of which is covered by Medicare) and to have limitations in activity as a result of chronic conditions (National Center for Health Statistics, 1986). The NIA report (1991, p. 30) suggests that more research is needed on the status of aging rural women—for example, the availability, use, and quality of health care and other services for women and aging rural women as resources for themselves and others.

Health of Older Women

Older women's health issues are enormous. Their increasing longevity places them at risk for multiple concurrent chronic illnesses. Arthritis, rheumatism, heart conditions, and hypertension combined are reported to limit some functioning by 64.7% of women versus 47.7% of men. Most of the morbidity of older women is due to chronic conditions—for example, arthritis; hypertension; osteoporosis and its sequelae; dementias; depression; urinary incontinence (UI); and vision, hearing, and foot problems. Three of these conditions are of particular concern to older women: depression, dementia, and UI.

The risk of major depression is 20% to 25% for women compared with 7% to 12% for men; 30% to 50% of the time it is underdiagnosed or undertreated. Among older women, who are at particular risk, factors that might confound the diagnosis of depression include dementia and side effects of frequently used medications, such as antihypertensives (Agency for Health Care Policy and Research [AHCPR], 1993). Restrictive insurance coverage for treatment of depression (medications and/or counseling) creates economic barriers to care for older women on fixed incomes.

The fourth leading cause of death among older adults is senile dementia of the Alzheimer's type (SDAT). The prevalence of severe dementia is estimated to be 7% for ages 75 to 84, and 25% beyond the age of 85 (Cross & Gurland, 1986). It is a primary diagnosis in 60% of residents in nursing homes, 70% of whom are old women. Although SDAT is more commonly seen in older women, it is unknown whether this is due to a gender difference or simply to the longevity of women (Butler, 1990). The long period of time between diagnosis and death, coupled with generally poor medical insurance coverage, makes the economic and psychological burdens on families of SDAT victims enormous.

Although not a disease, UI accounts for significant functional disability in older women. It is prevalent in 15% to 30% of persons over the age of 60 and is twice as likely in women. Depression, diminished social involvement, and restricted sexual activity are frequent consequences of UI. Transient UI is a common outcome of urinary tract infections, which are frequent among older women. Drugs commonly prescribed for women, such as antihypertensives and antidepressants, can also result in transient UI (AHCPR, 1992).

Older women are overrepresented in nursing homes; they have fewer financial resources and thus less access to health care. They are likely to make more physician and outpatient visits than older men (Soldo & Manton, 1985; Verbrugge & Wingard, 1987), use more prescription medications, and require more custodial services, both in institutions and in the home (Verbrugge, 1982). The current reimbursement system discriminates against women because of its heavy emphasis on acute illness and high-technology medical care. The two major sources of reimbursement for health care used by older women are Medicare and Medicaid. If these sources were, in fact, providing adequate coverage, older women would not be spending the same proportion of their income (15% or more) on health care currently as they did before the passage of Medicare in 1965 (Prospective Payment Assessment Commission, 1989). Medicare reimburses costs of hospitalization, skilled nursing and rehabilitation services, skilled home health services, physician costs, and laboratory costs done on an outpatient basis. However, each of these potentially reimbursable services has exceptions, copayments, deductibles, and other requirements that place considerable limitations on the coverage overall. In addition to these restrictions, Medicare does not cover, or covers in extremely limited ways, many important health care services, such as long-term care in nursing homes, medications prescribed for outpatients, hearing aids, eyeglasses, dentures, foot care, preventive health examinations, and outpatient psychotherapy. In fact, Medicare provides disproportionately better coverage for men, who are more likely to use acute services (which are covered by Medicare), than for women, whose needs are often for chronic care services (Sofaer & Abel, 1990). The feminization of poverty among older women, particularly women who live alone and for women of color, makes out-of-pocket costs for older women a critical issue (Sofaer & Abel, 1990; Stone, 1989). In an astute analysis of out-of-pocket costs for a variety of commonly occurring illnesses of older adults, Sofaer and Abel (1990) showed the bias of the health care reimbursement system toward men. Four of the 10 illnesses analyzed had high out-of-pocket costs: hypertension (63% paid by the patient), arthritis (73%), depression (89%), and stroke (52%). The first three are more common among women. One condition, breast cancer, had moderate out-of-pocket costs (35%). The remaining five illnesses were considered to have low out-of-pocket costs: pneumonia (16%), lung cancer (17%), heart attack (19%), enlarged prostate (21%), and fractured hip (25%). The first three of these occur more often in men, and one is exclusively a male condition. Fractured hips and hip replacements are more common among women. Even with various supplemental policies, which are intended to provide coverage for services not covered by Medicare, the results do not differ dramatically and the trends remain the same.

The Medicaid program is the primary source of health care coverage for the poor in America. Among older men and women (over 65 years), women represent 62% of those eligible for Medicaid. Medicaid coverage is thus both a class and gender issue, because more older women than men are likely to be poor (Muller, 1988).

Any discussion of reimbursement for health care services must acknowledge the out-of-control, spiraling cost of health care. A variety of strategies for containing costs have been proposed. Among these are various proposals for rationing health care on the basis of age (Callahan, 1987). Rationing health care on the basis of age must be carefully analyzed and recognition given to the fact that older women would bear the brunt of such rationing much more than older men (Jecker, 1991; McElmurry & Zabrocki, 1989). Jecker (1991) stated that although everyone recognizes the dilemmas of pitting one age group against another by age-based rationing of care, the inequalities produced between the sexes are more ethically troubling. These inequalities cannot be justified even when they benefit other segments of society at large.

Health Promotion

Lifestyle modifications are beneficial at all ages. Exercise, nutrition, and sexuality are three (of many) important components of a healthy lifestyle program for older women.

Exercise. Fewer than 10% of either men or women 65 years of age or older exercise on a regular basis. This is a fact in spite of growing evidence of the benefits of exercise, which have been shown to improve fitness, particularly strength and aerobic capacity; improve gait and balance; decrease pain in persons with arthritis; and result in modest improvement in cognition (Buchner, Beresford, Larson, LaCroix, & Wagner, 1992). Cardiorespiratory endurance, body agility, flexibility, body fat, and balance have improved among older women who engage in low-impact aerobic dance (Hopkins, Murrah, Hoeger, & Rhodes, 1990). The issue of long-term adherence to an exercise program needs further study. (See Chapter 13, "Exercise," for detailed discussion of exercise.)

Nutrition. For many women, both older and younger, the role of good nutrition is synonymous with weight control. Both women and men tend to gain weight as they age. For older women, this may be due in part to metabolism changes with menopause as well as reduced physical exercise (Burke & Raskind, 1991). Factors that enter into poor nutrition habits for older women are: living alone and thus eating alone, with the potential for less nutritious meals and more frequent snacking; having a low income and trying to conserve money by purchasing less fresh fruit and vegetables and more fast foods, which may be cheaper but also higher in fat and sodium. Some older women who live alone meet their social needs by joining other older women once or twice a week for a meal in a restaurant. Food prepared in restaurants is often high in fat and sodium, and vegetables are frequently overcooked, thus losing important vitamins and minerals. Older women need to be counseled regarding restriction of fats, cholesterol, and sodium; the need for adequate intake of fiber, potassium, vitamins, minerals, and proteins; and the importance of maintaining or increasing daily calcium for the maintenance of good health. Steen, Nilsson, Robertson, and Ostberg (1988) found that one third of retired women were below the recommended dietary allowances (RDA) for calcium and almost all women in the study were below the RDA for vitamin D (see Chapter 12).

Sexuality. Older women are capable sexual partners and competent physiologically and psychologically to establish meaningful sexual relationships. However, a number of factors influence their sexual abilities: normal physiological changes of aging, established behavioral patterns, illness, the availability of a satisfactory mate, and societal values. If a healthy older female has remained sexually active, is not inhibited by societal stereotypes and myths against sex with advanced age, and has a partner who has maintained sexual interests, it is likely that she will have continued satisfactory sexual relationships. A comprehensive life span discussion of sexuality is covered in Chapter 21, "Sexuality in Women's Lives."

During the past decade, more accurate information has emerged on older lesbian women. Older lesbian women have been a silent group whose sexual needs and special social situation have not been acknowledged. This group of older women is faced with the negative attitudes accompanying being old, being female, and being lesbian and are thus at great risk for discrimination in health care. Lesbian issues are covered more fully in Chapter 10, "Lesbian Health Care."

Successful Aging

Aging involves the process of loss, growth, and change. Success in the process depends on characteristics of the woman, her access to resources that promote health, and her ability to develop strategies for coping with loss and change. Coping with the changes that accompany aging involves some losses that may not be anticipated, but many of the normal psychological and physiological changes that affect older women may be predicted. If women are educated about such changes and given time to assimilate and plan for the process of transition from one phase of life to the next, the outcome of successful aging will be enhanced.

To promote growth and optimal aging, women must secure adequate information about their bodies as well as behavioral strategies that ensure a healthy lifestyle. This requires skills in information processing, decision making, and action. With adequate information and skills, and an environment that promotes physical, mental, economic, and social health, older women are in a position to maintain independence and achieve late-life goals.

In addition to their internal resources, most older persons require the support of others to meet the challenges of aging. Who will be the primary source of support to women as they age? Can older women depend on their families for continued support as they age, now and in the future? With changing social factors, such as increased population mobility, diminishing fertility, and increasing divorce rates, the likelihood of changing styles of family support is high. In response to these trends, older women are beginning to organize and develop strategies for supporting each other and promoting societal change.

The political power of the women's movement is a vehicle that can be used by aging women collectively. A coalition between older and younger women would be mutually beneficial for changing the stereotypes about older women originating from ageism and sexism. Through working together, women can strive to improve the quality of life for older women today and also for themselves as the older women of tomorrow.

This chapter focused on women in the later years of their lives. Physiological processes and physical and psychological changes affect the health of older women. These are modified by sociocultural factors that combine either to promote or hinder adaptation, growth, and change in the lives of aging women. Successful aging for women may be enhanced through individual behavior and action or through collective collaboration with other women by organizing and promoting strategies for change.

What has become crystal clear throughout these discussions is the paucity of research to support a scientific perspective on the health and well-being of older women. Research can expose and challenge the stereotypes that perpetuate ageism and sexism and can enlighten understanding of the process of normal aging among older people, especially women. Research can inform efforts to lift the burden of poverty, provide open access to adequate and appropriate health care, and enhance the overall well-being of older women.

References

Agency for Health Care Policy and Research. (1992). *Urinary incontinence in adults: Clinical practice guideline* (DHHS, PHS AHCPR Publication No. 92-0038). Washington, DC: Government Printing Office.

Agency for Health Care Policy and Research. (1993). *Depression in primary care: Detection and diagnosis* (DHHS, PHS AHCPR Publication No. 93-0550). Washington, DC: Government Printing Office.

Atchley, R. (1976). *The sociology of retirement.* New York: Wiley.

Atchley, R. (1989). A continuity theory of normal aging. *The Gerontologist, 29*(2), 183-190.

Belgrave, L., Haug, M., & G'omez-Belleng'e, F. (1987). Gender and race differences in effects of health and pension on retirement before 65. *Comprehensive Gerontology, 1*(3), 109-117.

Brody, E. (1985). Parent care as a normative family stress. *The Gerontologist, 25*(1), 19-29.

Buchner, D., Beresford, S., Larson, E., LaCroix, A., & Wagner, E. (1992). Effects of physical activity on health status in older adults. *Annual Review of Public Health, 13,* 469-488.

Burke, W., & Raskind, W. (1991). Preventive health care of older women. In M. Stenchever & G. Aagaard (Eds.), *Caring for the older woman* (pp. 55-120). New York: Elsevier.

Butler, R. (1990). Senile dementia of the Alzheimer's type (SDAT). In W. Abrams & R. Berkow (Eds.), *The Merck manual of geriatrics* (pp. 933-938). Rahway, NJ: Merck Sharp & Dohme Research Laboratories.

Butler, R., & Lewis, M. (1975). *Why survive? Being old In America.* New York: Harper & Row.

Callahan, D. (1987). *Setting limits: Medical goals in an aging society.* New York: Simon & Schuster.

Chatta, G., & Dale, D. (1991). Alterations of host-defense mechanisms and the susceptibility to infections. In M. Stenchever & G. Aagaard (Eds.), *Caring for the older woman* (pp. 37-55). New York: Elsevier.

Comfort, A. (1976). Age prejudice in America. *Social Policy, 7*(3), 3-8.

Commonwealth Fund Commission. (1988). *Aging alone: Profiles and projections.* Baltimore, MD: Author.

Coward, R., Lee, G., Dwyer, J., & Seccombe, K. (1993). *Old and alone in rural America.* Washington, DC: American Association of Retired Persons.

Cumming, E. (1975). Engagement with an old theory. *Aging and Human Development, 6*(3), 187-191.

Cumming, E., & Henry, W. (1961). *Growing old.* New York: Basic Books.

Department of Health and Human Services, Bureau of the Census. (1980). Life tables (Vol. II, Section V. Table 5-5). *Vital Statistics of the United States.* Washington, DC: Government Printing Office.

Department of Health and Human Services. (1984). *Normal human aging: The Baltimore longitudinal study of aging.* Washington, DC: Government Printing Office.

Department of Health and Human Services. (1990). *Health status of minorities and low-income groups* (3rd ed.). Washington, DC: Government Printing Office.

Dimond, M. (1989). Health care and the aging population. *Nursing Outlook, 37*(2), 76-77.

Estes, C. L. (1991). The Reagan legacy: Privatization, the welfare state, and aging. In J. Myles & J. Quadagno (Eds.), *States, labor markets, and the future of old age* (pp. 54-83). Philadelphia: Temple University Press.

Gleckman, R., & Hibert, D. (1981). Afebrile bacteremia: A phenomenon in geriatric patients. *JAMA, 248*(12), 1478-1481.

Havighurst, R. (1968). Personality and patterns of aging. *The Gerontologist, 8*(2), 20-23.

Hooyman, N., & Kiyak, A. (1988). *Social gerontology.* Newton, MA: Allyn & Bacon.

Hopkins, D., Murrah, B., Hoeger, W., & Rhodes, R. (1990). Effects of low-impact aerobic dance on the functional fitness of elderly women. *The Gerontologist, 30*(2), 189-192.

Jecker, N. (1991). Age-based rationing and women. *JAMA, 266*(21), 3012-3015.

Kane, R., Ouslander, J., & Abrass, I. (1989). *Essentials of clinical geriatrics* (2nd ed.). New York: McGraw-Hill.

Lewis, M. (1985). Older women and health: An overview. *Women and Health, 10*(2/3), 1-16.

Longino, C., & Kart, C. (1982). Explicating activity theory: A formal replication. *Journal of Gerontology, 37*(6), 713-722.

Lund, D. (1989). *Older bereaved spouses: Research with practical applications.* New York: Hemisphere.

Martin, G. (1992). Biological mechanisms of ageing. In J. G. Evans & T. F. Williams (Eds.), *Oxford textbook of geriatric medicine* (pp. 41-48). Oxford, UK: Oxford University Press.

McElmurry, B., & Zabrocki, E. (1989). Ethical concerns in caring for older women in the community. *Nursing Clinics of North America, 24*(4), 1041-1050.

Muller, C. (1988). Medicaid: The lower tier of healthcare for women. *Women and Health, 14*(2), 81-102.

National Center for Health Statistics. (1986). *Vital and health statistics* (Series 10, No. 160). Washington, DC: Government Printing Office.

National Institute on Aging. (1991). *Research on older women: Highlights from the Baltimore Longitudinal Study of Aging* (Document prepared for the National Advisory Council on Aging). Washington, DC: Government Printing Office.

Neugarten, B., Havighurst, R., & Tobin, S. (1968). Personality and patterns of aging. In B. Neugarten (Ed.), *Middle age and aging* (pp. 173-177). Chicago: University of Chicago Press.

Perales, C. (1988). Introduction. *Women and Health 14*(2), 1-20.

Prospective Payment Assessment Commission. (1989). *Medicare prospective payment and the American health care system: Report to the Congress.* Washington, DC: Government Printing Office.

Rabins, P. (1992). Cognition. In J. G. Evans & T. F. Williams (Eds.), *Oxford textbook of geriatric medicine* (pp. 463-479). Oxford, UK: Oxford University Press.

Rosenblatt, R., & Moscovice, I. (1982). *Rural health care.* New York: John Wiley.

Sofaer, S., & Abel, E. (1990). Older women's health and financial vulnerability: Implications of the Medicare benefit structure. *Women and Health, 16*(3/4), 47-67.

Soldo, B., & Manton, K. (1985). Health status and service needs of the oldest old: Current patterns and future trends. *Milbank Memorial Fund Quarterly, 63*(2), 286-319.

Steen, B., Nilsson, K., Robertson, E., & Ostberg, H. (1988). Age retirement in women: Dietary habits and body composition. *Comprehensive Gerontology, 2*(2), 78-82.

Stone, R. (1989). The feminization of poverty among the elderly. *Women's Studies Quarterly, 17*(1/2), 20-34.

U.S. Bureau of the Census. (1989). Projections of the population of the U.S. by age, sex and race: 1988-2080. *Current Population Reports* (Series P-25, No. 1018). Washington, DC: Government Printing Office.

U.S. Senate Special Committee on Aging. (1986). *Aging America: Trends and projections, 1985-1986.* Washington, DC: Government Printing Office.

U.S. Senate Special Committee on Aging. (1989). *Aging America: Trends and projections, 1989* (Serial 101-E, and U.S. Bureau of the Census, March 1988). Washington, DC: Government Printing Office.

Verbrugge, L. (1982). Women and men: Mortality and health of older people. In M. Riley, B. Hess, & K. Bond (Eds.), *Aging in society* (pp. 139-174). Hillsdale, NJ: Lawrence Erlbaum.

Verbrugge, L., & Wingard, D. (1987). Sex differentials in health and mortality. *Women and Health, 12*(2), 103-145.

Watson, W. (1982). *Aging and social behavior.* Monterey, CA: Wadsworth.

Zambrana, R. (1988). A research agenda on issues affecting poor and minority women: A model for understanding their health needs. *Women and Health, 14*(2), 137-160.

PART II

7

Women and Health Care

DEBBIE WARD

Women are redefining health. Women's work, interests, recreation, childbirth, menstruation, menopause, aging, sexuality, and body size and shape are all undergoing redefinition as women create their own health standards rather than accept others' definitions of appropriate beliefs, appearance, and behavior. Women are also redefining health care. In addition to revealing the aspects of personal and public health services, research, and health policies that do not address their views and needs, women have created alternative personal health services, conducted their own research on women's health, established a women's public health agenda, and wrought changes in American health policy.

A focus on and by women is bringing about profound alterations in health care. As feminists analyze health care delivery systems, structural changes are being instituted that meet human needs—from secure parking for night shift nurses and reimbursement for screening mammography to group counseling sessions by conference call for women caring for housebound, chronically ill family members and friends. As feminism has encouraged both genders to move beyond feminine and masculine stereotypes, the expressive capacities (empathy, emotional support, nurturance) of those who provide personal health services are receiving more attention. This new emphasis on the art of health care affects even the financing of health care: Federally set physician fee schedules, revamped by the valuation system called resource-based relative value scales, have provided increased payment for such cognitive services as taking a patient history, whereas payment for such technical procedures as sigmoidoscopy has been lowered (Hsiao, Braun, Dunn, & Becker, 1988).

Women no longer equate medical care with health. The potential for detrimental effects from medical intervention is widely recognized: The Dalkon shield is a concrete example. Feminist analysts recognize the focus on illness, not health, in the United States. Some conclude that the United States has an illness care nonsystem (Ward, 1990b), an irregularly controlled medical-industrial complex designed to profit from the illnesses of those who can pay while denying even the most basic care to those who cannot (Bullough & Bullough, 1982; Corea, 1977; Crane

& Kaye, 1986; Daly, 1978; Ehrenreich & English, 1978; Himmelstein & Woolhandler, 1989).

This chapter will survey women's health care. It will explore problems women have historically faced in receiving personal health services, as well as the influence that education for health professionals and research on women's health has had on the clinicians who care for women. Women's place in health research and health policy will be considered. Attempts to predict some future trends will conclude this survey.

Health Care: A Woman's Problem

The social and health sciences literature provides evidence of the complex role of gender in personal health services, in the education of health professionals, and in research on women's health. In the delivery of personal health services, investigators have found evidence of sexist bias in diagnosis, treatment, prescription of medications, and admission to hospital for psychiatric problems. Similarly, the diagnosis and treatment of women for a variety of medical and surgical conditions has also been gender biased, with strong evidence that gynecology and surgical practices, in particular, are affected.

Diagnosis

Psychiatric. Classic studies (Aslin, 1977; Broverman, Broverman, Clarkson, Rosenkrantz, & Vogel, 1970) demonstrated that women judged to behave in gender-appropriate ways were also judged to be psychologically less healthy than men and that the gender of a therapist can influence expectations about women's mental health. More recent work suggests continuing issues of bias in women's mental health. In a study of 25 *DSM-III* (*Diagnostic and Statistical Manual of Mental Disorders-Third Edition*) diagnoses among psychiatric patients during the intake process, men and women differed in frequency in 12 diagnoses; men were more likely to have substance abuse disorders and schizophrenia, for example, whereas women were more likely to manifest depression, anxiety, and especially phobias (Fabrega, Mezzich, Ulrich, & Benjamin, 1990). Whether the genders fall into gender-neutral diagnostic categories as a result of gender-neutral evaluations or are guided into gender-biased diagnoses as a result of gender-biased evaluations are important questions raised but not answered by such studies.

The intricate interweaving of socially constructed definitions of gender and their relation to diagnostic taxonomies is also illustrated by the controversy surrounding the inclusion of the diagnosis of masochistic personality disorder in the *DSM-III-R* (*Diagnostic and Statistical Manual of Mental Disorders-Third Edition-Revised*; American Psychiatric Association [APA], 1987). In the face of feminist criticism, the APA renamed the syndrome "self-defeating personality disorder," and listed it not as an established diagnosis but as a diagnosis still under consideration. Writing as a battered-women's therapist and advocate, Walker (1987) notes that what may be called self-defeating behavior—accommodating others, emphasizing relationships instead of independence—is culturally approved for women in general and may represent the behavior that provides the best coping strategy for many women, especially if they are battered.

Medical. An early study suggested that certain health problems specific to women are likely to be labeled psychogenic in origin despite evidence of organic causation (Lennane & Lennane, 1973). On the basis of such misdiagnoses, it was determined that practitioners may mismanage such ailments as dysmenorrhea, nausea during pregnancy, labor pain, and infantile behavioral disturbances. In contrast, McCranie, Horowitz, and Martin (1978) found no statistically significant differences by patient gender in physicians' assessments of severity or prognosis with and without treatment.

The AIDS epidemic has provided a troubling example of diagnostic delay by gender (Marte & Anastos, 1990). Ten years after identification of the disease, the diagnostic findings in HIV-positive women, which are hallmarks of disease (such as chronic vaginal infections and cervical dysplasia), had not been added to the nationally referenced lists put out by the Centers for Disease Control (CDC) (Smeltzer & Whipple, 1991). In 1992, the CDC proposed a revised definition of AIDS that would add three conditions—invasive cervical cancer, pulmonary tuberculosis, and recurrent pneumonia—to the list of 23 indicator conditions, such as Kaposi's sarcoma (*off our backs,* 1992).

Verbrugge's (1986) analysis of the results of the National Ambulatory Medical Care Survey indicates that women experience more daily symptoms, higher incidence of all types of acute conditions (except injuries at young ages), higher prevalence of nonfatal chronic diseases, more physician visits per year, and more hospital stays than do men. Even when reproductive events and disorders were removed from the analysis, this imbalance persisted. At the same time, Verbrugge found that men have a higher prevalence of principal fatal chronic diseases and higher limitation rates than do women. Women therefore suffer more frequent but less serious morbidity than do men. Verbrugge found that the types of diseases that men and women contracted revealed no significant difference by gender and concluded that the disease characteristic that differs between men and women is the frequency and not the type of illness, injury, health care, or mortality.

Overall, the evidence about medical diagnosis suggests not so much overt gender-based discrimination (over and above baseline bias) as a complex segregation of men and women into different health care consumers, the sources of which remain to be illuminated.

Treatment

Women enter the health care system via their reproductive organs: Obstetricians and gynecologists are their primary care providers. However, Verbrugge and Wingard (1987) found that even when pre- and postnatal visits are not counted, women use more outpatient services than do men and are more likely to have a regular source of health care than are men. Excluding admissions related to reproduction, women between the ages of 15 and 64 are hospitalized more often than men in the same age bracket (although these hospitalization rates are reversed after 65 years of age). For many women, health care does emphasize the reproductive system to the exclusion of other aspects of their health, but women as a group use in- and outpatient services of all types more than do men.

Missing from this analysis is the fact that women are primary care providers for children and thus familiarize themselves with the medical waters on their families' behalf, whereas men tend to go to doctors only for their own treatment. For men, clinical offices and the hospital are more alien environments. For some mothers who work at home, a visit to a doctor or even a hospital means at least in part a break from the seclusion of child care or an interaction with another adult, perhaps a sympathetic and caring adult. For a man, however, a trip to a clinician or a hospital not only threatens his independence but promises only waiting, confrontation with a problem preferably denied, and humiliating procedures that may even cause pain and steal him away from the refuge of work or other pursuits felt to be more gender appropriate than admitting to illness.

Admission and Referral for Psychiatric Treatment. Early studies of psychiatric treatment found evidence of gender bias. In a study of hospitalization for psychosis, investigators suggested that males are more likely to be directed to psychiatric treatment at younger ages and stay institutionalized longer than females because social tolerance of mental illness in men is more limited than for women (Tudor, Tudor, & Gove, 1977). In a 1990 study of the psychiatric intake process, women outnumbered men at presentation. But men were again found to be more severely symptomatic and have more accompanying problems (comorbidity) at intake than women (Fabrega et al., 1990). Instead of bearing out Tudor's (Tudor et al., 1977) interpretation, the preponderance of females in the 1990 study may demonstrate society's unwillingness to tolerate even slight degrees of deviance in women. It found that women enter treatment earlier than do men and that men may not seek treatment until they are very ill. Women and men exhibited simple diagnostic conditions equally, but men exhibited higher degrees of social impairment associated with complex clinical conditions, including such accompanying disorders as substance abuse.

Psychiatric Therapy. Women are subject to discrimination in the provision of psychiatric services, for instance when facilities for them are inadequate. More drug and alcohol treatment is available to men than to women. Over 75% of drug treatment slots in state programs were filled by men in 1987 (Butynski & Canova, 1988). Treatment programs for men are better than those for women, and yet not only do women suffer alcohol problems of equal severity, but their lower social and economic supports necessitate comprehensive treatment programs that are currently unavailable to them (Lex, Teoh, Lagomasino, Mello, & Mendelson, 1990).

The therapeutic process itself is subject to sexism. Mitchell (1974) and others have observed that Freudian theory and practice, which constitutes a major body of the psychotherapeutic canon, is itself antiwoman. In the growth of the psychoanalytic literature since the turn of the century, a recurrent theme has been the association of neurosis with feminism: "Many twentieth-century psychiatrists and psychologists claimed that feminist aspirations either resulted from or led to neurosis" (Stage, 1979, p. 228).

Drug Therapy. Sexism also contaminates the prescription of medications. More women than men are prescribed mood-altering drugs. Cooperstock (1971) suggests that because Western women are permitted greater freedom in expressing feelings than are men, women are more inclined to bring their emotional problems to the attention of their physicians. Because most physicians are male and embrace certain expectations about female behavior and adjustment, they tend to determine that women are more in need of such drugs than their equally troubled but more reticent male patients.

Physicians may discount women's symptoms and attempt to reduce their complaints by prescribing psychotropic drugs (Verbrugge & Steiner, 1981, 1985). Waldron (1977) concluded that physicians felt that "doing something" to decrease a patient's presenting symptom is easier than helping her to remedy the personal/social conditions that may promote the symptoms in the first place.

The conditions that lead women more than men to use medicaments of all types still await full explication. The historical development of women as herbalists clearly arose from their role as family nurse and healer (Ehrenreich & English, 1973). An argument can be made that faith in pharmaceutical therapy is a logical association with what has been called women's culture—a culture of connection and mutual aid rather than the individualism associated with male culture. Women would be more likely to use drugs of all types, from diet pills to megavitamins, whereas men are more apt to be socialized to ignore or endure symptoms such as low energy, despondency, or overeating.

Surgery. By 1980, the hysterectomy had become the most frequently performed major operation for women of reproductive years. The American College of Obstetricians and Gynecologists estimated that 15% of hysterectomies were performed to remove cancer, 30% to remove noncancerous fibroids, 35% for pelvic relaxation or prolapse, and 20% for sterilization (Scully, 1980).

A hysterectomy should not be performed as an elective procedure or when more conservative treatment will suffice, and yet it has been estimated that one third of the hysterectomies and one half of the cesarean sections performed in the United States were unnecessary (Seaman, 1972). More than twice as many hysterectomies are performed in the United States than in England and Wales. American physicians are more aggressive—less apt to consult and geographically concentrated so that pursuit of work is heightened—and the U.S. fee-for-service payment method provides an incentive toward surgery (Bunker, 1970).

Fisher (1986) found evidence of such prevailing paternalism in women's encounters with gynecologists. She observed physicians encouraging women to have hysterectomies that were not medically warranted and at the same time failing to encourage women at high risk for cervical cancer to have Pap smears. Communication was controlled by the physicians, who used their institutionally based authority to cement the asymmetry in the patient-doctor imbalance of power, to which preexisting gender and class differences already contribute.

Gynecology was one of the first specialty areas to fall under the scrutiny of women's health care analysts. Other surgical specialties are now beginning to be studied, including cardiovascular surgery. Although the risk of developing coronary heart disease has increased for women and decreased for men since 1950, women are less likely to be referred promptly for cardiac surgical consultation than are men (Tobin et al., 1987). And when hospitalized for presumed coronary heart disease, women undergo fewer diagnostic and therapeutic interventions than do men (Ayanian & Epstein, 1991). These differences could mean that women are not receiving full benefit from the clinical advances in cardiology or that men are undergoing more coronary procedures than optimal. The researchers point out, however, that the differences in care may be unrelated to the state of the art in cardiology because similar gender differences have been found in patients with end-stage kidney disease with regard to dialysis and transplantation.

Long-Term Care. Women are the recipients of some and the providers of most long-term care. The U.S. population is aging as a whole; at the same time, individuals are living longer

(Pifer & Bronte, 1986). Older women outnumber older men: The gender ratio for persons aged 65 to 69 is 81:100, males to females. For persons 85 and older, the gender ratio grows to 39:100 (U.S. Bureau of the Census, 1990). Nursing home populations are overwhelmingly female. Of older nursing home residents, 80% are women (Siegel & Taeuber, 1986). But only some 5% of the elderly live in institutions. A significant proportion of the elderly population are defined as frail (having limitation in one or more activities of daily living). According to the 1982 National Long Term Care Survey, frail elderly get necessary assistance not from institutions or agencies but from family members and friends. These caregivers are overwhelmingly female (Stone, Cafferata, & Sangl, 1986).

Populations other than the elderly also need long-term care: those with chronic mental and physical illnesses, the developmentally delayed, and disabled persons of all ages. The AIDS epidemic has brought new populations into chronic care: HIV-positive children and adults. Grandmothers are the caregiving population with increasing responsibility for the care of their HIV-positive and drug- and alcohol-affected grandchildren (Browne, 1991; Gross, 1991; Harrell, 1991).

Clancy and Massion (1992) conclude that barriers to quality health care for women persist. Finances are an initial set of hurdles; because of low income or lack of health insurance, women are significantly less likely than men to receive needed health care. Despite recent increases in Medicaid benefits to women and children, for example, 14 million women of reproductive age have no health insurance; 5 million have coverage that excludes prenatal care and delivery. Middle-aged and older women also experience gender-based barriers. Compared to men, they are twice as likely to have no insurance, less likely to obtain insurance through employment, and if insured, pay higher premiums than do men. Medicare coverage is biased against women, with better coverage for acute illnesses, such as lung cancer, found more commonly in men and poorer coverage for chronic illnesses common to women, such as breast cancer and arthritis. The authors suggest that this policy-based pattern of discrimination is augmented by gender bias and bad habits in provider practice, producing fragmented and duplicate services for women.

Sexism and the Education of Health Professionals

Analyses of professional education materials as well as influential advertising directed toward health professionals demonstrate this continuing gender bias. Early work demonstrated inaccurate information in medical texts concerning such subjects as the strength of women's sexual drives, the roles of the vagina and clitoris in orgasm, and the incidence and prevalence of female sexual dysfunction (Scully & Bart, 1973). One text portrayed women as inherently sick and stated that the feminine core consists of masochism, passivity, and narcissism. At the same time, the text advised physicians to counsel their women patients to simulate orgasms if they were not orgasmic with their husbands.

The authors of *A New View of a Woman's Body* (Federation of Feminist Women's Health Centers, 1981) countered such pseudoscience with pioneering basic research on the anatomy and physiology of the clitoris. They found it to be a vital sexual organ whose very existence was omitted from medical texts. Careful dissection-based drawings of the penis had been executed since Leonardo da Vinci's time, but textbook illustrations of women's genitals frequently excluded the clitoris altogether.

Health care textbooks have benefited from careful criticism. The pernicious effect of language in reinforcing stereotypes about women is well demonstrated (Spender, 1980). Sexist language is evident in the continuing use of the masculine pronoun for physicians, even in nursing textbooks, and in descriptions of how women are thought to believe and act (Roland, 1977). Textbooks and advertisements aimed at gynecologists reinforced status and intellectual asymmetry between patients and doctors (Fisher, 1986). "By controlling women and their reproductive capacities," wrote Fisher, "medical domination functioned to sustain male domination" (p. 160).

Journal Advertising. The advertising that appears in professional journals, especially for pharmaceuticals, obviously is intended to influence clinicians. Women pictured in medical journal advertisements are more often portrayed as mentally ill than are men; men are portrayed as physicians more than women are (Stockburger & Davis, 1978). In ads for mood-modifying drugs, women are featured (pictures are used less often in ads for other categories of drugs). In a set of advertisements, portrayals of patients as well as professionals adhered to stereotypical gender roles (Mant & Darroch, 1975). In the use of misleading images of women to sell drugs to male physicians, medical advertising may reflect medical practice (Smith & Griffin, 1977). A study of medical and nursing journal advertisements found that nurses were consistently portrayed as "sex objects, ornaments and as handmaidens to physicians" (Aber & Hawkins, 1992, p. 289).

Sexism and Research on Women and Health

Like health care practice, health research has also been affected by gender-based bias and stereotype. All aspects of the research process may be influenced, including the conceptual frameworks that form the theoretical basis for research, the selection of problems for study, funding, the logistics of research methodology, and the conclusions drawn from the results.

Conceptual Frameworks. The conceptual frameworks guiding research about women have their own historical context—the times in which the studies were conducted as well as the contemporaneous academic orientations.

Social science research, for example, has been predicated on certain beliefs about the social structure (Gouldner, 1970) of the family, such as the perception that children should be raised in families in which men perform the active, doing, instrumental roles, whereas women perform the feeling, "expressive" roles (Parsons & Bales, 1955). The effects of such a normative conceptual framework are evident in psychoanalytic research, in which illness in women has been equated with rejection of culturally defined roles, such as losing interest in housework. It can also be seen in the family care literature, in which women are automatically assigned nurturing roles in situations as different as family therapy and cardiac rehabilitation. Although women's interest in the caregiving aspects of family life is assumed, their interest in other family issues—economic health, for example—is ignored. Studies on the stress of chronic illness care, for example, routinely ask for women's responses on expressive items, whereas instrumental aspects of family life, such as finances, are left unstudied.

Women's health research remains illness-oriented and concerns itself not with health but with pathology (Litt, 1992). Such normal events as lactation, childbirth, menstruation, menopause, and female sexual response have frequently been approached in the context of dysfunction or pathology.

Topics for Study. The problems chosen for research also reflect widely held assumptions about women. Central among society's assumptions regarding women is the inherent otherness of women; in this context, normal, positive physiological functions are seen as pathological. Most menstrual cycle studies, for example, were designed to detect the problems women experience because they menstruate—for example, a hypothesized propensity for violent crimes or accidents. The positive effects of menstruation have been the subject of very few studies.

Diseases primarily affecting men have traditionally received a large share of researchers' attention. Serious and costly conditions such as osteoporosis that affect women have long been neglected. Osteoporosis was not studied until recently, despite clear evidence that hip fracture—only one of the consequences of increased bone fragility—is a leading cause of hospitalization, surgery, and nursing home placement among older women.

Coronary heart disease (CHD) affects both men and women. In fact, CHD is a leading cause of death in women, surpassing deaths from the top three cancers: lung, breast, and colon. In 1989, the National Heart, Lung and Blood Institute, which has funded most of the clinical trials on heart disease, broke tradition by funding its first women-only study, the Postmenopausal Estrogen Progestin Intervention (PEPI) trial to study the effects of prescribed hormonal treatment on the risk of CHD in women (Stefanick, 1992).

The choice of study problems is obviously related to the research perspectives and tools available and popular at the moment. A biomedical orientation to research has emphasized specialization and an orientation to microcellular and molecular events. Concentration on these aspects of illness ignores the final object of study: the total organism. Sophisticated instrumentation and specialization in research areas promote science that examines only a fragment of the patient, male or female, rather than the person as a whole. New methodologies (especially qualitative approaches), interdisciplinary research teams, and expanded venues for publication and discussion might encourage research directed at women as totalities.

Funding. To the extent that such large funding sources as the National Institutes of Health allocate scarce resources for research programs, they define the nature of research about women.

The peer review process exerts at least an indirect influence as well. For example, the predominantly male composition of the study sections that review proposals for scientific merit and allocation of funding certainly influences the types of research funded. Were it not for the increasing visibility of women on these bodies it is likely that the biomedical approach and the traditional orientations toward women's health would have continued unchallenged.

The medical research community—funding agencies, study sections, research teams, faculties of major medical centers, and editorial boards of journals—is dominated by males (Sechrest, 1975). The National Institutes of Health (NIH), supported by the tax dollars of male and female citizens, has seen only 13% of its research funds go to study the health problems of women (Litt, 1992). Under recent pressure from Congress, the NIH has been mandated to include women in NIH-funded research and has established a special Office of Women's Health Research.

The research efforts of the largest single group of health care professionals—nurses—were not organizationally included in the NIH until 1986, when the National Center for Nursing Research was established. By far the smallest of the institutes, the nursing center received 39 million dollars in 1992, which enabled it to fund 222 research grants. In contrast, the National Cancer Institute was allocated 1.2 billion dollars for over 4,000 projects; and the Institute of Allergy and Infectious Disease more than 600 million dollars to fund 1773 projects (NIH Research Grants, fiscal year 1992). In 1993, the Center for Nursing Research became a full-fledged Institute.

Sampling and Informed Consent. Women are not the only group who may be coerced into participation in research studies, but they deserve special attention from prospective researchers in regard to issues of power and information. Sechrest (1975) was an early reporter on the coercion and power that can be applied to foster women's participation in research projects. She noted that early research on oral contraceptives took advantage of relatively uninformed and low-resource Puerto Rican women who found few options for avoiding pregnancy. Financial incentives or provision of free medical care for women and their children may also be irresistible elements in recruiting.

Data Analysis, Interpretation, and Conclusions. Woods (1992) has made it clear that helpful research on women's health will not come about from old wine in new bottles. She advocates for a reformulation of science, and clear views of women's experiences through lenses ground by women. This could include qualitative methods of analysis, which are reaching new levels of rigor and reproducibility. It could include interpretation of biological uniqueness as a sign of health rather than deviance or illness. Menopause, for example, could be characterized as a beginning rather than an end (Banner, 1992). And reformulated science could include designing research for, rather than on, women, with liberating rather than oppressive results.

> Simply adding a cohort of women to a study designed to illuminate issues grounded in thinking about men or increasing the proportion of women researchers in a male-dominated field will not solve the problem of advancing a more complete understanding of women's health. What is necessary is a reexamination of the nature of science that will foster a better understanding of the health of the many populations of women and serve emancipatory ends. (Woods, 1992, p. 1)

Women's Health Care: Issues and Arenas

Personal Health Services

A notable shift in health care over the last few decades has been from a traditionally authoritarian manner of delivering personal health services to a pluralistic array of clinicians, healers, and approaches to cure and care (Lowenberg, 1989). Moving over time from word-of-mouth to the Yellow Pages, services as diverse as acupuncture and music therapy are entering the everyday consumer vocabulary. Although the evolution of some models of women's personal health care delivery has been the result of humanistic movements within some of the professions, women themselves have had a profound influence on the structure of personal health services. In some instances, such as the increasing use of midwives among families in rural Utah, traditional modes of health care, often culturally linked, have come into wider use (Sakala, 1988). In other instances, women created new types of services, such as self-help clinics, menstrual extraction groups, and homebirth services provided by lay women. In some cases, professionals took over women's efforts, creating modified forms of personal health services that remain firmly under the control of professionals (e.g., the development and promotion of homelike birthing rooms in hospitals).

Ruzek (1978) described four models of health care: the traditional authoritarian, traditional egalitarian, traditional feminist, and radical feminist. At one end of the spectrum is traditional authoritarian health care, in which authority and decision making are the sole province of physicians. In this model, the doctor-patient relationship is active-passive; minimal medical information is shared with the patient. Tasks are clearly delineated, and rigid distinctions are maintained between categories of workers. Professionals monopolize access to curatives. Out of a concern for the professional's convenience rather than the patient's, professionals exercise exclusive control over the management of space and time. Professionals promote the myth of risk-free care and, out of an assumption that patients are unable to weigh the risks involved, do not encourage patients to make decisions about their own care. This type of patient-professional relationship can be seen in some public and private hospitals, clinics, and private physician practices.

At the other end of the continuum is the radical feminist world of health care. In self-help clinics and lay midwife-attended homebirths, women are encouraged and expected to be responsible for their own health care, and professionals are employed primarily as consultants. Knowledge about health is shared by all participants, and everyone, including professionals, is expected to learn from one another. The division of labor is less hierarchic, with each participant in a self-help group observing, advising, treating, and being treated. Women are encouraged to rely less on pharmaceuticals and to use curatives regarded as natural and low risk. Professional control over such devices as diaphragms is questioned; some self-help groups assist women in fitting diaphragms and provide instructions for their use. The turf of self-help groups is variable, and self-help clinic personnel tend to minimize the distinction between patient and practitioner in the allocation of time and space, as well as in knowledge and authority.

Health care settings such as self-help clinics arose from the women's health movement, which Marieskind (1975) described as a grassroots organization dating from about 1970. Drawing parallels to the popular health movement of the mid-19th century, Marieskind saw modern interest in women's health linked to activism for political gains for women. Just as the popular health movement was associated with gaining the vote for women, so this century's women's health movement has been linked to a progressive, feminist, political and economic agenda (Leavitt, 1984). Ruzek (1978) and Marieskind reported some common features of women's health movement organizations: reduction in hierarchy, changes in the profit-making orientation, increased use of lay workers, involvement of clients in their own care, and a commitment to a feminist ideology.

Morgen and Julier (1991) revisited a sample of organizations arising from the women's health movement to document development and change over the decades since the late 1960s. They mailed questionnaires to 144 women's health clinics and advocacy and/or education organizations. The 35% return rate ($N = 50$) is in itself an indication of the change these organizations have undergone. The authors reported that a significant number of questionnaires were returned undelivered, indicating that the organization was no longer in existence (the actual number was not reported). Three quarters of the responding organizations described themselves as focused on prevention or self-care; two thirds identified themselves as ideologically feminist. Commitment to low-income and minority women was high: A majority of the organizations served poor and minority women either in excess of or in direct proportion to the percentage of low-income and minority women in their communities. These characteristics conform to much of the original expressed intent of the women's health movement. In contrast to the organizational mission, the organizational structures have tended to change over the decades, from egalitarian staff models (pay, for example, in some women's health clinics was equal for all workers) to more traditional ranking of workers and from consensus to hierarchical decision making. Staff hiring, training, and development continue to reflect feminist principles, such as diversity and group solidarity. This study suggests that the women's health movement continues to influence the delivery of health services and that, not without struggle, alternatives to the health business-as-usual continue their work. Developments in both professional and community arenas reflect the continuing influence of the women's health movement.

Nurse Practitioners. The nurse practitioner movement represents an important addition to the pluralistic U.S. health care labyrinth. Developed in the late 1960s, nurse practitioners are nurses with advanced training in the diagnosis and treatment of minor, acute, and chronic illness. They have evolved much as their original planners hoped they would (Lynaugh, 1986): Nurse practitioners provide primary care equal to, and in some cases better than, that provided by physicians (Office of Technology Assessment, 1986; Perrin & Goodman, 1978). In a study comparing nurse practitioner and physician care of hypertensive patients, patients of nurse practitioners had significantly greater reductions in blood pressure and weight (Ramsay, McKenzie, & Fish, 1982). Nurse practitioners work with poor and underserved populations, concentrate on patient education and advocacy as well as diagnosis and treatment, and have gained a high level of consumer confidence (Draye & Stetson, 1975; Levine, Orr, Sheatsley, Lohr, & Brodie, 1978).

Community Leadership. The Boston Women's Health Book Collective and the National Black Women's Health Project are two examples of groups arising from communities that are defining their own health concerns and seeking alternatives to paternalistic care bestowed from on high.

Our Bodies, Ourselves is the Book Collective's (1971/1993) most famous publication and represents a revolutionary and collective effort by women to answer questions about health issues for themselves. Having started as a mimeographed booklet in 1971, it has evolved into a regularly revised softcover book that has sold millions of copies.

Billye Avery, founder of the National Black Women's Health Project, joined with women in southeastern communities to address their own health problems through self-help chapters, educational presentations, a national newsletter, and national and local media productions and conferences. "We've worked on everyone else's issues; it's time to work on ours" is one of their slogans.

Public Health Services

Although women are directly affected by personal health services, they are just as surely but less obviously affected by the public health system.

The mission of public health services is the surveillance and promotion of the health of all people in the United States. Health care in the United States is private business; the government is less involved here than in most other industrialized countries (Jonas, 1986). But some elements of the health care system are government controlled: Military health care, including the Veterans' Administration hospital system, and the Indian Health Service are two examples of publicly run personal health care delivery systems. Women's health issues confront these systems with problems as various as domestic violence on military bases to fetal alcohol syndrome prevention on Native American reservations.

Two major divisions of the U.S. Department of Health and Human Services administer health programs: the Public Health Service and the Health Care Financing Administration. The Public Health Service has five major agencies, including the National Institutes of Health and the Health Resources and Services Administration. The federal health programs are enormously complex, primarily the result of the lack of centralized, rational planning. Although some analysts find beneficial the continuous creation of new programs in response to public demand in that it maintains the health system's link to reality, others fear the changing political tides that ebb and flow in funding and support.

A prime example of the variability of public funding and governmental support is the recent history of family planning, including access to contraception and abortion services. Despite a worldwide population explosion and a national explosion in the number of teen pregnancies over the past three decades, federal funding for international family planning has decreased and access to abortion services has been curtailed.

States and localities offer a highly variable range of public health services, from widely accepted traditional public health services—such as vital statistics, communicable disease control, environmental sanitation, and public health education—to providing personal health services of last resort to the poor and such special groups as the chronically mentally ill and persons with AIDS. These services, too, ebb and flow with unreliable funding, often affecting the services available to needy women, such as the county well-baby clinic and the public health nurse.

International Concerns. Criticisms of the U.S. health system's shortchanging of women can be voiced on an international level as well. Habitual regard of women solely as reproductive organisms has pervaded the health policy of many nations. National and international health policies have often centered on only this function—from outlawing abortion under pronatalist regimes to coercive sterilization and contraception in countries with exploding populations. At both extremes, the voices of the women themselves are infrequently heard. Women's health advocates and activists have important responsibilities to foster public involvement and to monitor international health efforts in adult and child health, workplace health and safety, contraception, and access to abortion. The focus on reproduction—to the exclusion of other important issues such as job creation, providing market access for women growers, sponsoring credit and loan mechanisms to women—calls for continuing advocacy and the development of new priorities.

Health Policy

Although researchers and feminist authors have seriously addressed the problems women encounter in personal health service interactions, only recently have they begun to explore the connections between policy and women's health. Labor and pension policy has been shown to be closely related to the relative poverty of older women and their unmet long-term care needs (Stone, 1986). The long-term care vacuum in the United States has been shown to demand a substantial subsidy in time and money from women who are the majority of caregivers to the frail elderly (Ward, 1990a). The absence of child care and parental leave similarly have been shown to affect women's health and well-being (Hartmann & Spalter-Roth, 1987). Even the health of women in prison, and in particular the effects on offenders' children of the increasing incarceration rates for women, are new subjects for analysis (Applebome, 1992). The widespread changes in health policy predicted for the decades ahead will be important concerns for women.

National Health Insurance. A current health policy issue that embodies a number of women's concerns is national health insurance. In marked contrast to the rest of the industrialized world, the United States has never made health care available to its citizenry in the same manner in which public education, for example, is—a right for all. The advent of national health insurance in the United States has not been brought about by a change in political culture but by the economic bottom line—the expense of 35 million Americans without health insurance and the growing cost, especially to the business sector, of providing employer-based insurance to the rest. At this writing, many states have instituted or are developing statewide health plans—for example, Oregon, Minnesota, Vermont, Colorado, and New York.

This state-by-state approach to the problem of access to health care is apt to continue and will substantially affect women's health issues. Advocates for women's health must carefully assess state and federal health insurance proposals. Attention must be paid to issues such as the scope of services to be reimbursed. Benefits must not be limited to illness care; illness prevention and health promotion services—adult health screening, worksite health and safety, contraceptive services, pelvic examinations, breast exams, pregnancy and childbirth care—are especially important for women and the children they tend. A health insurance plan that limits the number of providers would adversely affect women who tend to use more than one clinician—for example, a midwife and a family practitioner. Current debates over employer-based (as opposed to residency-based) insurance plans also affect women. Women's employment patterns are different from men's, with more interruptions for family care—children, spouses, and parents all receive the majority of their care from their mothers, spouses, and daughters. Can employer-based insurance accommodate the employment interruptions women need? Women's health activists and advocates must be prepared to work at both the state and national levels to ensure that plans now being written for financing health care meet women's real needs (see Table 7.1)

Table 7.1 A Woman's Scorecard for National Health Insurance Plans

	Response	
	Yes	*No*
1. Will privacy and confidentiality be assured to women who participate?		
2. Will the national health insurance plan provide for the following well-woman services?		
a. Screening for common gynecological problems (e.g., Pap smears, breast examinations)		
b. Care during pregnancy		
c. Childbirth care		
d. Treatment for common gynecological problems (e.g., dysmenorrhea, vaginal infections, menopausal symptoms)		
3. Will the plan cover a range of family planning services?		
a. Basic family planning counseling		
b. Prescription devices, drugs, implants, or injectables		
c. Female and male sterilization		
d. Pregnancy termination		
e. Infertility services		
4. Does the plan allow for choices of health care providers?		
a. Nurse midwives		
b. Social workers		
c. Nurse practitioners		
d. Nutritionists		
e. Physical therapists		
5. Is the use of traditional physician services required?		
6. Will the woman who chooses more than one source of care (e.g., an internist and a nurse midwife) be penalized?		
7. Does the plan allow for alternatives to the traditional medical care system?		
a. Birthing centers		
b. Women's health care providers		
8. Will the plan provide coverage for women who work at home?		
a. Will lower benefits be provided for women who work at home?		
b. Will the coverage be more restrictive?		
9. Will coverage be contingent on marital status?		
a. Will the plan cover single women to the same extent as married women?		
b. Will national health insurance coverage be protected in case a married woman becomes separated or divorced?		
c. Must the woman remain in contact with her spouse to receive benefits?		

The Future

The personnel, institutions, research, and policies particular to women's health care will undoubtedly reflect the broad changes taking place in all of health care in the 1990s and beyond. If burgeoning health care costs are controlled so that profits in the lucrative health care business will be reduced, target incomes of clinicians may decrease, and the pool of applicants for health care training will change. The numbers of female physicians will increase. Pressure is also being applied for fewer specialists and more general clinicians. To meet the demand for primary care clinicians, workers such as nurse practitioners will see their numbers grow. The demand for nurses will continue, with increased pressure to place a variety of workers—some with shorter and less costly education—at the bedside. The demand for nursing aides and assistants will also be influenced by the aging of our population; in-home assistance is an as-yet underdeveloped segment of the health care industry. Training and supervision of in-home caregivers will pose new challenges for managers of public and private home care agencies. The movement of health care out of institutions into the home may add additional pressure for change already underway in the nature of patient/provider arrangements, a change from hierarchical to mutual relationships. But this shift may also institutionalize women's role as family health provider, a role made even more demanding in the face of competing demands from out-of-home work.

Institutional changes now occurring will affect women's health care: the demise of small and rural hospitals; a move from private, independent physicians practices to health maintenance organizations and other group practices; the growth in home health care. The role of public health departments in women's health is yet to be determined. Long the provider of specific services, such as treatment for sexually transmitted disease, health departments may expand their personal health services, especially to women and children. Pilot projects in which public health and school nurses are the neighborhood primary care clinicians may foretell a future community-based system of care, particularly in low-income neighborhoods. Nurses, the single largest group of health care professionals, yet often the group least represented at policy and planning levels, could be an important group of women workers called on to shape the health care systems for the future (Ward, 1990b).

Improvements such as the federal requirement for women's participation in federally funded research may foster knowledge of women's health in the previously male-dominated world of biomedical research. Increased awareness of women's health issues has led to policy changes as diverse as funding for breast cancer research and new light on sexual harassment in the workplace.

Many state governments have expanded their Medicaid programs to include women and children not otherwise insured for health care. In keeping with the incremental nature of social policy change in this country and a history of distributing welfare resources group by group, rather than universally, women and children will continue to be a group readily identified as worthy of guaranteed health care. As states work on their individual health insurance plans, the need to design dependable basic, minimum sets of primary care services will include identification of appropriate primary care services specific to women. This could include a call for increased attention to preventive services for women, with the design and implementation of well-woman care that extends beyond its current class and economic boundaries to low-income women and women of color. Long-term care will continue to be considered a financial black hole for public money; the growth of the private insurance industry's marketing of long-term care insurance will call for careful scrutiny by prospective women buyers (Quinn, 1992).

It remains to be seen whether the net outcome of a focus on women's health on women's terms will be the institutionalization of their values, the co-optation of their health-related activities, or a useful, if often strained, dialectic between women's critique of the health care system and the traditional institutions it decries. But the attitudinal changes brought about among patients and practitioners, the alterations wrought in modes of health care delivery, the continuing examination of sexism in illness care, reassessment of the use of drugs and devices, and the movement of women's issues into the nation's health agenda demonstrate a vital and enduring impact on American health care.

References

Aber, C. S., & Hawkins, J. W. (1992). Portrayals of nurses in advertisements in medical and nursing journals. *Image, 24*(4), 289-291.

American Psychiatric Association. (1987). *Diagnostic and statistical manual of mental disorders* (3rd ed., rev.). Washington, DC: Author.

Applebome, P. (1992, November 30). U.S. prisons challenged by women behind bars. *New York Times*, p. A7.

Aslin, A. L. (1977). Feminist and community mental health center psychotherapists' expectations of mental health for women. *Sex Roles, 3*(6), 537-544.

Ayanian, J. Z., & Epstein, E. M. (1991). Differences in the use of procedures between men and women hospitalized for coronary artery disease. *New England Journal of Medicine, 325*(4), 221-225.

Banner, L. (1992). *In full flower: Aging women, power, and sexuality.* New York: Knopf.

Boston Women's Health Book Collective. (1993). *The new our bodies, ourselves.* New York: Simon & Schuster. (Original work published 1971)

Broverman, I. K., Broverman, D. M., Clarkson, F. E., Rosenkrantz, P. S., & Vogel, S. R. (1970). Sex role stereotypes and clinical judgements of mental health. *Journal of Consulting and Clinical Psychology, 34*(1), 1-7.

Browne, G. (1991). Having to parent again. *Iceberg, 1*(3), 1, 6.

Bullough, V. L., & Bullough, B. (1982). *Health care for the other Americans.* New York: Appleton-Century-Crofts.

Bunker, J. (1970). Surgical manpower: A comparison of operations and surgeons in the United States and in England and Wales. *New England Journal of Medicine, 282*(3), 135-144.

Butynski, W., & Canova, D. M. (1988). Alcohol problem resources and services in state supported programs, FY1987. *Public Health Reports, 103*(6), 611-620.

Clancy, C. M., & Massion, C. T. (1992). American women's health care: A patchwork quilt with gaps. *JAMA, 268*(14), 1918-1920.

Cooperstock, R. (1971). Sex differences in the use of mood modifying drugs: An explanatory model. *Journal of Health and Social Behavior, 12,* 238-244.

Corea, G. (1977). *The hidden malpractice: How American medicine treats women as patients and professionals.* New York: William Morrow.

Crane, S., & Kaye, P. (1986). *Conflicts in medicine, economics, and human values: The American health care system* [Position paper for the Subgroup on Health Policies, General Assembly of the Presbyterian Church]. Unpublished manuscript.

Daly, M. (1978). *Gyn/ecology: The metaethics of radical feminism.* Boston, MA: Beacon.

Draye, M. A., & Stetson, L. A. (1975). The nurse practitioner as economic reality. *Nurse Practitioner, 1*(2), 60.

Ehrenreich, B., & English, D. (1973). *Witches, midwives, and nurses: A history of women healers.* Old Westbury, NY: Feminist Press.

Ehrenreich, B., & English, D. (1978). *For her own good: 150 years of the experts advice to women.* New York: Anchor.

Fabrega, H., Mezzich, J., Ulrich, R., & Benjamin, L. (1990). Females and males in an intake psychiatric setting. *Psychiatry, 53*(2), 1-16.

Federation of Feminist Women's Health Centers. (1981). *A new view of a woman's body.* New York: Touchstone.

Fisher, S. (1986). *In the patient's best interest.* New Brunswick, NJ: Rutgers University Press.

Gouldner, A. (1970). *The coming crisis of Western sociology.* New York: Avon.

Gross, J. (1991, April 14). Help for grandparents caught up in drug war. *New York Times,* p. 12.

Harrell, D. C. (1991, February 26). Seniors bringing up juniors. *Seattle Post Intelligencer,* p. C1.

Hartmann, H., & Spalter-Roth, R. M. [Institute for Women's Policy Research]. (1987, October 29). *Costs to women and their families of childbirth and lack of parental leave.* Testimony before the Subcommittee on Children, Families, Drugs and Alcoholism, Committee on Labor and Human Resources, U.S. Senate.

Health Grants and Contracts Weekly [newsletter]. (1991, December 9). Alexandria, VA: Capitol Publications.

Himmelstein, D. U., & Woolhandler, S. (1989). A national health program for the United States. *New England Journal of Medicine, 320*(2), 102-108.

Hsiao, W. C., Braun, P., Dunn, D., & Becker, E. (1988). Resource-based relative values: An overview. *JAMA, 260,* 2347-2353.

Jonas, S. (1986). *Health care delivery in the United States.* New York: Springer.

Leavitt, J. W. (1984). *Women and health in America.* Madison: University of Wisconsin Press.

Lennane, K. J., & Lennane, R. J. (1973). Alleged psychogenic disorders in women: Possible manifestations of sexual prejudice. *New England Journal of Medicine, 288*(6), 288-292.

Levine, J. I., Orr, S. T., Sheatsley, D. W., Lohr, J. A., & Brodie, B. M. (1978). The nurse practitioner: Role, physician utilization, patient acceptance. *Nursing Research, 27,* 245-254.

Lex, B. W., Teoh, S. K., Lagomasino, I., Mello, N. K., & Mendelson, J. H. (1990). Characteristics of women receiving mandated treatment for alcohol or polysubstance dependence in Massachusetts. *Drugs and Alcohol Dependence, 25*(1), 13-20.

Litt, I. F. (1992). Letter from the director. *Stanford University Institute for Research on Women and Gender Newsletter, 16*(2), 1.

Lowenberg, J. S. (1989). *Caring and responsibility: The crossroads between holistic practice and traditional medicine.* Philadelphia, PA: University of Pennsylvania Press.

Lynaugh, J. (1986). The nurse practitioner: Issues in practice. In M. D. Mezy & D. O. McGivern (Eds.), *Nurses, nurse practitioners* (pp. 137-145). Boston: Little, Brown.

Mant, A., & Darroch, D. B. (1975). Media images and medical images. *Social Science and Medicine, 9,* 613-618.

Marieskind, H. I. (1975). The women's health movement. *International Journal of Health Services, 5*(2), 217-223.

Marte, C., & Anastos, K. (1990). Women—the missing persons in the AIDS epidemic. *Health/PAC Bulletin, 20*(1), 11-18.

McCranie, E. W., Horowitz, A. J., & Martin, R. M. (1978). Alleged sex-role stereotyping in the assessment of women's physical complaints: A study of general practitioners. *Social Science and Medicine, 12*(2A), 111-116.

Mitchell, J. (1974). *Psychoanalysis and feminism.* New York: Random House.

Morgen, S., & Julier, A. (1991). *Women's health movement organizations: Two decades of struggle and change.* Eugene, OR: University of Oregon, Center for the Study of Women in Society.

Office of Technology Assessment. (1986). *Nurse practitioners, physician assistants, and certified nurse midwives: A policy analysis* (Health Technology Case Study 37, OTA-HCS-37). Washington, DC: Government Printing Office.

Parsons, T., & Bales, R. F. (1955). *Family socialization and interaction process.* Glencoe, IL: Free Press.

Perrin, E., & Goodman, H. (1978). Telephone management of acute pediatric illness. *New England Journal of Medicine, 298,* 130-135.

Pifer, A., & Bronte, L. D. (1986). Squaring the pyramid. *Daedulus, 115*(1), 1-12.

Quinn, J. B. (1992, April 20). Policies for old-age care. *Newsweek,* p. 61.

Ramsay, J. A., McKenzie, J. K., & Fish, D. G. (1982). Physicians and nurse practitioners: Do they provide equivalent care? *American Journal of Public Health, 72*(1), 55-57.

Roland, C. G. (1977). The insidious bias of medical language. *Nursing Digest, 5*(1), 53-55.

Ruzek, S. B. (1978). *The women's health movement: Feminist alternatives to medical control.* New York: Praeger.

Sakala, C. (1988). Content of care by independent midwives: Assistance with pain in labor and birth. *Social Science and Medicine, 26*(11), 1141-1158.

Scully, D. (1980). *Men who control women's health.* Boston: Houghton Mifflin.

Scully, D., & Bart, P. (1973). A funny thing happened on the way to the orifice: Women in gynecology textbooks. *American Journal of Sociology, 78,* 1045-1050.

Seaman, B. (1972). *Free and female.* Greenwich, CT: Fawcett.

Sechrest, L. (1975). Ethical problems in medical experimentation involving women. In V. Olesen (Ed.), *Women and their health: Research implications for an era* (DHEW HRA 77-3138). Washington, DC: Department of Health Education and Welfare.

Siegel, J. S., & Taeuber, C. M. (1986). Demographic perspectives on the long-lived society. *Daedulus, 115*(1), 77-117.

Smeltzer, C., & Whipple, B. (1991). Women and HIV infection. *Image, 23*(4), 249-256.

Smith, M. C., & Griffin, L. (1977). Rationality of appeals used in the promotion of psychotropic drugs: A comparison of male and female models. *Social Science and Medicine, 11,* 409-414.

Spender, D. (1980). *Man made language.* London: Routledge & Kegan Paul.

Stage, S. (1979). *Female complaints: Lydia Pinkham and the business of women's medicine.* New York: Norton.

Stefanick, M. L. (1992). Postmenopausal hormone replacement and cardiovascular disease. *Stanford University Institute for Research on Women and Gender Newsletter, 16*(2), 2-3.

Stockburger, D. W., & Davis, J. O. (1978). Selling the female image as mental patients. *Sex Roles, 4*(1), 131-134.

Stone, R. (1986). *The feminization of poverty and older women.* Rockville, MD: National Center for Health Services Research and Health Care Technology Assessment.

Stone, R., Cafferata, G. L., & Sangl, J. (1986). *Caregivers of the frail elderly: A national profile.* Rockville, MD: National Center for Health Services Research and Health Care Technology Assessment, Division of Intramural Research.

Tobin, J. N., Wassertheil-Smoller, S., Wexler, J. P., Steingart, R. M., Budner, N., Lense, L., & Wachspress, J. (1987). Sex bias in considering coronary artery surgery: Evidence for referral bias. *Annals of Internal Medicine, 107*(1), 19-25.

Tudor, W., Tudor, J., & Gove, W. (1977). The effect of sex role differences on the social control of mental illness. *Journal of Health and Social Behavior, 18,* 98-112.

U.S. Bureau of the Census. (1990). *Statistical abstract of the United States: 1990* (110th ed.). Washington, DC: Government Printing Office.

Verbrugge, L. M. (1986). From sneezes to adieux: Stages of health for American men and women. *Social Science and Medicine, 22*(11), 1195-1212.

Verbrugge, L. M., & Steiner, R. P. (1981). Physician treatment of men and women—Sex bias or appropriate care? *Medical Care, 19,* 609-632.

Verbrugge, L. M., & Steiner, R. P. (1985). Prescribing drugs to men and women. *Health Psychology, 4*(2), 79-98.

Verbrugge, L. M., & Wingard, D. L. (1987). Sex differentials in health and mortality. *Women & Health, 12*(2), 103-143.

Waldron, I. (1977). Increased prescribing of valium, librium, and other drugs: An example of the influence of economic and social factors on the practice of medicine. *International Journal of Health Services, 7*(1), 91-94.

Walker, L. E. (1987). Inadequacies of the masochistic personality disorder diagnosis for women. *Journal of Personality Disorders, 1*(2), 183-189.

Ward, D. (1990a). Gender, time, and money in caregiving. *Scholarly Inquiry for Nursing Practice, 4*(3), 223-236.

Ward, D. (1990b). National health insurance: Where do nurses fit? *Nursing Outlook, 38*(5), 206-207.

Woods, N. F. (1992). Future directions for women's health research. *NAACOG's Women's Health Nursing Scan, 6*(5), 1-2.

8

Frameworks for Nursing Practice With Women

NANCY FUGATE WOODS

The frame of reference we use in delivering health care, if not in everyday living, influences how we think and what we do. Over the last three decades, there has been steadily increasing encouragement for clinicians to specify the frame of reference that guides how we deliver services to people and conduct inquiry, and educators have exposed their students to several theoretical orientations for nursing. Indeed, nursing has an identifiable metaparadigm that undergirds much of its theoretical writings. In this chapter, we will explore how that metaparadigm guides our thinking about women and the notions we have about their health care. We will begin with a discussion of feminism and feminist theory and inquiry as background against which to consider concepts central to nursing practice: the person, environment, health, and nursing. We will conclude by considering new models for health care for and with women that are informed by feminist perspectives.

Feminism and Feminist Theory

Feminism

The word *feminism* stimulates a variety of responses reflecting confusion and lack of awareness of the large body of feminist theory. It is not uncommon to find women and men who insist they are not "feminists" yet they advocate feminist agendas. For some, feminism conveys threatening images of a social order in which everything is different from the status quo. For others, feminism conveys promising images of a social order in which women and men would have political, economic, and social rights that are equal. Feminism, as it is currently defined, includes not only equality for women with men but changes in our social reality that some argue are linked to the possibility that earthly life can go on in the future. Indeed, Dinnerstein (1989) says that the question for women is "what kind of public power we want to share: the kind that is killing the world or the kind that is focussed on keeping the world alive" (p. 16). In linking feminism not only to change in our uses of gender but also to our reversal of our involvement in nuclear and ecological disaster, Dinnerstein points out the need for feminist survival activists who are concerned with more than equality with men. Today, feminists need to be concerned with rapid change: changes in which women become responsible for their self-creation and responsible for the preservation of the ecosphere—focusing their energy on protection of the life web for future generations.

Feminist Theory

Just as there is a range of definitions of feminism, there are many feminist theories or perspectives. Each attempts to describe women's oppression, explain its causes and consequences, and prescribe strategies for women's liberation. Some of the perspectives include liberal, Marxist, radical, psychoanalytic, socialist, existentialist, and postmodern feminist theory. Tong (1989) has reviewed how each offers a partial and provisional answer to the "woman question," each with its own perspective and implications for method.

Liberal Feminism. Liberal feminism is exemplified in works such as Mary Wollstonecraft's (1975) *A Vindication of the Rights of Woman* and John Stuart Mill's (1970) *On the Subjection of Women.* The work of the National Organization of Women in support of equal rights for women reflects contemporary liberal feminism. Central to the beliefs of liberal feminists is the assumption that women's subordination is rooted in customary and legal constraints blocking women's entrance and or success in the so-called public world. Because society has viewed women as being less important than men, women have been excluded from many arenas of public life. Liberal feminists advocate gender justice, making gender equity replace the politics of exclusion (Tong, 1989).

Marxist Feminism. Marxist feminists, exemplified in some of Angela Davis's (1981, 1989) works, believe it is impossible for anyone, especially a woman, to obtain genuine equal opportunity in a class society in which wealth is produced by many powerless for a powerful few. Tracing their works to Engels, Marxist feminists assert that women's oppression originates in introduction of private property. To eradicate women's oppression, Marxist feminists advocate replacing capitalism with a socialist system. In this new system, the means of production would belong to everyone, and women would no longer be economically dependent on men (Tong, 1989).

Radical Feminism. Radical feminists, as exemplified by Mary Daly (1978), Andrea Dworkin, Gena Corea, and Shulamith Firestone, believe the patriarchal system oppresses women. They advocate that a system characterized by power, dominance, hierarchy, and competition cannot be reformed but must be eradicated. It would not be sufficient to replace the legal and political structure. Social and cultural institutions, especially the family, the church, and the academy (academic institutions), would need to be replaced. Some radical feminists question the concept of "natural order" in which men are "manly" and women "womanly." Their goal is to overcome whatever negative effects this thinking about biology as destiny has had on women and men. Radical feminists assert that biology is not the only source of women's oppression; so are gender (masculinity, femininity) and sexuality (heterosexuality, homosexuality). Most radical feminists focus on ways in which gender and sexuality have been used to subordinate women to men. They support reproductive rights as a means of enhancing women's choices. Some advocate escaping the confines of heterosexuality through celibacy, autoeroticism, or lesbianism, emphasizing acceptance of women's own desires.

Psychoanalytic Feminism. Psychoanalytic feminist theorists believe that the centrality of sexuality arises out of Freudian theory and concepts, such as the Oedipus complex. Chodorow (1978, 1989) and Dinnerstein (1976, 1989) exemplify psychoanalytic feminist thought. Central to their work is the assumption that the root of women's oppression is embedded deeply within her psyche. These theorists recommend dual parenting and dual participation in the workforce as a means of solving women's oppression.

Existentialist Feminism. Work in this tradition is exemplified by Simone de Beauvoir's work, *The Second Sex* (1949). A central assumption is that women are oppressed by "otherness." In other words, women are oppressed because they are not men but the "other." Women's meaning is defined by men. These theorists assert that if woman is to become a self she must transcend the definitions, labels, and essences that limit her existence.

Socialist Feminism. Socialist feminist theory is exemplified in works such as Juliet Mitchell's (1971) *Woman's Estate* and Nancy Hartsock's (1983) *Money, Sex and Power.* Tong (1989) suggests that this group has woven together several strands of feminist theory. Socialist feminists assert that women's conditions are overdetermined by structures of production (from Marxist feminism), socialization of children (from liberal feminism), and reproduction and sexuality (from radical feminism). They believe that women's status and functions must be changed in all these structures. In addition, a woman's interior world must also be transformed (from psychoanalytic feminism), to be liberated from patriarchal thought that undermines her confidence (as emphasized by the existential feminists). Allison Jaggar pointed out the interrelationship of forms of women's oppression, emphasizing the concept of alienation: Under capitalism, everything (sex, work, and play) and everyone (family, friends) that could be a source of integration becomes a source of disintegration (Jaggar & Rothenberg 1984). Most socialist feminists maintain that only complex explanations can account for women's subordination and emphasize integration of women's lives and the usefulness of a unified feminist theory.

Postmodern Feminist Theory. Postmodern theorists challenge the existence and adequacy of a single specifically feminist standpoint. They assert that a synthesis of multiple theories is neither feasible nor desirable. Instead, they advocate that because women are many and not one, feminisms should be many and not one. Postmodern feminists emphasize differences such as those occurring at the intersections of gender, race, and class. Their orientation involves no single standpoint but several perspectives that can account for the experiences of difference: Black women's experiences are not white women's experiences. Recent works about black women challenge us to think about the specific life experiences of women and consequences for their well-being (Collins, 1989a, 1989b, 1991; Davis, 1981, 1989; Dill 1983, 1987; Gillespie, 1984; Gordon-Bradshaw, 1987; Herman, 1984; hooks, 1984; Lorde, 1984a, 1984b, 1988a, 1988b; B. Smith, 1982). Work about Hispanic women (Anzaldua, 1987; Apodaca 1977; Chavez, Cornelius, & Jones 1986; del Portillo, 1987; Ginorio & Reno, 1985; Hurtaldo, 1989; Moraga, 1983, pp. 90-144; Moraga & Anzaldua, 1983; Sanchez, 1984; Sanchez-Ayendez, 1989; Segura, 1989) Asian American (Chow, 1987; Tsutakawa, 1988) and Native American women (Hale, 1985; Witt, 1984) provide powerful accounts of issues central to women's lives, illustrating points of difference that may help account for health experiences.

Perspectives for Inquiry

Awareness of the multiple feminist theories provides a useful analytic schema for those interested in understanding women's lives and promoting women's health. Feminist theoretical orientations have influenced the process of inquiry about women and women's health. Some have asked what are the consequences of these theories for inquiry? What is a feminist research perspective? What are the consequences of a feminist perspective for health research or for knowledge about women's health? Is there a feminist method? If so, what is it? If not, is it sufficient simply to add women to research to answer feminist criticisms? Answers to these questions can influence development of research agendas for nursing and other health-related sciences, knowledge about women's health and policies regarding women's health care, and models for delivery of nursing and other types of health care.

Just as there is no single feminist theory, there is no single feminist method. As a basis for considering what feminist science is, Harding (1987) emphasized the interrelationship of method, methodology, and epistemology. *Method* refers to techniques for gathering evidence, such as by listening, observing, and examining historical traces. In contrast, *methodology* refers to the theory and analysis of how research should proceed. *Epistemology* refers to issues about what is adequate theory of knowledge and strategies that are acceptable for justification of a theory. Epistemological issues concern who can be a knower, what tests must be passed to legitimize knowledge, and what types of things can be known. Epistemological concerns are exemplified in the concern about whether subjective truth counts as knowledge.

Feminists claim that mainstream science had its origins in a masculine voice; that the history of science emerged from dominant gender, class, and racial groups; and that women have not been regarded as legitimate knowers. Most feminists would assert that adding women—as scientists, as participants in studies, and as contributors to knowledge—is not enough. Instead, contemporary feminist theorists have recommended new directions for the conduct of research.

Although concern for feminist methodology is relatively new in nursing science, MacPherson's (1983) recommendations and McBride and McBride's (1982) consideration of new paradigms for nursing research initiated early discussion of a topic that has persisted in our literature. Duffy (1985); Duffy and Hedin (1988); Campbell and Bunting (1991); Hall and Stevens (1991); Allen, Allman, and Powers (1991); and Parker and McFarlane (1991), among others, have contributed to a growing understanding of feminist research and its possibilities in nursing.

Origin of the Questions for Feminist Researchers

Contemporary feminists advocate finding new empirical and theoretical resources in women's lived experiences. They emphasize the importance of the origins of scientific "problems" or research questions. They believe the questions asked are at least as important as the answers to those questions. In a context of discovery (theory development) versus justification (theory testing), concern for the origin of the question is particularly important. Questions grounded in men's experiences as the norm are not likely to illuminate the nature of women's experiences. Moreover, questions not grounded in women's lived experiences are not likely to generate knowledge *for* women and probably do not generate valid knowledge *about* women (Duffy & Hedin, 1988; Klein, 1983).

Feminist researchers identify problems from the perspective of women's experiences, recognizing that there is no single woman's experience. That is, class, race, and culture must be considered within considerations of gender. Women's fragmented identities, such as African American feminist or Japanese American feminist, give rise to partial perspectives that allow a researcher to see phenomena from a viewpoint that is limited (Campbell & Bunting, 1991; Haraway, 1988).

In addition, feminist researchers are concerned with ways to change conditions rather than with merely discovering truth. It is not enough to describe women's oppression; it is also important to change the conditions that create and sustain it. This concern gives legitimacy to an action component as part of the research process, a concern for praxis as part of the research process. It follows that researchers should concern themselves with questions that women want answered (Lather, 1991).

Purposes of Feminist Science

The purposes of feminist science are to provide information *for* women rather than merely about women. The goal is seeking explanations for women that are liberating, that have the capacity to be used by women for women's good. Moreover, feminist researchers are explicit about their purpose, enhancing the well-being of women through providing information that has the possibility to be helpful to women themselves. They are also explicit about their politics, asserting the value systems that undergird their science rather than maintaining the pretense of objectivity.

Nature of the Subject Matter

The nature of the subject matter for feminist researchers may not differ dramatically from that concerning researchers with nonfeminist perspectives. Studying women is not new. Studying women from the perspective of their own experiences so that women can understand themselves and their world is a novel aspect of feminist research. For example, studying gender as a social construction rather than studying gender as a biological absolute illustrates an important distinction in feminist and nonfeminist research perspectives (Campbell & Bunting, 1991).

"Studying up" as well as "studying down" is both legitimate and necessary. For example, nurses cannot merely study the behavior of their women clients; to have more than a partial perspective of a phenomenon, it is also important for women to study nurses' behavior. A researcher is a situated knower, that is, an individual who can have only a partial perspective of a problem. Only through multiple perspectives can multiple truths inform a topic. A woman seeking health care, a nurse, and a biostatistician are each able to contribute a different, but partial, perspective on the problem. Together, these individual and partial perspectives do not constitute a whole but contribute a more complete understanding of the topic (Haraway, 1988).

Methods and Methodology

Harding (1987) suggested that it is the purpose of the inquiry, the alternative hypotheses being considered, and the relationship between the researcher and the person participating in the research that make feminist research distinctive. Because the frame of reference for women is relational and contextual, qualitative research methods often have been identified with feminist research (see MacPherson, 1983; McBride & McBride, 1982). Yet methods such as observation and listening are not bound to a certain philosophical stance: Methods do not drive the assumptions grounding the research. Although debates over appropriately feminist methods are likely to continue in nursing and other sciences, there are some common dimensions underlying the search for an appropriate methodology for feminist research. These grow from an understanding of epistemology in feminist theory (Campbell & Bunting, 1991).

Feminist researchers recognize the validity of women's perceptions as truth for them (Campbell & Bunting, 1991). Women are regarded as a legitimate source of knowledge, capable of telling about and reflecting on their own experiences. Women, themselves, then, are the appropriate participants in research about and for women.

Research participants are experts on their own lived experiences. Methods of inquiry that involve eliciting women's own perceptions about their experiences and their health yield appropriate information for feminist inquiry (Campbell & Bunting, 1991).

Because knowledge is relational, contextual research methods that acknowledge and reflect the importance of interrelationship between history and contemporary observations are essential. Moreover, both historical and concurrent events should be considered in designing, conducting, and interpreting research endeavors (Campbell & Bunting, 1991).

Boundaries between the personal and public or political spheres are artificial. Sharp dichotomies and boundaries should be carefully scrutinized in research involving women (and all humans). What is regarded as a personal problem may also be understood as a social or political problem (Campbell & Bunting, 1991).

Relationships between researchers and participants in studies should be nonhierarchical. *Participants* is an appropriate term to describe individuals who are actively engaged in studies. Indeed, the researchers can think of themselves as participants in a cooperative effort in which the researcher's role is helping produce knowledge that will be useful to the participants (Campbell & Bunting, 1991).

Interpretations of the data and conclusions by the researcher are validated by the participants and shared with them for their own use. Because the goal of the research is producing knowledge that will benefit the participants, they have a stake in interpreting the results (Campbell & Bunting, 1991).

Analyses

Cultural beliefs and behaviors shape the results of our analyses and interpretations. Paradoxically, introducing the subjective element into the analyses enhances the objectivity of the research by revealing to the public the point of view of the investigator. Reflexivity as a methodological feature involves looking at oneself as the researcher and examining one's own position and values relative to the participants in a study. Some recommend that researchers identify their age, ethnicity, and feminist stance in publications of their works (Reinharz, 1983).

Feminist researchers have suggested use of specific criteria for judging the adequacy of the analysis. We can ask the following:

1. Are women's experiences used as the test of adequacy of problems, concepts, hypotheses, research design, data collection, and interpretation?
2. Does the research project compare women with men or institutions that men control?
3. Does the researcher or theorist place herself in the same class, race, culture, and gender-sensitive critical plane as the people being studied?

Feminist Perspectives for Nursing Practice

Feminist perspectives for nursing practice mirror some of the major assumptions undergirding the family of feminist theories. Moreover, feminist perspectives point to the need to redefine the concepts central to nursing's conceptual models for practice. The metaparadigm reflected in most of nursing's theoretical works includes the concepts of the person, environment, health, and nursing. In the following discussion, we will explore each of these concepts as the basis for proposing a feminist model for nursing practice.

Person

In most theoretical formulations, the person who receives nursing care is central. Usually the person is conceived of as an individual as opposed to a member of a group of persons, family, or community. The most consistent view of the person emphasizes wholeness. Some conceive of wholeness or holism as meaning that the person is a bio-psycho-social-spiritual organism whose environment can be manipulated to maintain or promote health. The person is more than and different from the sum of her or his parts. Still others assert that the person and environment are inseparable: Considering the individual in isolation from the context is not possible (Chinn & Jacobs, 1987; Parse, 1987).

Feminist writings about women mirror many dimensions of contemporary nursing theorists' concepts of person. In fact, many revisionist accounts of women's development emphasize the importance of understanding women in the context of their social environments. Concepts of self, role, and body frequently appear in feminist writings about women's health. Consideration of these concepts as they inform nursing practice with women follows.

Self and Role. Self-in-relation theory, a product of thinkers such as Jean Baker Miller (1986), Nancy Chodorow (1989), and Carol Gilligan (1982) defines a woman's orientation to her relationships as a central, positive aspect of development beyond childhood. This body of theory emphasizes the differences between women and men in the strengths and vulnerabilities that develop out of their relational contexts and the norms that regulate their lives. A woman's concept of self is a relational self, one that exists in a web of relationships with others. Social intimacy organizes her experiences. Most women experience interdependence, not autonomy and separation, as is emphasized in theories about men's development.

Differentiation for women occurs within these ongoing relationships throughout life. Creativity, autonomy, competence, and self-esteem develop in a relational context. Indeed, relationships are essential for well-being and healthy development (Miller, 1986; Surrey, 1985). Development of a more complex sense of self in an increasingly complex web of relationships to others is the result (Miller, 1986). Developmental failure occurs not as a result of a failure to separate but as the result of a failure to remain connected while asserting a distinct sense of self (Gilligan, 1977). Indeed, Gilligan suggests that the relational self is foundational to a morality grounded in an ethic of care (Gilligan, 1982).

The dilemma for women arises from our social contexts. Women are simultaneously pushed to define themselves through relationships in a society that views orientation to relationships as a sign of dependence or immaturity and that values achievement over affiliation (Jack, 1987).

Body. At the same time that feminist theorists have constructed new visions of the self, they have considered the problems of "the body." Women have lived with the consequences of "biology as destiny" ideology. Their possibilities as humans have been defined by society's beliefs about what women can and should do based on their reproductive capacities. Biological essentialism refers to the assumption that the essence of a woman is her body and its bodily functions. Although feminists reject the assumptions of biological essentialism, some feminist theorists have focused on biological difference and women's reproductive roles without reducing women to an identity with their bodies. Insisting that gender differences are socially constructed, some have pointed out that women's perceptions of their bodies are culturally controlled. Throughout history, women have been considered to be ruled by their bodies, bodies that are seen as inherently unstable and weak. Biological difference has been and still is used to justify the subjugation of women.

Scheper-Hughes and Lock (1987) consider "three bodies": the individual body, referring to the lived experience of the body-self; the social body, referring to the representational uses of the body as a symbol with which to think about nature, society, and culture; and the body politic, referring to the regulation, surveillance, and control of bodies (individual and collective) in reproduction, sexuality, work and leisure, sickness, and other forms of human difference. The Cartesian legacy of separateness of the body and mind persists in health sciences literature about women. Separation of the self and the body, if not alienation of the body from the self, appears in women's descriptions of menstruation, menopause, labor, and birthing. Women describe these experiences as "something that happens to you," not as "something you do" (Martin, 1987). Women's conversations about their bodies reveal their beliefs that "your body needs to be controlled by your self" and that "your body sends you signals." This fragmentation and alienation in women's concepts of body and self link the notions that women have of their bodies to the social body and the body politic: Women's bodies have come to symbolize something that is separate from their person. The body politic has constructed ideas about women's bodies that allow them to be regulated in ways that disregard their attachment to personhood. Restricting attention to the nature of women's bodies, for example, by locating women's problems *in* their bodies, has served to deflect attention from the broader sociopolitical environments influencing women's health.

Environments

Women's environments are multidimensional, despite the fact that many nurse theorists restrict their concepts of environment to the immediate surroundings of the hospitalized individual (Chinn & Jacobs, 1987). Beginning with Nightingale's conception of the environment as the origin of health and health problems, nurse theorists focused on dimensions of the physical environment, such as air and water quality, cleanliness, and light. Over time, these concerns gave way to concern with the social environment and how it required adaptation if not accommodation of the individual.

Chopoorian (1986) points out that focusing almost exclusively on the adaptation of individuals to their environments has excluded concern for persons or groups who refuse to accommodate to their environments that present intolerable or unacceptable social, political, or economic circumstances. She encouraged analysis of the environment as a social, political, and economic world that influences both well-being of clients and nursing practice. She urged stretching beyond a concept of environments as client relationships to a conception of environments along dimensions of social, political, and economic structures producing class relationships, economic policies, and ideologies such as sexism, ageism, racism, and classism, all with the power to influence health (Chopoorian, 1986).

One consequence of nursing's limited view of environments is that persons must adjust, assimilate, or accommodate and that nurses support them in the process. Persons, not societal structures or institutions, are seen as the focus for change or adaptation. For example, when women are considered as members of a family, from a family systems perspective, emphasis is often on what is adaptive for the family system rather than for the individual woman (Allen, 1986). New works, such as those on women's friendships by Raymond (1986), provide evidence of women's ability to create socially supportive environments. Works of ecofeminists, encouraging women to renew their ties to the earth, link women to the life of the planet (Schuster, 1990).

Chopoorian (1986) urged nurses to assume activist roles, diagnosing and treating the root of health problems rather than human responses to them. Beginning by reconceptualizing the environment as social, political, and economic structures; social relationships; and everyday life, nurses would extend their arenas for intervention beyond the boundaries of health care institutions.

Chopoorian's urging to consider multiple dimensions of environments for human health is consistent with many feminist theories that link women's lives to social, political, and economic structures as context. Moreover, the emphasis on social relationships, including domination, power, and authority within organizations and families, leads one to examine exploitation of women and other forms of sexism and their relationships to women's health. Finally, emphasis on understanding everyday life for women and its meaning is consistent with feminist conceptions of the importance of women's lived experience.

Health

Health is another concept central to nursing's metaparadigm, a concept with many meanings. Judith Smith (1981) identified four models of health from published literature: the eudaemonistic, adaptive, role performance, and clinical models. The eudaemonistic model connotes exuberant well-being and the ability to actualize the self, whereas the adaptive model connotes health as flexible adjustment to the environment and the ability to cope with stressful events. The role performance model emphasizes health as performance of one's socially defined roles and the ability to engage in activities of daily living at an expected level. The clinical model emphasizes health as the absence of disease, symptoms, or bad feelings as well as the absence of need for medical care.

In spite of decades of research on women's health, there is no consensus on a definition of women's health to guide scientists and clinicians in their work. The U.S. Public Health Service Task Force on Women's Health Issues (1985) defined women's health issues from a statistical standpoint, including those "areas where circumstances for women are unique, the noted condition is more prevalent, the interventions are different for women than for men, or the health risks are greater for a woman than for a man" (p. 6). McBride and McBride (1982) examined the concept of women's health as it was used during the 1970s. They found a growing emphasis on women's health as more than reproductive health. Besides finding concern about the physical and psychological well-being of women, they found emphasis in health literature on (a) inclusion of women as participants in studies about health, (b) investigation of sociocultural factors leading to health problems, (c) analysis of unnecessary surgery for women, (d) examination of exclusion of women from decision-making and treatment choices, (e) recognition that males were not "the norm," (f) identification of sexist bias in therapy, and (g) recognition that women were worthy of serious scientific consideration. They found that a common theme in defining the focus of research on women's health was an emphasis on women's overall health concerns, not just reproduction. In addition, emphasis on the health consequences of changing sex roles for women was common in the 1970s and early 1980s. In short, they found evidence of interest in more than sex differences but no well-articulated frameworks for studying women's health. They concluded that the growing emphasis on women's health, as opposed to the diagnosis and treatment of women's diseases, implied a rejection of the traditional patriarchal medical model in favor of one generally concerned with attaining, retaining, and regaining health. They cautioned that women's health, at the core, meant taking women's lived experience as the starting point for all health efforts.

Despite widespread interest in women's health, few accounts of women's own perceptions have been published. When over 500 women participating in a women's health survey responded to the question "What does being healthy mean to you?" their statements reflected the four models of health that Judith Smith (1981) proposed. Moreover, women identified several dimensions of the eudaemonistic model of health as seen in Table 8.1. These dimensions span a wide range of being and doing, supporting the assumption that women themselves articulate the meaning of health for them.

Nursing

The final concept in nursing's metaparadigm is "nursing." Variously described in nursing's theoretical literature, nursing is conceived of as health promotion, care and cure of the sick, and prevention of illness. Some theorists conceive of the goal of nursing care as helping people adapt to their health-related situations. Other theorists have focused on the goal of nursing as promoting optimal quality of life from the person's own perspective. In this paradigm, the nurse focuses on guiding a person who determines the activities for changing health patterns. Outcomes of nursing practice are determined by the person who develops a plan for changing health patterns as they relate to the quality of his or her life (Parse, 1987).

The concept of caring has become part of nursing's ideology, if not an ethic. Among contemporary theorists, Watson (1990), Swanson (1990), and others have elucidated definitions and dimensions of caring as nurses practice it. Swanson (1990) defines caring as acting in a way that preserves human dignity, restores humanity, and avoids reducing persons to the moral status of object. Grounded in her studies of women, she has identified several dimensions of caring:

Knowing: striving to understand an event as it has meaning in the life of the person being cared for

Being with: being emotionally present to the person

Doing for: doing for the person as she would do for herself if it were possible

Enabling: facilitating the person's passage through life transitions and unfamiliar events

Maintaining belief: sustaining faith in the person's capacity to get through an event or

Table 8.1 Women's Health Images and Definitions

Clinical model	health as absence of illness, infrequency or absence of symptoms, freedom from addiction, ability to recover quickly from illness, absence of need for medical care or medication
Role performance model	health as ability to perform one's activities of daily living at an expected level
Adaptive model	health as ability to adjust flexibly to the environment and cope with stressful events
Eudaemonistic model	health as exuberant well-being, including the following dimensions: actualizing the self—reaching one's optimum, achieving one's goals practicing healthy lifeways—taking action to promote health or to prevent disease positive self-concept—feeling good about oneself, a positive sense of one's worth social involvement—ability to interact, love, care, enjoy relationships, and give and receive pleasure in relationships fitness—feelings of stamina and strength, being energetic and in good shape cognitive function—thinking rationally, being creative, having many interests, being alert and inquisitive positive mood—feeling positive affect, such as happiness, joy, affection, excitement, and exhilaration harmony—feeling spiritually whole, centered, in balance, and content

SOURCE: Adapted from Woods et al. (1989).

transition and to face a future of fulfillment (Swanson, 1990)

Caring, as central to nursing practice, has been the object of feminist analysis. MacPherson (1988) pointed out that a radical feminist analysis has yet to be integrated into thinking about caring and nursing. The concept of caring does not incorporate the concepts of patriarchy and misogyny to explicate health problems common to women, such as depression, nor does it inform nurses of uncaring roles, such as that of "token torturers," the witnessing and participating in unnecessary or harmful treatment of women (Daly, 1978). Moreover, socialist feminist critique has not led to incorporation of a focus beyond the individual to the social collective and an emphasis on the importance of caring as a societal responsibility, not an individual one. Visions of feminist nursing practice attempt to integrate these critical dimensions.

Feminist Models of Nursing Practice

Feminist nursing practice refers to nursing care that is informed by feminist theory. Within this perspective, women's health is more than reproductive health. Women's health care focuses on women's overall well-being and quality of life as women themselves define it. For example, women's experiences of role strain and anxiety about balancing their child care, care for an elderly parent, and work roles are not diagnosed as a problem to be located within the woman herself but are seen as arising within a nonsupportive social context (Sampselle, 1990).

Feminist Nursing Practice Values Women as Women

Men are not the "norm," and concern is about more than whether women are equal to men. A feminist perspective presupposes definitions of health and health care that are grounded in the woman's own perspective. Feminist practice rejects patriarchy that values men more than women and biological essentialism that restricts a woman's control of her reproductive functions. The use of inclusive language and demonstration of respect for women and their information about their health reflect feminist values. A woman's basis for being valuable to her society is not limited to her reproductive capacity. Moreover, feminist practitioners recognize that a woman's body belongs to her and is not owned by someone else or regarded only as a sexual object (Sampselle, 1990).

Range of Nursing Services

Western women have demonstrated their desire for health care that encompasses their total person, not simply their reproductive functions. Female consumers of health care have expressed a preference for a pluralism of health services and health care providers. The range of services they desire include the following:

- Care for menstrual cycle problems and menopausal problems
- General health promotion, including prevention, nutrition, sexual and exercise counseling, and counseling for eating disorders
- Services for chemical dependency
- Mental health services, especially for depression
- Occupational health and career counseling
- Stress management services
- Reproductive services, including infertility, contraception, and genetic counseling
- Family and marital counseling
- Help with problems of aging, including caretaker stress, transitions and loss, osteoporosis, and care for chronic illness
- Pregnancy and childbirth services, child care counseling
- Services for abused women, including women who have been sexually abused, battered, and raped
- Care for sexually transmitted diseases
- Cosmetic surgery
- Special services for adolescent women (Woods, 1985)

These services span women's lives, and few are encompassed within the traditional domain of obstetrics/gynecology (Woods, 1985). Although some of these services reflect women's concerns about reproductive issues, such as pregnancy and infertility care, many reflect a broader range of concerns regarding health, such as child care counseling and services for sexual abuse. Still others reflect social pressures for women to adapt to their environments, such as cosmetic surgery and stress management. These services do not adequately reflect the desires of women who are often invisible to the health care system: Those who are poor, those from underrepresented ethnic groups, and the elderly.

Goals of Feminist Practice

The goal of feminist nursing practice is to improve the lives of all women. Emancipatory feminist paradigms orient practice to praxis, active engagement and participation in the larger society. The notion of praxis reflects awareness that women are in the world and that their actions affect the world. Being actively engaged and participating in the larger society unites individual concerns with the concerns of all women. The goal of feminist practice thus transcends the boundaries of traditional practice, in which the client is an individual, and instead encompasses the well-being of all women.

Bermosk and Porter (1979) advocated a balanced complementarity in the relationships between nurse and women clients. In a symmetrical partnership, nursing care reflects these goals: (a) increasing women's awareness of their human wholeness, (b) promoting opportunities for women for expansion of their mind-body-spirit-environment interactions, (c) fostering women's willingness to take responsibility for and make decisions about their health, and (d) promoting women's effective participation with health care providers as facilitators of health.

In their model, the female client is seen as ever evolving, ever changing, and repatterning. Feminism is an integrative process that helps women expand their own consciousness about health and who they are. Promotion of health, in this model, is a function of transforming one's life through the expansion of one's consciousness rather than merely engaging in periodic medical checkups (Bermosk & Porter, 1979).

A Feminist Model for Nursing Practice for Women

Wilma Scott Heide (1985), a nurse and past president of NOW, characterized nursing as nurturance and nourishment of the whole person. She advocated a vision of health care in which power enabled the "self to be and become," not to control others. In her book, *Feminism for the Health of It,* she asserted that feminist values provide the experiential reality whereby health care encounters are affectively positive, conducive to healing and nurturing of positive self-images for both clients and practitioners. Like the self-help movement that provided women assertive nurturance based on discovery and sharing of knowledge and skills, nursing care can empower women through demystification and consciousness raising. Like the self-help model, a feminist nursing model can reflect valuing scientific knowledge as well as intuitive and experiential knowledge, can focus on the whole person in context, and can therapeutically empower women to experience wellness.

Ideology is central to feminist practice and reflects many themes. *An end to patriarchy* implies that the practitioner attempts to demystify health care in a way that values women's perspectives in the context of a partnership for health. Attempting to create interpersonal and social relations that enable protection and preservation of values that women guard should lead to recognition of the need for a "fundamentally transformed, nonexploitive social order." The dimensions of this order will be discovered through the exploration of women's own experiences when they are no longer devalued (Bricker-Jenkins & Hooyman, 1989).

Empowerment implies an enabling, nonviolent, problem-solving orientation to practice that occurs in an egalitarian relationship between a woman and a health professional. Empowerment involves liberating the energy of women and others in a way that uses that energy in a noncoercive fashion (Bricker-Jenkins & Hooyman, 1989).

Process as product reflects concern for the ends that are part of the means. The process of care itself is a product. Being "in process" means that conditions and consciousness are in constant flux. Caring involves mutually educating, democratizing, and enabling responsibility (Bricker-Jenkins & Hooyman, 1989).

The ideology that *the personal is political* implies that personal problems that women experience have historical, material, and cultural origins and dimensions. The way they feel about themselves has political origins. In addition, this principle implies that women change their world as they change themselves as they change the world. This awareness confirms that failure to act is to act. Moreover, women's interconnections with others make them responsible to others for their acts (Bricker-Jenkins & Hooyman, 1989).

Another dimension of feminist practice ideology is the notion of *unity/diversity*. This implies that diversity is a source of strength and growth. Although conflict in human relations is inevitable, peace is achievable. Sisterhood reflects the concern that none is free until all are free. Racism, classism, heterosexism, ableism, anti-Semitism, and other forms of oppression affect all. Valuing diversity is a beginning to creating conditions for peace (Bricker-Jenkins & Hooyman, 1989).

Validation of the nonrational is another dimension of feminist practice. This orientation allows for multiple competing definitions of problems, many "truths." It emphasizes women's ability to reconstruct their own experiences, to find a meaning of events that they alone can determine. For example, a woman may perceive that her mastectomy is not a sexual phenomenon but one that raises existential issues for her. The process of problem definition is recognized as subjective. Nonlinear, multidimensional thinking is encouraged (Bricker-Jenkins & Hooyman, 1989).

Finally, *consciousness raising and praxis* are central to a feminist model. The intended outcome of consciousness-raising is a new set of values, assumptions, and expectations. It is part of an evolving process of social change. Praxis references the component of feminist consciousness that leads to social transformation. An awareness of the reality that shapes women's lives becomes infused into public values. Reality is renamed according to women's own experience rather than grounded in the experiences of others. Recognition of the small group as a unit of social change is explicit. Self-help is one means of change, but it does not substitute for the provision of adequate services from the state. Struggles to implement values such as egalitarianism, consensus democracy, nonexploitation, cooperation, collectivism, diversity, and nonjudgmental spirituality are central to feminist practice (Andrist, 1988; Bricker-Jenkins & Hooyman, 1989; Sampselle, 1990).

Structure and Process of the Relationship

Caring for women occurs in the context of an egalitarian and collaborative relationship. This implies that the relationship is structured so that the professional power of the nurse is balanced with the power of the woman seeking health care. Mutual recognition of one another's expertise, sharing of information, and defining goals in collaboration are central elements of the process. Women are regarded as experts about their own bodies and self-care, and nurses are regarded as experts in the health problems populations of women experience and the processes that can be used to facilitate health. Information is shared freely between the nurse and the woman seeking care so that the woman herself can have as much of the necessary data as possible to make informed choices about her health. The woman seeking care is an active participant in her own self-health care, not a passive recipient. She alone makes decisions about her own self-care. The nurse as a consultant provides information to women about the full range of alternatives for health. The woman herself makes prescriptions for her own health on the basis of information about self-care options. She is part of a relationship in which she strives for health as she defines it.

The focus of the relationship is on the woman as a person, her "self" as she defines herself in the context of her lived experience. A woman seeking care is not defined simply in terms of her biological nature or her role. She is not seen as a mother simply because she seeks pregnancy care. She may define herself in terms of her roles as a care provider for an aging parent, a worker, a wife, or a mother, or perhaps all of these. She may not define herself in terms of any role but as feeling overwhelmed by obligation or challenged by her environment. She may be unable to define herself, unable to voice who she is.

Data to be collected relate to the woman herself, not only to her reproductive system structure and function. Data include potential or emergent health problems as defined by changing health patterns of populations of women and by the woman's own individual concerns. The woman herself provides her nurse with her own data regarding her health. She is invited to share the data she believes to be relevant. Nurses may point to other useful data to consider. This is in contrast to systems in which the nurse decides what data are relevant and the woman's only contribution is responding to nurse-initiated questions.

The goals for health care are set by the woman herself, and her nurse acts as a consultant. Nurses share their own impressions about possibilities and facilitate women's ability to perform processes important for self-care. This may involve helping women adapt their environments to support them rather than helping women adapt to their environments.

Evaluation of care is process oriented. The woman herself compares the goals she has set for herself with her own self-care agency, using process-oriented criteria. It is important for women to have an improved understanding of their health and self-care abilities as a result of their encounters with health care providers. Women should have an improved ability to collect data about their own health and make appropriate judgments based on the data. They should have expanded their ability to perform processes important to their self-care. Finally, women should have an improved capacity for making decisions about their health. This system of care rests on the assumption that women will have their values respected during encounters with health care professionals, and their health problems or concerns will be managed in a way that is congruent with their values.

Requirements for the Practitioner. Requirements for feminist practice include (a) identifying implications of the issues that arise for women, (b) recognizing patterns of institutionalized sexism and other oppressive ideologies and behaviors that create problems for all, but for women in particular, (c) developing strategies to remove material and ideological barriers to the fullest development of individuals and groups, and (d) recognizing that feminist nursing practice is political practice if it enables women to control the conditions of their lives by equalizing power relationships (Bricker-Jenkins & Hooyman, 1989).

Some feminists would insist that any specialized skills for assisting women with menstruation, orgasm, childbirth, and early abortion should be practiced by women only. Although this might ensure the representation of a greater number of women in some of the male-dominated health fields, one cannot assume that gender confers on the health practitioner freedom from sexism and sex role stereotyping. On the other hand, a woman should have access to a female health care provider if that is her preference. Moreover, men who practice women's health care will benefit from studying with and about women by gaining a more complete perspective of women's lives.

References

Allen, D. (1986). Nursing and oppression: "The family" in nursing texts. *Feminist Teacher, 2*(1), 15-20.

Allen, D., Allman, K., & Powers, P. (1991). Feminist nursing research without gender. *Advances in Nursing Science, 13,* 49-58.

Andrist, L. (1988). A feminist framework for graduate education in women's health. *Journal of Nursing Education, 27*(2), 66-70.

Anzaldua, G. (1987). *Borderlands/La frontera: The new mestiza.* San Francisco: Spinsters/Aunt Lute.

Apodaca, M. L. (1977). The Chicana woman: An historical materialist perspective. *Latin American Perspectives, 4*(1/2), 70-89.

Bermosk, L., & Porter, S. (1979). *Women's health and human wholeness.* New York: Appleton-Century-Crofts.

Bricker-Jenkins, M., & Hooyman, N. (1989). *Not for women only: Social work practice for a feminist future.* Silver Spring, MD: National Association of Social Workers.

Campbell, J., & Bunting, S. (1991). Voices and paradigms: Perspectives on critical and feminist theory in nursing. *Advances in Nursing Science, 13*(3), 1-15.

Chavez, L. R., Cornelius, W. A., & Jones, O. W. (1986). Utilization of health services by Mexican immigrant women in San Diego. *Women & Health, 11*(2), 3-20.

Chinn, P., & Jacobs, M. (1987). *Theory and nursing: A systematic approach.* St. Louis: C. V. Mosby.

Chodorow, N. (1978). *The reproduction of mothering: Psychoanalysis and the sociology of gender.* Berkeley: University of California Press.

Chodorow, N. (1989). *Feminism and psychoanalytic theory.* New Haven, CT: Yale University Press.

Chopoorian, T. (1986). Reconceptualizing the environment. In P. Moccia (Ed.), *New approaches to theory development* (pp. 39-54). New York: National League for Nursing.

Chow, E. N. (1987). The development of feminist consciousness among Asian American women. *Gender & Society, 1*(3), 284-299.

Collins, P. H. (1989a). A comparison of two works on black family life. *Signs, 14,* 875-884.

Collins, P. H. (1989b). The social construction of black feminist thought. *Signs, 14,* 745-773.

Collins, P. H. (1991). *Black feminist thought.* New York: Routledge.

Daly, M. (1978). *Gyn/ecology: The metaethics of radical feminism.* Boston: Beacon.

Davis, A. Y. (1981). *Women, race and class.* New York: Vintage.

Davis, A. Y. (1989). *Women, culture, and politics.* New York: Random House.

de Beauvoir, S. (1949). *The second sex.* New York: Bantam.

del Portillo, C. T. (1987). Poverty, self-concept, and health: Experience of Latinas. *Women & Health, 12*(3/4), 229-242.

Dill, B. T. (1983). Race, class, and gender: Prospects for an all-inclusive sisterhood. *Feminist Studies, 9*(1), 131-149.

Dill, B. T. (1987). The dialectics of black womanhood. In S. Harding (Ed.), *Feminism and methodology: Social science issues* (pp. 97-108). Bloomington: Indiana University Press.

Dinnerstein, D. (1976). *The mermaid and the minotaur: Sexual arrangements and human malaise.* New York: Harper & Row.

Dinnerstein, D. (1989). What does feminism mean? In A. Harris & Y. King (Eds.), *Rocking the ship of state: Toward a feminist peace politics* (pp. 13-24). Boulder, CO: Westview.

Duffy, M. E. (1985). A critique of research: A feminist perspective. *Health Care for Women International, 6,* 341-352.

Duffy, M., & Hedin, B. (1988). New directions for nursing research. In N. Woods & M. Catanzaro (Eds.), *Nursing research: Theory and practice* (pp. 530-539). St Louis: C. V. Mosby.

Gillespie, M. A. (1984). The myth of the strong black woman. In A. M. Jaggar & P. S. Rothenberg (Eds.), *Feminist frameworks: Alternative theoretical accounts of the relations between women and men* (2nd ed., pp. 32-35). New York: McGraw-Hill.

Gilligan, C. (1977). In a different voice: Women's conception of the self and of morality. *Harvard Educational Review, 47,* 481-517.

Gilligan, C. (1982). *In a different voice: Psychological theory and women's development.* Cambridge, MA: Harvard University Press.

Ginorio, A., & Reno, J. (1985). Violence in the lives of Latina women. *Working Together, 5*(5), 7-9.

Gordon-Bradshaw, R. H. (1987). A social essay on special issues facing poor women of color. *Women & Health, 12*(3/4), 243-259.

Hale, J. C. (1985). Return to the bear paw. In J. W. Cochran, D. Langston, & C. Woodward (Eds.), *Changing our power: An introduction to women's studies* (pp. 55-60). Dubuque, IA: Kendall/Hunt.

Hall, J., & Stevens, P. (1991). Rigor in feminist research. *Advances in Nursing Science, 13*(3), 16-30.

Haraway, D. (1988). Situated knowledges: The science question in feminism and the privilege of partial perspective. *Feminist Studies, 14*(3), 575-599.

Harding, S. (Ed.). (1987). *Feminism and methodology: Social science issues.* Bloomington: Indiana University Press.

Hartsock, N. (1983). *Money, sex and power.* Boston: Northeastern University Press.

Heide, W. S. (1985). *Feminism for the health of it.* Buffalo, NY: Margaretdaughters Press.

Herman, A. M. (1984). Still . . . Small change for black women. In A. M. Jaggar & P. S. Rothenberg (Eds.), *Feminist frameworks: Alternative theoretical accounts of the relations between women and men* (2nd ed., pp. 36-39). New York: McGraw-Hill.

hooks, b. (1984). The myth of black matriarchy. In A. M. Jaggar & P. S. Rothenberg (Eds.), *Feminist frameworks: Alternative theoretical accounts of the relations between women and men* (2nd ed., pp. 369-373). New York: McGraw-Hill.

Hurtaldo, A. (1989). Relating to privilege: Seduction and rejection in the subordination of white women and women of color. *Signs, 14*(4), 856-883.

Jack, D. (1987). Self in relation theory. In R. Formanek & A. Gurian (Eds.), *Women and depression: A lifespan perspective* (pp. 41-45). New York: Springer.

Jaggar, A. M., & Rothenberg, P. S. (1984). *Feminist frameworks: Alternative theoretical accounts of the relations between men and women* (2nd ed.). New York: McGraw-Hill.

Klein, K. (1983). How to do what we want to do: Thoughts about feminist methodology. In G. Bowles & R. D. Klein (Eds.), *Theories of women's studies* (pp. 88-104). Boston: Routledge & Kegan Paul.

Lather, P. (1991). *Getting smart: Feminist research and pedagogy with/in the postmodern.* New York: Routledge.

Lorde, A. (1984a). Scratching the surface: Some notes on barriers to women and loving. In A. M. Jaggar & P. S. Rothenberg (Eds.), *Feminist frameworks: Alternative theoretical accounts of the relations between women and men* (2nd ed., pp. 432-436). New York: McGraw-Hill.

Lorde, A. (1984b). *Sister outsider: Essays and speeches.* Trumansburg, NY: Crossing.

Lorde, A. (1988a). *A burst of light: Essays.* Ithaca, NY: Firebrand.

Lorde, A. (1988b). Age, race, class and sex: Women redefining difference. In C. McEwen & S. O'Sullivan (Eds.), *Out the other side* (pp. 269-276). London: Virago.

MacPherson, K. I. (1983). Feminist methods: A new paradigm for nursing research. *Advances in Nursing Science, 5*(2), 17-25.

MacPherson, K. (1988). Looking at caring and nursing through a feminist lens. In *Caring and nursing: Explorations in the feminist perspectives* (conference proceedings, pp. 25-55). Denver: University of Colorado School of Nursing.

Martin, E. (1987). *The woman in the body: A cultural analysis of reproduction.* Boston: Beacon.

McBride, A. B., & McBride, W. L. (1982). Theoretical underpinnings for women's health. *Women and Health, 6*(1/2), 37-53.

Mill, J. (1970). The subjection of women. In J. Mill & H. Mill (Eds.), *Essays on sex equality* (pp. 123-242). Chicago: University of Chicago Press.

Miller, J. B. (1986). *Toward a new psychology of women* (2nd ed.). Boston: Beacon.

Mitchell, J. (1971). *Women's estate.* New York: Pantheon.

Moraga, C. (1983). A long line of vendidas. In C. Moraga, (Ed.), *Loving in the war years: Lo que nunca paso por sus labios* (pp. 90-144). Boston: South End Press.

Moraga, C., & Anzaldua, C. (Eds.). (1983). *This bridge called me back: Writings by radical women of color.* New York: Kitchen Table/Women of Color Press.

Parker, B., & McFarlane, J. (1991). Feminist theory and nursing: An empowerment model for research. *Advances in Nursing Science, 13*(3), 59-67.

Parse, R. (1987). *Nursing science: Major paradigms, theories, and critiques.* Philadelphia: W. B. Saunders.

Raymond, J. G. (1986). *A passion for friends: Toward a philosophy of female affection.* Boston: Beacon.

Reinharz, S. (1983). Experiential analysis: A contribution to feminist research. In G. Bowles & R. Klein (Eds.), *Theories of women's studies* (pp. 162-191). Boston: Routledge & Kegan Paul.

Sampselle, C. (1990). The influence of feminist philosophy on nursing practice. *Image, 22*(4), 243-247.

Sanchez, C. L. (1984). Sex, class and race intersections: Visions of women of color. In B. Brant (Ed.), *A gathering of spirit* (pp. 150-155). New York: Sinister Wisdom.

Sanchez-Ayendez, M. (1989). Puerto Rican elderly women: The cultural dimension of social support networks. *Women & Health, 14*(3/4), 239-252.

Scheper-Hughes, N., & Lock, M. (1987). The mindful body: A prolegomenon to future work in medical anthropology. *Medical Anthropology Quarterly, 1*(1), 6-39.

Schuster, E. (1990). Earth caring. *Advances in Nursing Science, 13*(1), 25-30.

Segura, D. A. (1989). Chicana and Mexican immigrant women at work: The impact of class, race, and gender on occupational mobility. *Gender & Society, 3*(1), 37-52.

Smith, B. (1982). Black women's health: Notes for a course. In R. Hubbard, M. S. Henifin, & B. Fried (Eds.), *Biological woman—The convenient myth* (pp. 227-239). Rochester, VT: Schenkman.

Smith, J. (1981). The idea of health: A philosophical inquiry. *Advances in Nursing Science, 3*(1), 43-50.

Surrey, J. (1985). Self in relation: A theory of women's development. *Works in progress* (Paper 13). Wellesley, MA: Stone Center.

Swanson, K. (1990). Providing care in the NICU: Sometimes an act of love. *Advances in Nursing Science, 13*(1), 60-73.

Tong, R. (1989). *Feminist thought: A comprehensive introduction.* Boulder, CO: Westview.

Tsutakawa, M. (1988). Chest of kimonos—A female family history. In J. W. Cochran, D. Langston, & C. Woodward (Eds.), *Changing our power: An introduction to women's studies* (pp. 76-83). Dubuque, IA: Kendall/Hunt.

U.S. Public Health Service, Task Force on Women's Health Issues. (1985). *Women's health* (Vol. 2, PHS-85-50206). Washington, DC: Author.

Watson, J. (1990). Caring knowledge and informed moral passion. *Advances in Nursing Science, 13*(1), 15-24.

Witt, S. H. (1984). Native women today: Sexism and the Indian woman. In A. M. Jaggar & P. S. Rothenberg (Eds.), *Feminist frameworks: Alternative theoretical accounts of the relations between women and men* (2nd ed., pp. 23-31). New York: McGraw-Hill.

Wollstonecraft, M. (1975). *A vindication of the rights of women.* New York: Norton.

Woods, N. F. (1985). New models of women's health care. *Health Care for Women International, 6,* 193-208.

Supplemental Reading

Allen, D. (1985). Nursing research and social control: Alternative models of science that emphasize understanding and emancipation. *Image, 17*(2), 58-64.

Allen, D., Benner, P., & Dickelmann, N. L. (1986). Three paradigms for nursing research: Methodological implications. In P. Chinn (Ed.), *Nursing research methodology: Issues and implementation* (pp. 23-38). Rockville, MD: Aspen.

Allen, D., & Wolgram, B. (1988). Nursing, therapy, and social control: Feminist science and systems-based family therapy. *Health care for Women International, 9*(2), 107-124.

Ashley, J. A. (1976). *Hospitals, paternalism, and the role of the nurse.* New York: Teachers College Press.

Belenky, M. F., Clinchy, B. M., Goldberger, N. R., & Tarule, J. M. (1986). *Women's ways of knowing: The development of self, voice, and mind.* New York: Basic Books.

Bleier, R. (1986). *Feminist approaches to science.* New York: Pergamon.

Bowles, G., & Klein, R. D. (Eds.). (1983). *Theories of women's studies,* Boston: Routledge & Kegan Paul.

Campbell, J. (1981). Misogyny and homicide of women. *Advances in Nursing Science, 3*(2), 67-85.

Chinn, P., & Wheeler, C. (1986). Feminism and nursing. *Nursing Outlook, 33*(2), 74-77.

Connell, M. T. (1983). Feminine consciousness and the nature of nursing practice: A historical perspective. *Advances in Nursing Science, 5*(3), 1-10.

Connors, D. D. (1985). Women's "sickness": A case of secondary gains or primary losses. *Advances in Nursing Science, 7*(3), 1-17.

Cooper, R. (1986). The biological concept of race and its application to public health and epidemiology. *Journal of Health Politics, Policy and Law,* 11(1), 97-116.

Donovan, J. (1985). *Feminist theory: The intellectual traditions of American feminism.* New York: Frederick Ungar.

Dressel, P. L. (1988). Gender, race, and class: Beyond the feminization of poverty in later life. *The Gerontologist, 28*(2), 177-180.

Easterday, L., Papademas, D., Schorr, L., & Valentine C. (1987). The making of a female researcher: Role problems in field work. In M. J. Deegan & M. Hill (Eds.), *Women and symbolic interaction* (pp. 333-344). Boston: Allen & Unwin.

Fausto-Sterling, A. (1985). *Myths of gender: Biological theories about women and men.* New York: Basic Books.

Fee, E. (1981). Is feminism a threat to scientific objectivity? *International Journal of Women's studies, 4,* 378-392.

Fee, E. (1983). Women and health care: A comparison of theories. In E. Fee (Ed.), *Women and health: The politics of sex in medicine* (pp. 17-34). Farmingdale, NY: Baywood.

Flax, J. (1987). Postmodernism and gender relations in feminist theory. *Signs, 12,* 621-643.

Gates, H. (1989). The commoditization of Chinese women. *Signs, 14,* 799-832.

Gilligan, C., Ward, J. V., Taylor, J. M. (1989). *Mapping the moral domain.* Cambridge, MA: Harvard University Press.

Gould, K. H. (1989). A minority-feminist perspective on women and aging. In J. D. Garner & S. O. Mercer (Eds.), *Women as they age: Challenge, opportunity and triumph* (pp. 195-216). New York: Haworth.

Guillaumin, C. (1988, Fall). Race and nature: The system of marks. The idea of a natural group and social relationships. *Feminist Issues,* pp. 25-43.

Halpin, Z. T. (1989). Scientific objectivity and the concept of "the other." *Women's Studies International Forum, 12*(3), 285-294.

Harding, D., & Hintikka, M. (1983). *Discovering reality: Feminist perspectives on epistemology, metaphysics, methodology, and philosophy of science.* Boston: D. Reidel.

Harding, S. (1986). *The science question in feminism.* Ithaca, NY: Cornell University Press.

Harding, S. (1989). How the women's movement benefits science: Two views. *Women's Studies International Forum, 12*(3), 271-283.

Keller, E. F. (1985). *Reflections on gender and science.* New Haven, CT: Yale University Press.

Lugones, M. C., & Spelman, E. V. (1983). Have we got a theory for you! Feminist theory, cultural imperialism and the demand for "the woman's voice." *Women's Studies International Forum, 6*(6), 573-581.

MacPherson, K. (1988). The missing piece: Women as partners in feminist research. *Response, 11*(4), 19-20.

Marieskind, H. (1977). The women's health movement: Past roots. In C. Dreifus (Eds.), *Seizing our bodies: The politics of women's health* (pp. 3-12). New York: Vintage.

Markides, K. S. (1989). Aging, gender, race/ethnicity, class, and health: A conceptual overview. In K. S. Markides (Ed.), *Aging and health: Perspectives on gender, race, ethnicity, and class* (pp. 9-21). Newbury Park CA: Sage.

Mitchell, J., & Oakley, A. (1986). *What is feminism: A re-examination.* New York: Pantheon.

Padgett, D. (1989). Aging minority women: Issues in research and health policy. *Women & Health, 14*(3/4), 213-225.

Pratt, M. (1984). Identity skin blood heart. In E. Bulkin, M. Pratt, & B. Smith (Eds.), *Yours in struggle* (pp. 12-63). New York: Long Haul Press.

Riessman, C. K. (1987). When gender is not enough: Women interviewing women. *Gender & Society, 1*(2), 172-207.

Roberts, H. (1981). *Doing feminist research.* London: Routledge & Kegan Paul.

Rose, H. (1983). Hand, brain, and heart: A feminist epistemology for the natural sciences. *Signs: A Journal of Women in Culture and Society, 9*(1), 73-90.

Ruddick, S. (1989). *Maternal thinking.* Boston: Beacon.

Seaman, B. (1975) Pelvic autonomy: Four proposals. *Social Policy, 6*(2), 43-47.

Shaver, P., & Hendrick, C. (Eds.). (1987). *Sex and gender.* Newbury Park, CA: Sage.

Smith, B. (1988). Racism and women's studies. In J. W. Cochran, D. Langston, & C. Woodward (Eds.), *Changing our power: An introduction to women's studies* (pp. 7-9). Dubuque, IA: Kendall/Hunt.

Spelman, E. V. (1988). *Inessential woman: Problems of exclusion in feminist thought.* Boston: Beacon.

Spender, D. (1983). *Feminist theorists.* New York: Pantheon.

Suleiman, S. R. (Ed.). (1986). *The female body in Western culture: Contemporary perspectives.* Cambridge, MA: Harvard University Press.

Walker, A. (1983). *In search of our mothers' gardens: Womanist prose.* San Diego, CA: Harcourt Brace Jovanovich.

Walsh, M. R. (Ed.). (1987). *The psychology of women: Ongoing debates.* New Haven, CT: Yale University Press.

Weiler, K. (1988). *Women teaching for change.* New York: Bergin and Gawery.

White, E. C. (1994). *The black women's health book speaking for ourselves.* Seattle, WA: Seal Press.

Woods, N. F., Laffrey, S., Duffy, M., Lentz, M. J., Mitchell, E. S., Taylor, D., & Cowan, K. (1988). Being healthy: Women's images. *Advances in Nursing Science, 11*(1), 36-46.

Yamamoto, J. (1988). Mixed bloods, half breeds, mongrels, hybrids . . . In J. W. Cochran, D. Langston, & C. Woodward (Eds.), *Changing our power: An introduction to women's studies* (pp. 22-24). Dubuque, IA: Kendall/Hunt.

Zambrana, R. E. (1987). A research agenda on issues affecting poor and minority women: A model for understanding their health needs. *Women & Health, 12*(3/4), 137-160.

9

Well-Woman Assessment

LINDA WHEELER

Women are increasingly expecting health care that is based on their assessment of what they need and what facilitates their involvement in their own health care. Women visit health care providers for two reasons: to maintain their health and to resolve health problems. Nursing is uniquely suited to providing holistic care that incorporates these expectations. To do this, however, nurses must develop additional physical assessment and diagnostic skills and use those they already have more effectively to provide primary health care to women clients. Assessment skills and knowledge that nurses provide can enhance the collaboration between client and nurse to identify self-care assets and limitations. Well-woman assessment identifies present and potential health problems and areas for health promotion and maintenance in contrast to assessment directed toward the resolution of a specific health problem or illness. Both types of assessment include obtaining a health history, performing a physical examination, and requesting laboratory studies. Nurses have an essential role in interpreting and evaluating this information.

The health history is, in reality, the client's story. The role of the interviewer is to facilitate the telling of that story so that enough information is obtained to support or refute the initial hunches made as the clinician synthesizes the information presented. From the information obtained, the clinician formulates a list of possible problems, decides how to pursue the physical examination, and makes a preliminary determination of laboratory tests to request. Each activity contributes an essential component to the database.

This chapter suggests an approach to the health history. Areas to be addressed and specific ways to phrase questions at the initial and subsequent health care visit are offered. Supplemental inquiries appropriate for adolescents, and older, pregnant, and postpartum women also are presented. In addition, the chapter discusses components of the physical examination that are unique to women as well as commonly requested laboratory tests.

Health Assessment for All Women

Routine well-woman care usually occurs at 1- to 3-year intervals. When a thorough database has been obtained at the initial visit, information can be readily updated.

The health assessment begins with the health history. The traditional role of the interviewer who obtains the health history has been to focus on the presenting question or complaint, gathering information for preliminary hypotheses. In a broader sense, the health history should also be used to (a) appreciate the client from a biopsychosocial perspective, (b) understand the meaning of the problem(s) to the client, (c) identify the client's perception of her health as well as attitudes and values that may influence the management plan, (d) identify the client's risks for illness and/or disease, (e) identify health education needs, (f) provide emotional support, and (g) recognize areas in which referral is indicated.

The extent to which the health care provider achieves these goals will depend on her or his philosophy of health care. Although the amount of time available for the interview and the willingness of the client to respond to the questions asked also influence the outcome of the interview, it is primarily the attitude and values of the clinician that affect the quality of the information obtained. The likelihood of obtaining the requisite information is increased if time is taken at the beginning of the encounter to put the client at ease and allow her to tell her story with a minimum of interruption. After the story is told the clinician can begin asking questions generated by the client's description of her situation and the symptoms she reports (Smith & Hoppe, 1991).

By actively involving the client in data gathering and by acknowledging her many-faceted life, the likelihood of obtaining a complete story and gaining her cooperation in a plan of care is increased. For example, in a setting where the biomedical problem is the focus of care, a woman who complains of burning on urination and a vaginal discharge will probably receive medication that will cure her sexually transmitted disease. However, she also may be in an abusive relationship, a situation that may continue unless the nurse establishes a climate in which she is encouraged to recount all aspects of her life circumstances.

The ability of the nurse to elicit important information involves both art and science. It requires a substantial knowledge base about disease and its manifestation in women as well as a fascination with the lives of women and a concern for their well-being. Other helpful qualities include a willingness to express one's concern and a willingness to become involved. Such expressions may well be, in their own way, as valuable as antibiotics.

The skilled clinician values the emotional component of the client's life and uses interviewing techniques that assist the client in revealing the information that is needed. Actions likely to put the client at ease and establish rapport include (a) listening attentively to what is said and how it is said; (b) avoiding assumptions and judgments about personal issues such as lifestyle, sexual behavior, drug use, and emotional well-being; (c) being willing to work toward overcoming one's own personal reluctance to obtain a truly comprehensive health history; and (d) using facilitative interviewing techniques, such as encouraging nods, an open facial expression, and prompts such as "Go on" and "Tell me more."

It is not unusual for the nurse to be reluctant to ask important questions, particularly in private health care settings. In fact, hesitancy about asking so-called personal questions usually stems from nurses' own discomfort; for example, nurses may fear that asking about drug use will imply that a client is abusing drugs or that inquiring about her sexual partners will suggest that she is sexually promiscuous. Yet rapport is most rapidly established in an environment that demonstrates immediate concern for the whole person. The client who comes for assistance with a health problem expects the nurse to obtain all of the information requisite to a correct diagnosis. The client who comes for tests/procedures that will maintain her health expects the nurse to make recommendations about lifestyle that can affect her health. Cutting corners or not asking personal questions because of his or her personal discomfort does the client a disservice.

Health History

Whenever possible, the history should be obtained with the client fully clothed and should begin with introductions if the client is new to the setting. A few social amenities are always in order unless the client is in distress. New clients should be asked how they would like to be addressed. In some parts of the country, last names preceded by Ms., Miss, or Mrs. are preferred. In other parts of the country, use of first names is common. The client may wish to be called by a nickname. Some nurses feel it appropriate to call a client by her first name only when the nurse is also willing to be called by his or her first name.

When the client is accompanied by a partner, family member, or friend, she should be asked if she would like the accompanying person to participate in the interview. Inform the client that some of the information to be discussed is of a personal nature. If the client prefers to be accompanied during the interview, remember to ask for time alone with her before the conclusion of the visit. A statement such as, "I'd like to have a few minutes alone with each person I see. Would you excuse us for a few minutes, please?" may be used. This gives the nurse an opportunity to ask the client in private, "Is there anything else you think I should know in order to take good care of you?" Under these circumstances, the client may reveal a history of drug abuse, herpes, the relinquishment of a child, domestic violence, or some other information that she wishes to keep private.

Although the presence of the accompanying party is usually helpful to the client, his or her presence is not always beneficial or welcome. It may take some time for this fact to become obvious. When it does, the provider can say, "It is the practice of this office/clinic to spend a little time alone with each client. Would you excuse us for a few minutes please?" If an opportunity does not present itself to speak to the client alone, or if the accompanying party will not leave, a note should be made in the client's record to speak to the client by herself at another visit or to contact the client at home.

This section discusses the health assessment interview in some detail. Table 9.1, the Health History Form, lists specific areas of the well-woman health history. Information about initial and interval well-woman visits and suggestions for phrasing questions that provide lead-ins to lines of questioning for areas of a woman's life that are personal and sometimes sensitive are given. The phrasing of the questions should be adjusted to fit women of different cultures, social classes, ages, and geographical locations. Phrasing should also be adjusted for the comfort level of the interviewer as long as the goals of the health assessment are accomplished.

This type of interviewing is helpful to all women but may be particularly beneficial to disadvantaged women. Their dealings with the health care system are often irregular and fragmented. Those who care for them often do not understand why clients do not keep appointments, change health habits, take drugs that have been prescribed, or follow advice. Health care providers may not realize that disadvantaged clients often are unable to deal with a health care system that is complex and frequently does not address critical issues that affect use of a health care system. These include language barriers, cultural practices, access to providers, impersonal care, and health care costs.

Health care practitioners who recognize the importance of a truly comprehensive health assessment face the reality of needing to deliver care to a large number of women in a limited amount of time. Continual searching for creative ways to address this problem is in order. Nurses serving a population with high-level reading skills may wish to develop a form that clients can complete prior to their visit. Those serving a population with low-level reading skills may wish to train indigenous health workers to obtain some of the information. A close look at the organization of the health care setting and its associated rituals might free time that could be devoted to the health assessment.

Obtaining a good history is facilitated by providing the client with privacy while the history is obtained and the physical examination is performed. Assuring the client that the information given will be kept confidential and using language that the client understands help to ensure that accurate information will be provided. Speaking in a tone of voice that conveys respect and concern and providing enough time for the client to respond to questions also will facilitate obtaining a good history. Explaining why questions are being asked and allaying the client's anxiety about responding to personal/intimate questions are also useful in collecting a health history.

After the initial social amenities, the reason(s) the client is seeking care is identified. "How may I help you?" or "Why did you come to the clinic/office today?" can be used to start. She is then asked if there is anything else she would like to discuss. The client should then be given an opportunity to ask any questions she may have. This relieves her of having to try to remember the questions until later in the interview and indicates the health care provider's interest in her concerns. Let the client know how much time is available and the manner in which the visit will proceed.

text continued on page 149

Table 9.1 Health History Form

The health history suggests information that should be obtained at an initial well-woman visit. The information gathered assists the nurse in understanding a woman's life situation and how it affects her health. The form should be adapted to work setting and personal style. Categories of information and questions asked need not be asked in any special order. Rather, the form is more useful if questions flow from the client's responses and the feeling the nurse gets about how the interview is going.

I. Reason(s) for seeking care
   A. How can I help you today?
   B. Ask for a description of the problem, including the following:
      1. How long has it been present?
      2. What might have precipitated it?
      3. Remedies/treatment attempted and result
      4. Client's perception of the cause of the problem and treatment needed
II. Psychosocial/living situation
   A. Tell me a little about yourself and your life right now.
   B. How much stress are you under now?
   C. What are the major causes?
   D. Where do you get emotional support? Do you have a best friend? How about a family member you can call on for help or to talk to?
   E. On a scale of 1 to 10, how would you rate your relationships with your
      1. Partner
      2. Children
      3. Parents
      4. Siblings
      5. Friends
   F. What major losses have you had in your life (children, parents, partner, friends, abortion, miscarriage, jobs)?
   G. What do you think are your personal strengths? What do you do particularly well?
   H. On a scale of 1 to 10, how satisfied are you with your present life?
   I. What do you wish were different (if answer to H less than 10)?
   J. Do you have any special goals for the future?
   K. Have you ever been married? How many times?
   L. Has your partner ever been married? If yes, how many times?
   M. Does your partner have any children from previous relationships? If yes, does he or she have any involvement with that child/those children?
   N. Where are you living? How many people live with you? How many bedrooms and bathrooms are there? Are there any animals?
   O. How safe is the neighborhood where you live?
   P. How long have you lived there? Where did you live before? How long?
   Q. Is there anything you would like to change about your living situation?
III. Racial and ethnic background
   A. Where were you born?
   B. If the client was born in a foreign country, ask the following:
      1. How long have you been in the United States?
      2. What cultural practices should be honored?
IV. Religious preference
   A. Do you have a religious preference?
   B. Did you come from a strong religious background?
   C. How important is religion to you?
V. Work history
   A. Are you working for money now? If yes, what is your job?
   B. How many hours per week are you working? What hours do you work?
   C. Rate your job on a scale of 1 to 10.
   D. What would you like to change about your job?
   E. What is stressful? What is satisfying?

Table 9.1 Health History Form—Continued

F. What other jobs have you had?
G. Have you ever had a job that you would consider dangerous?

VI. Educational background and interests
- A. What was the last grade you finished in school? If the answer is lower than the 12th grade, ask the following:
  1. Why did you drop out?
  2. How were you doing at the time?
- B. Do you have any plans to return to school in the future?
- C. Do you have any hobbies?

VII. Menstrual history
- A. Age at menarche
- B. Frequency of cycles
- C. Duration of flow
- D. Quantity of flow
- E. Presence of cramps
- F. Use of pads or tampons
- G. Perimenstrual/menopausal symptoms
  1. Mood swings, irritability, tension
  2. Weight gain, swelling
  3. Depression, fatigue, crying
  4. Painful breasts, headache, cramps, backache
- H. LMP and LNMP or age at menopause
- I. Attitude toward menses/feelings about menopause

VIII. Obstetric history
- A. Gravida, para (mature, preterm, abortions, living child/ren)
- B. When
- C. Result
  1. Gestational ages
  2. Lengths of labor
  3. Birth weights
  4. Sex of each
  5. Names
  6. Antepartum (AP), intrapartum (IP), postpartum (PP) complications
  7. Present condition
  8. Whereabouts of child/ren
  9. Which children have the same father?
  10. Paternal involvement with child/ren if the father does not live in the home
  11. Feelings about labor/births
  12. Feelings about any perinatal loss
- D. Desire to be pregnant in future or have sterilization procedure
- E. Feelings about present number of children
- F. Problems achieving and/or completing pregnancy in past/at present?
  1. Etiology, if known
  2. Length of time to resolve problem or is it unresolved
  3. Treatment
  4. Result
  5. Emotional response

IX. Contraceptive history
- A. Are you sexually active now?
- B. If yes, are you using any birth control?
- C. If not using a method but sexually active, are you interested in a method?
- D. If not interested, "Can you tell me why?"
- E. If presently using a method, ask which one, how long, side effects, level of satisfaction.
- F. What other methods have you used? For how long? Ask about side effects, satisfaction, reason for discontinuing.

(continued)

Table 9.1 Health History Form—Continued

X. Family medical history (parents, grandparents, siblings)

Anemia	Kidney disease	Clotting problem
High blood pressure	Heart disease	Genetic problem
Diabetes	Hyperlipoproteinemia	Congenital anomaly
Cancer	Lung disease	Stroke
Tuberculosis	Depression	Alcoholism
Seizures	Mental illness	

XI. Personal medical history

A. Illnesses

Seizures	High blood pressure
Anemia	Blood clot
Headaches	Clotting problem
Cancer	Heart disease
Thyroid disease	Lung disease
Stroke	Lupus
Migraine	Diabetes
UTI (bladder or kidney infection)	

B. Gynecologic problems

DES daughter	UTI
Abnormal Pap	Pelvic pain
Pelvic infection	Urinary incontinence
Vaginal bleeding	Dyspareunia
Vaginal infection: malodor/pruritis/discharge	
STDs (syphilis, gonorrhea, chlamydia, herpes, condyloma, Hepatitis B)	

C. Injuries

D. Blood transfusion/blood products
   1. Type
   2. Year

E. Foreign travel

F. Allergies
   1. Drugs
   2. Food
   3. Environment

G. Surgery
   1. Type
   2. Year
   3. Sequelae

XII. Emotional history

A. What do you know about your own birth?
   1. What was your mother's labor like?
   2. Were there any problems?
   3. Were you healthy when you were born?

B. How would you describe your childhood?
   1. Were you an easy child or a difficult child?
   2. How did you get along with your brothers and sisters?
   3. Were you healthy?
   4. How did arguments get resolved?
      a) Between your parents
      b) Between you and your mother/father
      c) Between you and your siblings
      d) Were you ever called insulting names?
      e) Screamed or yelled at?
      f) Pushed or shoved?
      g) Slapped, kicked, punched
      h) Was your hair pulled?
      i) Was something ever thrown at you?

Table 9.1 Health History Form—Continued

j) Were you ever forced to have sex when you didn't want to?
k) Were you ever touched in ways that made you uncomfortable?
l) Were you beaten up/choked?
m) Were you ever threatened with a knife or a gun?
n) Did your parent(s) ever threaten to leave you or send you away?

C. Previous counseling
1. Years
2. Reasons
3. Results

D. History of depression, nervous or emotional problems, anxiety

E. History of abuse/domestic violence as an adult
1. How do you resolve arguments in your family now?
2. Since you've been away from home (or as an adult) has anyone called you insulting names?
a) Told you that you were worthless or put you down?
b) Screamed or yelled at you?
c) Pushed or shoved you?
d) Slapped, kicked, or punched you?
e) Pulled your hair?
f) Thrown something at you?
g) Forced you to have sex when you didn't want to?
h) Beaten you?
i) Choked you?
j) Threatened you with a weapon?
k) Has anyone ever threatened to leave you? Take your child/ren from you?
(1). If yes, were drugs or alcohol involved when this happened?
(2). Have you ever talked to anyone about these things? If yes, what were their responses?
l) Number of yelling fights in the last month?
m) Episodes of pushing, shoving, hitting? (If answer to any of *b* through *m* is positive, ask if she is safe now.)
n) Have you ever thought you are/were too hard on your child/ren? If yes, in what way?
o) How do you discipline your child/ren?
p) Do you feel comfortable leaving your child/ren with the other people in the house?

F. Have you ever been in foster care or had a child in foster care? If yes, reasons?

G. Fears/phobias

H. If you are adopted, thoughts about birth parents, efforts to "search."

XIII. Sexual history

A. Risk factors for AIDS
1. Are you sexually active now?
a) If no, is that a problem for you?
b) If no, have you had intercourse in the past?
2. Have your partners been men, women, or both?
3. Have you ever had sex with
a) More than 5 men in a year?
b) Someone who has been in jail?
c) More than 1 man at a time?
d) Someone who has had a blood transfusion or hemophilia?
e) Someone who has had a positive AIDS test?
f) Someone you think might have AIDS?
g) Someone who uses drugs? IV drugs? Cocaine?
4. Do you think any of your partners might have had sex with a prostitute or may have had sex with both men and women?
5. Have you ever been in a position where you traded sex for drugs, money, food, housing, or anything else?
6. Do you ever have sex when you are high (if history of drug use)?

(continued)

Table 9.1 Health History Form—Continued

7. Could it be that your current partner(s) is having sex with someone besides you?
8. Do/does your current partner/s have any symptoms of a genital infection—warts, blisters, sores, painful urination, penile discharge?

B. Sexuality/problems/concerns about sex
1. If you were rating the sexual part of your life on a scale of 1 to 10, where would you put it?
2. What would you change about it if you could?
3. Do you have any problems with orgasm? Desire? Frequency?
4. Do you climax (come)? If no, is that a problem for you?
5. Do you have any pain at the beginning of, during, or after having sex?
6. Has anything about your sex life changed significantly in the past few years?
7. Do you think there is anything your partner would like to change?

XIV. Lifestyle

A. Nutrition
1. Present weight
2. Is that what you usually weigh?
3. When was the last time your weight was checked?
4. If weight has changed either way, what is client's perception of what happened?
5. What would you like to weigh?
6. How often do you diet?
7. What type of diet do you go on?
8. Have you ever used diet pills?
9. History of eating disorder
10. How many glasses of water do you drink each day? How much milk? Coffee? Caffeinated or decaf? Tea? Soda? What type?
11. Use of snack foods
12. Diet restrictions/foods not eaten
13. Do you fast?
14. Use of vitamins
    a) Type
    b) Dose

B. Sleep
1. Hours per night
2. Frequency of naps
3. Problems with sleep? Insomnia?

C. Exercise
1. Type
2. Amount
3. Frequency

D. Environmental hazards: physical, chemical, biological
1. In the home
2. On the job

E. Smoking
1. Cigarettes per day
2. Age started
3. Attempts to quit
    a) Number
    b) How
4. Number of smokers in household
5. Is it a good time for you to stop?

F. Use of alcohol (liquor, beer, wine)
1. Do you drink anything alcoholic—liquor, beer, wine?
2. When do you drink?
3. What do you drink?
4. Do others encourage you to drink?
5. How old were you when you started drinking?

Table 9.1 Health History Form—Continued

6. Has anyone ever criticized your drinking? If yes, how did you feel about that?
7. Which family members drink a lot?
8. What does your partner think about your drinking?
9. How many drinks does it take before you feel high?
10. Have you ever thought you had a problem with drinking? If yes, what did you do about it?
11. If indicated, have you ever blacked out while drinking? Been in an accident? Lost a job or friends? Been arrested because of drinking?

G. Recreational drugs
1. What type of recreational drugs do you use?
2. Have you ever shot cocaine? Heroin? Amphetamines ("speed")?
3. Have you ever shot other IV drugs?
4. Have you ever used amyl nitrate ("poppers")?
5. Have you smoked marijuana? Crack?
6. When you do drugs, where do you do them?
7. Do you ever have sex when you are high?
8. How much are you using a week?
9. When do you use it?
10. Have you had any bad reactions to drugs? If yes, what happened?
11. Have you ever shared needles for drugs? Tattoos? Ear piercing? Skin popping? To take medicine? Anything else?
12. How old were you when you started using drugs?
13. Have you ever been in a drug treatment program? When? What type? Follow-up?
14. Have you had any drug-related accidents? Family problems? Job problems? Arrests?
15. Do you think you have a problem with drugs?

H. Over-the-counter drugs: Names and frequency of use
I. Prescription drugs, including mood elevators, tranquilizers, hormone therapy
J. Use of menstrual history calendar
K. Breast self-examination.
L. Immunizations: Polio, Rubeola, Diphtheria, Tetanus, Hepatitis B
M. Smoke detectors in home
N. Year of most recent cholesterol check? Result?
O. Year of most recent Pap smear?
P. Knowledge of risk factors for AIDS? What do you think about condoms?

XV. Is there anything else you think I should know about you to give you good care?

The importance of allowing the client time to tell her story cannot be overemphasized. Interruptions by the clinician during this phase should be minimal and primarily aimed at understanding the psychosocial context in which any presenting problem occurs.

Subsequent visits should begin by asking the client if she has any particular concerns. Ask her to tell you about her present life and how things have changed since the last visit. Problems noted at previous visits and goals that were established earlier should be discussed. New information about each of the above should be noted.

Identify any visits to another health care provider since the last encounter. Include the reason for seeking care, laboratory tests performed, medicines taken, and the outcome. Ask about illnesses and injuries for which the client did not seek medical care as well as over-the-counter medicine, vitamins, and herbs used in the interval.

Psychosocial Context

Although some situations require active questioning about the medical history before the client's story is told, an evaluation of the psychosocial situation obtained early in the interview is usually preferred. "Can you tell me a little more about yourself?" provides information to supplement that initially volunteered by the client.

Subsequent questions depend on how the client responds. "Tell me a little bit about your living situation" can lead to important information about who the client lives with, where they live, and the quality of the relationships in the home. Find out the type of dwelling, the number of people living there, its size, the kind and number of animals, the client's perception of whether or not the neighborhood is safe, and how frequently the family has moved. Identify the ages of those with whom the client lives and inquire about the health of each.

Replies to these questions may reveal homelessness, dangerous animals such as ferrets and pit bulls in homes with children, or the presence of a terminally ill family member who requires constant care. "What would you like to change about your living situation?" provides insight into the client's perception of her immediate environment.

Questions such as the following can elicit other important information: "How much stress are you under now? What is the best part of your life at this time? What is the most difficult part of your life?" Questions such as these give necessary information about the client's support system: "Who is the most important person in your life? Do you have a best friend or a family member you can call on for help or just to talk to?"

Asking the client to rate her relationships with key people on a scale of 1 to 10 is a useful way to make a preliminary determination of the quality of the relationships with significant people in her life: "On a scale of 1 to 10, with 1 being the worst and 10 being the best, how would you rate your relationship with your partner? How about your relationship with . . . ?" Insert the names of the people in the household and add the client's parents if they are alive. Include the client's children even if they no longer live at home. For example, a 36-year-old woman coming to the office/clinic for the first time and requesting her annual Pap smear can be asked, "And your parents, are they alive?" If the answer is yes, the nurse can continue, "How would you rate your relationship with your mother? Your father?" It is interesting to add, "What would it take to make it a 10?" At times an inconsistency can be noted between the rating given by the client and her tone of voice. A comment such as, "You say 8, but your voice doesn't sound like an 8," may make the client aware of what she would really like to say.

"Have you had any major losses in your life?" refers to loss of significant people, jobs, possessions, and dreams. If the client does not seem to understand the question, questions such as "Have you ever lost a child? A family member? A friend? How about a job? Have you moved frequently?" illustrate the point the clinician is trying to make.

Other questions also elicit clues to the life situation of the client: "What do you think you do especially well? What are you most proud of about yourself? Is there something you have done in the past that you are particularly proud of? On a scale of 1 to 10 how satisfied are you with your life right now? What do you wish were different? Are there some special things you want to do in the future?"

Marital status should be determined at some point in the interview. Although there are various ways to ask the question, it is important to use words that do not imply that marriage is the only desired state. Whereas, "Are you married?" is the common query, "Have you ever been married?" may be less emotionally tinged. If the client responds in the affirmative, the clinician can respond with, "Are you married or in a relationship now?" and move into the number of relationships for both the client and her partner. Children from previous relationships the partner has had should be determined. It is also helpful to identify whether or not there is any involvement between nonresident fathers and the children in the home and between the current partner and his or her children from previous relationships.

At the interval well-woman visit, clients should be asked if any of the relationships identified as important at a previous visit have changed. Are there new people in her life who are significant? Has the constellation of the household changed? Use the 1 to 10 scale again to inquire about relationships with family members. Inquire about school and job as appropriate.

Ask the client if she has lost anyone close to her or has moved to a new location. If she has moved, find out why and ask her to describe her new residence. Ask her to talk about stressors in her life and sources of emotional support. Ask also if new illness have been diagnosed in family members or friends. Has she taken on any new responsibilities, such as the care of a family member?

Racial and Ethnic Background

Identification of racial and/or ethnic heritage is necessary because of medical conditions found in certain groups and because an understanding of cultural practices can significantly improve care. Sickle-cell testing should be provided to women of African American descent, Tay-Sachs testing is appropriate for women of Eastern European Jewish descent, specifically Ashkenazic Jewish women, and testing for beta-thalassemia is appropriate for women of Mediterranean descent. In the United States, syphilis occurs 50 times more frequently in black women and 10 times more frequently in Hispanic women than in white women (Centers for Disease Control, 1991). Breast cancer survival in poor black women is very low compared to white women (Freeman & Wasfie, 1989), and hypertension is more prevalent in black women than in white women (Anastos et al., 1991).

"Where were you born?" is a helpful question for identifying ethnicity in some, but not all, situations. Certain diseases are endemic to particular regions of the world. Hepatitis B in Southeast Asian countries is an example. Medical problems that may need to be investigated include parasites, malaria, hepatitis, tuberculosis, and HIV infection. The latter is endemic in some countries.

Religious Affiliation

Religion that can dictate cultural practices may be a significant feature in the lives of clients, often influencing lifestyle practices such as dietary habits. As such, it is appropriate to ask, "Do you have a religious preference?" Whether the answer is "Yes" or "No," it is also helpful to inquire if the client comes from a strong religious background and the extent to which religion is important in the client's life at the present time.

Work History

A woman's job as homemaker and/or wage earner can be a source of danger, illness, and stress. For example, occupations such as those involving work on an assembly line or piecework in the garment industry have high rates of repetitive stress injuries, such as carpal tunnel syndrome. A job can also be a source of satisfaction and mental health.

Begin this section of the interview by asking the client, "What is your occupation?" or "What type of work do you do?" Be alert to those who respond, "I'm just a homemaker." A follow-up question might be "Why do you say just a homemaker?" Regardless of the response, follow with, "Is there something you would rather be doing now or in the future?"

Ask women who are wage earners about the number of hours per day or per week they work, the time at which the work is started and ends, and the amount of satisfaction and stress associated with the job. Difficulties associated with rotating shifts should be identified, as should any job-related hazards. Exposure to toxic chemicals, heavy lifting requirements, and work that involves physical danger should be noted.

Health care and public safety workers should be asked, "Are you afraid of contracting AIDS?" Either a positive or a negative response allows the clinician to pursue the client's knowledge about risks in her job setting and steps she takes to minimize that risk. (See Chapter 16, "Women in the Workplace," for a discussion of occupational risks and HIV infection.)

Educational Background and Interests

Determine the highest grade of schooling completed. Although years of schooling do not necessarily equate with reading skill, educational background does serve as a place to start for evaluating a client's ability to read—important information to consider when providing educational material for clients.

Menstrual History

The menstrual history begins with age at menarche and continues through the usual questions to determine frequency of cycles, days of flow, and amount of flow. This information provides baseline data that may influence method of birth control and allows for counseling about the fertile period of the cycle. Information about the menstrual cycle is found in Chapter 3, "Women's Bodies." Chapter 23, "Common Symptoms," provides a thorough discussion of assessment of gynecologic bleeding.

Women who menstruate should be asked about menstrual cramps and other perimenstrual symptoms such as mood swings, irritability, weight gain, depression, headaches, bloating, breast tenderness, and vomiting. Medicines used for symptom relief should be identified. Women with perimenstrual symptoms should be asked if they think they have premenstrual syndrome (PMS). Episodes of intermenstrual bleeding (IMB) should be noted because this can represent gynecologic abnormalities. IMB can also be related to hormonal contraception and the intrauterine device. Young teenagers, perimenopausal women, and postmenopausal women should be asked about their feelings in regard to the onset or the cessation of menses, as appropriate.

Women who menstruate should be asked about the first day of their last menstrual period (LMP) and the date of the last normal or usual (by their definition) menstrual period (LNMP). Knowledge of the client's place in the menstrual cycle may make pregnancy a possibility and allows the clinician to take appropriate care during the physical examination. For example, sometimes the breast examination may be deferred because of breast tenderness in early pregnancy.

At the interval visit, information about the client's menstrual cycle should be updated. The nurse should always be alert to the possibility of pregnancy when women are in the childbearing years. As women approach the perimenopausal years, the nurse should ask if they have given any thought to how this might affect their lives and how they feel about it. The nurse should also inquire about perimenopausal symptoms, such as hot flashes or flushes and vaginal dryness.

Obstetric History

When a woman is new to a clinic or office and the known intent of her visit is not prenatal, she should be asked, "Have you ever been pregnant?" If the response is "No," it is appropriate to ask, "Have you ever wanted to be pregnant?" Follow-up is indicated if the client responds in the affirmative.

Women who have been pregnant should be asked about each pregnancy. "How many times have you been pregnant?" is a good way to start. Determine when each pregnancy ended, the length of each, the outcome, and the year in which it occurred. For pregnancies with a gestational age greater than 20 weeks, include the length of the labor, birth weight, the sex of the child, medical complications, and the whereabouts of each living child. The client's feelings about each labor and birth may provide information that will be useful if another pregnancy is planned or occurs. The nurse might ask "When you recall that birth, what is it that you remember? What do you wish you could have changed about that birth?"

Knowing the names of the client's children allows the clinician to personalize care. The name of each should be recorded. When time allows, ask how each child was given her or his name. Determine where each child lives. Older children may live far away and not be available for certain types of support. Young children may be in foster care or living with their father somewhere else. A child may have been relinquished for adoption. When children are still in the home, the clinician should ask about the father of each child. When different fathers are identified, it is appropriate for the clinician to ask about the father's involvement in the child's life and how both the child and the client feel about the involvement or lack of it. Ask if the current partner has any other children from previous relationships.

This is often a good time to ask about children who spend part of their time in the client's home and part of the time elsewhere. "Do you have any other children—stepchildren, children you are no longer involved with?" may be appropriate to ask.

The health status of each child can provide helpful information, including potential areas of stress. For example, a child of any age who is seriously ill or has a chronic disease requiring family care can impose considerable stress on the client. An assessment of the client's relationship with each child using the 1 to 10 scale may also indicate areas of stress or support. If the children are school-age, the clinician should inquire about how the children are doing in school. Children with learning and/or behavioral problems also may pose considerable stress for the family.

The four-digit designation used to describe pregnancy outcome uses the letters *T*, *P*, *A*, and *L* (Tennessee Power and Light may be a helpful acronym). The *T* refers to term pregnancies (>37 weeks), the *P* to preterm births (<37 weeks), *A* to abortions (through 20 weeks), and the *L* to living children. Although helpful, this designation does not distinguish between ectopic pregnancies, spontaneous abortions, and elective abortions.

"How was/is it for you having this many children and boys and girls?" or "having no children?" gives the client an opportunity to express her feelings about her childbearing status.

Discuss any perinatal losses that may have occurred. Whether the loss was from an elective abortion, a miscarriage, an ectopic pregnancy, a midtrimester fetal death, a stillbirth at term, or a neonatal death, or the result of relinquishing a child for adoption, and whether or not the loss is recent or occurred many years ago, the client may still grieve. Many women who have had reproductive losses have never had a chance to discuss what happened and how they felt or how they are feeling with a caring person.

Women who have chosen to relinquish a child or terminate a pregnancy, even when the decision was felt to be a good one, can be sad and may benefit from the opportunity to talk about it. "Do you ever think about that child?" is a helpful way to begin. The person who responds affirmatively can be asked, "How was that for you?" and later, "How is that for you now?"

Women can also be asked if they ever tried unsuccessfully to obtain an abortion. Their feelings about this situation should be explored because many have not had the opportunity to share the terror and desperation that they felt.

Some women seeking health care will give a history of infertility. They should be asked to describe any therapy or procedures they underwent to resolve the problem and the results/consequences of each. Women who wish to become pregnant and have not been successful can be asked if they wish a referral to a specialist. Nurses should remember that loss is a pervading theme among women who are unable to conceive or carry a pregnancy that results in a living child. Acknowledgment of that loss is an important part of the health assessment.

Women who have had a cesarean section should be asked about that experience. Some women feel it is the only way to have a baby. Others are devastated and carry feelings of failure and anger with them for years. At times it is helpful to obtain the records of the surgery to help women piece together the events surrounding the birth.

Contraceptive History

Women of childbearing age should be asked if they are currently sexually active with a male partner. If the answer is "Yes," ask, "Are you or your partner using any method of birth control?" Those women not using a method should be asked if they are interested in one. If they are not interested, it is appropriate to determine the reason they are not contracepting. Occasionally, it is because their partner does not wish them to do so. Exploration of the quality of their relationship should occur in such circumstances.

The clinician should discuss methods of fertility control with women of childbearing age. Methods used, duration of use, side effects, complications, satisfaction with the method, and the reason for discontinuing use will be helpful to the clinician. Satisfaction with the present method, if one is being used, should be determined. It is appropriate to ask the satisfied client if she has thought of changing her method. This gives the clinician an opportunity to provide accurate information about other methods, thereby expanding the number of choices available. A woman who says she does not want more children should be asked if she or her partner (if she has one) has considered a sterilization procedure.

At the interval well-woman visit, clients in the childbearing years who are sexually active with a male partner should be asked about their present method of birth control, how they are using it, if any side effects are experienced, and level of satisfaction with the present method. Clients should be asked if they have thought about changing methods. When new methods become available, the clinician should be sure that this information is made available to clients. The nurse also reviews the client's future childbearing plans at this time: Does she wish any children/additional children/a sterilization procedure?

Family Medical History

The family medical history refers primarily to illnesses and diseases experienced by the client's parents, siblings, and grandparents. The history form (Table 9.1) lists common problems that may run in families. Genetic problems and congenital anomalies may be determined by asking, "Has anyone in your family had a child that was deformed or retarded?" Another useful question to ask is, "Is there anything strange or unusual that runs in the family?" It is important to ask all questions using words that the client will understand. These words vary from one population to another. When inquiring about mental illness in the family, use of the term *nervous breakdown* may mean more than mental illness. And some clients may understand *drinking problem* better than they understand or are willing to identify *alcoholism.*

Because depression is not an infrequent occurrence in women, the clinician must also ask about this entity. Chapter 15, "Mental Health," expands on the subject of depression and the consequences to the child raised in an environment where the mother was depressed. When women report a family history of depression, be sure to explore with the client what that experience has been like for her.

A family history of heart disease or breast cancer prior to the age of 50 requires exploration of the client's fears that the same thing could happen to her.

Personal Medical History

Physical assessment textbooks delineate questions to ask about the client's personal medical history. This section supplements that information by focusing on those elements particularly relevant to the health care of women. The client born between 1940 and 1965 should be asked if her mother took diethylstilbestrol (DES) while the client was in utero. Because DES affects the reproductive tract of babies in utero, DES daughters are at risk for vaginal adenocarcinoma and malformations of the uterus and cervix that are associated with preterm labor. The risk for adenocarcinoma lasts until these women are in their early 30s. Because DES was used at least until 1965, DES-related adenocarcinoma may be found through the year 2000 (Melnick, Cole, Anderson, & Herbst, 1987).

Sexually transmitted diseases (STDs) are of great concern to women because of their potential for infertility, chronic illness, and cancer. When a history of one or more STDs is given, determine when it happened, the treatment given, the follow-up that has occurred, the client's understanding of the consequences of the disease and how it is transmitted, and whether or not the sexual partner/s was/were treated and had appropriate follow-up. Chapter 24, "Sexually Transmitted Diseases," discusses the assessment, prevention, and treatment of these diseases.

Ask about the results of the most recent Pap smear and when it was obtained. Women with a history of condyloma or genital warts need to be followed up with interval (usually every 6 months) Pap smears. Determine if this is occurring or has occurred and, if not, provide counseling about the necessity of this health care practice.

Women who report having had genital herpes should be asked if the diagnosis was confirmed with laboratory testing. Without laboratory confirmation, the health care provider cannot counsel definitively on precautions to take to decrease the spread to sexual partners, the need for follow-up Pap smears, or the risk of transmission to newborns. A history of herpes requires inquiry about lesions induced by emotional stress and discussions about the stress-producing factors and ways to decrease them. (See Chapter 24 for specific suggestions.)

Urinary incontinence is a common problem for women over 60, possibly approximating 40% of that population (Diokno, Brock, Brown, & Herzog, 1986). Often, women are grateful that someone asks about this embarrassing problem. Additional information about assessment of common gynecologic problems is found in Chapter 23.

Surgical History. The surgical history should include information about the reason for surgery, the type of operation(s) performed, complications, and sequelae.

Emotional History

An assessment of the client's emotional well-being is as important as the assessment of her physical well-being. The questions listed in this and the next section of the history form (sexual history) require that the health care practitioner be able and willing to ask questions about intimate parts of the client's life. These questions may be embarrassing to the client and, possibly, the nurse. Often, the client will not volunteer information about emotional problems. The nurse can facilitate disclosure by gently probing into various facets of the client's life with specific questions.

If the client has previously identified any emotional problems or episodes of counseling, the nurse may ask for additional information by saying, "Tell me a little more about the situation you were in when you had counseling." When no previous problems have been identified, "I'd like to ask some questions about a different part of your life" will introduce this section. The nurse should begin with a question in an area that has little emotional charge for the interviewer. This question will vary from nurse to nurse. "Have you ever been depressed?" can be a starting point for some. Because this word is not understood by everyone, follow it with, "How about nervous or emotional problems, attacks of anxiety?"

Incidences of abuse are important to document. To begin this line of questioning, try, "How do you resolve arguments or differences of opinion in your family?" Follow with, "Have you ever been called insulting names?" After pausing for the client's response, continue with, "Have you ever been told you are worthless or been put down in any way? Have you been screamed or yelled at? Pushed or shoved? Slapped, kicked, or punched? Ever had your hair pulled? Something thrown at you? Have you ever been forced to have sex? Ever been assaulted? Have you ever been forced to do anything sexual you didn't want to do? Have you ever been beaten up? Choked? Threatened with a weapon, such as a knife or a gun? Has anyone ever threatened to leave you? Take your children from you?" Pause after each question to allow the client to respond to each. If the answer to any of these questions is yes, determine whether or not the problem is current. Ask, "How many yelling fights have you been in this past month? How many episodes of pushing, shoving, hitting? Has anyone been injured?" Additional discussion of this topic is found in Chapter 18, "Violence Against Women."

When the client is in an abusive situation, the clinician must assess the extent of the danger to the woman and others in the household. The client's immediate plans and resources should be identified. Nursing care of women in a violent situation, including references to appropriate resources, is found in Chapter 18.

During this section of the health assessment, the client may reveal physical, emotional, or sexual abuse as well as abuse in more than one area. A history of abuse as a child may also emerge. Women who disclose a history of sexual abuse as a child should be asked if it was by a family member (incest). The question is important to ask because incest is associated with sexual dysfunction and problems with intimate relationships (Lowery, 1987). Because treatment cannot occur until disclosure has taken place, the practitioner must be willing to ask the questions that might allow the client to ask for help and provide a setting in which discussion is facilitated.

Questions the nurse might ask include, "Have you ever talked with anyone about these things? What was their response? How are you feeling now?" Women who have not received counseling in regard to these issues can be asked, "Have you ever thought about counseling or about joining a support group?" If the response is "No," ask, "What would you think about that now?" Some women will reply that they think the issue is resolved and they don't need counseling. Some will say they are not ready. Others may feel that counseling is a good idea and will accept a referral. When the clinician feels that counseling is indicated but the client is uninterested, the clinician should place a notation in the record to bring this matter up at a later date. A client may be unwilling to pursue the matter for various reasons at this point in time but be able to respond otherwise at a different point in her life. Remember, too, that domestic violence can occur in homosexual relationships as well as in heterosexual ones.

It is also possible that the client has previously abused or is presently abusing her children. "Have you ever thought you were/are too hard with your children?" may address this possibility. If the client says "No," ask, "What do/did you use to discipline your children?" Follow-up questions will depend on the client's response. If the client says that she feels she has been too hard on the children, ask her, "In what way?" Depending on the answer, it may be appropriate to ask the client if she has ever thought she needed help learning some new approaches to parenting.

Asking if the client feels comfortable leaving the children alone with other people in the house may elicit her concern for possible abuse while she is away. Women who have in the past suspected that abuse was going on may feel guilty about not pursuing the matter or not doing something about it. They often appreciate a chance to talk about their feelings.

The client should be asked if she was ever in foster care or had a child placed in foster care. A positive response to either question indicates a need for further discussion. If she herself was in foster care, ask the client about the circumstances surrounding her placement, the length of time she was in care, the number of homes she was in, and her feelings about what happened. If one or more of her own children have been in foster care or are in foster care, ask the reasons, when the placement/s was/were made, future plans for the children, and her feelings about the reasons for placement as well as plans for having the children in the future.

Inquire about any particular fears or phobias the client might have. Although responses such as heights or needles may be elicited, occasionally a bizarre fear (e.g., inability to leave home without washing one's hands 10 times) indicative of psychiatric illness may be identified. (See Chapter 15 for further information.)

Women who were adopted should be asked if they ever wonder about their adoptive parents. They should be asked if they have thought about or think about looking for their birth parents. Answers to these questions may indicate how a woman feels about her adoptive status.

Sexual History

Information about a client's sexual practices is essential for risk assessment. Without this information, inadequate testing may be done, the sequelae of disease may threaten physical and emotional health, and the disease may be unnecessarily transmitted to others. Information obtained from the sexual history can lead to prevention and treatment of disease and an improvement in the quality of a sexual relationship. Accordingly, a sexual history should be a routine part of any health assessment.

Discomfort with the topic, an inadequate knowledge base, embarrassment about probing into this intimate area of the client's life, and fear of evoking an angry response from an offended client may prevent nurses from incorporating a sexual history into their history-taking practices. When the nurse acknowledges that her own attitudes prevent asking questions of a sexual nature, yet she recognizes the importance of this aspect of the health assessment, it may be helpful to begin obtaining sexual histories by asking only a few nonthreatening questions. For example, while gathering information about a woman's birth control method ask her if the method affected her sex life. If she responds "Yes," ask, "In what way?" Most clients are not only willing to respond to questions that are gently asked but also grateful for the information given by the health care provider.

The lead-in question for the sexual history can be preceded by a statement about why this information is important and why it has become routine to include it in a health assessment. Often, a statement is not necessary, particularly if the response to another question provides a natural lead-in to the sexual history. For example, a woman who reports a vaginal discharge can be asked if she has a new sexual partner. Whatever her response, the rest of the sexual history might be inserted at this point.

"Are you sexually active now?" is a general question that can establish a starting point for obtaining additional information. If the client's response is "No," follow with, "Is that a problem for you?" If the client admits to a problem, ask her to elaborate. In addition, if the client is not sexually active now, ask "Have you been sexually active in the past?" A "no" response should be followed again with a question designed to elicit the client's feelings about the situation.

The client who is or has been sexually active should be asked, "Have your partners been men, women, or both?" This question permits a preliminary assessment of risk for STDs. (See Chapter 24 for further discussion of this topic.)

The sexual history continues with questions about the quality of the sexual relationship. Some people may prefer to begin the sexual history with this information and move from there to assessing STD risk. An opening question could be "On a scale of 1 to 10, how satisfied are you with your sex life?" Those who rate it less than 10 can be asked, "What would it take to make it a 10?" Specific information can be obtained by asking, "Do you have an orgasm?" If no, ask whether or not this is a problem. Continue by asking questions about sexual desire, frequency of sexual activity, problems in these areas, and if she and her partner feel the same about what they do when they make love/have sex and how often they do it.

"Do you have any pain when you are having sex?" If the answer is "Yes," ask, "Does it occur at the beginning, during, or after?" Pain at the beginning of lovemaking is often due to a vaginal infection or inadequate foreplay and also may be associated with first vaginal intercourse. Dyspareunia, painful intercourse, is discussed in Chapter 21, "Sexuality in Women's Lives."

Additional helpful information may be obtained by asking the following: "Have you had a significant change in your sex life recently or in the last few years? Is there anything about your sex life that you would like to change? Do you think there is anything that your partner would like to change?"

At the interval well-woman visit, the nurse should ask the client if she has had any new sexual partners since the last visit. If she says yes, ask how she decided to engage in sex with the new person(s) and help her assess her risk for STDs (see Chapter 24). Ask how her sexual life has changed since her last visit. Use the 1 to 10 scale again. Is she having any problems with desire or pain? What would she like to change?

Lifestyle

The last part of the health assessment inquires about the client's health habits. Because clients rely on health care providers to recommend good health habits, this is an important part of health assessment. The nurse can begin with any aspect of lifestyle. Some areas may have been covered previously as opportunities for discussion arose.

Nutrition. The nurse may begin a nutritional history with "I see you weigh *XX* pounds. Is that your usual weight?" If this is not her usual weight, the nurse should inquire what her weight was the last time she weighed, when that was, and her perception of what has happened since then. A height/weight chart should be used to determine the appropriateness of the client's weight for her height. Women with an appropriate weight for height should be asked if they have ever been overweight or underweight.

The assessment continues by asking the following: "What would you like to weigh? Have you ever tried to lose weight? How often do you diet? What type of diet do you go on? Have you ever used diet pills? Are you dieting now?"

At some point in the interview, the client should be asked if she now has or has ever had an eating disorder. Identify anorexia nervosa and bulimia by name. Although these diseases occur at all socioeconomic levels, most cases of anorexia involve young women of high social class (Yates, 1989).

Other information about nutrition that may be helpful includes the amount and type of liquid consumed during the day, with specific questions being asked about soft drinks, coffee, tea, and milk; ask, too, about vitamin intake because some women consume vast quantities each day. Women should be asked about foods used for snacking, the amount of cholesterol and saturated fat in their diet, dietary restrictions for health or religious reasons, and foods not eaten because of food preferences. (See Chapter 12, "Nutrition," for additional information.)

Sleep. Asking about the number of hours of sleep per day may identify insomnia or excessive sleep and the possibility of depression or other emotional problems.

Exercise. Clients should be asked to describe the type, amount, and frequency of exercise in their lives. Nurses should inquire about exercise-related problems when clients are involved in an exercise program (see Chapter 13, "Exercise").

Environmental Hazards. Environmental hazards should be identified. Client awareness of hazards on the job site, at home, and in the community needs to be identified (see Chapter 16).

Immunizations. The nurse should ask when the client had her last tetanus injection and determine if women in their childbearing years have a positive rubella titer. An additional dose of measles vaccine may be indicated for children more than 13 years old and to young adults living and working in institutions, pregnant women excluded (Staff, 1989). A woman's risk for hepatitis B infection should be determined (see Chapter 24), and if she is at risk, her vaccination status should be ascertained.

Over-the-Counter Medicine. Nonprescription medicine that the client takes should be identified along with frequency of use and the reason for taking the medicine. Inappropriate use should be noted.

Prescription Medicine. Any prescription medicine should also be identified along with frequency of use, the medical indication, and the date the client was last seen by a health care provider. It may be helpful to ask specifically about certain drugs: "How about mood elevators? Tranquilizers? Hormones? When was the last time you had your prescription filled?"

Smoking. During a well-woman assessment, all women should be asked if they smoke or use other tobacco products. Once it has been determined that the client smokes, it is helpful to find out how long she has been smoking and to identify the number of times the client has tried to quit or cut down. If she has attempted to stop smoking, she should be complimented for trying and then asked, "Is this a good time for you to try again?" For women who have not tried to quit before, the nurse should ask "Is this a good time for you to stop or cut down?"

The National Cancer Institute recommends marking the charts of smokers with an identifier such as a sticker and adoption of "the four A's plan": (a) ask about smoking, (b) advise smokers to stop, (c) assist those willing to stop, and (d) arrange follow-up.

Alcohol. Although alcohol is a legal recreational drug, alcohol abuse is a major health problem for women. Accordingly, alcohol use by the client should be identified.

Begin this line of questioning by asking, "Do you drink anything alcoholic—liquor, beer, wine, wine coolers?" Specify beer and wine because some people do not consider them alcoholic. Women who deny drinking should be asked, "Has drinking ever been a problem for you?" If it has, ask the client when the problem occurred, what the circumstances were, and whether or not she participated in a treatment program.

If the client is currently drinking, identify when she drinks and what she drinks. Because clients frequently do not admit to all types of alcohol that they drink, add, "Do you drink *XXXX* (e.g., beer) too?" after the client identifies what it is that she drinks. Additional questions that can provide insight into the situation include the following:

- "Do others encourage you to drink?"
- "How old were you when you started drinking?"
- "Has anyone ever criticized you about your drinking?" If yes, ask, "How did you feel about that?"
- "Which family members drink a lot?"
- "What does your partner think about your drinking?"
- "How many drinks does it take before you feel high?"
- "Have you ever thought you have a drinking problem?" If yes, ask, "What did you do about it?"
- "Have you ever blacked out while drinking? Been in an accident while drinking? Been arrested because of drinking?"

When the clinician becomes aware of an alcohol problem early in the interview, it is often appropriate to ask this series of questions at that time. Because of differences between men and women in the metabolism of alcohol, women usually feel the effects of alcohol sooner than do men. A woman who states that it takes more than three drinks before she feels high probably has developed a tolerance to alcohol and has a drinking problem. The reader is referred to Chapter 22, "Drug Abuse Problems Among Women," for additional information.

Other Recreational Drugs. Use of illegal recreational drugs is costly, impairs judgment, endangers public safety, and contributes substantially to morbidity and mortality. Questions about illegal drug use logically follow those about alcohol use. Try, "Have you ever used recreational drugs, such as cocaine or amphetamines?" Although it may be necessary to use the colloquial name for these drugs, such as "speed" for amphetamines, use of the street name can trigger cravings in drug users and thus should be avoided if possible. Regardless of the response to the first question, continue asking about drugs by naming each one individually. "Have you ever used amyl nitrate ("poppers")? How about marijuana? Have you ever sniffed anything—how about cocaine? Glue? Ever shot IV drugs? How about heroin? Have you ever smoked crack?"

When the client admits to use of drugs, a form such as the screening questionnaire displayed in Table 9.2 may be helpful. The nurse should also determine when each drug was used and for how long. If the client is currently using drugs, estimate the frequency by asking, "How much are you using a week? When do you use it?" Ask her where she uses the drugs: at home, at the house of a friend, or elsewhere. Women who have children at home and who take drugs should be asked where the children are when the drugs are being used.

Also ask clients how old they were when they started using drugs and if they have ever had any drug-related accidents, family problems, job problems, or arrests. Continue with, "Have you had any bad reactions from drugs?" If yes, ask, "What happened?"

Ask the client if she has ever been in a drug treatment program, if it has not been previously identified. If yes, determine when, what type, and the result of treatment. Finally, ask the woman who still uses drugs how many people in the household are also drug users.

Women who use drugs may deny that a problem exists. People who smoke marijuana are particularly likely to feel this way even when they smoke it frequently. People addicted to other drugs may also deny that they have a problem. Brief risk intervention (BRI) is a technique developed to (a) help health care practitioners understand why some clients are unable to change their behavior and to (b) help clients understand that they have a problem when they are not able to see one.

When a practitioner perceives that a drug problem exists but the client does not, ask, "How would you know if it was a problem? What would have to happen for you to think it is a problem?" This may be enough for the client to see the situation in a new light. If she is able to see the problem, ask, "What are you ready to do

Table 9.2 Screening for Illicit Drugs

Drug	Age at First Use	How Often Used in Past Year	How Often Used This Month	Number of Times/ Day When Used
Wine				
Beer				
"Hard" liquor				
Tobacco				
Marijuana				
PCP (angel dust)				
LSD				
Tranquilizers				
Heroin				
Smoking cocaine (freebasing/crack)				
Sniffing/snorting cocaine				
Skin popping				
Other cocaine				
Speedball (heroin and cocaine)				
Codeine				
Methamphetamines (crystal/speed)				
Diet pills				
Methadone				
Other (please specify)				

NOTE: The questionnaire shown here can be used to assess a woman's use of illicit drugs.

about it? Do you know what your choices are?" Important for the clinician to understand at this point is that there may be too much loss involved for the client to take immediate action. Asking, "If you change this behavior, what will you lose?" may clarify the reality of the situation for both clinician and client.

The client who indicates readiness to change her behavior will probably need help at some time. Ask, "What do you need in order to do this?" Responses often require referral to other agencies because provision for housing, day care, and job skills training may be necessary.

A final question should be asked of women with a history of intravenous drug use (IVDU). "Have you ever shared needles for drugs? Tattoos? Ear piercing? Skin popping? To take medicine? For anything else?" The latter question should be asked of all clients because people in some cultures believe that injectable medicine such as antibiotics and some vitamins is always good for one's health, regardless of health status or problem.

Health Habits

The nurse should ask if her clients of childbearing age use a menstrual calendar. Menstrual-history calendars are charts on which women mark the days on which they experience vaginal bleeding. Each calendar provides space to record the menstrual cycle for one year. (See Chapter 14, "Fertility Control," for an example.)

Women should be asked if they perform monthly breast self-examination (BSE) and, if not, why not. If the woman does not practice BSE, information on why the practice is important and how to perform it should be offered. (See Chapter 28, "Problems of the Breast," for additional information.)

The nurse should ask if a woman has periodic evaluation of cholesterol and triglycerides. Cholesterol levels should be measured every 5 years in adults starting at the age of 20. Because cholesterol levels may be normal in some people while triglycerides are elevated, some clinicians advocate routine check of triglycerides as well as cholesterol. Adult clients should be asked the year of their most recent cholesterol determination. (See Chapter 12 for further discussion of this topic.)

Clients should be asked about safety practices in the home, including the use of smoke detectors, the availability of locked storage space for dangerous items when children are around, the presence of weapons, and hazardous living conditions. If indicated, other residential hazards such as wood stoves, unscreened fireplaces, and farm equipment should be reviewed.

All women should be asked if they have had periodic screening (Papanicolaou smear) for cervical cancer. No right answer exists as to how often to screen for cervical cancer, and recommendations range from yearly to every 2 to 3 years for women with no history of abnormal findings. Women with previous abnormal results should be screened yearly or more frequently. All women over the age of 40 should be asked about mammograms. (See Chapter 28 for additional information.)

Nurses must ascertain women's knowledge of risk factors for STDs. The information needed to accomplish this is found in Chapter 24.

Finally, the nurse should ask if there is anything else the client would like to relate or thinks the nurse should know to give her the best possible care. Occasionally, an important piece of information will be revealed.

During an interval well-woman exam, the nurse should follow up on deficiencies noted previously. To assess exposure to infectious diseases, ask about travel outside the United States. Inquire whether or not the client has dieted or changed an exercise program since her last visit. Inquire again about her personal use of alcohol and drugs as well as use by family members. If the client is sexually active and uses drugs, ask if she ever trades sex for drugs. The client should also be asked what else she would like to discuss.

Age-Related Considerations in Health Assessment

Adolescence

The adolescent history contains all of the elements identified in the general health assessment with some modifications made for age, life circumstances, and awareness of the behaviors and tasks of adolescence—namely, developing self-identity, seeking peer approval, being concerned with body image, experimenting with intense friendships, striving for independence, experimenting with behavior perceived to be adult, living in the present, and developing a value system.

Most female adolescents are uneasy about seeing a health care provider, often because they dread having a pelvic examination. Their apprehension can be eased by respecting their privacy and assuring them of confidentiality. When the adolescent client is accompanied by someone else, it is helpful to see the client alone initially to ask how much involvement she would like from the accompanying person. Giving the client additional time alone at the end of the visit also is appropriate. The following section includes suggestions for adapting the adult health assessment to adolescent girls. Specific adolescent well-woman health assessment considerations are outlined in Table 9.3.

Most adolescents experience some emotional turmoil as they pass through their adolescent years. Therefore, relationships at home and at school should be assessed. Helpful introductory questions include the following: "Where do you live? Who lives with you? How are things at home?" Asking "What would you like to change about the people you live with?" can evoke responses that provide insight into the family dynamics.

"Does anyone in the house have a problem with alcohol or drugs?" followed by, "How many people in the house use alcohol? How about drugs?" can lead to a discussion about drugs and the problems that might result from them.

Ask the client how she would describe her mother and father as parents and as disciplinarians. If the client is unable to respond to the question, ask, "Would you say she/he is fair, too strict, likes the other kids better, doesn't care

Table 9.3 Age-Related Health History Considerations

Adolescent Women	*Midlife/Older Women*
Assess preparation for, knowledge of, and feelings about menarche/menstruation.	Because vaginal bleeding/spotting after menopause indicates health problems, always ask about this.
Evaluate contraceptive use for consistency.	Assess for depression; incidence is high in elderly women.
Assess for suicide risk; incidence is high in adolescence.	Inquire about threats of or acts of violence toward woman; elder abuse is rising in the United States.
Inquire about presence of weapons in school and at home.	Continue substance abuse assessment, especially polysubstance and/or prescription medication abuse.
Begin substance abuse assessment in early teen years. Inquire about cigarettes and other tobacco use and drinking and driving.	Ask about vaginal lubrication, dyspareunia, and changes in sexual desire.
Specific body image areas to assess are dieting and tanning.	Ask about risk factors for breast cancer, cardiovascular disease, colon cancer, hyperlipidemia, and osteoporosis.
	Do a nutritional profile for prevention of obesity, hyperlipidemia, and osteoporosis.
	Ask about past, present hormonal therapy, and contraceptive method (midlife women).

NOTE: Elements of the well-woman health history may need to be modified for age-related reasons. Suggestions for adapting the adult woman health history for adolescents and midlife and older women are given.

about you, gives you support when you need it—those types of things?" If the clients' birth parents do not live together, ask about relationships with the noncustodial parent and what it is like having parents who do not live together. When stepparents are involved, include a discussion of relationships with them.

Identify disciplinary practices in the home by asking, "What happens if you do something you are not supposed to do?" Ask the client if she was spanked as a child and inquire if anyone hits her now. Ask how problems in the house are resolved and whether anything that happens in the house bothers her. Ask if her parents get along, if her siblings get along, and if she gets along with her siblings.

Ask the client if she is happy. It may be helpful to ask her to rate her feelings about school, friendships, and life in general on a scale of 1 to 10. Questions that can be asked to help understand her life circumstances include: "What do you think about school this year? What grade are you in? What are your grades like? Do you make friends easily? Do you have a best girlfriend? How about a boyfriend? Do you ever worry about boyfriends? Do you ever worry about being gay? Have you ever thought about running away from home? Have you ever thought about killing yourself? Have you ever been depressed? Has anyone ever touched you in a way that makes you feel uncomfortable? Have you ever been raped or assaulted? Do you think you have ever been emotionally abused?" Positive responses to any of these questions must be pursued.

Other questions about school should address participation in extracurricular activities and educational plans for the future. Girls who have dropped out of school should be asked to talk about their reasons for dropping out and plans they might have for returning.

Midlife and Older Women

History collected from a perimenopausal woman should be specific as to the risk factors associated with this phase in her life. Special attention is paid to the breast and to cardiovascular, musculoskeletal, endocrine, and genitourinary systems. Women should be asked about medication use; particularly important is past or current hormonal therapy. A substance abuse history should always be obtained, because midlife and older women are at high risk for alcohol and drug dependency, and many providers assume that there is no risk in this age group. A family history of colon cancer, breast cancer, hyperlipidemia, or heart disease is important when assessing risk and suggests appropriate physical examinations and laboratory studies. Women should be asked about risk factors for osteoporosis (see Chapter 5, "Midlife Women's Health").

A nutritional profile is important in the prevention of osteoporosis and risk of coronary heart disease. A number of dietary factors are linked to osteoporosis, including low calcium intake, lack of vitamin D, and a history of high intake of foods that impair absorption of calcium. These include foods high in phosphorus or fiber, such as carbonated drinks and meats, and excessive amounts of fats, chocolate, and caffeine. Because the relationship between obesity and risk of coronary heart disease has been well established, identifying obesity in a midlife woman is important.

An obstetric and gynecologic history should be gathered. During the perimenopausal years, women have little difficulty providing details about their gynecologic and obstetric experiences or the age at which menopause occurred. In the late menopausal period this information may not be remembered as clearly. A sexual history with specific inquiries regarding vaginal lubrication, dyspareunia, and changes in sexual desires should be done. (See Chapter 21 for information on obtaining a sexual history.) Although ovulation becomes less frequent in the premenopausal years, conception is possible until menses have been absent for 1 year. Therefore, when appropriate, the practitioner should ascertain what method of contraception the client is using.

Review of Systems

The initial part of the health assessment contributes information about many aspects of the client's life. From the information gained, the practitioner begins a list of problems. The next part of the history is a review of the body's major functional systems. The clinician refines the list of possibilities and gains information that may have been missed initially. Physical assessment textbooks discuss this aspect of the history.

Physical Examination

Many excellent physical assessment textbooks describe the physical and pelvic examinations. Only the pelvic examination is discussed here because it is not always a part of a physical assessment course. "The pelvic" is almost always a dreaded experience. It can sometimes be made tolerable and even fun by making it an educational experience. With the client in a semi-Fowler's position, offer her a hand mirror and ask her to place it between her legs while you point to her labia, urethra, clitoris, vagina, perineum, and rectum. Both anatomical and more common terms can be used. *Outer* and *inner lips* instead of *large* and *small lips* can be used to describe the labia because the labia majora can be smaller than the labia minora. The client can rest the mirror on her abdomen to facilitate relaxation during insertion of the speculum. Once the cervix is found, the client replaces the mirror between her legs. Usually some adjustment of the light will be necessary for good visualization. If the cervix is posterior, elevate the speculum handle. The section, "Assessing the Female Genitalia," page 179, describes the pelvic examination in detail.

Laboratory Studies

An integral part of well-woman assessment, laboratory tests are used to confirm information gathered from a thorough history taking and physical examination. Laboratory tests are used for periodic screening of asymptomatic women for certain conditions or illnesses—for example, a Pap smear; for confirmation of a diagnosis suggested by history or physical exam as with a pregnancy test or clean catch urine culture; and to monitor improvement or document cure as with a repeat gonorrheal culture. Recommended screening laboratory tests for nonpregnant adult women are found in Table 9.4. Laboratory tests for specific health problems or illnesses are discussed in the appropriate chapters.

Health Assessment of the Pregnant Woman

The health assessment of pregnant women should include the same information obtained

Table 9.4 General Laboratory Examinations: Adult Women

Tests	*19-39 Years*	*40-64 Years*	*65+ Years*	*Comments*
Cholesterol	Every 4-5 years*	Every 3 years*	Yearly	*More often, plus HDL/LDL, if elevated
Papanicolaou smear	Every 1-3 years*	Every 1-3 years*	*	*High risk, every 3-12 months
Fasting glucose	*	*	*	*High-risk individuals
Mammogram		*	*	Every 1-2 years beginning at age 50; age 35 for those at increased risk
Urine dipstick			*	
Fecal occult blood		*	*	Yearly; begin at age 45-50. Some authorities recommend only for high-risk persons.
Thyroid function test		*		

SOURCES: Adapted from U.S. Preventive Services Task Force (1989); Sloane, Slatt, and Curtis (1993); and Rosen (1990).

when a nonpregnant woman presents for care. As in the adolescent history, some points should be emphasized. It is helpful to begin by asking the client how she feels about being pregnant and what she knows about her own birth. For example, What does her mother remember about her labor? The birth? Was she afraid? Were there any problems with her birth? Did anything unusual happen to her mother? To her? Was she healthy? These questions may provide information about what the client expects about her own childbirth experiences. Often, women know little about their birth, and it is fun and sometimes revealing for them to discuss their birth with their mother. If their birth mother is dead or estranged from the client, another family member may be able to supply helpful information.

Work History

Four areas of work may be hazardous to pregnant women: (a) jobs involving exposure to toxic chemicals, (b) jobs that require prolonged standing, (c) jobs that require heavy lifting, and (d) jobs with potential for impairing physical balance in the second half of pregnancy. Anesthetic gases, chemical sterilants, antineoplastic agents, semiconductor chips, and some substances used in chemical laboratories have been implicated as teratogens. The reader is referred to Chapter 16 for additional information on this topic. Nurses should make note of the client's employment history and be alert for new developments. Always ask the client if she is aware of exposure to potentially dangerous chemicals because health care providers are not always aware of use of these agents in a particular workplace.

Menstrual History

The menstrual history assumes great importance in pregnancy because the last menses is used to calculate gestational age. Accurate determination of gestational age is imperative because fetal growth assessments and postdates (after estimated date of delivery) testing are based on it. Reliable dating is facilitated when the client arrives knowing the first day of her LMP. Unfortunately, recording of menstrual cycles is not the norm and, therefore, accurate determination of LMP may require some time. It is time well spent, however, when compared with the time that might be required in the future trying to decipher gestational age.

The estimated date of delivery (EDD) can be calculated by using Naegele's rule: Add 7 days to the first day of the last normal menstrual period and subtract 3 months. However, irregular or prolonged menstrual periods or a known single sexual exposure can cause variations from this estimate. Avoid using gestation calculators to determine the EDD because they may overestimate the due date by 1 to 4 days. This becomes important when a decision must be made about when to begin postdates testing. In decreasing levels of accuracy, criteria for estimating date of delivery are as follows:

- Basal body temperature with coital record
- Ultrasound between 7 and 10 weeks menstrual age, documenting crown-rump length
- Serum HCG
- Urine pregnancy testing
- Two ultrasounds prior to 26 weeks gestation
- Last menstrual period in which cycle is normal and regular (Aumann & Baird, 1993)

Obstetric History

The obstetric history is of major importance at the initial prenatal visit because some complications, such as preterm labor and postpartum depression, are likely to recur. The emotional consequences of a poor outcome or problems in a previous pregnancy may also affect the way a woman experiences her current pregnancy. For example, a woman whose first labor was unusually long may anticipate a recurrence and be fearful throughout the pregnancy. A woman who miscarried at 16 weeks may not be able to think about the child she carries in her womb until the pregnancy progresses beyond 16 weeks. Nurses alert to the connection between prior problems and stress in the current pregnancy can provide factual information and support to help alleviate fear and anxiety. They can also identify women at particular risk and arrange for them to receive care in the most appropriate setting.

The obstetric history was discussed in detail previously. Other information that becomes important when a pregnancy actually exists includes parity, method of delivery, and intrapartal problems. Grand multiparity, often defined as more than five births, has traditionally been looked upon as a cause of malpresentation, dysfunctional labor, and postpartum hemorrhage. A recent study from Israel, where the researchers were able to separate grand multiparity from socioeconomic status, found that women having their sixth or greater child were not at inherent risk (Eidelman, Kamar, Schimmel, & Bar-On, 1988).

Method of delivery is important because previous cesarean section requires special care when vaginal delivery is to be attempted. Many clinicians now encourage vaginal delivery after cesarean section if the hospital is able to respond quickly should uterine rupture occur.

Intrapartal complications that are likely to recur should be noted. These include shoulder dystocia and postpartum hemorrhage caused by uterine atony. Hemorrhage caused by lacerations is not likely to occur again unless the bleeding was the result of a coagulation disorder.

Contraceptive History

The contraceptive history can contribute to accurate dating of the pregnancy. Because cessation of oral contraceptive use may result in a postpill amenorrhea, pregnancy may occur prior to the resumption of spontaneous menses. Women who report stopping "the pill" and becoming pregnant before menstruating will benefit from an ultrasound obtained for dating purposes. Women who have regularly used reliable barrier methods may be able to contribute helpful dating information. If they remember not using the method or a method accident such as condom breakage, dating the occurrence may pinpoint conception.

Family Medical History

The main concern about the family medical history is hereditary disease. Other diseases, such as breast cancer, may mean the client herself could develop these conditions, but they are usually of no import if the client herself does not have them during the pregnancy. Infectious diseases, however, such as tuberculosis or Hepatitis B in a family member require appropriate testing and counseling.

A diagnosis of severe preeclampsia or pregnancy-induced hypertension (PIH) in the client's mother or sisters should be noted because this disease seems to have a hereditary component (Chesley & Cooper, 1986; O'Brien, 1990). Consequently, all instances of elevated blood pressure in the client's mother or sisters during their pregnancies should be noted.

Personal Medical History

Aspects of the client's medical history that are important are those in which the maternal medical condition may be exacerbated or the disease may affect the growing fetus. Conditions that should be noted include STDs, DES exposure, seizures, diabetes, hypertension, thyroid disease, lupus erythematosus, cardiac conditions, anemia, history of thrombus or coagulation disorders, mental illness, and previous injuries.

The presence of any STDs, including herpes, condyloma accuminatum, HIV infection, gonorrhea, chlamydia, syphilis, and Hepatitis B should be determined and treated. (Chapter 24 provides information on the assessment and management of pregnant women who have an STD).

Pregnant women who are DES daughters are at risk for preterm labor, in part probably associated with structural abnormalities. A history of seizures should be identified because they may become more frequent during pregnancy. Dilantin, a drug often used for seizure control, is teratogenic.

All pregnant women should be screened initially for diabetes and glucose intolerance in pregnancy. High blood glucose levels in early pregnancy may cause fetal anomalies. Without appropriate blood sugar control in the second half of pregnancy, macrosomia may occur. Large (> 9 lbs) babies can cause traumatic delivery leading to maternal and newborn injury. Mothers with long-standing and/or severe diabetes may have growth-retarded infants, and their own disease may worsen significantly with pregnancy.

The presence of preexisting hypertension is always assessed. Women with existing hypertension are at risk for developing superimposed preeclampsia. Their babies are at risk for developing intrauterine growth retardation because of impaired uterine blood flow.

Women who are hypothyroid may deliver babies with congenital hypothyroidism, a condition associated with mental retardation. A history of hypothyroidism requires that maternal thyroid levels be evaluated each trimester because thyroid medication may need to be initiated or adjusted. Women with lupus have an increased incidence of growth-retarded babies. Their own disease process may be accelerated.

Maternal heart disease may also result in a growth-retarded baby, and maternal symptomatology may intensify. When the maternal disease is congenital, babies may also have congenital cardiac problems. Fetal echocardiograms aid in-utero diagnosis. Certain types of anemia, such as the thalassemias, are hereditary. Any anemia may worsen in pregnancy. Although iron deficiency anemia rarely affects the fetus, it does affect the mother's ability to withstand unusual blood loss after delivery. Women previously diagnosed with iron deficiency anemia may not have resolved the problem.

The hypercoagulability that occurs in pregnancy increases the risk of a blood clot for women who have had previous thrombotic episodes. Blood dyscrasia may cause bleeding problems at the time of birth and during the postpartum period. Thus the client is asked if she has ever had a bleeding problem, such as placenta previa, during a previous pregnancy, labor, or delivery.

Medicines used in the treatment of mental illness are often teratogens. Lithium, for example, is known to cause fetal anomalies. Consequently, mentally ill pregnant women who take psychotropic drugs need to be identified. At times, it is possible to decrease the dosage of the psychotropic agent or change the prescription altogether. A second concern when mental illness is present in a pregnant woman is the woman's ability to parent.

Women who have had pelvic or upper-leg injuries that might interfere with fetal descent should be identified. X-rays taken in association with the injury should be obtained.

Emotional History

For most women pregnancy is as much an emotional experience as it is a physical one, and for many, it is much more of an emotional experience. Consequently, an assessment of emotional well-being is a critical part of the initial prenatal assessment. An assessment of physical safety for women living in abusive environments is essential. Physical abuse does not stop because women are pregnant. In fact, the abuse may increase. Blows to the abdomen in the second half of pregnancy may cause placental abruption, threatening the lives of both mother and baby. Women should be asked to call the health care provider if any trauma to the abdomen occurs. Questions about their safety and their readiness to move to a safer environment should be asked at each visit. An essential component of the emotional history for pregnant women is a discussion of previous birth experiences. It can occur at any time during the interview.

Often it is a good way to begin the data gathering. "When you remember your other pregnancies and births, what are the things that come to mind?" may evoke forgotten memories. "Do you think that anything that happened then will influence this pregnancy and birth?" may also yield helpful information. Ask about each pregnancy individually.

Lifestyle

Nutrition. A nutrition questionnaire is often helpful in assessing food intake during pregnancy. Foods and beverages commonly consumed by the groups of people served in the ambulatory care setting can be listed to be circled by the client prior to the health assessment interview or be done verbally when the client cannot read. Pictures or drawings may also be used. Additional questions can address financial ability to purchase food; resources for supplementing the food budget, such as the women, infants, and children (WIC) program, food banks, and church programs; eating habits (e.g., frequency of meals); symptoms that interfere with eating (e.g., nausea and heartburn); and foods avoided because of religious customs/prohibitions or ethnic beliefs about what is appropriate for pregnant women to eat. Additional information regarding pregnancy and nutrition is found in Chapter 12.

Exercise. Determine the amount and type of exercise the client is getting. The effect of exercise on pregnancy is discussed in Chapter 11. Exercise also increases the risk of accidents, and each pregnant woman's potential for exercise-associated accidents and injuries should be assessed.

Smoking. Smoking is clearly associated with reduced birth weight (see Chapter 19, "High-Risk Childbearing"). The nurse walks a delicate line between encouraging women to stop smoking or cut down and inducing anxiety in women who find quitting impossible or personally undesirable. Nicotine chewing gum is contraindicated in pregnancy at the present time because it has not been clinically tested in pregnant women.

Alcohol. Alcohol consumption during pregnancy may cause fetal alcohol syndrome (FAS) (see Chapters 19 and 22). Unfortunately, the association between the amount of alcohol and the appearance of FAS, as well as the association between gestational age at which alcohol abuse occurs and development of FAS, remains unknown. Determination of the client's alcohol consumption during pregnancy is essential for good care. Both the amount consumed and the frequency of consumption should be noted. Refer to the initial history form (Table 9.1) for appropriate questions.

History of the Present Pregnancy

Data about the current pregnancy is needed to differentiate between serious conditions that require further investigation and those that constitute the "common discomforts" of pregnancy. Areas that should be addressed are discussed next and include questions about possible complications, conditions that may cause intense discomfort, fetal movement, drug use, sexual activity, and emotional well-being.

Headaches. Headaches occur frequently in pregnant women. Although they are often related to stress, the origin of most remains unknown. When headaches occur late in pregnancy, the clinician must always consider a diagnosis of preeclampsia and inquire about other symptoms of this disease: visual disturbances, epigastric pain, and right, upper quadrant pain. Headaches that increase in frequency, duration, or intensity and those not relieved by rest or simple medication require further investigation. Occasionally, brain tumors are the cause.

Nausea/Vomiting. Nausea and vomiting in the first trimester are usually "morning sickness," one of the common discomforts of pregnancy. Because it occurs frequently in early pregnancy, health care providers can overlook the disruption it may cause for a woman and for her family, particularly when the activities of daily living aggravate the symptoms. Unusual patterns, associated symptomatology, or prolongation of the period of vomiting past the first trimester must be investigated.

Heartburn. Heartburn due to the decreased stomach emptying time, displacement of the stomach upward late in pregnancy, and subsequent regurgitation and reflux of stomach contents can be a source of misery to pregnant women. It can also be a signal of worsening preeclampsia.

Pain in Chest, Abdomen, Back, and Legs. Chest pain may be indicative of a pulmonary embolus or myocardial infarction. Abdominal pain early in pregnancy may be a symptom of ectopic pregnancy or abortion. Uterine fibroids may also cause abdominal pain during pregnancy as the growing uterus stretches the tumor and uterine muscle. Late in pregnancy, abdominal pain may be caused by placental abruption. At any time throughout gestation, a pregnant woman may have appendicitis, pancreatitis, a twisted ovary, a bowel obstruction, gallstones, or any other condition that occurs in nonpregnant women. Back pain of obstetric significance involves the costovertebral angle, the site of pain when pyelonephritis is present. Leg pain may be indicative of thrombophlebitis. Look for redness, warmth, tenderness, and swelling.

Vaginal Discharge. Vaginal discharge commonly increases toward the end of pregnancy and at times is heavy enough to require panty liners for protection. This discharge must be differentiated from that caused by a sexually transmitted disease, amniotic fluid, and vaginitis. The latter usually causes malodor and/or pruritus. Wet smears will help identify vaginitis as the cause; cervical cultures can identify chlamydia and gonorrhea; and a positive nitrazine test, vaginal pooling, and ferning can identify amniotic fluid.

An increase in vaginal discharge may also presage preterm labor. Therefore, the clinician should inquire about concurrent contractions, cramping, and pelvic pressure when increased discharge is reported prior to term. Occasionally, persistent vaginal discharge is due to infection resulting from penile-vaginal contact after anal intercourse. History taking in such instances should include a question about anal intercourse (Cohall & Warren, 1991).

Vaginal Bleeding. Vaginal bleeding must always be taken seriously. In early pregnancy it can be a symptom of abortion or ectopic pregnancy. Later, it may be a symptom of abruptio placentae or placenta previa. A small amount of bleeding may occur at the time of implantation, with cervicitis, after a Pap smear, after coitus, or subsequent to a digital cervical examination. Because of the potential seriousness of vaginal bleeding, each episode should be reported by the client and investigated by the health care provider.

Constipation and/or Diarrhea. Constipation occurs frequently in pregnancy, even in the first trimester. Occasionally, it is so severe that a fecal impaction occurs. It may even be impossible to insert a vaginal speculum because the rectum full of feces encroaches on the vagina.

Diarrhea is usually the result of an infectious process but it can also be a symptom of Crohn's disease (inflammatory bowel syndrome) or AIDS. When questioning the client about episodes of diarrhea, be sure to determine her definition because some women refer to diarrhea as frequent stools.

Edema. Most pregnant women experience some degree of edema. Lower extremity edema occurs in up to 90% of women with normal pregnancies, and 50% report edema of the fingers. The most significant edema is that occurring in the face or dependent edema in significant amounts (i.e., 3+ to 4+ on a scale of trace to 4+). The subjective nature of evaluating for edema must be recognized.

Urinary Tract Infection (UTI) Symptoms. UTIs are relatively common in pregnant women (see Chapter 23 for a discussion of assessment and treatment of these conditions). Any client report of urgency, burning on urination, or voiding in small amounts requires laboratory testing of a urine specimen. A clean-catch, midstream specimen should be obtained for urinalysis and/or culture. If the client has already voided, do not ask her to drink water so that she will be able to void quickly, because a dilute urine sample may be misleading.

Fever. Data on fever in pregnancy is practically nonexistent. No particular temperature is known to cause fetal anomaly or fetal death. It is good practice, however, to record known instances of fever in pregnancy in the client's record. Because many clients do not have a thermometer at home, the first prenatal visit is a good time to suggest that one be obtained. It will be invaluable in following illness in the child and can be used, meanwhile, for maternal purposes.

Contractions. Uterine contractions begin early in pregnancy but are not usually perceived by the mother until much later. Occasional contractions occurring before term and felt by the mother are usually benign. Unfortunately, it is often difficult to differentiate between benign contractions and those that result in cervical effacement, dilatation, and delivery of a preterm child. More than six contractions per hour or contractions occurring at 10-minute intervals or less require evaluation for cervical change. Women who are 24 weeks pregnant should be counseled about the signs of preterm labor.

Fetal Movement. A moving fetus is a healthy fetus. The date of quickening (first movement felt) should be noted, and the clinician should inquire about fetal movement at each prenatal visit. Unfortunately, the exact number of movements likely to predict a compromised fetus is unknown. The current recommendation is that mothers notify their health care provider if the fetus moves fewer than 10 times in a 12-hour period. This number is far below the daily normal range. (See Chapter 19 for a discussion of fetal movement assessment.)

Sexual Activity. Inquiries about sexual activity should be made at the first prenatal visit. Women who are sexually active should be asked if they are having any problems or have any questions. "Most women have questions about sex during pregnancy," lets the client know that the clinician is open to questions. Ask women who are not sexually active why it is that they are not having intercourse. Some women, of course, will be without a partner. Others may appreciate an opportunity to discuss problems that have arisen.

When pregnancy is normal, vaginal intercourse may continue until labor begins, bleeding occurs, or membranes rupture. However, maternal discomfort and male fears of harming the baby may result in cessation of sexual activity before this time. Women who have been asked to observe "pelvic rest" have been known to awaken in the midst of an orgasm (personal communication to author from client). It is helpful if the nurse asks if the client has experienced orgasm during sleep when she has been asked to abstain from orgasm. The nurse can then provide reassurance that this can happen and that there is nothing that the client can do to prevent it, thus alleviating guilt that might exist. All women need to be cautioned not to allow their partner to blow air into their vagina during intercourse, an uncommon practice that has been reported to cause air emboli that results in maternal death.

Emotional Well-Being. An assessment of emotional well-being includes an evaluation of how the client seems to be bonding to her unborn child. Questions that can facilitate this evaluation include, "Do you ever think about this baby?" If "yes," "What do you think about? What do you think about when you picture yourself as the mother of this child? How do you feel when the baby moves?" Some activities may help the mother attach to her baby while it is still in utero. A discussion about the size of the fetus and what it is able to do as the pregnancy progresses is often fun. Pictures of the fetus at various gestational ages are usually of interest.

Prescription, Over-the-Counter, and Illicit Drugs. Ask the client what medicine she has taken since the beginning of the pregnancy. Be vigilant for drugs known to be teratogens. Determine the client's use of illicit drugs. While asking a pregnant client questions about drug use, it is essential that the nurse remain aware of personal biases. Nurses often believe that illicit drug use in pregnancy does not occur in women obtaining care from private physicians. The result is that the women using drugs in these settings are overlooked.

Laboratory Tests

Certain tests are indicated for all pregnant women and are routinely performed at the initial prenatal visit. The need for other studies is determined by a woman's history, physical examination, and health status throughout her pregnancy. These are listed in Table 9.5.

The urine culture will identify asymptomatic bacteriuria, a UTI that may go unnoticed because of unaccompanying symptoms. The diagnosis of asymptomatic bacteriuria is based on colony counts greater than 100,000 in urine specimens obtained by the clean-catch method, except when *Escherichia coli* is the identified pathogen. Asymptomatic bacteriuria in this case is diagnosed from smaller colony counts. It is important to remember that colony counts are influenced by voiding frequency, diuresis, urine Ph, drugs, and food. Acidic urine inhibits bacterial replication.

Continuing Health Assessment During Pregnancy

Pregnant women are seen at intervals throughout the pregnancy to evaluate fetal growth and fetal well-being, screen for maternal disease and obstetric problems, promote a healthy lifestyle, answer questions, provide support, assess readiness for birth and parenthood, and refer as necessary to community resources. The intervals at which return visits should be scheduled have not been studied, but, traditionally, they have occurred every 4 weeks until 28 weeks gestation, every 2 weeks from the 28th to the 36th week of gestation, and weekly thereafter until delivery. New guidelines from the Public Health Service (PHS) Expert Panel on Content of Prenatal Care (1989) suggest a visit schedule for healthy women that decreases the number of total visits and differentiates between nulliparas and multiparas. The model also emphasizes an attention to health promotion and emotional concerns of clients to complement the typical emphasis on measurement of selected parameters. Table 9.6 outlines the PHS recommended visit schedule for healthy pregnant women.

Maternal Well-Being

Maternal well-being is evaluated at each visit by (a) asking the prenatal screening questions described earlier, (b) measuring blood pressure, (c) examining a urine specimen for protein and sugar, and (d) comparing weight with norms for gain in pregnancy.

Measurement of Blood Pressure. Blood pressure elevations may be indicative of chronic hypertension and/or PIH. Accurate determination of blood pressure is a critical feature of prenatal care. Accordingly, measures known to obtain accurate readings should be observed. These include use of an appropriately sized cuff and regularly scheduled equipment maintenance. Ideally, blood pressure measurements obtained throughout pregnancy are compared with a prepregnant measurement. When a pregnant woman is new to a health care setting, the nurse lacks the advantage of knowing the client's prepregnant blood pressure. In these instances, an accurate first-visit measurement is particularly important. It is often useful to obtain prenatal blood pressures personally. In a busy setting with many blood pressures obtained by a person assigned specifically to this task, hurried readings may be taken, resulting in significant elevations being missed.

Blood pressure readings in pregnancy should be made with the client in a sitting position. The same arm should be used each time. Elevated readings should not be ignored. Measurements obtained with the client in a side-lying position can give false reassurance that the blood pressure is in the normal range.

A midtrimester measurement of the mean arterial pressure (MAP) should be obtained. MAP is calculated by adding the diastolic pressure (DP) to one third of the pulse pressure, which is systolic pressure (SP) minus DP:

$$MAP = DP + (SP-DP)/3$$

A rise of 20 mg Hg in the MAP is thought to be ominous, and a MAP of 100 is abnormal. A MAP of 105 indicates hypertension (Knuppel & Drukker, 1993).

Checking a Urine Specimen. A random urine specimen is traditionally tested at each prenatal visit for the presence of protein and/or sugar. Protein may indicate preeclampsia, renal disease, or a urinary tract infection. Sugar may indicate diabetes. The PHS Expert Panel on Content of Prenatal Care (1989) felt that routine urine testing is not required at any time during pregnancy for low-risk pregnant women. If the nurse chooses to continue performing the urine dipstick test, a 1-hour glucose screening test should be ordered whenever glucosuria occurs. This holds true even if the client has recently consumed foods high in glucose, because it is not possible to determine whether the glucosuria is due to altered carbohydrate metabolism or to a lowered renal threshold.

Evaluating Weight Gain. Weight grids can provide a visual picture of weight change in pregnancy (see Chapter 12). Although the typical pattern of weight gain associated with good fetal outcome is a gradual, steady increment, the actual rate of desired gain is not well defined. Poor weight gains may indicate a poorly growing fetus or inadequate maternal nutrition. Large gains may indicate preeclampsia or macrosomia. Although clinical usefulness of this information has recently been questioned (Dawes & Grudzinskas, 1991), many clinicians continue to use

Table 9.5 Laboratory Examinations: Pregnant Women

Tests	*Initial Visit*	*26-30 Weeks*	*36 Weeks*	*Further Assessment Needed*
Blood tests				
Complete blood count				
Hemoglobin (Hgb)	X	X	X*	Hgb < 10g/dl *Not recommended by Expert Panel
Hematocrit (Hct)	X	X	X*	Hct 32% or more *Not recommended by Expert Panel
White blood cell count	X			15,000 mm or more
Differential smear	X			Cellular abnormalities and/or decreased platelets
Blood Group				
Rh factor	X			Mother Rh negative; partner Rh negative or unknown
Antibody screen	X	*	*	Significant titer as defined by local laboratory *For Rh negative women only
Rubella titer	X			Titer less than 1:8 or significant rise in titer
Sickle-cell screen	X*			Positive for trait or anemia; partner should be tested *Done when history indicates
Tay-Sachs screen	X*			Carrier *Done when history indicates
Maternal serum alpha-fetoprotein (MSAFP)	*			Counsel at initial visit; done between 15-20 weeks; significant if > 2.0 MoMs
Random blood glucose	X*	X	X	140 mg/dl or greater *Expert panel recommends at 24-28 weeks; authorities differ as to need for all women; some only for high risk
Oral glucose tolerance test (OGTT)	*	*	*	*Done if random blood glucose is elevated above 140 mg/dl
Syphilis serology	X		X*	Positive; some authorities recommend repeat only if high risk
Hepatitis B	X		*	Positive; repeat if high risk
Human immunovirus (HIV)	X			Positive; offer to all women
Urine tests				
Culture for bacteria	X			Positive
Urine glucose and protein				
Cervical tests				
Papanicolaou smear	X*			Positive *Unless tested in past year
Gonorrheal culture	X		*	Positive *Repeat for high-risk individuals
Chlamydial culture or rapid screen	X			Positive *Repeat for high-risk individuals
Skin test tuberculosis	X*			Positive *Expert Panel recommends for high-risk women only
Illicit drug screen	X			(Offer)

SOURCES: Adapted from Public Health Service Expert Panel on Content of Prenatal Care (1989) and Aumann and Baird (1993).

Table 9.6 Public Health Service Recommended Schedule of Prenatal Visits

New guidelines from the Public Health Service Expert Panel on the Content of Prenatal Care suggest the following visit schedule for healthy pregnant women. These guidelines represent a decrease in the number and frequency of visits traditionally suggested. They are only for healthy pregnant women; women experiencing a high-risk pregnancy will be seen more frequently.

Nulliparas	*Multiparas*
First visit: 6-8 weeks	First visit: 6-8 weeks
Second visit: within 4 weeks of previous visit	Second visit: 14-16 weeks
Third visit: 14-16 weeks	Third visit: 24-28 weeks
Fourth visit: 24-28 weeks	Fourth visit: 32 weeks
Fifth visit: 32 weeks	Fifth visit: 36 weeks
Sixth visit: 36 weeks	Sixth visit: 39 weeks
Seventh visit: 38 weeks	Seventh visit: 41 weeks
Eighth visit: 40 weeks	
Ninth visit: 41 weeks	

SOURCE: Adapted from Public Health Service Expert Panel on Content of Prenatal Care (1989).

the information as a rough estimate of fetal growth.

Laboratory Tests

At approximately 28 weeks gestation, all clients should be screened for gestational diabetes with a 1-hour glucose screen. A flavored drink containing 50 grams of glucose is swallowed, and blood is drawn 1 hour later. Most institutions set the cutoff for normal glucose at 135 to 140 mg/dl. A 3-hour glucose tolerance test is performed when higher values occur. The test should be preceded by a 3-day diet high in carbohydrates. Economic status may preclude consumption of the recommended diet. In such instances, clients should be asked to eat four slices of bread each day for 3 days in addition to their regular food intake. This will approximate the required carbohydrate intake and increase the likelihood of accurate test results.

Women with very high glucose levels on the screening test are not given the 3-hour test because it uses 100 grams of glucose, a load not appropriate to a woman with impaired glucose metabolism.

Selected tests are routinely performed in some settings at 36 weeks gestation. The tests most often repeated are for STDs and anemia. Cultures for gonorrhea and chlamydia are obtained, and blood tests for syphilis, hepatitis B, and HIV may be performed.

Although it is common to retest for anemia at this time, it is probably better to perform this test before 28 weeks gestation because maximum hemodilution occurs between 28 and 34 weeks. The clinician could be misled by the results. Retesting prior to 28 weeks also allows time for a diagnostic workup and treatment should a true anemia be diagnosed.

Fetal Well-Being Assessment

Fetal well-being is evaluated by counting fetal heart tones, asking about fetal movement, and by measuring fundal height. Normal fetal heart tones have a regular rhythm and can be heard beating 120 to 160 times per minute. Fetal heart tones can usually be heard with a doppler-type instrument at 10 to 12 weeks gestation and with a fetoscope at 17 to 20 weeks gestation. Failure to hear fetal heart tones at these times may indicate an error in dates or fetal demise. An irregular rhythm requires further evaluation, usually with a fetal echocardiogram. Because the heart is very small in a first-trimester fetus, the chances of hearing the heart beat with a doppler-type instrument will increase if the instrument is slowly rotated 360 degrees at each position.

A heart beat of less than 100 beats per minute (bpm) may be a sign of a congenital heart block. Tachycardia (>160 bpm) may be a sign of congestive heart failure. With high or low rates, differentiation of maternal and fetal heart beats may be achieved by palpating the maternal pulse while listening to the fetal heart rate with a Doppler-type instrument or a fetoscope.

An active fetus is a healthy fetus. An inactive fetus may or may not be healthy. All high-risk pregnant women should be asked to count fetal movements each day. In addition, women who report that the fetus does not seem to be active and women approaching a gestational age of 41 ½ weeks should be asked to concentrate on fetal movement twice each day. If the fetus moves five times before 60 minutes has elapsed, counting can be discontinued. It should be resumed in approximately 12 hours. If the fetus does not move five times in an hour, electronic fetal monitoring should occur. Although the exact number of movements necessary to ensure that the fetus is healthy has not been determined, the minimum number of movements generally accepted is 10 in a 12-hour period. This number is well below the average number of movements made by a healthy fetus each day. (See Chapter 19 for additional discussion of fetal movement as an indicator of fetal well-being.)

The height of the maternal fundus should be noted at each visit beginning with the 16th week of gestation. At this time, the top of the uterus should be halfway between the top of the symphysis pubis and the umbilicus. At 20 weeks, the uterus should be at the umbilicus. These guidelines seem to hold true despite the wide individual variation in the length of the maternal abdomen. After 24 weeks gestation, fundal height should be measured in centimeters from the top of the symphysis to the top of the fundus. If the fundus grows steadily after 24 weeks and is within 2 centimeters of the gestational age, the fetus is usually growing well. When there is a discrepancy of 4 centimeters or more, an ultrasound examination should be obtained. Although a dating error is the most common explanation of the difference, oligohydramnios (decreased amounts of amniotic fluid), polyhydramnios (excess amniotic fluid), intrauterine growth retardation, malpresentation, and multiple gestation may also be present.

The value of the fundal height measurement in assessing fetal growth diminishes after 36 weeks gestation. Measurements that continue rising and coincide with increasing gestational age pose no problem. But measurements that show no growth in fundal height after this time may leave the clinician unable to determine whether or not this is a cause for concern or whether the fetus is merely low in the maternal pelvis. In addition, in some women, the fetus is difficult to palpate or outline, leaving the clinician either worrying or requesting an ultrasound that, in hindsight, was unnecessary. Continuing maternal weight gain and an active fetus are reassuring that the fetus is growing and is well.

To avoid being influenced by gestational age when measuring fundal height, place the side of the measuring tape that is measured in centimeters directly on the maternal abdomen. When gestational age is known and the centimeter markings on the measuring tape can be seen, the clinician may be more likely to try for a measurement approximating the gestational age.

Screening Questions

At each visit, information obtained by asking the prenatal screening questions previously described can be helpful in evaluating the physical and emotional status of the client. Health education and counseling should be discussed as appropriate at prenatal visits. Table 9.7 summarizes important prenatal markers, identifies times at which selected testing is indicated, and recommends topics for discussion at selected prenatal visits.

Special Considerations for the Postpartum Client

Traditionally, the postpartum checkup is scheduled 6 weeks after delivery. The focus of the examination is an evaluation of the reproductive organs and assessment of any episiotomy or laceration repair. Awareness of the emotional significance of this period makes the postpartum checkup an ideal time to evaluate other aspects of the new mother's life.

No one really knows exactly when the postpartum checkup should occur. Some schedule the visit at 4 weeks postpartum in hopes that the mother will have begun using a method of birth control, which can also be assessed. The advantage of scheduling the checkup later is that Pap smears obtained at 8 weeks increase the accuracy of interpretation.

Trade-offs will be found regardless of when the examination is scheduled. Telephone calls and home visits prior to the checkup can provide support and identify early problems. Either may be particularly valuable for women having their first baby; experiencing psychosocial stress; having a history of previous postpartum depression; having conditions interfering with activities of

Table 9.7 Key Moments in Prenatal Care

1. First visit (6-10 weeks) Blood pressure Cervical length and dilatation Genetic problems	2. 16-18 weeks Maternal serum alpha-fetoprotein Body image Early pregnancy classes Quickening
3. At 20 weeks Weight gain Fetal heart tone with fetascope Quickening	4. 22-26 weeks Cervical check if nullipara or history of preterm labor Cervical check for history of preterm labor Stressors Preterm labor instruction
5. At 28 weeks Body image Preeclampsia labor instruction Dreams 1-hour glucose screen Antibody screen if Rh negative/RHO Gam Fetal movement Childbirth education	6. At 36 weeks Presentation Labor fears Consider retest for syphilis hepatitis B gonorrhea chlamydia hematocrit Layette Fetal movement instructions Birth plan

daily living, such as large and painful hemorrhoids; breast-feeding for the first time or having problems with a crying baby.

The postpartum assessment consists of a postpartum history, an abbreviated physical examination, and laboratory studies that should, at the minimum, include a Pap smear. At times, problems identified prenatally or intrapartally will need laboratory follow-up. Referrals to specialists or community agencies may be needed.

The labor/delivery/postpartum records should be reviewed if available. If the records are not available, ask the client if anything happened during the labor or birth that requires follow-up. For example, gestational diabetes should disappear after delivery. A postprandial blood glucose is often ordered to be sure that a true diabetic state does not exist. Hematocrits may or may not be ordered. They are almost always normal at the postpartum examination.

Table 9.8 outlines questions to identify physical and emotional problems that may be present. Areas of assessment include emotional status, weight and body image, parenting concerns, employment, infant feeding, and sexual activity. Health practices since delivery, such as selecting sexual partners, medication use, and substance use, are assessed.

Women should be asked about bleeding and spotting since delivery. When more than one perineal pad is saturated in an hour, bleeding is excessive. Pain should be described: "Where is it? What type is it? How long does it last? Is it getting worse? Are there any associated signs and symptoms? What have you done for it? What do you think is the cause?" The main causes of pain after discharge from the hospital/birth center are due to lacerations/episiotomy and infections of the uterus, urinary tract, and breasts.

Ask, "Have you taken any medicine since the baby was born? Have you been to a clinic, hospital, or emergency room?" to identify problems that may have occurred since discharge from the hospital/birth center.

The incredible demands of being a new mother affect her relationship with her baby. Accordingly, nurses should attempt to determine from all new mothers their feelings about the baby and being a mother. "How is being a mother compared with what you thought it would be? In what ways is it harder?" Asking if the baby is hard or easy as well as asking the mother for other words to describe her infant can be helpful. The nurse should ask how the baby was named and who named the child, "Is there anything

text continued on page 176

Table 9.8 Postpartum History

I. Screening for physical well-being
   A. How are you feeling?
   B. Are you still bleeding/spotting? (frequency, amount)
   C. Have you had any pain?
   D. Any vaginal discharge?
   E. How about feeling tired?
   F. Have you taken any medicine since the baby was born?
   G. Have you been to a clinic/hospital/emergency room?
   H. Was there anything that happened when you were pregnant or during your labor that needs to be followed up?

II. Screening for psychosocial well-being
   A. How are you doing emotionally?
   B. How would you describe your disposition? Have you been irritable? Scared? Overwhelmed? Hard to get along with? Angry? Satisfied? Excited? Happy?
   C. What is hardest for you now?
   D. How many times have you cried?
   E. How is your appetite?
   F. How much sleep are you getting?
   G. Do you think you've changed in any way since the baby was born?
   H. Has anything changed between you and your partner?
   I. What do you need most right now?
   J. What do you wish your partner would do for you?
   K. Is there anything you wish your partner would stop doing?
   L. What is the nicest thing that anyone has done for you since the baby was born?
   M. When you remember your labor and birth, what things stand out for you?
      1. How was your labor different from what you expected?
      2. How was your behavior different from what you wanted?
      3. What are you proud about?
      4. Is there anything you wish you had done differently?
      5. Is there anything you wish you could change about your labor?
      6. What about the birth itself? What memories do you have?
      7. Is there anything you would like to change?
      8. Was there anything about yourself that surprised you? What about your partner/others who were with you? Anything about the baby that surprised you?
   N. What do you like best right now about yourself, your partner, the baby?
   O. How is being a mother compared with what you thought it would be?
   P. Would you say you have a hard baby or an easy baby?
      1. Why do you say that?
      2. How else would you describe your baby?
      3. Have you had any thoughts about hurting the baby?
      4. Have you been afraid that anyone else might hurt the baby?
   Q. What name did you give the baby?
      1. Who picked the name?
      2. Why did you decide on that name?

III. Concerns about weight/body image
   A. How do you feel about your present weight?
   B. Do you still feel you would like to weigh ______ (refer to initial history)?
   C. How important is it that you get to your ideal weight?
   D. Do you have a time frame in mind for getting there?
   E. Have you thought about how you are going to get there? What type of help do you think you might need?
   F. What has your partner said about your weight?
      1. Have there been any comments made about how you look?
      2. If yes, how did that make you feel?
      3. Have you felt afraid of your partner?

IV. Are you working for money?
   A. If yes, what do you do?
   B. What hours do you work? What days? What shift?
   C. On a scale of 1 to 10, how do you feel about working? About this particular job?

Table 9.8 Postpartum History—Continued

- D. Do you have any plans to change this situation in the future?
- E. What do you do for child care? How do you feel about this arrangement?

V. How are you feeding your baby?
- A. If breast-feeding
  1. How is it going for you?
  2. Did you have any initial problems?
  3. Are you having any problems now?
  4. What do you do about leaking?
  5. How does your partner feel about your breast-feeding?
  6. Do you nurse in public? How is that for you?
  7. Has your partner tasted the milk? If yes, how was that for him? for you?
  8. How long do you think you might like to nurse?
  9. Is there anything that might interfere with that?
  10. How have your other children reacted?
- B. If tried breast-feeding, but now bottle-feeding
  1. How was breast-feeding for you?
  2. How do you feel about having given breast-feeding a try?
  3. How do you feel about bottle-feeding?
  4. What has your partner had to say about the change? Your family?
  5. Did you have any breast discomfort/pain when you changed?
  6. If yes, what did you do about it? Did you ask for advice on what to do?
  7. How important was it to you to breast-feed? If important, what information/support might have been helpful to you?

VI. Have you made love (had sex) yet?
- A. If not, why is that?
- B. If yes, how did it go?
- C. Were you afraid of anything?
- D. Was there anything different about making love now compared to before you were pregnant or before the baby was born?
- E. Did your partner say anything about its being different?
- F. Was there any discomfort/pain?
  1. If yes, when did it occur?
  2. Was this pain that you have had before?
  3. What do you think was/is the cause of the pain?
  4. What have you done about it? Has that helped?
- G. Are you having any problems now?
  1. How about *wanting* to make love? Has that been a problem?
  2. What about vaginal dryness?
  3. What about not being able to find time?
- H. Have you climaxed?
  1. If no, is this a problem for you?
  2. If yes and client is breast-feeding, did your milk let down? How was that for you? For your partner?

VII. Birth control—Have you used any birth control?
- A. What type?
- B. How often?
- C. How are you using it?
- D. How do you feel about that method? How does your partner feel about it?
- E. Do you think you will want to change your birth control method soon? Later on?
- F. Is there anything that would keep you from using this method successfully?
- G. Do you think you will want more children in the future?
- H. If no, have you thought about having your tubes tied?

VIII. Health practices
- A. Do you have a new sexual partner?
- B. If sexually active, are you having sex with more than one person?
- C. What drugs have you used since the baby was born?
  1. How often?
  2. Did you have sex when you were high?

(continued)

Table 9.8 Postpartum History—Continued

- D. How many times have you used alcohol since the birth of the baby?
    1. What did you drink?
    2. When?
    3. How much?
    4. Did anyone encourage you to drink?
    5. Who was with you?
- E. Are you smoking?
    1. How much?
    2. How about marijuana?

IX. Health education
- A. Are there any questions you want to ask today?
- B. Here is a list of things parents sometimes want information about. Tell me if any of these interest you.
    1. Smoking cessation programs
    2. Drug and alcohol programs
    3. Risks for AIDS
    4. Weight control ideas
    5. How to get back into shape
    6. Working and breast-feeding
    7. How to parent an infant
    8. How to parent toddlers, etc.
    9. Anger control
    10. How to use a menstrual calendar
    11. Support groups: new moms, rape victims, children of alcoholics, sexual abuse, emotional abuse, physical abuse

about this baby you don't like or you have a hard time with? What would you change about him or her if you could?"

Identification of the new mother who is depressed and development of a plan to ameliorate the symptoms is essential. Women at risk for developing depression in the postpartum period are those who have experienced a depressive episode previously and those with a family history of depression (Unterman, Posner, & Williams, 1990). Women who report crying a lot, not eating, and sleeping either a lot or a little should be noted. Other important symptoms are negative feeling states, anxiety, insomnia, fatigue, anger, and irritability (Affonso, Lovett, Paul, & Sheptak, 1990). The nurse can ask directly, "Are you depressed?" Most mothers who are depressed know that they are and will discuss it readily. They may not, however, volunteer that they are.

Depressed mothers often perceive their baby as difficult (Whiffen, 1988). Ask, "How would you describe your baby?" If depression is suspected, continue with, "Have you thought of hurting the baby?" When the response is "Yes," ask the mother if she has tried to harm the baby or is afraid she will harm the baby. Immediate intervention or referral may be necessary. Culturally appropriate ways of alleviating this distress and supporting women through difficult emotional times need to be identified and developed.

"What do you think you do best as a mother?" and "Is there anything you are working on?" can initiate a discussion of the client's feelings about herself as a parent.

Most women are anxious to lose the weight they gained while pregnant. This seems to happen most easily for women who were underweight at conception. See Table 9.8 for specific ways to assess weight and body image concerns. Help her to be realistic and provide counseling when necessary if she has chosen a potentially dangerous diet plan. Occasionally, an underweight woman will wish to retain the weight she gained during her pregnancy. This is often difficult and usually requires the help of a nutritionist/dietitian.

Questions regarding employment are directed at discovering how mothers who are or will be working for money feel about employment while their baby is small and also helping the client think through her arrangements for child care. Health care providers often have personal feelings either for or against particular mothers being employed. Providers should be aware of these feelings and allow each woman to sort out for herself what is in the best interest of herself and her family.

It is important for the nurse to know how her client is feeding her baby so that the practitioner can become aware of problems that may occur in the initial days and weeks. Nurses can set up early intervention programs that may decrease the numbers of women who switch to bottle-feeding. Women who have stopped breast-feeding should be asked when they stopped, why they stopped, and who they turned to for help if they were experiencing problems. Advice about the resumption of penis-in-vagina intercourse varies widely. Despite evidence that many women resume intercourse before the 6-week postpartum examination and have no problems as a result, many practitioners still ask women to avoid intercourse until the postpartum checkup or, in women without any laceration/episiotomy repair, until lochia stops. Lochia, however, persists longer than most practitioners think; for example, normal loss of lochia serosa has been documented beyond 60 days after delivery (Oppenheimer, Sherriff, Goodman, Shah, & James, 1986).

The nurse can begin assessment of sexual activity by asking the client if she has had intercourse/made love/had sex since the baby was born. If she has not, ask, "Why is that?" If she is ready to be sexually active again, ask if she is afraid of anything. Many women will be afraid of pain. Whether or not the experience will be painful will depend on the type and extent of lacerations/episiotomy, the technique used for repair, the amount of vaginal lubrication that occurs, the client's emotional state, and previous experiences with intercourse. Breast-feeding women may report less lubrication as well as decreased desire for sex.

Ask breast-feeding women who do climax whether or not their milk "let down." If milk did appear, ask, "How was that for you? For your partner?" Many women and their partners are unprepared for the spurt of milk that may accompany orgasm. They often appreciate being informed of this possibility ahead of time so that the woman can wear a bra or protect the place of lovemaking. If you did not inquire previously about whether the partner tasted the breast milk, this is a good time to ask. Tasting of the breast milk by the partner is a common practice, yet many women feel guilty about it.

Birth control is often discussed with women before they are discharged from the setting where they gave birth. At the postpartum checkup many women will already be taking an oral contraceptive. See Chapter 14, for information about the oral contraceptive and other methods of family planning. Assessment questions are found in Table 9.8.

Women who are not using a method of birth control at the time of their postpartum checkup may expect a method to be suggested at the time of the examination. Intrauterine devices may be inserted and diaphragms fitted at this time. Ask the client if she thinks she will want more children in the future. Ask women who had a tubal ligation while in the hospital how they feel about their decision.

The nurse should inquire about health practices since delivery. Some postpartum clients will have a new sexual partner or will anticipate a new partner in the future. In these cases, review safe sex guidelines. When appropriate, offer the client condoms before she leaves the ambulatory care setting.

Inquire about prescription, over-the-counter, and illicit drugs taken since the baby was born. Counseling about drugs while breast-feeding is appropriate. Women who do not consider marijuana a drug may continue to smoke it while breast-feeding. Women have also smoked crack and used other forms of cocaine while breast-feeding. All of these practices are unsafe. Inquire also about consumption of alcohol. Beer and other forms of alcohol are no longer recommended to encourage milk production or maternal relaxation.

The postpartum assessment will need to be adjusted for women who have experienced a perinatal loss. Emphasis should be on the client's emotional state. Although great strides have been made toward recognizing the importance of grieving, routine prescription of activities thought to be helpful in the resolution of grief, such as seeing or holding her dead baby or waiting for her grief to be "resolved" before conceiving again, may be harmful. In addition, not everyone goes through the grieving process in the stages generally reported in the literature (Levy, 1992). Each perinatal loss should be approached from the unique circumstances women bring as individuals to any given situation.

Conclusion

Provision of holistic health care to women requires comprehensive well-woman assessment. It is based on data from a health history, physical examination and laboratory studies. During a well-woman assessment, the nurse should obtain information about the client's past and present health status, lifestyle behaviors, and family relationships. In this chapter, an approach for gathering and interpreting this data for all women was presented. In addition, information specific to adolescents and childbearing women was given. Components of the physical examination unique to women were discussed and interpretation of common laboratory studies provided. It is hoped that this framework for assessment will assist practicing nurses in the provision of care to their women clients.

References

Affonso, D. D., Lovett, S. T., Paul, S. M., & Sheptak, S. (1990). A standardized interview that differentiates pregnancy and postpartum symptoms from perinatal clinical depression. *Birth, 17*(3), 121-130.

Anastos, K., Charney, P., Charon, R. A., Cohen, E., Jones, C. Y., Marte, C., Swiderski, D. M., Wheat, M. E., & Williams, S. (1991). Hypertension in women: What is really known. *Annals of Internal Medicine, 111*(4), 287-293.

Aumann, G. M.-E., & Baird, M. M. (1993). Risk assessment for pregnant women. In R. A. Knuppel & J. E. Drukker (Eds.), *High-risk pregnancy: A team approach* (pp. 8-35). Philadelphia: W. B. Saunders.

Centers for Disease Control. (1991). Primary, secondary syphilis—U.S., 1981-1990. *Morbidity and Mortality Weekly Report, 40*, 314-323.

Chesley, L. C., & Cooper, D. W. (1986). Genetics of hypertension in pregnancy: Possible single gene control of pre-eclampsia in the descendants of eclamptic women. *British Journal of Obstetrics and Gynecology, 93*, 898-908.

Cohall, A. T., & Warren, A. (1991, January). Persistent vaginal discharge in a sexually active adolescent female. *Journal of Adolescent Health*, pp. 58-59.

Dawes, M. G., & Grudzinskas, F. (1991). Pregnancy measurement of maternal weight during pregnancy. Is this a useful procedure? *British Journal of Obstetrics and Gynecology, 98*, 189-194.

Diokno, A. C., Brock, B. M., Brown, M. B., & Herzog, A. R. (1986). Prevalence of urinary incontinence and other urological symptoms in the noninstitutionalized elderly. *Journal of Urology, 136*, 1022-1025.

Dykers, J. R. (1988). Wet-mount examination for the diagnosis of trichomoniasis. *JAMA, 259*, 3560-3561.

Eidelman, A. L., Kamar, R., Schimmel, M. S., & Bar-On, E. (1988). The grandmultipara: Is she still a risk? *American Journal of Obstetrics and Gynecology, 158*(2), 389-392.

Freeman, H. P., & Wasfie, T. J. (1989). Cancer of the breast in poor black women. *Cancer, 63*, 2562-2569.

Knuppel, R. A., & Drukker, J. (1993). Hypertension in pregnancy. In R. A. Knuppel & J. E. Drukker (Eds.), *High-risk pregnancy: A team approach* (pp. 468-517). Philadelphia: W. B. Saunders.

Levy, I. G. (1992, February/March). *Perinatal loss. A critique of current hospital procedure.* Paper presented to the American Society for Psychosomatic Obstetrics and Gynecology, Seattle, WA.

Lowery, M. (1987). Adult survivors of childhood incest. *Journal of Psychosocial Nursing, 25*(1), 27-31.

Melnick, S., Cole, P., Anderson, D., & Herbst, A. (1987). Rates and risks of diethylstilbestrol-related clear-cell adenocarcinoma of the vagina and cervix: An update. *New England Journal of Medicine, 316*(9), 514-516.

Murphy, P. A. (1990). Laboratory testing. In R. Lichtman & S. Papera (Eds.), *Gynecology well-woman care* (pp. 1-54). Norwalk, CT: Appleton & Lange.

O'Brien, W. F. (1990). Predicting preeclampsia (review). *Obstetrics and Gynecology, 17*, 3.

Oppenheimer, L. W., Sherriff, E. A., Goodman, J. D. S., Shah, D., & James, C. E. (1986). The duration of lochia. *British Journal of Obstetrics and Gynecology, 93*, 754-757.

Public Health Service Expert Panel on Content of Prenatal Care. (1989). *Caring for our future: The content of prenatal care.* Washington, DC: Public Health Service.

Rosen, M. (1990). Health maintenance strategies for women of different ages. *Obstetrics and Gynecology, 17*, 673-694.

Sloane, P. D., Slatt, L. M., & Curtis, P. (1993). *Essentials of family medicine.* Baltimore, MD: Williams & Wilkins.

Smith, R. C., & Hoppe, R. B. (1991). The patient's story: Integrating the patient and physician-centered approaches to interviewing. *Annals of Internal Medicine, 111*(6), 470-477.

Staff. (1989, July 28). Measles revaccination. *Medical Letter, 31*, 69-70.

Unterman, R. R., Posner, N. A., & Williams, K. N. (1990). Postpartum depressive disorders: Changing trends. *Birth, 17*(3), 131-137.

U.S. Preventive Services Task Force. (1989). *Guide to clinical preventive services.* Baltimore, MD: Williams & Wilkins.

Whiffen, V. E. (1988). Vulnerability of postpartum depression: A multivariate study. *Journal of Abnormal Psychology, 97*(4), 467-474.

Yates, A. (1989). Current perspectives on the eating disorders: 1. History, psychological, and biological aspects. *Journal of the American Academy of Child and Adolescent Psychiatry, 28*, 813-823.

ASSESSING THE FEMALE GENITALIA

There are two components to assessing the female genitalia: inspection and palpation done during the speculum and bimanual examinations. In addition, various smears and cultures, notably the Papanicolaou smear, gonorrheal culture, and chlamydia culture may be collected. Wet smears used to detect some vaginal infections may also be collected during the examination. This examination is always done with gloved hands. Areas near the anus should not be palpated until assessment completion to decrease the possibility of spreading fecal material to the vagina and urethra. Each step of the procedure should be explained prior to its initiation.

External Genitalia and Speculum Examination

1. To avoid startling the client tell her that she will feel you touching her before doing so. First touch her thigh and then her external genitalia. Examine the external genitalia, noting any vular lesions, growths, discharge, edema, discoloration, varicosities, or trauma. Tell the client you will place a finger just inside her vagina. Next gently spread the labia majora with the left hand, insert the right index finger into the vagina about 1.5 inches to 2 inches, and turn the finger upward (see Figure 9.1).

Milk the urethra and Skene's glands gently by exerting upward pressure on the urethra. Culture any discharge (see Figure 9.2).

2. Rotate the index finger downward and, using the thumb and index finger, palpate the areas of Bartholin's glands (at the 5 o'clock and 7 o'clock positions) in the vaginal walls. The areas should feel smooth with no swelling, masses, or tenderness (see Figure 9.3).

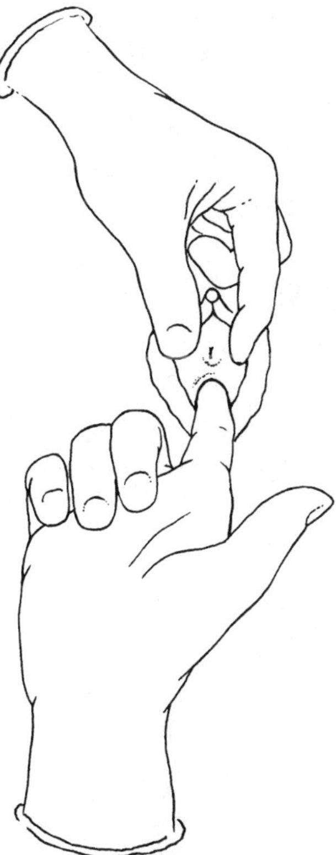

Figure 9.1.

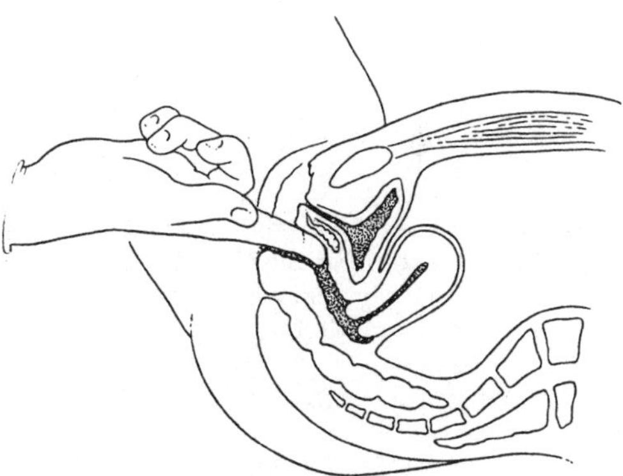

Figure 9.2.

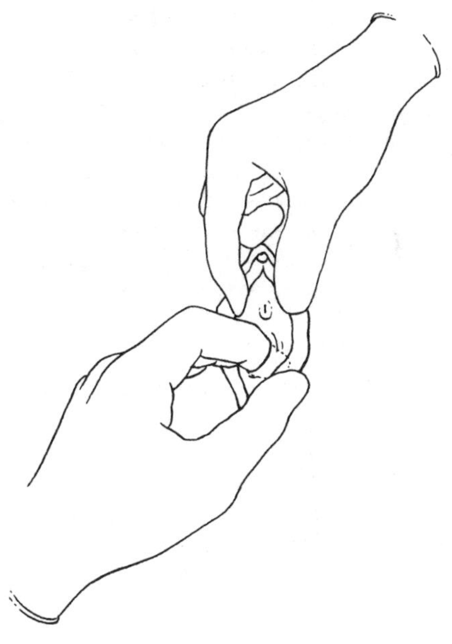

Figure 9.3.

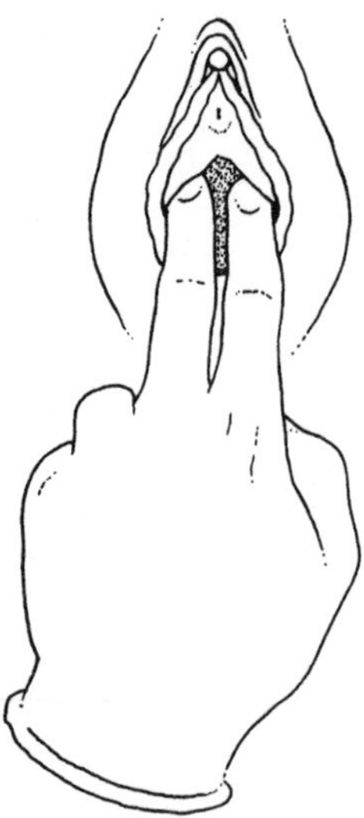

Figure 9.4.

3. Tell the client that you will place a second finger in her vagina. Insert two fingers into the vagina and ask the client to bear down (see Figure 9.4). Some slight muscle bulging is normal. Horizontally ridged tissue anteriorly is cystocele, whereas posterior tissue is rectocele. Assess vaginal tone by having the client tighten her vaginal muscles around your two fingers.

4. Select an appropriately sized speculum, usually a Pederson (A) if the client has never had a vaginal birth, a Graves (B) speculum if she has had a vaginal delivery (see Figure 9.5). The speculum should be warm. Lubrication may not be necessary for women in their childbearing years. If a lubricant is needed, warm water is preferred. It is helpful to recall that the vagina extends diagonally toward the spine. Again reminding the client that you will be touching her, place the index and middle finger of one hand inside the vagina to spread it apart about 1 inch (2.5 cm). Exert downward pressure with the fingers. Simultaneously use the opposite hand to introduce the closed speculum over the spread fingers (see Figure 9.6A). This maneuver bypasses the sensitive urethra adjacent to the anterior vaginal wall. Hold blades closed with the index and middle fingers of the introducing hand. Be sure the opening you have made is wider than the speculum.

5. Once the blades have passed the introitus, remove the fingers, exerting downward pressure. Maintain downward and posterior pressure on the blades until the instrument is completely inserted (see Figure 9.6B).

6. Open the speculum blades and look for the cervix. If you can't see it, reposition the speculum more anteriorly, posteriorly, or laterally until the complete cervix appears. Occasionally, the speculum will need to be removed, the cervix located digitally, and the speculum reinserted. Tell the client when the

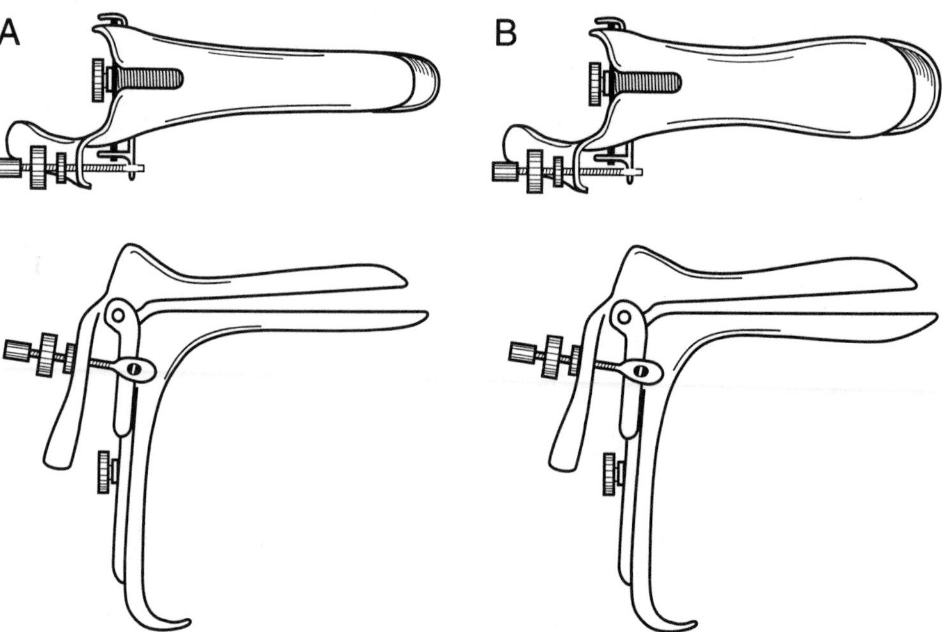

Figure 9.5.

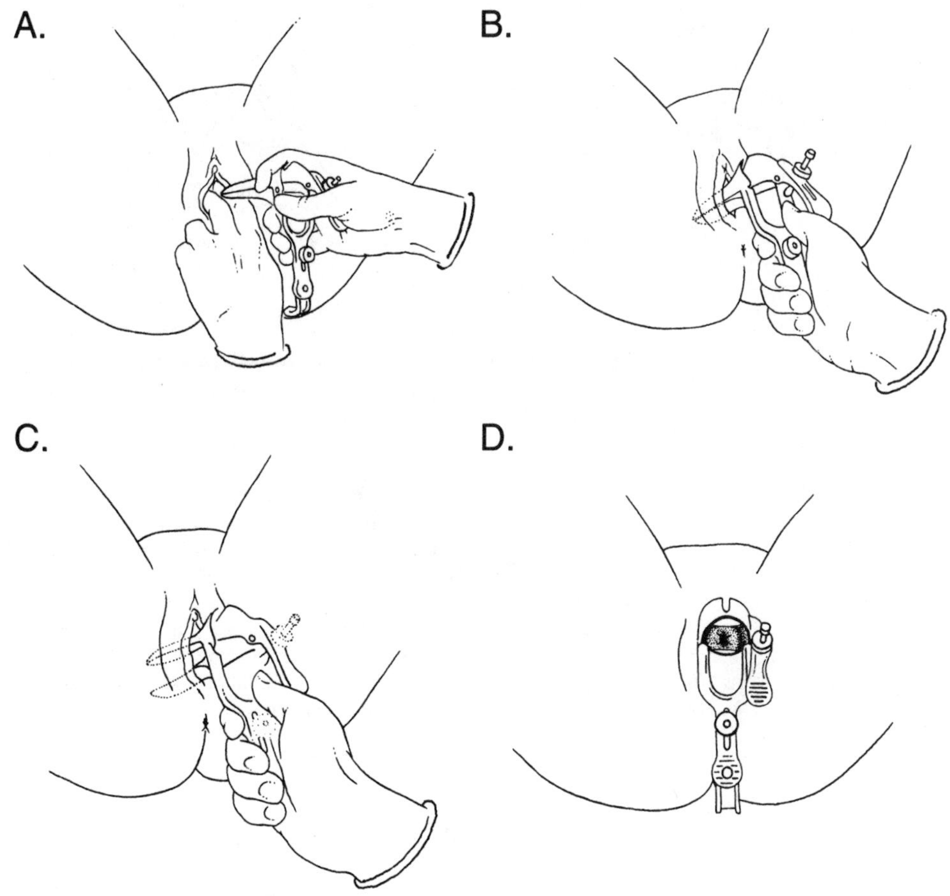

Figure 9.6. Procedure for Speculum Examination

speculum will be removed or reinserted (see Figures 9.6C and 9.6D).

To fix the blade of the metal speculum in the open position, tighten the thumbscrew. During speculum repositioning maneuvers, remind the client to relax as much as she can. The cervix will be more posterior with the anteverted or anteflexed uterus and more anterior with the retroverted or retroflexed uterus. (Figures 9.7 and 9.8 show the cervix as it appears through the speculum.)

The cervix should be shiny pink. However, it may be pale if the woman is anemic or menopausal. Pregnancy gives a bluish purple cast. The cervix, with a diameter of about 3/4 inch to 1 1/4 inches (2 to 3 cm) projects about 1/4 inch to 1 1/4 inches (1 to 3 cm) into the vagina.

Assess for abnormalities. Growths, lesions, mucopurulent discharge, or abnormal color require further evaluation.

7. After inspecting the cervix, obtain an endocervical specimen for the Pap smear by inserting an endocervical brush, the longer serrated edge of a spatula, or a cotton swab about 1/8 inch (0.5 cm) into the cervical os and rotating the instrument 360 degrees clockwise (see Figure 9.9). Then smear the specimen onto a glass slide with a smooth, painting motion. Too much pressure may destroy cells. Spray the slide with a cytological fixative agent within 10 seconds of smearing.

8. Obtain a specimen from the ectocervix (outer area of the cervix) with the curved end of the spatula. Place the curved end of the spatula in the os, apply gentle pressure while rotating the

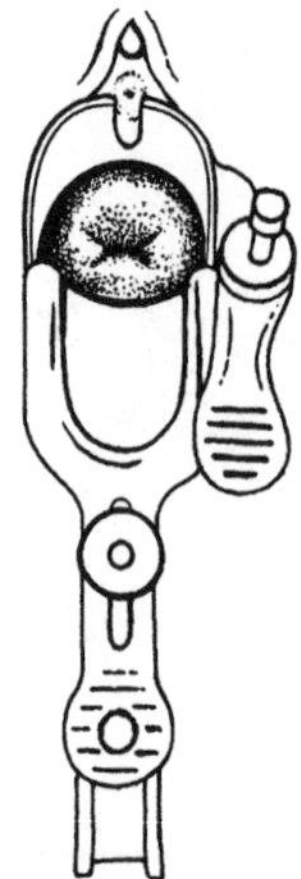

Figure 9.7. View Through a Speculum

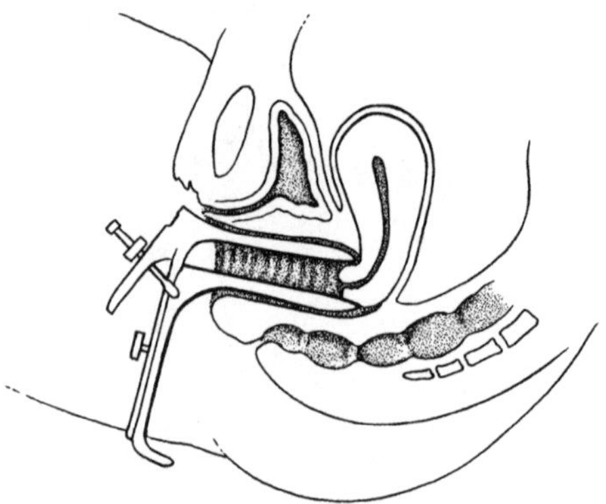

Figure 9.8. Cross-Sectional View Through a Speculum

spatula 360 degrees, transfer the scrapings to a second slide, and spray the slide with fixative. In some settings, both the endocervical and ectocervical specimens are placed on a single slide. Regardless, the procedure is the same.

If the client has no cervix, as after a complete hysterectomy, scrape the vaginal cuff and obtain a vaginal pool specimen from the posterior vaginal fornix with a cotton-tipped applicator. If the client has dry mucosa, the applicator tip can be moistened with normal saline solution. Prepare the slide specimen as described previously. Slides must be labeled to indicate where the specimen came from.

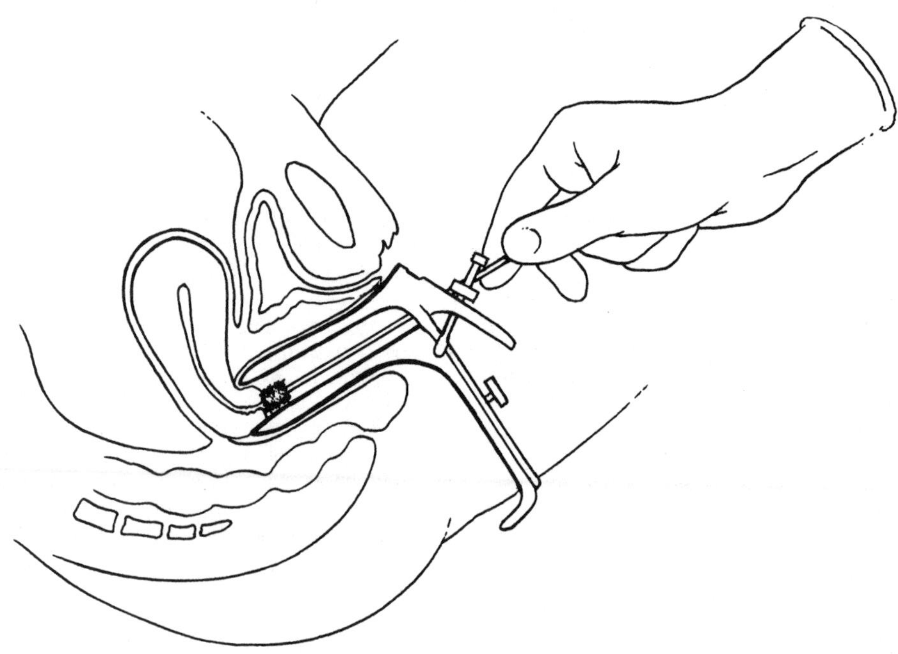

Figure 9.9. Technique for Obtaining an Endocervical Specimen for a Pap Smear

When a client reports vaginal itching or malodorous discharge, obtain a wet smear. This procedure is described in "Preparation of a Wet Smear" below.

9. After collecting all specimens, unlock the speculum thumbscrew. Rotate the blades 90 degrees while on the cervix to inspect the anterior and posterior vaginal wall. (Speculum rotation is not necessary with a plastic speculum because it allows observation through the clear plastic.) Women with adequate estrogen levels have pink, moist, rugose vaginal walls.

The speculum blades will close just before the distal ends reach the area adjacent to the introitus. Place the speculum into a soaking solution or container or discard if it is disposable.

Bimanual Palpation

Following the speculum examination, a bimanual examination is performed to assess internal genitalia (vagina, cervix, uterus, fallopian tubes, and ovaries) and evaluate pelvic support. Palpation provides information regarding size, shape, consistency, position, mobility, tenderness, nodules, masses, and anatomical landmarks. To perform this part of the assessment of female genitalia, palpate the internal genitalia as follows. Use the dominant hand internally for the most comfortable approach, but try the other hand if this seems awkward.

1. Lubricant comes in a multi-use or single-use tube or foil packet and may be squeezed onto a disposable gauze or paper square for easy use. Never touch a multitube end with your gloved

Preparation of a Wet Smear

The wet smear or wet mount is the most useful technique available for the diagnosis of some vaginal infections. The procedure for performing this diagnostic tool is described below. Chapters 23 and 24 describe the organisms commonly found using the wet smear technique.

Collect vaginal discharge with a cotton swab or Pap smear spatula and place it in a tube containing 1 ml of normal saline. Vigorously mix discharge with the saline.

Place a drop of the specimen solution on two glass swabs.

Add a drop of KOH (potassium hydroxide) to one slide and immediately sniff for the characteristic "fishy" odor of bacterial vaginosis (whiff test). Some clinicians prefer to place a drop of KOH on the vaginal discharge that pools in the speculum blade and perform the whiff test this way.

Examine the normal saline slide within 2 minutes under an ordinary light microscope at low power. Trichomonads lose motility rapidly under the hot light of the microscope; thus a cover slip should not be placed until the initial evaluation has been done. This routine will yield a higher percentage of wet smears positive for trichomonas infection.

Move the slide until a general impression of number of squamous cells is obtained. Normal vaginal epithelial cells are flat with sharp clear edges. Switch to a higher power; it may be necessary to increase the amount of light slightly.

Evaluate the normal saline slide for bacteria, white blood cells, clue cells, trichomonas, and Candida. Clue cells or epithelial cells covered with bacteria obscuring the edges of the cell and giving the cell a granular appearance are strongly suggestive of bacterial vaginosis. White blood cells are found in small numbers in normal vaginal discharge. The entire slide should be scanned to evaluate the specimen thoroughly because vaginitis may have more than one cause.

The KOH slide is examined next to evaluate for Candida or yeast infection. If hyphae are found, switch to high power to confirm impression.

Microscopic examination is facilitated by using subdued light and a lowered condenser for a wet specimen.

SOURCES: Murphy (1990) and Dykers (1988).

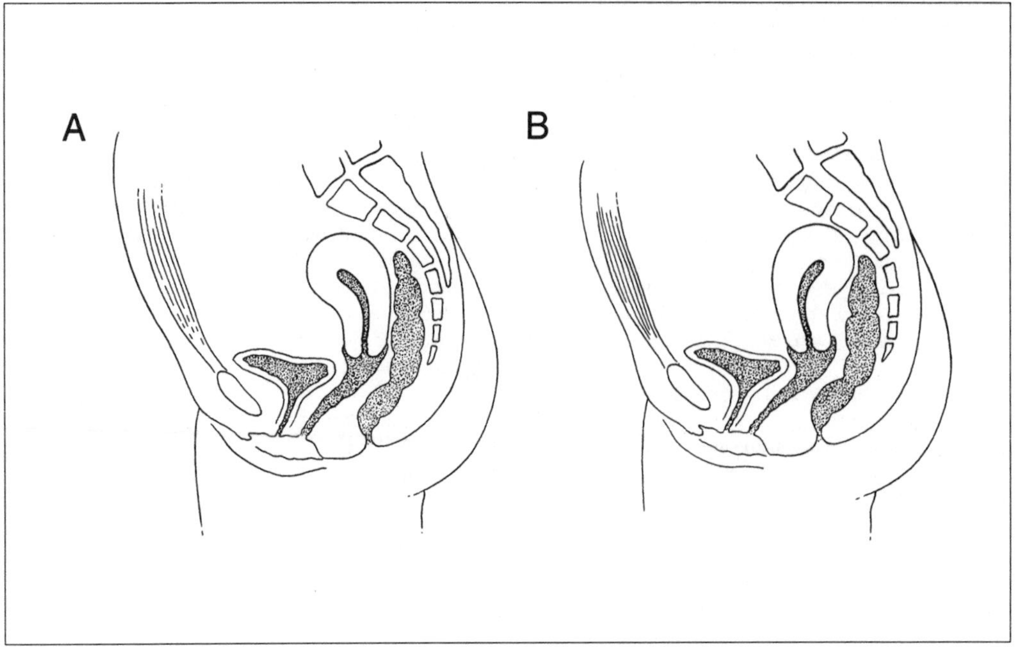

Figure 9.10.

fingers; instead, allow the lubricant to drop freely onto the fingers. Discard single-use tube or packet after one use.

Lubricate the index and middle fingers of the examining hand. Advise the client that you are going to place two fingers in her vagina to palpate her cervix, uterus, and ovaries. Introduce the fingers into the vagina. With the thumb abducted to avoid the clitoris, palpate the vaginal wall with the palmar surfaces of the fingers, rotating them as necessary (see Figure 9.10). Rugae, a normal finding, feel like small ridges running concentrically around the vaginal wall. Note any nodules, tenderness, or other abnormalities. A client with a small vaginal opening may need to be examined with one finger.

The cervix, usually in the midline, points anteriorly, posteriorly, or midplane. Cervical position generally relates to uterine position. For example, a posterior cervix typically appears with an anteverted/antiflexed uterus (see Figure 9.10a), an anterior cervix with a retroverted/ retroflexed uterus (see Figure 9.10b). A cervix positioned to the right or left may indicate an abdominal mass shifting the uterus—and the cervix—to one side. Tenderness upon cervical movement may signal ectopic pregnancy or pelvic inflammatory disease (PID) (see Chapter 23).

2. Insert your fingers deeper until the cervix is located with the palmar surface of the fingers (see Figure 9.11). Feel its surface and run the fingers around its circumference. Gently move the cervix from side to side 1/2 inch to 3/4 inch (1 to 2 cm). This should not be painful to the client. Assess the shape, position, and consistency of the cervix. It should feel firm, smooth, mobile, and nontender when moved and touched. The cervix of a prepubescent girl and an older woman typically is smaller and usually recessed. A pregnant woman's cervix usually is softened and enlarged by the third trimester.

3. Position the second hand for examination of the uterus. Place it on the abdomen. Leave the index and middle fingers of the examining hand in the vagina. Bring the external hand down toward the symphysis pubis and inward toward the internal hand to trap the uterus for examination (see Figure 9.12).

Examine the uterus for position, shape, consistency, tenderness, mobility, and surface regularity. Flexion indicates that the uterus is bent upon itself. Midplane position means the long axis of the uterus is parallel to the long axis of the body. Also note whether the uterus lies midline or deviates to the left or right of the pelvis.

Determine whether the uterus is of normal size or enlarged. The normal nonpregnant uterus is small, fitting comfortably under the symphysis pubis in the pelvis. It is not palpable by

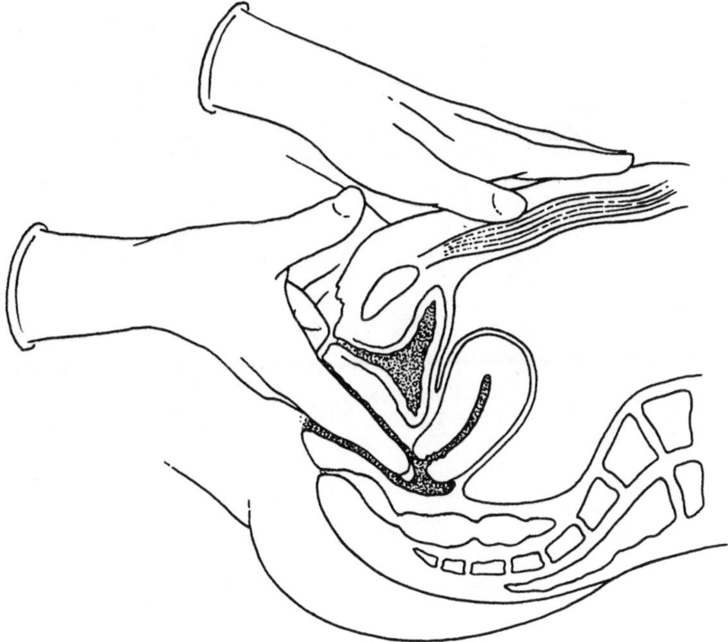

Figure 9.11.

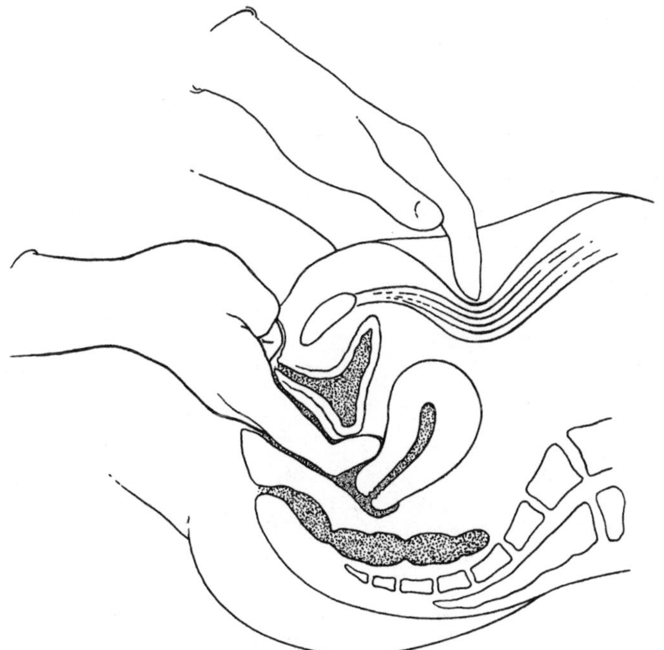

Figure 9.12.

abdominal examination. In postmenopausal women, the uterus normally is smaller than before menopause. An enlarged uterus is generally due to pregnancy, fibroid tumor, adenomyosis (uterine mucosal tissue growth into the uterine wall or oviducts), or carcinoma. If the uterus is enlarged, estimate its size in weeks of gestation (e.g., 12 weeks).

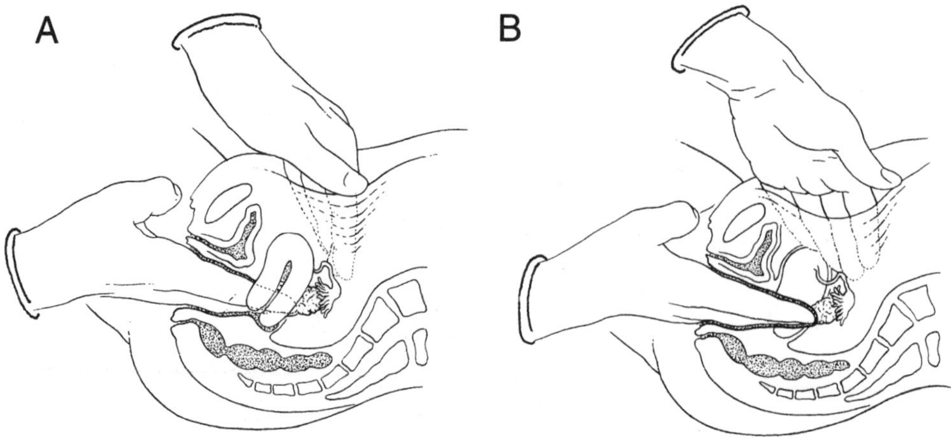

Figure 9.13. Assess the Ovaries

Unless an abnormality or pregnancy changes its shape, the uterus is pear shaped and symmetrical. Sometimes, however, the body of the uterus is small and feels like a soft walnut. Note any deviations such as a protruding mass on the fundal surface. A heart-shaped uterus may indicate a bicornate, or horned, uterus.

The muscular composition of the uterus typically makes it feel firm and smooth. A soft uterus suggests pregnancy; an irregular surface suggests fibroids. Severe tenderness may indicate PID or adenomyosis. The ligaments suspending the uterus in the pelvis allow slight mobility. Limited mobility may indicate a pathological condition such as adhesions, infection, or carcinoma.

4. Assess the right and left ovaries. Place the internal fingers to the side of the uterus that has just been palpated. Then lift the internal fingers as the external fingers press down and inward toward the symphysis pubis. This maneuver traps the ovary and any masses between the fingers (see Figure 9.13). Repeat the maneuver on the left side.

The ovaries should be mobile, oval, firm, and smooth. They are 1¼ inch × ¾ inch × ¼ inch (3 × 2 × 0.5 cm) and shaped like almonds. They may be sensitive to palpation. The ovaries of prepubescent and postmenopausal women should not be palpable. An ovary larger than 2 inches (5 cm) is abnormal and must be evaluated further. Normal fallopian tubes have a very small diameter and are not palpable or sensitive. Ectopic pregnancy or infection may cause sufficient enlargement so as to cause the tube to be palpable.

5. To prepare for rectovaginal examination, change the glove on the internal hand. This prevents transfer of vaginal organisms into the rectum. The rectovaginal assessment should be a part of most pelvic examinations.

Explain the procedure to the client. Lubricate the fingers with a water-soluble lubricant. To relax the client's anal sphincter and allow easy entry of the examining finger, ask the client to bear down as if to have a bowel movement. Assure her she will not. As she bears down, carefully insert the middle finger into the rectum. Be sure to look for the opening. Do not rely on touch alone (see Figure 9.14).

Inspect for hemorrhoids or other painful areas and avoid these lesions when inserting the finger. As the index finger is inserted into the vagina, tell the client to stop bearing down and relax. Place the vaginal finger under the cervix to keep it from being confused with a retroverted uterus.

No masses or nodules should be felt by the rectal finger. The rectovaginal assessment provides a more complete evaluation of the posterior side of the uterus.

After withdrawing the gloved finger from the rectum, check it for stool color and note any blood. Test for occult blood if the woman is over

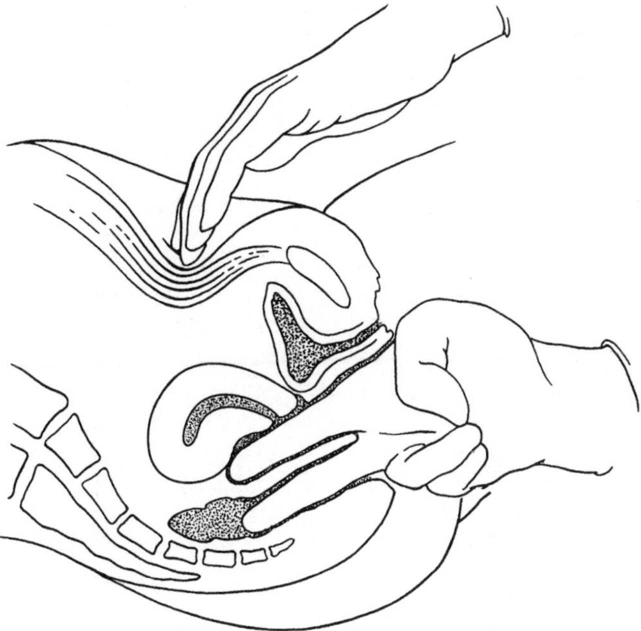

Figure 9.14. Rectovaginal Examination

40 or if you see tarry black stool (a possible sign of gastrointestinal bleeding) on the glove.

When the examination is complete, clean the perineal area with tissue from front to back to remove excess lubricant. Help the client to a sitting position and give her additional tissue or cleansing wipe for additional cleansing if necessary. Wash your hands.

10

Lesbian Health Care

SHARON DEEVEY

Looking at the historical development of research on lesbians and their communities, we learn how new categories of persons and experiences get incorporated into social science [and health care]: First they are not seen; then they are found deviant (and viewed as exotic); then they are defended; and finally when perceived as sufficiently ordinary, they are included with the rest of what is partly understood (Krieger, 1982).

Introduction

In the past, nurses were at a disadvantage in their efforts to provide knowledgeable and culturally sensitive nursing care for lesbian women. Nursing education gave them limited information about lesbian health concerns and life experiences, and many lesbians preferred to remain hidden and to pass for heterosexual in settings they perceived to be unsafe. Because lesbians rarely disclosed much personal information, their parents, coworkers, and health care providers usually remained ignorant of the complexity of lesbian lives or denied that lesbians exist.

Today, however, health care professionals are becoming increasingly aware of lesbian and gay (male homosexual) issues, and lesbian women who formerly were "not seen" or were "found deviant" are coming to be perceived as more "ordinary."

This chapter introduces the nurse to the health concerns of lesbian women. Here, health is considered to be more than the absence of disease. It is seen broadly as a sense of physical, emotional, and social well-being. The chapter assumes that nursing care includes psychosocial interventions and client teaching as well as physical care in hospitals and other settings. It also assumes that continual interaction between the individual and the environment significantly affects health.

The chapter explores three aspects of lesbian health: individual, family, and community health. For each of these aspects, the chapter addresses assessment, nursing care, and resources. It also examines the special issues of age, substance abuse, violence, and bereavement. It concludes with an overview of the controversies and challenges of lesbian research and identifies various topics for future research into lesbian health.

Barriers to Care

For lesbian women, barriers to health care have two main causes. First, many health care professionals are prejudiced or uninformed about lesbian life. Second, lesbian women commonly hesitate to share personal information (Deevey, 1993).

Prejudice of Health Care Professionals

Prejudice against lesbians and gays is known as *homophobia* or *heterosexism* (Stevens & Hall, 1991). Weinberg (1972) first defined homophobia as acute feelings of discomfort in the presence of people known to be homosexual. In popular usage, the term *homophobia* currently refers to a broad spectrum of negative feelings, attitudes, behaviors, and institutional sanctions against lesbians and gays.

Neisen (1990) and Pharr (1988) explain the parallels between racism, sexism, and heterosexism. Like the white race and the male sex, heterosexual orientation has been assumed superior and has been reinforced by legal and religious institutions in American society. Although these racist, sexist, and heterosexist assumptions are changing gradually, many health care professionals continue to carry such assumptions into their practice.

Lesbian women are acutely sensitive to language and behaviors that signal danger or safety on issues of sexual orientation. Health care professionals who use the term *homosexual* rather than *lesbian* or *gay* or who assume heterosexuality by asking "Are you married?" rather than "Who is your major support?" are seen as threatening or homophobic. Those who pull away from or suddenly avoid touching the client when she mentions her lesbian sexual orientation are immediately recognized as prejudiced.

Historically, nursing literature described homosexuality as pathological (Bieber, 1969), and homophobia among nurses was common (White, 1979). Randall (1989) recently found that half of her sample of Bachelor of Science in Nursing (BSN) educators "indicated that lesbianism is not a natural expression of human sexuality" and one fourth "would have difficulty communicating with a woman they knew to be a lesbian." Schwanberg (1985, 1990) reported that the number of articles reflecting negative attitudes toward lesbian and gay clients has increased recently in the medical and psychiatric literature.

However, a more positive view of lesbians and gays gradually is becoming more common in the nursing literature. Several pioneering articles have urged nurses to improve their care of lesbian and gay clients (Deevey, 1990; Irish, 1983; Kus, 1990; Stephany, 1988). Sharkey (1987) encouraged the nursing profession to be more supportive of its own lesbian and gay members. Textbooks on public health nursing (Roberts, 1985) and women's health nursing (Holmes, 1982; LoBiondo-Wood, 1986; Morrison, 1986; Williamson, 1986) have offered affirmative and practical information on lesbian health. The number of nursing journal articles about lesbians has increased, especially since the 1980s. These articles have addressed topics such as lesbian parenting (Harvey, Carr, & Bernheine, 1989; Olesker & Walsh, 1984; Wismont & Reame, 1989; Zeidenstein, 1990), stress and coping (Gillow & Davis, 1987), coming out (Deevey, 1993; Kus, 1985), and aging (Deevey, 1990). Affirmative information about lesbians also is beginning to appear in medical (Gartrell, 1981), social work (Hidalgo, Peterson, & Woodman, 1985; Maggiore, 1988), and women's studies (Hitchcock, 1989b; Rothblum & Cole, 1989; Shaw, 1989) literature.

Professional nursing organizations have shown some leadership in urging culturally sensitive care of lesbian and gay clients. The American Nurses' Association (ANA, 1976) included the lesbian and gay population in a bibliography of minority groups in nursing. In response to the acquired immunodeficiency syndrome (AIDS) crisis, the ANA (1985) issued its "Statement on Health Care for a Population at Risk" that acknowledged the "continuing discrimination in health care experienced by members of the gay/lesbian population." The statement also affirmed that "the gay/lesbian population has a right to quality health care." Sigma Theta Tau (1987) included "lesbian/gay lifestyles" as an area for research in its 1987 Directory of Nurse Researchers. However, the questionnaire for the upcoming edition of the directory included the category "homosexual," but omitted the more affirmative term *lesbian*.

In 1979, Sharon Kowalski and Karen Thompson fell in love and began to share their lives. They knew little about lesbian culture and told no one about their relationship.

In 1983, Sharon was severely injured when her car was struck by a drunk driver. Karen stayed by Sharon's side constantly during her coma and the first months of her recovery from a severe brainstem injury. Then Sharon's parents told Karen to stop visiting. In the hope that Sharon's parents would understand the importance of her love to Sharon and her recovery, Karen decided to disclose the true nature of their relationship. Instead, Sharon's parents took out an injunction to block Karen's access to Sharon. This revelation was done on the advice of the hospital psychologist.

During the next 8 years, Karen fought a prolonged legal battle against Sharon's parents to be allowed to visit and care for Sharon. In a legal decision, *In re Guardianship of Sharon Kowalski*, the Minnesota Court of Appeals finally awarded guardianship to Karen over the ongoing objections of Sharon's parents. The court ruled that Karen had demonstrated that she was best able to care for Sharon.

Figure 10.1. Case in Point: Thompson and Kowalski

Hesitancy to Disclose Information

Lesbian women say that "the most serious health issue for lesbians is that too often we don't feel comfortable or safe seeking care when we need it (until an emergency arises) because of the ignorance, anti-woman, and anti-lesbian attitudes we encounter in most of the medical system" (Boston Women's Health Collective, 1993, p. 190).

According to various authorities (Cochran & Mays, 1988; Hitchcock, 1989a; Johnson & Guenther, 1987; Stevens & Hall, 1988), many lesbians are hesitant to come out (disclose their sexual orientation). As one lesbian explains,

> I would not come out in a medical situation unless there were compelling reasons to do so, because in the "patient" role I have so little power and am especially vulnerable to harassment. So I practice in advance how to maintain my privacy and still get the care I need. (Boston Women's Health Collective, 1993, p. 190)

Lesbian women may avoid discussing their true relationships because they fear isolation from their loved ones in emergency rooms and intensive care units (Barrett, 1989, chap. 34). If parents or other members of the family of origin are hostile to or unaware of the lesbian relationship, the health care professional may support only the traditional family, isolating the lesbian client from her real support system: her family of choice. Karen Thompson (Thompson & Andrzejewski, 1988) is an example of a lesbian who was denied access to her injured lover as well as the opportunity to care for her (see Figure 10.1).

Individual Health Issues

Nurses commonly provide care for lesbians who seek emergency assistance, symptom management, routine physical assessment, or health information. Physiologically, lesbians are no different than other women. However, many health care scholars and practitioners believe that culture and stress interact with health in ways that are not well understood and that these can affect lesbian health. This section addresses the issues that may affect a lesbian client's health and identifies related nursing care and resources.

Assessment

Lesbian women are a minority group whose culture sometimes is hidden. They are stressed by their devalued status within the majority culture. To provide culturally sensitive nursing care for a lesbian client, the nurse must determine how the client copes with her devalued status. The following questions help provide this information:

- How does the client feel about her lesbian identity?
- How well does she manage information about her sexual orientation?
- How knowledgeable is she about lesbian identity development? Health risks? Local health care providers? Support groups?

However, these questions are rarely answered in an initial or brief health care visit because of

Table 10.1 Risks and Benefits of Disclosure

To help a lesbian client decide whether to disclose her sexual orientation, the nurse should explore with her the potential risks and benefits of disclosure listed below.

Risks
- Loss of employment
- Avoidance by family of origin
- Loss of support from religious community
- Legal sanctions (homosexuality is illegal in 23 states, and lesbians could be arrested for consensual sexual acts)

Benefits
- Improved self-esteem
- Freedom from living a lie
- Improved communication with heterosexuals

Table 10.2 Stages of Lesbian Identity Development

According to Cass (1979), lesbian identity develops through the six stages listed below. The accompanying statements are examples that reflect a woman's growth in each stage. The nurse uses this information in assessment of his or her clients.

Stage of Development	*Representative Statement*
Confusion	"I thought I was like everyone else, but now I'm afraid I might be a lesbian."
Comparison	"No one could guess I'm a lesbian. I can't stand being different."
Tolerance	"I'm OK about my lesbian life, but I sure hate those drag queens and diesel dykes."
Acceptance	"I'm fairly active in the local lesbian community. I told my mom and one straight friend about myself."
Pride	"I thank the goddess every day that I'm a lesbian. Straight people are so weird."
Synthesis	"I'm very open about being a lesbian. I get a lot of support from all the gay and straight people in my life."

time limitations and the lesbian's possible distrust of the health care system. If the client is extremely fearful or guarded, the nurse should not ask these questions directly, unless the client initiates a discussion of lesbian issues. Instead, the nurse should be sensitive to the risks and benefits of disclosure, informed about the stages of lesbian identity development, and aware that a lesbian in any stage of identity development may seek health care (see Tables 10.1 and 10.2).

Because, typically, sexual orientation is not assessed and recorded in the client's health history, a full and accurate description of lesbian health currently is not available. However, the following information is known about the physical and mental health issues of lesbian women. (For specific information about age, substance abuse, violence, and bereavement, see the "Special Health Issues" section of this chapter.)

Physical Health

The first research on lesbian physical health focused on sexually transmitted diseases (STDs). Because the STD rate is high in gays, many people assumed it would be high in lesbian women also. However, researchers found that lesbian women had very low rates of STDs (Johnson, Smith, & Guenther, 1987; Robertson & Schachter, 1981).

Lesbian women have been considered to be at low risk for AIDS. However, little actually is known about transmission of the AIDS virus during lesbian sex. The Centers for Disease Control (CDC) keeps statistics about male-male and female-male sexual transmission of AIDS but does not record data about female-female transmission (Leonard, 1990). Also, AIDS may be underdiagnosed in all women because until late 1992 the CDC list of opportunistic infections that determine a diagnosis of AIDS had been developed exclusively from male clients. Many women with human immunodeficiency virus (HIV) who die of gynecologic infections are not counted as AIDS victims because they never developed the diseases found in HIV-positive men, such as pneumocystic pneumonia or Kaposi's sarcoma. (See Chapter 24, "Sexually Transmitted Diseases," for further discussion of women and HIV infection.)

Most of the current information about other aspects of physical health is anecdotal. Winnow (1989/1990) observed that lesbians have high rates of breast and cervical cancer, Epstein-Barr virus infection, multiple sclerosis, and environmental illnesses such as allergies. The apparently high cancer rate has been attributed to delay in seeking care because of fear of health care system prejudice and lack of routine gynecologic examinations because contraception is not needed. It also may stem from lack of breastfeeding, a factor that may help prevent breast cancer.

Usually, sign language translation and wheelchair access are provided at lesbian community events. This may reflect a higher incidence of disability or a higher consciousness about disability among lesbians (Browne, 1985).

Mental Health

The effect of prejudice and minority stress on lesbian mental health is not understood fully. Minority stress occurs in a lesbian woman when she constantly receives negative messages from the environment about her identity and is burdened by the attacks and the need to avoid or respond to them (Brooks, 1981). However, some research has begun to illuminate lesbian mental health issues.

Bradford and Ryan (1988) found that 75% of 1,917 lesbians had sought mental health counseling of some type. Indeed, extensive literature exists on the special challenges and controversies of counseling lesbians (Brown, 1989; Hall, 1985; Klein, 1986; Moses & Hawkins, 1982; Stein & Cohen, 1986; Ward, 1988/1989).

The exact incidence of schizophrenia and bipolar illness in lesbian women is unknown. In current practice, however, many psychiatrists diagnose lesbian clients with borderline personality disorder—a pervasive pattern of instability of mood, interpersonal relationships, and self-image beginning by early adulthood and present in a variety of contexts (American Psychiatric Association, 1987, p. 346).

Some evidence suggests that the rates of suicide and depression are two to seven times higher in lesbians and gays than in heterosexuals (Rofes, 1983; Saunders & Valente, 1987). These high suicide and depression rates may reflect a response to constant shaming. Women who are labeled as perverted or disgusting may have great difficulty achieving a sense of self-worth and mental well-being.

Nursing Care

The nurse can eliminate threats to lesbian safety and self-esteem by avoiding the assumption of heterosexuality and the use of homophobic language. By carefully listening to and observing a female client, the sensitive nurse should be able to detect guardedness or hesitancy about discussing family and social support, which may help identify the client as a lesbian.

Providing information, assistance, and care in a warm, supportive environment may help the lesbian client discuss her presenting problem and her often-unspoken lesbian concerns. Recent publications on lesbian health prominently displayed on the nurse's bookshelf may encourage comfort and disclosure in the lesbian client (Bradford & Ryan, 1988; Hepburn & Gutierrez, 1988; Kus, 1990; O'Donnell, Loeffler, Pollock, & Saunders, 1979; Shernoff & Scott, 1988).

When caring for lesbian clients, confidentiality is an important issue. Information leaks about sexual orientation can endanger the lesbian client's employment, ties with her family of origin, and sense of safety. If the client is extremely private, the nurse should respect her unwillingness to discuss her sexual orientation by maintaining strict confidentiality and omitting information about lesbian issues from her chart. In general, the nurse should allow the lesbian client to set the pace in sharing personal information. An off-the-record discussion of the options and implications of various levels of openness can be helpful. Together, the nurse and client can determine how much openness the client finds comfortable; can assess the probable effects of disclosure in the client's workplace, family, and community; and can rehearse the communication of disclosure.

Nurses caring for women clients have a responsibility to examine their beliefs about lesbian women because these can affect the care they provide. The nurse who considers lesbianism a radical lifestyle may be surprised to find some lesbian women somewhat rigid and hesitant to take risks. Lesbian women who have been traumatized by rejection or have experienced violence from their families or from strangers in the street may overcompensate by being conformist in almost everything except their sexual orientation.

The nurse should respect the challenge that lesbian women face in seeking physical and mental health in a hostile environment. To feel safe, lesbians use various coping strategies, such as denial, substance abuse, confrontation, and humor. The nurse who supports directness and laughter will contribute to lesbian health.

The nurse who becomes an advocate for lesbian clients may experience direct homophobic attacks. The nurse may be shunned or questioned about his or her sexual orientation, and efforts to provide accurate information about lesbian women and gays may be ignored or condemned. Therefore, each nurse must assess his or her skills, support network, and working environment before deciding to be a client advocate.

Resources

The nurse can teach lesbian clients about a wide spectrum of resources for individual physical and mental health. For a lesbian woman who feels alone, the nurse may suggest contacting local networks of lesbian support groups and social organizations, attending sports events, and visiting lesbian bookstores. For a client who requests an openly lesbian or gay physician, therapist, or other healer, the nurse can refer her to a local lesbian and gay hotline, lesbian and gay civil rights group, lesbian and gay support group in a health care facility, or lesbian and gay health clinic. For general information, the nurse may refer the client to the National Lesbian and Gay Health Foundation, which publishes research on lesbian health and sponsors an annual lesbian and gay health conference. (For more information, see "Resources for Lesbian Health," p. 205.)

Family Health Issues

Family nursing is concerned with family processes and the interactions of family members. Family nursing practitioners concentrate on the interactions between or among family members or between the family and others outside the family (Feetham, 1984). Bozett (1987) notes that the traditional family structure, which consists of a breadwinner (father), housewife (mother), and two or more children, is found in only 13% of families. Therefore, he urges nurses to define the family as "who the patient says it is." Bozett also encourages nurses to confront outmoded "immediate family only" hospital policies, which ignore the various family structures in the United States today. To help the nurse understand lesbian family health, this section explains how to assess family health issues and discusses related nursing care and resources.

Assessment

The word *family* may have many meanings for a lesbian woman. It sometimes is used as a code word for sexual orientation. For example, a lesbian woman may ask, "Is she family?" when inquiring if another woman is lesbian. Also, lesbian and gay marches and music festivals sometimes are referred to as family reunions.

Lesbians usually distinguish between their family of origin (parents, siblings, and other relatives) and their family of choice (lesbian partner, children, ex-lovers, friends, and animals that constitute the lesbian family household and extended primary network). Children, whom Maggiore (1988) calls the family of procreation, may enter a lesbian's life from a previous heterosexual relationship or by alternative insemination, adoption, or coparenting of a lover's children.

The lesbian family may take many forms. For example, it may be a childless adult couple, a communal nonmonogamous trio, a single mother with children, a couple caring for aging parents or ill friends, or an individual who lives alone and keeps in close touch with a lover, friends, and her family of origin. Anthropologists Riley (1988) and Weston (1988) have studied kinship networks among lesbians and gays. They determined that the lovers, ex-lovers, and friends of these individuals played the roles filled by spouses, siblings, and cousins of heterosexual individuals.

Irish (1990) stresses the importance of correctly identifying the actual sources of support for lesbian and gay clients who seek health care. To do this, the nurse needs the answers to these questions:

- Who counts as family? The lover or partner? The family of origin? Friends? Ex-lovers? Gay men? Children?
- How well do the family members communicate?
- How supportive of each other are the family members?
- How do family members feel about lesbian issues? How do they manage information about their lesbian family member with people outside of the family? How knowledgeable are they about resources for lesbian families?

One problem complicates the answers to these questions: Lesbian families may define themselves differently in different settings. For example, a lesbian couple with a child by alternative insemination may proclaim themselves a lesbian family to their trusted friends but may present themselves as a single mother with a helpful friend in potentially threatening situations. The parents of one of the women may consider themselves proud grandparents in an extended lesbian family; the parents of the other may worry about their unwed daughter and may never have heard of the word *lesbian*.

Communication between a lesbian and her family of origin can be problematic (Fairchild & Hayward, 1979; Griffin, Wirth, & Wirth, 1986). Although parental disowning of a lesbian daughter seems to be less common now than it was in the past, many lesbians never risk discussing their lives with their parents and siblings. Many live far from their family of origin and lead double lives, sharing few details or feelings with family members. In doing so, they sacrifice honesty and emotional depth for safety. Some women tell their parents that they are lesbian, and the topic never is mentioned again by either the woman or her parents or both. Others feel sure their parents "know, but don't want to know."

Borhek (1983) recommends that lesbians carefully consider the decision to come out to their family of origin, prepare themselves for a variety of possible responses, rehearse the communication, and realize that parents will need to grieve the loss of the child they thought they knew. Neisen (1987) also emphasizes how families of origin grow through the process of grieving, finding support, and finally accepting their lesbian family member.

Researchers have found lesbian couples to be similar to heterosexual couples in commitment and areas of conflict (e.g., money, sex, work) (Clunis & Green, 1988; Peplau, Cochran, & Padesky, 1978; Tanner, 1981). Some have noted differences from heterosexual couples because both lesbian partners are socialized as nurturers and noninitiators (Nichols, 1982) and because lesbian couples receive limited social support for their relationship (Kurdek, 1988). As a result, lesbian couples may have difficulty with fusion as a couple or with maintaining a long-term relationship.

Lesbian women sometimes disagree about the ideal form of lesbian family. Berzon (1988) encourages lesbians to form permanent partnerships similar to marriage; others emphasize the diversity and creativity of complex lesbian families, which sometimes include more than one lover (Kassoff, 1988), friends (Loulan, 1987, "Passionate Friendships"), and ex-lovers (Becker, 1988).

Lesbian women usually use the term *lover* to refer to a person with whom they have had a short-term or long-term relationship, but substitute the words *partner*, *friend*, or *roommate* when speaking to heterosexuals who may associate the term *lover* with short-term relationships only. Feminists condemn the terms *butch* and *femme*, and lesbians consider the words pejorative when used by heterosexuals. However, the terms recently have been reclaimed as part of lesbian culture and sexuality (Loulan, 1990; Nestle, 1981). Therefore, they may be considered negative or positive terms, depending on who uses them.

Health care professionals should not assume that lesbians are childless. Almvig (1982), Kehoe (1989), and Deevey (1990) found that about one third of older lesbians had children by previous heterosexual relationships. Among younger lesbians, children were mainly the result of alternative insemination and intentional pregnancy by brief heterosexual encounter (Eskenazi, Pies, Newsletter, Shepard, & Pearson, 1989; Pies, 1985; Pollach & Vaughn, 1987).

Lesbian women with children may face special problems. Some may lose custody of their children in conservative communities. Others may find that their adolescent children have difficulty coping with homophobia in themselves and in their peers (Deevey, 1989).

Gay men may be among the closest family and friends of lesbians, especially among the older generation who socialize in private clubs and those in urban lesbian and gay communities since the AIDS epidemic. Throughout the country, many lesbian women have organized support for gays with AIDS and have been touched by the numerous deaths and the homophobic backlash caused by the AIDS epidemic (Machs & Ryan, 1988). However, many feminist lesbian women believe in separatism and avoid contact with men. They are angry that so many lesbian women work actively in AIDS organizations and ignore issues that are a much greater threat to lesbians, such as breast cancer (Winnow, 1989/1990).

Nursing Care

The family nurse can contribute to lesbian family health by providing information to counter ignorance and negative stereotypes about lesbian life, by affirming individual differences, and by teaching family members how to manage conflict. Because their unique ties to both communities provide them with unique experiences, openly lesbian and gay health care professionals can be particularly helpful to families who have no direct experience with lesbian culture (Stephany, 1988).

In some families, poor communication and keeping secrets are the norm. If these patterns are detected, the nurse can teach all family members how to improve their listening and communication skills. This should help the family deal with conflict over sexual orientation and many other issues.

Resources

Depending on the client's needs, the nurse can make referrals to support groups for parents of lesbians and gays or for lesbian and gay parents. For a lesbian client considering parenthood, the nurse may refer her to local and national resources for alternative insemination and for anticipatory guidance on such issues as coparenting, disclosure of sexual orientation to children, and coping with school authorities.

Community Health Issues

In community health nursing, population groups are the focus of nursing care (Anderson, McFarlane, & Helton, 1986; Shamansky & Pesznecker, 1981). This section assesses the issues that may affect the lesbian community and its interactions with the heterosexual community. Then it identifies related nursing care and resources.

Assessment

To evaluate lesbian community health, the nurse should assess regional, racial or ethnic, religious, and workplace issues.

Regional Variations

Various estimates have been made of the extent and distribution of lesbian populations. A study by Kinsey, Pomeroy, Martin, and Gebhard (1953) estimated that 4% to 5% of American women were primarily or exclusively "homosexual" at the time of the research. More recently, women who identify themselves as lesbians have been more visible and vocal (Troiden, 1988).

In the United States, lesbian community competence (ability of a community to meet the sometimes conflicting needs of its members) varies greatly by region (Goeppinger, Lassiter, & Wilcox, 1982). In some geographical areas, such as San Francisco, lesbian women are extremely open about sexual orientation and have access to extensive lesbian-specific and mainstream community legal and health care resources. In many midsized cities, some lesbian women may interact in the larger lesbian community only at concerts and festivals. In some rural locales, lesbians may be isolated from each other and, to find others like themselves, they may have to drive many miles to small-city bars where they can be sure that a given woman is lesbian. The power and intensity of homophobic violence also varies enormously by region and by institution in a given community. Lesbian women have more options for interaction with other lesbian women and openness about their sexual identity in more competent communities.

Anecdotal evidence suggests that many rural lesbians migrate to urban areas, where greater diversity, increased anonymity, and more established lesbian organizations offer a supportive climate. Recent efforts to organize lesbian and gay services in rural communities may change this relocation pattern (D'Augelli & Hart, 1987).

Experts disagree about the effects of the interaction of a prejudiced majority and a stigmatized minority on both groups. Some argue that the strongest lesbian communities exist where prejudice is greatest because the need for secrecy and mutual support generates committed alternative institutions. Others believe the strongest lesbian communities exist where openness on lesbian issues is the norm and where openly lesbian and gay people are well integrated into mainstream institutions.

To understand the effect of community issues on lesbian health in a specific region, the nurse should consider two sets of assessment questions. The first set assesses the local heterosexual population within which lesbian women live:

- What is the level of prejudice toward lesbian women? What is the level of support for lesbians?
- How diverse is the community in terms of race, ethnicity, religion, economics, and other characteristics?
- What prolesbian or antilesbian policies are stated by local institutions, such as religious groups, schools, and employers? To what extent are these policies enforced?

The second set of questions applies to the local lesbian community:

- What are the local lesbian and gay organizations and businesses?
- How diverse is the lesbian community in terms of race, ethnicity, religion, economics, and other characteristics?
- How visible and self-accepting are most lesbian women in the area?

The nurse can answer the first set of questions by doing research in local libraries and monitoring the local media. The nurse also may obtain information on lesbian and gay organizations and diversity from local gay hotlines, national lesbian directories such as *Gaia's Guide*, and local lesbian and gay civil rights organizations, which are listed under social services in the telephone directory.

Race and Ethnicity

Lesbian women who belong to populations stigmatized by race or ethnic origin face additional challenges (Garcia, Kennedy, Pearlman, & Perez, 1987; Morales, 1990). Lesbian women of color report triple jeopardy because of their race, sexual orientation, and gender. The white lesbian community may be prejudiced against lesbians of color; the culture of origin may consider lesbianism to be white decadence; and men of all races may see them as they see all women—as heterosexual sex objects.

Religious Influences

Lesbian women report a wide range of religious upbringing (Beck, 1982; Curb & Manahan, 1985). Historically, established churches have been among the most homophobic religious institutions (Clark, Brown, & Hochstein, 1990; Ritter & O'Neill, 1989). Today, however, many of these churches and temples provide support groups for lesbian and gay parishioners, including the Catholic, Episcopal, Lutheran, and Unitarian churches and the Society of Friends (Hasbany, 1989/1990). Many lesbian women also seek alternatives, such as the national lesbian and gay church (Metropolitan Community Church), women's spirituality groups, feminist theology, or New Age religions (Heyward, 1987).

Workplace Issues

The workplace is the community institution where many lesbian women spend most of their public time, and the process of managing information about their lives in that setting is an ongoing challenge (Levine & Leonard, 1984; Schmitz, 1988). To feel secure in the workplace, some lesbians may need to spend energy guarding their safety or to limit their options for a full range of employment or advancement.

Hall (1986) encourages lesbians who are closeted in the workplace to find ways to manage their discomfort about deception rather than risk being fired or harassed by disclosing their sexual orientation. Managing discomfort can include dissociation from lesbian culture, avoidance of straight coworkers, or token or partial disclosure (e.g., coming out to only a few individuals).

Despite high educational levels, many lesbians are underemployed because of sexist policies that block the promotion of women or because lesbians avoid seeking promotions for fear that greater responsibility will threaten their carefully guarded privacy (Stewart, 1991). Schneider (1987) found that employment settings where lesbians safely could be open were low paid and primarily female, did not involve child supervision or care, and had a human service focus.

Nursing Care

The community health nurse can contribute to the health of the lesbian—and heterosexual—populations by becoming politically active at the local and national level. For example, the nurse may advocate more humane laws regarding sexual orientation, support political candidates who affirm lesbians and gays, and confront antilesbian prejudice and ignorance with courage and accurate information. To provide this type of communitywide care, the nurse should teach other health care professionals about lesbian issues and refer them to local lesbian and gay community resources as needed.

Resources

For more information about lesbian community health, the nurse may rely on organizations that represent culturally diverse groups within the lesbian community and nationally distributed publications that list resources in local lesbian and gay communities (see the appendix to this chapter).

Special Health Issues

Besides being knowledgeable about the individual, family, and community health concerns of lesbians, the nurse should be aware of four special issues—age, substance abuse, violence, and bereavement—and their potential effects on lesbian health. To familiarize the nurse with these issues, this section explains how to assess special health issues and discusses related nursing care and resources.

Assessment

When assessing lesbian clients and families, the nurse may need to ask specific questions about age, substance abuse, violence, and bereavement.

- Is the client or family aware of special problems and resources for elderly or adolescent lesbian women?
- Is the client or family aware of special problems and resources for lesbian women who abuse substances or are recovering from substance abuse?
- Is the client or family aware of special problems and resources for lesbian women survivors of hate crimes, rape, incest, or partner abuse?
- Is the client or family aware of special problems and resources for lesbian women who are dying or bereaved?

Age

A lesbian's age contributes to her view of her sexual orientation and to the world's view of her. Therefore, the concerns of elderly and adolescent lesbians may vary greatly.

Elderly Lesbian Women. Many older lesbian women recognized their sexual orientation when the social sanctions against homosexuality were severe (Adelman, 1986; Kehoe, 1989; Sang, Warshow, & Smith, 1991). Therefore, some who have been lesbians all their lives hesitate to label themselves as such and do not participate in lesbian community activities. Others who raised children and grandchildren before coming out are among the most militant lesbian activists.

Friend (1987) believes that older lesbians are well qualified to cope with the stresses of aging because of their extended social networks, ability to cope with crises, and gender role flexibility.

In San Francisco and New York, federally funded agencies, such as Gay and Lesbian Outreach to Elderly (GLOE) and Senior Action in a Gay Environment (SAGE), offer social services for elderly lesbians and gays (Barracks & Jarratt, 1980). The National Association for Lesbian and Gay Gerontology serves as a clearinghouse of information on the older lesbian population.

Adolescent Lesbian Women. Heterosexual adults have greater difficulty accepting lesbianism in adolescents than in adults (Herdt, 1989). In the past, lesbians who came out as teenagers reported significant isolation, harassment, and sometimes suicidal despair as adults condemned their lesbian feelings or tried to change their behavior through psychiatric hospitalization (Hepburn & Gutierrez, 1988).

Now, some youth services and special programs, such as New York's Harvey Milk High School for lesbian and gay students, are becoming available for adolescent lesbians and gays. Also, health care professionals are being urged to be more sensitive to the problems these adolescents face by providing peer support groups and access to lesbian and gay literature, lesbian Big Sister programs, and educational materials for parents (Bidwell, 1988; Cates, 1987; Coleman & Remafedi, 1989).

Substance Abuse

Substance abuse is a serious problem in lesbian communities (Finnegan & McNally, 1987; Glaus, 1989; Kus, 1990; Nicoloff & Stiglitz, 1987). Several reasons may explain its prevalence. In some areas, lesbian bars are the only safe places to socialize, leading patrons to frequent exposure to alcohol. Also, lesbians may use alcohol and mood-altering drugs to numb lesbian feelings that they don't want to face or to numb the anguish of rejection by heterosexuals. On the other hand, denial of the pain of social rejection by some lesbians may contribute to a denial of substance abuse.

Because of these links to lesbian feelings and because lesbian women may avoid dealing with substance abuse by blaming the straight world for their problems, Finnegan and McNally (1987) believe a link exists between substance abuse and lesbian identity development. They suggest that sobriety and lesbian self-acceptance may be interdependent.

Of lesbian women, 30% are believed to abuse alcohol compared to 10% of the general population (Deevey & Wall, 1992; Hall, 1990). McKernan and Peterson (1989) found that lesbian and gay alcohol use does not taper off in the late 20s and early 30s, as it typically does in heterosexuals.

Recovery in a 12-step program for alcohol or drug abuse, overeating, and codependency is widespread in lesbian communities (Swallow, 1983). Most treatment programs do not address problems specific to lesbian women or other women. Without addressing these topics, relapse is common. Fortunately, some specialized resources are available. In many parts of the country, the Alcoholics Anonymous (AA) central office can refer a client to local AA meetings for women or for lesbians and gays. Other recovery groups can be located through lesbian and gay hotlines and bookstores. Lesbian and gay residential treatment programs, such as the Pride Institute in Minnesota, emphasize confronting homophobia and the effect of the AIDS epidemic on lesbian and gay recovery (Ratner, 1988). The National Association of Lesbian and Gay Alcoholism Professionals meets annually and publishes a national directory of related services.

Violence

Lesbian women may experience violence from hate crimes, rape, incest, and partner abuse. In the past, hate crimes against lesbian women and gays were underreported because of the fear of reporting attacks to the same police who raided lesbian and gay establishments (Comstock, 1989; Herek, 1989). Now, the National Gay and Lesbian Task Force has a hate crime hotline, and legislators in several states are discussing laws that mandate statistical monitoring of lesbian and gay hate crimes. Lesbian women and gays would be protected by these ethnic intimidation laws, which would increase penalties for crimes committed out of hatred against racial, religious, or sexual minorities compared to crimes that are committed as random acts of violence.

Lesbian women may experience rape and incest (Orzek, 1989). In fact, Brannock and Chapman (1990) found that reported rates of rape and incest were the same for lesbian and heterosexual women in a matched nonclinical sample. Partner abuse also is a problem in lesbian communities (Hart, 1986). Lesbian women commonly have difficulty getting support services to cope with the traumatic sequelae of these types of violence because rape crisis centers and battered women's shelters are unfamiliar with their needs. However, in some locations, support groups are available for lesbians who have experienced partner abuse.

Bereavement

Since the beginning of the AIDS epidemic, lesbian women and gay men have learned the brutal lessons of bereavement (Schindelman & Schoen, 1988). Yet little is known specifically about the lesbian experience of death, dying, and bereavement (Saunders, 1990).

A lesbian woman's obituary may say, "She left no survivors" (Grenwald, 1990). In reality, however, she may be survived by a large, hidden network of loved ones. The folksinger Judy Small recently wrote a song called "No Tears for the Widow," which contrasted the social support her mother experienced as a widow with the isolation her lesbian friend experienced after the death of her life partner.

Although informal support during lesbian bereavement is reported in community literature (Butler, 1989), no national resources currently exist in this area.

Nursing Care

Before providing care for a lesbian client, the nurse must be aware of his or her feelings about age, substance abuse, violence, and bereavement so that personal responses to these issues do not interfere with nursing care. If the lesbian client is young (e.g., the nurse's teenage daughter) or old (e.g., the grandmother) or a violent alcoholic (e.g., the father), countertransference may occur (Boden, 1988). Countertransference happens when the nurse's feelings about his or her life experiences affect the clinical response to the client. If the nurse is unresolved about sexuality and sexual orientation, the client's lesbianism may cause personal conflict in the nurse. Paying attention to feelings of discomfort and discussing them with colleagues or supervisors will contribute to personal growth and improved nursing care.

Resources

The nurse may call on various national and local organizations for information about age, substance abuse, and violence in the lesbian community. The nurse also may refer the lesbian client to appropriate resources for assistance with these issues (see the appendix to this chapter).

Lesbian Health Research

Many authors recommend a spectrum of lesbian health topics for further research. Lesbian topics offer the nurse researcher challenging theoretical questions, a surprisingly large interdisciplinary literature, a wide choice of methodologies, and great potential for generating new knowledge.

The theoretical challenge involves rethinking the concepts of gender and sexuality, which commonly are taken for granted. It also requires participation in intellectual debates about the biological and social determinants of human behavior throughout the life span (Epstein, 1987; Weeks, 1987; Weinrich, 1987).

The nurse researcher can draw on data from various disciplines and data sources. Researchers and theorists have approached lesbian issues from the perspectives of pathology (DeCecco, 1987), sociobiology (Money, 1987), feminism (Rich, 1980), sociology (Risman & Schwartz, 1988), politics (Rubin, 1984), and culture (Newton, 1988). Methodological approaches have been empirical (Wells & Kline, 1987), phenomenological (Hunnisett, 1986), and ethnographic (Wolf, 1979). In addition to published research, the nurse researcher can use new computer databases to locate unpublished dissertations and theses on lesbian topics. A rich ethnographic lesbian community literature is available in lesbian, gay, and feminist bookstores in many cities.

However, bias is a problem in lesbian health research. Morin (1977) notes a significant homophobic bias in medical research that assumes psychopathology in lesbians. More recent, affirmative lesbian research may be biased, overlooking accuracy in an attempt to improve the safety and civil rights of a stigmatized population.

Sampling problems can also occur in lesbian health research. As DeSantis (1990) noted in her research with undocumented aliens, representative sampling is impossible with certain vulnerable populations. Suppe (1985) argues that accurate research in lesbian and gay communities is impossible for male heterosexual investigators and for lesbian and gay researchers who have recently disclosed their sexual orientation because they all tend to share the homophobic biases of the mainstream heterosexual culture.

Conclusion

By providing quality care to lesbian women, the nurse gains an opportunity to think beyond stereotypes and grow beyond fear. Pheterson (1986) believes that attitudes of domination based on race, sex, religion, and sexual orientation damage the prejudiced individual as well as the individual who is despised for being different. The nurse who is open to learning about those who are different will gain new information, improved professional skills, and greater self-awareness. In growing beyond homophobia, the nurse can provide care for lesbian women in full appreciation of the courage and diversity of this vulnerable population.

References

BARRIERS TO CARE

American Nurses' Association. (1976). *Minority groups in nursing: A bibliography*. Kansas City, MO: Author.

American Nurses' Association. (1985). *Statement on health care for a population at risk*. Kansas City, MO: Author.

Barrett, M. B. (1989). *Invisible lives: The truth about millions of women-loving women*. New York: William Morrow.

Bieber, I. (1969). Homosexuality. *American Journal of Nursing*, *69*(12), 2637-2641.

Boston Women's Health Collective. (1993). Loving women: Lesbian life and relationships. In J. Pincus & W. Sanford (Eds.), *The new Our Bodies, Ourselves* (pp. 177-203). New York: Simon & Schuster.

Cass, V. C. (1979). Homosexual identity formation: A theoretical model. *Journal of Homosexuality*, *4*(3), 219-235.

Cochran, S. D., & Mays, V. M. (1988). Disclosure of sexual preference to physicians by black lesbian and bisexual women. *Western Journal of Medicine*, *149*, 616-619.

Deevey, S. (1990). Older lesbian women: An invisible minority. *Journal of Gerontological Nursing*, *16(5)*, 35-39.

Deevey, S. (1993). Lesbian self-disclosure: Strategies for success. *Journal of Psychosocial Nursing*, *31*(4), 21-26.

Gartrell, N. (1981). The lesbian as a "single woman." *American Journal of Psychotherapy*, *35*(4), 502-516.

Gillow, K. E., & Davis, L. L. (1987). Lesbian stress and coping methods. *Journal of Psychosocial Nursing*, *25*(9), 28-32.

Harvey, S. M., Carr, C., & Bernheine, S. (1989). Lesbian mothers: Health care experiences. *Journal of Nurse-Midwifery*, *34*(3), 115-119.

Hidalgo, H., Peterson, T. L., & Woodman, N. J. (1985). *Lesbian and gay issues: A resource guide for social workers*. Silver Spring, MD: National Association of Social Workers.

Hitchcock, J. (1989a). Bibliography: Lesbian health. *Women's Studies*, *17*(1/2), 139-144.

Hitchcock, J. (1989b). *Personal risking: The decision-making process of lesbians regarding self-disclosure of sexual orientation to health care providers*. Unpublished doctoral dissertation, University of California, San Francisco.

Holmes, M. A. (1982). Lesbian health care. In L. J. Sonstegard, K. M. Kowalski, & B. Jennings (Eds.), *Women's health: Ambulatory care* (pp. 207-220). New York: Grune & Stratton.

Irish, A. C. (1983). Straight talk about gay patients. *American Journal of Nursing*, *83*(8), 1168-1170.

Johnson, S. R., & Guenther, S. M. (1987). The role of "coming out" by the lesbians in the physician-patient relationship. *Women and Therapy*, *6*(1/2), 231-238.

Krieger, S. (1982). Lesbian identity and community: Recent social science literature. In E. B. Freedman, B. C. Gelpi, S. L. Johnson, & K. M. Weston (Eds.), *The lesbian issue: Essays from* Signs (pp. 223-240). Chicago: University of Chicago Press.

Kus, R. J. (1985). Stages of coming out: An ethnographic approach. *Western Journal of Nursing Research*, *7*(2), 177-198.

LoBiondo-Wood, G. (1986). Health education for the homosexual female. In V. M. Littlefield (Ed.), *Health education for women: A guide for nurses and other health professionals* (pp. 252-267). Norwalk, CT: Appleton-Century-Crofts.

Maggiore, D. J. (1988). *Lesbianism: An annotated bibliography and guide to the literature, 1976-1986*. Metuchen, NJ: Scarecrow.

Morrison, E. (1986). Lesbians. In D. K. Kjervik & I. M. Martinsen (Eds.), *Women in health and illness: Life experience and crises* (pp. 60-66). Philadelphia: W. B. Saunders.

Neisen, J. H. (1990). Heterosexism: Redefining homophobia for the 1990s. *Journal of Gay and Lesbian Psychotherapy*, *7*(3), 21-35.

Olesker, E., & Walsh, L. V. (1984). Childbearing among lesbians: Are we meeting their needs? *Journal of Nurse-Midwifery*, *29*(5), 322-329.

Pharr, S. (1988). *Homophobia: A weapon of sexism*. Inverness, CA: Chardon.

Randall, C. E. (1989). Lesbian phobia among BSN educators: A survey. *Journal of Nursing Education*, *28*(7), 302-306.

Roberts, S. J. (1985). Gay health issues. In L. L. Jarvis (Ed.), *Community health nursing: Keeping the public healthy* (pp. 679-693). Philadelphia: F. A. Davis.

Rothblum, E. D., & Cole, E. (Eds.). (1989). *Loving boldly: Issues facing lesbians*. New York: Harrington Park Press.

Schwanberg, S. L. (1985). Changes in labeling homosexuality in health sciences literature: A preliminary investigation. *Journal of Homosexuality*, *12*(1), 51-73.

Schwanberg, S. L. (1990). Attitudes toward homosexuality in American health care literature, 1983-87. *Journal of Homosexuality*, *19*(3), 117-136.

Sharkey, L. (1987). Nurses in the closet: Is nursing open and receptive to gay and lesbian nurses? *Imprint*, *34*(3), 38-39.

Shaw, N. S. (1989). New research issues in lesbian health. *Women's Studies*, *17*(1/2), 125-137.

Sigma Theta Tau. (1987). *Directory of nurse researchers*. Indianapolis, IN: Author.

Stephany, T. M. (1988). Lesbian nurse. *Nursing Outlook*, *36*(6), 295.

Stevens, P. E., & Hall, J. M. (1988). Stigma, health beliefs, and experiences with health care in lesbian women. *Image*, *20*(2), 69-73.

Stevens, P. E., & Hall, J. M. (1991). Critical, historical, analysis of the medical construction of lesbianism.

International Journal of Health Sciences, 21(2), 291-307.

Thompson, K., & Andrzejewski, J. (1988). *Why can't Sharon Kowalski come home?* San Francisco: Spinsters/Aunt Lute.

Weinberg, G. (1972). *Society and the healthy homosexual.* New York: St. Martin's.

White, T. A. (1979). Attitudes of psychiatric nurses toward same sex orientations. *Nursing Research, 28*(5), 276-281.

Williamson, M. (1986). Lesbianism. In J. Griffith-Kenney (Ed.), Contemporary women's health: A nursing advocacy approach (pp. 278-296). Menlo Park, CA: Addison-Wesley.

Wismont, J. M., & Reame, N. E. (1989). A lesbian childbearing experience: Assessing developmental tasks. *Image, 21*(3), 137-141.

Zeidenstein, L. (1990). Gynecological and childbearing needs of lesbians. *Journal of Nurse-Midwifery, 35*(1), 10-18.

INDIVIDUAL HEALTH ISSUES

American Psychiatric Association. (1987). *Diagnostic and statistical manual of mental disorders* (3rd ed., rev.). Washington, DC: American Psychiatric Press, Inc.

Bradford, J., & Ryan, C. (1988). *The national lesbian health care survey: Final report.* Washington, DC: National Lesbian and Gay Health Foundation.

Brooks, V. R. (1981). *Minority stress and lesbian women.* Lexington, MA: D. C. Heath.

Brown, L. (1989). Beyond thou shalt not: Thinking about ethics in the lesbian therapy community. *Women & Therapy, 8*(1/2), 13-25.

Browne, S. E. (1985). Social networks, social support, and general well-being of lesbians with chronic illness or hidden disabilities. *Dissertation Abstracts International, 46*(5), 1510-B. (University Microfilms No. ADG85 13655 8511)

Hall, M. (1985). *The lavender couch: A consumer's guide for lesbians and gay men.* Boston: Alyson.

Hepburn, C., & Gutierrez, B. (1988). *Alive and well: A lesbian health guide.* Freedom, CA: Crossing Press.

Johnson, S. R., Smith, E. M., & Guenther, S. M. (1987). Comparison of gynecologic health problems between lesbians and bisexual women: A survey of 2,345 women. *Journal of Reproductive Medicine, 32*(11), 805-811.

Klein, C. (1986). *Counseling our own: The lesbian/gay subculture meets the mental health system.* Seattle, WA: Consultation Services Northwest.

Kus, R. J. (Ed.). (1990). *Keys to caring: Assisting your gay and lesbian clients.* Boston: Alyson.

Leonard, Z. (1990). Lesbians in the AIDS crisis. In ACT/UP New York Women and AIDS Book Group (Ed.), *Women, AIDS, and activism* (pp. 113-118). Boston: South End Press.

Moses, A. E., & Hawkins, R. O. (1982). *Counseling lesbian women and gay men: A life-issues approach.* St. Louis: C. V. Mosby.

O'Donnell, M., Loeffler, V., Pollock, K., & Saunders, Z. (1979). *Lesbian health matters!* Santa Cruz, CA: Santa Cruz Women's Health Center.

Robertson, P., & Schachter, J. (1981). Failure to identify venereal disease in a lesbian population. *Sexually Transmitted Diseases, 8*(2), 75-76.

Rofes, E. E. (1983). *I thought people like that killed themselves: Lesbians, gay men, and suicide.* San Francisco: Grey Fox Press.

Saunders, J., & Valente, S. M. (1987). Suicide risk among gay men and lesbians: A review. *Death Studies, 11*(1), 1-23.

Shernoff, M., & Scott, W. A. (1988). *Sourcebook on lesbian/gay health care* (2nd ed.). Washington, DC: National Lesbian and Gay Health Foundation.

Stein, T. S., & Cohen, C. J. (Eds.). (1986). *Contemporary perspectives on psychotherapy with lesbians and gay men.* New York: Plenum Medical.

Ward, J. M. (1988/1989, Winter). Therapism and the taming of the lesbian community. *Sinister Wisdom,* pp. 33-41.

Winnow, J. (1989/1990, Winter). Lesbians' evolving health care: Our lives depend on it. *Sinister Wisdom,* pp. 53-62.

FAMILY HEALTH ISSUES

Almvig, C. (1982). *The invisible minority: Aging and lesbianism.* Syracuse, NY: Utica College of Syracuse University.

Becker, C. S. (1988). *Unbroken ties: Lesbian ex-lovers.* Boston: Alyson.

Berzon, B. (1988). *Permanent partners: Building gay and lesbian relationships that last.* New York: E. P. Dutton.

Borhek, M. V. (1983). *Coming out to parents: A two-way survival guide for lesbians and gay men and their parents.* New York: Pilgrim Press.

Bozett, F. W. (1987). Family nursing and life-threatening illness. In M. Leahey & L. Wright (Eds.), Families and life-threatening illness (pp. 2-25). Springhouse, PA: Springhouse Corporation.

Clunis, D. M., & Green, G. D. (1988). *Lesbian couples.* Seattle, WA: Seal Press.

Deevey, S. (1989). When mom or dad comes out: Helping adolescents cope with homophobia. *Journal of Psychosocial Nursing, 27*(10), 33-36.

Deevey, S. (1990). Older lesbian women: An invisible minority. *Journal of Gerontological Nursing, 16(5),* 35-39.

Eskenazi, B., Pies, C., Newsletter, A., Shepard, C., & Pearson, K. (1989). HIV serology in artificially inseminated lesbians. *Journal of Acquired Immune Deficiency Syndrome, 2*(2), 187-193.

Fairchild, B., & Hayward, N. (1979). *Now that you know: What every parent should know about homosexuality.* New York: Harcourt Brace Jovanovich.

Feetham, S. L. (1984). Family research: Issues and directions in nursing. In H. H. Werley & J. J. Fitzpatrick (Eds.), *Annual review of nursing research* (pp. 3-25). New York: Springer.

Griffin, C. W., Wirth, M. J., & Wirth, A. G. (1986). *Beyond acceptance: Parents of lesbians and gays talk about their experiences.* Englewood Cliffs, NJ: Prentice Hall.

Irish, A. C. (1990). Incorporating the client's support system into the plan of care. In R. J. Kus (Ed.), *Keys to caring: Assisting your gay and lesbian clients* (pp. 19-27). Boston: Alyson.

Kassoff, E. (1988). Nonmonogamy in the lesbian community. *Women and Therapy, 8*(1/2), 167-182.

Kehoe, M. (1989). *Lesbians over 60 speak for themselves.* New York: Harrington Park Press.

Kurdek, L. A. (1988). Perceived social support in gays and lesbians in co-habiting relationships. *Journal of Personality and Social Psychology, 54*(3), 504-509.

Loulan, J. (1987). *Lesbian passion: Loving ourselves and each other.* San Francisco: Spinsters/Aunt Lute.

Loulan, J. (1990). *The lesbian erotic dance: Butch, femme, androgyny, and other rhythms.* San Francisco: Spinsters.

Machs, J., & Ryan, C. (1988). Lesbians working in AIDS: An overview of our history and experience. In M. Sherhoff & W. A. Scott (Eds.), *The sourcebook on lesbian/gay health care* (2nd ed., pp. 198-201). Washington, DC: National Lesbian and Gay Health Foundation.

Maggiore, D. J. (1988). *Lesbianism: An annotated bibliography and guide to the literature, 1976-1986.* Metuchen, NJ: Scarecrow.

Neisen, J. H. (1987). Resources for families with a gay/lesbian member. *Journal of Homosexuality, 14*(1/2), 239-251.

Nestle, J. (1981). Butch-femme relationships: Sexual courage in the 1950s. *Heresies 12, 3*(4), 21-24.

Nichols, M. (1982). The treatment of inhibited sexual desire (ISD) in lesbian couples. *Women and Therapy, 1*(4), 49-66.

Peplau, L. A., Cochran, S., & Padesky, C. (1978). Loving women: Attachment and autonomy in lesbian relationships. *Journal of Social Issues, 34*(3), 7-27.

Pies, C. (1985). *Considering parenthood: A workbook for lesbians.* San Francisco: Spinsters.

Pollach, S., & Vaughn, J. (Eds.). (1987). *Politics of the heart: A lesbian parenting anthology.* Ithaca, NY: Firebrand.

Riley, C. (1988). American kinship: A lesbian account. *Feminist Issues, 8*(2), 75-94.

Stephany, T. M. (1988). Lesbian nurse. *Nursing Outlook, 36*(6), 295.

Tanner, D. M. (1981). *The lesbian couple.* Lexington, MA: Lexington Books.

Weston, K. M. (1988). Contesting the meaning of kinship: Discourse among lesbians and gays in the United States. *Dissertation Abstracts International, 49*(12), 3776A. (University Microfilms No. 890 6772)

Winnow, J. (1989). Lesbians' evolving health care: Our lives depend on it. *Sinister Wisdom, 39,* 53-62.

COMMUNITY HEALTH ISSUES

Anderson, E., McFarlane, J., & Helton, A. (1986). Community as client: A model for practice. *Nursing Outlook, 34*(5), 220-224.

Beck, E. T. (Ed.). (1982). *Nice Jewish girls: A lesbian anthology.* Trumensburg, NY: Crossing Press.

Clark, J. M., Brown, J. C., & Hochstein, L. M. (1990). Institutional religion and gay/lesbian oppression. In F. W. Bozett & M. B. Sussman (Eds.), *Homosexuality and family relations* (pp. 265-284). New York: Harrington Park Press.

Curb, R., & Manahan, N. (1985). *Lesbian nuns: Breaking silence.* New York: Warner.

D'Augelli, A. R., & Hart, M. M. (1987). Gay women, men, and families in rural settings: Toward the development of helping communities. *American Journal of Community Psychology, 15*(1), 79-93.

Garcia, N., Kennedy, C., Pearlman, S. F., & Perez, J. (1987). The impact of race and culture differences: Challenges to intimacy in lesbian relationships. In Boston Lesbian Psychologies Collective (Ed.), *Lesbian psychologies* (pp. 142-160). Urbana: University of Illinois Press.

Goeppinger, J., Lassiter, P. G., & Wilcox, B. (1982). Community health is community competence. *Nursing Outlook, 30*(8), 464-467.

Hall, M. (1986). The lesbian corporate experience. *Journal of Homosexuality, 12*(3/4), 59-75.

Hasbany, R. (1989/90). *Homosexuality and religion.* New York: Haworth.

Heyward, C. (1987). Heterosexist theology: Being above it all. *Journal of Feminist Studies in Religion, 3*(1), 29-38.

Kinsey, A. C., Pomeroy, W. B., Martin, C. E., & Gebhard, P. H. (1953). *Sexual behavior in the human female.* Philadelphia: W. B. Saunders.

Levine, M. P., & Leonard, R. (1984). Discrimination against lesbians in the work force. *Signs, 9*(4), 700-710.

Morales, E. S. (1990). Ethnic minority families and minority gays and lesbians. In F. W. Bozett & M. B. Sussman (Eds.), *Homosexuality and family relations* (pp. 217-239). New York: Harrington Park Press.

Ritter, K. Y., & O'Neill, C. W. (1989). Moving through loss: The spiritual journey of gay men and lesbian women. *Journal of Counseling and Development, 68*(1), 9-15.

Schmitz, T. J. (1988). Career counseling implications with the gay and lesbian population. *Journal of Employment Counseling, 25*(2), 51-56.

Schneider, B. E. (1987). Coming out at work: Bridging the private/public gap. *Work and Occupations, 13*(4), 463-487.

Shamansky, S. L., & Pesznecker, B. (1981). A community is . . . . *Nursing Outlook, 29*(3), 182-185.

Stewart, T. A. (1991, December 16). Gay in corporate America. *Fortune*, pp. 42-54.

Troiden, R. R. (1988). *Gay and lesbian identity: A sociological analysis*. Dix Hills, NY: General Hall.

Weinberg, G. (1972). *Society and the healthy homosexual*. New York: St. Martin's.

SPECIAL HEALTH ISSUES

Adelman, M. (1986). *Long-time passing: Lives of older lesbians*. Boston: Alyson.

Barracks, B., & Jarratt, K. (Eds.). (1980). *Sage writings: From the lesbian and gay men's writing workshop at Senior Action in a Gay Environment*. New York: Teachers and Writers Collaborative.

Bidwell, R. J. (1988). The gay and lesbian teen: A case of denied adolescence. *Journal of Pediatric Health Care*, *2*(1), 3-8.

Boden, R. (1988). Countertransference responses to lesbians with physical disabilities and chronic illnesses. In M. Shernoff & W. A. Scott (Eds.), *The sourcebook on lesbian/gay health care* (pp. 119-122). Washington, DC: National Lesbian and Gay Health Foundation.

Brannock, J. C., & Chapman, B. E. (1990). Negative sexual experiences with men among heterosexual women and lesbians. *Journal of Homosexuality*, *19*(1), 105-110.

Butler, S. (1989). Living in sacred time: Journal of a survivor. *Outlook: National Lesbian and Gay Quarterly*, *1*(4), 68-73.

Cates, J. A. (1987). Adolescent sexuality: Gay and lesbian issues. *Child-Welfare*, *66*(4), 353-364.

Coleman, E., & Remafedi, G. (1989). Gay, lesbian, and bisexual youth: A critical challenge to counselors. *Journal of Counseling and Development*, *68*(1), 36-40.

Comstock, G. D. (1989). Victims of anti-gay/lesbian violence. *Journal of Interpersonal Violence*, *4*(1), 101-106.

Deevey, S., & Wall, L. J. (1992). How do lesbian women develop serenity? *Health Care for Women International*, *13*(2), 199-208.

Finnegan, D. G., & McNally, E. B. (1987). *Dual identities: Counseling chemically dependent gay men and lesbians*. Center City, MN: Hazelden.

Friend, R. A. (1987). The individual and social psychology of aging: Clinical implications for lesbians and gay men. *Journal of Homosexuality*, *14*(1-2), 307-331.

Glaus, K. O. (1989). Alcoholism, chemical dependency, and the lesbian client. In E. D. Rothbaum & E. Cole (Eds.), *Loving boldly: Issues facing lesbians* (pp. 131-144). New York: Harrington Park Press.

Grenwald, M. (1990, January). In memory of the voices we have lost. *Lesbian Herstory Archives Newsletter*, p. 6.

Hall, J. M. (1990). Alcoholism and lesbians. Developmental, symbolic interactionism, and critical perspectives. *Health Care for Women International*, *11*(1), 84-107.

Hart, B. (1986). Lesbian battering: An examination. In K. Lobel (Ed.), *Naming the violence: Speaking out about lesbian battering* (pp. 173-189). Seattle, WA: Seal Press.

Hepburn, C., & Gutierrez, B. (1988). *Alive and well: A lesbian health guide*. Freedom, CA: Crossing Press.

Herdt, G. (Ed.). (1989). *Gay and lesbian youth*. New York: Harrington Park Press.

Herek, G. M. (1989). Hate crimes against lesbians and gay men: Issues for research and policy. *American Psychologist*, *44*(6), 948-955.

Kehoe, M. (1989). *Lesbians over 60 speak for themselves*. New York: Harrington Park Press.

Kus, R. J. (1990). Alcoholism in the gay and lesbian communities. In R. J. Kus (Ed.), *Keys to caring: Assisting your lesbian and gay clients* (pp. 66-81). Boston: Alyson.

McKernan, D. J., & Peterson, P. C. (1989). Alcohol and drug abuse among homosexual men and women: Epidemiology and population characteristics. *Addictive Behaviors*, *14*, 545-553.

Nicoloff, L. K., & Stiglitz, E. A. (1987). Lesbian alcoholism: Etiology, treatment and recovery. In Boston Lesbian Psychologies Collective (Ed.), *Lesbian psychologies* (pp. 283-293). Urbana: University of Illinois Press.

Orzek, A. M. (1989). The lesbian victim of sexual assault: Special consideration for the mental health professional. In E. D. Rothblum & E. Cole (Eds.), *Loving boldly: Issues lesbians face* (pp. 107-117). New York: Harrington Park Press.

Ratner, E. (1988). A model for the treatment of lesbian and gay alcohol abusers. *Alcoholism Treatment Quarterly*, *5*(1/2), 25-46.

Sang, B., Warshow, J., & Smith, A. J. (1991). *Lesbians at midlife: The creative transition*. San Francisco: Spinsters.

Saunders, J. M. (1990). Gay and lesbian widowhood. In R. Kus (Ed.), *Keys to caring* (pp. 224-243). Boston: Alyson.

Schindelman, E., & Schoen, K. (1988). Gay and grieving: Bringing grief out of the closet. In M. Shernoff & W. A. Scott (Eds.), *The sourcebook on lesbian/gay health care* (pp. 114-118). Washington, DC: National Lesbian and Gay Health Foundation.

Swallow, J. (Ed.). (1983). *Out from under: Sober dykes and our friends*. San Francisco: Spinsters/Aunt Lute.

LESBIAN HEALTH RESEARCH AND CONCLUSION

DeCecco, J. P. (1987). Homosexuality's brief recovery: From sickness to health and back again. *Journal of Sex Research*, *23*(1), 106-114.

DeSantis, L. (1990). Fieldwork with undocumented aliens and other populations at risk. *Western Journal of Nursing Research*, *12*(3), 359-372.

Epstein, S. (1987). Gay politics, ethnic identity: The limits of social construction. *Socialist Review*, *17*(3/4), 9-54.

Hunnisett, R. J. (1986). Developing phenomenological methods for researching lesbian existence. *Canadian Journal of Counseling*, *20*(4), 255-268.

Money, J. (1987). Sin, sickness, or status: Homosexual gender identity and psychoneuroendocrinology. *American Psychologist, 42*(4), 384-399.

Morin, S. F. (1977). Heterosexual bias in psychological research on lesbianism and male homosexuality. *American Psychologist, 32*(8), 629-637.

Newton, E. (1988). Of yams, grinders, and gays: The anthropology of homosexuality. *Outlook: National Lesbian and Gay Quarterly, 1*(1), 28-37.

Pheterson, G. (1986). Alliances between women: Overcoming internalized oppression and internalized domination. *Signs, 12*(11), 146-160.

Rich, A. (1980). Compulsory heterosexuality and lesbian existence. *Signs, 5*(4), 631-660.

Risman, B., & Schwartz, P. (1988). Sociological research on male and female homosexuality. *Annual Review of Sociology, 14*, 125-147.

Rubin, G. (1984). Thinking sex: Notes for a radical theory of the politics of sexuality. In C. S. Vance (Ed.), *Pleasure and danger* (pp. 261-318). Boston: Routledge & Kegan Paul.

Suppe, F. (1985). The Bell and Weinberg study: Future priorities for research on homosexuality. In N. Koertge (Ed.), *Philosophy and homosexuality* (pp. 69-97). New York: Harrington Park Press.

Weeks, J. (1987). Questions of identity. In P. Caplan (Ed.), *The cultural construction of sexuality* (pp. 31-51). London: Tavistock.

Weinrich, J. D. (1987). *Sexual landscapes: Why we are what we are, why we love whom we love*. New York: Scribner's.

Wells, J. W., & Kline, W. B. (1987). Self-disclosure of homosexual orientation. *Journal of Social Psychology, 127*(2), 191-197.

Wolf, D. G. (1979). *The lesbian community*. Berkeley: University of California Press.

RESOURCES FOR LESBIAN HEALTH

The nurse may contact the following resources for more information about lesbian health or may refer the lesbian client to them for further assistance with individual, family, community, or special health concerns.

Individual Health

American Association of Physicians for Human Rights
Lesbian Physicians Annual Conference
P.O. Box 14366
San Francisco, CA 94144

Association of Lesbian and Gay Psychologists
2336 Market Street, No. 8
San Francisco, CA 94114

Dykes, Disability, and Stuff Newsletter
P.O. Box 6194
Boston, MA 02114

Fenway Community Health Center
16 Haviland Street
Boston, MA
617-267-7573

The Mautner Project for Lesbians With Cancer
P.O. Box 90437
Washington, DC 20090

National Lesbian and Gay Health Foundation
P.O. Box 65472
Washington, DC 20035
202-797-3708

Whitman-Walker Clinic
1407 S Street NW
Washington, DC 20009
202-797-3585

Family Health

Gay and Lesbian Parents Coalition International
P.O. Box 50360
Washington, DC 20091
202-583-8029

Lambda Legal Defense and Education Fund
666 Broadway
New York, NY 10012
212-995-8585

Lesbian Mothers National Defense Fund
P.O. Box 21567
Seattle, WA 98111
206-325-2643

National Center for Lesbian Rights
1370 Mission Street, 4th floor
San Francisco, CA 94103
415-621-0674

Parents and Friends of Lesbians and Gays (PFLAG)
P.O. Box 27605
Washington, DC 20038-7605
202-638-4200

Community Health

Fan the Flames Feminist Bookstore
65 South 4th Street
Columbus, OH 43215

Gaia's Guide (international lesbian directory)
c/o Bookpeople
2929 Fifth Street
Berkeley, CA 94710
415-655-0364

Lesbian Connection (newsletter)
Ambitious Amazons
P.O. Box 811
East Lansing, MI 48823
517-371-5257

LLEGO (Latino/a Lesbian and Gay Organization)
P.O. Box 44483
Washington, DC 20026
202-544-0092

National Coalition for Black Lesbians and Gays
P.O. Box 19248
Washington, DC 20036
202-265-4736

Outlook: National Lesbian and Gay Quarterly
2940 16th Street, Suite 319
San Francisco, CA 94103
415-626-7929

Special Issues

Alpatha Healing Center (substance abuse and violence resources)
815 North High Street
Columbus, OH 43215
614-294-7979

Gay and Lesbian Adolescent Social Services (GLASS)
8235 Santa Monica Blvd., No. 214
West Hollywood, CA 90046

Gay and Lesbian Outreach to Elderly (GLOE)
1853 Market Street
San Francisco, CA 94103

Golden Threads (friendship club for lesbians over age 50)
P.O. Box 3177
Burlington, VT 05401

Harvey Milk High School
Hetrick-Martin Institute
401 West Street
New York, NY 10014
212-633-8920

The Lesbian Caucus
Mass Coalition of Battered Women Service Groups
107 South Street, Fifth Floor
Boston, MA 02111
617-426-8492

National Association for Lesbian and Gay Gerontology (NALGG)
1290 Sutter Street, Suite 8
San Francisco, CA 94109

National Association of Lesbian and Gay Alcoholism Professionals (NALGAP)
204 West 20th Street
New York, NY 10011
212-713-5074

National Gay and Lesbian Task Force
Anti-Violence Project
1317 U Street
Washington, DC 20009
202-332-6483

Pride Institute
14400 Martin Drive
Eden Prairie, MN 55344

Senior Action in a Gay Environment (SAGE)
208 West 13th Street
New York, NY 10011

Youth Services Department
Gay and Lesbian Community Service Center
1213 N. Highland Ave.
Los Angeles, CA 90038
213-633-8920

PART III

11

Health Protection and Health Promotion for Women

ELLEN SULLIVAN MITCHELL

Health is a central concept of nursing practice and is essential to the identity of the nursing profession. Numerous health professions claim to focus on the health of their clients but tend to have a narrower, less integrated view of health than does nursing—that is, some focus only on illness, others only on wellness, and some only on one part of the client. What distinguishes nursing from the other health professions is (a) the integration of the biological and psychosocial world of the client (Shaver, 1985); (b) the integration of illness and wellness dimensions as they affect the client's health; (c) the awareness of the interaction between clients and their environment as it contributes to health; and (d) a focus on the client as a whole, whether the client is the individual, the family, or the community. From this perspective, nursing has an important role to play in helping to achieve the health goals of our nation (U.S. Department of Health and Human Services, 1990).

Optimum health is achieved through a variety of health care goals. These practice goals include helping the client to restore health, to maintain health, to protect health, and to promote health. The particular health care goals selected by the nurse for any one client is dependent on the clinician's model of health and scope of practice as well as the health status and needs of the client. How the health care goals are achieved is guided by the particular intervention model endorsed by the nurse. The purpose of this chapter is to review several models of health that guide practice and then to describe several health promotion and health protection models. The emphasis will be on the individual woman as the client.

Models of Health

Health is a concept as old as modern nursing. It has its roots in the nursing profession in the work of Florence Nightingale (Nightingale, 1860/ 1969) and in the brave efforts of Lillian Wald and the Henry Street Visiting Nurse Service in New York City beginning in the late 19th century (Christy, 1970). The focus of these nursing giants was not just on the treatment of disease and illness, for there was very little to offer in those days, but mainly on helping people improve their living

Table 11.1 Definitions Related to Health and Illness

Health—The state whereby level of disease, illness, and wellness are integrated to produce optimal biological, psychological, sociocultural, and spiritual functioning of a client. In Healthy People 2000 (U.S. Department of Health and Human Services, 1990), good health is said to come from the reduction of unnecessary suffering, illness, and disability and from an improved quality of life measured by a sense of well-being.

Wellness—The degree to which self-care behaviors in interaction with the environment enhance or damage health. Wellness, a component of health but not synonymous with health, focuses on client self-care behaviors that affect health.

Illness—The response of an individual to disease.

Disease—Any alteration in the functional or structural integrity of the mind or body.

Health restoration—Those activities of the clinician aimed at diagnosing or treating the disease and the illness state of the client, such as prescribing an antibiotic for endometritis or obtaining blood pressure from a woman with pregnancy-induced hypertension.

Health maintenance—Clinician activities focused on early detection and prevention of disease, such as giving immunizations, obtaining Pap smears, or ordering a screening mammogram. Health restoration and health maintenance involve the activities of the health care provider on behalf of the client with a focus on either the diagnosis, treatment, or prevention of disease.

Health protection—The acquisition of new self-care behaviors or the cessation or avoidance of existing self-care behaviors to prevent or treat disease. Examples of health protection include teaching breast self-examination, encouraging clients to seek age- and gender-appropriate screening, teaching effective communication skills, and smoking cessation counseling.

Self-care—Behaviors performed by the client rather than the clinician.

Health promotion—The maintenance or improvement of existing self-care behaviors that promote growth, human potential, and quality of life and are directed toward high-level wellness. The primary focus of health promotion is wellness (Brubaker, 1983; Pender, 1987), such as helping a woman develop a physical fitness program, teaching a pregnant woman about optimal nutrition, or leading a group of women in values clarification to assist in decision making about lifestyle. Health protection and health promotion center around self-care behaviors of a woman within the context of her environment and require some element of motivation to be achieved. The role of the clinician is assisting the client with the behavior change.

SOURCE: Pender, N. J. (1987). *Health Promotion in Nursing Practice* (2nd ed.) Norwalk, CT: Appleton & Lange. Rerpinted with permission.

conditions, their nutrition, their shelter, and their spirit. This heritage of viewing the whole person in interaction with his or her environment, as well as focusing on promoting and protecting health, is the central core of nursing practice today.

Issues Related to Definitions of Health

Numerous definitions of health proposed over the years have generated several major issues: (a) whether *disease* and *illness* are equivalent terms, (b) whether *health* and *wellness* are synonymous, and (c) whether health and disease and illness are part of the same continuum. It is important for the clinician to resolve these definitional issues about health because the way health is defined influences the selection of health care goals and the particular model of practice used to achieve those goals (see Table 11.1).

Defining Disease and Illness. Disease and illness are used interchangeably in many definitions of health. Exceptions are those definitions that differentiate the client's personal perspective of health, called the *emic* dimension, from the clinician's perspective, called the *etic* dimension (Tripp-Reimer, 1984). In this definition, the emic dimension is referred to as illness and the etic dimension as disease. Some define disease as a functional or structural disturbance of the body and illness as the state of being of the person in response to the disease (Edelman & Mandle, 1990). According to the latter perspective, disease is viewed as the objective experience (signs) of a biological or psychological disturbance and illness as the subjective experience (symptoms or response to symptoms) of that alteration (see Table 11.1).

Defining Wellness and Health. Wellness is equated with health in many definitions of health, whereas disease and illness are treated as something different (Dunn, 1959; Oelbaum, 1974; Pender, 1987; World Health Organization [WHO], 1947). Most definitions of wellness do not include disease and illness states. Wellness most frequently includes how well people take care of themselves, how constructively they use their minds, how effectively they express their emotions, how concerned they are with their environment, and how creatively they are involved with those around them (Ryan & Travis, 1981). Wellness in this sense means moving to a higher potential of functioning or to optimal health (Edelman & Mandle, 1990). The problem with using wellness synonymously with health is that disease and illness are then something separate from health. This way of defining health does not permit the integration of disease and illness into an evaluation of the health status of a client. For example, if health and wellness were synonymous, which implies that disease is not part of the definition, both a person with a disease and another without disease who engaged in self-care behaviors that enhanced health would be said to have the same state of health. Are both of these people just as healthy? Without a definition of health that includes disease state, they would be evaluated equally.

Single-Dimension Models of Health

World Health Organization Definition. The third issue involved in the definition of health is whether health and disease or illness are part of the same continuum, with health at one end and disease or illness at the other end—that is, whether a single dimension or continuum of health exists. An example of a single-continuum definition of health was proposed by WHO (1947). In the WHO definition, health is described as "a state of complete physical, mental and social well-being, and not merely the absence of disease or infirmity." A single dimension of health raises the question of whether health is something different from, but interrelated with, disease or illness. Prior to the WHO definition in 1947, health was commonly referred to as the absence of disease, which meant that, to be healthy, the focus of action was on eliminating the disease. The WHO definition continued to reflect health as a single dimension but did add a level of complexity by stating that being disease free was not enough to be healthy. It was the first definition to integrate illness and well-being into a concept of health by including the positive health goals of complete physical, mental, and social well-being. However, even though it shifted the focus more toward achieving general well-being, it still implied that a healthy state could not exist in the presence of disease because disease was at one end and well-being at the other end.

Dunn's Model of Health. Dunn (1959) further developed the WHO definition by describing the positive health goal as peak wellness. In the Dunn model, death and peak wellness are at opposite ends of a horizontal continuum. Peak wellness was viewed as a level of functioning in which the potential of the client is maximized. Dunn incorporated more complexity into a definition of health than did the WHO definition by the addition of a vertical axis reflecting the influence of the environment on the ability to achieve peak wellness (see Figure 11.1). The most positive outcome resulting from the interaction of the two axes was called high-level wellness. Although the Dunn model has two axes, it still depicts disease and wellness on a single continuum and therefore does not allow for the simultaneous existence of disease and wellness. Both of these single-dimension models of health, the WHO model and the Dunn model, with health or wellness at one end and illness, disease, or death at the other end of a continuum, are called *clinical models of health* (Smith, 1981). The health care goals for a clinical model of health are health restoration and health maintenance because they emphasize the diagnosis and treatment of disease.

Other Single-Dimension Models. Many other single-dimension models of health exist. The role performance model (Parsons, 1958) defines health as the degree to which people perform their roles in life. The adaptation model (Dubos, 1965; Roy, 1984) views a healthy person as one who can engage in adaptive behavior to interact effectively with the physical and social environment. In the clinical model of health, the healthy person is free of disease or disability. Finally, the eudaemonistic, general well-being or the self-actualization model (Maslow, 1970; Smith, 1981) defines health as the realization of self-fulfillment and complete development. In all but the clinical model, the role of disease or illness is not addressed. The drawback of these

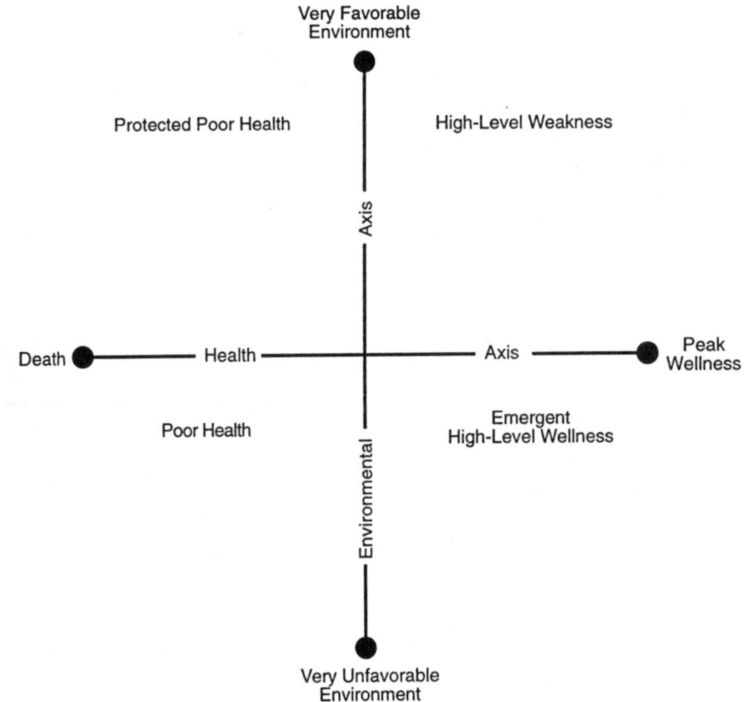

Figure 11.1. The Health Grid: Its Axes and Quadrants
SOURCE: U.S. Department of Health, Education and Welfare, Public Health Service, National Office of Vital Statistics.

single-dimension models is that they do not permit the type of assessment of a client that integrates the disease, illness, and wellness state of that client. The focus of these single-dimension models is either on altering the disease and illness or on enhancing wellness but not on all components together. Placing disease and wellness at opposite ends of a continuum fragments the person and does not permit a holistic view of the person's health status. In treating a woman as a whole person with a disease, one cannot separate biological alterations and the response to them from the self-care behaviors that contribute to wellness.

Multidimensional Models of Health

In an attempt to overcome the deficiencies of the single-continuum definition of health, several authors have proposed models that integrate disease, illness, and wellness into a multidimensional interactive model (Oelbaum, 1974; Orem, 1985; Pender, 1987; Shaver, 1985; Wu, 1973). However, none of the existing multidimensional models of health provides a specific framework for guiding the assessment of the health status of the client as well as the selection of health care goals to guide intervention.

The Integrated Health Model. A model of health that builds on that of Pender (1987), Shaver (1985), Oelbaum (1974), and Dunn (1959) was developed by the author. This integrated model places disease and illness state on one continuum and level of wellness on the other continuum (see Figure 11.2). Health is a dynamic state in which the extent of disease and illness and level of wellness are integrated. The goal of the clinician is to help the client move toward the most positive state of health possible. Disease, illness, and health-damaging behaviors are viewed as threats to health. This integrated model of health expands on earlier models by providing a framework on which the clinician and client can determine which health care goals are most appropriate for the client. Using this model, the clinician can determine the client's need for health maintenance, health promotion, health protection, and health restoration, as well as determine which goals take priority.

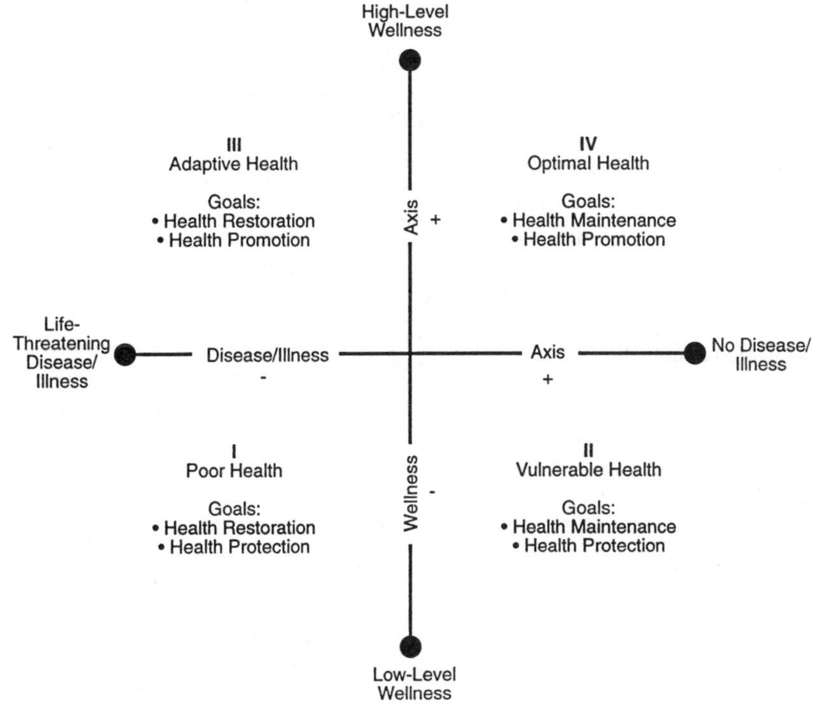

Figure 11.2. Integrated Health Model
SOURCE: Developed by the author.

The integrated health model (IHM; see Figure 11.2) consists of two intersecting dimensions, disease/illness and wellness, which together constitute the state of health of the individual. In this model, the terms *illness* and *disease* are used together on the same continuum with different but related meanings. Disease represents alterations in functional and structural integrity, whereas illness corresponds to the response of the client to the disease. For example, for a woman with endometriosis, the disease is endometrial tissue implanted outside the uterus, whereas the illness is the pain she experiences, her inability to obtain adequate sleep as a result of the pain, and her fear of infertility. On the horizontal disease/illness continuum of the model, there is a positive half and a negative half with all levels of disease included. In the positive half, there is no disease, risk of disease, minor acute disease, and stable uncomplicated chronic disease. Complicated chronic disease, unstable disease, and life-threatening disease occur in the negative half. The primary focus of the clinician on this axis is the diagnosis and treatment of disease and illness by the clinician. This continuum by itself represents a clinical model of health. The aim of this dimension is attainment of the highest degree of integrity of the body, mind, and spirit and indicates the health care goals of health restoration and health maintenance.

Health restoration is defined as the health care goal of reestablishing health by engaging in such activities as life support, rehabilitation, and diagnosis and treatment of illness and disease. For a woman with pelvic inflammatory disease, this might include interventions such as use of antibiotics and monitoring of signs and symptoms. Health maintenance is the health care goal of preserving health by targeting specific diseases. Health maintenance includes prevention of disease and early detection of disease through screening and risk assessment. Examples of health maintenance activities are conducting breast examinations, screening for sexually transmitted diseases, obtaining Pap smears, osteoporosis and cardiac disease risk assessment, ordering mammograms, and administering immunizations. Within the IHM, health maintenance and health promotion differ. Health maintenance does not include nursing interventions that focus on changing the behavior of the client as does health promotion. The focus is on the clinician's activities related to disease and illness. This is an important point because different theoretical models guide the nursing interventions involved in health maintenance and health promotion.

The vertical wellness dimension of the model is the second critical dimension of health. This continuum goes from low-level wellness in the negative half of the continuum to high-level wellness in the positive half. This dimension includes self-care behaviors involved in nutrition, rest, physical activity and fitness, elimination, family planning, substance use, stress management, communication, and socialization, to name a few. The focus of nursing intervention within this axis is to help the client either maintain or enhance positive lifestyle behaviors or to avoid potentially harmful ones. Thus the emphasis is on lifestyle or self-care behaviors of the client that can affect the wellness level and not on a specific disease or illness response, even if disease is present. This view of wellness as a part of health but separate from disease is consistent with earlier work on wellness (Ardell, 1979; Brubaker, 1983; Clark, 1986). Lifestyle refers to those activities that have a significant impact on health that are part of a person's daily pattern of living (Wiley & Camacho, 1980).

A low level of wellness is recognized by the predominance of health-damaging behaviors and is in the negative or lower half of the wellness continuum. Health-damaging behaviors include smoking, drug and alcohol abuse, sedentary lifestyle, overwork, unsociable behavior, interpersonal conflict, unhealthy eating habits, chronic tension, lack of seat belt use, avoidance of health screening, unsafe sex practices, and nonadherence to a therapeutic regimen for disease treatment. The health care goal indicated by the presence of health-damaging behaviors is health protection. Health protection is defined as the health care goal of conserving, guarding, or defending health by the cessation or avoidance of behaviors that impede progress toward high-level wellness. Even though health protection involves preventing disease and illness, as does health maintenance, it is not part of the disease/illness continuum. The reason for this is that in the IHM, health protection focuses on self-care behaviors that are dependent on the motivation of the client, whereas health maintenance as a health care goal focuses on behaviors of the clinician that are guided by the clinical decision-making process as well as those of the client. Both are different but important in the health care of the client.

High-level wellness is in the positive or upper half of the wellness continuum and is apparent by the predominance of behaviors that enhance health. Health-enhancing behaviors include those aimed at improving health above a maintenance level and at taking positive action toward higher wellness. The health care goal indicated by these health-enhancing behaviors is health promotion, which focuses on advancing health and increasing well-being through positive experiences and growth. Behaviors involved in health promotion include positive lifestyle habits, relaxation, fitness, pleasure, positive mood, loving, being creative, and being in harmony with oneself and others (Maslow, 1970; Pender, 1987; Smith, 1981; Woods et al., 1988). Pender (1987) stated that health-enhancing behaviors are directed toward maintaining or improving personal fulfillment, self-actualization, and level of well-being by promoting change, growth, and maturation. The focus of assessment on the wellness dimension of the IHM is the negative or positive quality of the client's self-care behaviors and how they actually or potentially can affect the integrity of the mind, body, and spirit.

At all times, the selection of specific health care goals is influenced by the clinician's definition of health. For example, if health is viewed as the absence of disease, then health restoration and health maintenance goals would predominate. If health is considered a single continuum with disease and wellness at opposite ends of the poles, then health protection, with its additional component of self-care behaviors, would be added to the goals of care and a high level of wellness could not exist in the presence of any disease. For all four health care goals to become part of nursing practice, a model of health such as the IHM, which integrates disease, illness, and wellness, is needed.

In the IHM, the intersection of the disease/illness and wellness dimensions creates four health status quadrants (see Figure 11.2). The particular quadrant that represents the health status of the client is determined by a thorough assessment of the disease and illness state and level of wellness. It then guides nursing intervention by indicating the appropriate health care goals to pursue. Quadrant I represents poor health status with the wellness level and the disease and illness state in the negative half of each dimension. An example is a woman with unstable diabetes who abuses alcohol and engages in no regular exercise. Quadrant II describes vulnerable health status in which the client's wellness level is in the negative portion, and the disease/illness state is in the positive end of the continuum. An example of vulnerable health is a woman with a urinary tract infection who smokes and has unsafe sex practices. Adaptive health status, Quadrant III, represents a positive level of wellness with the disease/illness state in the negative portion of the continuum. For example, a woman with unstable hypertension and coronary artery disease who eats balanced low-sodium, low-fat meals, exercises regularly, has a normal weight, and has a satisfactory social network would be represented by Quadrant III. Finally, Quadrant IV represents optimal health status with a positive wellness level and the disease/illness state in the positive portion of the continuum. An example is a woman whose mother had breast cancer, who does monthly breast self-examination (BSE), has regular checkups, eats well-balanced meals, has a positive self-concept, and feels self-fulfilled.

Each quadrant in the IHM has implications for specific health care goals as well as for providing direction for movement toward a higher level of health. Placement in a particular quadrant is dependent on the assessment of all disease and illness states of the client as well as all self-care behaviors, both health enhancing and health damaging. The type and quality of self-care behaviors and their potential negative or positive contributions to wellness are assessed to place a client at a point on the wellness continuum. Placement on the disease/illness continuum is determined by the amount, complexity, and stability of disease present; the risk of disease; the potential seriousness of the disease; and the amount and type of illness resulting from disease. The point where the wellness and disease/illness assessments intersect determines the health status of the client—that is, into which quadrant the client fits as a result of the assessment.

All four health status quadrants influence the health care goals that guide nursing intervention. The key is the location of the health status of the client within one of the four quadrants in the model. In Quadrant IV (optimal health), health promotion and health maintenance are the appropriate health care goals. In Quadrant III (adaptive health), health promotion and health restoration are the focus of the intervention, with health restoration possibly predominating over health promotion if the situation warrants. Within Quadrant II (vulnerable health) health maintenance and health protection need to be considered. Finally, in Quadrant I (poor health) health protection and health restoration are important, with the possibility of interventions focused on health restoration taking precedence over health protection, depending on the severity and extent of the disease and illness.

In addition to indicating goals for appropriate nursing intervention, the placement of the client into one of the four health status quadrants offers guidance in determining the appropriate direction for improving the health status of the client. For example, the woman with the urinary tract infection in an earlier example who had vulnerable health (Quadrant II) could be helped to move to optimal health (Quadrant IV) by treating her infection, discussing ways to prevent a recurrence, and helping her to stop smoking and to use condoms. If only her disease were treated, she would remain in Quadrant II although in a more positive location along the disease and illness continuum as her infection resolved. Optimal health, Quadrant IV, may not be an appropriate goal for everyone: For example, for a woman with uncontrolled diabetes who is in poor health (Quadrant I), initially it may be more appropriate to focus on controlling the disease and encouraging health maintenance behaviors, thus aiming for vulnerable health (Quadrant II). Later, as her disease stabilizes, optimal health may be a more appropriate goal, which can be reached by adding health protection goals to her plan of care. If her life is chaotic, she has limited personal and social resources, and she is doing the best she can within her circumstances, the highest point in Quadrant II may be the most reasonable goal for her.

Models of Health Protection and Health Promotion

Several models of practice exist that can guide the nurse clinician in health care delivery. The particular model selected will be greatly influenced by the model of health the clinician believes in. Models of health protection and health promotion serve as a framework and guide to the clinician when focusing on the wellness dimension of health. The clinical decision-making model is the framework that guides the clinician when the focus is on the diagnosis and treatment of disease and illness. In this section, several health protection and health promotion models will be described. Each model, in a different way, attempts to account for motivational factors that affect self-care behavior change related to health. Although the emphasis of this book is on women, models of health protection and health promotion are not unique for women because they were developed for men and women. Nevertheless, self-care models are important for providers of women's health care because women are more self-care oriented than men (Hibbard & Pope, 1987; Lantz, 1985). Women either have been the focus of studies or have been included in studies along with men to predict specific self-care behaviors using the health belief model (HBM) (Fulton et al., 1991; Lashley, 1987; Williams, 1991), the planned behavior model (Saltzer, 1981; Schifter & Ajzen, 1985), the relapse prevention model (RPM) (Abrams et al., 1987; Curry, Marlatt, Gordon, & Baer, 1988), the self-regulation model (SRM) (Johnson & Lauver, 1989), Orem's self-care model (Denyes, 1988; Fitzgerald, 1980; Harper, 1984; Oakley, Denyes, & O'Connor, 1989; Whetstone & Reid, 1991), and the health promotion model (HPM) (Duffy, 1988; Duffy & MacDonald, 1990; Gillis & Perry, 1991; Pender, Walker, Sechrist, & Frank-Stromborg, 1990). Studies are still needed to test these models of health protection and health promotion for gender differences.

The models of care with a predominant focus on health protection are the HBM (Becker, 1974), the planned behavior model (Ajzen, 1985), and the RPM (Marlatt & Gordon, 1985). Models that account for health promotion are the SRM (Kanfer, 1980), the self-care model (Orem, 1985), and the HPM (Pender, 1987). Two concepts important to several of the models, self-efficacy expectations (Bandura, 1977) and levels of prevention (Leavell & Clark, 1965), will be discussed first because they are important in understanding the models.

Self-Efficacy Expectations

Self-efficacy expectations is a concept central to several models of health protection and health promotion. Bandura (1977) described and developed this concept as part of his social learning theory (Bandura, 1977; Strecher, DeVellis, Becker, & Rosenstock, 1986). Self-efficacy is the appraisal by a person that by using their available skills they can act competently and cope effectively with a situation (Bandura, 1977). Self-efficacy plays an important role in the initiation and maintenance of behavior change (Strecher et al., 1986). Behavior change and maintenance of that change are influenced by a person's expectations about the outcomes of the behavior change and the expectations of one's ability to engage in or execute the behavior change. For example, whether a woman's smoking behavior will change or not is determined by how skillful she perceives she is regarding her ability to stop smoking (efficacy expectations) in addition to how much she believes her efforts will produce the desired results (outcome expectations).

Levels of Prevention

Levels of prevention are frequently mentioned in the nursing literature as a way of labeling different goals of health care. The focus of levels of prevention is on the natural history of a disease and the point at which health care intervention might prevent the next stage of the disease (Leavell & Clark, 1965). Within this concept, there are three levels of prevention: primary, secondary, and tertiary. Primary prevention consists of interventions aimed at preventing the occurrence of disease. Examples are immunizations against specific diseases, smoking cessation, and prenatal care. Within the IHM, primary prevention is part of the health care goals of health maintenance and health protection, depending on whether the nurse clinician directly provides the intervention to prevent disease (giving an immunization) or assists the client to alter her own behavior to prevent disease, such as smoking cessation, avoiding risky behaviors, or obtaining an adequate calcium intake. Primary prevention plays a major role in health protection but only a minimal role in health maintenance as defined in the IHM. In other words, it is the client who is most directly involved in prevention of disease (primary prevention) as part of health protection. The clinician's role is an indirect one through coaching, teaching, and counseling the client.

Primary prevention is not the same as primary care, yet the two concepts are often confused with each other. Primary care refers to a specific type of health care delivery system, which includes interventions aimed at primary prevention. However, primary care is also involved with secondary and tertiary prevention. Also, other health care systems in addition to primary care, such as hospital-based care, provide primary prevention interventions.

Secondary prevention focuses on early detection and early treatment of disease. Prevention here is used in the sense of preventing the progress of the disease by taking prompt action. Secondary prevention includes screening for disease for early diagnosis and treating disease promptly. Common examples are ordering mammography, obtaining Pap smears, teaching women to perform BSE, seeking health care for screening, and early treatment of a disease. The dimension of secondary prevention that focuses on screening for early detection of disease is part of health maintenance and health protection. The dimension of secondary prevention that involves early treatment of disease is part of health restoration. The clinician plays a major role in secondary prevention that is part of health maintenance. The third level of prevention is tertiary prevention. Tertiary prevention involves those activities that focus on prevention of complications and rehabilitation to minimize disability. Disease is present but cannot be cured, so prevention of complications and further disability is the goal. This third level of prevention fits within the health restoration goal on the disease/illness continuum because it focuses on the diagnosis and treatment of disease and prevention of complications.

In summary, both primary and secondary prevention involve health maintenance and health protection depending on whether the client or the clinician is performing the behavior. In addition, secondary prevention involves health restoration, as does tertiary prevention. Because the levels of prevention relate to disease, health promotion, which does not focus on disease, is not involved. Looked at another way, health maintenance involves both primary and secondary prevention with secondary prevention playing a major role. Health protection involves all three levels of prevention, and health restoration involves both secondary and tertiary prevention.

Health Protection Models

Health Belief Model. The HBM is widely used in nursing, as well as in other health-related disciplines. Originally, the HBM was developed by social psychologists as a model to explain and predict the likelihood of behavior directed toward prevention or early detection of a specific disease, such as obtaining immunizations, participating in tuberculosis and cervical cancer screening, and having health check-ups (Becker, 1974). Within the framework of the IHM, the HBM is a guide to health protection. It has been used to explain and predict behaviors involved in smoking cessation, dietary alteration, and seat belt use. The predominant focus of this model is primary and secondary prevention. The basic premise of the HBM is that the likelihood of taking health-related action is influenced by attitudes and beliefs that motivate behavior. The model depicts the likelihood of performing a recommended health behavior as the interaction between perceptions of susceptibility to disease, seriousness of disease, and threat of disease, as well as the perception of the benefits of action when weighed against barriers to those actions. Self-efficacy is a component of perceived barriers. All perceptions in the model are modified by demographic characteristics, personal and social factors, prior knowledge of and experience with the disease, and cues to action found in the environment (Becker, 1974). The most frequent type of study testing the HBM that involves women is the study about frequency of BSE. Consistently perceived barriers predict this health protection behavior (Fulton et al., 1991; Lashley, 1987). This is also a consistent finding in studies that include both men and women or men only (Janz & Becker, 1984). The HBM has been most useful for predicting behaviors when attitudes and beliefs are predominantly involved in the decision to take action, such as seeking immunizations or screening procedures. It has not been as successful at predicting habitual health behaviors, such as brushing one's teeth or smoking cigarettes; when the goal of action is not directly related to physical health, such as dieting to look more attractive, which is health promotion; or when forces outside the individual, such as economic or environmental factors, are major barriers to action (Janz & Becker, 1984). Although the HBM has been widely tested and used in nursing, it is not a model that predicts health-promoting behavior—that is, enhancing health by promoting general well-being.

Planned Behavior Model. Another model that can guide health protection behaviors is Ajzen's model of planned behavior (Ajzen, 1985), which is an extension of the reasoned action model (Ajzen & Fishbein, 1973). In the planned behavior model, subjective norms or social approval, personal attitudes, and perceived control are central. The basic assumption of this model is that intention or motivation to perform a behavior precedes actual performance. Within this model, subjective norms, which are beliefs about the standards or expectations of others, guide acceptable behavior. These normative beliefs determine whether a behavior is perceived as socially acceptable or not. This social approval dimension of the model is related to the perceived benefits and barriers dimensions of the HBM (Janz & Becker, 1984). The personal dimension of the model is reflected in the attitudes of the individual toward the specific behavior and in perceptions of personal control. These personal factors include whether a favorable attitude exists about a specific behavior achieving a desired outcome, the value of the outcome to the individual, and the perception of ease or difficulty in achieving the desired outcome (Fleury, 1992). Thus, for a woman at risk for osteoporosis, if exercising is perceived as socially acceptable, if it is viewed as an important component of risk reduction, if there is a strong desire to avoid osteoporosis, and if establishing an exercise program seems feasible, then the intention of engaging in regular exercise will be strong. The planned behavior model has been used to explain motivation to lose weight, to exercise, and to adhere to a postmyocardial infarction regimen. However, it does not account for the influence of past experience, habit, and health outcome values on motivation (Fleury, 1992).

Relapse Prevention Model. A third health protection model is the RPM developed by Marlatt and colleagues (Marlatt & Gordon, 1985). This model emphasizes tertiary prevention because it has mainly been applied to addictive behaviors when abstinence is the goal—alcoholism, drug addiction, and nicotine addiction—and to overeating when moderation is the goal. The RPM is a cognitive-behavioral approach aimed at avoiding or ceasing a health-damaging behavior. This model, which draws heavily on self-efficacy theory, predicts the probability of relapse when the person is exposed to a high-risk situation. This model can be used to guide intervention through anticipatory guidance of the client who is attempting to abstain from alcohol, drugs, and nicotine or to moderate food intake. There are three stages involved in preventing relapse: (a) motivation and commitment to change, (b) initial behavior change, and (c) maintenance of change. During the first stage, the clinician helps the client develop methods to enhance motivation and screens the client to identify likelihood of success. During the second stage, when the treatment program is initiated, the RPM includes helping the client to analyze factors that contribute to relapse, to use cognitive restructuring, and to develop coping skills to deal with high-risk situations. Within the third stage, or the maintenance stage, the model includes the need to help the client with self-monitoring; developing social support; and making general lifestyle changes, such as relaxation training and exercise (Brownell, Marlatt, Lichtenstein, & Wilson, 1986).

Most of the studies testing the RPM have included both men and women. In one study about smoking cessation comparing the RPM and traditional contracting and abstinence, women who used the RPM intervention were more successful after 1 year than the women who used the more traditional approach. For men in the study, the findings were the opposite. The men did better with the traditional approach (Curry, Marlatt, Gordon, & Baer, 1988). In one study about gender differences and smoking relapse, women relapsers exhibited more stress and less confidence in their coping abilities than did the men (Abrams et al., 1987). More work is needed to determine whether gender-specific RPMs are needed.

The three health protection models described earlier focus on different aspects of what motivates behavior change that is centered around the prevention, early detection, or treatment of disease. The HBM has the broadest applicability for health protection because it accounts for all three levels of prevention. However, different models are needed to explain motivation to engage in behaviors that are focused on personal growth, self-fulfillment, and quality of living because different motivational mechanisms are involved (Pender, 1987).

Health Promotion Models

Self-Regulation Model. One health promotion model is the SRM, developed by Kanfer (1980) to explain the process by which a person manages his or her own behavior. The SRM model focuses on the influence of the self, with the clinician providing support during the development of needed self-regulation skills. Within this model, self-regulation is influenced by self-monitoring, self-evaluation, and self-reinforcement.

Self-monitoring exists when a person deliberately and carefully pays close attention to his or her own behavior by asking "What am I doing?" Frequently, this is accomplished by some means of observing and recording behavior. Self-evaluation then occurs when the person weighs the behavior against expectations of what should be occurring and finds a discrepancy. The question asked here is, "What should I do?" The third phase, self-reinforcement, occurs when behaviors are initiated to correct any discrepancy between what is happening and what should be happening. Interventions focus on helping a person become more efficient in each of the three stages of the model.

Orem's Self-Care Model. Self-care is a concept that is an important part of nursing intervention and is a major component of both health protection and health promotion. From an intervention perspective, it is helping people help themselves or enhancing the capacity of the client to help him- or herself. The most widely reported model of self-care was developed by Orem (1985). In the Orem model, self-care represents the actions performed by a person to maintain life, health, and well-being. When a health care need is not met (self-care deficit), whether in the areas of basic physiological needs or activities of daily living (universal requisites), growth and development (developmental requisites), or disease/illness (health deviation requisites), nursing intervention is indicated. The type of intervention depends on any difference (self-care deficit) between a specific need of the client (self-care requisite), what is required to meet the need (self-care demand), and the ability of the client to meet that need (self-care agency). When a self-care deficit exists, the clinician (nursing agency) assists the individual with interventions focused on health education, guidance, support, and consultation to help the client to overcome the deficit and actively participate in his or her own care (Orem, 1985).

The self-care model can be used for health protection and health restoration, as well as for health promotion. Most of the research to date based on this model is focused on health protection and health restoration (Chang, Uman, Linn, Ware, & Kane, 1985; Fitzgerald, 1980). More focus is needed to test the model in terms of health promotion self-care behaviors (Hartweg, 1990). It is a model appropriate for health protection when the self-care requisites are within the domain of health deviations and the interventions needed are of a supportive-educational nature. It is appropriate for health restoration when the needs are health deviations, but the interventions indicated are the direct provision of nursing care to the client (compensatory nursing). The self-care model does not account for motivational factors that affect behavior change.

Pender's Health Promotion Model. A model that explains motivation to engage in health-enhancing behavior in a comprehensive way is the HPM, developed by Pender (1987; see Figure 11.3). It is an adaptation of the HBM, incorporating self-efficacy and elements of the planned behavior model and the self-care model. The HPM model explains the likelihood of engaging in behaviors such as regular physical exercise, healthy eating, developing social support, and using relaxation techniques (Pender, 1987). Within the model (see Figure 11.3) the primary motivational mechanisms for acquiring and maintaining health-promoting behaviors are cognitive and perceptual factors. These motivational factors, which directly influence the likelihood of engaging in health-promoting behaviors, are (a) importance of health, (b) perceived control of health, (c) perceived self-efficacy, (d) a personal definition of health, (e) perception of health status, (f) perceived benefits of the health-promoting behavior, and (g) perceived barriers to the health-promoting behavior. These cognitive-perceptual motivational factors can be modified by demographic and biological characteristics, expectations of others, and environmental and behavioral factors, such as availability of alternatives and previously acquired knowledge and experience. Also, affecting the likelihood to act are internal and environmental cues, such as awareness of the potential for growth, advice from others, and mass media materials. The HPM expands on the HBM by incorporating five cognitive and perceptual factors. These additions, the essence of health promotion, are the importance of health, perceived control of health, perceived self-efficacy, definition of health, and perceived health status. The HPM does not include the three disease-oriented factors of the HBM, perceived susceptibility to disease, seriousness of disease, and threat of disease. For this reason, the HPM is truly a model to guide health promotion activities. Research with women to test and refine this model has focused on exercise (Gillis & Perry, 1991), self-actualization, and interpersonal support (Duffy, 1988). Research testing this model has also been done

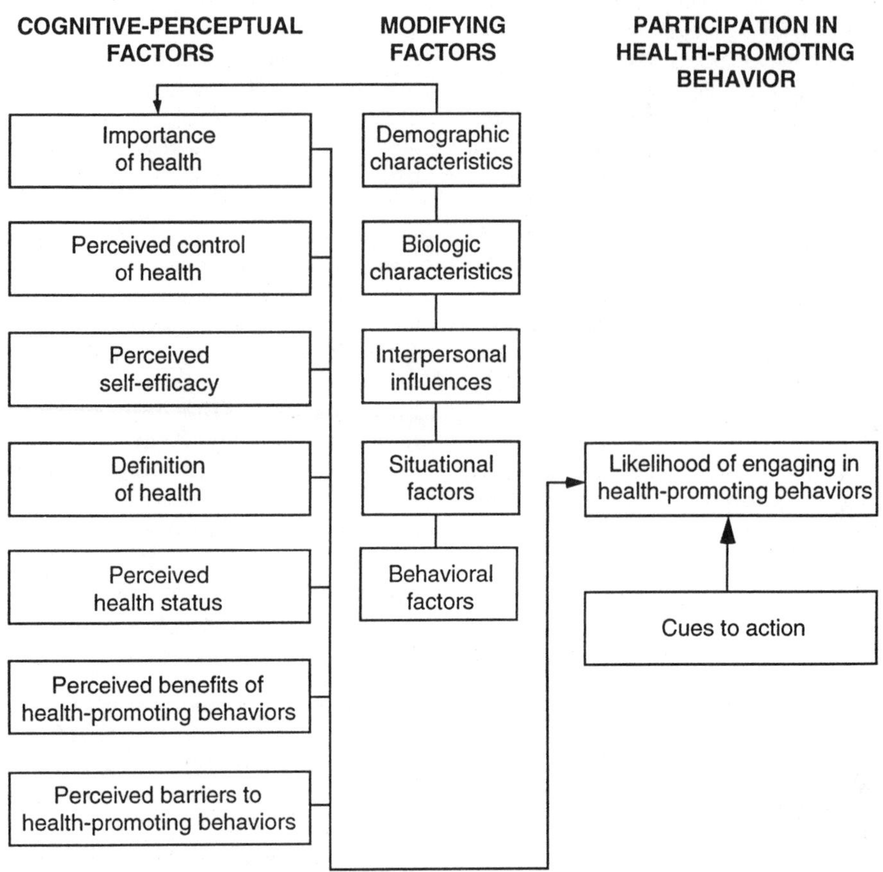

Figure 11.3. Health Promotion Model
SOURCE: Pender, N. J. (1987). *Health Promotion in Nursing Practice* (2nd. ed.). Norwalk, CT: Appleton & Lange. Reprinted with permission.

with men and women to determine predictors of health promotion behaviors (Pender et al., 1990; Weitzel, 1989). Further research is needed to determine if there are gender differences for this model. Data are also needed to identify which health promotion activities the model explains and predicts the best. One of the drawbacks of this model is its complexity. It is very difficult to test the entire model with the number of variables it contains. As further research is conducted, ideally it will be refined, and only the most predictive variables will be retained.

Conclusion

A theoretical framework of health and models of care to guide nursing interventions provides an important foundation for nurse clinicians as providers of health care for women. Through use of these models, the clinician's practice remains grounded in nursing and the integration of practice and research can become a reality. However, in the delivery of care to women, a strong foundation in nursing practice is not enough. The clinician also needs a strong philosophy of health care for *women* on which to build a nursing practice. Women's health care clinicians need to be continually aware of what it means to be a woman from both the social and biological perspective. Valuing a woman for herself, as an equal participant in society and in health care, without applying stereotypes regarding female and male roles or behavior is critical. Also extremely important is maintaining a sensitivity to possible negative consequences of sexism and gender role stereotyping.

This includes alertness for any signs of abuse or violence experienced by the woman such as rape, battering, or harassment, and a sensitivity to excessive demands placed on the woman because she is a woman, whether at home or in the workplace. With a strong philosophy of health, with models of health care to guide practice, and with a sensitive and caring attitude about women, the nurse clinician is equipped to provide high-quality women's health care.

References

Abrams, D. B., Monti, P. M., Pinto, R. P., Elder, J. P., Brown, R. A., & Jacobus, S. I. (1987). Psychosocial stress and coping in smokers who relapse or quit. *Health Psychology, 6,* 289-303.

Ajzen, I. (1985). From intentions to actions: A theory of planned behavior. In J. Kuhl & J. Beckman (Eds.), *Action control: From cognition to behavior* (pp. 11-39). New York: Springer-Verlag.

Ajzen, I., & Fishbein, M. (1973). Attitudinal and normative variables as predictors of specific behaviors. *Journal of Personality and Social Psychology, 27*(1), 41-57.

Ardell, D. (1979). The nature and implications of high-level wellness, or why "normal health" is a rather sorry state of existence. *Health Values: Achieving High Level Wellness, 3*(1), 17-24.

Bandura, A. (1977). Self-efficacy: Toward a unifying theory of behavioral change. *Psychological Review, 84,* 191-215.

Becker, M. H. (1974). *The health belief model and personal health behavior.* Thorofare, NJ: Charles B. Slack.

Brownell, K. D., Marlatt, G. A., Lichtenstein, E., & Wilson, G. T. (1986). Understanding and preventing relapse. *American Psychologist, 41,* 765-782.

Brubaker, B. H. (1983). Health promotion: A linguistic analysis. *Advances in Nursing Science, 5*(3), 1-14.

Chang, B. L., Uman, G. C., Linn, L. S., Ware, J. E., & Kane, R. L. (1985). Adherence to health care regimens among elderly women. *Nursing Research, 34*(1), 27-31.

Christy, T. E. (1970). Portrait of a leader: Lillian D. Wald. *Nursing Outlook, 18*(3), 50-54.

Clark, C. (1986). *Wellness nursing: Concepts, theory, research and practice.* New York: Springer.

Curry, S. J., Marlatt, G. A., Gordon, J., & Baer, J. S. (1988). A comparison of alternative theoretical approaches to smoking cessation and relapse. *Health Psychology, 7,* 545-556.

Denyes, M. J. (1988). Orem's model used for health promotion: Directions from research. *Advances in Nursing Science, 11*(1), 13-21.

Dubos, R. (1965). *Man adapting.* New Haven, CT: Yale University Press.

Duffy, M. E. (1988). Determinant of health promotion in midlife women. *Nursing Research, 37,* 358-362.

Duffy, M. E., & MacDonald, E. (1990). Determinant of functional health of older persons. *The Gerontologist, 30,* 503-509.

Dunn, H. L. (1959). High-level wellness for man and society. *American Journal of Public Health, 49,* 786-792.

Edelman, C. L., & Mandle, C. L. (1990). *Health promotion throughout the life span.* St. Louis: C. V. Mosby.

Fitzgerald, S. (1980). Utilizing Orem's self-care nursing model in designing an educational program for the diabetic. *Topics in Clinical Nursing, 2*(2), 57-65.

Fleury, J. (1992). The application of motivational theory to cardiovascular risk reduction. *Image, 24,* 229-239.

Fulton, J. P., Buechner, J. S., Scott, H. D., DeBuono, B. A., Feldman, J. P., Smith, R. A., & Kovenock, D. (1991). A study guided by the health belief model of the predictors of breast cancer screening of women ages 40 and older. *Public Health Reports, 106,* 410-420.

Gillis, A., & Perry, A. (1991). The relationships between physical activity and health-promoting behaviours in mid-life women. *Journal of Advanced Nursing, 16,* 299-310.

Harper, D. C. (1984). Application of Orem's theoretical constructs to self-care medication behaviors in the elderly. *Advances in Nursing Science, 6*(3), 29-46.

Hartweg, D. L. (1990). Health promotion self-care within Orem's general theory of nursing. *Journal of Advanced Nursing, 15*(1), 35-41.

Hibbard, J. H., & Pope, C. R. (1987). Women's roles, interest in health and health behavior. *Women & Health, 12*(2), 67-102.

Janz, N. K., & Becker, M. H. (1984). The health belief model: A decade later. *Health Education Quarterly, 11*(1), 1-47.

Johnson, J. E., & Lauver, D. R. (1989). Alternative explanations of coping with stressful experiences associated with physical illness. *Advances in Nursing Science, 11*(2), 39-52.

Kanfer, F. H. (1980). Self-management methods. In F. H. Kanfer & A. P. Goldstein (Eds.), *Helping people change* (pp. 334-389). New York: Pergamon.

Lantz, J. M. (1985, July). In search of agents of self-care. *Journal of Gerontological Nursing,* pp. 10-14.

Lashley, M. E. (1987). Predictors of breast self-examination practice among elderly women. *Advances in Nursing Science, 9*(4), 25-34.

Leavell, H. R., & Clark, H. P. (1965). *Preventative medicine for the doctor in his community.* New York: McGraw-Hill.

Marlatt, G. A., & Gordon, J. R. (1985). *Relapse prevention.* New York: Guilford.

Maslow, A. (1970). *Motivation and personality.* New York: Harper & Row.

Nightingale, F. (1969). *Notes on nursing: What it is and what it is not.* New York: Appleton. (Original work published 1860)

Oakley, D., Denyes, M. J., & O'Connor, N. (1989). Expanded nursing care for contraceptive use. *Applied Nursing Research, 2*(3), 121-127.

Oelbaum, C. H. (1974). Hallmarks of adult wellness. *American Journal of Nursing, 74,* 1623-1625.

Orem, D. E. (1985). *Nursing: Concepts of practice.* New York: McGraw Hill.

Parsons, T. (1958). Definitions of health and illness in light of American values and social structure. In E. G. Jaco (Ed.), *Patients, physicians, and illness* (pp. 165-187). New York: Free Press.

Pender, N. J. (1987). *Health promotion in nursing practice.* Norwalk, CT: Appleton & Lange.

Pender, N. J., Walker, S. N., Sechrist, K. R., & Frank-Stromborg, M. (1990). Predicting health-promoting lifestyles in the workplace. *Nursing Research, 39,* 326-332.

Roy, C. (1984). *Introduction to nursing: An adaptation model.* Englewood Cliffs, NJ: Prentice Hall.

Ryan, R. S., & Travis, J. W. (1981). *The wellness workbook.* Berkeley, CA: Ten Speed Press.

Saltzer, E. B. (1981). Cognitive moderators of the relationship between behavioral intentions and behavior. *Journal of Personality and Social Psychology, 41,* 260-271.

Schifter, D. E., & Ajzen, I. (1985). Intention, perceived control, and weight loss: An application of the theory of planned behavior. *Journal of Personality & Social Psychology, 49,* 843-851.

Shaver, J. (1985). A biopsychosocial view of human health. *Nursing Outlook, 33*(4), 186-191.

Smith, J. A. (1981). The idea of health: A philosophical inquiry. *Advances in Nursing Science, 3*(1), 43-50.

Strecher, V. J., DeVellis, B. M., Becker, M. H., & Rosenstock, I. M. (1986). The role of self-efficacy in achieving health behavior change. *Health Education Quarterly, 13*(1), 73-91.

Tripp-Reimer, T. (1984). Reconceptualizing the construct of health: Integrating emic and etic perspectives. *Research in Nursing and Health, 7*(2), 101-109.

U.S. Department of Health and Human Services. (1990). *Healthy people 2000.* Washington, DC: Government Printing Office.

Weitzel, M. H. (1989). A test of the health belief model with blue collar workers. *Nursing Research, 38*(2), 99-104.

Whetstone, W. R., & Reid, J. C. (1991). Health promotion of older adults: Perceived barriers. *Journal of Advanced Nursing, 16,* 1343-1349.

Wiley, J. A., & Camacho, T. C. (1980). Lifestyle and future health: Evidence from the Alameda County study. *Preventive Medicine, 9*(1), 1-21.

Williams, A. B. (1991). Women at risk: An AIDS educational needs assessment. *Image, 23,* 208-213.

Woods, N. F., Laffery, S., Duffy, M., Lentz, M. J., Mitchell, E. S., Taylor, D., & Cowan, K. A. (1988). Being healthy: Women's images. *Advances in Nursing Science, 11*(1), 36-46.

World Health Organization. (1947). *Constitution.* Geneva: Author.

Wu, R. (1973). *Behavior and illness.* Englewood Cliffs, NJ: Prentice Hall.

12

Nutrition

BONNIE WORTHINGTON-ROBERTS

From beginning to end, the life cycle of the woman is a fascinating sequence of events. From the moment of fertilization through the stages of growth, development, maturation, and aging, the interactions between genes and environment determine the details of the process. The importance of the genetic base cannot be ignored, but it is clear that an assortment of environmental factors have the potential of significantly modifying the course of events. This chapter focuses on the contributions that diet and nutrition make to the developmental process and to the prevention and management of selected acute and chronic diseases.

The Nutrients—A Brief Review

Survival requires not only oxygen and water but food as well. Food provides the energy required to support the life-sustaining processes; it also contains the materials needed to build and maintain all body cells. These materials are referred to as *nutrients;* each plays a role in ensuring that the biochemical machinery of the human body runs smoothly.

Nutrients are classified into six categories (see Table 12.1), including the energy-yielding nutrients (carbohydrates, lipids, and proteins), vitamins, minerals, and water. Their basic features include the following:

1. Carbohydrates contain carbon, hydrogen, and oxygen combined in small molecules called sugars and large molecules represented mainly by starch.
2. Lipids (fats and oils) contain carbon, hydrogen, and oxygen, as carbohydrates do, but the amount of oxygen is much less. Triglyceride is the main form of food fat.
3. Proteins contain carbon, hydrogen, nitrogen, oxygen, and sometimes sulfur atoms arranged in small compounds called *amino acids.* Chains of amino acids make up dietary proteins.
4. Vitamins are organic compounds that serve to catalyze or support a number of biochemical reactions in the body.
5. Minerals are inorganic compounds that play important roles in metabolic reactions and

Table 12.1 Essential Nutrients in the Human Diet

Energy Nutrients					
Carbohydrate	*Fat (lipid)*	*Protein (amino acid)*	*Vitamins*	*Minerals*	*Water*
Glucose (or a carbohydrate that yields glucose)	Linoleic acid (omega-6) Linolenic acid (omega-3)	Histidine	A	Arsenic	Water
		Isoleucine	D	Boron	
		Leucine	E	Calcium	
		Lycine	K	Chloride	
		Methionine	Thiamin	Chromium	
		Phenylalanine	Riboflavin	Copper	
		Threonine	Niacin	Cobalt	
		Tryptophan	Pantothenic acid	Fluoride	
		Valine	Biotin	Iron	
			B-6	Magnesium	
			B-12	Manganese	
			Folate	Molybdenum	
			C	Nickel	
				Phosphorus	
				Potassium	
				Selenium	
				Silicon	
				Sodium	
				Sulfur	
				Zinc	

serve as structural compounds of body tissue, such as bone.

6. Water is vital to the body as a solvent and lubricant and as a medium for transporting nutrients and waste.

Nutritional Needs of Women Throughout the Life Cycle

Satisfactory nutrition is required to support normal fertility and reproduction and to reduce risk of developing both acute and chronic diseases. Poor nutrition can shorten the length of a woman's reproductive life span and reduce its efficiency. The undernourished woman will experience menarche later and menopause earlier than a well-nourished women will. She will have a higher frequency of irregular and anovulatory cycles and may stop menstruating completely if undernutrition is severe enough. When pregnant, she has a higher probability of miscarriage or stillbirth. After delivery, lactational amenorrhea may last longer and result in longer birth intervals than those of a well-nourished woman.

Given the influence that adverse nutritional states have on a woman's ability to conceive and bear healthy children, it is crucial that nursing practitioners make interconceptual nutritional teaching a part of established health care for women. Interconceptual care is defined as specific maternal and child health practice that applies the principle of the periodic health examination throughout the entire cycle of human reproduction. It begins with birth and extends through infancy, childhood, adolescence, and young adulthood to conception, then resumes following delivery and continues until the next conception or menopause occurs. The long-term nutritional history of the mother is as important to fetal outcome as diet is during pregnancy.

Infancy and Childhood

The nutritional needs of the infant and child do not differ according to sex. Both sexes need a diet that is nutritionally adequate in all respects to meet their continuing needs for physical growth and development. Nutritional status and food habits developed in infancy and childhood may have far-reaching effects on adult nutritional status and eating patterns. The girl who is overfed as an infant or young child may find she has a problem with obesity throughout her adult life. Malnutrition begun in the early years will affect reproductive ability and outcomes and general health as an adult. Learned behavior about food and eating will affect nutritional status throughout life.

Adolescence

With the onset of adolescence, special dietary considerations emerge. Adolescence is a unique period of change. Increased nutrients are needed to meet accelerated physical growth needs; therefore, increased amounts of food are needed. The adolescent's specific nutritional needs relate directly to the timing and extent of the pubertal growth spurt (see Chapter 3). The character and timing of physical growth and sexual maturation differ greatly from individual to individual; however, in general, linear growth is not complete in the adolescent female until 4 years after menarche.

Generally, the increased energy requirements needed during rapid growth periods are met without concentrated effort on the adolescent's part. Appetite usually increases, and increased food intake is the normal response. One factor that can adversely affect this is the pressure many teenage girls feel to be "fashionably" thin. In an effort to achieve this, many girls severely limit their food consumption to levels far lower than are needed to meet normal growth demands. The long-term effects of caloric restriction by teenage girls are not presently known. It has been hypothesized that effects will be directly related to the time in the growth period when caloric restriction is imposed. If it occurs at the height of the rapid growth period, normal growth of the skeletal system may be compromised and the long bones particularly affected; the dimensions of the pelvic girdle will also be adversely affected. Caloric restriction after the growth spurt will not be as devastating; however, nutritional status may be poor and tolerance to stress and disease lower.

Protein deposition and nitrogen retention are greatest during the period of most active growth in adolescence and slow down as growth slows. Most studies indicate that, generally, protein intake exceeds recommended levels (see Table 12.2). Usually, protein makes up at least 10% of all calories consumed, and, frequently, the proportion is higher. Most adolescent girls prefer protein foods with low caloric intake. Often diets are reasonably high in protein but low in calories so that some dietary protein is used for energy, leaving less for building body tissues. For this reason adolescent girls should be encouraged to choose foods that contain enough energy to allow for an adequate amount of protein for tissue synthesis.

Iron needs for the adolescent girl are large because of the iron necessary for enlarging muscle mass and blood volume. Extra iron is needed to maintain adequate iron stores. Additional stress is placed on the girl by body iron losses during menstruation. The recommended daily allowance (RDA) for adolescent girls and women is 15 mg daily of iron; this amount will allow buildup of sufficient iron stores, although it may be difficult to obtain because dietary sources of iron are limited. Several studies have noted that iron consumption is often less than the RDA; although the incidence of iron deficiency anemia is low, the problem of low iron stores is widespread.

Calcium absorption and retention increase prior to menarche and the growth spurt. This is necessary if adequate mineralization of the skeleton is to take place. Teenage diets frequently appear to be low in calcium. The restricted diets that many adolescent girls eat often contain inadequate amounts of vitamins and trace minerals, particularly vitamin A.

The emotional and psychological growth that takes place during adolescence also influences nutritional status. As she seeks to establish her own identity, the adolescent tests, rejects, and/or accepts her parents' values and beliefs. Dietary habits may be challenged because parents advocate them. Often, teenagers are told to eat something because it is good for them, whether they like it or not. Adolescents usually do not experience the nutritional disaster predicted by their parents if they practice poor food habits. As long as they feel well, they are not concerned about nutrients. Many adolescents have a sense of invulnerability about their bodies; they find it difficult to imagine long-term adverse effects.

Peers and peer activities are essential for adolescents. Often, these activities revolve around fast-food places and result in the ingestion of empty calories, which replace balanced meals. Peer reinforcement of slimness as a valued objective can result in fad diets and severe caloric restrictions. These behaviors are even common among adolescent girls who are not overweight.

Food is only one component of an active life; what teenagers need and will eat is not always

Table 12.2 Recommended Dietary Allowances for Women Through the Life Cycle

Age (years) or Condition	*Energy (kcals)*	*Protein (g)*	*Fat Soluble Vitamins*		*Water Soluble Vitamins*				*Minerals*			
			Vitamin A (μg RE)	*Vitamin D (mg α-TE)*	*Vitamin C (mg)*	*Vitamin B_6 (mg)*	*Folate (μg)*	*Vitamin B_{12} (μg)*	*Calcium (mg)*	*Magnesium (mg)*	*Iron (mg)*	*Zinc (mg)*
11-14	2,200	46	800	10	50	1.4	150	2.0	1,200	280	15	12
15-18	2,200	44	800	10	60	1.5	180	2.0	1,200	300	15	12
19-24	2,200	46	800	10	60	1.6	180	2.0	1,200	280	15	12
25-50	2,200	50	800	5	60	1.6	180	2.0	800	280	15	12
51+	1,900	50	800	5	60	1.6	180	2.0	800	280	10	12
Pregnant	+300	60	800	10	70	2.2	400	2.2	1,200	320	30	15
Lactating	+500	65	1,300	10	95	2.1	280	2.6	1,200	355	15	19

SOURCE: National Research Council (1989).

available at the times and places where they do eat. Irregular eating habits are characteristic of most adolescents. Teenagers tend to eat more than three times a day. Girls appear to eat more often than boys. The obese eat less frequently and tend to skip breakfast. Snacking is a normal pattern of teenagers and should be used in meal planning; typically, at least one fourth of all calories come from snacks.

Young Adulthood (Before Menopause)

Nutritional demands of the young adult woman are less than those of the adolescent due largely to the completion of physical growth (Newman & Lee, 1991). However, maintenance of fertility and general health require continued attention to meeting calorie and nutrient requirements (see Table 12.3). It is well known that women who engage in aggressive weight loss programs may gradually disturb the normal process of ovulation and menstruation. This condition is well known in women who suffer anorexia nervosa, but it is also observed in women following less rigorous weight loss regimens (Stewart, Robinson, Goldbloom, & Wright, 1990; Wynn & Wynn, 1990). Other dietary factors, such as carotene, may be responsible for impaired fertility. High circulating levels of carotene in the blood have been reported to be associated with amenorrhea in women whose diets included many carotene-rich foods. Infertility in European women has been reported among those using tanning pills containing carotene. Reducing the intake of carotene from either source reportedly leads to restoration of normal menstrual patterns. Whether other dietary factors have similar effects is yet to be determined (Reid & VanVugt, 1987).

Recently, interest has emerged in the role that caffeine might play in the promotion of infertility. To date, available data are inconclusive (Joesoef, Beral, Rolfs, Aral, & Cramer, 1990; Wilcox, Weinberg, & Baird, 1988). Wilcox et al. (1988) studied 104 healthy women who for 3 months had been attempting to become pregnant; they were interviewed about their use of caffeinated beverages, alcohol, and cigarettes. In their subsequent cycles, women who consumed more than the equivalent of 1 cup of coffee per day were half as likely to become pregnant as women who drank less; a dose-response effect was apparent. However, Joesoef et al. (1990) examined the association between time to conceive reported by 2,817 women who had recently had a liveborn child and consumption of coffee, tea, and cola drinks. No evidence of an adverse effect of caffeine was found. Clearly this issue is unresolved.

Many questions remain about the relationship of obesity to ovulatory dysfunction (Reid & VanVugt, 1987). The fact that most obese women remain fertile suggests that obesity per se is not the sole explanation for the disordered menstrual function and fertility in some obese women. Current evidence suggests the existence of a more complex pathophysiological mechanism involving changes in sex hormone-binding globulin, altered ovarian and adrenal androgen production, changes in peripheral aromatization of androgens to estrogen, and inappropriate gonadotropin secretion. Weight reduction may improve the endocrine state.

Despite over 50 years of research on the etiology and treatment of premenstrual syndrome (PMS), the underlying mechanisms remain poorly understood (Casey & Dwyer, 1987). Methodological problems have plagued studies, preventing consistency in results of similar treatments. An operational definition of PMS does not exist. Symptomatic women have been studied in treatment trials without regard to their symptom typology. Because it is apparent that different symptoms may have distinct etiologies, this may partially explain why single-focus treatment trials have failed to yield consistent results. Also significant is the unusually high placebo response to interventions, reportedly from 40% to 80%.

Although there are many attractive theories and a multiplicity of nutritional, drug, and psychotherapeutic treatments, evidence that they are effective is weak. There is no proof that PMS is caused by a poor diet or vitamin/mineral deficiency or that it can be prevented or cured by dietary therapy (Casey & Dwyer, 1987). Although limited evidence suggests that moderate doses (50 mg/day) of vitamin B_6 may reduce emotional symptoms (depression, irritability, tiredness) (Doll, Brown, Thurston, & Vessey, 1989), confirmation of this finding is required. In any case, megadoses of vitamin/mineral supplements should be avoided. The best advice for women is to follow these dietary guidelines for Americans (U.S. Department of Agriculture, 1990):

- Eat a variety of foods.
- Maintain a healthy weight.

Table 12.3 Daily Food Guide for Women

			Recommended Minimum Servings		
			Nonpregnant		Pregnant/
Food Group	*One Serving Equals*		*11-24 years*	*25+ years*	*Lactating*
Protein foods Provide protein, iron, zinc, and B vitamins for growth of muscles, bone, blood, and nerves. Vegetable protein provides fiber to prevent constipation.	*Animal protein* 1 oz. cooked chicken or turkey 1 oz. cooked lean beef, lamb, or pork 1 oz. or ¼ cup fish or other seafood 1 egg 2 fish sticks or hot dogs 2 slices luncheon meat	*Vegetable protein* ½ cup cooked dry beans, lentils, or split peas 3 oz. tofu 1 oz. or ¼ cup peanuts, pumpkin seeds, or sunflower seeds 1 ½ oz. or ⅓ cup other nuts 2 tbsp. peanut butter	5 A half serving of vegetable protein daily	5	7 One serving of vegetable protein daily
Milk products Provide protein and calcium to build strong bones, teeth, healthy nerves, and muscles, and to promote normal blood clotting.	8 oz. milk 8 oz. yogurt 1 cup milk shake 1½ cups cream soup (made with milk) 1 ½ oz. or ½ cup grated cheese (cheddar, Monterey Jack, mozzarella, or Swiss)	1½-2 slices presliced American cheese 4 tbsp. parmesan cheese 2 cups cottage cheese 1 cup pudding 1 cup custard or flan 1 ½ cups ice milk, ice cream, or frozen yogurt	3	2	3
Breads, cereals, grains Provide carbohydrates and 8 vitamins for energy and healthy nerves. Also provide iron for healthy blood. Whole grains provide fiber to prevent constipation.	1 slice bread 1 dinner roll ½ bun or bagel ½ English muffin or pita 1 small tortilla ¾ cup dry cereal ½ cup granola ½ cup cooked cereal	½ cup rice ½ cup noodles or spaghetti ¼ cup wheat germ 1 4-inch pancake or waffle 1 small muffin 8 medium crackers 4 graham cracker squares 3 cups popcorn	7 Four servings of whole-grain products daily	6	7
Vitamin C-rich fruits and vegetables Provide vitamin C to prevent infection and to promote healing and iron absorption. Also provide fiber to prevent constipation.	6 oz. orange, grapefruit, or fruit juice enriched with vitamin C 6 oz. tomato juice or vegetable juice cocktail 1 orange, kiwi, or mango ½ grapefruit, cantaloupe ½ cup papaya 2 tangerines	½ cup strawberries ½ cup cooked or 1 cup raw cabbage ½ cup broccoli, brussels sprouts, or cauliflower ½ cup snow peas, sweet pepper, or tomato puree 2 tomatoes	1	1	1

(continued)

- Choose a diet low in fat, saturated fat, and cholesterol.
- Choose a diet with plenty of vegetables, fruits, and grain products.
- Use sugar in moderation.
- Use salt and sodium only in moderation.
- If you drink alcoholic beverages, do so in moderation.

Table 12.3 Daily Food Guide for Women—Continued

Food Group	*One Serving Equals*		*Recommended Minimum Servings* — *Nonpregnant* *11-24 years*	*25+ years*	*Pregnant/ Lactating*
Vitamin A-rich fruits and vegetables Provide beta-carotene and vitamin A to prevent infection and to promote wound healing and night vision. Also provide fiber to prevent constipation.	6 oz. apricot nectar or vegetable juice cocktail 3 raw or ¼ cup dried apricots ¼ cantaloupe or mango 1 small or ½ cup sliced carrots 2 tomatoes	½ cup cooked or 1 cup raw kale ½ cup cooked greens ½ cup pumpkin, sweet potato, winter squash, or yams	1	1	1
Other fruits and vegetables Provide carbohydrates for energy and fiber to prevent constipation.	6 oz. fruit juice (if not listed above) 1 medium or ½ cup sliced fruit (apple, banana, peach, pear) ½ cup berries (other than strawberries) ½ cup cherries or grapes ½ cup pineapple ½ cup watermelon	¼ cup dried fruit ½ cup sliced vegetable (asparagus, beets, green beans, celery, corn, eggplant, mushrooms, onion, peas, potato, summer squash, zucchini) ½ artichoke 1 cup romaine	3	3	3
Unsaturated fats Provide vitamin E to protect tissue.	½ med. avocado 1 tsp. margarine 1 tsp. mayonnaise 1 tsp. vegetable oil	2 tsp. salad dressing (mayonnaise-based) 1 tbsp. salad dressing (oil-based)	3	3	3

SOURCE: Adapted from Maternal and Child Health Branch, Department of Health Services (1991).

Women should also participate in regular exercise and enjoy daily periods of relaxation and stress reduction. Perhaps during the next decade the complex hormonal relationships associated with this "popular" syndrome will be better understood.

Besides fertility and PMS, nutrition-related issues of relevance to premenopausal women include pregnancy, lactation, weight control, eating disorders, and the prevention of disease. Pregnancy, lactation, weight control, and eating disorders will be addressed in detail later in this chapter. Several aspects of disease prevention are discussed here.

Bone Health. Many questions remain to be answered about the relative importance of specific nutrients in achieving peak bone mass and reducing risk of developing osteoporosis (Anderson, 1990; Cauley et al., 1988; Holbrook, Barrett-Connor, & Wingard, 1988; Smith, Gilligan, Smith, & Sempos, 1989). Important questions include the following: (a) What daily level of calcium intake is associated with the achievement of maximum augmentation in bone density? (b) At approximately what age is peak bone density achieved? (c) What is the relative importance of weight-bearing exercise in the development of peak bone mass and in retarding the normal process of bone resorption later in life? (d) What is the relative importance of vitamin D in optimizing bone development in the young adult years? (e) How significant is the level of protein in positively or negatively affecting bone health? and (f) Is caffeine or any other dietary constituent detrimental to the development of peak bone mass or the maintenance of bone later in life?

Evidence does exist for a strong hereditary role in the development of bone mass in women, independent of the consumption patterns of calcium and other nutrients (Lutz & Tesar, 1990; Pollitzer & Anderson, 1989; Seeman et al., 1989). It appears that dietary factors, physical activity, and hormonal determinants can modulate or fine-tune the genetically predetermined quantity, size, and shape of bone. Only with relatively recent noninvasive measurement techniques has it been possible to begin to assess the relative influences of hereditary versus environmental factors. The next decade should yield an abundance of new information about the interactions of these many factors in bone development and the maintenance of bone health. In the meantime, a strong case can be made for counseling women to select food rich in calcium and vitamin D. Avoiding excessive use of alcoholic beverages also is well advised because alcohol has been clearly shown to interfere with the bone-remodeling process.

Breast Cancer. The alarming increase in the incidence of breast cancer in many countries has intensified interest in discovering preventive strategies (International Agency for Research on Cancer, 1987). Considerable effort has been made to explore the potential danger or value of specific dietary components. Today, results are sufficiently inconsistent to propose dietary or supplementation strategies for breast cancer risk reduction. However, because both animal studies and descriptive epidemiological investigations support an association between increased dietary fat intake and increased risk of breast cancer, some public health spokesmen have urged high-risk women to moderate their intake of fat (Buell, 1973; Carroll, 1986; Goodwin & Boyd, 1987; Hirayama, 1978; Howe et al., 1990; Jones et al., 1987; Kelsey & Berkowitz, 1988; Prentice et al., 1989; Rohan & Bain, 1987; Willett et al., 1987). Although the last word is certainly not in on the merits of this dietary focus for cancer prevention, its potential value for reduction in cardiovascular disease risk and obesity is worth keeping in mind. Overall emphasis on complex carbohydrates and de-emphasis on dietary fats is a justifiable dietary guideline for women of reproductive age.

Cardiovascular Disease. Heart disease is the second leading cause of death for women by the age of 40; it is the leading cause of death by the age of 67. Although much research has focused on the value of diet and/or drug intervention for cholesterol lowering in men, very little attention to the merits of these approaches has been given to women. As of the early 1990s, substantial U.S. federal dollars have been allocated to this cause. In the meantime, because moderation in the intake of fat makes sense for a variety of reasons, this effort seems reasonable until additional research data are available.

Pregnancy

Today, maternal nutrition is considered critically important to both mother and fetus. The risks for preterm and growth-retarded infants are so well documented that low birth weight in itself is considered an unfavorable outcome of pregnancy. It has been estimated that between 10% and 20% of all low-birth-weight infants are the result of intrauterine growth retardation—that is, the infant experienced malnutrition in utero. Fetal malnutrition is defined as a reduction in maternal supply or placental transport of nutrients so that fetal growth is significantly restricted. A number of factors influence fetal growth; maternal malnutrition is but one of these, however crucial.

The timing and duration of nutritional restriction are significant. During the embryonic stage of fetal development, cells differentiate into three germinal layers. Growth during this time occurs only by an increase in the number of cells. The fetal stage is the time of most rapid growth. During this time, growth is almost continuous and is accompanied by increase in cell size. Most organ cells continue to proliferate after birth. It is thought that growth in cell size begins at around 7 months gestation and can continue for 3 years after birth. Given this sequence of growth, it is possible to suggest the effects malnutrition might have at different stages of gestation. During the embryonic phase, a severe limitation in nutrients could have teratogenic effects, causing malformation or death. Although malnutrition occurring after the third month of gestation would not generally have teratogenic effects, it could cause fetal growth retardation. During the last trimester, nutritional needs are at a peak as cells increase in both size and number. Poor nutrition in the latter stages of pregnancy affects fetal growth, whereas malnutrition in the early months affects embryonic development and survival.

In addition to the relationship between nutritional status and fetal outcomes of pregnancy, nutritional status has an effect on maternal well-being. Nurses need to know specific nutritional requirements of pregnancy so that they can advise clients to meet their nutritional needs (see Table 12.3).

Table 12.4 Estimated Components of Weight Gain During Pregnancy (in pounds)

Infant at birth	7 ¾
Placenta	1 ½
Increased maternal blood volume	6
Increased maternal tissue fluid	3
Increased size of maternal uterus	2
Increased size of maternal breasts	3
Fluid to surround infant in amniotic sac	2
Mother's fat stores	4 ¾
Total	30

Table 12.5 Recommended Total Weight Gain Ranges for Pregnant Women,[a] by Prepregnancy Body Mass Index (BMI; weight/height[b])

	Recommended Total Gain	
Weight-for-Height Category	*kg*	*lb*
Low (BMI < 19.8)	12.5-18	28-40
Normal (BMI of 19.8-26.0)	11.5-16	25-35
High[c] (BMI > 26.0-29.0)	7-11.5	15-25

SOURCE: Institute of Medicine (1990).
a. Young adolescents and black women should strive for gains at the upper end of the recommended range. Short women (< 157 cm or 62 in.) should strive for gains at the lower end of the range.
b. Body mass index (BMI) is calculated using metric units wt·kg/m^2.
c. The recommended target weight gain for obese women (BMI > 29.0) is at least 6.0 kg (15 lb).

Weight Gain During Pregnancy

There is general agreement that the optimal weight gain in pregnancy follows a pattern, showing little gain in the first trimester, a rapid increase in the second, and some slowing in rate of increase in the third. Most of the weight gain associated with the products of conception takes place in the second half of pregnancy, while maternal stores are laid down very rapidly before midpregnancy, then slow down and appear to stop before term. By the time of delivery, the weight gain can be accounted for in the fetus, placenta, amniotic fluid, maternal blood, maternal extracellular fluid, maternal breast and uterus, and maternal fat (see Table 12.4). The latter represents an emergency energy reserve to be drawn on in case of food deprivation during either pregnancy or lactation.

Monitoring weight gain during the course of pregnancy serves to estimate the adequacy of pregnancy progress, including dietary sufficiency. Review of new information about weight gain associated with optimum pregnancy outcome has yielded a set of guidelines for subgroups of American women (see Table 12.5) (Institute of Medicine, 1990). The recommendation for women of normal body weight for height (greater than 62 in) is 25 to 35 pounds; other specific recommendations have been developed for women who are underweight, overweight, short, and of very young age. Several newly designed weight gain charts for clinical use with pregnant women have become available (see Figure 12.1). Each of these charts is considered useful as a monitoring tool but none is based on longitudinal evaluation of a large group of pregnant women.

The client who enters pregnancy significantly under- or overweight is at risk. Prepregnant weight and pregnancy weight gain exert independent and additive influences on birth weight. The importance of adequate nutrition before conception and during pregnancy has already been established. Deviations in weight gain are common problems in obstetric practice. The following definitions have been suggested:

Underweight—prepregnant weight of 10% or more below standard weight for height and age

Overweight—prepregnant weight of 20% or more above standard weight for height and age

Extremely overweight (obese)—prepregnant weight of 35% or more above standard weight for height and age

Inadequate gain—less than 2.2 lbs per month in second and/or third trimester

Excessive gain—more than 7 lbs gained in 1 month

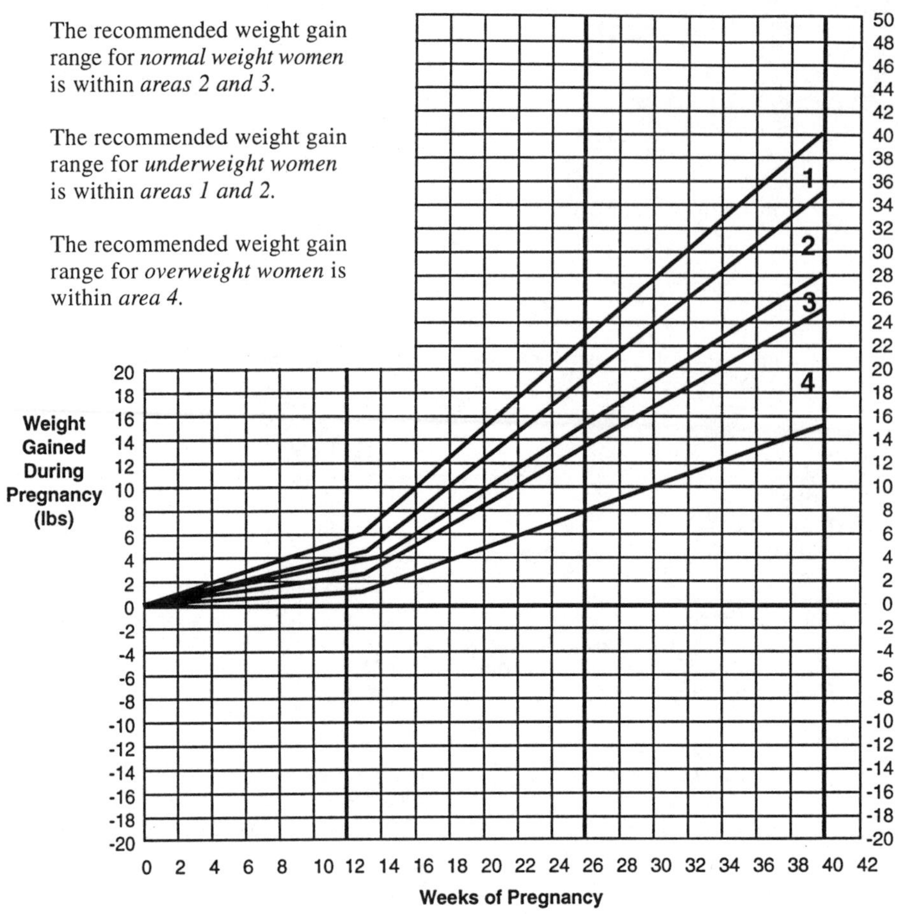

Figure 12.1. A "Modern" Weight Gain Chart for Pregnant Women[a]
SOURCE: *Great Beginnings*. Courtesy of NATIONAL DAIRY COUNCIL.®
a. Based on the 1990 recommendations from the National Academy of Sciences.

The obese pregnant client is at increased risk for several complications. If a women is obese, the chance of her having hypertension of pregnancy is increased severalfold. She is also at greater risk for diabetes during pregnancy. Obesity probably increases her chance of pyelonephritis and breech presentation. In the primigravida, obesity appears to increase the risk of dystocia and cesarean section; these risks are not increased in the multigravida.

In the past, caloric restriction has been advocated for the obese pregnant client, to hold weight constant or even lose weight during pregnancy. The pregnant woman may see pregnancy as a time to get rid of excess pounds. This is no longer considered advisable in any circumstances.

Weight loss or no weight gain during pregnancy brings serious risks. Insufficient intake of nutrients at crucial developmental stages may result in infants with a defect or low birth weight. Marked caloric restriction, even if adequate protein is provided, may result in use of protein for energy, making it unavailable for tissue growth and repair and fetal needs. In addition, when maternal intake is severely restricted, maternal fat stores are catabolized to meet energy requirements, resulting in ketosis and ketonuria. Maternal ketonuria may be associated with neurological damage to the fetus. Pregnancy should never be viewed as a convenient or easy time to correct maternal obesity.

Table 12.6 Sample Menus for Pregnant or Lactating Females—"Best" Choices

Meal	*Day 1*	*Day 2*
Breakfast	1 cup oatmeal ⅛ cup raisins 12 oz. nonfat milk	1 sl. whole wheat toast 1 tsp. margarine ¾ cup shredded wheat 12 oz. nonfat milk ½ cup strawberries, raw
Snack	6 oz. fresh orange juice	3 cups popcorn, plain
Lunch	Chili made from 3 oz. lean ground round ½ cup kidney beans, cooked ¼ cup onions, cooked 2 sl. whole wheat bread 1 cup romaine lettuce 1 tbsp. Italian dressing	¾ cup corn chowder 1 sl. whole-grain rye bread 2 oz. lean roast beef
Snack	½ cup prunes, cooked	
Dinner	3 oz. turkey, dark meat 1 cup brown rice, cooked ½ tsp. margarine ½ cup peas, frozen ½ cup spinach, fresh cooked ½ tsp. olive oil plus garlic powder (on spinach) 1 whole wheat roll 1 tsp. margarine	4 oz. white fish, cooked 2 whole wheat rolls 1 tsp. margarine ½ cup beet greens, fresh cooked 1 cup cabbage, raw, shredded 2 tsp. salad dressing (mayonnaise-type)
Snack	12 oz. nonfat milk	¾ cup corn flakes

SOURCE: Adapted from Maternal and Child Health Branch, Department of Health Services (1991).

The undernourished woman begins her pregnancy with inadequate stores to meet the increased nutritional demands. The additional metabolic needs of pregnancy, nausea and vomiting in early pregnancy, and the psychological adjustments to pregnancy may all compound the problem. The principal hazard is delivery of a low-birth-weight infant. The underweight category includes those women who seem uninterested in food and those who do not understand the link between food and health. The underweight woman should be considered at high risk and encouraged to gain as much as she can within reasonable limits.

There appears to be a relationship between excessive weight gain in pregnancy and subsequent obesity. This is significant, given that obesity is a common, serious condition in American women. It is likely that some women become obese because excessive fat is laid down during pregnancy and is not lost between pregnancies; there is an additive effect in successive pregnancies. Gestational obesity often results from misguided eating habits, "eating for two," and cravings. For this reason it may be sensible to limit weight gain to some degree. However, severe caloric restrictions or fad diets are not indicated; rather, a diet soundly based on the basic food groups and relatively free of empty calories is needed (see Table 12.6).

Calories

Growth is a process that requires energy. Therefore, additional calories, above those required for maintenance, are needed during periods of growth. Table 12.2 gives the recommended dietary allowances for calories that provide optimal weight gain at various ages; meet growth needs of the fetus, placenta, and associated maternal tissues; and take care of the increased maternal basal metabolism. Caloric needs may often be partially offset by decreased activity. Calories are essential in protecting protein. If caloric intake is not adequate for energy needs, protein will be used for energy and thus be unavailable for growth.

Caloric restriction in pregnancy is a firmly rooted dictum not based on scientific fact. Earlier, it was thought that dietary restrictions limiting caloric intake would help prevent maternal complications. Numerous studies of experimental animals subjected to dietary restrictions during pregnancy have demonstrated profound negative effects on maternal physiological adjustments and fetal growth and development.

Protein

Protein needs are increased in pregnancy. Protein is essential for synthesis of hemoglobin and provides the nitrogen and amino acids essential for forming body tissue. Protein intake should be increased from about 46 to 50 gm to 60 gm per day in pregnancy. The pregnant adolescent often needs even more protein to sustain her during a period of rapid growth for herself as well as her fetus.

Sodium

The restriction of sodium in the pregnant woman's diet was standard practice for decades. It has been recognized, however, that the healthy pregnant woman retains salt normally and to restrict her salt intake may be dangerous. There is a positive sodium balance in normal pregnancy, resulting from significant changes in renal and hormonal function. The glomerular filtration rate increases by 50% in early pregnancy and remains elevated until late in the third trimester, filtering sodium into the renal tubules. At the same time progesterone exerts a salt-losing action in the kidneys, retarding absorption of filtered sodium through the renal tubules.

In the absence of some compensatory mechanism, electrolyte imbalance can occur. The renin-angiotensin-aldosterone system acts as a compensatory mechanism in normal pregnancy. Renin, a proteolytic enzyme of the kidneys that acts on circulating plasma renin substrate, causes the release of angiotensin. Angiotensin, in turn, stimulates the adrenal cortex to secrete aldosterone, which counterbalances the salt-losing tendencies of progesterone. Urinary excretion of dietary sodium is decreased as a result of increased renin and aldosterone secretion.

Sodium is conserved to meet the additional amounts needed for expanded tissue and fluid compartments. Therefore, sodium retention is an expected component of normal pregnancy. To maintain fluid balance and osmotic integrity when sodium is retained, water must be retained as well. This retained water will contribute significantly to weight gain. Salt-restricted diets used to be routinely prescribed to prevent or treat what is now thought to be a normal physiological component of pregnancy. It appears that rigorous sodium restriction so severely stresses the physiological mechanism of sodium conservation that it causes the system to break down; then blood volume cannot be expanded and hyponatremia develops in fluid and tissues.

Iron and Folic Acid

Pregnancy imposes a severe burden on the maternal hematopoietic system. Normal hematopoiesis requires a nutritionally adequate diet. Hemoglobin is a complex molecule of protein and iron. To produce it, there must be protein to provide essential amino acids and sufficient additional iron. Various vitamins and minerals, such as copper, zinc, folic acid, and vitamin B_{12}, are needed to serve as cofactors in synthesis of heme and globin. The limiting factor in the synthesis of hemoglobin is usually the availability of iron.

The requirement for iron during pregnancy is less than 1 gm (see Table 12.7); fetal needs are approximately 300 mg at term, and the iron lost at delivery through the placenta, umbilical cord, and maternal blood account for another 100 to 500 mg. Dietary iron intake provides only slightly more than the amounts lost through stool, urine, and skin. The average healthy young American woman has approximately 300 mg of iron stores. A significant proportion of women enter pregnancy with minimal iron stores, usually because of menstrual blood loss or previous pregnancy. Because the demand for iron during pregnancy is sizable and many women begin pregnancy with limited iron stores, it is currently recommended that all pregnant women take a low-level iron supplement, especially during the latter half of pregnancy; 30 mg of elemental ferrous iron is recommended daily (Institute of Medicine, 1990).

Anemia is a relatively common complication of pregnancy because the small amounts of usable dietary iron ingested combined with low iron storage cannot meet the increased need for iron. Anemia is defined as a hemoglobin lower than 11 gm/100 ml during the 1st and 3rd tri-

Table 12.7 Iron "Cost" of a Normal Pregnancy

Iron contributed to the fetus	200-370 mg
Iron in placenta and cord	30-170 mg
Iron in blood lost at delivery	90-310 mg
Total	320-850 mg[a]

SOURCE: Adapted from Bothwell, Charlton, Cook, and Finch (1979).
These figures are in addition to the normal excretory loss of 0.5 to 1.0 mg/day and ignore the demand during the second half of pregnancy for iron to support the expansion of red blood cell mass. This latter amount (200-600 mg) is not included as an iron "cost" because it is largely conserved (and not lost from the body) when the red blood cell mass returns to normal after delivery.

mesters and less than 10.5 gm/100 ml during the 2nd trimester. For women who are anemic according to the definition that follows, supplemental iron should be given in therapeutic doses of a total of 60 to 120 mg per day, in divided doses, along with 300 μg foliate daily. The National Academy of Sciences Committee on Nutrition in Pregnancy and Lactation (Institute of Medicine, 1990) also suggests that when therapeutic levels (> 60 mg/day) of iron are given, supplementation with 10 mg of zinc and 1 mg of copper is desirable. The effectiveness of this therapy should be monitored at subsequent prenatal visits. If anemia persists after treatment, inquiries should be made about compliance with iron supplementation, and there should be further laboratory evaluation. If anemia is reversed, iron administration at a lower dose of 30 mg daily can be resumed.

Excessive iron supplementation should be avoided for several reasons. First, supplemental iron is known to be associated with gastrointestinal discomfort in a number of individuals. Second, iron is known to inhibit zinc absorption if consumed at a ratio higher than 2:1. In a Colorado study (Hambidge, Krebs, Sibley, & English, 1987), women taking daily supplements of 150 mg or more of iron had plasma zinc levels significantly lower than those of women taking smaller amounts of iron.

Other Minerals

Increased calcium is needed during pregnancy for fetal bone development; calcium deposition in fetal bones and teeth is most active during the last trimester. At birth, the infant has accumulated approximately 25 grams. The current RDA for calcium during pregnancy is 1,200 mg—a level 400 mg higher than that recommended for the mature nonpregnant woman. The degree to which the maternal skeleton suffers from demineralization if calcium consumption is low is largely unknown because extensive adjustments in calcium metabolism routinely occur during pregnancy. At this point, it is purely speculative to propose that osteoporosis in later life is associated with reproduction in the face of suboptimal dietary calcium.

Whether or not calcium status is etiologically related to the development of pregnancy-induced hypertension is currently the subject of much debate. Several studies have been conducted to determine if calcium supplementation reduces the incidence of this problem. Results to date suggest beneficial effects from calcium supplementation. A large, multicenter trial is scheduled in the United States to further explore the role that calcium might play in this mysterious prenatal condition.

Although available data are insufficient to support routine calcium supplementation for the prevention of osteoporosis, prenatal nutrition counseling should certainly address dietary strategies to meet calcium needs. Dairy products obviously represent a major source of dietary calcium, but a variety of other nondairy sources can make significant contributions. In situations in which milk intolerance severely limits intake of dairy products, consideration should be given to the prescription of a calcium supplement. This is particularly important for women under 25 years of age whose dietary calcium intake is less than 600 mg per day. In such cases, a supplement of about 600 mg daily is appropriate (Institute of Medicine, 1990).

Although data from animal models convincingly show that maternal zinc deficiency is associated with abnormal fetal development and prolonged labor, epidemiological and clinical reports involving pregnant women are less convincing. Even still, such reports do exist (Hambidge, Neider, & Walravens, 1975; Jameson,

Table 12.8 Relationship Between Plasma Zinc and Antenatal and Intrapartum Complications

	Plasma Zinc		
	Low (n = 144) (%)	*High (n = 135) (%)*	*p Value (%)*
Mild toxemia	5.6	0.7	0.02
Vaginitis	12.6	4.4	0.01
Postterm > 42 weeks	4.2	0	0.01
Prolonged latent phase	2.8	0	0.05
Protracted active phase	28.7	18.2	0.04
Labor > 20 hours	6.3	1.5	0.03
Second stage > 2.5 hours	6.3	0.7	0.01
Lacerations > 3rd degree	7.0	1.5	0.02

SOURCE: Adapted from Lazebnik, Kuhnert, Kuhnert, and Thompson (1988).

1976; Soltan & Jenkins, 1982). Recently, zinc status was evaluated in 279 pregnant women at delivery and subsequently compared with the incidence of complications during the antenatal period and major dysfunctional labor patterns (see Table 12.8). Low levels of plasma zinc were associated with more complications in the prenatal and intrapartum periods. The authors suggest that suboptimum zinc nutrition or abnormal zinc absorption/metabolism may directly affect pregnancy course and outcome (Lazebnik, Kuhnert, Kuhnert, & Thompson, 1988).

Several efforts have been made to examine the impact of zinc supplementation on the course and outcome of human pregnancy. Low-income Mexican American women supplemented with 20 mg of zinc daily had a lower incidence of pregnancy-induced hypertension than did unsupplemented women; no difference in other complications was associated with zinc supplementation (Hunt et al., 1984). Seven Scandinavian women (Jameson, 1981) with low serum zinc concentrations were supplemented with zinc (90 mg daily) during the latter 6 to 16 weeks of pregnancy. At delivery, these women had shorter labors and less blood loss than did 13 similar unsupplemented women, 6 of whom experienced severe hemorrhage with uterine atony. In a further study, half of the women with serum zinc concentrations less than the mean 65 μg/dl at week 14 of pregnancy were given 45 mg of zinc daily. Of 69 unsupplemented women, 33 had normal deliveries compared with 40 of 64 supplemented women. Normal pregnancy outcomes resulted from only 26% of the pregnancies in which serum zinc at week 14 was less than the mean and declined thereafter (Jameson, 1981). Even though these observations are interesting and suggest that continued attention to the role of zinc in the reproductive process is justified, routine prescription of zinc supplements for pregnant women has not been proposed by any recognized professional committee or government agency.

Iodine is an essential component of the thyroid hormones and is an essential nutrient for women. The need can easily be met by using iodized salt. Various other minerals, such as copper and magnesium, have been found to be essential.

Folic Acid

Folic acid requirements are increased during pregnancy because of augmented maternal erythropoiesis and fetal and placental growth. Folic acid is an essential coenzyme in purine and pyrimidine metabolism and in DNA synthesis. Megaloblastic anemia, the principal effect of folic acid deficiency, is not as common as iron deficiency anemia, but it does occur in high-risk clients, such as those of low socioeconomic status and those with a multiple pregnancy or chronic hemolytic anemia.

Although folic acid supplementation is deemed unnecessary as a routine, it should be considered when dietary intake is low or when the woman has chronic hemolytic anemia, has a multiple pregnancy, or is on anticonvulsant medication. The recommended level of supplementation is 300 μg daily (Institute of Medicine, 1990).

The role of folic acid deficiency (or deficiency of some other vitamin) in the etiology of neural tube defects is presently a subject of considerable research focus. Smithells et al. (1980, 1981, 1983), Sheppard et al. (1989), and Laurence, James, Miller, Tennant, and Campbell

(1981) in Northern Europe have suggested that periconceptional multivitamin or folic acid supplementation of women with previous neural tube defect offspring is associated with significant reduction in recurrence of the problem. In the Smithells et al. studies, women who had previously given birth to an infant with a neural tube defect were provided an iron and multivitamin supplement (with folic acid) and directed to take it three times daily for no fewer than 28 days prior to conception, until the second missed menstrual period. The control group did not follow this protocol; these women either declined to participate in the study or were already pregnant. Significantly more infants with neural tube defects were produced by the controls.

Research in the United States has yielded conflicting results. Mulinare, Cordero, Erickson, and Berry (1988) completed a retrospective project using data from the Atlanta Birth Defects Case Control Study. Periconceptional multivitamin use was assessed in mothers of babies with neural tube defects and in mothers of control infants; an apparent protective effect of periconceptional multivitamin use was reported. Similarly, Milunsky et al. (1989) examined the relation of multivitamin intake in general, and folic acid in particular, to the risk of neural tube defects in 23,491 women cohorts undergoing maternal serum alpha-fetoprotein screening or amniocentesis around 16 weeks of gestation. The prevalence of neural tube defect was 3.5 per 1,000 among women who never used multivitamins before and after conception or who used multivitamins before conception only. The prevalence of neural tube defect for women who used folic acid-containing multivitamins during the first 6 weeks of pregnancy was substantially lower—0.9 per 1,000. For women who used multivitamins without folic acid during the first 6 weeks of pregnancy and women who used multivitamins containing folic acid beginning at 7 or more weeks of pregnancy, the prevalences were similar to that of the nonusers, and the prevalence ratios were close to 1.0. However, Mills et al. (1989) conducted a similar study involving women from Illinois and California. In this study, periconceptional use of multivitamins or folate-containing supplements was not associated with a decreased risk of having an infant with a neural tube defect. A randomized controlled supplementation trial currently underway in Northern Europe may clarify the role of vitamin deficiency in the etiology of neural tube defects (Wald, 1984).

Because the relationship between folic acid deficiency and neural tube defects is still unclear, routine recommendation of folic acid supplementation for prevention of these congenital malformations is unjustified. However, as mentioned before, women whose folic acid status is suspect are good candidates for folate supplements (300 μg/day). In addition, some clinicians feel that women who have delivered infants with neural tube defects previously (or have had prenatal diagnosis of these malformations) should be told that folic acid supplementation *might* reduce their risk of recurrence in subsequent pregnancies if the supplement is taken in the periconceptional period.

Vitamin A

Excessive consumption of vitamin A appears to be teratogenic. At least seven case reports of adverse pregnancy outcome have been associated with a daily ingestion of 25,000 international units (IUs) or more (Rosa et al., 1986). These data derive from 11 adverse drug reaction reports associated with the use of vitamin A during pregnancy that were filed with the Food and Drug Administration (FDA). Almost all of the FDA cases are brief retrospective reports of malformed infants or fetuses exposed to supplements of at least 25,000 IUs per day of vitamin A during pregnancy. In addition, epidemiological evidence indicates that the drug isotretinoin (used for treatment of cystic acne) causes major malformations involving craniofacial, central nervous system, cardiac, and thymic changes (Benke, 1984; Lammer et al., 1985); isotretinoin is a vitamin A analogue. The Teratology Society (1987) urges that women in their reproductive years be informed that the excessive use of vitamin A shortly before and during pregnancy could be harmful to their babies. This group also suggests that manufacturers of vitamin A-containing supplements should lower the maximum amount of vitamin A per unit dosage to 5,000 to 8,000 IU and identify the source of vitamin A to indicate that consumption of excessive amounts of vitamin A may be hazardous to the embryo or fetus when taken during pregnancy and that women of childbearing age should consult their physicians before consuming these products.

Table 12.9 Current Supplementation Recommendations for Pregnant Women From the National Academy of Sciences, 1990

Nutrient	*Candidates for Supplementation*	*Levels of Nutrient Supplementation*
Iron	All pregnant women (2nd and 3rd trimesters)	30 mg ferrous iron daily
Folic acid	Pregnant women with suspected dietary inadequacy of folate	300 μg/day
Vitamin D	Pure vegetarians and others with low intake of vitamin D-fortified milk	10 μg/day
Calcium	Women under age 25 whose daily dietary calcium intake is less than 600 mg	600 mg/day
Vitamin B_{12}	Complete vegetarians	2 μg/day
Zinc/copper	Women under treatment with iron for iron deficiency anemia	15 mg Zn/day
Multivitamin-mineral supplements	Pregnant women with poor diets who are considered high risk: multiple gestations, heavy smokers, alcohol/drug abusers, others	Preparation containing iron—30 mg zinc—15 mg copper—2 mg calcium—250 mg vitamin B_6—2 mg folate—300 μg vitamin C—50 mg vitamin D—5 μg

SOURCE: Institute of Medicine (1990).

Other Vitamin Issues

The physiological and metabolic demands of pregnancy quite logically increase the daily requirements for most vitamins (see Table 12.1). Fortunately, the American diet offers ample opportunity to fulfill these estimated needs; however, limited food intake or poor dietary choices over time may compromise vitamin status. Women with such dietary practices are reasonable candidates for prenatal vitamin/mineral supplements. Specific vitamin/mineral supplements are also justified for pure vegetarians and women whose use of calcium-rich foods is limited (see Table 12.9). It is true, however, that the consequences of specific vitamin deficiencies and excesses during human pregnancy are poorly understood.

Specific Dietary Problems in Pregnancy

Pregnancy-Induced Hypertension (PIH)

The cardinal symptoms of PIH are hypertension, proteinuria, and edema, usually occurring after the 20th week of gestation (Worthington-Roberts & Williams, 1989). This condition is unique to pregnancy and "cured" only by the termination of the pregnancy. It is almost always seen in the course of the first pregnancy and most frequently affects women at reproductive age extremes (under 20 or over 35). Criteria for diagnosing this disorder include the following:

Hypertension: 140/90 or increase of 30 mm Hg systolic or 15 mm Hg diastolic above woman's usual baseline; at least two observations at 6 or more hours apart

Proteinuria: 500 mg or more in 24-hour urine collection or random 2+ protein; develops late in course of PIH

Edema: Significant; usually in hands and face; if left unattended, convulsions may occur; can be fatal to either mother or baby

The etiology of PIH has been a mystery for many years. Although a number of theories have been proposed and carefully examined, the precise cause of this common disorder of pregnancy is still unknown. Even still, the notion that nutritional deficiency is responsible has been suggested a number of times. This idea is based in part on the observation that PIH frequently occurs in women of lower socioeconomic status. Clear scientific data confirming a role of malnutrition in the establishment of this disorder are presently lacking.

Although we have no guaranteed strategies involving dietary manipulations that will prevent PIH, it is clear that management of the woman who develops this condition requires nutritional support. Sodium restriction to prevent edema is now known to be unnecessary; in fact, this practice is best described as obsolete. If proteinuria has been an ongoing problem, replacing that protein loss is important. A high-quality diet with plenty of protein is the best recommendation for the preeclamptic patient.

Bulimia

The woman with a history of bingeing and vomiting is clearly at risk for adverse pregnancy outcome. Because most bulimics are not underweight and amenorrheic, they are as fertile as other "healthy" women. Because bulimia is a relatively recently described disorder, very few observations have been reported about pregnancy course and outcome. The limited database suggests that with aggressive counseling to motivate the mother to place the health of the fetus first, binge/vomiting episodes can be markedly reduced. The course of pregnancy appears to be relatively normal when these efforts are effective. Of great importance, however, is the need to prepare the bulimic mother for successful parenting. Avoidance of restrictive feeding patterns is obviously a message that must be emphasized.

Diabetes

Pregnancy is a diabetogenic event. To care for the pregnant woman with diabetes, the nurse needs an understanding of the metabolic states of pregnancy and the way in which diabetes affects and alters these. In pregnancy, energy needs and fuel requirements to meet these needs are increased. Glucose is a primary fuel, particularly for the growing fetus. The fetal uptake rate of glucose is at least twice that of an adult. To meet fetal needs, glucose is transferred rapidly from the mother to the fetus through simple diffusion and active transport. Although glucose crosses the placental barrier, insulin does not, and the fetus is dependent on its own supply for development. Maternal fasting blood glucose levels drop as a result of rapid fetal uptake of glucose and glucose precursor amino acids. The drop in maternal blood levels decreases the fasting insulin levels, which leads to starvation ketosis. The next response of the mother to even brief fasting is hypoglycemia, hypoaminoacidemia, hypoinsulinemia, and finally hyperketonemia. The ketones can be taken by the fetus as an alternative fuel source; however, this carries a risk of fetal brain damage. Changes in maternal fasting glucose levels result not only from fetal demands but also from increased secretion of placental hormones. Normal glucose tolerance is maintained, however, by increased maternal secretion of insulin.

The normal energy metabolism of pregnancy and the maternal-fetal relationship have certain implications for the person with diabetes. During the first half of pregnancy the increased transfer of maternal glucose to the fetus along with the often lowered food intake because of nausea and vomiting may result in reduced insulin requirements. The decreased availability of maternal circulatory blood glucose may create a decreased need for insulin. In the second half of pregnancy the diabetogenic effects of the placental hormones override the continuous fetal drain of glucose so that insulin requirements are increased by as much as 65% to 70%. At the same time that insulin efficiency is decreased, the tendency to ketoacidosis is increased because blood glucose levels do not increase markedly. The pregnant diabetic may have ketonuria reflecting starvation ketosis or diabetic ketosis. It is essential that the practitioner be able to differentiate between the two.

Diet is critical in the management of the pregnant woman who has diabetes. Energy input or calories must balance energy needs to reach and maintain ideal weight. During pregnancy, total energy needs are determined by maternal-fetal growth demands and overall increased metabolic needs.

The recommended daily dietary intake for the pregnant woman with insulin-dependent diabetes is estimated on the basis of prepregnancy body weight status (see Table 12.10), which is approximately 35 calories per kg of ideal weight or between 2,200 and 2,400 calories (Gabbe, 1985). Distribution of calories is typically 20% from protein, 30% from fat, and 50% from carbohydrate. Distribution of the carbohydrate throughout the day is typically 25% in the morning, 25% at midday, 5% midafternoon, 30% evening, and

Table 12.10 Recommended Energy Intake for the Pregnant Diabetic

Prepregnant Weight Status	*Kcal/kg/day*[a]	*Kcal/lb/day*[a]
Normal range	36	16
Underweight	45-50	20-23
Obese	25-30	11-20
Adolescent (< 15 years of age)	45	20

SOURCE: Adapted from Nelson and Kilbury (1987).
a. Pregnant body weight.

15% bedtime. This pattern may vary depending on the type and schedule of insulin administration.

Maintenance of satisfactory control of blood glucose levels during pregnancy is associated with a marked improvement in pregnancy course and outcome. Rates of congenital malformations, spontaneous abortion, and macrosomia are much reduced; these improvements are directly related to reduced perinatal mortality. In fact, with the gradual improvements in the management of diabetic pregnancies over the past 50 years, an impressive decline in perinatal mortality rate has been recorded in the United States, Canada, and Europe (see Figure 12.2) (Centers for Disease Control, 1990).

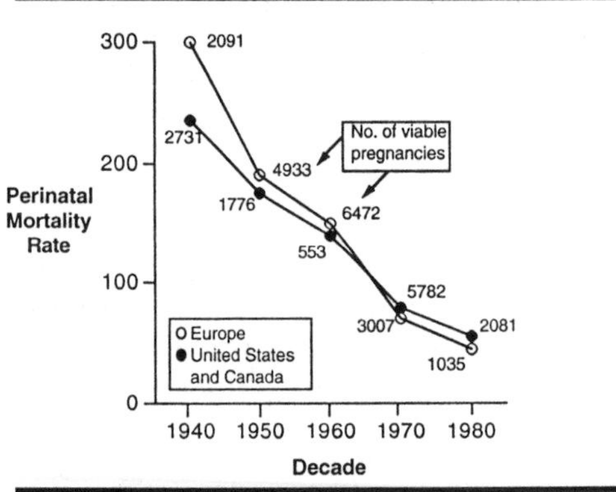

Figure 12.2. Decrease in Rates of Perinatal Mortality (Late Fetal and Early Neonatal Deaths per 1,000 Births) Among Infants Born to Women With Insulin-Dependent Diabetes[a]

SOURCE: Centers for Disease Control (1990).
a. Determined by hospital-based reports by decade: United States, Canada, and Europe (Austria, Belgium, Denmark, Federal Republic of Germany, Finland, France, German Democratic Republic, Italy, Netherlands, Norway, Sweden, Switzerland, and the United Kingdom), 1940-1988.

A program of outpatient care has become the rule rather than the exception in the management of the pregnancy complicated by insulin-dependent diabetes mellitus. Sometimes hospitalization is required early in gestation to assess the patient's vascular status and to provide patient education. Outpatient visits are usually scheduled at 1- to 2-week intervals. The log of glucose values kept by the patient is carefully reviewed at each visit. Patients are also encouraged to telephone their physician if episodes of hyperglycemia or hypoglycemia occur. Careful monitoring of established retinopathy or nephropathy is necessary, and serum alpha-fetoprotein levels may be obtained in the second trimester to screen for neural tube defects.

In the case of the woman with gestational diabetes, focus on diagnosis and management is directed toward the last half of pregnancy (American Diabetes Association, 1985). A well-ordered screening program must be established to detect this disorder. In the past, screening was based on recognized historical or clinical clues, including a family history of diabetes, delivery of a macrosomic baby, an infant with malformation, or an unexplained stillborn, or presence of obesity, hypertension, or glycosuria. However, screening only these patients is now recognized to be inadequate. Up to 50% of women who go on to develop gestational diabetes will fail to manifest these clues. Therefore, it is now recommended that all pregnant patients should be screened at approximately 24 to 28 weeks gestation using a 50-gm oral glucose load followed by a glucose determination 1 hour later. Patients need not be fasting when the screening test is performed. If the screen is abnormal, that is, a plasma value of greater than 140 mg per dl, an oral glucose tolerance test is scheduled. Selected high-risk patients, those with gestational diabetes in a previous pregnancy or women who demonstrate carbohydrate intolerance while using oral contraceptives, may be screened earlier in pregnancy. Similarly, if the initial screen at 24 to 28 weeks is negative, but the patient is thought to be at great risk for gestational diabetes, a repeat test should be scheduled at 32 weeks.

Once the diagnosis of gestational diabetes has been established, patients are started on a diet that excludes simple sugars and contains approximately 2,000 to 2,500 calories daily distributed in three meals and a bedtime snack. Fasting and postprandial glucose levels should be evaluated at 1- and 2-week intervals until delivery. Use of insulin is not routine, but it may be necessary in some cases.

Pica

Pica is the general term for the habit of eating nonfood substances (Horner, Lackey, & Kolasa, 1991). Substances linked with pica in the United States include clay, starch, chalk, and unusual quantities of ice. Pica is found in all ages and both sexes; however, the practice is most common in pregnant women. The underlying cause of pica is unknown. Pica is associated with a higher incidence of malnutrition. There is also a strong link between pica and iron deficiency; however, the exact relationship is not clear.

Pica is thought by some researchers to cause anemia by binding dietary iron, making it useless to the body. Clay with a high cation exchange capacity effectively blocks iron absorption. Magnesium oxide found in antacids used for pica prevents iron absorption. It has also been suggested that nonfood substances take the place of iron-containing foods, causing anemia. For example, laundry starch provides empty calories, thus decreasing hunger; but these are calories without iron. Other researchers believe that depleted iron stores lead to pica—that pica is a consequence, not a cause, of iron deficiency.

The reasons for pica have not been clearly identified. One important factor is culture and tradition. In a study in Alabama it was determined that women ate substances such as clay, cornstarch, flour, and baby powder because they believed these substances would relieve nausea, prevent vomiting, relieve dizziness, cure swelling, relieve headaches, and make sure the children were attractive. Other women have reported a belief that clay contains substances that are beneficial for the child.

Pica is potentially dangerous for both the woman and her baby. The ingestion of empty calories instead of foods containing essential nutrients can lead to malnourishment. Anemia is commonly associated with pica, as already noted. Intestional and pyloric obstruction in the mother, prematurity, preeclampsia, and perinatal mortality have all been linked to pica during pregnancy.

It is not easy to discourage ingestion of nonfood substances by those pregnant women who practice it. For the nurse, the most immediate need is to identify pica. Often, direct questions about diet will uncover the fact. An open-ended question about cravings or eating unusual substances is most likely to detect pica. The nurse should determine how much is being eaten, why it is being eaten, and when the woman practices pica. With this information and a thorough dietary assessment, the nurse can begin nutrition education. She needs to provide the client with in-depth nutritional guidance, including explanations of the significance of good diet and the potential harm current eating practices may cause.

Food Taboos

Superstitions and taboos about food are as old as human life (Carruth & Skinner, 1991). Pregnancy seems to be a time of great concern about food taboos, with strong connotation as to what is beneficial or harmful. When these taboos are grounded in ignorance, they can have a deleterious effect on the pregnant client's diet. Many superstitions have been associated with protein and protein-rich foods. For example, milk would supposedly cause cancer if you were pregnant, and pork and fish would "rot" the uterus. Cheese was thought to cause "dry labor," as were peanuts. Green leafy vegetables were taboo because they would "mark the baby." From these examples, it is easy to see why dietary inadequacies of protein, calcium, iron, and vitamins A and C might occur. Although poor nutrition is most often the result of nutritional ignorance, specific food dislikes, unavailability, superstition, and bizarre food traditions can be significant.

Lactose Intolerance

The majority of the world's population is able to digest varying quantities of milk because of low levels of activity of the lactose enzyme. The mother who says she just cannot drink milk because it makes her sick may be lactose intolerant.

This trait does not appear to be modifiable because it is based on genetic predisposition.

Lactase is the enzyme responsible for the hydrolysis of lactose into glucose and galactose. If lactose is not broken down, it enters the large intestine undigested, where it pulls water from the surrounding tissue into the intestinal lumen. It is also fermented by bacteria present in the colon, producing organic acids, carbon dioxide, and hydrogen. These cause the symptoms of lactose intolerance—abdominal cramps, bloating, diarrhea, and flatulence.

Because milk is a major dietary source of calcium and vitamin D, poor tolerance of it poses a substantial challenge in meeting recommended levels of consumption of these nutrients in particular. Women who cannot or will not drink milk should be advised of alternative foods. Fermented dairy products, including yogurt and cheese, are excellent sources of calcium that contain substantially less lactose than does milk. Often, these foods can be tolerated to some degree by lactose intolerant women. In addition, it is now possible to purchase lactose hydrolyzed milk in the dairy section of most grocery stores; the lactose has been largely broken down by the addition of lactase enzyme. Women can also make their own lactose hydrolyzed milk by purchasing a commercial lactase enzyme product and adding it to regular milk at home. Milk with the lactose hydrolyzed is nutritionally comparable to milk without this treatment. (A word of caution—sweet acidophilus milk is not low in lactose. It is essentially 2% milk to which a culture of *Lactobacillus Acidophilus* has been added.)

When calcium needs cannot be met by dietary manipulation, calcium supplements provide a reliable source of calcium. Some supplements also contain vitamin D. The other nutrients obtained through consumption of dairy products, however, will not be derived from these supplemental sources. Thus supplements are opted for only when dietary solutions cannot be found.

Adolescent Pregnancy

When pregnancy occurs in adolescence, there are potential physical and psychological risks. Adolescence is a period of rapid growth and development that requires substantial nutritional intake. Increased amounts of food are needed, as well as specific nutrients related to pubertal growth spurts. Teenagers who become pregnant in the 4 years following menarche are at biological risk because they are anatomically and physiologically immature. Pregnancy may occur before skeletal growth, most particularly of the pelvis, is completed. In addition, nutritional states at conception and during pregnancy determine in part the nutritional state and reproductive capability of the subsequent generation. These may be compromised in the adolescent who is pregnant.

Caloric needs are usually greater during pregnancy and during adolescence. This assumes additional significance in light of teenagers' widespread practice of dieting. Protein needs are also high for the pregnant teenager to meet both her own and her baby's growth needs. The need is intensified for the teenager who has a poor nutritional history. A protein intake of at least 60 gm per day is recommended. More calcium is needed to provide for fetal skeletal development and to prevent compromising the maternal skeleton by demineralization. Iron needs are at least 15 mg per day. Adequate nutritional intake of all other vitamins and minerals, as outlined in Table 12.1, is recommended.

A number of researchers have attempted to describe the nutritional status of pregnant adolescents. Growth retardation related to poor nutrition is not common in North America. Neither is there much evidence from biochemical measurements of nutritional status that serious malnutrition exists. Observations suggest, however, that suboptimum dietary practices are widespread. Iron deficiency is relatively common, and nutrients frequently consumed at less than recommended levels include vitamins A, C, and B_6, folic acid, and riboflavin and the minerals calcium and zinc. When supplements are recommended for pregnant teens, their use is best described as erratic.

Given the pregnant adolescent's increased nutritional needs to provide optimal growth conditions for herself and her offspring, and given the fact that adolescents frequently do not meet their needs for several essential nutrients, it is imperative that the nurse encourage positive nutritional patterns for the adolescent. This requires an individualized approach to the problem for each girl.

Nursing Implications

Nutritional counseling is an integral component of comprehensive nursing care for the maternity client. Counseling begins with an in-depth assessment of maternal nutrition early in prenatal care and proceeds to individualized

Table 12.11 Nutritional Risk Factors

Factor	*Significant*
Age	The adolescent whose reproductive biological age (chronological age minus menarche age) is less than 3 is at particular risk because of her own growth needs. Adolescent pregnancy may also be associated with emotional, financial, and educational risks. Advanced age may be associated with high parities. Age of menarche is significant in that it can be delayed by poor nutrition.
Reproductive performance	Short interconceptual periods are a risk factor, particularly when coupled with high parity. Past obstetric history of abortions, poor weight gain, anemia, generalized edema, stillbirth, toxemia, low-birth-weight infants, and premature labor are also factors.
Chronic systemic illness	Anemia, thyroid dysfunction, diabetes, chronic infection, malabsorption syndromes, and severe emotional/psychosocial problems constitute risk factors, as do drugs used to treat these illnesses that may interfere with nutrition.
Weight	Low pregnant weight or low weight (less than 85%) for height may indicate long-term nutritional inadequacy. Inadequate weight gain during pregnancy is a risk factor, as is obesity above 120% of standard weight for height.
Unusual nutritional patterns	Food fads and/or constant dieting can result in inadequate food intake. Pica is a special risk. Special dietary restrictions owing to ethnic or cultural factors may also cause nutrition problems.
Substance abuse	Use of tobacco, drugs, or alcohol may decrease nutrition intake and directly affect fetal growth and development.
Economic deprivation	Inability to purchase inadequate amounts of the required nutrients and chronic, low-level nutritional inadequacy constitute risks.

guidance based on the assessment. Three basic methods of assessment will provide the data necessary to determine nutritional needs. These are (a) a thorough history, (b) a physical examination, and (c) laboratory tests. Primary factors included in the basic history are age, marital status, previous obstetric history, and prior medical, social, personal, and nutritional histories. The nurse should be able to recognize factors that place the client at nutritional risk, collect a nutrition history, perform selected physical examination procedures, and interpret laboratory tests to assess nutritional adequacy.

Many factors may place the pregnant woman at increased nutritional risk (see Table 12.11). The presence of one or more of these indicates a need for a more intensive nutritional assessment than that provided by routine history, physical examination, and laboratory tests. The information gathered from carefully taken medical, obstetric, and personal histories is a good way to begin determining the client's nutritional risk.

The diet history is an indispensable component of nutritional assessment, yet it is rarely a routine component of clinical practice. This may result from lack of training and experience, time constraints, or lack of recognition of its value. A diet history need not be time-consuming, and it can be both informative for the practitioner and educational for the client. The process is begun by collecting some general data. The pregnant woman is first a person with specific attitudes toward food, emotional responses to food, cultural beliefs about food, and knowledge about nutrition that must be explored. It is also important to know how she views health, being pregnant, and bearing a child. It is important to explore her cultural beliefs about food, particularly in relation to appropriate foods during pregnancy. Determining her birthplace and early childhood home can help identify cultural food influences. The nurse needs to identify the value that food holds for the client in terms of nutritional status, appetite, and emotional significance. Inquiry should be made as to the influence of economic factors on food selection, storage, and preparation. It is helpful to know how much control the pregnant woman has over food preparation and purchasing. The expectant mother's education and occupation should be

Name____________________ Address____________________

Race ____________________ Age ______ Height ______ Weight ______

Vitamin or mineral supplements taken ____________________

Salt intake: light, moderate, or heavy

Foods eaten in last 24 hours

Kind and amount of food and drink (List main foods in mixed dishes)	Number of servings				
	Milk	Meat	Veg/ fruits	Bread cereal	Misc. (list)
Morning					
Midmorning					
Noon					
Afternoon					
Evening					
Before bed					

Total servings eaten	______	______	______	______
Recommended servings	______	______	______	______
Comparison	______	______	______	______

What food and drink do you think people should have to keep healthy?

Figure 12.3. Twenty-Four-Hour Diet History

noted. Any special practices, food allergies or intolerances, and medication or supplements routinely taken must be ascertained.

Once the nurse has gathered the requisite background information, a specific diet history should be obtained. A technique suited to many types of clinical practice is the 24-hour recall. It is relatively accurate, simple, and brief and does not require a lot of experience to use it. Figure 12.3 is an example of a 24-hour recall diet history form. During the process of taking a diet history, much valuable information about the woman's level of nutritional knowledge and tips for counseling methods can be obtained. In addition to the types of food eaten, amounts and methods of preparation should be recorded. At times, it is useful to supplement the 24-hour recall with a 7-day list of foods eaten.

A thorough general physical examination is a standard component of prenatal care. Unfortunately, physical evidence of poor nutrition usually appears relatively late and is often nonspecific and subtle. The practitioner needs to be careful to distinguish between nutritionally significant findings and normal maternal physiological changes during pregnancy (for example, dependent edema or gingival hyperplasia).

Table 12.12 Serum Nutrient Levels in Pregnant and Nonpregnant Women

Nutrient	*Normal Pregnancy Range*	*Nonpregnancy Range*
Total protein	6.5-8.5g/1,000 ml	6.0-8.0
Albumin	3.5-5.0 g/100 ml	3.0-4.5
Glucose	< 100 mg/100 ml	< 120
Cholesterol	120-190 mg/100 ml	200-325
Vitamin A	20-60 μg/100 ml	20-60
Carotene	50-300 μg/100 ml	80-325
Ascorbic acid	0.2-2.0 μg/100 ml	0.2-1.5
Folic acid	5-21 μg/100 ml	3-15
Calcium	4.6-5.5 mEq/L	4.2-5.2
Iron/iron-binding capacity	< 50/250-400 μg/100 ml	> 40/300-450

SOURCE: National Research Council (1978).

Perhaps the single most significant physical finding indicating nutritional adequacy is weight—both prepregnant weight and gain during pregnancy. Clients who weigh less than 90% or more than 120% of the standard weight for height require intensive individualized nutrition counseling. In addition, poor weight gain during pregnancy or sudden, excessive bursts of weight gain can indicate nutritional problems.

More objective precise information about nutritional status can be obtained from laboratory assessments. Laboratory tests often reflect poor nutrition well before it is clinically evident. Interpretation may be difficult because established norms for pregnant women are not always available. Table 12.12 summarizes those laboratory tests that appear to be of some assistance.

Once all baseline data from the physical, dietary, and general history and laboratory studies have been gathered, evaluation of the client's nutritional status may be done jointly by the nurse and client. The diet is analyzed to determine its adequacy to meet the increased nutritional needs of pregnancy. Using a food chart, the diet is analyzed for calories, protein, calcium, iron, and key vitamins and minerals. The diet is then compared with the recommended dietary allowances for pregnancy (see Table 12.1). These findings along with laboratory data and physical findings will identify the strengths and weaknesses of the expectant mother's diet and nutritional status. From this point, nutritional counseling may proceed.

Many expectant mothers are interested and motivated to make the changes needed in their diets. For these women, providing information initially and following up at subsequent prenatal visits is usually all that is required. There is a second group—those women who are either not able, interested, or willing to change their diets—who may require the nurse's most creative intervention to motivate them to improve their diets.

Nutrition counseling begins with the individual woman and is tailored to meet her needs. The goals should be clearly identified, realistic, and challenging yet attainable. Nutritional instruction must be meaningful and not beyond the client's ability to comprehend. New material is built on what is already known so that it is readily associated. Using a variety of teaching aids increases the likelihood of understanding and remembering. Material that can be taken home, such as pamphlets, can be used for continued reference.

The Daily Food Guide for Women (Table 12.3) is an excellent guide for well-balanced nutrition. It is a foundation on which nutritional counseling is built. From this foundation, the nursing practitioner can help the pregnant woman or couple convert recommended dietary allowances into specific amounts and types of food.

Individual prenatal nutritional counseling should include reinforcement of good food habits as well as new information. The nurse can strengthen good habits by pointing out the relationship of positive food practices to nutritional needs in pregnancy, by reviewing the reasons for the increased nutritional needs, and by giving warm praise for good habits. Nutritional deficiencies can be corrected in a constructive manner by helping the client identify the difficulties herself and the reasons for them. This can be followed by exploring possible alternative solutions to the problem. The woman should participate in the determination of nutritional assets and the diagnosis of nutritional deficits. She devises her own plan of care, thus enhancing self-care activities and the possibility of effecting positive change.

During pregnancy, ethnic variations in diet can prevent optimal nutrition. The practitioner needs to be familiar with cultural variations in diet and potential problems.

Vegetarian diets are becoming increasingly numerous for a variety of socioeconomic, cultural, religious, and personal reasons. Limited intake of protein can create hazards for the fetus and mother. There are three basic types of vegetarians: (a) pure vegetarians, who exclude all animal foods; (b) lacto-vegetarians, who allow the inclusion of dairy products; and (c) lacto-ovo-vegetarians, who include eggs and dairy products in the diet. In all three diets, meat and poultry are excluded, but all types of fruits, vegetables, legumes, grains, and nuts are allowed. Obviously, the more limited the diet, the more hazardous it is.

Vegetarians can have nutritionally adequate diets when they consume wide varieties of grains, legumes, fruits, vegetables, nuts, seeds, milk and milk products, and eggs in the right combinations. Potential problems in pregnancy result from inadequate intake of protein and calories, vitamin B_{12}, vitamin D, riboflavin, calcium, and iron.

If dairy products are eaten, vitamin B_{12}, vitamin D, riboflavin, and calcium needs will be met. It is possible to plan a vegetarian diet that is adequate for all nutrients. To ensure an adequate diet, the consumption of milk, milk products, and eggs should be encouraged. Meat is replaced with a generous intake of legumes, nuts, and meat analogues made from wheat and soy products. The milk group is replaced by greater amounts of low-fat milk and milk products, such as cheese and cottage cheese. Food intake should increase slightly—fruits and vegetables are used to make up the needed caloric intake, so the amounts selected are important. Vegetarians who adhere to the strictest form of the diet should usually take calcium, vitamin B_{12}, and vitamin D supplements. Iodized salt should be used and iron supplements prescribed.

In all cases of nutritional counseling, it is mandatory that food plans be realistic. For most women, minimal guidance and assistance will result in a diet sufficient to meet their needs. For those women with real dietary problems and/or substantial pregnancy risks, careful supportive counseling is essential. Some type of follow-up support and evaluation must be a part of the ongoing nursing care. In all cases, nutritional counseling will reduce risk of poor pregnancy outcome.

Lactation

Well over 50% of women in North America decide to breast-feed their infants for at least several months (Institute of Medicine, 1991). Interest in breast-feeding began to rise in the early 1970s and peaked at about 1982. Since then, there has been a modest drop in interest in this mode of infant feeding; the reasons for this recent decline are uncertain, but it is speculated that the demands placed on the working woman are important contributors to this trend.

Nutritionally speaking, lactation places a greater nutritional stress on a woman than any other time in the postadolescent years. The typical mother who is nursing one infant produces about 750 ml of milk daily; this milk not only contains 500 calories but also contains significant amounts of other nutrients. Maintenance of an adequate supply of high-quality milk is a well-established physiological priority. If the mother's diet is poor, she will drain her own nutritional reserves to ensure that the nursing infant does not suffer.

The amount of extra nutrition required by the lactating woman depends directly on the amount of milk that is produced. The RDAs for lactation are based on the milk production of the "average" American woman. An additional 500 calories is recommended in the daily diet along with extra amounts of nutrients. Obviously, these numbers are underestimates for women who are extremely active or nursing more than one infant. Likewise they are overestimates for women who become very sedentary or who provide much supplemental formula to their infants.

The postpartum pattern of weight loss during lactation varies greatly from one woman to another. Many women gradually lose 1 to 2 pounds per month while breast-feeding. Others, however, seem to be very resistant to weight loss during this time. It seems likely that this difference relates to the level of daily calorie intake; proof that this is in fact always the case is not available.

The nurse who counsels lactating women should be prepared to provide information on a wide array of topics. Early on, women need assistance in dealing with the "mechanical" issues, such as sore nipples, engorgement, leaking, and the like. Dietary advice should include recommendations about reasonable ways to meet increased needs, particularly of key nutrients such as calcium. Dieting should be discouraged because it may interfere with the establishment and/or maintenance of lactation. Reminders about ingestion of plenty of fluid may be in order, especially in hot climates, where risk of dehydration is increased.

Lactating mothers are likely to inquire about a number of other concerns about breast-feeding in general or about diet/nutrition issues related to their health or that of their infants. Examples of such topics include the following:

1. Nutrient supplementation of the breast-feeding baby: Vitamin D and fluoride usually are advised.
2. Allergic reaction of the baby to a compound in breast milk: Most babies tolerate breast milk very well. A minority, however, may demonstrate an adverse reaction to a diet-derived component in breast milk. Cow's milk protein is reportedly the major culprit. If this problem occurs, a lactating woman should be advised to avoid the potentially problematic food and assess the behavior of the infant during the next few days. If maternal dietary change seems to be beneficial to the health of the infant, consideration should be given to diet or supplement strategies that will ensure health maintenance of the mother.
3. Contaminants in breast milk: The lactating woman is often exposed to a variety of non-nutritional substances that may be transferred to her milk. Such substances include drugs, environmental pollutants, viruses, caffeine, and alcohol. Although moderate amounts of many of these agents are believed to pose no risk to nursing infants, some substances provoke concern because of known or suspected adverse reactions.
4. The AIDS virus and breast milk: Evidence suggests that the AIDS virus can be transmitted from mother to infant through breast milk. This recent finding has provoked much concern from the standpoint of providing appropriate advice about infant feeding to high-risk women. Should one encourage or discourage breast-feeding by such women? The current thinking in the United States is that breast-feeding should be discouraged when a woman is known to carry this virus. The World Health Organization, however, supports the concept that infants in many developing countries run greater risks of dying of diarrheal disease if they are not breast-fed than of developing AIDS from breast milk exposure. Debate on this issue continues around the world. In the meantime, breast milk banks are taking special precautions to screen out donors who potentially could contribute virus-contaminated specimens; samples are also pasteurized sufficiently to destroy viruses that might be present.

The Postmenopausal Years

Nutritional needs of older women relate directly to the size of the lean body mass, the level of physical activity, and the presence or absence of diseases that modify the efficiency of digestion, absorption, or metabolism. Active women involved in regular rigorous physical fitness programs, for example, generally have greater nutritional needs than do sedentary women with limited muscle mass. On the other extreme, women with chronic gastrointestinal disorders associated with periodic diarrheal episodes may have substantially elevated nutritional needs due to excessive nutrient losses. Because the aging process is known to affect the efficiency of digestion, absorption, and metabolism in some individuals, it is easy to understand why the aging female population is such a diverse group.

As a general rule, as women age they tend to decrease their level of physical activity and gradually lose lean body mass. This phenomenon results in a gradual reduction in daily calorie requirements. Because need for other nutrients generally does not decrease to the same extent, if at all, older women are faced with a situation of meeting their nutritional needs within the framework of lower calorie meals and snacks. Failure to achieve this adjustment in dietary patterns is associated with either excessive calorie intake and weight gain or the gradual development of specific nutrient deficiencies. Either circumstance increases the risk that quality of life will deteriorate prematurely.

Of particular concern to the postmenopausal woman is the prevention of debilitating sequelae related to aging bone loss. Although it is known that the process of bone resorption is normal following menopause, reducing the rapidity with which this occurs is a primary focus of health care for women of this age. The value of estrogen administration appears to be well established, especially for high-risk women. The role that calcium in the diet or calcium supplementation plays in these preventive efforts has been the subject of much research. The bulk of the evidence leads to the conclusion that satisfactory dietary or supplemental calcium retards the rate of postmenopausal bone loss. It does not appear to be as effective as estrogen in so doing, but it is better than the alternative diet that is low in calcium and/or inadequate in calcium supplementation (Horsman, Gallagher, Simpson, & Nordin, 1977; see Chapter 5 for further information).

Table 12.13 Eating Disorders Diagnostic Criteria

Anorexia Nervosa

1. Refusal to maintain body weight over a minimal normal weight for age and height—for example, weight loss leading to maintenance of a body weight 15% below that expected or failure to make expected weight gain for period of growth, leading to a body weight 15% below that expected.
2. Intense fear of gaining weight or becoming fat, even though underweight.
3. Disturbance in the way in which one's body weight, size, or shape is experienced—for example, the person claims to "feel fat" even when emaciated, believes that one area of the body is "too fat" even when obviously underweight.
4. In females, absence of at least three consecutive menstrual cycles when otherwise expected to occur (primary or secondary amenorrhea). (A woman is considered to have amenorrhea if her periods occur only following hormone—e.g., estrogen—administration.)

Bulimia Nervosa

1. Recurrent episodes of binge eating (rapid consumption of a large amount of food in a discrete period of time).
2. A feeling of lack of control over eating behavior during the eating binges.
3. Regularly engaging in self-induced vomiting, fasting, or vigorous exercise to prevent weight gain.
4. A minimum average of two binge eating episodes a week for at least 3 months.
5. Persistent overconcern with body shape and weight.

Eating Disorder Not Otherwise Specified

1. Having average weight and no binge eating episodes but frequently engaging in self-induced vomiting for fear of gaining weight.
2. All of the features of anorexia nervosa in a female except absence of menses.
3. All of the features of bulimia nervosa except the frequency of binge eating episodes.

SOURCE: Reproduced with permission from *Nutrition and Eating Disorders* copyright © 1989, Quest Publishing Company, 1351 Titan Way, Brea, CA 92621, (714) 738-6400.

The nurse who is caring for the postmenopausal woman should encourage attention to nutrient-dense food choices. Moderation in consumption of fatty foods goes a long way in achieving this goal. A number of useful educational materials are available for use in counseling or for distribution to clients. Specific mention of calcium-rich foods is of particular importance. If dairy products are viewed as an undesirable option in the diet, recommendation of an appropriate calcium supplement should be considered.

Eating Disorders Common to Women

Although eating disorders have long been recognized as relatively common among women in developed countries, increased attention has been devoted to these problems during the past decade. With both anorexia nervosa and bulimia nervosa, early diagnosis and prompt, aggressive intervention are necessary to minimize morbidity.

Anorexia Nervosa

Anorexia nervosa is an illness that usually occurs in girls shortly after puberty or later in adolescence (Herzog & Copeland, 1985). It is characterized by self-imposed weight loss, amenorrhea, and a distorted attitude toward eating and body weight (see Table 12.13). Accounts of women who refused to eat have appeared throughout the history of Western civilization, and it is likely that some of these women suffered from anorexia nervosa. In 1689, Dr. Morton, a British physician, reported two patients, one male and one female, who suffered from "nervous consumption." In 1874, a physician named the disorder anorexia nervosa, describing it as extreme emaciation associated with increased activity, episodes of binge eating, amenorrhea, and low body temperature. Epidemiological studies in the United States and Europe have documented an increased incidence in young women over the past 20 years. Data from hospitalized cases and psychiatric registers in the United States and Western Europe have shown a rate of about 15 per 100,000 women; among the most susceptible group, females aged 15 through 24 years, a rate of 76 per 100,000 was reported in the early 1980s. However, numerous cases of new onset anorexia in older women have been identified and described.

The specific cause of anorexia nervosa still is unknown but most scientific evidence suggests that there is an interaction of biological and psychosocial factors. A genetic component is strongly suggested by the observation that the disorder is much more common in pairs of identical twins than in pairs of fraternal twins. It is well documented that there is a disturbance in the hypothalamic-anterior pituitary-gonadal axis, but it is likely that this disturbance is secondary to malnutrition. Whatever the cause (Gold et al., 1986), the chronic dieting appears to trigger a process of continuous weight loss and hypometabolic adaptation in vulnerable individuals, leading to a vicious cycle that becomes self-perpetuating.

The girl who typically develops anorexia nervosa is conscientious, intensely achievement oriented, and perfectionistic. Family interactional patterns characterized by enmeshment or overinvolvement, overprotectiveness, rigidity, and poor conflict resolution have been implicated; however, a great variety of family dynamic patterns have been described in these families. Social influences, expressed in the cultural obsession with thinness, undoubtedly have a powerful bearing on the development of this disorder. The biologically vulnerable girl is set up to react to these pressures (Health and Public Policy Committee, 1986).

The typical progress of an anorexic is that of gradual self-starvation, which may begin with apparently normal concern about dieting. Food restriction becomes more and more stringent and often is accompanied by increasing exercise. Concerns about the pubertal changes in body shape become exaggerated, leading to deterioration of self-image. As weight loss becomes an obsession, social withdrawal and alienation from family members results. Symptoms of depression eventually ensue, but denial of any problem and resistance to medical examination and treatment is commonplace.

The medical complications largely relate to the progressive starvation. Anemia and hypoproteinemia are common, but classic vitamin deficiencies are late in developing if they develop at all (Palla & Litt, 1988). Gastrointestinal complications, including decreased motility and atonic gut, may occur. Prolonged reduction in estrogen levels leads to reduction in bone mineral mass and, ultimately, osteoporosis, even in young individuals (Rigotti, Nussbaum, Herzog, & Neer, 1984; Treasure & Russell, 1984). Serious electrolyte imbalances can occur when vomiting, laxative, or diuretic abuse are practiced. Muscular weakness, cardiac arrhythmias, and renal impairment may occur. These complications can lead to cardiac and renal damage or to sudden death.

A major difficulty in managing the patient with anorexia nervosa is that the patient often denies the extent of her illness and is thus unwilling to accept treatment. A family member may bring the young woman to the physician's office against her will. Typically, she enjoys the control she seems to have over her life through maintenance of slimness by marked limitation in food intake. Interference with this established routine is viewed as unwarranted, if not frightening.

Initially, it may be helpful to educate the patient about the disorder. A reminder about the disruptions of daily life associated with anorexia may ring true. The patient may eventually be willing to acknowledge problems with concentration on school or work, depression, isolation from peers, sleep disorders, and physical complaints, such as hair loss or cold intolerance. Long-term complications, including osteoporosis with an increased risk of bone fracture, should be discussed.

Most patients are handled on an outpatient basis, but, occasionally, hospitalization is necessary. Medical indications for hospitalization include severe emaciation, hypokalemia, hyponatremia, and an abnormal electrocardiogram. Recurrent use of syrup of ipecac can be toxic to the muscular system. Cardiomyopathy, if present, may be life threatening, and hospitalization is indicated. Psychiatric indications for hospitalization include moderate to severe depression because risk of suicide is greatly increased. Inability to function in the home, school, or workplace is also an indication for inpatient treatment. Failure of outpatient treatment after 3 months should suggest the need for hospital care. Some clinicians recommend immediate hospitalization after any recurrence of an eating disorder.

Regardless of the treatment location, there is now consensus that most patients require a multidimensional approach that addresses both the physiological and psychological manifestations of the illness. Resumption of normal eating patterns is the major goal of treatment, leading eventually to the restoration of desirable body weight. Some controversy exists about how rapidly weight should be restored, but thus far research that declares that slow weight gain is better or worse than more rapid weight augmentation is insufficient. It is clear that the younger the patient, the more important it is to involve the family in treatment.

In the outpatient setting, the physical condition is monitored by the patient's primary physician. A nutritionist can assist with meal planning. A psychiatrist provides psychotherapy and, if necessary, adjunctive medication. In the inpatient setting, the treatment team is expanded. It should include an occupational therapist, who will develop productive activities that reduce obsession with body image. The nursing staff can provide a social structure that will assist the patient's integration into a therapeutic milieu. Some nurses should be "administrative" and monitor weight, food consumption, and activity. Other nursing personnel should assume a supportive role and provide a sympathetic outlet for the patient's conflicts.

A significant complication of anorexia nervosa is its chronicity. It has been estimated that about 15% to 30% remain chronically ill, even after lengthy treatment programs. Some of the chronically ill patients develop bulimia nervosa (episodic binge eating, vomiting, and purging). Death may occur from electrolyte imbalance, or it may be a late outcome due to chronic starvation. These statistics are unlikely to change significantly until comparative research on different treatment regimens is completed. Ideally, within the next decade, proven treatment strategies will be widely available. (Psychotherapy is discussed in detail in Chapter 15.)

Bulimia Nervosa

Bulimia nervosa was first described as a distinct psychiatric illness in 1979; it has therefore been the focus of research for a fairly brief period of time. No population-based epidemiological survey has specifically examined the prevalence of bulimia nervosa; published studies to date have focused on college students, high school students, and other nonrandom samples. Reports of prevalence have varied greatly, largely because of the differing definitions applied to the disorder (Drewnowski, Hopkins, & Kessler, 1988; Katzman, Wolchick, & Braver, 1984; Kurtzman, Yager, & Landsverk, 1989; Mintz & Betz, 1988; Pyle et al., 1983; Schotte & Stunkard, 1987). Episodes of binge eating, for example, reportedly occur in 26% to 79% of women. If more stringent criteria are used, such as the requirement that binge eating be coupled with self-induced vomiting or laxative abuse, the prevalence rate drops to between 1% and 3% for young women and is probably more representative of the disorder (see Table 12.13) (Kirkley, 1986).

The mean age of onset of this disorder is about 19 years, a time when many young women leave home to attend college or to join the workforce. This transitional time in life appears to be one of very high risk for the development of problematic eating behaviors. Available evidence suggests that patients with bulimia nervosa are symptomatic for about 6 years before seeking help. Often, treatment is sought to deal with the secondary symptoms that frequently develop, such as medical complications, depression, impaired job performance, or poor school performance.

The binge/purge behavior often leads to the development of a "chipmunk-like" face due to swelling of the parotid glands. The swelling is secondary to frequent contact with acidic gastric contents, which also causes etching and later rotting of the inner aspects of the teeth. Bulimic patients who induce emesis with a finger in the throat may also present with chemical scarring over the dorsum of one hand. Abdominal distention is a frequent complaint, and weight fluctuations of 10 pounds or more are not uncommon. Diuretics, laxatives, and high-fiber foods may all be consumed inappropriately. Routine laboratory analysis may reveal hypokalemia and metabolic alkalosis. An elevated serum cholecystokinin level is considered by some to be a marker for bulimia nervosa. Signs and symptoms of bulimia are summarized in Table 12.14 (Palla & Litt, 1988).

Most bulimic patients can be treated effectively on an outpatient basis. This mode of management is cost-effective, less socially disruptive, and is less stigmatizing. Moreover, lessons learned in an outpatient setting are more likely to correlate to the normal surroundings compared with those learned in a novel hospital environment.

In general, two forms of therapy have been used in the treatment of the patient with bulimia nervosa. The first is antidepressant treatment using a variety of drugs, including tricyclics, heterocyclics, and monoamine oxidase inhibi-

Table 12.14 Signs and Symptoms of Bulimia

Abdominal distention
Abdominal striae
Anal tear and fissures
Binge eating
Diuretic abuse
Elevated serum cholecystokinin level
Emesis
High-fiber diet
Laxative abuse
Parotid enlargement (bilateral)
Postbinge depression
Scarring of dorsum of one hand
Teeth etched or rotting on inner aspects
Weight fluctuating by 10 or more pounds in a 1-month period

tors; the second is psychotherapy involving behavioral and cognitive-behavioral techniques. Most of the antidepressant drugs suppress bulimic symptoms, but the majority of patients continue to have some bulimic episodes; for this reason, some clinicians question the merits of pharmacotherapy. Psychotherapeutic approaches vary considerably in duration and theoretical framework but overall are allied with considerable success. (See Chapter 15 for discussion of psychotherapy.)

Nutrition intervention for the bulimic patient (Story, 1986) includes components best described as education, self-monitoring, and meal planning (see Table 12.15). Patients are taught to eat regular meals because bulimia nervosa is characterized by episodes of fasting as well as binge eating and vomiting. Keeping a food diary may help improve the frequency and severity of bulimic behaviors. Structured meal-planning experiences are quite effective in helping bulimics eat balanced meals. Many patients respond better if they are allowed to exclude certain "high-risk binge foods" from their diet early in the course of treatment. These foods are reintroduced later so that the "feared foods" concept is not continued. The goal is to help patients learn that they can eat any food they choose in reasonable amounts, as long as their diet is balanced and adequate in quantity.

While patients are working to overcome their purging practices, attention should be given to weight maintenance. Weight and calorie changes are best addressed at a later point but a rigidly structured diet may *never* be indicated because of high risk of failure. Most patients with bulimia have a long history of failed weight loss attempts and another experience of that nature may perpetuate the binge/purge cycle and further decrease their self-esteem. Patients are best encouraged to let their care provider know when they are ready for a food plan and for assistance in using it as a guideline.

Suggestions for Those With Anorexia Nervosa

- Eat small frequent meals to help reduce bloating.
- Eat a moderate amount of fat—enough to meet taste and nutritional needs, because fat slows the emptying of food from the stomach and may make you feel uncomfortable.
- Eat foods cold or at room temperature to lessen early feelings of fullness (satiety).
- Eat finger foods or snacks.
- Eat high-fiber foods from the bread/starch group to encourage good bowel habits.
- Limit fruits and vegetables because the soluble fiber they contain slows the emptying of food from the stomach and may make you feel bloated.
- Limit caffeine intake because it may interfere with normal appetite patterns.
- Take a multivitamin-multimineral supplement, as recommended by your doctor or nutrition counselor (Patterson, Whelan, Rock, & Lyon, 1989, p. 16).

Suggestions for Those With Bulimia Nervosa

- Avoid "trigger foods" (those you associate with a binge) at first. These can be reintroduced later in your treatment. Instead, eat a nutrient-dense replacement that has some of the same pleasant characteristics.
- Eat three planned meals a day, rather than smaller, more frequent meals, if reducing exposure to food will help you avoid binges.
- Eat foods that require the use of utensils rather than eating finger foods. This will slow eating time and help increase meal satiety.
- Include generous portions of carbohydrate-containing foods.
- Include low-calorie items in each meal, such as vegetables, broth-based soup, salad, and/or fruit, to prolong the mealtime.

Table 12.15 General Protocol for Outpatient Dietary Management of Bulimia

Education	*Weight Issues*	*Food Diary*	*Dietary Plan*
Aim: To inform/educate patient about bulimia and its consequences.	Aim: To reduce preoccupation and overconcern with body weight and develop an acceptance of normal body weight.	Aim: To gain a thorough understanding of patient's current eating habits.	Aim: To help patient gain control and establish a pattern of regular eating.
1. Patient education begins early in treatment and continues throughout.	1. Any desired weight loss must be delayed until after the bulimic/ purging behaviors are under control and a normal eating pattern has been established.	1. Upon entering the program, patients are given forms and instructed to keep a structured food diary of quantities of all foods eaten, eating environment, accompanying thoughts, feelings, and binge/purge episodes.	1. The dietary plan is three structured meals a day with one or two snacks eaten irrespective of patient's appetite and at the same time each day (when possible).
2. Topics covered include a. Physical and health risks of bulimia and purging. b. Physiological and psychological effects of starvation. c. Ineffectiveness of various purging techniques in controlling weight. d. Role of body fat in normal development. e. Basic information on energy and nutrient processes. f. Identifying misconceptions and dysfunctional attitudes about food, eating, and dieting.	2. For bulimics entering treatment in a starvation state, reversal of starvation must occur before psychotherapy begins.	2. The diary is kept throughout treatment until eating habits are under control and is useful in monitoring progress and making dietary recommendations.	2. Patients are taught to use food lists for meal planning. Diet sizes are based on calorie levels needed to maintain current weight (minimum of 1,200 kcal per day).
	3. Patients are instructed not to weigh themselves and are weighed once a week by a treatment team member.		3. Patients are taught behavior strategies to help regulate eating.
	4. Help patients accept a normative weight for themselves and give up an unrealistically thin body weight.		4. Patients are advised to preplan meals.
	5. The concept of a normal "weight range" of 3-6 pounds is stressed.		5. Patients are initially told to avoid foods that are binge items. After treatment has progressed, those foods should be reintroduced into their diets as possible.

SOURCE: Adapted from Story (1986).

- Include adequate fat, which slows the emptying of food from the stomach, thus increasing meal satiety.
- Eat a variety of foods at each meal.
- Eat all meals and snacks sitting down.
- Include hot or warm foods, rather than eating just cold or room temperature foods.
- Plan meals ahead using a food diary.
- Use foods that are naturally divided into portions, such as one potato (rather than rice or pasta); 4- and 8-ounce containers of yogurt, ice cream, or cottage cheese; precut steaks or chicken parts; and frozen dinners and entrees (Patterson, Whelan, Rock, & Lyon, 1989, p. 17).

Obesity and Weight Management

Definition of Overfatness

The term *obesity* refers to the condition of excessive body fatness, but different definitions exist that consider body weight, body fat, fat distribution, and age of onset. Using body weight as a criterion, overweight can be defined as weighing 10% to 20% more than desirable body weight. Obesity is then defined as weighing over 20% more than desirable body weight. To further define obesity, weighing 20% to 40% more than desirable body weight represents mild obesity, weighing 41% to 99% more than desirable body weight represents moderate obesity, and weighing more than twice desirable body weight represents severe (morbid) obesity. Most causes of obesity in North America are of the mild form and are associated with little health risk. Approximately 0.2% of cases are severe, a circumstance carrying a 12-fold increase in health risk (Bray, 1987).

The term *desirable body weight* was first used in 1959 by the Metropolitan Life Insurance Company who developed the most widely used height and weight table in the United States. The 1959 version is still in use but some care providers have accepted the 1983 revised guidelines for clinical use (see Table 12.16). These tables list for any height the weight that is associated with maximum life span, but they do not identify the weight that will make one the healthiest while alive. Other nagging problems also exist. For one, the table's data are derived only from purchasers of life insurance; this means that poor people and many minorities are underrepresented. Second, smokers are included in the table; they have both lower body weights and earlier ages of death often related to lung cancer and heart disease. The table may therefore overestimate the best weight for maximum longevity. The Metropolitan Life height and weight table should therefore be used cautiously as a rough guideline in estimating appropriateness of body weight.

Other height and weight tables are available, including those generated by the National Health and Nutrition Examination Survey (NHANES I) (Table 12.17). Unlike the Metropolitan Life tables, which refer only to people under 60, the NHANES I table can be used for elderly people. The Andres Table (Table 12.18) can be used with healthy elderly people; it allows for a gradual increase in body fat as one ages through adulthood.

Enthusiasm has developed in recent years for using body mass index (BMI) to define obesity. BMI is calculated by dividing the person's weight in kilograms by his or her height in meters squared. Health risks from obesity begin when the BMI exceeds about 25. A BMI above 30 is often used as the cutoff for obesity. About 10% to 14% of North Americans exceed this value.

Methods are available for estimating body fatness directly rather than just assessing weight for height. The most widely used method measures skin-fold thicknesses. Because more than half of body fat lies under the skin, the thickness of the fat layer can be measured at specified sites using a special caliper. Data obtained can then be compared with age- and sex-specific standards. Other methods for measuring body fat storage directly have recently become available. One of these methods is bioelectrical impedance, a technique using a low-energy current. Because fat resists the flow of electricity, the analyzers in the device convert body electrical resistance into an estimate of the percentage of the body that is fat. Another method uses infrared light interactions with the fat and protein in arm muscle. A device about the size of a flashlight is held on the biceps muscle for several seconds while total body fat is estimated.

A recent trend has been to estimate the distribution of fat stores as well as the level of body fatness (Bjorntorp, 1987; Campaign, 1990; Fujioka, Matsuzawa, Tokunaga, & Tarui, 1987). This step is helpful in predicting the health risks of obesity in individuals. Risks to health appear to be greater when the preponderance of fat is

Table 12.16 Suggested Weights for Adults

	Weight (lb.)[b]			
	19-34 Years		*35 Years and Over*	
Height[a]	*Midpoint*	*Range*	*Midpoint*	*Range*
5′0"	112	97-128	123	108-138
5′1"	116	101-132	127	111-143
5′2"	120	104-137	131	115-148
5′3"	124	107-141	135	119-152
5′4"	128	111-146	140	122-157
5′5"	132	114-150	144	126-162
5′6"	136	118-155	148	130-167
5′7"	140	121-160	153	134-172
5′8"	144	125-164	158	138-178
5′9"	149	129-169	162	142-183
5′10"	153	132-174	167	146-188
5′11"	157	136-179	172	151-194
6′0"	162	140-184	177	155-199
6′1"	166	144-189	182	159-205
6′2"	171	148-195	187	164-210
6′3"	176	152-200	192	168-216
6′4"	180	156-205	197	173-222
6′5"	185	160-211	202	177-228
6′6"	190	164-216	208	182-234

SOURCE: U.S. Department of Agriculture amd U.S. Department of Health and Human Services, Home and Garden Bulletin No. 232, *Nutrition and Your Health: Dietary Guidelines for Americans*, 3rd ed. (Washington, DC: U.S. Government Printing Office, 1990).

NOTE: The higher weights in the ranges generally apply to men, who tend to have more muscle and bone; the lower weights more often apply to women, who have less muscle and bone. The higher weights for people aged 35 and older reflect recent research that seems to indicate that people can carry a little more wieght as they grow older without added risk to health.

a. Without shoes.

b. Without clothes.

distributed in the abdominal region (upper body and android obesity, "apple" shape) rather than around the hips and thighs (lower body or gynecoid obesity, "pear" shape) (see Figure 12.4). Hypertension, non-insulin-dependent diabetes mellitus, cardiovascular disease, and possibly breast cancer (Ballard-Barbash et al., 1990; Folsom et al., 1990) reportedly are more common in individuals with upper-body obesity. The basis for this phenomenon is currently the subject of much research; it has been proposed, however, that the androgen-driven upper body fat sets off a metabolic derangement involving increased lipolysis and hyperinsulinemia.

The ratio of waist circumference (at the level of the umbilicus) to hip circumference greater that 0.9 in men and 0.8 in women indicates android obesity. Only a small percentage of women have android obesity.

Significance of the Problem

Obesity is a serious health problem in North America and is considered to be one of the most important nutritional diseases in Western societies (NIH Consensus Development Conference, 1985). The goal of maintaining an ideal or desirable

Table 12.17 Desirable Weight[a] for Men and Women Aged 20 to 74 Years, by Height: United States, 1971-1974

Height (inches)[b]	*Weight (pounds)*[c]	
	Men	*Women*
57	—	113
58	—	117
59	—	120
60	—	123
61	—	127
62	136	130
63	140	134
64	145	137
65	150	140
66	155	144
67	159	147
68	163	151
69	168	154
70	173	158
71	178	—
72	182	—
73	187	—
74	192	—

SOURCE: National Health and Nutrition Examination Survey (1979).
a. Based on average weights estimated from regression equation of weight per height for men and women aged 20 to 29 years.
b. Height measured without shoes.
c. Clothing ranged from 0.20 to 0.62 lbs., which was not deducted from weight shown.

Table 12.18 Andres Table for Adults and the Elderly—Age-Specific Weight-for-Height Tables[a]

Height	*Weight range for men and women by age (years) in pounds*				
ft-in	*25*	*35*	*45*	*55*	*65*
4-10	84-111	92-119	99-127	107-135	115-142
4-11	87-115	95-123	103-131	111-139	119-147
5-0	90-119	98-127	106-135	114-143	123-152
5-1	93-123	101-131	110-140	118-148	127-157
5-2	96-127	105-136	113-144	122-153	131-163
5-3	99-131	108-140	117-149	126-158	135-168
5-4	102-135	112-145	121-154	130-163	140-173
5-5	106-140	115-149	125-159	134-168	144-179
5-6	109-144	119-154	129-164	138-174	148-184
5-7	112-148	122-159	133-169	143-179	153-190
5-8	116-153	126-163	137-174	147-184	158-196
5-9	119-157	130-168	141-179	151-190	162-201
5-10	122-162	134-173	145-184	156-195	167-207
5-11	126-167	137-178	149-190	160-201	172-213
6-0	129-171	141-183	153-195	165-207	177-219
6-1	133-176	145-188	157-200	169-213	182-225
6-2	137-181	149-194	162-206	174-219	187-232
6-3	141-186	153-199	166-212	179-225	192-238
6-4	144-191	157-205	171-218	184-231	197-244

SOURCE: Data are from Andres, R., Gerontology Research Center, National Institute of Aging, Baltimore, MD.
a. Values in this table are in pounds for height without shoes and weight without clothes. To convert inches to centimeters, multiply by 2.54; to convert pounds to kilograms, multiply by 0.455.

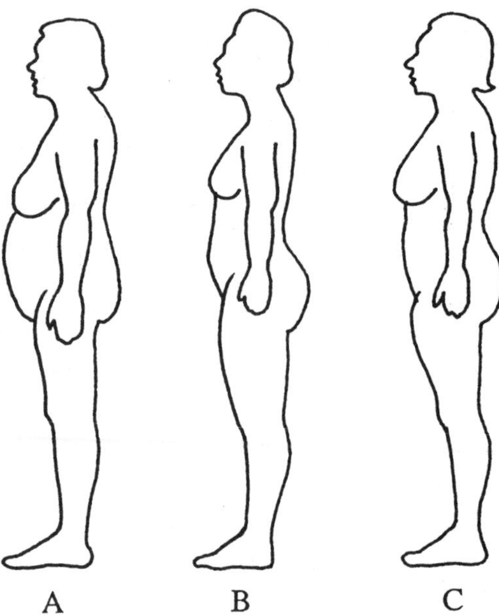

Figure 12.4. Classification of Body Fat Distribution by Photographic Assessment

NOTE: Shape A = android or central fat, primarily associated with males; Shape B = gyenecoid or peripheral body fat, primarily associated with females; Shape C = intermediate, somewhere between the other two types.

body weight has appeared in every set of health and nutrition recommendations published by governmental and not-for-profit organizations. Despite this prudent recommendation, the prevalence of obesity among Americans has remained unchanged or even increased in some demographic subgroups. Data from the second NHANES (1976-1980) estimated that nearly 1 of 4 adults is overweight and 1 of every 10 is severely overweight (National Center for Health Statistics, 1987). Females are more overweight than males, and black females are more overweight than white females.

Effort has recently been made to determine how the incidence of obesity has changed over time among adults in the United States (Williamson, Kahn, Remington, & Adra, 1990). A cohort of 9,862 men and women, aged 25 to 74 at baseline and 86% of whom were white, were identified from NHANES 1 and remeasured after 6.7 to 12.6 years. The authors defined major weight gain as an increase in BMI of > 5 kg/m^2 and overweight as a BMI of > 27.8 kg/m^2 for men and > 27.3 kg/m^2 for women. Overall, the authors found that BMI increased in men and women aged 25 to 54 years and decreased thereafter. Only 38% to 43% of men and 30% to 35% of women maintained their weight within 1 kg/m^2 of BMI. The incidence of major weight gain was greatest in the youngest age groups and approximately twice as high in women as in men (8.4% vs. 3.9%). Most significantly, women aged 24 to 44 years who were overweight at baseline had the highest incidence (14.2%) of major weight gain. Furthermore, the peak incidence of becoming overweight also occurred in the 35- to 44-year age group. Ethnic differences in body weight were more apparent among women. In addition to having higher mean BMI at baseline, young black women were 30% to 40% more likely to have experienced a major weight gain and nearly twice as likely to become overweight over the 10 years as white women.

Comparison of three successive prevalence studies conducted in the United States has revealed some alarming trends. Over a 20-year period, mean BMI has increased for both white and black women aged 18 to 34 years. The black/white differences seen in body weight have also persisted over this period. In addition, there has been an increased shift in the proportion of young adult women who are overweight and severely overweight.

The etiology for the age, gender, and racial differences in BMI and weight gain has been investigated in several population studies. In general, the prevalence of obesity in women varies inversely with socioeconomic status and educational level. However, these behavioral variables explain only a small portion of the difference; thus other unmeasured genetic and environmental influences are involved.

Consequence of Obesity

The hazards associated with the obese state are familiar to almost everyone. Diseases that occur more frequently in obese women include hypertension, coronary heart disease, thrombophlebitis, diabetes mellitus, gallbladder disease, osteoarthritis, and some cancers (including breast cancer). Obese individuals also are at greater risk for accidents, emotional disorders, and social discrimination. Menstrual abnormalities and ovarian dysfunction are more common in obese women, and they also carry a greater risk of adverse pregnancy course and outcome.

One positive circumstance for heavier women is their reduced risk of developing osteoporosis. It is speculated that the constant weight borne by the skeletal system helps maintain bone density to some degree over the years. It is also true that women with a distinct gynecoid distribution of fat are much less likely to suffer from many of the metabolic disorders mentioned earlier (Campaign, 1990).

Etiologic Factors

Many factors interplay in the process by which an individual becomes obese and then maintains that weight. Consideration of these factors is valuable in understanding the obese person and in designing effective treatment. Factors that should be assessed include (a) medical evaluation of physical health and documentation of metabolic aberrations, (b) history of weight gain, (c) measurement of the extent of the obesity (BMI, skin-fold measurements, fat tissue biopsy, if available), (d) family attitudes, (e) the role of the obese person in the family, (f) emotional and psychological status (self-concept and body image, self-esteem), (g) eating behavior (binges, eating at night, usual eating pattern, eating for emotional reasons), (h) activity and exercise habits, (i) social relationships, (j) motivation, and (k) reasons for desiring weight loss.

The importance of genetics in the establishment of this problem is now widely appreciated (Garn, 1986; Poehlman et al., 1986; Price, 1987; Price, Cadoret, Stunkard, & Troughton, 1987; Stunkard, Foch, & Hrubec, 1986; Stunkard et al., 1986), but eating behavior and exercise patterns clearly modify the extent of fat deposition (Ravussin, Lillioja, Anderson, Christian, & Borgardus, 1986; Van Itallie, 1986). Although it is known that weight loss is achievable through a variety of means, it is still unclear why maintenance of weight loss is so difficult for most people. Efforts are being made to define specific metabolic differences between lean and obese individuals (Elliot, Goldberg, Kuehl, & Bennett, 1989; Kern, Ong, Saffari, & Carty, 1990). Attention is also being given to identifying the means by which the "fat pad" communicates with the brain to ensure that the genetically mandated level of fatness is maintained over time. Pharmaceutical companies are investing heavily in research directed toward the development of drugs that will reduce appetite effectively or otherwise prevent or treat obesity (Rock & Coulston, 1988; Sullivan & Garrattini, 1985). Some experts say that by the year 2000, one or more such products may be available to the general public.

In a nutshell, our understanding of energy balance goes something like this. Energy balance depends on calorie input and calorie output; excessive input or decreased output will increase energy stores, primarily in adipose tissue. Many factors influence the desire to eat. Hunger is a sign of the physiological drive to find and eat food; appetite represents the psychological drive to find and eat food. When both of these drives are satisfied, the state of satiety is said to exist. Centers in the brain interact with other groups of cells in the brain and liver that participate in the complicated network of messages that control hunger and satiety. There are specific sites in the brain and other organs that, when stimulated, greatly affect (increase or decrease) the desire to seek and eat food. Many hormones and hormonelike compounds have been identified as potentially influential in affecting feeding behavior and satiety.

Most adults maintain a relatively stable body weight over months and years. The mechanism by which this takes place is unknown but the "comfort zone" for an individual has been referred to as the *set point.* It has been proposed that a compound (specifically a protein) is produced by adipose cells and released into the bloodstream to provide a communication link between adipose cells and the brain, allowing for body weight regulation. There is sound evidence that body weight is regulated. Loss of weight to a level below the set point, for example, is known to be associated with a defensive response; basal metabolic rate goes down, adipose tissue fat-synthesizing enzyme (lipoprotein lipase) levels go up, and constant hunger sets in. Over time, these effects usually lead to regain of the weight that was originally lost. Successful maintenance of body weight below the set point therefore is "painful" and requires much patience and perseverance.

Management Strategies

Although achieving and maintaining a reduced level of body fatness is known to be difficult, it is not impossible. Success is often associated with a pattern of gradual weight loss accompanied by a strong motivation to resist caloric temptations. Most successful weight management programs consist of three components: a sensible diet, an individualized exercise schedule, and a food habit management thrust.

A sound weight loss diet should include attention to a number of issues. Specifically, the following characteristics are desirable:

1. The diet should meet nutritional needs, except for calories.
2. The diet should allow adaptations to individual habits and tastes.
3. Slow and steady weight loss should be stressed.
4. The diet should minimize hunger and fatigue.
5. The diet should contain readily available foods.
6. The diet should be socially acceptable.
7. The diet should help change problem eating habits.
8. The diet should improve overall health.

Although moderation in total caloric intake is the primary concern, achieving this goal can usually be simplified by paying specific attention to moderating consumption of fat. Not only is dietary fat calorically dense, but it is very efficiently converted into body fat; only about 3% to 5% of the ingested calories are burned in the process. On the other hand, about 25% of ingested carbohydrate calories are burned in the process of laying down fat.

The importance of regular physical activity in a program of weight management cannot be overemphasized. Not only does exercise burn calories, but it also maintains or even increases lean body mass. Lean tissue is metabolically active 24 hours per day; the larger the lean body mass (which is mostly skeletal muscle), the higher the resting metabolic rate. The significance of this augmented metabolic rate is by no means trivial. The number of calories expended meeting resting needs each 24-hour day, 365 days per year, can make a major contribution to the energy expenditure side of the equation.

Long-term success in managing body weight usually involves a behavior modification effort. Close look at lifestyle and environment should be followed by definition of problem periods and behaviors and development of strategies to change them permanently. Psychologists use terms such as *chain-breaking, stimulus control, cognitive restructuring, contingency management,* and *self-monitoring* when discussing behavior management (Brownell, 1984):

Chain-breaking is breaking the link between two or more behaviors that encourage overeating, such as snacking while watching TV.

Stimulus control has to do with altering the environment to minimize the stimuli for eating, for example, removing foods from sight and storing them in the kitchen cabinet.

Cognitive restructuring means changing one's frame of mind regarding eating; for example, instead of using a difficult day as an excuse to overeat, substitute other pleasures for rewards, such as a relaxing walk with a friend.

Contingency management is forming a plan to respond to an environment where overeating is likely, such as when snacks are within arm's reach at a party.

Self-monitoring refers to tracking foods eaten and conditions affecting eating; actions are usually recorded in a diary, along with location, time, and state of mind. This is a tool that helps a person understand more about his or her eating habits.

Books and classes on behavior modification (specifically, food habit management) are widely available. In the end, however, dieters must analyze their own particular shortcomings and sensitize themselves to facets of their lifestyle that make dieting difficult. A written plan of action may be useful. Social support is always valuable. A system of rewards for both short-term and long-term successes may add incentive.

Even motivated dieters will periodically experience a lapse in their planned weight management routine. Such lapses should be viewed as expected and not as signals that failure is imminent. Plans for dealing with lapses can be made in advance. Encouragement from self and others to "stay calm" and "return to the original plan" may help prevent a true relapse in the weight control program.

Is Prevention of Obesity Possible?

Although level of body fatness is a characteristic that appears to be embedded in one's genes, it is certainly possible to create a lifestyle that limits the expression of this trait. In fact, because this "gene for obesity" seems to be widespread, conscientious efforts to develop a lifestyle emphasizing wise food choices and regular aerobic exercise make much sense. Establishing a "fat-minimizing" routine in childhood is in order. Aggressive thrust in this direction over the next several decades might reverse the trend toward rising adiposity, which has been evident for so long.

References

American Diabetes Association. (1985). Summary of recommendations from the Second International Workshop-Conference on Gestational Diabetes Mellitus. *Diabetes, 34*(Suppl. 2), 123-126.

American Psychiatric Association. (1987). *Diagnostic and statistical manual of mental disorders* (3rd ed., rev.). Washington, DC: Author.

Anderson, J. (1990). Dietary calcium and bone mass through the lifecycle. *Nutrition Today, 25*(2), 9-14.

Ashwell, M., Chinn, S., Stalley, S., & Garrow, J. S. (1978). Female fat distribution: A photographic and cellularity study. *International Journal of Obesity, 2,* 289-302.

Ballard-Barbash, R., Schatzkin, A., Carter, C., Kannel, W., Kreger, B., D'Agostino, R., Splansky, G., Anderson, K., & Helsel, W. (1990). Body fat distribution and breast cancer in the Framingham Study. *Journal of the National Cancer Institute, 82,* 286-290.

Benke, P. J. (1984). The isotretinoin teratogen syndrome. *JAMA, 251,* 3267-3269.

Bjorntorp, P. (1987). Classification of obese patients and complications related to the distribution of surplus fat. *American Journal of Clinical Nutrition, 45*(Suppl. 3), 1120-1125.

Bothwell, T. H., Charlton, R. W., Cook, J. D., & Finch, C. A. (1979). *Iron metabolism in man.* Cambridge, MA: Blackwell.

Bray, G. A. (1987). Obesity—A disease of nutrient or energy balance? *Nutrition Reviews, 45*(2), 33-43.

Brownell, K. D. (1984). The spychology and physiology of obesity: Implications for screening and treatment. *Journal of the American Dietetic Association, 84*(4), 404-414.

Buell, P. (1973). Changing incidence of breast cancer in Japanese-American women. *Journal of the National Cancer Institute, 51,* 1479-1483.

Campaign, B. N. (1990). Body fat distribution in females: Metabolic consequences and implications for weight loss. *Medical Science in Sports and Exercise, 22,* 291-297.

Carroll, K. (1986). Experimental studies of dietary fat and cancer in relation to epidemiologic data. *Progress in Clinical and Biological Research, 222,* 231-248.

Carruth, B. R., & Skinner, J. D. (1991). Practitioners beware: Regional, differences in beliefs about nutrition during pregnancy. *Journal of the American Dietetic Association, 91,* 435-440.

Casey, V., & Dwyer, J. (1987). Premenstrual syndrome: Theories and evidence. *Nutrition Today, 22*(6), 4-12.

Cauley, J., Gutai, J., Kuller, L., LeDonne, D., Sandler, R., Sashin, D., & Powell, J. (1988). Endogenous estrogen levels and calcium intake in postmenopausal women. *JAMA, 260,* 3150-3155.

Centers for Disease Control. (1990). Perinatal mortality and congenital malformations in infants born to women with insulin-dependent diabetes mellitus—United States, Canada and Europe, 1940-1988. *JAMA, 264,* 437-441.

Doll, H., Brown, S., Thurston, A., & Vessey, M. (1989). Pyridoxine (vitamin B_6) and the premenstrual syndrome: A randomized crossover trial. *Journal of the Royal College of General Practitioners, 39,* 364-368.

Drewnowski, A., Hopkins, S., & Kessler, R. (1988). The prevalence of bulimia nervosa in the U.S. college student population. *American Journal of Public Health, 78,* 1322-1325.

Elliot, D., Goldberg, L., Kuehl, R., & Bennett, W. (1989). Sustained depression of resting metabolic rate after massive weight loss. *American Journal of Clinical Nutrition, 49*(1), 93-96.

Fujioka, S., Matsuzawa, Y., Tokunaga, K., & Tarui, S. (1987). Contribution of intraabdominal fat accumulation to the impairment of glucose and lipid metabolism in human obesity. *Metabolism, 36*(1), 54-59.

Gabbe, S. G. (1985). Management of diabetes mellitus in pregnancy. *American Journal of Obstetrics and Gynecology, 153,* 824-830.

Garn, S. (1986). Family-line and socioeconomic factors in fitness and obesity. *Nutrition Reviews, 44,* 381-386.

Gold, P., Gwirtsman, H., Avgerinos, P., Nieman, L. K., Gallucci, W. T., Kaye, W., Jimerson, D., Ebert, M., Rittmaster, R., Loriaux, D. L., & Associates. (1986). Abnormal hypothalamic-pituitary-adrenal function in anorexia nervosa. *New England Journal of Medicine, 314,* 1335-1342.

Goodwin, P., & Boyd, N. (1987). Critical appraisal of the evidence that dietary fat intake is related to breast cancer risk in humans. *Journal of the National Cancer Institute, 79,* 473-485.

Hambidge, K. M., Krebs, N. E., Sibley, L., & English, J. (1987). Acute effects of iron therapy on zinc status during pregnancy. *Obstetrics and Gynecology, 70,* 593-596.

Hambidge, K. M., Neider, K. H., & Walravens, P. A. (1975). Zinc, acrodermatitis and congenital malformations. *Lancet, 1,* 577.

Health and Public Policy Committee, American College of Physicians. (1986). Eating disorders: Anorexia nervosa and bulimia. *Annals of Internal Medicine, 105,* 790-794.

Herzog, D., & Copeland, P. (1985). Eating disorders. *New England Journal of Medicine, 313,* 295-303.

Hirayama, T. (1978). Epidemiology of breast cancer with special reference to the role of diet. *Preventive Medicine, 7*(2), 173-195.

Holbrook, T., Barrett-Connor, E., & Wingard, D. (1988). Dietary calcium and risk of hip fracture: 14 year perspective population study. *Lancet, 2,* 1046-1049.

Horner, R. D., Lackey, C. J., & Kolasa, K. (1991). Pica practices of pregnant women. *Journal of the American Dietetic Association, 91,* 34-38.

Horsman, A., Gallagher, J. C., Simpson, M., & Nordin, B. E. C. (1977). Prospective trial of O-estrogen and calcium in postmenopausal women. *British Medical Journal, 2,* 789-792.

Howe, G., Hirohata, T., Hislop, G., Iscovich, J., Yuan, J., Katsouyanni, K., Lubin, F., Marubini, E., Modan, B., Rohan, T., Toniolo, P., & Shunzhang, Y. (1990). Dietary factors and risk of breast cancer: Combined analysis of 12 case-control studies. *Journal of the National Cancer Institute, 82,* 561-569.

Hunt, I. F., Murphy, N. J., Cleaver, A. E., Faraji, B., Swenseid, M. E., Coulson, A. H., Clark, V. A., Browdy, B. L., Cabalum, M. T., & Smith, J. C. (1984). Zinc supplementation during pregnancy: Effects of selected blood constituents on progress and outcome of pregnancy in low-income women of Mexican descent. *American Journal of Clinical Nutrition, 40,* 508-521.

Institute of Medicine. (1990). *Nutrition during pregnancy: Weight gain and nutrient supplements.* Washington, DC: National Academy Press.

Institute of Medicine. (1991). *Nutrition during lactation.* Washington, DC: National Academy Press.

International Agency for Research on Cancer. (1987). *Cancer incidence in five continents* (Vol. 5, IARC Scientific Publication No. 88). Lyon: Author.

Jameson, S. (1976). Effects of zinc deficiency on human reproduction. *Acta Medica Scandinavica,* (Suppl. 593), 5-64.

Jameson, S. (1981). Zinc and pregnancy. In J. O. Nriagu (Ed.), *Zinc in the environment: Part II. Health effects* (pp. 183-197). New York: John Wiley.

Joesoef, M., Beral, V., Rolfs, R., Aral, S., & Cramer, D. (1990). Are caffeinated beverages risk factors for delayed conception? *Lancet, 1,* 136-137.

Jones, D., Schatzkin, A., Green, S., Block, G., Brinton, L., Ziegler, R., Hoover, R., & Taylor, P. (1987). Dietary fat and breast cancer in the National Health and Nutrition Examination Survey I Epidemiologic Follow-up Study. *Journal of the National Cancer Institute, 79,* 465-471.

Katzman, M., Wolchick, S., & Braver, S. (1984). The prevalence of frequent binge eating and bulimia in a nonclinical college sample. *International Journal of Eating Disorders, 3,* 53-62.

Kelsey, J. L., & Berkowitz, G. S. (1988). Breast cancer epidemiology. *Cancer Research, 48*(20), 5615-5623.

Kern, P., Ong, J., Saffari, B., & Carty, J. (1990). The effects of weight loss on the activity and expression of adipose-tissue lipoprotein lipase in very obese humans. *New England Journal of Medicine, 322,* 1053-1059.

Kirkley, B. G. (1986). Bulimia: Clinical characteristics, development and etiology. *Journal of the American Dietetic Association, 86,* 468-475.

Kurtzman, F., Yager, J., & Landsverk, J. (1989). Eating disorders among selected female populations at UCLA. *Journal of the American Dietetic Association, 89,* 45-53.

Lammer, E. J., Chen, D. T., Hoar, R. M., Agnish, N. D., Benke, J. J., Braun, J. T., Curry, C. J., Fernhoff, P. M., Brix, A. W., Lott, I. T., Richard, L. M., & Sun, S. C. (1985). Retinoic acid embryopathy. *New England Journal of Medicine, 313,* 837-841.

Laurence, K. H., James, N., Miller, M. H., Tennant, G. B., & Campbell, H. (1981). Double-blind randomized controlled trial of folate treatment before conception to prevent recurrence of neural-tube defects. *British Medical Journal, 282,* 1509-1511.

Lazebnik, N., Kuhnert, B. R., Kuhnert, P. M., & Thompson, K. L. (1988). Zinc status, pregnancy complications and labor abnormalities. *American Journal of Obstetrics and Gynecology, 158,* 161-166.

Lutz, J., & Tesar, R. (1990). Mother-daughter pairs: Spinal and femoral bone densities and dietary intakes. *American Journal of Clinical Nutrition, 52,* 872-877.

Mills, J. L., Rhoads, G. G., Simpson, J. L., Cunningham, G. C., Conley, M. R., Lassman, M. R., Walden, M. E., Depp, O. R., Hoffman, H. J., & National Institute of Child Health and Human Development Neural Tube Defects Study Group. (1989). The absence of a relation between the periconceptional use of vitamins and neural tube defects. *New England Journal of Medicine, 321,* 430-435.

Milunsky, A., Jick, H., Jick, S. S., Bruell, C. L., MacLaughlin, D. S., Rothman, K. J., & Willett, W. (1989). Multivitamin/folic acid supplementation in early pregnancy reduces the prevalence of neural tube defects. *JAMA, 262,* 2847-2852.

Mintz, L., & Betz, N. (1988). Prevalence of correlates of eating disordered behaviors among undergraduate women. *Journal of Counseling Psychology, 35,* 463-471.

Mulinare, J., Cordero, J. F., Erickson, J. D., & Berry, R. J. (1988). Periconceptional use of multivitamins and the occurrence of neural tube defects. *JAMA, 260,* 3141-3145.

National Center for Health Statistics. (1987). Anthropometric reference data and prevalence of overweight, United States 1976-1980. *Vital and health statistics* (Series 11, No. 238; DHHS Publication No. 87-1688). Washington, DC: Government Printing Office.

National Institutes of Health Consensus Development Conference. (1985). Health implications of obesity. *Annals of Internal Medicine, 103,* 1073-1077.

National Research Council. (1978). *Laboratory studies of nutritional status in pregnancy.* Washington, DC: National Academy Press.

National Research Council. (1989). *Recommended dietary allowances* (10th ed.). Washington, DC: Academy Press.

Nelson, P. A., & Kilbury, A. (1987). Nutritional support of pregnant diabetic patients. In B. S. Nuwayhid, C. R. Brinkman, & S. M. Lieb (Eds.), *Management of the diabetic pregnancy* (pp. 168-213). New York: Elsevier.

Newman, V., & Lee, D. (1991). Developing a daily food guide for women. *Journal of Nutrition Education, 23*(2), 76-82.

Palla, B., & Litt, I. F. (1988). Medical complications of eating disorders in adolescents. *Pediatrics, 81,* 613-623.

Patterson, C. M., Whelan, D. P., Rock, C. L., & Lyon, T. J. (1989). *Nutrition and eating disorders.* Van Nuys, CA: PM, Inc.

Poehlman, E., Tremblay, A., Despres, J., Fontaine, E., Perusse, L., Theriault, G., & Bouchard, C. (1986). Genotype-controlled changes in body composition and fat morphology following overfeeding in twins. *American Journal of Clinical Nutrition, 43,* 723-731.

Pollitzer, W., & Anderson, J. (1989). Ethnic and genetic differences in bone mass: A review with an hereditary vs. environmental perspective. *American Journal of Clinical Nutrition, 50,* 1244-1259.

Prentice, R., Kakar, F., Hursting, S., Sheppard, L., Klein, R., & Kushi, L. (1989). Aspects of the rationale for the Women's Health Trial. *Journal of the National Cancer Institute, 80,* 802-814.

Price, A. (1987, January). Genetics of human obesity. *Annals of Behavioral Medicine,* pp. 9-14.

Price, R., Cadoret, R., Stunkard, A., & Troughton, E. (1987). Genetic contributions to human fatness: An adoption study. *American Journal of Psychiatry, 144,* 1003-1008.

Pyle, R., Mitchell, J., Eckert, E., Halvorson, P., Newman, P., & Goff, G. (1983). The incidence of bulimia in freshman college students. *International Journal of Eating Disorders, 2,* 75-85.

Ravussin, E., Lillioja, S., Anderson, T., Christian, L., & Bogardus, C. (1986). Determinants of 24-hour energy expenditure in man. *Journal of Clinical Investigation, 78,* 1568-1578.

Reid, R., & VanVugt, D. (1987). Weight-related changes in reproductive function. *Fertility and Sterility, 48,* 905-913.

Rigotti, N., Nussbaum, S., Herzog, D., & Neer, R. (1984). Osteoporosis in women with anorexia nervosa. *New England Journal of Medicine, 311,* 1601-1606.

Rock, C., & Coulston, A. (1988). Weight control approaches: A review by the California Dietetic Association. *Journal of the American Dietetic Association, 88,* 44-51.

Rohan, T. E., & Bain, C. J. (1987). Diet in the etiology of breast cancer. *Epidemiologic Reviews, 9,* 120-145.

Rosa, F. W., Wilk, A. L., & Kelsey, F. O. (1986). Teratogen update: Vitamin A congeners. *Teratology, 33*(3), 355-364.

Schotte, D., & Stunkard, A. (1987). Bulimia vs. bulimic behaviors on a college campus. *JAMA, 258,* 1213-1216.

Seeman, E., Hopper, J., Bach, L., Cooper, M., Parkinson, E., McKay, J., & Jerums, G. (1989). Reduced bone mass in daughters of women with osteoporosis. *New England Journal of Medicine, 320,* 554-558.

Sheppard, S., Nevin, N., Seller, H., Wild, J., Smithells, R., Read, A., Harris, R., & Fielding, D. (1989). Neural tube defect recurrence after "partial" vitamin supplementation. *Journal of Medical Genetics, 26,* 326-329.

Smith, E., Gilligan, C., Smith, P., & Sempos, C. (1989). Calcium supplementation and bone loss in middle-aged women. *American Journal of Clinical Nutrition, 50,* 833-842.

Smithells, R., Nevin, N., Seller, M., Sheppard, S., Harris, R., Read, A., Fielding, D., Walker, S., Schorah, C., & Wild, J. (1983). Further experience of vitamin supplementation for prevention of neural tube defect recurrences. *Lancet, 1,* 1027-1030.

Smithells, R., Sheppard, S., Schorah, C., Seller, J., Nevin, N., Harris, R., Read, A., & Fielding, D. (1980). Possible prevention of neural-tube defects by periconceptional vitamin supplementation. *Lancet, 1,* 339-340.

Smithells, R., Sheppard, S., Schorah, C., Seller, J., Nevin, N., Harris, R., Read, A., & Fielding, D. (1981). Apparent prevention of neural tube defects by periconceptional vitamin supplementation. *Archives of Diseases in Childhood, 56,* 911-918.

Soltan, M., & Jenkins, M. (1982). Maternal and fetal plasma zinc concentration and fetal abnormality. *British Journal of Obstetrics and Gynecology, 89*(1), 56-58.

Stewart, B., Robinson, G., Goldbloom, D., & Wright, C. (1990). Infertility and eating disorders. *American Journal of Obstetrics and Gynecology, 163,* 1576-1577.

Story, M. (1986). Nutrition management and dietary treatment of bulimia. *Journal of the American Dietetic Association, 86,* 517-519.

Stunkard, A., Foch, T., & Hrubec, Z. (1986). A twin study of human obesity. *Journal of the American Dietetic Association, 256,* 51-54.

Stunkard, A., Sorengen, T., Hanis, C., Teasdale, T., Chakaborty, R., Schull, W., & Schulsinger, F. (1986). An adoption study of human obesity. *New England Journal of Medicine, 314,* 193-198.

Sullivan, A., & Garrattini, S. (Eds.). (1985). *Novel approaches and drugs for obesity.* Lancaster, PA: Technomic.

Teratology Society. (1987). Teratology Society position paper: Recommendations for vitamin A use during pregnancy. *Teratology, 35,* 269-275.

Treasure, J., & Russell, G. (1987). Reversible bone loss in anorexia nervosa. *British Medical Journal, 295,* 474-475.

U.S. Department of Agriculture. (1990). *Dietary guidelines for Americans* (DHHS Home and Garden Bulletin No. 232). Washington, DC: Government Printing Office.

U.S. Department of Health, Education, and Welfare. (1979). *National Health and Nutrition Examination Survey.* Health Services and Mental Health Administration, Centers for Disease Control, Atlanta, GA.

Van Itallie, T. (1986). Bad news and good news about obesity. *New England Journal of Medicine, 314,* 239-240.

Wald, N. (1984). Neural tube defects and vitamins: The need for randomized clinical trial. *British Journal of Obstetrics and Gynecology, 91,* 516-523.

Wilcox, A., Weinberg, C., & Baird, D. (1988). Caffeinated beverages and decreased fertility. *Lancet, 2,* 1453-1455.

Willett, W., Stampfer, M., Colditz, G., Rosner, B., Hennekens, H., & Speiker, F. (1987). Dietary fat and the risk of breast cancer. *New England Journal of Medicine, 316,* 22-28.

Williamson, D., Kahn, H., Remington, P., & Adra, R. (1990). The 10-year incidence of overweight and major weight gain in U.S. adults. *Archives of Internal Medicine, 150,* 665-672.

Worthington-Roberts, B., & Williams, S. (1989). *Nutrition in pregnancy and lactation.* St. Louis, MO: C. V. Mosby.

Wynn, A., & Wynn, M. (1990). The need for nutritional assessment in the treatment of the infertile patient. *Journal of Nutritional Medicine, 1,* 315-324.

13

Exercise

CHERYL A. CAHILL

Over the last decade, regular physical exercise has been recognized to be to an essential component of a healthy lifestyle. Regular exercise has been shown to improve cardiopulmonary function, skeletal and muscle integrity, and psychological well-being. Epidemiological studies of the effects of exercise on disease prevention and longevity of life are less conclusive, but the evidence to date suggests that regular physical activity can prevent and control coronary heart disease, hypertension, non-insulin-dependent diabetes, osteoporosis, obesity, and mental health problems (Harris, Caspersen, DeFriese, & Estes, 1989). Because much of the research involving the effects of exercise has been conducted on men, the particular benefits to women's health are not well understood. This chapter includes a review of the effects of exercise on the psychophysiological well-being of women and a discussion of therapeutic exercise programs for women.

Metabolic Effects of Exercise

Exercise increases metabolic demands for nutrients and oxygen accompanied by needs to eliminate metabolic wastes and heat within skeletal muscle cells. The systemic effects of exercise are related to physiological mechanisms governing delivery of oxygen and nutrients to individual muscle cells. Regular exercise results in more efficient oxygen and nutrient use by the skeletal muscle cell and improved capacity of oxygen and nutrient delivery systems to meet added demands. Cardiopulmonary fitness is equivalent to the overall capacity of an individual to accomplish work while efficiently using oxygen. A clear understanding of the way muscle cells use oxygen and nutrients is essential for the nurse who may prescribe exercise for a client.

Skeletal Muscle Cell Metabolism

Although exercise depends on adequate functioning of the musculoskeletal system under the control of the nervous system, nearly every other physiological function is affected by exercise as well. Understanding muscle cell function and metabolism is at the core of understanding the physiological consequences of exercise. The overall function of a muscle cell is to shorten and lengthen in response to neurological stimulation. Coordinated shortening or contraction of skeletal muscle followed by lengthening or relaxation results in functional movement.

There are two basic muscle fiber types. Type 1, slow-twitch muscle cells have high oxidative capacity, which means that this type of cell has a greater capacity to produce adenosine triphosphate (ATP) via aerobic pathways. Type 2, fast-twitch fibers, have a greater capacity to produce ATP by the anaerobic process of glycolysis. Type 2 fibers may be most useful at the onset of exercise before the cardiorespiratory system has been able to adequately supply the Type 1 muscles with oxygen. The distribution of muscle cell types within an individual is genetically determined. The contractile qualities and glycolytic capacities of each cell are also genetically conferred. A program of exercise can influence the oxidative capabilities of the cell. After a program of physical training, the number of mitochondria in muscle cells has been reported to increase (Ryan, 1990). The number of slow-twitch muscle fibers also increases.

The primary compound used by the skeletal muscle cell for energy is ATP. In the mitochondria, ATP supplies energy when it is converted to adenosine diphosphate (ADP) and phosphate. In the process of this conversion, electrons are released by ATP and used in various biochemical reactions. In the muscles, electron transfer is a major component of contraction. Thus ATP is a source of energy because of its capacity to provide electrons or energy for other biochemical reactions. ATP is derived in the cell from glucose and other nutrients.

The biochemistry of ATP production differs with the amount of oxygen available. In the absence of oxygen, anaerobic mechanisms produce ATP. In anaerobic glycolysis, the 6-carbon sugar, glucose, is cleaved into two 3-carbon molecules of pyruvic acid or pyruvate. Pyruvate is then converted into lactic acid and released into the extracellular fluid. Glycolysis is a very inefficient use of glucose, yielding only about 5% of the ATP that could be produced in the presence of oxygen. There are limited quantities of glucose and ATP stored in muscle cells, and these substrates are quickly exhausted. Therefore, anaerobic production of ATP does not supply adequate energy to muscles to sustain activity for long periods of time.

Aerobic production of ATP will sustain activity (see Figure 13.1). When adequate supplies of oxygen are available, glucose, pyruvic acid, and other nutrients are converted to acetyl CoA. Acetyl CoA passes into the mitochondria, where it is catabolized into carbon dioxide, water, and ATP. The biochemical production of ATP from acetyl CoA is known as the Kreb's cycle. Of the ATP used, 90% is produced by this very important process.

Increased muscle activity stimulates glycolysis. As long as adequate amounts of oxygen are available, pyruvate produced by glycolysis is converted to acetyl CoA, which provides the energy needed by the muscle via the Kreb's cycle. However, if muscle activity exceeds the capacity of the cardiopulmonary system to provide sufficient oxygen, pyruvate is converted to lactic acid.

Nutrient and Oxygen Delivery to Skeletal Muscle Cells During Exercise

Because the capacity of the muscle cell to work is based on availability of ATP, and ATP is most plentiful when oxygen is available, the amount of oxygen used indicates the effectiveness of the cardiorespiratory system to meet oxygen and nutrient needs. Oxygen consumption (VO_2) is a function of heart rate, stroke volume, and arterial and venous oxygen concentration differences. The ability of the cardiopulmonary system to meet the need for oxygen and nutrients during exercise may be referred to as maximum aerobic capacity.

Gender differences in the maximum aerobic capacity have been noted in adults but are not observed in children. Smaller hearts, lower hemoglobin levels, lower blood volume, and smaller lung size contribute to lower maximum aerobic capacity in women (Harris, 1991). Yet well-trained women athletes may demonstrate superior maximum aerobic capacity when compared to sedentary men. The considerable overlap in maximum aerobic capacity among women and men of varying fitness levels and sizes suggests that women should not be excluded from activities based on this gender difference. Evidence suggests that women and men adapt to endurance training in exactly the same way (Pollock

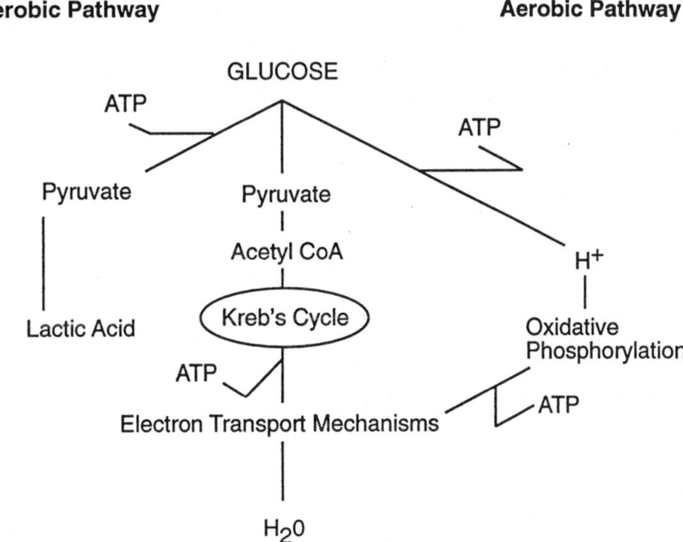

Figure 13.1. The Metabolism of Glucose
NOTE: The metabolism of glucose is dependent on the amount of oxygen available. The left side of the figure illustrates the anaerobic pathway. The remainder illustrates the aerobic pathway. ATP produced by glucose catabolism is used by the electron transport mechanisms of the muscle cell for energy during contraction. Note that the aerobic pathway is much more efficient than the anaerobic, producing considerably more ATP.

& Wilmore, 1990), indicating that similar training activities may be used with both sexes.

Because heart rate increases as the intensity of muscle activity increases, the amount of work that can be accomplished is limited by the capacity to increase heart rate. The maximum heart rate attainable by a healthy individual is dependent on age. A rough estimate of maximal heart rate can be calculated by subtracting the individual's age from 220. So, at age 40, a healthy individual will reach maximal exercise capacity when the heart rate is 180. However, the individual would be unable to maintain that level of activity for very long.

Stroke volume, that is, the amount of blood ejected from the left ventricle during systole, increases with exercise as well. The maximal increase in stroke volume occurs at approximately 50% of maximal heart rate. In the 40-year-old, that would correspond to a pulse of 90 beats per minute. Stroke volume increases very little beyond that point, probably because of the shortened diastolic filling time at rapid heart rates. Increases in stroke volume are due to increased cardiac muscle contractility during exercise.

The net effect of increased heart rate and stroke volume is increased cardiac output, which means that the rate at which oxygen and nutrients are supplied to the muscles is increased. To further enhance the delivery of essential substrates during exercise, blood flow is redirected to those organs requiring additional oxygen. Blood flow increases to large muscle groups, the lungs, and the myocardium. Blood flow to the skin also increases to assist with temperature regulation. Flow is maintained to the brain but is reduced to the gastrointestinal tract. In addition to cardiac changes, systolic blood pressure increases with little change in diastolic blood pressure in healthy adults. Concurrent with changes in the cardiovascular system, respiratory rate and blood flow to the lungs increase. Oxygen diffusion increases in the lung as well as at the cell level. The overall effect of these actions is to ensure adequate delivery of oxygen and nutrients to skeletal muscle cells in maintaining aerobic glucose metabolism.

Exercise Effects on Glucose Metabolism

Glucose use can increase as much as 20-fold over basal rates during exercise and accounts for 25% to 40% of the energy used (Leon, 1989). Despite this remarkable demand, exercise does not result in marked reduction in blood glucose levels. Increased demands for fuel by skeletal muscles during exercise are met by activation of several mechanisms that provide carbohydrates and fats as metabolic substrates. At the onset of exercise, the primary fuel used by the cell is stored glycogen. Because this reserve is limited, continued exercise requires resupply of glycogen and glucose to the cell. An additional source of energy is supplied by the mobilization of lipids from adipose tissue for conversion to glucose and subsequent catabolism in the cell.

The liver plays a key role in maintenance of adequate supplies of glucose during exercise. Initially, increased glucose is provided to the cells by increased production of glucose from hepatic stores of glycogen. These stores are limited, and prolonged exercise results in an accelerated rate of production of glycogen to replenish supplies. Gluconeogenesis uses pyruvate, lactate, and some amino acids to produce glycogen, which is then converted to glucose by glycogenolysis. Conversion of lipids and fatty acids to glucose and subsequent metabolism of it by the cell contributes to two major positive effects of exercise on reducing cardiovascular risk factors, weight loss and reduced plasma concentrations of lipoproteins and triglycerides.

Depletion of glycogen stores in both the muscles and the liver stimulates production of the enzyme glycogen synthase (Bak, Jacobsen, Jorgensen, & Pedersen, 1989). This enzyme appears to be responsible for increased non-insulin-dependent uptake of glucose by skeletal muscle cells. Increased activity of this enzyme persists up to 48 hours after strenuous exercise stops (Leon, 1989; Rogers, 1989). Evidently, during this time depleted cellular stores of glycogen are replenished. Highly trained athletes are reported to have lower resting insulin levels and enhanced tolerance to glucose loading, which may reflect increased glycogen synthase levels.

At rest, glucose metabolism is dependent on adequate supplies of insulin. Exercise has been shown to increase glucose uptake by skeletal muscles (Sahlin, 1990), whereas plasma levels of insulin fall. Reductions in plasma insulin levels are related not only to increased non-insulin-dependent skeletal muscle uptake of glucose, thereby reducing the demand for insulin, but also to increased insulin receptor activity (Leon, 1989). The combination of these two mechanisms facilitates delivery of glucose to the muscle cell; however, for the diabetic, special consideration must be given to maintenance of glucose metabolism during exercise.

Several investigators have considered exercise-induced changes in carbohydrate metabolism within the context of the pathophysiology of diabetes mellitus. Type I or insulin-dependent diabetes mellitus (IDDM) results from severe insulin deficiency associated with failure to produce biologically active insulin. Treatment requires supplementing endogenous insulin with various injected forms of the hormone. Adequate control of carbohydrate metabolism is difficult in IDDM. Increased non-insulin-dependent uptake of glucose consequent to vigorous exercise may require modification of the usual insulin dose (Wasserman & Abumrad, 1989). In general, a reduction in insulin dosage and the added ingestion and continual availability of carbohydrates are wise precautions for individuals with IDDM to take when exercising at strenuous levels (Ekoe, 1989). These aspects must be considered when prescribing or supervising a program of exercise for IDDM patients.

Type II or non-insulin-dependent diabetes mellitus (NIDDM) is associated with decreased availability of biologically active insulin. Treatment of this condition is usually limited to dietary regulation, weight loss, and possibly oral hypoglycemic drugs. Several investigators have considered the effects of exercise on glucose metabolism in these individuals as possible preventive measures or treatments for NIDDM. The effect of exercise most intriguing to these investigators is the apparent effect of exercise in increasing insulin receptor activity. One characteristic of Type II diabetes may be that the insulin receptor becomes insensitive or resistant to the effects of insulin. Increasing the activity of the receptor thus reduces resistance to insulin and normalizes insulin-mediated glucose metabolism. Rogers (1989) has reported that normalization of the glucose tolerance test was achieved in a group of mildly non-insulin-dependent diabetic men but only after 12 months of fairly intense physical activity. The glucose tolerance test was normal if it was administered within 18 hours of the last exercise period. Pasternostro-Bayles, Wing, and Robertson (1989) reported that beneficial alterations in glucose metabolism could be induced by moderate exercise performed for 20 to 40 minutes. Women in this study with mild Type II diabetes walked vigorously for 20 to 40 minutes and demonstrated lowered blood glucose levels. However, the ingestion of a meal eliminated the effect. These data suggest that exercise can increase insulin effectiveness with NIDDM, but the short duration of the effect and the level of exercise demanded could limit therapeutic usefulness. Because obesity is a common complication in NIDDM, regular moderate activity may prove useful in modulating weight.

Exercise Effects on Calcium Metabolism

Weight-bearing exercise has been shown to play a significant role in the development and maintenance of the skeletal system. Experiments conducted by the National Aeronautics and Space Administration on the effects of weightlessness on muscle function and bone changes have demonstrated that even short periods of nonweight-bearing inactivity can result in profound demineralization of the bone. Loss of mineral content of bone has been associated with aging in both women and men. Women seem to experience more problems associated with demineralization or osteoporosis. Clinical problems include greater incidence of fractures, particularly of the hip, and severe pain from osteoporosis of the spine.

Explanations for the apparent sex differences in bone loss with age are unclear. Because osteoporosis is a major clinical problem of postmenopausal women, a role for estrogen in modulating bone mineral content has been proposed (Bunt, 1990). Correlational studies of the relationship between bone mass and estrogen levels are inconclusive and contradictory, although the evidence seems to favor the conclusion that adequate levels of estrogen and calcium are essential in maintaining bone density. The major evidence for this conclusion is that osteoporosis is associated with anorexia nervosa. Young women who are both anorexic and amenorrheic demonstrate the most dramatic loss of bone mass (Bachrach, Guido, Katzman, Litt, & Marchas, 1990). Bunt (1990) has also reported that conditioned women athletes with exercise-related amenorrhea also demonstrate less bone mass than do athletes who menstruate regularly.

The role of exercise without regard to estrogen levels is a little clearer. Birge and Dalsky (1989) have reported that prospective studies have shown that regular weight-bearing exercise has a role in preventing age-related osteoporosis. Chow, Harrison, and Dornan (1989) have reported that exercise improved or arrested bone mass loss in 80% of patients who exercised. The effect of 1 hour per day of vigorous walking on the bone density of the neck of the femurs of 141 women demonstrated a significant increase in bone density after 1 year (Zylstra, Hopkins, Erk, Hreshchyshyn, & Anbar, 1989). Smith, Gilligan, McAdam, Ensign, and Smith (1989) reported that exercise prevented bone loss but did not increase bone density. After reviewing the literature and analyzing the results and effectiveness of research design and data analysis, Block, Smith, Friedlander, and Genant (1989) concluded that "exercise may have only limited value in protecting bone mass in the short term" (p. 17). Therefore, prescription of regular exercise for all clients to prevent osteoporosis may be premature. This conclusion is supported by a study of the bone density of apparently normally ovulating premenopausal women, including a group of women runners and a group of women marathon runners reported by Prior, Vigna, Schechter, and Burgess (1990). There were no significant differences in the amount of bone loss experienced in 1 year across groups. Women with the greatest amount of bone loss were those who experienced ovulatory disturbances reflected in shortened luteal phases or anovulation.

Caution must be used when prescribing exercise for individuals with osteoporosis because of the increased risk of bone fracture. Also, consideration of strength and postural stability must be included when recommending increased activity for the elderly or frail person. In all cases, for exercise therapy to affect bone density, adequate nutritional intake of calcium must be ensured.

Exercise Effects on Lipid Metabolism

There are two major forms of cholesterol, low-density lipoprotein cholesterol (LDL-C) and high-density lipoprotein cholesterol (HDL-C). Total cholesterol (TC) content of plasma is the sum total of LDL-C and HDL-C. LDL-C plays a significant role in the development of atheroma. As a category, these lipoproteins bind to specific receptors on the intima of the arteries and disrupt smooth muscle growth (Upton, 1990). The net effect is histological transformation of the normal intima to an atheroma. The HDL-C, on the other hand, is protective of the cardiovascular system. Molecules of HDL-C bind to specific receptors in the liver and facilitate removal of cholesterol from peripheral tissues. The

Table 13.1 Recommended Cholesterol Norms

	Desirable	*Borderline High*	*High*
Total cholesterol	Less than 200 mg/dl	200 mg/dl to 239 mg/dl	240 mg/dl or higher
Low-density lipoproteins	Less than 130 mg/dl	130 mg/dl to 159 mg/dl	160 mg/dl or higher
High-density lipoproteins	Greater than 35 mg/dl	Less than 35 mg/dl	Less than 35 mg/dl

SOURCE: Report of the National Cholesterol Education Program Expert Panel on Detection: Evaluation and Treatment of High Blood Cholesterol in Adults (1988).

proportion of HDL-C to TC levels is inversely proportional to the risk of cardiovascular disease. That is, the greater the percentage of TC that is of the HDL-C type the lower the risk of cardiovascular disease. Modification of dietary intake of cholesterol and saturated fats will help to lower cholesterol levels and lower weight.

Studies in both women and men demonstrate that a program of moderate exercise maintained over time effectively lowers blood cholesterol levels. The data are mixed as to differential effects on HDL-C and LDL-C and effects associated with sex differences. In sedentary premenopausal women, TC levels are generally lower with a higher proportion of HDL-C than in age-matched sedentary men (Boyd & McGuire, 1990). In both women and men, a program of moderate exercise will lower TC and increase the ratio of HDL-C to TC (Jula, Ronnemaa, Rastas, Karvetti, & Maki, 1990; Lokey & Tran, 1989). The change in the ratio of HDL-C to TC translates into an improved cardiovascular risk index. The mechanism by which exercise affects cholesterol blood levels is not clear. Lokey and Tran (1989) conducted a meta-analysis of the available data regarding the effects of exercise on women's lipid profile. The results demonstrate that exercise reduces TC and triglyceride levels and improves the ratio of HDL-C to TC, but there is no reduction of LDL-C cholesterol or an increase in HDL-C. Initiation of a regular program of exercise is generally accompanied by a reduction in body weight and, in many cases, a general improvement in health practices. Many who are motivated to begin a fitness program are also motivated to stop or reduce smoking and to choose a healthier diet. Therefore, differentiating the effect of exercise from other lifestyle changes on lipid profiles is difficult.

The degree to which exercise effectively reduces cholesterol is dependent on the state of the individual at the outset of therapy. Individuals with the worst lipid profiles have the greatest need for improvement and respond rather quickly to intervention. However, significant improvement in very high-risk individuals may take several months. Ideally, TC levels should be maintained below 200 mg per dl with a high percentage of HDL-C ("Report of the National Cholesterol Education Program Expert Panel," 1988). Triglyceride and LDL-C levels should be reduced as much as possible (see Table 13.1). Estrogen levels play an important role in modifying lipid metabolism, particularly that related to HDL-C production.

Sex differences in lipid metabolism are mediated by the effects of estrogen. Premenopausal women are reported to have higher concentrations of HDL-C than do age-matched males. Women who smoke effectively eliminate any positive effect of estrogen on cholesterol levels and increase their risk of cardiovascular disease to that of men (Bush, 1990; Cohn, Brand, & Hulley, 1989). Postmenopausal women are reported to have cholesterol profiles similar to those of men. Presumably, estrogen levels of the nonsmoking premenopausal woman influence lipid metabolism to favor HDL-C.

The effects of oral contraceptive agents have been extensively studied. An increased risk of cardiovascular disease has been associated with the use of high-dose progesterone contraceptive pills (Boyd & McGuire, 1990; Clarkson, Adams, Kaplan, Shively, & Koritnik, 1989). Lipid metabolism is influenced by progesterone levels. Reformulation of oral contraceptives to contain lower doses of progesterone has apparently eliminated the risks previously associated with use of the "pill" (Derman, 1990). Because exercise positively affects cholesterol levels, women who use the birth control pill should be encouraged to exercise. Whether or not exercise alone is sufficient to prevent or overcome the negative effects of progesterone is not known. Women who take high doses of progesterone are at risk of developing hypercholesterolemia. Nurses and other health care providers should monitor plasma lipid levels and encourage healthy lifestyles that should include regular moderate exercise.

The importance of understanding the interaction between estrogen levels, lipid metabolism, and exercise is underscored by a study of highly trained women athletes. Lamon-Fava et al. (1989) studied the lipid profiles of 25 women runners and 36 age-matched nonexercising women. Nine of the women runners had exercise-induced amenorrhea. Normally menstruating athletes had lower TC levels and higher HDL-C to TC ratios and lower LDL-C and triglyceride levels than did sedentary women. In contrast, the amenorrheic runners' lipid profiles were comparable to those of the nonexercising control group. They also demonstrated lower estradiol levels than did the menstruating runners. Thus amenorrhea accompanied by decreased endogenous estrogen negated the positive effects of strenuous exercise on lipids.

Improvement of Cardiovascular Risk Factors

Cardiovascular disease is the number-one cause of death of both American women and men. General health indices and practices that reflect increased probability that an individual will develop cardiovascular disease include elevated TC; high concentrations of LDL-C and proportionally lower concentrations of HDL-C; high concentrations of triglycerides in plasma; high-fat, low-fiber diet; smoking; sedentary lifestyle; and alcohol ingestion (Cohn et al., 1989). Many of these risk factors can be minimized or eliminated by modification of lifestyle.

In addition to the positive effects of modulating lipid metabolism, exercise can reduce the risk of cardiovascular disease by directly affecting the heart muscle, improving vasculature of the skeletal muscle, and lowering blood pressure. These and other cardiovascular adaptations occur to varying degrees in individuals who engage in aerobic exercise. The extent of the changes are related to genetic characteristics, the intensity and frequency of the exercise, and the length of time that the exercise program is followed. There is evidence that responses may be different between women and men and across the life span (Abbott et al., 1989; Wilson, 1987). The effects of a program of regular moderate physical activity may produce less dramatic changes in the anatomy of the cardiovascular system, but the overall reduction in cardiovascular risk factors is unequivocal.

Although increases in the thickness of the left ventricular walls appear to be limited to those athletes who engage in very strenuous activity, such as weight lifting, changes in heart function are evident after adherence to a program of regular moderate aerobic exercise over time (Gibbons & Blair, 1989). Generally, increased cardiovascular fitness is accompanied by slowing of the heart rate at rest. To maintain adequate cardiac output in the face of decreased heart rate, the ventricular diameter of the fit individual may be larger than nonconditioned control subjects. The increase is not clinically significant and should not be confused with pathological dilation of the ventricle. Because ventricular capacity increases, end diastolic volume increases. During systole, increased ventricular volume translates to increased stroke volume. The net result is no change in cardiac output despite lower heart rate.

Some changes in the vasculature have been attributed to physical conditioning. Kramsch, Aspen, Abramowitz, Kreimendahl, and Hood (1981) have reported that the diameter of coronary arteries of conditioned monkeys is larger. Increases in the number of capillaries per muscle cell is reported to increase with aerobic conditioning. These changes, coupled with diversion of blood flow from inactive organs, such as the gut, ensure adequate perfusion of muscles. Thus necessary substrates to maintain activity reach the most active muscles, and waste products of metabolism are removed.

Several investigators have reported that a program of moderate exercise can reduce blood pressure in mildly hypertensive individuals ("1988 Report of the Joint Committee," 1988). Significant differences in the blood pressure of adolescents have been reported in relation to aerobic fitness (Harshfield et al., 1990). Of particular interest in this study was the finding that sedentary African American youngsters had significantly higher blood pressure than did fit African American children or sedentary white children. In an intervention study reported by Danforth et al. (1990), a 12-week program of regular aerobic physical activity at school resulted in significant reductions in both systolic and diastolic blood pressures in the African American group. These data suggest that increased incidence of hypertension in African Americans begins early in life. Effective interventions to control cardiovascular disease and stroke in the African American population should target youngsters and emphasize healthy lifestyles.

Pulmonary Effects of Exercise

As muscle activity increases, the demand for oxygen increases and the amount of carbon dioxide to be excreted increases. To meet these increased demands, blood flow to the lungs increases during exercise. Increased ventilation of the alveoli is the consequence of increased respiratory rate. Increased rate is not accompanied by increased tidal volume, however. Concurrent with increased ventilation and perfusion, an increase in oxygen diffusion rate is observed. The net effect of these physiological additive mechanisms is supplying adequate oxygen to the red blood cells for transport to the skeletal muscles. Carbon dioxide is excreted. The ability of these cardiac and pulmonary mechanisms to supply nutrients and oxygen to the working muscles and to rid the body of the waste products of metabolism is of central importance to cardiopulmonary fitness. In fact, enhancement of these mechanisms is the contribution of regular physical exercise to fitness and health.

Measures of Cardiopulmonary Fitness

The best measure of an individual's work capacity is the determination of oxygen consumption at maximal activity (VO_2max). VO_2max can be measured directly while an individual exercises on a treadmill or stationary bike. The actual value may be compared to a normative predicted value based on age, sex, and usual level of activity. Comparison of these two values may be used as an indicator of cardiorespiratory fitness. An individual whose actual VO_2max is less than the predicted level can improve to achieve or exceed predicted VO_2max by maintaining a regular exercise program.

Several methods that estimate VO_2max have been developed. Direct measurement involves determination of the amount of oxygen extracted from inspired air. VO_2max is expressed as milliliters of oxygen per minute. Because individuals with large muscle mass have higher VO_2max values, VO_2max is usually divided by the person's weight in kilograms. The result is expressed as milliliters of oxygen per kilogram of body weight per minute. This measurement is generally taken in the final minutes of maximal exertion.

A second measure of cardiopulmonary fitness is the anaerobic threshold (AT). The AT is the point during exercise at which the demand for oxygen exceeds the capacity to deliver. This point is characterized by an increase in lactic acid in the plasma and muscle fatigue. Comparison of AT and VO_2max would give a fairly accurate indication of the amount of work an individual could sustain without experiencing muscle fatigue and lactic acid buildup. The average AT is 47% to 64% of actual VO_2max, although this may be somewhat higher in trained athletes. Therefore, one could expect an individual to maintain exercise at 50% to 60% of VO_2max. Some researchers have argued that the AT is a better measure of cardiopulmonary fitness for the general population because it reflects the individual's ability to sustain aerobic metabolism during exercise. This number may be useful when suggesting an exercise regimen for a client.

Effects of Exercise on Neuroendocrine Regulatory Mechanisms

In 1973, a receptor specific for opiatelike substances was isolated from animal tissue (Pert & Snyder, 1973; Simon, Hiller, & Edelman, 1973). Subsequently, substances that had the same biological effects as morphine were isolated (Cox, Opheim, Teschmacher, & Goldstein, 1975; Hughes et al., 1975; Terenius, 1975). These small peptides were dubbed endorphins. Scientists eager to understand the biological significance of these discoveries began vigorous campaigns to explore roles in pain perception, analgesia, and some psychiatric disorders (Madden, Akil, Patrick, & Barchas, 1977; Watson, Akil, Berger, & Barchas, 1979). Scientists have come to appreciate the complex role that endorphins and similar substances play in modulating neuroendocrine function and behavior. Research in this rich area has forced a reexamination of the traditional view that the nervous system is independent of the endocrine system and especially the parochial view that psychological and behavioral aspects of human function are independent of biological influences.

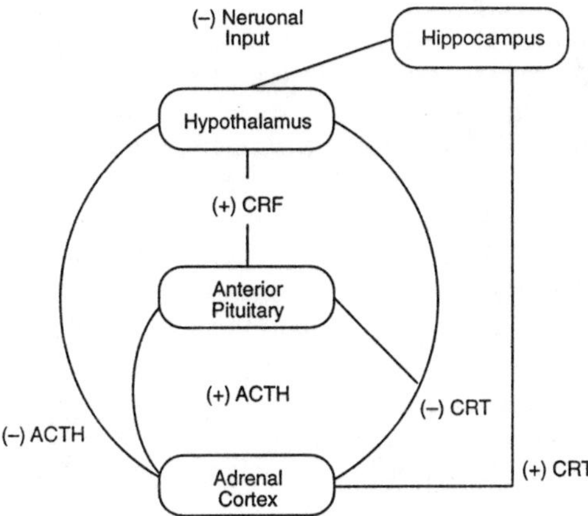

Figure 13.2. The Hypothalamic/Pituitary/Adrenal Axis

NOTE: The hypothalamic/pituitary/adrenal axis is activated by stress and exercise. The hypothalamus secretes corticotropin factor (CRF). CRF stimulates secretion of adrenocorticotropin hormone (ACTH) and β-endorphin-like immunoreactive peptides by the anterior pituitary. ACTH stimulates secretion of cortisol (CRT) from the adrenal cortex. Increased levels of ACTH feedback to the hypothalamus to inhibit further production of CRF, and CRT feeds back to the anterior pituitary and the hypothalamus to inhibit ACTH and CRF. These feedback loops are slow-acting, taking several hours to affect ACTH levels. CRT activates a neuronal loop from the hippocampus, a central nervous system structure, to the hypothalamus, inhibiting CRF secretion. The CRT hippocampal loop is fast-acting, causing ACTH levels to decrease within several minutes.

Evidence that exercise can modulate mood gives support to the notion that regulation of the nervous and endocrine systems is linked to behavior. Vigorous aerobic activity elicits many of the same neurological and endocrine responses observed in stress. Particularly, the autonomic nervous system is activated to regulate the cardiovascular system. Increased secretion of catecholamines and glucocorticoids modulate energy metabolism in preparation for increased energy demanded by the fight- or the flight-response. One of the endorphins, beta-endorphin (β-END), is increased in plasma by exercise (Mesaki et al., 1989). Analgesic effects of exercise seem to be modulated by endorphinergic mechanisms as the effects are reversed and prevented by naloxone, an opiate antagonist. Furthermore, stress-induced analgesia and analgesia secondary to electrical stimulation of the brain are accompanied by increased concentrations of endorphins in the terminals of endorphinergic neurones in the brain, known to be involved in pain transmission and perception. Cerebral spinal fluid from the fourth ventricle of the brain contains higher concentrations of endorphins as well (Akil, Richardson, Hughes, & Barchas, 1978; see Figure 13.2).

β-END is a potent endorphin that is synthesized from a precursor, proopiomelanocorticotropin (POMC). POMC is also the precursor for adrenocorticotropin hormone (ACTH). ACTH is released from the anterior pituitary in response to stress. In response to increased plasma levels of ACTH, the adrenal cortex increases secretion of cortisol, a glucocorticoid hormone involved in regulation of glucose and carbohydrate metabolism. Because ACTH and β-END are cosynthesized from the same precursor and costored in the anterior pituitary, they are coreleased (Guillemin et al., 1977). Plasma β-END levels, therefore, increase in response to stress. Paulev et al. (1989) and others have reported that naloxone increases postexercise muscle pain, suggesting that increased endorphin activity during exercise is involved in modification of pain perception. Animal studies that include concurrent measurement of plasma and central nervous system levels of endorphins support the notion that stress causes increased production and release of endorphins from brain and pituitary, resulting in analgesia (Akil, Mayer, & Liebeskind, 1976).

Effects of Exercise on Menstrual Function

Modulation of the endocrine mechanisms regulating the menstrual cycle has been associated with athletic training in some women. Although the mechanisms associated with this phenomenon are not precisely known, hints from the effects of stress and vigorous aerobic exercise suggest some possibilities. The menstrual cycle is regulated by the hypothalamic/pituitary/ovarian (gonadal) axis (see Figure 13.3). As in the stress axis, neuronal input from limbic structures and the diencephalon of the brain participates in the regulation of the menstrual cycle. Research on the nonhuman primate suggests that the basal medial hypothalamus serves as a "transducer" that integrates signals from the brain and the endocrine system to regulate menstrual cycles (Ferin, 1984). Maintenance of cyclicity, menstruation, and fertility is achieved by precise secretory patterns of gonadotropin-releasing hormone (GnRH). The secretory pattern of GnRH is modulated by estrogen and

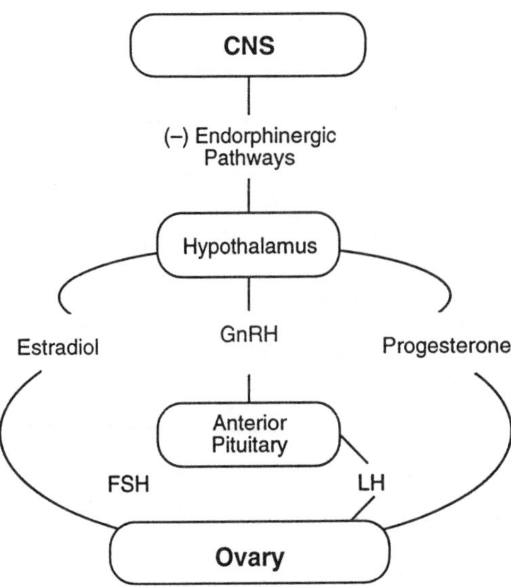

Figure 13.3. The Hypothalamic/Pituitary/Ovarian Axis

NOTE: The hypothalamic/pituitary/ovarian axis regulates the menstrual cycle. The hypothalamus secretes gonadotropin-releasing hormone (GnRH) in varying amounts and patterns. The specific pattern is determined by the relative amounts of estradiol and progesterone. Estradiol is highest during the follicular phase of the cycle. During this time, GnRH stimulates the secretion of follicle stimulating hormone (FSH). In response to this hormone, the ovary increases production of estradiol. At midcycle, GnRH stimulates the production of luteinizing hormone (LH). LH causes ovulation, and progesterone is produced by the ovary.

progesterone levels. Endogenous opiate secretion at the level of the hypothalamus also influences GnRH secretory patterns (Seifer & Collins, 1990; Veldhuis, 1990).

Stress has been associated with disturbances in the menstrual cycle. Therefore, menstrual abnormalities associated with exercise stress may be associated with concomitant secretion of opioids that disrupt the GnRH pattern. In addition to pituitary sources of β-END, neurons in the hypothalamus produce β-END. Studies of the concentrations of β-END in hypophyseal blood of female monkeys indicate that β-END levels change during the menstrual cycle. Levels are elevated during the luteal phase when GnRH secretion is at its lowest (Weherenberg, Wardlaw, Frantz, & Ferin, 1982). Supporting an inhibitory role for β-END in regulation of GnRH is the finding that administration of opiates or opioids results in decreased gonadotropin secretion. Administration of naloxone, an opiate antagonist, during the luteal phase causes gonadotropin levels to increase (Ropert, Quigley, & Yen, 1981). Further bolstering the evidence suggesting that opioids play some role in regulating the menstrual cycle is anatomical evidence that both the neurons that produce hypothalamic β-END and those that produce GnRH originate on the arcuate nucleus of the hypothalamus (MacLusky, Naftolin, & Leranth, 1988). Taken as a whole, these data serve to support the notion that synergy exists between endorphinergic stress mechanisms and gonadotropin mechanisms of the hypothalamus. Endorphinergic mechanisms of the hypothalamus may be the link between the stress axis and the gonadal axis.

Amenorrhea has been associated with strenuous physical training in a small percentage of women athletes. Loucks, Mortola, Girton, and Yen (1989) studied stress and gonadal axes hormones in athletic women. Significant differences in luteinizing hormone (LH) pulsatile patterns and cortisol levels were found in amenorrheic athletes. The amenorrheic athletes demonstrated fewer pulses of LH at more irregular intervals than did menstruating athletic women or sedentary control women. Both the amenorrheic and menstruating athletes demonstrated higher early-morning cortisol levels, which persisted throughout the day in the amenorrheic women, but no differences in ACTH levels between groups were noted. To determine the response patterns of the system to regulatory hormones, GnRH and CRF were administered. The menstruating athletes demonstrated reduced responsiveness to GnRH as evidenced by lower levels of FSH. In contrast, the amenorrheic group demonstrated increased secretion of LH in response to GnRH. Both the amenorrheic and menstruating athletes demonstrated less responsivity to CRF by lower levels of ACTH secretion. However, both groups demonstrated greater responsivity of the adrenal cortex by proportionally greater levels of cortisol in response to ACTH increases. In this study, women athletes with regular menstrual cycles were found to have shorter luteal phases and lower levels of progesterone than did the sedentary control group. Kaiserauer, Snyder, Sleeper, and Zierath (1989) also reported lower progesterone levels in amenorrheic runners and shorter luteal phases in regularly menstruating runners. Schweiger et al. (1989) studied gonadotropin secretion in a convenience sample of normally menstruating women. On the basis of serum sex steroid levels and luteal phase length, the subjects were divided into three groups. Group A consisted of 27 women with luteal phase lengths of 9 days or longer and normal levels of ovarian hormones. Group B consisted of 16 women with normal estrogen levels but lower progesterone levels and luteal phase length of less than 9 days. Group C had lower estrogen levels. Risk factors identified with membership in either Group B or Group C were intermittent dieting and vigorous exercise. These data support the argument that vigorous athletic training influences menstrual cycle regularity and may affect fertility as well. Mitigating evidence that not all athletes engaged in similar training programs experience amenorrhea suggests that some women may be more susceptible to gonadal disruption (Loucks, 1990). Those factors that confer vulnerability remain to be fully characterized. Estok, Rudy, Kerr, and Menzel (1993) investigated the effects of varying running intensities and duration on menstrual-cycle characteristics. The study included three groups of women runners and a group of women who did not run. When runners were compared to nonrunners, runners demonstrated shorter luteal phases and a greater incidence of ovulatory disturbances. The one incident most frequently associated with these menstrual disturbances in addition to running was a history of skipping periods between menarche and 18 years of age.

Effects of Exercise on Psychological Well-Being

The effects of regular aerobic exercise on psychological factors such as well-being and depression have been reported to range from very positive to negative. In samples from the general population, regular exercise has been shown to decrease anxiety and lift depression scores in individuals who had higher than average scores on these variables (Steptoe, Edwards, Moses, & Mathews, 1989). In others whose scores were average, no differences in these parameters were noted. These data lead to the speculation that in an average population, exercise may serve to protect the individual from depression and anxiety.

Studies of highly trained individuals have resulted in some fascinating paradoxical findings. Raglin (1990) has reported that overtraining, which might be required for endurance athletes, can lead to mood disturbances. Furthermore, some individuals may become "addicted" to vigorous exercise. Gauvin (1990) has reported that some regular exercisers feel that something is missing from their lives when they skip their daily exercise sessions. In extreme cases, individuals may exercise even though they are hurt. An attractive explanation for these findings is associated with the finding that exercise can cause endogenous opiate (endorphin) levels to increase and that omission of vigorous exercise leads to decreased levels of opioids and withdrawal symptoms. This hypothesis remains to be firmly established.

Effects on Menstrually Related Symptoms

Of American women of childbearing age, 50% to 90% report distress ranging from mild dysphoria to significant discomfort associated with different phases of the menstrual cycle (Halbreich, Alt, & Paul, 1988). A typical pattern of perimenstrual symptoms includes appearance of mild to severe symptoms during the week prior to the onset of menses and during the first few days of menses followed by profound relief from symptoms during the follicular phase.

Several investigators have reported that the type and severity of symptoms reported by some women are linked to stress levels. The relationship between neuroendocrine mechanisms associated with stressful events and release of CRF and β-END, which may alter the GnRH oscillating signal of the gonadal axis, provides the linkage between behavior and physiological mechanisms of the menstrual cycle.

To date, studies of hormones from both the stress axis and the gonadal axis have not clearly demonstrated significant differences in levels associated with the menstrual cycle. Some researchers have reported differences in levels of estrogen, progesterone, and cortisol levels, and still others report no absolute differences in levels. These confounding and contradictory findings may be associated with research paradigm inadequacies associated with subject selection. Furthermore, most studies report only baseline levels of stress hormones. If stress axis and/or gonadal axis disregulation is a characteristic of the biobehavioral bases of menstrually related symptoms, the disregulatory events are likely transient because menstrually related symptoms are not associated with infertility or menstrual pathology. Putative transient changes would be most evident during neuroendocrine responses to challenges or stressors.

Although theoretical evidence exists to suggest that exercise should have a positive effect by reducing menstrually related symptoms, few studies have been done to validate its usefulness. Kuczmierczyk (1989) has reported positive effects in a single case study in which exercise was prescribed as part of a multimodal therapy for severe symptoms. Exercise was studied as a component of the effectiveness of self-care measures in relieving menstrually related symptoms by Kirkpatrick, Brewer, and Stocks (1990). In this quasi-experimental study, self-care measures were reported to be effective in preventing and alleviating menstrually related symptoms. Taylor (1991) reported that women with depressive-type menstrually related symptoms who participated in a program of treatment that included exercise, group support, and stress reduction strategies reported improvement in symptoms. Because these studies included exercise as a component of a broader therapeutic plan, the unique contribution of exercise remains unclear. Yet several articles in journals targeted to clinicians include exercise as a recommended intervention. Because exercise in moderation represents minimal risk to an otherwise healthy young-adult to middle-aged population, continued inclusion in the therapeutic plan for perimenstrual symptoms is appropriate.

Exercise in Pregnancy and Lactation

Pregnancy and lactation are events in some women's lives that require special consideration regarding the amount and type of exercise. Consideration of cardiovascular changes associated with pregnancy includes increased cardiovascular load due to increased weight and vascular volume. Some have suggested that superimposing vigorous aerobic exercise could overtax the system and cause problems for the mother as well as the fetus. However, the overwhelming evidence suggests that if the woman engaged in regular aerobic exercise prior to her pregnancy, she may safely continue through her pregnancy. Women who exercise regularly are reported to have shorter labors and fewer operative deliveries (Beckmann & Beckmann, 1990; Oldridge & Streiner, 1990).

Animal research has indicated that hyperthermia may cause defects in the development of the fetal nervous system (Wolfe et al., 1989). Because excessive aerobic exercise can increase core body temperature enough to cause teratology, some have suggested that exercise may have negative effects on the fetus. To date, concerns about birth defects associated with thermal reactions in human populations have not been supported by research. However, women who engage in strenuous physical exercise during pregnancy should be carefully monitored. Weight control, one of the most positive effects of exercise in the nonpregnant population, may cause some difficulties during pregnancy. Pregnant women who gain little weight tend to have smaller babies. Low birth weight has been associated with health and development problems in childhood. Clapp and Capeless (1990) have reported that aerobic exercise above minimal training levels results in fetal growth restriction associated with reduced neonatal fat mass. In contrast, Beckmann and Beckmann (1990) report no adverse effects on the fetus with nonendurance exercise antepartum. Other investigations support the safety of moderate aerobic exercise during pregnancy for the fetus (Jette, Sidney, & Blumchen, 1990; Klebanoff, Shiono, & Carey, 1990; Oldridge & Streiner, 1990). The only contraindication to aerobic exercise for the woman experiencing a normal pregnancy is associated with pregnancy-related compromise of the cardiovascular system. Late in pregnancy, the position of the baby may interfere with respiratory reserves. Complications of pregnancy such as hypertension and fluid retention may compromise the woman's ability to exercise.

In general, a commonsense approach to exercise during pregnancy should prevail (Wolfe et al., 1989). If a woman has been exercising regularly prior to pregnancy, there is little risk associated with continuing with it. However, changes in balance due to added body weight and changes in posture may influence a pregnant woman's ability to continue to perform certain actions. Activities that require agility may result in greater risk for falling and injury during pregnancy. Authors have reported that activities requiring prolonged standing or that are performed in the upright posture may place the mother at risk for premature labor (Klebanoff et al., 1990). Generally, women who are pregnant should monitor their responses to and comfort during all activities and avoid those that are uncomfortable.

Special thought should be given to the type of exercise program initiated during pregnancy. Women should be advised to be very cautious because injury during initiation of a program of regular exercise is more likely. Changes in the physiological function associated with pregnancy may influence exercise capacity. Increased circulating blood volume and weight gain may result in increased challenge to the cardiopulmonary system during exercise. Activities that were easily tolerated prior to pregnancy may be too much during pregnancy. The best program of exercise for formerly sedentary women during pregnancy is conservative and includes regular monitoring of the mother and the fetus.

There is no evidence that suggests that exercise negatively affects lactation. One study reported that lactating women who exercised regularly produced more milk (Lovelady, Lonnerdal, & Dewey, 1990). In addition to lactation postpartum, exercise may have a positive effect on mood, reducing the risk of postpartum depression and perhaps reducing the fatigue reported to accompany the postpartum period.

Effects on Menopausal Symptoms

Transition from regular fertile menstrual cycles to cessation of menstruation is a time of significant endocrine readjustment. Some hormonal alterations profoundly affect physiological mechanisms that influence women's health patterns. In other sections of this chapter, the effects of reduced estrogen levels associated with the perimenopausal period and menopause and the usefulness of regular exercise as an adjunctive or palliative treatment for changes in lipid metabolism and subsequent risks for cardiovascular disease and changes in bone metabolism and osteoporosis were discussed. Associated with reduction in estrogen levels is vasomotor instability, which is manifested as "hot flashes." The first sign of transition to menopause for many women is the discomfort of a hot flash.

Women describe the experience in two phases. First, they report feeling "different," which is reminiscent of the aura reported to be prodromal to some epileptic seizures. This nonspecific ubiquitous experience is followed by vasodilation accompanied by increased pulse rate, a sensation of extreme heat, and, in some cases, sweating. The mechanisms underlying the vasomotor event of the hot flash are not well understood. Evidence to date suggests vasodilation of cutaneous capillaries accompanied by increased perspiration and heart rate are peripheral compensatory responses to hypothalamic thermodisregulation (Ravnikar, 1990). During a hot flash, the core body temperature decreases. In an attempt to equalize the peripheral temperature with the core temperature, cutaneous vessels dilate to promote heat loss and perspiration increases.

Mood changes are often associated with complaints of hot flashes. Hot flashes often occur at night and interfere with normal sleep patterns. In addition, alterations in sleep quality have been associated with estrogen deficiencies. Perimenopausal women experience less rapid eye movement sleep, which may explain the increased complains of irritability and fatigue (Ravnikar, 1990). Those placed on estrogen replacement therapy experience more rapid eye movement sleep and fewer sleep disturbances (Erlik et al., 1981). Exercise as a treatment for vasoactive symptoms has not been studied; however, the positive effects of exercise on mood and sleep patterns may prove helpful for perimenopausal women.

Therapeutic Programs of Exercise

The characteristics of a therapeutic exercise plan vary with the situation that prompts the intervention. Obviously, strenuous exercise would be contraindicated in an individual recovering from a heart attack or surgery. The American Heart Association (Fletcher, Froelicher, Hartley, Haskell, & Pollack, 1990) and the American College of Sports Medicine (Pate et al., 1991) have published guidelines for exercise testing and prescription of exercise plans for both health promotion and therapeutics.

Nurses and other health professionals who will be monitoring and prescribing exercise plans for large numbers of individuals are encouraged to seek special training and certification. The American College of Sports Medicine has identified a specific curriculum to prepare professionals for this role (Pate et al., 1991). The program is not limited to physicians and includes added experience and information on testing procedures and endurance training methods. In this section, general guidelines integrating the recommendations of the American Heart Association and the American College of Sports Medicine for exercise program requirements for health promotion in healthy young adults will be presented.

The decision to begin a program of regular exercise is one that should be encouraged. The purposes of the exercise prescription are to improve cardiovascular fitness, promote health, and prevent injury during exercise. The positive effects of exercise have been discussed previously, but there are risks to be considered as well. The first step in the prescriptive process, obviously, is assessment of the possible risks to the individual. Factors most likely to influence risk are age, presence of heart disease, and the intensity of the exercise to be done. The American Heart Association recommends that any individual beginning a program of physical fitness training visit a health professional for a physical examination. Individuals under 40 years of age should be evaluated for cardiovascular disease. In this age group, cardiovascular disease is usually congenital in nature. Those with murmurs or other abnormal findings on examination should defer participation in exercise programs until full evaluation of the nature and extent of the disorder is completed. Particular attention should be paid to resting blood pressure. Those with significant elevations in blood pressure should seek treatment before beginning the exercise regimen. Those with major coronary risk factors but who are apparently asymptomatic should have an exercise stress test before beginning a strenuous program of exercise. Similarly, for individuals over 40 years of age, the American Heart Association recommends an exercise stress test (Fletcher et al., 1990).

Additional information about the usual level of leisure time and occupational activity will guide the nurse's recommendation of the amount and intensity of exercise needed to minimize coronary artery disease risks and to improve fitness. Adequate occupational activity that contributes to reduction of cardiovascular risk is difficult to define. An example of the required amount of occupational activity "is a job that requires lifting loads of 20 pounds or more at least once an hour throughout the day or consistently moving loads of any size from one place to another without the assistance of mechanical devices" (Fletcher et al., 1990, p. 2307). One hour or more of low- to moderate-intensity walking as part of a job is sufficient to confer some degree of protection from coronary artery disease as well. Individuals whose jobs are not as physically demanding as those described need to exercise during part of their leisure time activities.

On the basis of the completed assessment, individuals can be assigned to a specific activity classification that has been recommended by the American Heart Association (Fletcher et al., 1990). The system provides guidance in determining risks associated with exercise and suggests activity guidelines, monitoring requirements, and amount of supervision needed to engage safely in exercise. Class A includes apparently healthy individuals under 40 years of age and apparently healthy individuals over 40 years old with normal exercise tests. The other classes include individuals with known cardiovascular disease with increased risk associated with exercise. Those involved in prescription of exercise for these individuals are encouraged to review the material. Discussion of exercise in this population of women is beyond the scope of this chapter.

Even though there are gender-related differences in the risks for coronary heart disease, most studies have focused on men. Studies of the effects of exercise on reducing the risk of disease have been done on men and have excluded women. Therefore, specific recommendations of the amount and intensity of exercise needed by women are not available. Those for men will be applied to women until more research is done (Fletcher et al., 1990). In general, exercise sufficient to consume 700 calories per week is recommended to maintain minimum fitness and provide health benefits. Activity should be performed on at least three nonconsecutive days per week. This level of activity could be achieved by walking a total of 20 miles per week at a slow to moderate rate. Fitness can be increased above minimal levels if additional exercise expending more calories is done. However, there is no evidence that fitness is improved or that greater protection from disease can be achieved by an exercise program that expends more than 2,000 calories per week.

Endurance or cardiovascular exercises are dynamic activities involving alternating contraction and relaxation of large muscle groups. Walking, running, swimming, and cycling are examples of endurance exercises. Exercise should be done a minimum of three times per week for at least 20 to 30 minutes. The American Heart Association suggests an intensity of 50% to 60% of VO_2max to achieve positive effects at this frequency (Fletcher et al., 1990). Each exercise session should be preceded and followed by 5 to 10 minutes of low-intensity exercise. Less strenuous activity performed for longer periods has been shown to be of some benefit. However, as cardiovascular fitness improves, individuals should be encouraged to increase the intensity of the activity.

Selection of Specific Activities

Selection of specific activities will necessitate setting realistic goals for the program. Consideration should be given to the current fitness status of the person. An individual who is initiating a program will have different needs than one wishing to improve or maintain physical status. The American College of Sports Medicine (Pate et al., 1991) has identified three stages of the aerobic exercise prescription. The initial stage includes low-intensity exercise intended to minimize muscle soreness and reduce the risk of injury. This stage lasts 4 to 6 weeks, after which the participant progresses to the conditioning stage. During this stage, intensity and duration of activity are increased at the same general pace that the individual adapts to the program. After the first 6 months of the conditioning program, the individual advances to the maintenance stage of the program. At this point, the participant's original goals should be reviewed and a specific exercise program designed.

Selection of aerobic endurance activities is necessary to improve cardiovascular fitness. Aerobic endurance activities may be divided into three groups on the basis of interindividual variability in caloric expenditure and the potential for maintaining a constant rate of energy expenditure (Pate et al., 1991). Group 1 activities show little interindividual variability in energy expenditure and can be maintained at a fairly constant level of intensity. Group 1 activities include walking and jogging. Group 2 activities demonstrate greater interindividual variability, but a specific individual may maintain a relatively stable level of intensity. These activities require some degree of skill and include swimming and cross-country skiing. In the last group, Group 3, activities are highly variable and include dancing and racquetball. Selection of Group 1 activities, therefore, would be most appropriate for the initial stage of an exercise program, in which better control of intensity is required to minimize injury and excessive fatigue. Personal preference and enjoyment may determine the usefulness of Group 2 and 3 behaviors.

Ensuring that the exercise prescription includes activities of sufficient intensity to improve fitness is essential. Exercise intensity may be prescribed as a percentage of an individual's functional capacity. The American Heart Association Guidelines suggest 40% to 90% of VO_2max. The easiest and cheapest measure of cardiovascular response to exercise is the pulse rate. Because there is a linear relationship between heart rate and VO_2 during exercise, a target heart rate corresponding to 40% to 90% of VO_2 can be selected. Seventy percent to 85% of maximal heart rate is equal to 60% to 80% of VO_2 max. Individuals should perform the particular exercise with sufficient vigor to increase heart rate to 60% to 70% of maximal heart rate. If the person has had a maximal exercise test, this value can be read from a graph of heart rate and VO_2. Most apparently, healthy young adults will not require this test. Other methods to determine target heart rate include calculations based on the difference between resting heart rate and maximal heart rate or simply taking a percentage of the maximal heart rate. Maximal heart rate tables are available. These tables are adjusted for gender, age, and usual activity. Another simple method of calculating maximal heart rate is subtracting the individual's age in years from 220. For an individual of 20, for example, maximal heart rate is 200. Therefore, that individual's heart rate should be raised to 100 to 120 to achieve positive effects. Heart rate should be maintained at that rate for 15 to 60 minutes three times per week.

Some individuals are not able to achieve and maintain target heart rates in the initial stage of the exercise regime. For those individuals, subjective assessment of the amount of effort required to maintain the activity may be used as an indication of therapeutic effect. The Borg Scale is an example of a rating of perceived effort (RPE) scale. There are two types of Borg scales. One is a 15-point numerical scale ranging from 6 to 20. The other is a 10-point numerical scale ranging from 1 to 10. The RPE response to exercise is highly correlated with cardiovascular and metabolic measures of exercise intensity (Pate et al., 1991). On the 15-point scale, a score of 12 or 13 corresponds to 60% of the desired heart rate. Similarly, a score of 4 to 6 on the 10-point scale would be sufficient. This method is attractive because it is easy to use and, over time, the individual learns to assess the effectiveness of the exercise on the basis of self-appraisal.

No matter how positive the benefits of an action may be, an individual will not continue an activity that causes pain or discomfort. In addition, excessive exercise in the early stage of a program can cause injury to the participant. Over time, capacity to exercise will increase as cardiovascular fitness improves. Individuals should be encouraged to increase the length of the exercise session gradually and to maintain effort at a moderate level. In a walking program, for example, individuals might begin by walking 1 mile in 15 minutes. Over the course of several weeks, they could increase the distance they walk to 4 miles in 30 to 40 minutes. This would constitute a brisk pace, which will likely challenge the cardiopulmonary system, improve lipid metabolism, and may reduce the percentage of body mass that is fat. Selection of activities that sufficiently tax the cardiovascular system and are enjoyable are key to maintaining the program throughout the life span.

Those interested in more details regarding specific exercise plans are encouraged to review the guidelines published by the American Heart Association (Fletcher et al., 1990) and the American College of Sports Medicine (Pate et al., 1991). These publications include tables of the energy expended by different activities and specific recommendations for therapeutic plans for patients after myocardial infarction, heart surgery, and other medical conditions influencing fitness activities.

Adherence to Therapeutic Exercise Plans

Evidence of the positive effects of exercise on the health and well-being of women should convince even the most dedicated couch potato to change her lifestyle to include regular moderate aerobic exercise. However, altering one's lifestyle is easier said than done. Because the positive health benefits of exercise are dependent on adherence to a long-term program of regular exercise, the clinician must balance the need for therapeutic effects with the likelihood of adherence. Several researchers have tried to identify personality characteristics of those individuals who are likely to succeed (Adame, Johnson, Cole, Matthiasson, & Abbas, 1990; Conway, 1989). The data are mixed and suggest that predictability of adherence based on personality characteristics is low. Other researchers have considered program characteristics that are most likely to result in adherence (Gleichmann et al., 1989).

The clinician must work closely with the client to develop a program that fits with the lifestyle and preferences of the client. Selection of an activity that serves to improve cardiovascular fitness and is enjoyable is essential to success. The physical abilities of the individual will influence the type of program selected. Care must be taken to avoid prescription of activities that may expose the individual to risks of injury. The older woman with a history of osteoporosis and postural instability probably should not be encouraged to perform activities that require weight shifting and balance. Sasaki et al. (1989) reported that mild exercise has a positive effect on the lipid profiles of participants. The easiest and possibly the most acceptable activity that has been shown to improve cardiovascular fitness is walking. Walking for 20 to 40 minutes at a moderate pace three times per week has been shown to have therapeutic effects on lipid profiles and the cardiovascular system (Morey et al., 1989). In some communities, problems associated with inclement weather and safety issues have been addressed by the formation of clubs that meet at the local shopping mall to walk.

Organized exercise similar to the mall walkers clubs has been shown to improve adherence to a program of exercise (Dalsky, 1990; Gleichmann et al., 1989). The comradery associated with group activities motivates some to attend sessions. Support and encouragement from fellow exercisers may also contribute to greater effort to extend capabilities. In addition, each member may informally share strategies that improve health.

Transformation within a culture is difficult, particularly when it requires abandonment of long-standing habits. Studies suggest that as children age they adopt increasingly sedentary lifestyles. The change is most evident when a girl reaches adolescence. Cultural norms that suggest that it is not feminine to be physically active may influence changes in a girl's behavior. The effect of a lifelong sedentary lifestyle on life span and health in later years could be disastrous. Children from lower socioeconomic groups and particularly minority children are at risk for significant cardiovascular disease in adulthood. Therefore, the clinician who is concerned with health promotion and maintenance may be well advised to concentrate some effort toward children, particularly young girls, and encourage the development of positive health habits including regular aerobic exercise.

Summary

Advances in technology have made the lives of the average American physically less challenging than they were even a generation ago.

The same technology has brought with it increasingly complex and demanding lifestyles that are challenging and stressful. Lack of physical fitness and increased stress levels have been associated with increased cardiovascular disease and cancer, which are the major causes of early death and illness. Regular exercise has been shown to improve health and prevent disease. Although the American health care system remains focused on an illness model, nursing has long addressed prevention and promotion as an aspect of our expertise. Therefore, the nurse involved in health promotion must consider prescription of physical exercise as an essential adjunct to other treatment modalities.

References

Abbott, R. D., Levy, D., Kannel, W. B., Castelli, W. P., Wilson, P. W., Garrison, R. J., & Stokes, J. (1989). Cardiovascular risk factors and graded treadmill exercise endurance in healthy adults: Framingham Adult Offspring Study. *American Journal of Cardiology, 63*(5), 342-346.

Adame, D., Johnson, T., Cole, S., Matthiasson, H., & Abbas, M. (1990). Physical fitness in relation to amount of physical exercise, body image, and locus of control among college men and women. *Perception and Motor Skills, 70*(3, pt. 2), 1347-1350.

Akil, H., Mayer, D. G., & Liebeskind, J. C. (1976). Antagonism of stimulation produced analgesia by naloxone. *Science, 191,* 961-962.

Akil, H., Richardson, D. E., Hughes, J., & Barchas, J. D. (1978). Enkephalin-like material elevated in ventricular cerebral spinal fluid of pain patents after analgetic focal stimulation. *Science, 20,* 463-465.

Bachrach, L. K., Guido, D., Katzman, D., Litt, I. F., & Marchas, R. (1990). Decreased bone density in adolescent girls with anorexia nervosa. *Pediatrics, 86*(3), 440-447.

Bak, J., Jacobsen, U., Jorgensen, F., & Pedersen, O. (1989). Insulin receptor function and glycogen synthase activity in skeletal muscle biopsies from patients with insulin-dependent diabetes mellitus: Effects of physical training. *Journal of Clinical Endocrinology and Metabolism, 69*(1), 158-164.

Beckmann, C., & Beckmann, C. (1990). Effect of a structured antepartum exercise program on pregnancy and labor outcome in primiparas. *Journal of Reproductive Medicine, 35*(7), 704-709.

Birge, S., & Dalsky, G. (1989). The role of exercise in preventing osteoporosis. *Public Health Reports, 104*(Suppl.), 54-58.

Block, J., Smith, R., Friedlander, A., & Genant, H. (1989). Preventing osteoporosis with exercise: A review with emphasis on methodology. *Medical Hypotheses, 30*(1), 9-19.

Boyd, N., & McGuire, V. (1990). Evidence of association between plasma high-density lipoprotein cholesterol and risk factors for breast cancer. *Journal of the National Cancer Institute, 82*(6), 460-468.

Bunt, J. C. (1990). Metabolic actions of estradiol: Significance for acute and chronic exercise responses. *Medicine and Science in Sports and Exercise, 22*(3), 286-290.

Bush, T. (1990). The epidemiology of cardiovascular disease in postmenopausal women. *Annals of the New York Academy of Science, 592*(5), 263-271.

Chow, R., Harrison, J., & Dornan, J. (1989). Prevention and rehabilitation of osteoporosis program: Exercise and osteoporosis. *International Journal of Rehabilitation Research, 12*(1), 49-56.

Clapp, J. F. III, & Capeless, E. L. (1990). Neonatal morphometrics after endurance exercise during pregnancy. *American Journal of Obstetrics and Gynecology, 163*(6), 1805-1811.

Clarkson, T. B., Adams, M. R., Kaplan, J. R., Shively, C. A., & Koritnik, D. R. (1989). From menarche to menopause: Coronary artery atherosclerosis and protection in cynomolgus monkeys. *American Journal of Obstetrics and Gynecology, 160*(5), 1280-1285.

Cohn, B., Brand, R., & Hulley, S. (1989, May). Correlates of high density lipoprotein cholesterol in women studied by the method of co-twin control. *American Journal of Epidemiology, 129*(5), 988-999.

Conway, T. L. (1989). Behavioral, psychological, and demographic predictors of physical fitness. *Psychological Report, 65*(3), 1123-1135.

Cox, B. M., Opheim, K. E., Teschmacher, H., & Goldstein, A. A. (1975). Peptide-like substance from pituitary that acts like morphine: 2. Purification and properties. *Life Sciences, 16,* 1777-1782.

Dalsky, G. P. (1990). Effect of exercise on bone: Permissive influence of estrogen and calcium. *Medicine and Science in Sports and Exercise, 22*(3), 281-285.

Danforth, J., Allen, K., Fitterling, J., Danforth, J., Farrar, D., Brown, M., & Drabman, R. (1990). Exercise as a treatment for hypertension in low-socioeconomic-status black children. *Journal of Consulting and Clinical Psychology, 58*(2), 237-239.

Derman, R. (1990). Oral contraceptives and cardiovascular risk. Taking a safe course of action. *Postgraduate Medicine, 88*(4), 119-122.

Ekoe, J. (1989). Overview of diabetes mellitus and exercise. *Medicine and Science in Sports and Exercise, 21*(4), 353-355.

Erlik, Y., Tataryn, I. V., Meldrum, D. R., Lomax, P., Bayorek, J. G., & Judd, H. L. (1981). Association of waking episodes with menopausal hot flashes. *JAMA, 245,* 1741-1744.

Estok, P. J., Rudy, E. B., Kerr, M. E., & Menzel, L. (1993). Menstrual response to running: Nursing implications. *Nursing Research, 42*(3), 158-165.

Ferin, M. (1984). Endogenous opioid peptides and the menstrual cycle. *Trends in Neuroscience, 6*(6), 194-196.

Fletcher, G. F., Froelicher, V. F., Hartley, L. H., Haskell, W. L., & Pollock, M. L. (1990). Exercise standards: A statement for health professionals from the American Heart Association. *Circulation, 82*(6), 2286-2322.

Gauvin, L. (1990). An experiential perspective on the motivational features of exercise and lifestyle [see comments]. *Canadian Journal of Sport Science, 15*(1), 51-58.

Gibbons, L. W., & Blair, S. N. (1989). Healthy adults. In B. A. Franklin, S. Gordon, & G. C. Timmis (Eds.), *Exercise in modern medicine* (pp. 22-43). Baltimore, MD: Williams & Wilkins.

Gleichmann, U. M., Phillippi, H. H., Gleichmann, S. I., Laun, R., Mellwig, K. P., Frohnapfel, F., & Liebermann, A. (1989). Group exercise improves patient compliance in mild to moderate hypertension. *Journal of Hypertension, 7*(Suppl. 3), S77-S80.

Guillemin, R., Vargo, T., Rossier, J., Minich, S., Ling, N., Rivier, C., Vale, W., & Bloom, F. (1977). Beta-endorphin and adrenocorticotropin are secreted concomitantly by the pituitary gland. *Science, 197,* 1367-1368.

Halbreich, U., Alt, I. H., & Paul, L. (1988). Premenstrual changes impaired hormonal homeostasis, endocrinology of neuropsychiatric disorders. *Neurologic Clinics, 6*(1), 173-194.

Harris, D. V. (1991). Special considerations for the female athlete. In W. A. Grana & A. Kalenak (Eds.), *Clinical sports medicine* (p. 68). Philadelphia, PA: W. B. Saunders.

Harris, S., Caspersen, C., DeFriese, G., & Estes, E. J. (1989). Physical activity counseling for healthy adults as a primary preventive intervention in the clinical setting. *JAMA, 261*(24), 3588-3598.

Harshfield, G., Dupaul, L., Alpert, B., Christman, J., Willey, E., Murphy, J., & Somes, G. (1990). Aerobic fitness and the diurnal rhythm of blood pressure in adolescents. *Hypertension, 15*(6, pt. 2), 810-814.

Hughes, J., Smith, T., Kosterlitz, H., Feathergill, L., Morgan, B., & Morris, H. (1975). Identification of two related pentapeptides from the brain with potent opiate agonist activity. *Nature, 259,* 577.

Jette, M., Sidney, K., & Blumchen, G. (1990). Metabolic equivalents (METS) in exercise testing, exercise prescription and evaluation of functional capacity. *Clinical Cardiology, 13*(8), 555-565.

Jula, A., Ronnemaa, T., Rastas, M., Karvetti, R., & Maki, J. (1990). Long-term non-pharmacological treatment for mild to moderate hypertension. *Journal of Internal Medicine, 227*(6), 413-421.

Kaiserauer, S., Snyder, A., Sleeper, M., & Zierath, J. (1989). Nutritional, physiological, and menstrual status of distance runners. *Medicine and Science in Sports and Exercise, 21*(2), 120-125.

Kirkpatrick, M., Brewer, J., & Stocks, B. (1990). Efficacy of self-care measures for premenstrual syndrome (PMS). *Journal of Advanced Nursing, 15*(3), 281-285.

Klebanoff, M. A., Shiono, P. H., & Carey, J. C. (1990). The effect of physical activity during pregnancy on preterm delivery and birth weight. *American Journal of Obstetrics and Gynecology, 163*(5), 1450-1456.

Kramsch, D. M., Aspen, A. J., Abramowitz, A., Kreimendahl, T., & Hood, W. B. (1981). Reduction of coronary atherosclerosis by moderate conditioning exercise in monkeys on an atherogenic diet. *New England Journal of Medicine, 305,* 1484-1489.

Kuczmierczyk, A. (1989). Multi-component behavioral treatment of premenstrual syndrome: A case report. *Journal of Behavioral Therapy and Experimental Psychiatry, 20*(3), 235-240.

Lamon-Fava, S., Fisher, E., Nelson, M., Evans, W., Millar, J., Ordovas, J., & Schaefer, E. (1989). Effect of exercise and menstrual cycle status on plasma lipids, low density lipoprotein particle size, and apolipoproteins. *Journal of Clinical Endocrinology and Metabolism, 68*(1), 17-21.

Leon, A. S. (1989). Patients with diabetes. In B. A. Franklin, S. Gordon, & G. C. Timmis (Eds.), *Exercise in modern medicine* (pp. 118-155). Baltimore, MD: Williams & Wilkins.

Lokey, E., & Tran, Z. (1989). Effects of exercise training on serum lipid and lipoprotein concentrations in women: A meta-analysis. *International Journal of Sports Medicine, 10*(6), 424-429.

Loucks, A. (1990). Effects of exercise training on the menstrual cycle: Existence and mechanisms. *Medicine and Science in Sports and Exercise, 22*(3), 275-280.

Loucks, A., Mortola, J., Girton, L., & Yen, S. (1989). Alterations in the hypothalamic-pituitary-ovarian and the hypothalamic-pituitary-adrenal axes in athletic women. *Journal of Clinical Endocrinology and Metabolism, 68*(2), 402-411.

Lovelady, C., Lonnerdal, B., & Dewey, K. (1990). Lactation performance of exercising women. *American Journal of Clinical Nutrition, 52*(1), 103-109.

MacLusky, N., Naftolin, F., & Leranth, C. (1988). Immunocytochemical evidence for direct synaptic connections between corticotrophin-releasing factor (CRF) and gonadotropin-releasing hormone (GnRH)-containing neurons in the preoptic area of the rat. *Brain Research, 439*(1-2), 391-395.

Madden, J., Akil, H., Patrick, R., & Barchas, J. D. (1977). Stress induced parallel changes in central opioid levels and pain responsiveness in the rat. *Nature, 265,* 358-360.

Mesaki, N., Sasaki, J., Motobu, M., Nabeshima, Y., Shoji, M., Iwasaki, H., Asano, K., & Eda, M. (1989). Effect of naloxone on hormonal changes during exercise. *Nippon Sanka Fujinka Gakkai Zasshi, 41*(12), 1991-1998.

Morey, M. C., Cowper, P. A., Feussner, J. R., DiPasquale, R. C., Crowley, G. M., Kitzman, D. W., & Sullivan, R. J., Jr. (1989). Evaluation of supervised exercise program in a geriatric population. *Journal of the American Geriatric Society, 37*(4), 348-354.

The 1988 Report of the Joint Committee on Detection, Evaluation, and Treatment of High Blood Pressure.

(1988). *Archives of Internal Medicine, 148*(5), 1023-1038.

Oldridge, N. B., & Streiner, D. L. (1990). The health belief model: Predicting compliance and dropout in cardiac rehabilitation. *Medicine and Science in Sports and Exercise, 22*(5), 678-683.

Pasternostro-Bayles, M., Wing, R. R., & Robertson, R. J. (1989). Effects of life-style activity of varying duration on glycemic control in type II diabetic women. *Diabetes Care, 12*(1), 34-37.

Pate, R. R., Blair, S. N., Durstine, J. L., Eddy, D. O., Hanson, P., Smith, L. K., & Wolfe, L. A. (1991). *Guidelines for exercise testing and prescription* (American College of Sports Medicine). Philadelphia: Leon & Febiger.

Paulev, P., Thorbll, J., Nielsen, U., Kruse, P., Jordal, R., Bach, F., Fenger, M., & Pokorski, M. (1989). Opioid involvement in the perception of pain due to endurance exercise in trained man. *Japanese Journal of Physiology, 39*(1), 67-74.

Pert, C. B., & Snyder, S. (1973). Opiate receptor: Demonstration in nervous tissue. *Science, 179,* 1011-1014.

Pollock, M. L., & Wilmore, J. M. (1990). *Exercise in health and disease* (2nd ed., pp. 139-140). Philadelphia, PA: W. B. Saunders.

Prior, J. C., Vigna, Y. M., Schechter, M. T., & Burgess, A. E. (1990). Spinal bone loss and ovulatory disturbances. *New England Journal of Medicine, 323*(18), 1221-1227.

Raglin, J. (1990). Exercise and mental health. Beneficial and detrimental effects. *Sports Medicine, 9*(6), 323-329.

Ravnikar, V. (1990). Physiology and treatment of hot flashes. *Obstetrics and Gynecology, 75*(Suppl. 4), 3s-7s.

Report of the National Cholesterol Education Program Expert Panel on Detection, Evaluation and Treatment of High Blood Cholesterol in Adults. (1988). *Archives of Internal Medicine, 148,* 36-69.

Rogers, M. (1989). Acute effects of exercise on glucose tolerance in non-insulin-dependent diabetes. *Medicine and Science in Sports and Exercise, 21*(4), 362-368.

Ropert, J. F., Quigley, M. E., & Yen, S. S. C. (1981). Endogenous opiates modulate pulsatile luteinizing hormone release in humans. *Journal of Endocrinology and Metabolism, 52*(3), 583-585.

Sahlin, K. (1990). Muscle glucose metabolism during exercise. *Annals of Medicine, 22*(3), 85-89.

Sasaki, J., Urata, H., Tanabe, Y., Kinoshita, A., Tanaka, H., Shindo, M., & Arakawa, K. (1989). Mild exercise therapy increases serum high density lipoprotein 2 cholesterol levels in patients with essential hypertension. *American Journal of Medical Science, 297*(4), 220-223.

Schweiger, U., Laessle, R., Tuschl, R., Broocks, A., Krusche, T., & Pirke, K. (1989). Decreased follicular phase gonadotropin secretion is associated with impaired estradiol and progesterone secretion during the follicular and luteal phases in normally menstruating women. *Journal of Clinical Endocrinology and Metabolism, 68*(5), 888-892.

Seifer, D., & Collins, R. (1990). Current concepts of beta-endorphin physiology in female reproductive dysfunction. *Fertility and Sterility, 54,* 5.

Simon, E. J., Hiller, J. M., & Edelman, I. (1973). Stereo specific binding of the potent narcotic analgesic (3H) etorphine to rat brain homogenate. *Proceedings of the American Academy of Science, 70,* 1947-1949.

Smith, E., Gilligan, C., McAdam, M., Ensign, C., & Smith, P. (1989). Deterring bone loss by exercise intervention in premenopausal and postmenopausal women. *Calcified Tissue International, 44*(5), 312-321.

Steptoe, A., Edwards, S., Moses, J., & Mathews, A. (1989). The effects of exercise training on mood and perceived coping ability in anxious adults from the general population. *Journal of Psychosomatic Research, 33*(5), 537-547.

Taylor, D. L. (1991, October). *Therapeutic response patterns and clinical indicators for evaluating nursing interventions directed to a theme perimenstrual negative affect: Results from a longitudinal clinical trial* (abstract). Paper presented at the International Nursing Research Conference, Los Angeles.

Terenius, L. (1975). Comparison between narcotic "receptors" in the guinea-pig ileum and the rat brain. *Acta Pharmacologica, 37,* 211-221.

Upton, G. (1990). Lipids, cardiovascular disease, and oral contraceptives: A practical perspective. *Fertility and Sterility, 53*(1), 1-12.

Veldhuis, J. D. (1990). The hypothalamic pulse generator: The reproductive core. *Clinical Obstetrics and Gynecology, 33*(3), 538-550.

Wasserman, D., & Abumrad, N. (1989). Physiological bases for the treatment of the physically active individual with diabetes. *Sports Medicine, 7*(6), 376-392.

Watson, S. J., Akil, H., Berger, P., & Barchas, J. D. (1979). Some observations on opiate peptides and schizophrenia. *Archives of General Psychiatry, 36,* 35-41.

Weherenberg, W. B., Wardlaw, S. L., Frantz, A., & Ferin, M. (1982). Beta-endorphin in hypophyseal portal blood: Variations throughout the menstrual cycle. *Endocrinology, 111,* 879-881.

Wilson, P. F. (1987). The epidemiology of hypercholesterolemia. *American Journal of Medicine, 87*(Suppl. 4A), 5S-13S.

Wolfe, L., Hall, P., Webb, K., Goodman, L., Monga, M., & McGrath, M. (1989). Prescription of aerobic exercise during pregnancy. *Sports Medicine, 8*(5), 273-301.

Zylstra, S., Hopkins, A., Erk, M., Hreshchyshyn, M., & Anbar, M. (1989). Effect of physical activity on lumbar spine and femoral neck bone densities. *International Journal of Sports Medicine, 10*(3), 181-186.

14

Fertility Control

JOELLEN HAWKINS
PEGGY S. MATTESON
ELEANOR SMITH TABEEK

The availability of relatively safe, inexpensive, and accessible contraceptive methods allows women to postpone pregnancy, alter the timing between pregnancies, or avoid pregnancy completely. By giving women a way to plan their children's births, contraception can also help increase their health and that of their family members.

Health care professionals who care for women must be prepared to assist them with contraception, if requested. As an aid, this chapter provides a basic understanding of contraception by exploring historical and social factors, current patterns and practices, and decision making related to contraception. It then describes common family planning services and details the various contraceptive methods. The chapter concludes with a brief look at future contraceptive methods.

Historical and Social Context

No scientific breakthrough has significantly altered as many women's lives as the discovery of safe, effective contraceptive methods. Before these methods were available, women suffered chronic illness, fatigue, and even death from unpreventable pregnancies (Cooke & Dworkin, 1979). Multiple pregnancies and unspaced births not only negatively affected women's physical health but also reduced their economic productivity, leading to increased dependence on others and unfulfilled potential.

Today, a sexually active heterosexual, bisexual, or lesbian woman can affect her physical, educational, and socioeconomic destiny—and that of her family—by choosing to use contraception. By using a highly effective contraceptive method, she reduces the risk of unplanned pregnancy, which enables her to plan her family along with other aspects of her life (Jones, Forrest, Henshaw, Silverman, & Torres, 1988).

The ability to prevent or defer childbearing allows a woman to pursue educational opportunities and participate in the labor force. It also may broaden her outlook when considering other life opportunities. Because a planned birth can be integrated into a woman's career or job more readily than an unplanned birth, a planned birth has fewer negative effects on her employment (Smith-Lovin & Tickamyer, 1978). Some women use contraception successfully to take advantage of educational and employment opportunities. Others are not as successful. Instead, they learn by experience that few things change a woman's life as much as the fear of conception or the reality of an unintended pregnancy.

Although information about contraception has been available since the precolonial period, American women could not always take advantage of it because of social or political constraints.

Precolonial America

Before Europeans colonized the New World, Native American women attempted to control their fertility. They used various herbs and roots, abstained from sex for 9 days following the onset of menses, and prolonged lactation to prevent conception. They also induced abortion occasionally (Himes, 1936, p. 213). In more recent oral histories, Native American women told of their knowledge of preventing pregnancy and inducing abortion, usually with plants. For example, Salish women drank a contraceptive made of dogbane roots and water.

Some Native Americans held magical beliefs about conception related to disposal of the placenta. For example, the Paiute believed that barrenness would result from burying the placenta upside down or allowing it to be eaten by animals. The Lummi believed that further conceptions would not occur if the placenta was hurled into a river or ocean eddy and twisted by it (Niethammer, 1977).

The Puritan Ethic

European settlers in the American colonies brought with them the sexual mores and practices of their homelands. For example, the Puritans in the Plymouth Colony used coitus interruptus (withdrawal of the penis immediately before ejaculation) to prevent pregnancy. Other European settlers brought a Christian morality that viewed sex as sinful. In fact, a perceptive Hopi interpreter of Native American ceremonies confessed that he edited the old Hopi stories because "I knew the whites can see more sin than pleasure in sex" (Himes, 1936).

Children as an Economic Asset

An economy based on agriculture and a high infant mortality rate curbed interest in contraception for many European settlers. They saw advantages in having large families to help clear the land, plant and tend crops, and process the products into goods for family consumption or trade with Europe. To ensure that at least some children would survive to adulthood, women tended to have many children. The price on their health was high: Many women died during childbirth or died later from the effects of multiple pregnancies. When they died, their husbands usually remarried and had more children.

In some states, slave owners pressured African American women to produce children to work on the plantations or to be sold for profit. The horror of seeing one's child sold motivated many of these women to try to avoid pregnancy. Because magical, medicinal, and mechanical contraceptive methods were practiced in Africa (Himes, 1936), women slaves may have been aware of them as part of their cultural heritage and used them to prevent pregnancy.

Victorian America

By the late 19th century, women had become idealized. Middle-class women, in particular, were seen as "sweet, untouchable guardians of morality, whose distaste for sex led to an explosive increase in prostitution" (Tannahill, 1980, p. 347). Freed from constant work by the industrial revolution, middle-class and upper-class women hired servants to do domestic chores and turned their efforts toward moral causes. However, poorer women continued to work long hours on farms, in factories, or in homes as domestic servants.

Typically illiterate, lower-class women could obtain contraceptive information only by word of mouth. Although most middle-class and upper-class women could read and use contraceptive information, efforts to disseminate such information were hampered by religious beliefs that abstinence was the only acceptable contraceptive method. Also, several states passed legislation that outlawed the dissemination of birth control information and contraceptive devices (Gieg, 1972). For example, in 1879, Massachusetts law prohibited the sale, loan, or exhibition of any article used to induce abortion or prevent conception as well as the publication of any information leading to pregnancy termination or prevention (Gieg, 1972). (This law was not abolished until 1967.)

Sanger and the Birth Control Movement

Early in the 20th century, Margaret Sanger began the modern birth control movement. Born in 1879, she dedicated herself to this work after seeing her mother die from tuberculosis and the burden of bearing 11 children and after observing women from New York's Lower East Side die from childbirth or illegal abortions. She completed nursing school at White Plains Hospital, New York, in 1902.

Inspired by Emma Goldman, the first American nurse to lecture on birth control, Sanger began to publish information about women's reproductive concerns in 1912. Her first efforts were a series of articles describing puberty and the functions of a woman's body for the *Call,* a socialist newspaper (Gordon, 1990). These articles were the basis for *What Every Girl Should Know,* a pamphlet published in 1915 and later published as a book (Sanger, 1920a). The first issue of *The Woman Rebel* was published in March 1914. In the same year, Sanger prepared the pamphlet *Family Limitation* and organized a committee called the National Birth Control League. She fled to England in October to avoid prosecution for violating the Comstock Law (federal law that prohibited the mailing of obscene material, which included birth control information and devices [Tannahill, 1980]). In England, Sanger met C. V. Drysdale, head of the international birth control movement, and Havelock Ellis, author of *Studies in the Psychology of Sex.* Then she visited Holland, where she learned how to fit pessaries (now known as diaphragms) and studied that country's birth control clinic system.

On October 16, 1916, Sanger and her sister Ethel opened the Brownsville Clinic in Brooklyn, America's first birth control clinic. The clinic provided birth control information and education, although this was illegal at the time. From 1916 to 1934, Sanger established birth control clinics, published birth control articles and pamphlets in defiance of the Comstock Law, worked to change birth control laws, organized the American Birth Control League (1921), attended national and international conferences on birth control, lectured around the world, and was jailed more than once for her activities. In 1922, she engaged Dr. Dorothy Bocker to run a Clinical Research Bureau. The next year, she hired Dr. James F. Cooper to lecture to physicians across the United States about birth control. She smuggled pessaries into the United States through her husband's factory in Canada until 1925, when she convinced two of her supporters to found the Holland-Rantos Company and begin U.S. production. In 1926, she traveled to London, Paris, and Geneva to prepare for an international meeting in 1927, which led to the formation of the International Union for the Scientific Investigation of Population Problems (Himes, 1936). In 1928, she resigned as president of the American Birth Control League but continued to edit the *Birth Control Review* until 1929, when she withdrew from the league and the paper. In April of that year, police raided the Clinical Research Bureau (because this type of research was also considered in violation of the Comstock Law), but Sanger did not give up.

The 1930s brought some victories for the birth control movement. In the summer of 1930, the Seventh International Birth Control Conference was held under Sanger's leadership. In 1934, Sanger went to Russia to gather data about the birth control movement there. The next year, she attended the All-India Women's Conference, met Ghandi, and gave 64 lectures across India. In 1936, Congress revised the Comstock Act, redefining obscenity to exclude birth control information and devices. One year later, the American Medical Association resolved that contraception was a legitimate medical service. By 1938, more than 300 clinics were operating in the United States. In 1939, the American Birth Control League and the Voluntary Parenthood League merged and named Sanger honorary president.

Throughout the 1950s, Sanger continued to promote birth control. In 1952, she persuaded Katherine McCormick, widow of the founder of International Harvester, to fund the research that produced the oral contraceptive. She also traveled to India to help organize the International Planned Parenthood Federation; the next year in Stockholm, Sanger was elected president of this organization. In 1959, 80-year-old Sanger attended the International Conference on Population in New Delhi, where she met Nehru. She died in 1966 in Tucson (Douglas, 1970; Gordon, 1990; Gray, 1979; Lader, 1955; Marlow, 1979; Sanger, 1920b, 1931, 1938; Sicherman, Green, Kantor, & Walker, 1980).

The New Feminism

While Sanger was establishing birth control clinics, other women were working to obtain the vote, which they finally gained with the passage of the 19th Amendment in 1920. The suffrage movement reflected women's growing desire to claim their place as fully contributing members of society. World War I (1914-1921) gave women opportunities for paid employment in nursing, munitions factory work, and other fields. This reinforced the desire to control other aspects of their lives, including fertility.

During this period, some advocates saw birth control as a tool not only for limiting pregnancies but also for promoting social revolution. They believed the solution to many social problems, such as poverty and limited resources, lay in population control (Gordon, 1990). Thus most birth control advocates were social radicals; some were also socialists or political radicals.

After World War I, women returned to work in the home, and the birth control movement changed considerably. As health care professionals made birth control an integral part of their practice, they moved it into the mainstream of society. Birth control, which had begun as a radical social movement, shifted decisively into the medical arena, ensuring medical control of contraception. Medical control was synonymous with middle-class and upper-class control, giving contraception a taint of ethnic genocide that survives even in the 1990s. If contraceptive information and methods had been controlled by radical feminists and socialists, such as Emma Goldman, the story might have evolved very differently. For example, contraceptive information and methods might have been in the hands of women users rather than physicians (Gordon, 1990).

The recent efforts of feminists to wrest control of contraception from physicians have their roots in the birth control movement of the 1920s and 1930s. In the 1990s in the United States, the most effective contraceptive methods—intrauterine devices (IUDs), oral contraceptives, and hormonal implants and injectibles—remain under physician control. As nurses in expanded roles gain prescription-writing privileges, control of these methods passes to health care professionals other than physicians and into the hands of more women. Interestingly, in many other countries, control of these methods rests with the women who use them or with health care professionals other than physicians.

Contraceptive Patterns and Practices

Sexual beliefs and practices of women in their childbearing years can influence patterns of contraceptive use as well as the number of planned and unplanned pregnancies.

Sexual Beliefs and Practices

Since the Kinsey report (Kinsey, Pomeroy, Martin, & Gebhard, 1953) released documentation that some women masturbated, had premarital sexual experiences, and were orgasmic, the American public has lived through the baby boom of the 1950s, when many women returned or stayed home to raise families; the new wave of feminism of the 1960s, beginning with Betty Friedan's (1963) *Feminine Mystique;* and the sexual revolution of the 1970s. (See Chapter 21, "Sexuality in Women's Lives," for in-depth discussion on this topic.)

While feminism was gaining popularity, scientists were developing oral contraceptives, which promised freedom from unwanted pregnancy in a pill—a contraceptive method totally dissociated from intercourse. However, physicians controlled this method as well as abortions, which were legalized in 1973. (For more information about abortions, see Chapter 20, "Unwanted Pregnancy.") To counter medical control of women's bodies, the Boston Women's Health Book Collective published *Our Bodies, Ourselves* in 1969, and self-help groups sprang up in the 1970s. At the same time, many authors addressed the "new sexuality" of women, allegedly discovered during the sexual revolution. Thus, while women worked for liberation from feminine stereotypes, they experienced a bombardment of expectations about their sexuality. The role of superwoman took on new qualities: Not only were American women expected to be faultless wives, mothers, and career women, but they were also supposed to fulfill all of their partner's sexual fantasies. However, the sexual revolution did not relieve women of the burden of contraception. Even today, most sexually active women of childbearing age make all decisions about contraception.

Patterns of Contraceptive Use

In 1989, of the 57.9 million women of reproductive age, approximately 35 million (60%) were using some form of contraception (Horton, 1992). The method chosen depends greatly on the woman's age, race, marital status, and socioeconomic status. For example, a black, single teenager might choose the oral contraceptives, whereas an older married woman with three children might elect to have a tubal ligation or have Norplant inserted.

Forrest (1987) reports that sexually active women of childbearing age have used an average of 2.8 contraceptive methods. Reasons for switching methods are many and complex. However, they frequently reflect women's concerns about the health risks of the contraceptive method rather than the risks of an unintended pregnancy (Silverman, Torres, & Forrest, 1987), even though virtually any method is safer than none at all. Women may choose a method based on incomplete information rather than on balanced facts. Some may choose not to use contraception at all because of fear of the adverse effects of various methods (Ory, Forrest, & Lincoln, 1983).

Contraceptive use is relatively low in the United States. Only 60% of women of childbearing age currently use contraception in contrast to 65% in the Netherlands and 70% in Great Britain. Among developed countries, the United States has the highest pregnancy rate (2.6 per woman), and more than half of the pregnancies are unintended (Jones et al., 1988). Most of these pregnancies result from sporadic use of contraception or use of an ineffective method or no method (Jones et al., 1988).

The Department of Health and Human Services funded three cycles of the National Survey of Family Growth, conducted between 1973 and 1988. Using a structured interview format, researchers asked women which contraceptive method (or methods) they used since their last pregnancy or first intercourse and which method they currently used (Grady, Hayward, & Florey, 1988).

From this national survey, contraceptive use can be estimated. Among single women, oral contraceptives were the method of choice, followed by condoms. The increased risk of acquired immunodeficiency syndrome (AIDS) in the 1980s may account for the rise in popularity of condoms, particularly among single women. Among all women, IUD use declined, possibly because some IUDs were removed from the market in the 1980s as patents ran out, and the remainder were restricted for use in women who had completed their families or who did not wish to have children. The percentage of women choosing sterilization has increased from 25.7% of all women in 1982 to 28.3% in 1988 (U.S. Bureau of the Census, 1991).

Unintended Pregnancies

The U.S. rate of unintended pregnancies is higher than that of most other developed countries. Compared to 19 other Western countries, the United States ranks in the middle (6th) for total fertility rate (average number of children per woman) but is higher than most (3rd) of the other countries for total abortion rate (average number per woman) and pregnancy rate (births plus abortions). Unplanned births and abortions are common, meaning that the unintended pregnancy rate is relatively high, especially for women under age 25.

The proportion of women using one of the three most effective methods (sterilization, oral contraceptive, and IUD) is much lower in the United States than in other countries (Jones et al., 1988). For example, only 37.4% of women in the United States use the most effective contraceptive methods, compared with 52% of women in Great Britain and 56.3% in the Netherlands. Use of these most effective methods requires access to health care. Unlike in other countries, access to health care in the United States depends greatly on ability to pay and proximity to a health care facility. Thus unintended pregnancies and limited access to health care seem inextricably connected.

Contraceptive Decision Making

From menarche to menopause, women must make decisions about their fertility, including if, how, and when they will regulate it. Women may choose to abstain from intercourse, engage in intercourse and risk pregnancy, or engage in intercourse and prevent pregnancy by using contraception.

Making a decision about contraception is more than selecting among attractive alternatives. It requires strategies and compromises that satisfy personal, social, cultural, and interpersonal needs influenced by constraints, opportunities, values, and norms.

Deciding to Use Contraception

Decision models assume that an individual's choices are determined by beliefs about their consequences and perceptions of their advantages and disadvantages. Although individuals try to make the best possible choices, they can be hampered by the complexity of the situation, conflicting beliefs and motives, misinformation, social constraints, and intrapsychic conflicts (Adler, 1979). When making a decision, an individual's values and perceptions of probable outcomes are valid, even if they are not objective or consistent with cultural values. Because of this, some investigators believe that the decision not to use contraception can be sensible even when pregnancy is not intended. In fact, it may be based on a decision model in which a woman decides that benefits associated with not using a contraceptive outweigh the risks associated with pregnancy (Luker, 1978). (Additional information on this topic is found in Chapter 20.)

Every decision has antecedents and consequences. Antecedents initiate the decision-making process. They are the events or incidents that cause doubt, wavering, debate, or controversy. They lead to searching for options, followed by a gathering of information about these options. Before a decision is made, the feasibility of each option is examined and evaluated and the possible risks and consequences of each option are considered. Consequences are the events or incidents that result from the decision.

When a decision is made, stabilization occurs because the decision ends the doubt, wavering, debate, or controversy. Then the individual may affirm the decision by implementing it, affirm it but postpone implementation, reverse it, or reconsider it and make new decisions as circumstances and desires change.

For example, a woman is considering switching from an oral contraceptive to a cervical cap. She may have used other contraceptive methods in the past and probably will consider them along with the cervical cap and other methods. Then she compares the cap's advantages and disadvantages with those of the other options. After considering the consequences of using the cap, such as use must be closely linked to intercourse, neccessity of inserting device in her body, and messiness of the method, she decides to use this contraceptive method. After choosing the cervical cap, the woman might consider the consequences of that decision on her relationship with her partner, the need to learn insertion and removal techniques, and other consequences unique to her lifestyle and roles.

Influences

Before deciding to use contraception, a woman must perceive herself as sexually active and at risk for becoming pregnant. A sexual self-concept is correlated strongly with contraceptive use (Winter, 1988). The decision to use contraception may be influenced by many factors, such as age, family patterns of health care, advice from health care professionals, cultural background, socioeconomic status, locus of control, knowledge of pregnancy risks, availability of contraception, approach to risk taking, and relationship with partner (Winter, 1988).

Inadequate or incorrect knowledge about conception leads women to miscalculate or underestimate their risk of pregnancy. Women may obtain this knowledge from friends, classes, books, magazines, family members, or sexual partners. Misinformation from any source can place a woman at risk. For example, a woman may risk pregnancy by not using contraception because her partner believes he is infertile.

Communication about sexual and other matters between partners tends to be related to contraceptive use: More communication is associated with more use of contraception and sometimes with use of more effective contraception (Burger & Inderbitzen, 1985). The partner's attitude also may influence contraceptive use in other ways. For example, one may threaten to leave if the woman uses contraception; another may threaten to leave if she becomes pregnant.

Statements from family members and friends may affect a woman's decision. Most adolescents who attend family planning clinics have the support of their friends or mothers in seeking contraception, but few have the support of both (Nathanson & Becker, 1986). Some women feel that family members, friends, or society in general would disapprove and thus may be less likely to use contraception.

Past experiences with contraception can determine which methods a woman will consider. So can the past experiences of family members and friends. Adverse effects from previous methods can affect a woman's choice of contraceptive method, as can the degree to which these effects interfered with her self-image, sexual expression, or lifestyle.

Choices

A woman's choice of contraceptive method results from her expectations about the method and her feelings about those expectations (Miller, 1986). A woman selects a method because it is available and because she believes it will prevent pregnancy. In making her choice, she uses the decision-making process described earlier. She may do this many times during her childbearing years.

Changes

A woman's opinions about contraceptive methods may change with her age, relationship, number of children, plans for future children, and experience with a method (Forrest & Fordyce, 1988). For example, a woman who used a barrier method during the years she was actively planning her family, may decide on a tubal ligation when she decides her family is complete. A woman who used oral contraceptives during the years she was sure she did not want children may switch to condoms and foam while she prepares to attempt conception. At any time, she may stop using a method because it does not meet her expectations, because it becomes unavailable, or because her situation changes.

Deciding to Collaborate With a Health Care Professional

Some women control their fertility without the assistance of a health care professional. They do not feel a need for educational services or prescription methods. Favorable attitudes toward methods are a prerequisite for contraceptive use and for seeking assistance from a provider when the woman believes she needs input from a professional to choose a method or have access to a prescription method (Silverman et al., 1987).

Other women see a health care professional, obtain a contraceptive method, and never return. If the prescription expires or the method needs replacement, they may discontinue it rather than return to the health care professional. Still other women switch from one health care professional to another for various reasons. To help maintain women's contraceptive use over time, nurses providing family planning services should promote quality interactions with clients. The quality of the interaction between nurses and their clients can positively or negatively affect women's level of contraceptive use over time.

Special Considerations for Adolescents

Unintended pregnancy is a greater problem in the United States than in any other developed country, especially among adolescents. To try to prevent pregnancy, adolescents typically depend on over-the-counter methods and natural methods, such as coitus interruptus or natural family planning methods. They commonly delay seeking contraceptive care because they fear that their confidentiality will not be maintained and their parents will discover their sexual activity.

When an adolescent chooses a health care professional, her criteria are likely to be confidentiality, a staff who cares about adolescents, and geographic proximity (Zabin & Clark, 1981). An adolescent expects confidentiality. However, her chances of finding confidential services may be slim, especially in a community with few alternatives. Health care professionals' beliefs may prevent them from condoning the adolescent's sexual behavior. One in four physicians will not provide contraceptives to minors without parental consent (Forrest, 1988).

When the parent and adolescent come together for care, they may have different agendas. The parent may want the health care professional to stop the adolescent from being sexually active; the adolescent simply may want to obtain a contraceptive method. The parent may wish to be informed of all findings and treatments, whereas the adolescent may not want her parents to be informed at all.

Deciding Not to Use Contraception

More than 3 million women in the United States risk unintended pregnancy each year (Klein, 1984). In addition, although nearly 90% of ever-married women report that their pregnancies were wanted, one in four of these were mistimed (Horton, 1992). Lack of contraception does not necessarily imply a wish for pregnancy, because many women feel as ambivalent about pregnancy as they do about contraception.

Luker (1978) asserts that women and health care professionals make disparate decisions about contraception because of their different perspectives. Health care professionals view the risk of pregnancy from unprotected intercourse as a known probability (statistical concept); women view it as an uncertainty or unknown. Using a rational decision-making process, women weigh the advantages and disadvantages of contraception against the advantages and disadvantages of pregnancy. Thus cost-benefit analysis (weighing of advantages and disadvantages of not using a contraceptive and becoming pregnant) determines the woman's decision to use contraception or not.

> When a woman cannot completely suppress her wish to become pregnant in spite of important situational constraints, when a woman loses the psychological energy that is continuously required to avoid conception, or when a woman feels the urge to use becoming pregnant as a way of dealing with certain negative feelings about herself, then her contraceptive practice tends to become inconsistent. (Miller, 1986, p. 427)

The woman's perceived risks of conception, her attitudes toward contraception, her interaction with the things and people associated with the method, and her partner's attitude may lead to the decision not to use contraception. Partner disapproval of contraception, in particular, can tip the balance in favor of the decision not to use contraception.

Rates of contraceptive nonuse are 80% higher among poor women than they are among women with higher incomes (Forrest, 1988). Research by Forrest (1988) has suggested, however, that cost is not a cause of contraceptive nonuse; rather, the cause lies with inadequate delivery of contraceptive services and restricted access to the most effective methods.

Special Considerations for Adolescents

The rate of contraceptive nonuse among sexually active adolescents is more than twice that of sexually active women in their early 20s (Forrest, 1988). According to Kisker (1985), adolescents cite these reasons for nonuse:

- They do not expect to have intercourse.
- Their partner objects to contraception.
- They believe that contraception is wrong or dangerous.
- They do not know which contraceptive methods exist or where to obtain them.
- They feel that contraceptives are too difficult or unpleasant to use.

Burke (1987) also notes that the adolescent male's beliefs and expectations about intercourse may not match those of his woman partner, placing her at risk for unintended pregnancy. For example, men may expect to have intercourse more often than do their female partners.

Family Planning Services

Various providers offer a range of family planning services such as counseling, prescribing oral contraceptives, fitting diaphragms or inserting the Norplant system in different settings, and using different educational materials and techniques. When assisting clients with family planning decisions, providers' styles may be paternalistic, maternalistic, or participatory.

Settings, Materials, and Techniques

Facilities that offer family planning services should offer clients free access to current developments in the field through state-of-the art media. They should be open at convenient hours for all consumers. These facilities should welcome the client's partner and, with the client's permission, encourage his participation in method selection and educational sessions.

The facility should be conducive to teaching and learning. Its waiting and counseling rooms should be large enough to permit various seating arrangements for several people. To promote teaching and learning, it should have adequate lighting and ventilation. Because individuals have different learning styles and educational backgrounds, various teaching methods should be used, such as one-to-one discussions and group sessions. Also, appropriate educational materials should be used, such as up-to-date printed materials, audiovisual materials, hands-on displays, and interactive computer software (Tabeek, 1990).

Changing from the present technically oriented family planning care delivery system to an educational delivery system with product and nonproduct methods of contraception requires fertility awareness education as the basis for all contraception. Fertility awareness assists women in becoming more knowledgeable regarding their bodies and how methods work to prevent conception. Increased client involvement and control over method selection may increase the client's use of the method she chooses.

The current system of delivering family planning services is not meeting the needs of all consumers. Drastic change in the system is unlikely, however, unless consumers demand more from the system. Client education may help solve this problem. However, changing the knowledge, attitudes, and behaviors of some family planning providers presents a greater challenge. Fortunately, most of them are enthusiastic about the future of family planning and eager to participate in new care delivery systems and to integrate new methods into their practice (Tabeek, 1990).

Providers

Various health care professionals offer family planning services. Specialists and general physicians, nurses, nurse practitioners, and nurse-midwives provide these services in private practices, clinics, and family planning agencies. Nursing roles range from teaching and counseling to direct hands-on care, such as inserting IUDs and contraceptive implants, fitting diaphragms and caps, and prescribing oral contraceptives. These nurses commonly assist the client with decision making by giving information and answering questions about prescription and over-the-counter methods as well as sterilization procedures.

Social workers, counselors with various educational backgrounds, health educators, and lay volunteers may also be part of the family planning team in private practices, clinics, and family planning agencies. All health care providers bring their personal agendas, biases, values, and cultures to the care setting, affecting care delivery and client interactions. The style of care delivery ranges from giving a method to a woman and assuming she will use it, to being a partner in decision making.

Different providers have different interaction styles when caring for clients who are making choices about their health. Providers with a paternalistic style assume they know what is best and make decisions for the client. They commonly use statements that begin with "I will . . . " and "You will . . . " Providers with a maternalistic style attempt to influence the client's choices and gain her acquiescence by stating the consequences of an action, rather than the alternatives to it. This focuses on potential outcomes and the effects of the client's choice on herself or others. They commonly use statements that begin with "If you don't . . . , then . . . " Providers of both styles focus on outcomes and attempt to gain the client's compliance with their predetermined goals.

Providers with a participatory style demonstrate respect for the client's autonomy and ability to make decisions. They focus on the process the client uses to reach a decision, presenting alternatives and urging her to participate in the decision. They use statements that begin with "What do you think about . . . ?" or "We can talk about . . . " (Taylor, Pickens, & Geden, 1989).

The client's needs and concerns are more likely to emerge in participatory interactions than in maternalistic or paternalistic ones. As Orne and Hawkins (1985) point out, "Providers must avoid the temptation to prescribe 'for clients.' Clients must make their own informed choice in collaboration with providers; they should feel supported in their right to choose" (p. 33).

Contraceptive Methods

For most American women, fertility regulation is a major concern. Ideally, they should be taught about their bodies before menarche (onset of menses), and learn about the developmental changes of puberty and the signs of fertility. After menarche, they may begin the journey along the sometimes tortuous path of decision making about contraception. During the childbearing years, they may decide the number and timing of any pregnancies they choose to have.

Table 14.1 Efficacy of Family Planning Methods (in percentages)

Method	*Theoretical Effectiveness*	*Use Effectiveness*
Oral contraceptives—combination	99.30	75-96
Oral contraceptives—progestin only	96.25-98.9	75-96
IUD	97-99	90-97
Diaphragm	97	80-85
Cap	96	82.6-93.6
Spermicides	96	60
Condoms	97-98.5	64-97
Condom and spermicide	99	95
Sponge	89-90.8	84.5-86.7
Implants	99.3	99
Natural family planning		
Mucus	98	75-90
Basal temperature	98	94
Symptothermal	98	90
Calendar	98	75
Sterilization—women	99.092	99.092
Sterilization—men	99.086	99.086
Female condom	97.5	87.6
Injectable contraceptive	99.7	99.3

SOURCE: Adapted from Hawkins, Roberto, and Stanley-Haney (1993).
NOTE: Failure rates vary from reference to reference and, within those references, may be based on one or several studies with widely varying populations and sample sizes. Thus it is not possible to say with certainty how effective a method is.

Before deciding to use a particular contraceptive method, a client should weigh the method's effectiveness against its risks (if any), advantages, disadvantages, and adverse effects. She also should consider any contraindications that may exist (see Tables 14.1 and 14.2). The effectiveness of various contraceptive methods can vary greatly. Each method has a theoretical effectiveness (effectiveness under ideal laboratory conditions, which depends solely on the method and not the human user) and use effectiveness (effectiveness under real life or human conditions, which allows for the user's carelessness or error as well as method failure). Table 14.1 indicates both types of effectiveness for each contraceptive method. The health care professional may use this information when counseling a client about contraceptive choices and risks. Table 14.2 summarizes the advantages, disadvantages, contraindications, and adverse effects of various barrier, chemical, hormonal, and intrauterine contraceptive methods.

When a client seeks assistance with family planning, the health care provider should perform a complete assessment, including a detailed health history and physical assessment with a pelvic examination and Papanicolaou (Pap) test (Nurses Association of the American College of Obstetricians and Gynecologists [NAACOG], 1991). Usually, this assessment is performed annually, although it may be done more or less frequently for some women. (See Chapter 9, "Well-Woman Assessment," for examples of the assessment process.) An important component of the initial assessment process is the client's personal and identifying information (for an example, see Figure 14.1).

On the basis of assessment findings and the client's preferences, the health care professional should assist with decision making. After the client selects a contraceptive method, she should receive appropriate care and client education (for a guide to general care, see Figure 14.2). Specific nursing care related to each method is discussed in this section.

Fertility Awareness Methods

The cornerstone of fertility regulation, fertility awareness, is the basis for understanding all contraceptive methods, especially the fertility awareness (natural family planning) methods. This information assists the client in knowing when or if she ovulates. Therefore, the health care professional should explore a client's awareness of her fertility patterns and provide additional information, if needed, before assisting

text continued on page 295

Table 14.2 Comparison of Contraceptive Methods

Advantages and Disadvantages	*Contraindications*	*Adverse Effects*
Fertility awareness method: All		
Advantages • Use no artificial means • Are accepted by all religions • Require little or no equipment • Can be started or stopped as needed • May be used for contraception or conception Disadvantages • Are user dependent • Need partner cooperation • Require abstinence during fertile period • Require client teaching	• Lack of motivation • Unwillingness to check fertility signs	• None
Barrier method: Diaphragm		
Advantages • May be inserted up to 4 hours before intercourse • May remain in place for up to 24 hours • Provides some protection against sexually transmitted diseases (STDs) • May be used as needed Disadvantages • Can stay in place 24 hours but has to be inserted before intercourse to be effective • Requires application of additional spermicide after 4 hours • Requires fitting	• Sensitivity to rubber • Anatomical characteristics such as malpositioned uterus • History of toxic shock syndrome (TSS)	• Allergic response to rubber or spermicide • Recurrent cystitis • Foul-smelling discharge if diaphragm remains in place too long • TSS • Rectal or bladder pressure with chronic constipation
Barrier method: Cervical cap		
Advantages • May be inserted any time • Offers some STD protection • May remain in place for up to 48 hours • Does not require application of additional spermicide for repeat intercourse • May be used as needed except during menses Disadvantages • Can stay in place 48 hours but has to be inserted before intercourse to be effective • Requires fitting • Cannot be used during menstruation • Requires follow-up Papanicolaou (Pap) test at 3 months	• Unavailability of correct size • Anatomical characteristics that preclude fitting, such as malshaped cervix	• Allergic response to rubber or spermicide • Abnormal Pap test results • TSS

(continued)

Table 14.2 Comparison of Contraceptive Methods—Continued

Advantages and Disadvantages	*Contraindications*	*Adverse Effects*
Barrier method: Vaginal sponge Advantages • May be inserted up to 1 hour before intercourse • Available over the counter • Some protection against STDs • Requires no additional spermicide for repeat intercourse • May remain in place for up to 24 hours • May be used as needed Disadvantages • Can stay in place 24 hours but has to be inserted before intercourse to be effective • Must be wet before insertion • Cannot be used during menstruation • May be used once only	• Sensitivity to spermicide • Inability to learn to insert or remove the sponge	• Allergic response to spermicide • TSS
Barrier method: Male Condom Advantages • Can be used as needed • Available over the counter • Protects against STDs • May be used as needed • Available with lubricant, spermicide, ribbing, reservoir tip, or coloring and in natural membrane or latex Disadvantages • Must be put on before intercourse • Must be put on erect penis • Decreases tactile sensations • Can be used once only	• Sensitivity to rubber	• Allergic response to rubber • Psychological impotence
Barrier method: Female condom Advantages • Temporary method • Use only as needed • One time use only • Protection against STDs, AIDS Disadvantages • Use dependent • Requires partner cooperation • Teaching necessary	• Sensitivity to lubricant • Sensitivity to polyurethane	• Allergic reaction to lubricant • Allergic reaction to polyurethane
Chemical method: Spermicidal foam Advantages • May be used as needed • Available over the counter • Some protection against STDs • Available in multiple-use or prefilled, single-use forms	• Sensitivity to spermicide or carrier	• Allergic response to spermicide or carrier

Table 14.2 Comparison of Contraceptive Methods—Continued

Advantages and Disadvantages	*Contraindications*	*Adverse Effects*
Disadvantages • Must be reapplied for each act of intercourse • Must be inserted before intercourse • Must be inserted with an applicator		
Chemical method: Spermicidal jelly or cream Advantages • Some protection against STDs • May be used as needed • Available over the counter • Available in different flavors and colors Disadvantages • Must be reapplied for each act of intercourse • Must be inserted before intercourse • Must be inserted with an applicator	• Sensitivity to spermicide or carrier • Allergic response to spermicide or carrier	
Chemical method: Spermicidal suppository Advantages • Some protection against STDs • Available over the counter • May be used as needed Disadvantages • Must be reapplied for each act of intercourse • Must be inserted into vagina • Must be inserted before intercourse • Can be used only once	• Sensitivity to spermicide	Allergic response to spermicide
Chemical method: Foaming tablet Advantages • Some protection against STDs • Available over the counter • May be used as needed Disadvantages • Must be reapplied for each act of intercourse • Must be inserted into the vagina • Can be used only once	• Sensitivity to spermicide	• Allergic response to spermicide • Chemical/allergic reactions
Chemical method: Vaginal film Advantages • Some protection against STDs • May be used as needed • Available over the counter • May be inserted 5 to 90 minutes before intercourse Disadvantages • Must be reapplied for each act of intercourse • Must be inserted into vagina	• Sensitivity to spermicide or film gel	• Allergic response to spermicide or film gel

(continued)

Table 14.2 Comparison of Contraceptive Methods—Continued

Advantages and Disadvantages	*Contraindications*	*Adverse Effects*
Hormonal method: Oral contraceptive		
Advantages • Use is unrelated to intercourse • Highly effective • Protects against pelvic inflammatory disease (PID), ovarian and endometrial cancer, benign breast tumors, endometriosis, osteoporosis, rheumatoid arthritis, and uterine fibroids • Relieves dysmenorrhea and menorrhagia • Reduces the risk of anemia Disadvantages • Must be taken daily at the same time • Depends on correct use by women • Requires a prescription • Requires user not to smoke • Must be taken daily for protection regardless of need	Absolute contraindications • Thromboembolic episodes • Cerebrovascular accident (CVA) • Coronary artery disease • Breast cancer • Estrogen-dependent cancer • Benign or malignant liver tumor, impaired liver function, or history of these • Pregnancy Relative contraindications • Severe vascular headaches • Family history of cardiovascular disease or death caused by myocardial infarction (MI) under age 50 • History of diabetes, gall bladder disease, acute mononucleosis, or sickle-cell disease • Long leg cast (possible thrombosis) • Scheduled surgery • Seizure disorder • Age (over age 35 in a smoker, or over age 40 in a nonsmoker)	• Breakthrough bleeding • Headaches • Hypertension • Increased appetite • Weight gain • Fluid retention • Depression or mood changes • Chloasma • Thromboembolic episode • Exacerbation of acne • CVA • MI • Exacerbation of varicosities • Liver and gallbladder disease • Mastalgia • Galactorrhea • Decreased libido • Drug interactions • Chlamydial cervicitis
Hormonal method: Contraceptive implant		
Advantages • Offers long-term protection • Allows restored fertility when removed • Unrelated to intercourse • Is in place when needed or not Disadvantages • Requires surgical insertion and removal by a trained health care professional • May be visible when implanted	Absolute contraindications • Pregnancy • Thromboembolic episode • Undiagnosed genital bleeding • Acute liver disease • Breast cancer Relative contraindications • History of MI, headaches, depression, severe acne, ectopic pregnancy, CVA, or angina • Hyperlipidemia • Long-term use of antiepileptics • Abnormal findings on breast examination or mammogram • Diabetes • Hypertension	• Infections at insertion site • Inability to place correctly in women • Inability to tolerate symptoms such as spotting or hypermenorrhea • Hypermenorrhea • Headaches • Weight change • Mastalgia • Galactorrhea • Exacerbation of acne • Irregular menses
Hormonal method: Injectable Depo-Provera®		
Advantages • Temporary, long-term method • Reversible method • No relation to intercourse • Confidential method • No estrogen	• Known or suspected pregnancy • Undiagnosed vaginal bleeding • Known or suspected breast malignancy • Active thrombophlebitis or current or past history of thromboembolic disorders or CVA	• Animal studies suggest a possible link with cancers of cervix, liver, and breast • Weight gain • Long-term use related to osteoporosis • Menstrual irregularity • Headaches

Table 14.2 Comparison of Contraceptive Methods—Continued

Advantages and Disadvantages	*Contraindications*	*Adverse Effects*
Disadvantages • Requires screening and physical exam • Injection every 3 months • Health care follow-up • Annual Pap smear and breast examination	• Liver dysfunction or disease	• Known sensitivity to Depo-Provera® or any of its ingredients • Tiredness, weakness • Depression • Postuse infertility of about 9 months • Thromboembolic disorder, visual disturbances, migraine headaches • Ectopic pregnancy • Leg cramps, vaginitis • Nausea • Thinning of hair • Breast pain, pelvic pain • Bloating or edema • Hot flashes • Decreased libido • Backache • Leukorrhea • Acne, rashes
Intrauterine device (IUD)		
Advantages • Use is unrelated to intercourse • Low risk of client error Disadvantages • Must be inserted and removed by a health care professional • Must be replaced once every year (progestin IUD) or 6 years (copper IUD) • Requires regular checking of strings to determine if the IUD is in place	Absolute contraindications • Pregnancy • Acute PID • Gonorrhea Relative contraindications • History of ectopic pregnancy • Multiple partners • Anatomic anomalies, such as a malpositioned uterus • Nulliparity or concern for future fertility • Impaired immune response • Chlamydia infection • Impaired coagulation • Gynecologic malignancy • Anemia • Abnormal Pap smear tests indicating infection, cervical intraepithelial neoplasia, or malignancy • History of gonorrhea • Allergy to copper	• PID • IUD expulsion • Allergic response to copper • Increased menstrual bleeding • Abdominal cramping • Ectopic pregnancy • Uterine perforation or IUD embedding in uterus • IUD migration into pelvis
Sterilization		
Advantages • Permanent Disadvantages • Is permanent • Requires surgery • Requires anesthesia	• Desire to bear children • Menopause • History of extensive pelvic surgery • Adhesions	• Post-tubal-ligation syndrome with symptoms such as menstrual irregularities, dysmenorrhea, and pelvic pain • Postoperative complications • Complications of anesthesia

SOURCE: Adapted from Hawkins, Roberto, and Stanley-Haney (1993).

with the selection of a contraceptive method (Tabeek, 1990).

Fertility awareness education refers to imparting information about male and female reproductive anatomy and physiology, primary and secondary signs of fertility, and cyclic changes in these signs. All fertility awareness methods use this information, as well as knowledge of

PERSONAL DATA

Today's date ______________________

Last name ______________________ First name ______________________

Street address ______________________

City/State/Zip ______________________

Date of birth ______________________ Age ____________

Marital status: Single ______ Divorced ______ Widowed ______
Married ______ Separated ______

Occupation ______________________ Religion ______________________

CONFIDENTIALITY INFORMATION

For medical reasons, we sometimes need to contact clients. This does not happen often, but when it does, we must be able to reach you. Please provide the following information for contacting you.

TO CONTACT ME BY TELEPHONE FOR IMMEDIATE EMERGENCY NOTIFICATION (check one):

______ It is not a problem for me. Telephone: ______________________

______ To protect my confidentiality, please say that ______________________ called ("Florence," for example. I will know that means to call the health care facility.)

Telephone: ______________________

______ Please leave a message for me with (name) ______________________

who is my (relationship) ______________________ Telephone: ______________

TO CONTACT ME BY MAIL FOR ROUTINE FOLLOW-UP (check one):

______ It is not a problem for me. You may address mail to me at home.

______ To protect my confidentiality, please use the name and address of my (relationship) ______________________

Name ______________________

Street ______________________

City/State/Zip ______________________

Figure 14.1. Sample Client Personal Data Form
NOTE: For a client who requests assistance with contraception, personal data should be obtained using a form like the sample shown above.

female fertile and infertile phases and their relationship to male fertility, and require abstinence from vaginal-penile intercourse during the fertile phase to prevent conception. Because these methods are unmodified by chemical, mechanical, or other artificial means, they represent a natural way to regulate fertility (New England Natural Family Planning, undated).

Fertility awareness methods include the calendar, ovulation (cervical mucus), basal body temperature (BBT), symptothermal, and lactational amenorrhea methods (LAM). Except for LAM, these methods use normal signs and symptoms of ovulation and the menstrual cycle to prevent or achieve pregnancy (Martin, 1981; NAACOG, 1983). However, the client must observe several cycles to understand and recognize her fertile and infertile phases.

Ovulation Method

This method is based on detecting signs and symptoms of ovulation through regular observation of cervical mucus, which is produced by tiny cells in the cervix. Throughout the menstrual cycle, cervical mucus changes. Immediately after the menstrual period, cervical mucus

ASSESSMENT

Subjective data

- Social history: Age, occupation, relationship status, number of partners, and other lifestyle considerations
- Personal habits: Smoking, alcohol use, and use of prescription, over-the-counter, and recreational drugs
- Personal health care: Diet, exercise, and use of personal hygiene products
- Reproductive history: Pregnancies and their outcomes
- Medical and surgical history: Acute and chronic diseases, infections, or illnesses; injuries; allergies; hospitalizations; surgeries; and blood transfusions
- Gynecologic history: Vaginitis, sexually transmitted diseases, contraceptive use, date and description of last menstrual period, description of normal menstrual cycles
- Family history: Medical, surgical, and gynecologic history

Objective data

- Vital signs: Height and weight
- Systems assessment: Reproductive system and breasts; immune, cardiovascular, respiratory, gastrointestinal, integumentary, and nervous systems, as needed
- Diagnostic tests: Hematocrit, hemoglobin level, urinalysis, cholesterol screen, total lipid level, gonorrhea culture, chlamydia screen, mammography, and other tests as prescribed

Review and analysis

- Client's choice of and access to method
- Suitability of method based on subjective and objective data
- Nursing diagnoses that derive from the data

CARE

Initial care and teaching

- Provide information about the method through group or individual teaching, using written materials, audiovisual materials, and hands-on learning and practice.
- Give feedback on practice.
- Involve the partner (if desired by the client).
- Identify support available to address questions and concerns.
- Discuss access to the method. Be sure to address obtaining a prescription or supplies, locating places to purchase supplies, and reviewing choices available.
- Describe self-care and care for the equipment, such as cleaning the diaphragm or cap.
- Discuss return visits for a pelvic examination and Papanicolaou test and for checking, removing, replacing, or changing the method.

Follow-up care and evaluation

- Assess the client's satisfaction with and use of the method.
- Review the client's continuing candidacy for the method.
- Identify and manage adverse effects or problems caused by the method and the client's perception of them.
- Evaluate the client's desire to continue or discontinue the method.

Figure 14.2. Nursing Care for a Client Who Requires Contraception

NOTE: When assisting a client who requests contraception, the nurse can use this guide to assess the client and provide appropriate care. It is intended to be used with Table 14.2, "Comparison of Contraceptive Methods," and the information on specific management strategies for each method.

SOURCE: Adapted from Hawkins, Roberto, & Stanley-Haney (1994).

is scant, and the client should notice vaginal dryness for a few days. Then mucus is present for a few days, in which the client should feel vaginal wetness. After this, mucus becomes clear (as differentiated from milky white, translucent, or creamy color) and stretchy, similar to raw egg white. The client should notice increased wetness or a slippery sensation. The peak day of wetness signals ovulation. After this day, the mucus starts to lose its slippery, wet quality and becomes cloudy and sticky until the next menstrual period. (See Chapter 3, "Women's Bodies," for additional information on ovulation and the attendant physical changes.)

To use the ovulation method, the client should check her cervical mucus daily to determine the peak day of wetness, which indicates ovulation—and fertility. During ovulation, cervical mucus nourishes sperm, facilitates their passage into the intrauterine cavity, and probably helps select sperm of the highest quality. However, the peak day is obvious only the day after it occurs, when the mucus becomes less slippery and stretchy.

The client can check her mucus in several ways, depending on her level of comfort with her body. She can wipe a folded piece of toilet tissue across her vaginal opening and then feel whether the tissue slides across easily or sticks. If mucus is present, she can place it between her fingers and check its wetness and stretchiness (spinnbarkheit). As an alternative, she can check these characteristics by holding the toilet tissue with both hands and pulling it apart (Tabeek, 1991).

Basal Body Temperature Method

This method is based on the temperature change triggered by the progesterone surge that occurs when the ovum leaves the ovary. To use this method, the client takes her temperature at rest at the same time every day, using a basal thermometer calibrated in 10ths of a degree. Then she documents her daily temperature on a BBT chart, noting any variations. During ovulation, the temperature typically rises up to 1° above the preovulatory BBT. (See Chapter 3 for additional information and illustration of this topic.) To prevent conception, the client should abstain from intercourse until after 3 days of temperature rise. Infections, illnesses, and other conditions such as fatigue, anxiety, sleeplessness, some medications, use of an electric blanket, or a heated water bed also can increase the temperature. Therefore, applying the rules for taking and interpreting the BBT are crucial to the effectiveness of this method.

Symptothermal Method

This method relies on identifying the primary signs of fertility: changes in cervical mucus, BBT, and the position, consistency, and opening of the cervix. Like cervical mucus and BBT, the cervix changes throughout the menstrual cycle. As ovulation approaches, the cervix becomes softer, and changes position from posterior to midline, and the os dilates slightly. After ovulation, it reverts to its preovulatory state. While squatting or standing with one foot on a stool or chair, the client may place a finger in her vagina and feel for position, softness, or firmness.

The symptothermal method also uses observation for secondary signs of fertility: cyclic breast, skin, hair, mood, and energy changes; vaginal aching; spotting; pelvic pain or aching; and mittelschmerz (abdominal pain during ovulation). By charting the primary and secondary signs, the client can detect her fertile phase with great accuracy and can prevent or achieve conception (see Figure 14.3).

Electronic devices, such as Bioself 110 and interactive computer programs, are available to teach fertility awareness methods. The Bioself 110 is intended to simplify and improve the use of the ovulation, BBT, and symptothermal methods. Tests of its effectiveness showed that the infertile phase was identified correctly in 93.3% of 178 cycles. The device is easier to use than these methods and provides a simple aid to couples who wish to achieve or avoid pregnancy (Orouin, Labrecque, Rioux, Gingras, & Spieler, 1988).

Although the Bioself 110 and other commercial devices can make natural methods easier to use, they may have some drawbacks. For example, they introduce a profit motive to a natural phenomenon. Also, their existence suggests that their use will make the method more effective, which is untrue because most women can accurately monitor and make decisions about their fertility without technology.

Lactational Amenorrhea Method

After decades of skepticism in the United States, LAM is becoming more popular as a fertility awareness method. This method is based on the fact that the length of postpartal amenorrhea is affected directly by the duration of lactation.

Postpartal amenorrhea varies among different populations. In general, it is shorter than the duration of lactation in populations that use prolonged breast-feeding (Diaz, 1989). In the United States, however, breast-feeding patterns (duration and amount) vary widely and are affected by women's multiple roles, including that of employee. Introduction of solid food or supplementary formula, which can be influenced by the client's sociocultural group and culture of origin, can also affect the duration of amenorrhea by influencing how often a mother breast-feeds. Most important to breast-feeding and amenorrhea is the infant's sucking pattern. In a recent study, the contraceptive effectiveness of LAM during the first 6 postpartal months compared

Daily observation chart no. 10 Month Aug. - Sept.
Name ______ Age 24
Address ______ Phone ______
City ______ State ______ Zip ______
Year 1994
Previous cycle variation 27-35
Cycle variation base on 12 recorded cycles
This cycle: 32 days

Sept. 1

Day of cycle	1	2	3	4	5	6	7	8	9	10	11	12	13	14	15	16	17	18	19	20	21	22	23	24	25	26	27	28	29	30	31	32	33
Menstruation	X	X	X	X	X																												
Coitus record																																	
Day of month																																	
Disturbances																																	
99.0																																	
98.8																		•			•	•		•	•	•	•	•	•	•	•		
98.6																	•		•	•			•									•	
98.4	•															•																	•
98.2		•		•		•			•		•	•	•	•	•																		
98.0			•		•		•	•		•																							
97.8																																	
97.6																																	
97.4																																	
97.2																																	
97.0																																	
99.0																																	
98.8																																	
98.6																																	
98.4																																	
98.2																																	
98.0																																	
97.8																																	
97.6																																	
97.4																																	
97.2																																	
97.0																																	
Mucus						d	d	d	d	d	d	d	d	w	w	w	w	w	d	d	d	d	d	d	d	d	d	d	d	d	d	d	M
Peak or last day																		P	1	2	3	4											
Cervix						•	•	•	•	•	•	•	•	•	•	•	o	O	•	o	o	•	•	o	•								
Notes: spotting, schedule changes, pains, moods, etc.																		pain														spotting	

Peak day refers to the last day of the fertile mucus before it begins to dry up.

Temperature: usual time 6:30 a.m.
Oral X Rectal ______ Vaginal ______

Key

Mucus:
P = peak mucus
D = dryness on labia
W = wetness on labia
M = ordinary, no particular consistency
T = tacky
S = smooth, slippery, stretchy
C = clear
O = opaque
Y = yellow

Stretch in inches
Quantity: 0, +, ++, +++

Cervix:
• = closed
O = open
F = firm
L = low
S = soft
H = high

Figure 14.3. Sample Symptothermal Chart
NOTE: The symbols shown in the key are all those that a woman might use in charting primary and secondary signs of fertility.

favorably with that of modern contraceptives (Diaz, 1989). Therefore, a client who plans to breast-feed should receive information about LAM to consider along with information about other fertility awareness methods.

Barrier Methods

Although most barrier methods are used with chemical spermicides, they also act, in part, as a mechanical barrier to sperm trying to reach the uterus. Barrier methods include the diaphragm, cervical cap, vaginal sponge, and condom. All four date from centuries past; their current forms reflect advances in materials and knowledge of fertilization.

Diaphragm

The diaphragm has existed for more than a century. The original rubber diaphragm was invented by a German physician in 1838 but did not gain much of a following until Karl Hasse introduced it in Holland in the late 19th century. Because Hasse used the pseudonym Mensinga to protect his reputation, the diaphragm became known as the Mensinga diaphragm or Dutch cap (Connell, Grimes, & Manisoff, 1989). In the early 1900s, Margaret Sanger introduced the diaphragm to the United States through her birth control clinics. Vulcanization of rubber made the diaphragm a more practical contraceptive device by making mass production practical and affordable. When used with the spermicidal jelly that became available in the 1920s, the diaphragm became one of the most popular methods (Glazer, 1965).

Modern diaphragms, which vary most in type of spring and size are available in four types—flat spring, coil spring, arcing spring, or bow-bend—and in sizes that range from 55 to 105 mm in diameter. The color (pale to dark pinkish-beige) and consistency (very thin to thick) of their rubber varies by type and manufacturer (see Figure 14.4).

The diaphragm has two modes of action. It forms a partial mechanical barrier to sperm, and it holds a spermicidal agent against the cervix to stop sperm that circumvent the diaphragm. Therefore, the diaphragm is designed for use with spermicidal jelly or cream. The Milex diaphragm has a cuff inside the rim, which, according to its manufacturers, enhances the mechanical barrier (Hawkins, Roberto, & Stanley-Haney, 1993).

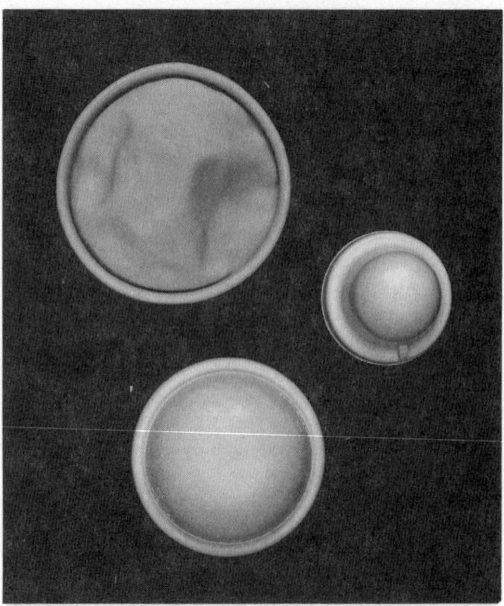

Figure 14.4. Sample Diaphragms

As with other contraceptive methods, the diaphragm's use effectiveness is lower than its theoretical effectiveness. This reflects the human involvement required by this method—and the resulting risk of human error. Effectiveness is reduced if the diaphragm is not used each time vaginal intercourse occurs, if it is used without spermicide, if it does not remain in place for several hours after intercourse, if the woman douches, if the diaphragm is dislodged during or after intercourse, or if it has a hole (Hawkins et al., 1993).

Before using the diaphragm, the client or her partner must prepare it with spermicidal jelly or cream (1% or 2% spermicide concentration), insert it correctly to cover the cervix completely, and remove it 6 to 8 hours after the last act of intercourse (for illustrations, see Figures 14.5a and b). The diaphragm can be left in place for up to 24 hours but should be removed for cleaning and spermicide renewal.

The client may choose spermicidal cream or jelly according to her preference. Made by many manufacturers, cream and jelly come in various flavors and colors, including white cream and clear jelly. Some health care professionals recommend application of a tablespoon of spermicide to the outside of the diaphragm when it has been in place for more than 4 hours before penetration or when intercourse is repeated. The client can do this with her fingers or an applicator, without removing the diaphragm.

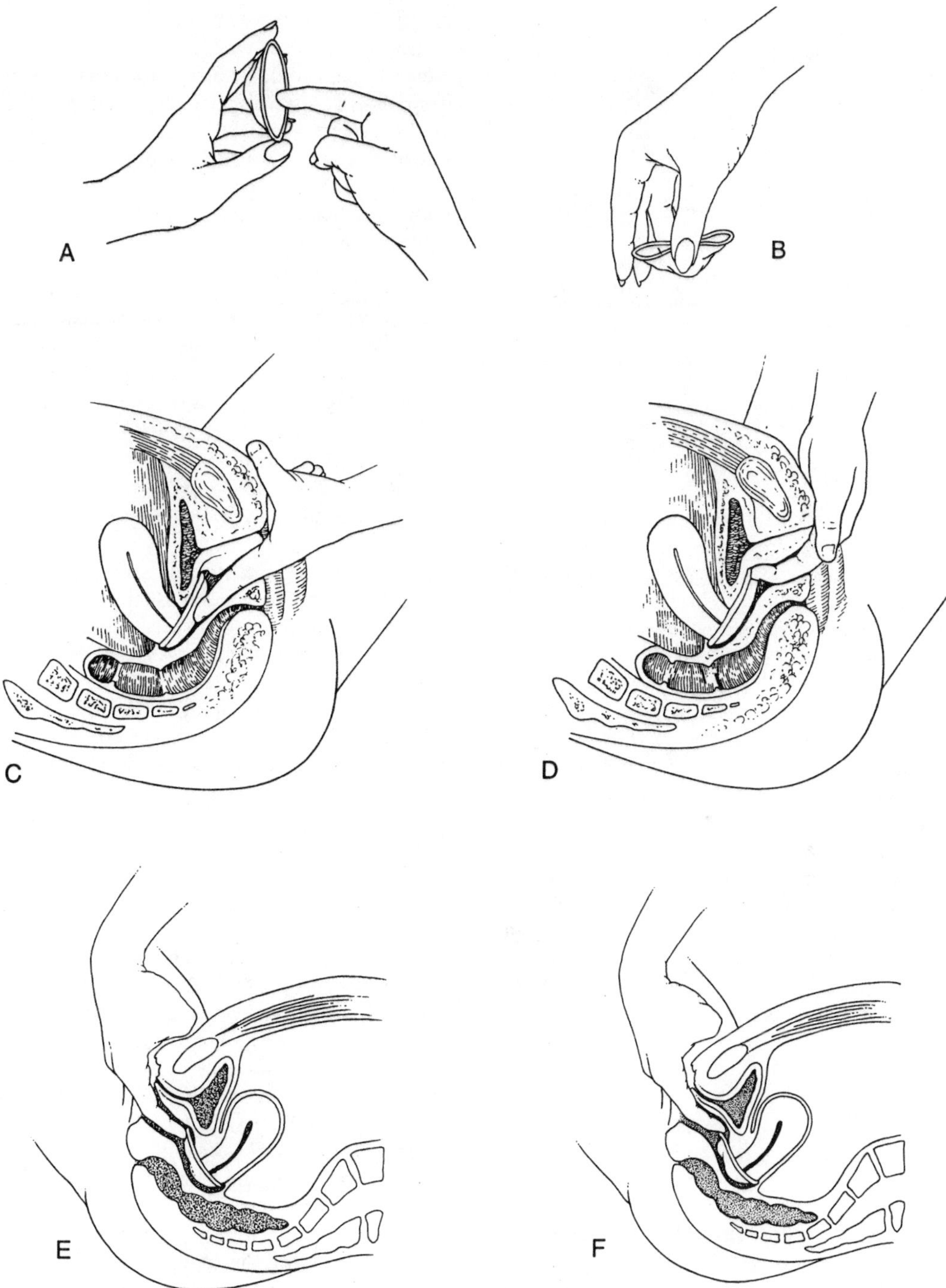

Figure 14.5a. Diaphragm Use

Diaphragm Insertion

The client should find a comfortable position for diaphragm insertion. After applying spermicide to the diaphragm (A), she should fold it in half (B) and push it up above the pubis (C and D).

Diaphragm Removal

When the client is ready to remove the diaphragm, she should hook a finger behind the front rim of the diaphragm (E) and gently pull it forward and out (F).

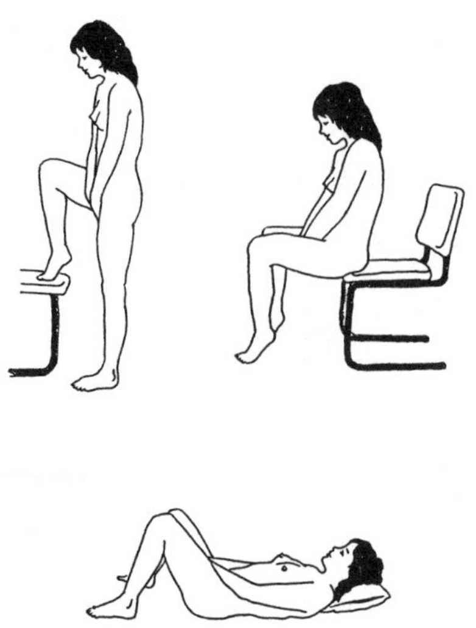

Figure 14.5b. Diaphragm Use—Positions for Diaphragm Insertion: Leg Up, Edge of a Chair, and Reclining

NOTE: To use a diaphragm effectively, the client must insert and remove it properly. When in place, the diaphragm should fit correctly, covering the cervix snugly.

Although clinical practice commonly requires the fit of a diaphragm to be checked when the client loses or gains 10 to 15 pounds, some research suggests that the woman's perception of a change is more likely to predict altered fit (Kugel & Verson, 1986). Many clinicians suggest that the fit be checked annually during the client's health assessment and Pap test and once after each pregnancy, but not earlier than 6 weeks after delivery.

Cervical Cap

In the late 1980s, the Food and Drug Administration (FDA) approved the cervical cap, which had been considered an experimental device for more than a decade (Klitsch, 1988). First invented in New York in 1860 by Dr. Edward Bliss Foote, the cervical cap fell into disuse in the United States due to birth control laws that made them unavailable. However, it was used widely in Central Europe. Early caps were made of gold, silver, platinum, stainless steel, aluminum, or celluloid. Modern caps are made of rubber or lucite (Glazer, 1965).

Only one type of cervical cap, the Prentif cap, currently is available in the United States. It comes in four sizes—22, 25, 28, and 31 millimeters—and should be used with a higher concentration of spermicide (2%) than the diaphragm. Under current FDA guidelines, the cap must remain in place for 8 to 12 hours after the last intercourse but can remain in place for up to 48 hours (Cervical Cap, Ltd., 1988; Lamberts (Dalston) Limited, 1988).

The cervical cap is held against the cervix by suction, providing a partial mechanical barrier against sperm. Also, the cap holds spermicide against the cervical os, so sperm that circumvent the cap are halted by the spermicide. Because of the risk of toxic shock syndrome (TSS) during menses and dislodgement or suction disruption by menstrual flow, the cap cannot be used during menses. Therefore, many women use a diaphragm instead of a cap during menses (Secor, 1991).

Only 50% to 60% of women can be fitted with a cervical cap. To accommodate one of the available caps, the woman's cervix must protrude into the vagina at least 1.5 cm and should be 1.0 to 2.5 cm wide (Secor, 1991). A cap can be custom made from an impression taken with materials used for dental impressions, but only a few health care professionals are offering this option now (Moore, 1990).

Vaginal Sponge

The vaginal sponge is a modern version of an old contraceptive method. During ancient Egyptian and Roman times, women placed sea sponges soaked with vinegar or lemon juice in the vagina to prevent pregnancy. They also used tampons of cotton or other materials in a similar manner (Glazer, 1965). In 1983, the FDA approved the vaginal sponge (Kafka & Gold, 1983), which is made of polyurethane impregnated with the spermicide nonoxynol-9 and has a loop for easy removal.

Before inserting the sponge, the client must wet it to activate the spermicide. Then she places it in the vagina over the cervix. The sponge must remain in place for at least 6 hours after intercourse but can remain in place for up to 24 hours. Because it has enough spermicide to last 24 hours, the client does not need to apply additional spermicide for repeat intercourse (McClure & Edelman, 1985).

The client may have problems with the sponge. She may have difficulty placing it over the cervix, find it difficult to remove, tear the sponge by pulling too vigorously, or visualize the sponge getting lost in her vagina or uterus. Most of these problems can be resolved by teaching the client to squat and bear down when inserting or removing the sponge, explaining basic reproductive anatomy, and providing reassurance.

Many health care professionals recommend using a condom with the sponge to increase its contraceptive efficacy. They also suggest that the client use another method during menses because of the risk of TSS.

Male Condom

The condom is the only barrier method currently available for males. In 1564, the Italian anatomist Fallopius (discoverer of the fallopian tubes) first suggested the use of linen covers for the penis as protection against sexually transmitted diseases (STDs). Subsequently, condoms were used not only for protection from infection but also as badges of rank or honor, for decoration or modesty, or as amulets for fertility (Himes, 1936). By the 18th century, condoms were used to prevent conception. Made of animal membrane, they were waterproof and protected against penetration of sperm and some micro-organisms (Gordon, 1990).

Today's condoms are made of latex or natural lamb membrane. They are available with or without lubricant, spermicide, ribbing, or a reservoir tip and come in various colors and sizes, such as snug fit, large, extra large, and jumbo (see figure 14.6). The Centers for Disease Control (CDC) state that only latex condoms or latex condoms with nonoxynol-9 can protect against human immunodeficiency virus (HIV) transmission by vaginal or rectal intercourse (Meisenhelder & LaCharite, 1989). Although this protection is not absolute, it is the best available.

Since the advent of oral contraceptives, knowledge about condom use seems less widespread. Yet women purchase more than 40% of condoms, indicating their interest in protecting themselves (Hatcher et al., 1990). Therefore, client teaching about condom use may be extremely helpful. (See Chapter 24, "Sexually Transmitted Diseases," for related information.)

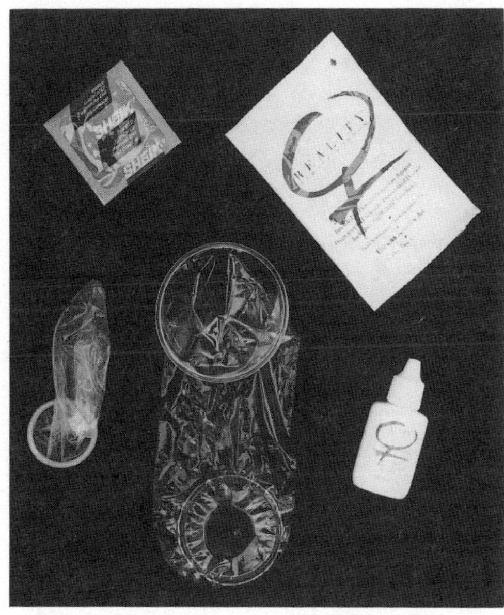

Figure 14.6. Male and Female Condoms

Vaginal Condom

The female condom, with the brand name Reality,™ was approved for marketing in the United States by the Food and Drug Administration (FDA) in 1993. This barrier device is made of polyurethane and is a soft sheath open on one end and closed on the other. At each end is a flexible ring. One is used to insert the device and hold it over the cervix and the other ring remains outside the vagina, covering the labia. The condom is prelubricated, disposable, and intended for one-time use only. As a barrier method of contraception, it also offers protection against STDs and AIDS. As with other barrier methods, this protection is relative (Trussel, Sturgen, Strickler, & Dominik, 1994; Wisconsin Pharmacal Company, 1994) (see Figures 14.6 and 14.7).

Chemical Methods

Several types of chemical methods may be used for contraception. They all may be used alone, but some are designed for use with a barrier method, such as the diaphragm, cervical cap, or vaginal sponge. The latter are not nearly as effective when used alone.

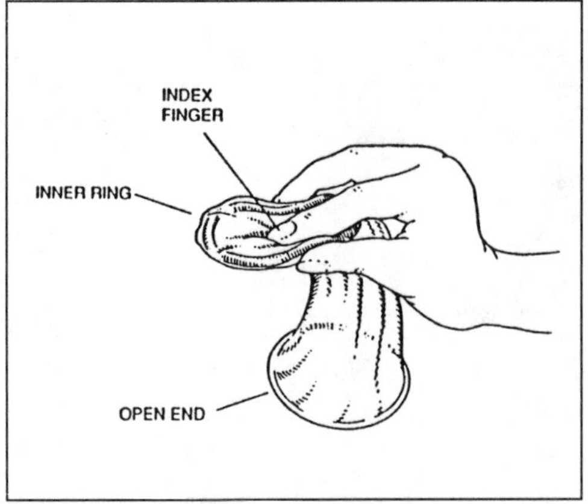

A. Inner ring is squeezed for insertion.

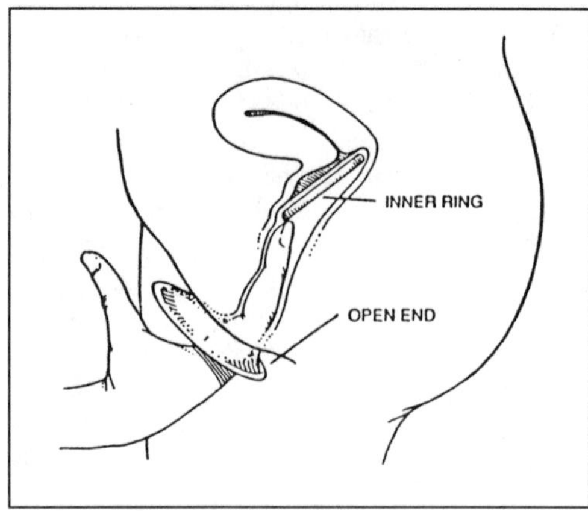

C. Inner ring is pushed up as far as it can go with index finger.

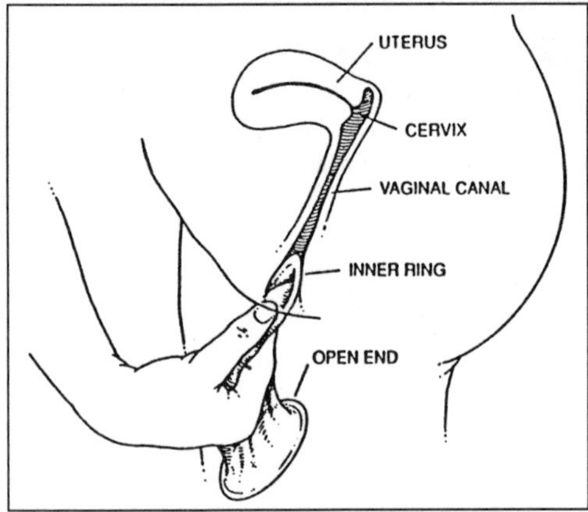

B. Sheath is inserted, similarly to a tampon.

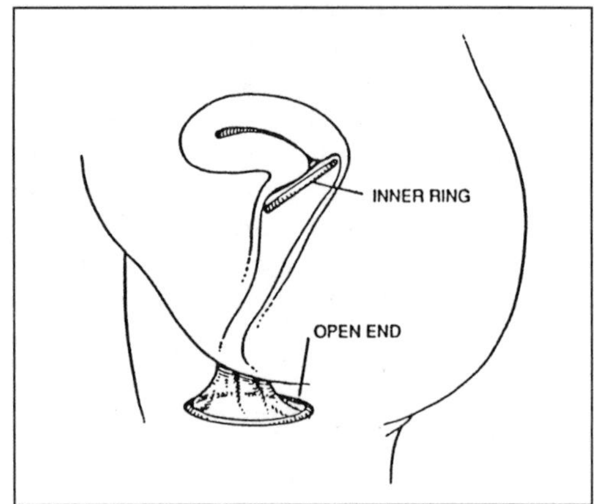

D. Condom is in place.

Figure 14.7. Female Condom Insertion and Positioning
SOURCE: Reality.

Spermicidal Jelly, Cream, and Foam

All contraceptive jellies and creams have a carrier substance and a spermicidal agent, usually nonoxynol-9. The carrier substance may be colored or flavored. Sensitivity to one carrier substance does not preclude use of the method; switching brands may eliminate the problem. The spermicide concentration varies with the brand and product from 1% to 5%.

Jellies and creams are inserted in the vagina with a reusable plastic or cardboard inserter or a disposable, prefilled one that is designed for a single use. They must be put into the vagina no more than 1 hour before intercourse and must be reapplied before each subsequent act of vaginal intercourse.

Spermicidal foams are similar to creams and jellies, except that they are designed to be used alone, without a barrier method. They all contain nonoxynol-9 in concentrations varying from 8% to 12.5% and are available in prefilled applicators or in canisters with reusable plastic applicators. Although marketed for use alone, foams are most effective when used with a condom. Like creams and jellies, foams should be applied no more than 1 hour before intercourse and should be reapplied before repeat intercourse (see Figures 14.8 and 14.9).

Other Chemical Methods

Other chemical contraceptive methods include vaginal suppositories, tablets, and film. Of the

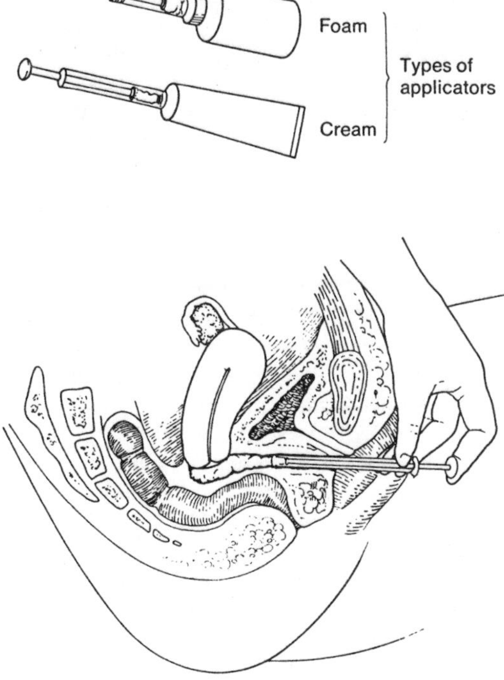

Figure 14.8. Inserting a Spermicidal Agent

various contraceptive suppositories sold in the United States, all contain the spermicidal agent nonoxynol-9 in concentrations from 2% to 10%. Some are waxy and melt in the vagina, releasing the spermicide. Others require a chemical reaction to release it. To ensure that the spermicide is dispersed and effective, the client should read and follow the manufacturer's instructions for the particular product because the waiting time before intercourse can vary. The client should insert another suppository before each act of vaginal intercourse.

Vaginal foaming tablets are commonly used in other parts of the world, and the spermicide in these tablets recently was approved for use in the United States. Like some suppositories, the tablets require a chemical reaction in the vagina to activate the spermicide. Some women complain of a sensation of heat, which can decrease use of this method.

Vaginal contraceptive film uses a 28% concentration of nonoxynol-9 for its spermicide. The film dissolves in 5 minutes or less after insertion in the vagina. Dispensed in 5-cm × 5-cm squares that are 80 microns thick, it can be folded and rolled over a fingertip (finger should be dry) for insertion (Apothecus, 1989). Some women have used film in a diaphragm instead of jelly or cream, although this may affect the diaphragm's effectiveness because the film may not coat its interior

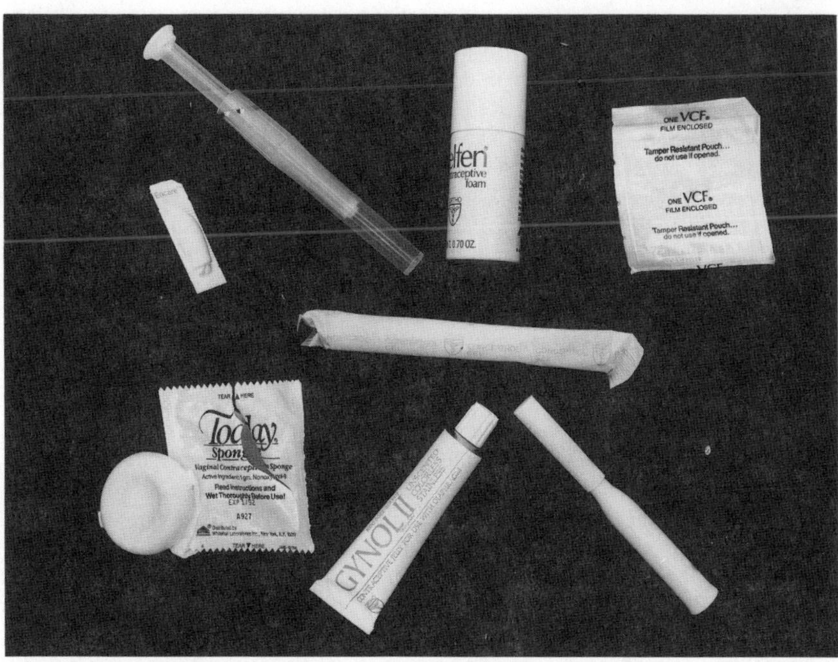

Figure 14.9. Sample Spermicidal Jelly, Cream, Foam, Sponge, and Film

thoroughly. The spermicide is effective for 2 hours, after which another film should be inserted.

Hormonal Methods

These methods include oral contraceptives, morning-after contraceptives, injectables, and contraceptive implants.

Oral Contraceptive

All oral contraceptives are composed of synthetic hormones. The discovery of progesterone and estrogens in the 1930s and the synthesis of these hormones in the 1950s led to the development of this hormonal method (Kistner, 1968; Rock, 1963).

Two basic types of oral contraceptives are currently used in the United States: the combination pill and the progestin-only pill. The combination pill uses one of two types of synthetic estrogen (ethinyl estradiol or mestranol) and one of seven types of synthetic progestin (norethindrone, ethynodiol diacetate, levonorgestrel, norethindrone acetate, norgestimate, or norgestrel). Doses range from 20 to 50 mcg of desogestrel estrogen and from 0.05 to 2.5 mg of progestin.

Progestins vary in estrogenic effect (acting like estrogen, the predominant female hormone) and androgenic effect (acting like androgen, the predominant male hormone). So if a client develops adverse reactions to the progestin in one oral contraceptive, she may be able to take a different oral contraceptive safely.

Oral contraceptive formulations vary. Some products contain the same formulation in all 21 pills; others have a biphasic or triphasic formulation. For example, one biphasic product has 0.5 mg of progestin in the first 10 pills and 1.0 mg in the remaining 11, creating two phases. In one triphasic product, the first 6 pills have 0.5 mg of progestin and 30 mcg of estrogen, the next 5 have 0.75 mg and 40 mcg, and the last 10 have 0.125 mg and 30 mcg, respectively (see Table 14.3; see also Dickey, 1994).

Combination oral contraceptives are available in many brands and formulations, but they all share the same underlying principle: They supress ovulation through the combined actions of estrogen and progestin. Protocols for starting an oral contraceptive depend on the manufacturer's recommendation and whether the woman is experiencing regular cycles or recently has given birth or had an abortion. The client takes one pill at the same time each day for 21 days and then takes no pills for 7 days or takes a placebo or iron pill each day for 7 days. During the last 7 days, the client experiences withdrawal bleeding, which ranges from spotting to several days of bleeding similar to her regular menses. (The endometrial stimulation from the synthetic estrogen and progestin produces sufficient lining to produce withdrawal bleeding.)

Current oral contraceptives provide much lower hormone doses than the original oral contraceptives. To maintain plasma hormone levels with these new contraceptives, manufacturers suggest that they be taken at the same time each day. Adverse effects and contraceptive failures are more common when the administration time varies by more than 1 hour. The most common adverse effect is breakthrough bleeding (bleeding that occurs while taking combination oral contraceptives). The health care professional should teach the client the importance of taking the pills on time and the actions to take if she forgets a pill (Connell, 1990a; Hawkins et al., 1995) (see Figure 14.10).

Because each oral contraceptive has a standardized formula, they do not accommodate individual needs. Therefore, a client may ovulate because the formula does not supply sufficient hormones to suppress ovulation. She is unlikely to become pregnant, however, because the oral contraceptive makes the endometrium relatively unreceptive to implantation and thickens the cervical mucus, inhibiting sperm migration.

Because oral contraceptives are highly effective, they would be ideal if they posed no dangers. However, they can cause annoying adverse effects and can be life threatening for some clients. Therefore, the health care professional should be aware of adverse effects and absolute and relative contraindications. Discussion of the management of adverse effects is beyond the scope of this book. (For sources of information on this topic, see the references for this section.)

Oral contraceptives pose these cardiovascular risks: thromboembolism, hemorrhagic and embolic cerebrovascular accident, myocardial infarction, hypertension, vascular headaches, and arterial conditions, such as subarachnoid hemorrhage and mesenteric artery thrombosis (Connell, 1990a). Careful screening and monitoring of clients taking oral contraceptives can reduce these risks considerably. Yet these cardiovascular risks are several times higher dur-

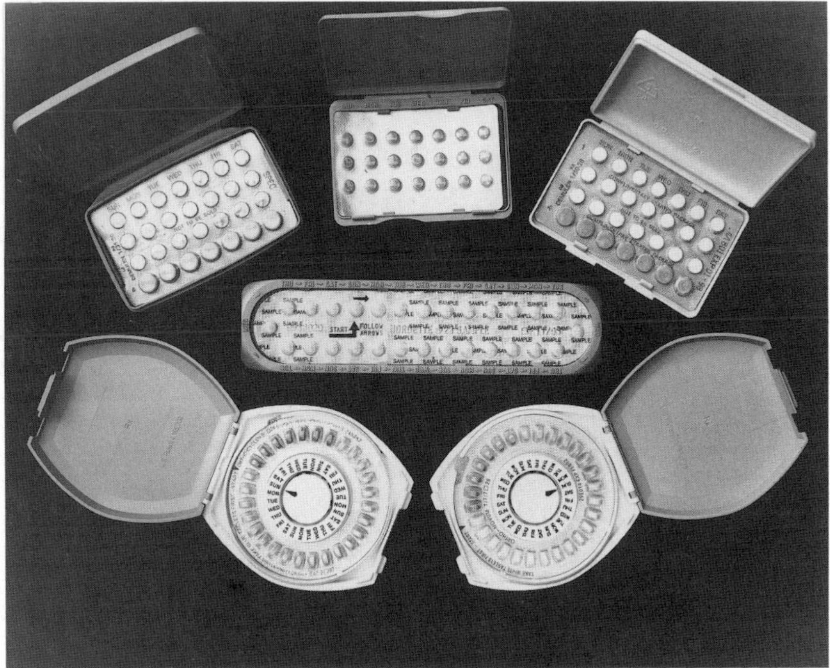

Figure 14.10. Sample Oral Contraceptives

ing pregnancy than they are during oral contraceptive use, and pregnancy creates other risks for women (Ory et al., 1983). Smoking and increased age may increase the cardiovascular risks of oral contraceptives, although evidence suggests that clients over age 35 who do not smoke and have no personal or family history of cardiovascular disease can take oral contraceptives safely (Mishell, Connell, Haney, Hodgen, & Speroff, 1990).

The effects of oral contraceptives on the liver and gallbladder also are significant. Clients with acute or chronic liver disease or a history of idiopathic jaundice of pregnancy probably should not take these drugs because they induce changes in hepatic excretory function. Oral contraceptives are also associated with hepatocellular adenoma, a rare nonmalignant liver tumor (Connell, 1990a). Like pregnancy, oral contraceptive use appears to induce gallbladder disease in some clients. However, no one knows whether gallbladder disease would have occurred in these clients if they had not been pregnant or taken oral contraceptives.

Oral contraceptives can affect carbohydrate metabolism and induce lipid and endocrine changes (Connell, 1990a). Although these alterations are not life threatening, they warrant monitoring in any client taking an oral contraceptive. The health care professional and client should consider these adverse effects when discussing the appropriateness of an oral contraceptive. Preexisting conditions, such as hypertension or diabetes, might contraindicate oral contraceptive use or, at least, require close follow-up.

Benefits of oral contraceptives may include relief of dysmenorrhea and menorrhagia and reduced risk of benign breast tumors, benign and malignant ovarian tumors, endometrial carcinoma, endometriosis, osteoporosis, rheumatoid arthritis, and uterine fibroids (Connell, 1990a; Ory, Forrest, & Lincoln, 1983). Current data conflict about the effects of oral contraceptives on breast cancer. Some reports say they increase the risk of cancer; others say they protect against it (Hatcher et al., 1990).

Although oral contraceptives protect against pelvic inflammatory disease (PID), they seem to heighten the risk of chlamydial cervicitis by an unknown mechanism. However, they do not increase the risk for chlamydial PID (Grimes, 1987). Therefore, clinical management should include screening clients at risk for chlamydia, such as those with the following:

text continued on page 311

Table 14.3 Formulas of Common Oral Contraceptives

	Progestin Content (mg)							Estrogen Content (mcg)			
Brand Name	*Estrogenic Effect 0.25 Norethindrone Androgenic Effect 1.6*	*Estrogenic Effect 0.86 Ethynodiol Diacetate Androgenic Effect 1.0*	*Estrogenic Effect 0.38 Norethindrone Acetate Androgenic Effect 2.5*	*Estrogenic Effect 0 Norgestrel Androgenic Effect 7.6*	*Estrogenic Effect 0 Norgestimate Androgenic Effect 1.9*	*Estrogenic Effect 0 Levonorgestrel Androgenic Effect 8.3*	*Estrogenic Effect 0 Desogestrel Androgenic Effect 3.4*	*Mestranol*	*Ethinyl Estradiol*	*Number of Hormonal Pills*	*Number of Other Pills*
Brevicon-21	0.5								35	21	
Brevicon-28	0.5								35	21	7 Inert
Demulen 1/35-21 & 28		1.0							35	21	7 Inert
Demulen-21		1.0							50	21	
Demulen-28		1.0							50	21	7 Inert
Desogen							0.15		35	21	7 Inert
Genora 0.5/35	0.5								35	21	7 Inert
										21	
Genora 1/35	1.0								35	21	7 Inert
									35	21	
Genora 1/50	1.0								50	21	7 Inert
									50	21	
Janest 28	0.5 mg (7 days) 1.0 mg (14 days)								35	21	7 Inert
Loestrin 1/20			1.0						20	21	7 Iron
Loestrin 1.5/30			1.5						30	21	7 Iron
Lo/Ovral				0.3					30	21	
Lo/Ovral-28				0.3					30	21	7 Inert
Modicon-21	0.5								35	21	
Modicon-28	0.5								35	21	7 Inert
Nelova 1/35E	1.0								35	21	7 Inert
Nelova 0.5/35E	0.5								35	21	7 Inert
Nelova 1/50	1.0								50	21	7 Inert
Nelova 10/11 (NEE 10/11 same)	1.0 (10 days) 0.5 (11 days)								35	21	7 Inert

Norcept E 1/35	1.0								35	21	7 Inert
Nordette 21 & 28						0.15			30	21	7 Inert
(Levelen same)											
(Levoar 0.15/30)						0.15			30	21	7 Inert
										28	
Norethin 1/50M	1.0							50		21	7 Inert
NEE 0.5/35	0.5								35	21	7 Inert
NEE 1/35	1.0								35	21	7 Inert
Norinyl 2 mg	2.0							100		20	
Norinyl 1 + 50/21	1.0							50		21	
Norinyl 1 + 50/28								50		21	7 Inert
Norlestrin 2.5/50-21	1.0		2.5						50	21	
Norlestrin 2.5/50-FE			2.5						50	21	7 Iron
Norlestrin 1/50-21			1.0						50	21	
Norlestrin 1/50-28			1.0						50	21	7 Inert
Norlestrin 1/50-FE			1.0						50	21	7 Iron
Ortho-Cept							0.15		30	21	7 Inert
Ortho-Cyclen					0.250				35	21	7 Inert
Ortho-Novum 1/35/28	1.0								35	21	7 Inert
Ortho-Novum 1/35/21	1.0								35	21	
Ortho-Novum 10/11/21											
White tablets	0.5								35		
Peach tablets	1.0										
Ortho-Novum 10/11/28											
White tablets	0.5								35		7 Inert
Peach tablets	1.0							50		21	
Ortho-Novum 1/50-21	1.0							50		21	7 Inert
Ortho-Novum 1/50-28	1.0							50		21	7 Inert
Ovcon-35	0.4								35	21	7 Inert
Ovcon-50	1.0								50	21	7 Inert
Ovral				0.5					50	21	
Ovral-28				0.5					50	21	7 Inert
Ovulen 21		1.0						100		21	
Ovulen 28		1.0						100		21	7 Inert
MINI											
Micronor	.35									28	
Nor-Q-D	.35									42	
Ovrette					0.075					28	

(continued)

Table 14.3 Formulas of Common Oral Contraceptives—Continued

	Progestin Content (mg)							Estrogen Content (mcg)			
Brand Name	*Estrogenic Effect 0.25 Norethindrone Androgenic Effect 1.6*	*Estrogenic Effect 0.86 Ethynodiol Diacetate Androgenic Effect 1.0*	*Estrogenic Effect 0.38 Norethindrone Acetate Androgenic Effect 2.5*	*Estrogenic Effect 0 Norgestrel Androgenic Effect 7.6*	*Estrogenic Effect 0 Norgestimate Androgenic Effect 1.9*	*Estrogenic Effect 0 Levonorgestrel Androgenic Effect 8.3*	*Estrogenic Effect 0 Desogestrel Androgenic Effect 3.4*	*Mestranol*	*Ethinyl Estradiol*	*Number of Hormonal Pills*	*Number of Other Pills*
TRIPHASICS											
Triphasil 21 28						0.050					
(Tri-levelen same)											
						(6)			30		
						0.075					
						(5)			40		
						0.125					7 Inert
						(10)			30	21	
Ortho-Novum 7 7/7/21	0.5 (7)								35	21	
Ortho-Novum 7 7/7/28	0.75 (7)								35	21	7 Inert
	1.0 (7)										
Tri-Norinyl21	0.5 (7)								35	21	
Tri-Norinyl28	1.0 (9)								35	21	7 Inert
	0.5 (5)										
Tri-Cyclen	0.180 (7)								35	21	7 Inert
	0.215 (7)										
	0.250 (7)										

SOURCE: Adapted from Goldzieher (1989); Hatcher et al. (1994); Ory, Forrest, and Lincoln (1983). Used with permission from Hawkins et al. (1995).
NOTE: The nurse practitioner or other health care professional can use this table in prescribing an oral contraceptive. In other settings, the nurse may use this chart as an adjunct to the facility's protocol for managing clients who are using oral contraceptives as a contraceptive method.

- Multiple partners
- One partner who is not mutually monogamous
- A new partner
- Clinical symptoms of cervicitis
- Pap smear indicative of inflammatory changes (cervicitis)
- Other types of STDs (Hawkins et al., 1993)

Weighing of risks and benefits against the contraindications and adverse effects is part of the decision-making process for the client with her health care professional. If she selects an oral contraceptive, management includes periodic reassessments. A typical management plan includes a follow-up visit after 3 months to assess for adverse effects and monitor blood pressure, one at 6 months for a similar assessment and a breast and bimanual examination, and one every 6 months thereafter for a complete health assessment with an annual Pap smear test (Hawkins et al., 1995) (see Table 14.4). Because oral contraceptives are drugs, they can interact with other drugs. The client should be instructed to consult her health care professional about interactions with any prescription or over-the-counter drugs.

Injectable Contraceptives

The injectable contraceptive, Depo-Provera®, is a synthetic hormonal substance (depot-medroxyprogesterone acetate) that acts by blocking gonadotropin, thus preventing ovulation from occurring. It also decreases sperm penetration through cervical mucus, decreases tubal motility, and causes endometrial atrophy, preventing implantation. Depo-Provera® is injected intramuscularly every 3 months into the muscle of the upper arm or buttocks. Research on the contraceptive has been conducted in countries around the world for well over a decade. It was approved by the FDA for marketing in the United States beginning in January of 1993.

Depo-Provera works by suppressing ovulation for 3 months through inhibition of gonadotropin production. It offers a reversible method that is long-term and disconnected from the act of intercourse. Its administration can be highly confidential, so the woman need not reveal that she is using this method. For women who are estrogen sensitive or have contraindications to methods containing estrogen, Depo-Provera offers a possible alternative.

As with most chemical methods, there are contraindications to its use. These include known or suspected pregnancy, undiagnosed vaginal bleeding, known or suspected breast malignancy, active thrombophlebitis, current or past history of thromboembolic disorders or a cerebral vascular accident, liver dysfunction or disease, or known sensitivity to Depo-Provera or any of its ingredients. (If a woman has had an allergic reaction to local anesthesia at the dentist, she may also have a reaction to Depo-Provera because it has the same carrier substance.)

Screening for relative contraindications is also important. These include a family history of breast cancer, an abnormal mammogram, fibrocystic breast disease, breast nodules or lumps, bleeding from nipples, kidney disease, irregular or scanty menses, high blood pressure, migraine headaches, asthma, epilepsy, diabetes or a family history of diabetes, a history of depression, and regular use of other prescription drugs because of possible interactions. Decisions should be made on a case-by-case basis with consultation with the woman's other health care providers as appropriate.

Depo-Provera is injected intramuscularly in one 150-mg dose every 3 months for as long as contraceptive effect is desired (in gluteal or deltoid muscle in the first 3 days of the menstrual cycle [after onset of menses] and within 5 days postpartum, or if breast-feeding, at 4-6 weeks postpartum). If the time between injections is greater than 14 weeks, a sensitive pregnancy test is done before administration. Women are advised to use a backup contraceptive method for 2 weeks after the first injection. Depo-Provera has some side effects and dangers as shown in Table 14.2 ("Hormonal Contraception, 1987; Kaunitz, 1993; Policar, 1993; Upjohn, 1992; Wymelenberg, 1990).

Morning-After Contraceptive

Administered shortly after unprotected, midcycle intercourse, this contraceptive is effective because estrogens prevent pregnancy when taken during ovulation (Connell, 1990a). Diethylstilbestrol (DES) is the only FDA-approved morning-after contraceptive. Up to 48 hours after unprotected, midcycle intercourse (but preferably within 12 to 24 hours), the client receives 25 mg of DES twice a day for 5 days to prevent ovum implantation. Adverse effects include nausea,

text continued on page 315

Table 14.4 Management of Common Adverse Effects of Oral Contraceptives[a]

Sign or Symptom	*Probable Cause*	*Management*
Nausea, abdominal pain	Use of a high-estrogen oral contraceptive	• Switch the client to a low-estrogen oral contraceptive or to one with a different type of estrogen. • Oral contraceptive administration on an empty stomach • Gastrointestinal virus or reaction to food
Headaches[b]	Use of a high-estrogen oral contraceptive	• Switch the client to a low-estrogen oral contraceptive.
	Severe migraine that existed before the client began taking an oral contraceptive	• Discontinue the oral contraceptive. • Consult with the physician.
	Fatigue, stress, lack of sleep (when headaches existed before the client began taking an oral contraceptive)	• Obtain a detailed history to identify the cause.
	Excessive television viewing, inadequate light for reading, or television viewing (when headaches existed before the client began taking an oral contraceptive)	• Obtain a detailed history. • Refer the client to an eye examination. • Teach the client about related health habits, such as stress management, adequate light for reading.
	Premenstrual tension	• Obtain a detailed history, particularly noting the timing of headaches in relation to the menstrual period.
	Vision problems with headaches	• Monitor the client's blood pressure regularly. • Perform an eye examination. • Refer the client to a neurologist to rule out CNS pathology.
	Anemia	• Check the client's hematocrit and hemoglobin level. • Obtain a dietary history. • Teach the client to eat a well-balanced diet.
Weight gain	Use of a progestin-dominant oral contraceptive, which increases appetite	• Switch the client to an estrogen-dominant or a low-androgen or a low-estrogen oral contraceptive.
	Unbalanced diet	• Obtain a complete dietary history. • Provide nutritional counseling and teaching.
	Hypertension and edema	• Monitor the client's blood pressure regularly. • Discontinue the oral contraceptive if necessary. • Consult with the physician.
	Stress or life events	• Counsel the client about stress management.
Weight loss	Poor appetite	• Obtain a detailed history to determine the cause.
	Limited time to eat	• Obtain a detailed history. • Counsel the client about nutrition and stress management. • Assist with priority setting.
	Stress or life events	• Counsel the client. • Teach the client appropriate health habits.
	Disorder such as anemia, tuberculosis, or hyperthyroidism	• Obtain a detailed history. • Perform a complete physical assessment. • Order appropriate diagnostic tests. • Consult with the physician.

Table 14.4 Continued

Sign or Symptom	*Probable Cause*	*Management*
	Use of a high-estrogen oral contraceptive (usually accompanied by nausea and vomiting)	• Considering switching to low-estrogen oral contraceptive.
	Fear of oral contraceptive adverse effects	• Explore the client's fears and degree of comfort with the method. • Discuss alternatives and assist with decision making.
	Imagined weight loss	• Compare the client's current and previous weights. • Obtain a detailed diet history.
Fatigue	Anemia	• Assess the client's hematocrit and hemoglobin level. • Obtain a dietary history. • Teach the client to eat a well-balanced diet.
	Infection	• Obtain a detailed history. • Perform a complete physical assessment. • Consult with/refer to the physician.
	Overwork, lack of sleep, poor dietary habits, or insomnia	• Obtain a detailed history. • Perform a complete physical assessment. • Help the client to take time for rest. • Refer the client for counseling or other assistance. • Teach client stress management techniques.
Spotting	Improper self-administration of the oral contraceptive	• Obtain a history of oral contraceptive use, including missed or late pills. • Reassure the client that spotting is a common adverse effect.
	Vaginitis or cervical ectropion	• Perform a pelvic examination, obtaining smears and cultures as needed. • Advise the client to have a Papanicolaou test annually.
	Gynecologic disorder, such as polyps, cysts, tumors, or diethylstilbestrol (DES) exposure	• Obtain a detailed history, particularly noting DES exposure in utero and gynecologic disorders or surgery.
	Use of an oral contraceptive	• Switch the client to an oral contraceptive that provides increased estrogen in the early cycle (pills 1 to 14) and increased progestin in the late cycle (pills 15 to 21).
Amenorrhea	Improper self-administration of the oral contraceptive (starting a new 21-day on day 22)	• Review proper administration of the prescribed oral contraceptive.
	Pregnancy	• Review the client's use of the prescribed oral contraceptive. • Assess for other signs of pregnancy such as fatigue, headaches, breast tenderness. • Perform a pelvic examination. • Perform a pregnancy test.
	Prolonged use of an oral contraceptive	• Switch the client to a higher-estrogen oral contraceptive for a few months. • Advise the client to use another contraceptive method for a few months. • Reassure the client that some women have no withdrawal bleeding when taking certain oral contraceptive formulas. • Order endocrine tests (see amenorrhea in Chapter 23).

(continued)

Table 14.4 Continued

Sign or Symptom	*Probable Cause*	*Management*
	Frequent, strenuous exercise	• Assess the client's percentage of body fat.
Milky breast discharge	Use of an oral contraceptive	• Obtain a detailed history. • Switch the client to a different oral contraceptive.
	Pregnancy	• Perform a pregnancy test. • Perform a pelvic examination.
	Breast stimulation, such as sucking or squeezing the nipples, especially during the postpartal period or after therapeutic abortion	• Suggest other forms of sexual stimulation until the discharge ceases.
	Pituitary disorder	• Determine the client's prolactin level. • Consult with the physician.
	Use of drugs, such as tranquilizers, heroin, and morphine	• Obtain a detailed drug history. • Consult with the physician.
	Breast disorder	• Teach client to do breast self-examination. • Inspect and palpate the client's breasts. • Order a mammogram for the client.
Chloasma	Use of a high-estrogen oral contraceptive	• Switch the client to a low-estrogen oral contraceptive.
	Pregnancy	• Perform a pregnancy test. • Perform a pelvic examination.
	Endocrine disorder or systemic lupus erythematosus	• Obtain a detailed history. • Perform a complete physical assessment. • Consider consulting with the physician.
Scant menstrual bleeding	Prolonged use of an oral contraceptive, especially a high-androgen formula	• Switch the client to a high-estrogen oral contraceptive.
	Pregnancy	• Perform a pregnancy test. • Perform a pelvic examination.
Skin rash	Use of an oral contraceptive	• Obtain a detailed history of the rash in relation to oral contraceptive use. • Switch the client to a different oral contraceptive. • Consult with the physician.
	Infection, allergy, syphilis, or other communicable disease	• Perform a complete physical assessment. • Order laboratory tests to help identify the cause. • Consult with the physician.
Fluid retention	Renal, vascular cardiac disease	• Obtain a detailed history. • Perform a complete physical assessment • Consult with the physician.
	Use of a high-estrogen oral contraceptive	• Switch the client to a low-estrogen pill. • Advise the client to consider another contraceptive method.
Hair loss	Use of damaging hair products, curling irons, dyes, straighteners, or a wig	• Obtain a detailed history of hair loss pattern.
	Postpartal physiological effects	• Reassure the client that hair loss is cyclic and temporary.
	Use of a high-progestin, highly androgenic oral contraceptive	• Switch the client to a less androgenic oral contraceptive.
	Endocrine disorder, cancer, or sexually transmitted disease (STD)	• Obtain a detailed history.
Decreased libido	Fatigue or stress	• Perform a complete physical assessment. • Consult with the physician. • Obtain a detailed history. • Counsel the client about stress management.

(continued)

Table 14.4 Continued

Sign or Symptom	*Probable Cause*	*Management*
		• Teach the client about appropriate health habits. • Refer the client for counseling as indicated.
	Use of a high-progestin oral contraceptive	• Switch the client to a low-progestin, estrogen-dominant oral contraceptive.
	No orgasms	• Review with the client anatomy and physiology of sexual responses. • Talk to the client about the role of foreplay in sexual response.
Excessive bleeding	Use of a high-estrogen oral contraceptive	• Switch the client to a low-estrogen, high-progestin oral contraceptive.
	PID, vaginitis, myomata, pelvic pathology, DES exposure	• Obtain a detailed history. • Perform a complete physical assessment. • Order laboratory tests (smears, cultures). • Perform a pregnancy test. • Consult with the physician.
Dyspareunia	Pelvic, vaginal, or cervical disorder, such as PID, STD, or vaginitis	• Perform a pelvic examination. • Consult with the physician.
	Scant lubrication or genital irritation from clothing, soap, deodorant, or douche	• Obtain a detailed history. • Teach the client about sexual arousal, use of lubricants, and avoidance of irritants.
	Severe uterine retroversion or retroflexion	• Suggest more comfortable positions for intercourse.
Vaginal discharge	Use of a high-estrogen oral contraceptive	• Change to different formulation of oral contraceptive.
	Vaginitis, local irritation, cervicitis, STD, or PID	• Perform a pelvic examination. Obtain smears and cultures for testing. • Consult with the physician.
Hirsutism	Use of high-progestin, highly androgenic oral contraceptive	• Change formulation of oral contraceptive.
	Endocrine disorder or polycystic ovaries (Stein-Leventhal syndrome)	• Obtain a detailed history. • Perform a complete physical assessment. • Consult with the physician.
Oily scalp and skin or acne	Use of a high-progestin, highly androgenic oral contraceptive	• Switch client to different formulation of oral contraceptive.
	Poor hygiene	• Teach the client the importance of good hygiene.
Depression or lability	Use of high-estrogen, high-progestin oral contraceptive	• Switch the client to a low-estrogen, low-progestin oral contraceptive. • Discuss the possibility of using another contraceptive method.
	Fatigue and stress	• Obtain a detailed emotional history and information on lifestyle and habit. • Counsel the client about lifestyle, stress management, and habits. • Refer the client for counseling, and stress management.

NOTE: This table can help the nurse practitioner or other health care professional determine if certain signs and symptoms indicate the adverse effects of an oral contraceptive or reflect another problem. It can also assist in managing these effects and problems appropriately. Nurses must follow facility protocol for managing such complaints.
a. For extensive discussion of management of adverse effects of oral contraceptives, see Hatcher et al. (1994).
b. For headache workup with oral contraceptive, see Hawkins, Roberto, and Stanley-Haney (1995).

vomiting, and breast tenderness. Because of reproductive tract defects in those who are exposed to DES in utero, the client should be offered the option of pregnancy termination if DES morning-after therapy fails (Connell, 1990a).

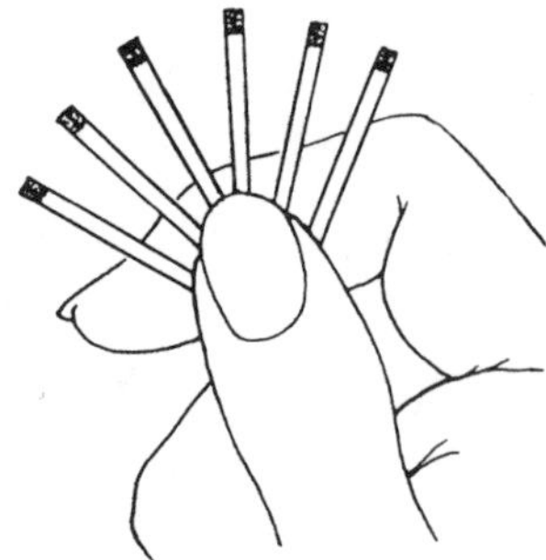

Figure 14.11. Contraceptive Implants
Only one implant, Norplant, is currently available in the United States. Its six tubes, filled with synthetic progestin, are implanted in the client's upper or lower arm. After insertion they are not visible.

Oral contraceptives may also be used as morning-after contraceptives, although they have not received FDA approval yet for this use. Planned Parenthood Affiliates in the United States have approved this usage since 1988. In a study of morning-after contraceptives, women received two doses, 12 hours apart, of an oral contraceptive that contained 1 mg of progestin and 100 mcg of ethinyl estradiol. Of the 51% who experienced adverse effects, 30% reported nausea and 20% reported nausea and vomiting. The failure rate was 2% ("Postcoital Pill," 1988). The regimen used in the study, the Yuzpe method, has been used in Canada since 1974.

Several other drugs can also be used for postcoital contraception. Danazol™ given in a 400- to 600-mg dose and repeated in the same dosage 12 hours later will inhibit implantation. Ideally, this regimen should be given within 72 hours of unprotected intercourse, and within 24 hours is ideal. Estrone (brand name, Ogen™) can be given in a 5-mg, oral, twice-a-day regimen for 5 days. RU 486 is also effective postcoital but has not received FDA approval in the United States (Schnare, 1993).

Contraceptive Implants

First proposed in 1967, contraceptive implants received FDA approval in 1990 but had been used for more than 20 years in other countries (Klitsch, 1983). The FDA-approved product, Norplant, consists of flexible, nonbiodegradable, hollow, Silastic™ tubes filled with the synthetic progestin, levonorgestrel. Each tube is 34 millimeters long. Six tubes are placed under the skin on the inside of the upper or lower arm and can remain in place for up to 5 years, releasing progestin at a constant rate. The progestin suppresses ovulation, thickens and reduces the amount of cervical mucus, and suppresses endometrial proliferation. Effectiveness rates are comparable to those of the IUD ("Injectables and Implants," 1987). Norplant failures are rare (Hatcher et al., 1990).

Norplant-2, a two-rod system that lasts at least 3 years, is under investigation in the United States and could gain approval in the next few years. Norplant-2 differs from Norplant in the number and character of the implants. Its two rods are solid Silastic™ and each measures 44 millimeters ("Injectables and Implants," 1987).

Besides performing a complete health assessment, the health care professional should teach the client about the method, especially about insertion and removal (Hawkins et al., 1995). The implants must be replaced after 5 years, but they can be removed at any time, restoring fertility. Insertion and removal are office procedures that require local anesthesia and a small incision. Therefore, they must be done by health care professionals with special preparation (see Figure 14.11).

Intrauterine Methods

These contraceptive methods have a long history. Ancient Turks and Arabs put stones in their camel's uteruses to prevent pregnancy. Intrauterine stems, rings, and pessaries were used in Europe during the 19th century and possibly as early as the 11th century (Connell, 1990b; Glazer, 1965). However, none of these was a lasting success because of risk of infection.

The IUD first described by Richter in 1909 was a ring-shaped device made of silkworm gut. Since then, various shapes, including rings, loops, spirals, T-shapes, and 7-shapes, and materials, including silver, copper, and plastic, have been used (Hatcher et al., 1990). These early IUDs caused problems, such as infection, perforation of the uterus and other pelvic organs, heavy bleeding, cramping, ectopic pregnancy, and infertility. Individual and class action suits against the manufacturer of the Dalkon shield because it caused infection and other adverse effects resulted in its removal from the market in 1974. The Lippes Loop and Saf-T-Coil were removed in 1984 and 1985, although they still had FDA approval. The Copper T (Cu-T) and Copper 7

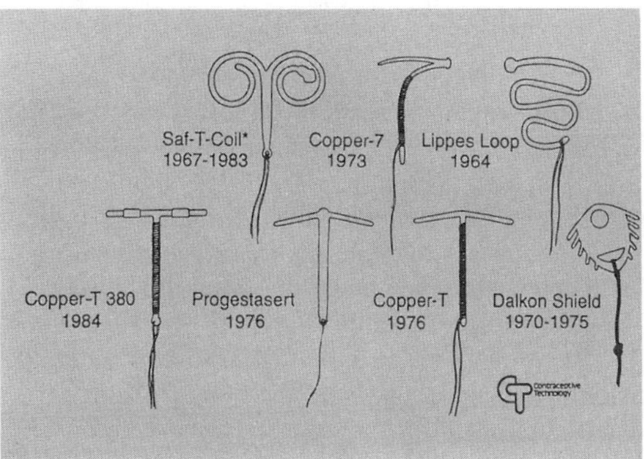

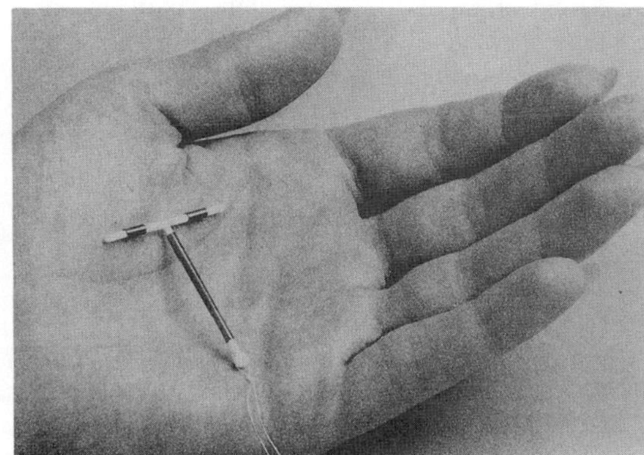

Figure 14.12. Sample Intrauterine Devices
Although many intrauterine devices (IUDs) have been withdrawn from the market, these IUDs are still available. NOTE: CU-7 is still marketed outside the United States.

(Cu-7) were removed from the market in 1986 when their patents expired (Connell, 1990b). The Progestasert remained on the market, and a new generation of copper devices replaced the Copper T and the Cu-7. Many of these devices remain in use around the world (see Figure 14.12).

IUDs are not abortifacients; they prevent pregnancy through several mechanisms of action. Some may set up a local sterile inflammatory response, changing the cellular composition of the endometrium. These changes may cause phagocytosis of the sperm or the blastocyst, prevent implantation, or disrupt the implantation site. Copper devices may exert a local effect on the endometrium by interfering with various enzyme systems. Devices containing progesterone may stimulate decidual and secretory changes (Connell, 1990b).

Progestasert, the first hormonal device impregnated with synthetic progestin, is still available. Because the progestin lasts only 1 year, the device must be replaced annually. The newest copper device, ParaGard T380A, can remain in place for 6 years ("Six-Year Contraceptive," 1990). This third generation, T-shaped, copper device has copper on the stem and both arms, unlike its predecessors the Cu-7 and Copper T, which have copper on the stems only (for illustrations, see Figure 14.12). Guidelines, for example, those outlined by Hatcher and associates (1990), are strict for receiving an IUD: Only a client who has completed her family or wants no children is eligible. Also, the health care professional and client must consider her lifestyle and other criteria, and the client must sign a lengthy consent form. The cost of an IUD is relatively high, which covers liability insurance. Nevertheless, many clients believe the IUD is the best contraceptive choice based on all the factors that they must consider (Hawkins et al., 1995).

Sterilization

Sterilization of men and women is the most popular contraceptive method in the United States today (Hatcher et al., 1990). It is considered permanent, although it may be reversed in a small percentage of clients. The decision to end fertility permanently requires a careful review of all alternatives and full information about the risks of surgery.

Female Sterilization

Female sterilization techniques are discussed in Chapter 26, "Reproductive Surgery." Sterilization involves a decision by the client to seek a permanent solution to fertility regulation. A client may seek tubal ligation because she (a) has used one or more contraceptive methods; (b) is dissatisfied with available methods; (c) has experienced method failure; (d) has medical contraindications for one or more methods; (e) has psychosocial contraindications for one or more methods, such as unwillingness to use, fear of use, or method unacceptability to partner; (f) desires to end fertility and have no more children (or no children); (g) is premenopausal and has had no menstrual periods for 1 year or less;

or (h) is experiencing problems with one or more methods (Hawkins et al., 1995).

When assisting the client with this decision, the health care professional should ask about prior use of contraceptive methods, desired family size, cultural beliefs about sterilization, family attitudes toward sterilization, knowledge about sterilization procedures, and history of previous pelvic surgery, such as oophorectomy (removal of one or both ovaries), salpingectomy (removal of one or both fallopian tubes), laparoscopy, or tubal reconstruction.

The nurse must have current information on the prerequisites or guidelines used by the medical profession for sterilization. Voluntary sterilization is legal in all 50 states. Guidelines set by the Department of Health, Education and Welfare ("Sterilization of Persons," 1978) to ensure informed consent for federally funded sterilizations include the following:

- A full explanation of the procedures, including risks and benefits, must be provided to the client.
- A statement about the permanent nature of the surgery must be presented to the client.
- The physician must wait 30 days after the client has given consent before performing the sterilization.
- The consent form must be in the woman's native language or an interpreter must be provided.

In addition, there are some restrictions on federal funds for minors (under the age of 21) and mentally incompetent women. Even when federal funds are not used, many hospitals and physicians have similar restrictions. A husband's consent is not legally required in most states; however, to avoid potential legal actions, many physicians try to obtain the husband's consent.

Although reanastomosis (surgical rejoining) of the fallopian tubes is possible, the success rate is not high, so the client should consider sterilization permanent. The request rate for reanastomosis ranges from 0.1% to 1.0%, but the success rate varies depending on the extent of tubal damage as does the resulting pregnancy rate and risk of ectopic pregnancy. (See Chapter 25, "Infertility," for related discussion of this topic.)

Consent procedures for sterilization vary from state to state and from institution to institution. In some states, the husband must consent to sterilization of his wife, but the reverse is not true. Therefore, the health care professional must be aware of all consent procedures that apply.

Male Sterilization

Male sterilization (vasectomy) involves location and surgical resection of the vas deferens. Although the procedure can be reversed, the success rate varies, so vasectomy should be considered permanent. Several means of occluding the vas deferens are under investigation and, when approved, may offer a greater chance of successful reversal.

The procedure for male sterilization is much shorter (15 to 30 minutes) than that for female sterilization. It can be done in an ambulatory setting with local anesthesia. Recovery is rapid and sutures are absorbed in 1 to 2 weeks. Most protocols require two follow-up visits (usually at 6 and 12 weeks) that include semen analysis to check for aspermia. Until the analysis shows no sperm, the couple should use another contraceptive method for vaginal-penile intercourse.

Death rates from vasectomy remain consistent at 0.1 per 100,000, compared to 4.0 per 100,000 for tubal ligation, making vasectomy much less risky. Morbidity is also lower because vasectomy does not require intra-abdominal surgery or general anesthesia.

Future Contraceptive Methods

Barrier, chemical, hormonal, and intrauterine contraceptive methods are under investigation in the United States and around the world. New barrier methods for women and men protect against not only pregnancy but also STDs. New male barrier methods include a water-soluble or spermicidal condom, which basically is a male form of contraceptive film (Connell, 1990c).

Researchers are investigating chemical contraceptive methods, such as enzyme-inhibiting spermicides and substances that coagulate sperm immediately after ejaculation. They are also studying ways to alter cervical mucus so that it will inhibit sperm movement.

Scientists are exploring new hormonal contraceptives, such as biodegradable implants that release progestin and dissolve over time, injectable microspheres and microcapsules that release hormones for months and then dissolve, and vaginal rings that remain in place for up to 3 months and release progestin. They are also developing vaginal rings impregnated with sperm antibody or estrogen and progestin.

Widely used in other parts of the world, long-acting and monthly injectable contraceptives are under study for contraceptive use in the United States. Transdermal delivery of contraceptive hormones through a skin patch shows some promise. With this method, the client applies one patch each week for 3 weeks. During the fourth week, she uses no patch and experiences withdrawal bleeding (Franklin, 1990; "Injectables and Implants," 1987; Wymelenberg, 1990).

Various contraceptive methods are being developed for men. An oral contraceptive for men has been found to interfere with spermatogenic cell maturation. However, it produces adverse effects, such as nephrotoxicity, which have not yet been reduced with different formulations. A removable intraluminal device for the vas deferens may be marketed to produce temporary sterility. New versions of the contraceptive film, in the form of penile caps, should be in clinical trials shortly. Weekly testosterone injections hold promise as a male contraceptive method. In clinical trials, their mean time for effective suppression is 120 days; their mean recovery time 3.7 months. These injections suppress sperm production completely, giving protection superior to the IUD, oral contraceptive, and condom ("Weekly Testosterone Injections," 1991).

A new IUD, the CuFix 390, consists of a string of hanging copper rings. It already is being used abroad, but its manufacturer may not seek licensure in the United States because of liability concerns (Connell, 1990b; Monier & Laird, 1989; Wymelenberg, 1990).

Although user acceptability of a contraceptive method seems critical to its acceptance and success, little research explores this issue. An interdisciplinary committee on contraceptive development recently told the FDA, "An expanded understanding of the 'user perspective' is required. Too often methods fail and expose the user to the medical risks associated with pregnancy and childbirth because they are too expensive, too difficult to use, or have unacceptable side effects" (Kaeser, 1990, p. 133).

References

HISTORICAL AND SOCIAL CONTEXT

Cooke, C., & Dworkin, S. (1979). *The MS guide to woman's health.* New York: Anchor.

Douglas, E. T. (1970). *Margaret Sanger: Pioneer of the future.* New York: Holt, Rinehart & Winston.

Gieg, D. M. (1972). The birth control movement in Massachusetts: Its early history, 1916-1931. *Essays and Studies by Students of Simmons College, 30*(2), 1-5.

Gordon, L. (1990). *Woman's body, woman's right.* New York: Penguin.

Gray, M. (1979). *Margaret Sanger.* New York: R. Marek.

Himes, N. E. (1936). *Medical history of contraception.* New York: Schocken.

Jones, E. F., Forrest, J. D., Henshaw, S. K., Silverman, J., & Torres, A. (1988). Unintended pregnancy, contraceptive practice, and family planning services in developed countries. *Family Planning Perspectives, 20*(1), 53-67.

Kinsey, A. C., Pomeroy, W. B., Martin, C. E., & Gebhard, P. H. (1953). *Sexual behavior in the human female.* New York: Pocket Books.

Lader, L. (1955). *The Margaret Sanger story.* Garden City, NY: Doubleday.

Marlow, J. (1979). *The great women.* New York: Galahad.

Niethammer, C. (1977). *Daughters of the earth.* New York: Collier.

Sanger, M. (1920a). *What every girl should know.* New York: Belvedere.

Sanger, M. (1920b). *Woman and the new race.* New York: Truth Publishing.

Sanger, M. (1931). *My fight for birth control.* New York: Maxwell.

Sanger, M. (1938). *Margaret Sanger: An autobiography.* New York: Dover.

Sicherman, B., Green, C. H., Kantor, I., & Walker, H. (1980). *Notable American women: The modern period.* Cambridge: Harvard University Press.

Smith-Lovin, L., & Tickamyer, A. (1978). Nonrecursive models of labor force participation, fertility behavior and sex role attitudes. *American Sociological Review, 43*(4), 541-557.

Tannahill, R. (1980). *Sex in history.* New York: Stein & Day.

CONTRACEPTIVE PATTERNS AND PRACTICES

Forrest, J. D. (1987). Has she or hasn't she? U. S. women's experience with contraception. *Family Planning Perspectives, 19*(3), 133.

Forrest, J. D. (1988). The delivery of family planning services in the United States. *Family Planning Perspectives, 20*(2), 88-98.

Forrest, J. D., & Fordyce, R. R. (1988). U.S. women's contraceptive attitudes and practice: How have they changed in the 1980s? *Family Planning Perspectives, 20*(3), 112-118.

Friedan, B. (1963). *The feminine mystique.* New York: Dell.

Grady, W. R., Hayward, M. D., & Florey, F. A. (1988). Contraceptive discontinuation among married women in the United States. *Studies in Family Planning, 19*(5), 227-235.

Horton, J. A. (1992). *The women's health data book.* Washington, DC: Jacob's Institute of Women's Health.

Jones, E. F., Forrest, J. D., Henshaw, S. K., Silverman, J., & Torres, A. (1988). Unintended pregnancy, contraceptive practice, and family planning services in developed countries. *Family Planning Perspectives, 20*(1), 53-67.

Kinsey, A. C., Pomeroy, W. B., Martin, C. E., & Gebhard, P. H. (1953). *Sexual behavior in the human female.* New York: Pocket Books.

Ory, H. W., Forrest, J. D., & Lincoln, R. (1983). *Making choices: Evaluating the health risks and benefits of birth control methods.* New York: Alan Guttmacher Institute.

Silverman, J., Torres, A., & Forrest, J. D. (1987). Barriers to contraceptive services. *Family Planning Perspectives, 19*(2), 94-102.

U.S. Bureau of the Census. (1991). *Statistical abstract of the United States: 1991* (111th ed.). Washington, DC: Government Printing Office.

CONTRACEPTIVE DECISION MAKING

Adler, N. (1979). Decision models and population research. *Journal of Population, 2*(3), 187-202.

Burger, J., & Inderbitzen, H. (1985). Predicting contraceptive behavior among college students: The role of communication, knowledge, sexual activity and self-esteem. *Archives of Sexual Behavior, 14*(4), 343-350.

Burke, P. J. (1987). Adolescents' motivation for sexual activity and pregnancy prevention. *Issues in Comprehensive Pediatric Nursing, 10*(2), 161-171.

Forrest, J. D. (1988). The delivery of family planning services in the United States. *Family Planning Perspectives, 20*(2), 88-98.

Forrest, J. D., & Fordyce, R. R. (1988). U.S. women's contraceptive attitudes and practice: How have they changed in the 1980s? *Family Planning Perspectives, 20*(3), 112-118.

Horton, J. A. (1992). *The women's health data book.* Washington, DC: Jacob's Institute of Women's Health.

Kisker, E. (1985). Teenagers talk about sex, pregnancy, and contraception. *Family Planning Perspectives, 17*(2), 83-90.

Klein, L. (1984). Unintended pregnancy and the risks/safety of birth control methods. *JOGNN, 13*(2), 287-289.

Luker, K. (1978). *Taking chances: Abortion and the decision not to contracept.* Berkeley: University of California Press.

Miller, W. B. (1986). Why some women fail to use their contraceptive method: A psychological investigation. *Family Planning Perspectives, 18*(1), 27-32.

Nathanson, C. A., & Becker, M. H. (1986). Family and peer influence on obtaining a method of contraception. *Journal of Marriage and the Family, 48*(3), 513-525.

Silverman, J., Torres, A., & Forrest, J. D. (1987). Barriers to contraceptive services. *Family Planning Perspectives, 19*(2), 94-102.

Winter, L. (1988). The role of sexual self-concept in the use of contraceptives. *Family Planning Perspectives, 20*(3), 123-127.

Zabin, L., & Clark, F. (1981). Why they delay: A study of teenage family planning clinic patients. *Family Planning Perspectives, 13*(4), 205-217.

FAMILY-PLANNING SERVICES

Orne, R., & Hawkins, J. W. (1985). Reexamining the oral contraceptive issues. *JOGNN, 14,* 30-36.

Tabeek, E. (1990). Mainstreaming of natural methods of family planning in selected family planning agencies that receive Title X funding. In J. Wang, P. Simoni, & C. Nath (Eds.), *Proceedings of the West Virginia Nurses Association 1990 research symposium* (pp. 423-427). Charleston: West Virginia Association Research Conference Group.

Taylor, S., Pickens, J., & Geden, E. (1989). Interactional styles of nurse practitioners and physicians regarding patient decision making. *Nursing Research, 38*(1), 50-55.

CONTRACEPTIVE METHODS

Apothecus. (1989). *Vaginal contraceptive film.* Oyster Bay, NY: Author.

Cervical Cap, Ltd. (1988). *The cervical cap.* Los Gatos, CA: Author.

Connell, E. B. (1990a). Hormonal contraception. In N. G. Kase, A. B. Weingold, & D. M. Gershenson (Eds.), *Principles and practice of clinical gynecology* (2nd ed., pp. 993-1019). New York: Churchill Livingstone.

Connell, E. B., Grimes, D. A., & Manisoff, M. E. (1989). *The contraceptive diaphragm.* New York: Healthcare Communications.

Diaz, S. (1989). Determinants of lactational amenorrhea. *International Journal of Gynecology and Obstetrics* (Suppl. 1), 83-89.

Dickey, R. P. (1994). *Managing contraceptive pill patients* (8th ed.). Durant, OK: Essential Medical Information Systems.

Forrest, J. D., & Fordyce, R. R. (1988). U.S. women's contraceptive attitudes and practices: How have they changed in the 1980's? *Family Planning Perspectives, 20*(3), 112-118.

Glazer, N. (1965). A history of mechanical contraception. *Medical Times, 93*(8), 865-869.

Goldzieher, J. W. (1989). *Hormonal contraception.* Dallas, TX: Essential Medical Information Systems.

Grimes, D. A. (1987). Preventing pregnancy—and STDs. *Dialogues in Contraception, 2*(2), 1-8.

Hatcher, R., Stewart, F., Trussell, J., Kowal, D., Guest, F., Stewart, G. K., & Cates, W. (1990). *Contraceptive technology 1990-1992* (15th ed.). New York: Irvington.

Hatcher, R. A., Trussell, J., Stewart, F., Stewart, G. K., Kowal, D., Guest, F., Cates, W., & Policar, M. S. (1994). *Contraception technology* (16th ed.). New York: Irvington.

Hawkins, J. W., Roberto, D., & Stanley-Haney, J. L. (1995). *Protocols for nurses in gynecologic settings* (5th ed.). New York: Tiresias.

Hawkins, J. W., Roberto, D., & Stanley-Haney, J. L. (1993). *Protocols for nurses in gynecologic settings* (4th ed.). New York: Tiresias.

Himes, N. E. (1936). *Medical history of contraception.* New York: Schocken.

Hormonal contraception: New long-acting methods. (1987). *Population Reports, 15*(1), K69-K75.

Injectables and implants. (1987). *Population Reports,* Series K (3).

Kafka, D., & Gold, R. B. (1983). Food and Drug Administration approves vaginal sponge. *Family Planning Perspectives, 15*(3), 146-148.

Kaunitz, A. M. (1993). DMPA: A new contraception option. *Contemporary OB/GYN-NP, 1*(1), 5-12.

Kistner, R. W. (1968). *The pill.* New York: Delacorte.

Klitsch, M. (1983). Hormonal implants: The next wave of contraceptives. *Family Planning Perspectives, 15*(5), 239-243.

Klitsch, M. (1988). FDA approval ends cervical cap's marathon. *Family Planning Perspectives, 20*(3), 137-138.

Kugel, C., & Verson, H. (1986). Relationship between weight change and diaphragm size change. *JOGNN, 15*(2), 123-129.

Lamberts (Dalston) Limited. (1988). *The Prentif cavity-rim cervical cap for contraceptive use.* Luton, UK: Author.

Martin, M. C. (1981). Natural family planning and instructor training. *Nursing and Health Care, 2*(10), 554-563.

McClure, D. A., & Edelman, D. A. (1985). Worldwide method effectiveness of the Today vaginal contraceptive sponge. *Advances in Contraception, 1,* 305-311.

Meisenhelder, J. B., & LaCharite, C. L. (1989). *Comfort in caring: Nursing the person with HIV infection.* Boston: Scott, Foresman.

Mishell, D. R., Connell, E., Haney, A., Hodgen, G., & Speroff, L. (1990). Oral contraception for women in their 40s. *Journal of Reproductive Medicine, 35*(Suppl. 4), 447-481.

Moore, R. A. (1990). Ask the experts. *NAACOG Newsletter, 1973-1988, 17*(12), 24.

New England Natural Family Planning. (undated). *New England natural family planning standards.* (Available from New England Natural Family Planning, 2121 Commonwealth Ave., Brighton, MA 02135)

Nurses Association of the American College of Obstetricians and Gynecologists. (1983). *Natural family planning.* Washington, DC: Author.

Nurses Association of the American College of Obstetricians and Gynecologists. (1991). *Standards for obstetric, gynecologic, and neonatal nursing* (4th ed.). Washington, DC: Organization for Obstetric, Gynecologic, and Neonatal Nurses.

Orne, R., & Hawkins, J. W. (1985). Reexamining the oral contraceptive issues. *JOGNN, 14,* 30-36.

Orouin, J., Labrecque, M., Rioux, J., Gingras, S., & Spieler, J. (1988). Effectiveness of the Bioself 110. In *Proceedings of the fifth national and international symposium on natural family planning* (pp. 59-63). Los Angeles: Los Angeles Regional Family Planning Council.

Ory, H. W., Forrest, J. D., & Lincoln, R. (1983). *Making choices: Evaluating the health risks and benefits of birth control methods.* New York: Alan Guttmacher Institute.

Policar, M. S. (1993, February 18). [Unpublished speech]. Presented to Planned Parenthood Federation of America, Philadelphia.

Postcoital pill: Rate of success seems high, but side effects common. (1988). *Family Planning Perspectives, 20*(3), 149.

Rock, J. (1963). *The time has come.* New York: Avon.

Schnare, S. (1993). Postcoital contraception. *Contemporary OB/GYN-NP, 1*(1), 3-4.

Secor, R. M. C. (1991). Cervical cap. In J. W. Hawkins, D. Roberto, & J. L. Stanley-Haney (Eds.), *Protocols for nurse practitioners in gynecologic settings* (3rd ed., pp. 38-49, 205-212). New York: Tiresias.

Six-year contraceptive now available for women. (1990). *NAACOG Newsletter, 17*(12), 14.

Tabeek, E. (1990). Mainstreaming of natural methods of family planning in selected family planning agencies that receive Title X funding. In J. Wang, P. Simoni, & C. Nath (Eds.), *Proceedings of the West Virginia Nurses Association 1990 research symposium* (pp. 423-427). Charleston: West Virginia Association Research Conference Group.

Tabeek, E. (1991). Natural family planning. In J. W. Hawkins, D. Roberto, & J. L. Stanley-Haney (Eds.), *Protocols for nurse practitioners in gynecologic settings* (3rd ed., pp. 52-54, 216-234). New York: Tiresias.

Trussel, J., Sturgen, K., Strickler, J., & Dominik, R. (1994). Comparative contraceptive efficacy of the female condom and other barrier methods. *Family Planning Perspectives, 26*(2), 66-72.

Upjohn Pharmaceutical Company. (1992). Manufactor's literature on Depo-Provera.

Wisconsin Pharmacal Company. (1994). *Reality female condom status.* Chicago: Author.

Wymelenberg, S. (1990). *Science and babies: Private decision, public dilemmas.* Washington, DC: National Academy Press.

FUTURE CONTRACEPTIVE METHODS

Connell, E. B. (1990b). Barrier methods of contraception. In N. G. Kase, A. B. Weingold, & D. M. Gershenson (Eds.), *Principles and practice of clinical gynecology* (2nd ed., pp. 981-991). New York: Churchill Livingstone.

Connell, E. B. (1990c). Intrauterine devices. In N. G. Kase, A. B. Weingold, & D. M. Gershenson (Eds.), *Principles and practice of clinical gynecology* (2nd ed., pp. 1021-1042). New York: Churchill Livingstone.

Franklin, M. (1990). Recently approved and experimental methods of contraception. *Journal of Nurse-Midwifery, 35*(6), 365-375.

Injectables and implants. (1987). *Population reports* (Series K, No, 3). Washington, DC: Government Printing Office.

Kaeser, L. (1990). Contraceptive development: Why the snail's pace? *Family Planning Perspectives, 22*(4), 131-133.

Monier, M., & Laird, M. (1989). Contraceptives: A look at the future. *American Journal of Nursing, 89*(4), 496-499.

Sterilization of persons in federally assisted family planning projects. (1978, November 8). *Federal Register,* pp. 52146-52175.

Weekly testosterone injections suppress sperm production, may provide effective contraception. (1991). *Family Planning Perspectives, 23*(2), 86-87.

Wymelenberg, S. (1990). *Science and babies: Private decision, public dilemmas.* Washington, DC: National Academy Press.

15

Mental Health

ANNE HOPKINS FISHEL

Patterns of mental illness vary for women and men (Russo, 1990). Gender differences are illustrated well by the National Institute of Mental Health (NIMH) Epidemiological Catchment Area (ECA) project, a community-based survey conducted between 1980 and 1984 of a probability sample of more than 18,000 adults that used the Diagnostic Interview Schedule (DIS) to generate DSM-IV diagnoses. The study was independently conducted at five United States sites: New Haven, Connecticut; Baltimore, Maryland; St. Louis, Missouri; Durham, North Carolina; and Los Angeles, California. In the 6 months preceding the study, phobias (anxiety disorders) were the most prevalent among women, followed by major depression without grief and dysthymia (mood disorders), and obsessive-compulsive disorders (anxiety disorder). For men the most common diagnosis was alcohol abuse/dependence, followed by phobia, drug abuse/dependence, and, finally, dysthymia (Taube & Barrett, 1985). There were substantial gender differences in prevalence rates of lifetime diagnoses: Women clearly predominated in diagnoses of major depression and phobias, whereas men predominated in antisocial personality disorder and alcohol abuse/dependence (Robins et al., 1984).

Although not as prevalent, eating disorder and dissociative identity disorder (DID) (formerly multiple personality disorder) are clearly gender related. For example, 90% of all patients diagnosed with anorexia nervosa are female, and DID is thought to occur from three to nine times more frequently in females than in males (American Psychiatric Association [APA], 1994).

This chapter focuses on mental health problems prevalent among women: anxiety disorders, including panic attacks and obsessive-compulsive disorders; post-traumatic stress disorders linked to rape and other violence; mood disorders, particularly depression; eating disorders; and dissociative identity disorders. Discussion of recommended health policy for women, feminist therapy models, and a women's mental health research agenda concludes the chapter.

Table 15.1 Anxiety Symptoms

Trembling or feeling shaky	Muscle tension
Restlessness	Easy fatigability
Palpitations	Sweating or cold clammy hands
Dry mouth	Dizziness or lightheadedness
Nausea or diarrhea	Flushes or chills
Frequent urination	Trouble swallowing
Feeling keyed up or on edge	Exaggerated startle response
Difficulty concentrating	Irritability
Trouble falling or staying asleep	Shortness of breath or smothering sensations

Defining characteristics for nursing diagnosis of anxiety include (in descending order of validation): anxiety, apprehension, worry, increased tension, fear of unspecific consequences, distress, feeling scared, restlessness, focus on self, facial tension, extraneous movement, and difficulty in cognitive functioning.

SOURCE: Adapted from Whitley (1989).

Anxiety Disorders

Anxiety is a common experience for most women. Talking with another person to decrease anxiety is the healthiest approach. When felt anxiety becomes intolerable, however, defensive mechanisms are used to control the anxiety. The cost of the relief from the felt experience of intense anxiety is a disorder such as phobia or obsessive-compulsive disorder. Post-traumatic stress disorder is a frequent aftermath of an anxiety experience induced by rape or family violence. The essential feature of an anxiety disorder is unrealistic or excessive anxiety and worry about life circumstances and/or finances (for no good reason), for at least 6 months or longer (APA, 1994). The afflicted person experiences at least six anxiety symptoms (see Table 15.1). With such symptoms it is easy to understand why women go to their nurse practitioner or family physicians for help with what they perceive as physical problems. It is equally important to remember that if they come to the nurse with these symptoms, a thorough physical examination must be done to rule out a physical illness.

Panic Disorders With or Without Agoraphobia

Definition

Diagnostic criteria for panic disorder include recurrent, unexpected panic attacks (discrete periods of intense fear or discomfort) followed by a month of at least one of the following: persistent fear of having another attack, worry about the consequences of the attack (e.g., losing control, "going crazy,"), and a change in behavior (APA, 1994). Also four of the following symptoms must have developed during at least one of the attacks: dyspnea, dizziness or faintness, palpitations, trembling, sweating, choking, nausea, depersonalization (feeling of unreality and alienation from oneself), paresthesias, flushes or chills, chest pain, fear of dying, fear of going crazy. Panic attacks usually last minutes or, more rarely, hours. The attacks are unexpected in that they do not occur immediately before or on exposure to a situation that almost always causes anxiety. Panic attacks typically begin with the sudden onset of intense apprehension, fear, or terror. Often there is a feeling of impending doom.

Agoraphobia meets the criteria for panic disorder and, in addition, includes a fear of being in places or situations from which escape might be difficult or embarrassing or in which help might not be available. As a result of this fear, the person restricts travel, needs a companion when away from home, or endures agoraphobic situations despite intense anxiety (APA, 1994). The main fears are of going out of the house alone (on the street, to movies, to shop, and so on); closed spaces (e.g., being in elevators or standing in line); traveling in trains, buses, subway, and planes; and being on bridges, in a crowd, or in tunnels (APA, 1994).

Incidence

Panic symptoms are experienced by about 10% of adults during their lifetime (Weissman,

1990). The full-blown panic disorder is less common: Approximately 1% of adults meet the criteria in any 6-month period. Phobias were the leading diagnosis for women in the ECA study. The rates of agoraphobia are considerably higher than for panic disorder, between 2% and 5% for 6-month prevalence. Prevalence rates of agoraphobia were 2 to 4 times higher in women than in men and less educated and nonwhite persons (Weissman, 1990). Agoraphobia and panic disorders are more common among urban than rural residents (Weissman, 1990).

Researchers investigating a large randomized sample of "healthy" college students showed that approximately 12% had experienced at least one unexpected panic attack, and 2.36 met DSM-III-R (APA, 1987) criteria for panic disorder, with women reporting a higher panic frequency than did men (Telch, Lucas, & Nelson, 1989).

Etiology

Fodor (1974) suggests that (a) phobic symptoms, particularly those of agoraphobia, are associated with extreme helplessness and dependency and appear to be related to societal role expectations for women, (b) the feeling of being dominated in a relationship with no outlet for assertive behavior may further enhance the development of agoraphobia, and (c) the agoraphobic response is an extreme and exaggerated extension of the stereotypic feminine role. Phobias in women have been described as their "declaration of dependence." According to Miller (1973), phobic women use marriage to get themselves taken care of. Young women who were independent, self-sufficient, and capable somehow change after marriage and develop phobias to conform to societal role expectations for married women.

Biology provides another explanation, especially for panic attacks. Given intravenously, sodium lactate induced panic in 64% of patients (and 34% of controls) (Maser & Woods, 1990). Noradrenergic function may be abnormally regulated in patients with panic disorders. Neuropeptides such as corticotropin-releasing hormone may also be implicated. Probably biological events act in concert with psychological factors creating a neurobiopsychology basis for panic (Maser & Woods, 1990).

Assessment Techniques

Peplau (1963) produced the classic work on anxiety for nursing using an interpersonal theoretical model (Sullivan, 1953). Several validating studies have been completed on the nursing diagnosis of anxiety (Whitley, 1989) (see Table 15.1 for anxiety symptoms).

When a nursing diagnosis of anxiety has been made, the level must be evaluated. With mild or moderate degrees of anxiety, nurses can use the motivation triggered by anxiety to engage the client in talking through and problem solving to change her life situation.

An assessment for panic disorder with agoraphobia includes a comprehensive, multifaceted evaluation outlining an individual's strengths as well as difficulties and includes goal setting, intervention strategies, and treatment effects (Laraia, Stuart, & Best, 1989). Assessment of phobic avoidance includes three main fear response modalities: motor behavior, physiological processes, and thoughts.

Nursing Interventions With Anxiety

Using Peplau's theory (1963), a nurse would ask the woman to describe one situation in which she felt anxious, including what preceded the feelings. Focus next would center on what the client expected to happen and what happened instead. Anxiety occurs when one's needs or expectations are not met. After helping the client clarify which needs were not met, it is necessary to think of ways the client can express her needs more clearly to others or change the nature of her needs if they are unreasonable. For example, women may expect men to meet all of their needs. Not only is that unrealistic, but often men are not aware of what women need because women have not been able to express themselves—and when they do, men do not always understand them. As women get clearer about what they need from people, and as they experience some success in expressing their needs, anxiety can be prevented.

Anxiety management training has been developed to treat both specific and generalized anxiety, and its effectiveness has been demonstrated (Childs-Clarke, Whitfield, Cadbury, & Sandu, 1989). Assertiveness training (discussed in the section on depression) can also help to reduce anxiety.

To lower anxiety, Knowles (1981) recommends round breathing (with mouth closed, breathe in and out in such a fashion that there is no pause at the beginning or end of each respiration) and breath holding (take a very deep breath and hold it for the count of three, then as you slowly release this breath, say to yourself, "Relax").

Cognitive therapy is superior to behavioral therapy in the treatment of performance anxieties, such as giving a piano recital or taking an exam (Hickey & Baer, 1988). It is based on the maladaptive cognitions theory; that is, people (especially women) behave on the basis of misconceptions and unrealistic thought patterns (Beck & Greenberg, 1974). The therapist allies herself with the client against the symptoms. Laraia et al. (1989) describes self-statement training, which consists of three steps: (a) the identification of negative self-statements; (b) recognition of the role that negative self-statements play in influencing self-concept, behavior, and mood; and (c) replacing negative self-statements with positive self-statements that help the patient cope with high levels of anxiety (e.g., "Anxiety won't kill me").

Drug Treatment of Anxiety. The benzodiazepines have been the standard drugs used in the treatment of most anxiety disorders and are preferable to barbiturates or meprobamate in terms of safety (in case of overdose), abuse liability, and (probably) the risk of physical dependence (Cole, 1988). Usually, benzodiazepines are prescribed only for a few weeks and then withdrawn gradually to deter physical dependence. Their use in anxiety disorders is usually limited to an environmentally induced crisis. Four or five of the lowest dosage pills a week, however, probably will not lead to physical dependence (Cole, 1988). Early in treatment, women should be warned about the potentiation of the benzodiazepine by alcohol and should be cautioned against operating complex machinery, including automobiles.

Alprazolam is becoming increasingly popular for generalized anxiety disorder. Physical dependence is a major disadvantage. Beta-adrenergic blocking drugs such as propranolol decrease tremor and heart rate and are useful in women whose anxiety manifests itself in shakiness and palpitations. They are widely used for performance anxiety by musicians and actors and students about to take examinations (Cole, 1988). Sometimes clonidine is useful, but it is relatively sedative and tends to cause moderate anticholinergic side effects (Cole, 1988). Buspirone (Buspar) is a newer antianxiety drug that shares no common feature with the benzodiazepines or the hypnotics. It probably works through serotonergic or dopaminergic mechanisms. It does not appear to cause physical dependence.

Treatment of Panic Disorder

The combined use of pharmacological agents and psychotherapy is used to treat panic disorders. Medications are used to block panic attacks and calm the anticipatory anxiety, and psychotherapy is used to alleviate the underlying cause of anxiety and help the individual deal with the psychosocial effect of the disorder (Wood, 1990). Pharmacological agents used in treating panic disorders include benzodiazepines, tricyclic antidepressants, and MAO inhibitors. The different psychotherapeutic approaches that have been used include supportive psychotherapy, cognitive therapy, and behavioral therapy. Although controversy exists about the relative merits of medications and behavioral therapy, most therapists prefer to use some combination of both (Dilsance, 1989; Hickey & Baer, 1988; Wood, 1990).

In the treatment of panic disorder without agoraphobia, the use of a benzodiazepine, either alprazolam or clonazepam, and perhaps the concomitant use of either imipramine or phenelzine sulfate for the rapid control of anxiety symptoms is recommended (Wood, 1990). In addition, supportive psychotherapy or cognitive therapy is recommended. The best drug treatment for panic agoraphobia comprises antidepressants such as imipramine and phenelzine, or trazodone and alprazolam (Cole, 1988).

Psychological Treatment of Panic-Related Avoidance Behavior. Usually behavioral therapies are emphasized rather than purely supportive or cognitive approaches (Wood, 1990). The dominant treatment technique for agoraphobia and most other phobias is exposure therapy (Laraia et al., 1989). In vivo exposure therapy has the patient contact fear-eliciting stimuli in real-life situations. The rate of exposure to fearful stimuli can be gradual, starting on the least fearful end of a fear hierarchy and slowly working up, or it can be extremely rapid, by starting with the most feared situations (Laraia et al., 1989). The 1980 National Institute of Mental Health Conference on anxiety disorders concluded that exposure treatments produce the most consistent improvement in anxiety and phobic disorders (Hickey & Baer, 1988). Implosive therapy involves the presentation of highly anxiety-provoking imagery (individualized for each phobic patient) in as vivid a manner as possible. The therapist discourages the person from escaping the scene to avoid the stimuli.

Sometimes flooding is more effective with agoraphobia. Flooding involves prolonged exposure to the feared situation so that the client can "learn" that horrible imagined consequences do not come to pass (President's Commission on Mental Health, 1978b). Reinforced practice allows the client to make gradual repeated approaches toward the phobic situation with permission to turn back whenever the level of anxiety becomes too high (Laraia et al., 1989). Relaxation tapes may be used, and the therapist is very liberal with praise about the client's increasing autonomy. The client also may be asked to record phobic occurrences during the week, what was done to overcome fears, and what set them off (Fodor, 1974).

Group Therapy for Agoraphobia. One of the major functions of any therapeutic intervention for agoraphobia is exposure to the feared stimulus (Brehony, 1987). Group in vivo exposure has been an effective procedure that may enhance cost-effectiveness as well as provide additional therapeutic advantages over individual sessions. Structured groups showed greater symptomatic improvement and social cohesion and had fewer dropouts and relapses than did unstructured groups at 6-month follow-up (Brehony, 1987).

For many years, agoraphobia has been a closet disorder. Culturally disempowered people, especially agoraphobic women, have come to accept the notion that they exist as solitary freaks unable to cope with the world or even simple tasks in any normal, productive fashion. Group experiences with other women with similar problems demand a personal paradigm shift. It no longer becomes possible to believe that one is entirely alone when confronted by other people experiencing a similar phenomenon (Brehony, 1987). Insight or understanding is not enough in overcoming agoraphobia. Individuals must behaviorally confront the situations and feelings that terrify them. From a behavioral perspective, exposure to the feared situations causes "extinction" of the conditioned response. The group often evolves into several subgroups that are labeled "buddy systems" (Brehony, 1987). For example, one woman who could drive but could not eat out in a restaurant paired up with another woman who found restaurants to be no problem but could not drive. They recognized the need to confront the fears and organized strategies so that they could confront them together.

As a larger goal of empowerment, it is important that the agoraphobic woman learn that there are a number of things she can do to control panic attacks. Three panic management techniques are (a) diaphragmatic breathing—taking a deep breath, holding it to the count of five, and slowly exhaling; (b) staying in the present with what's happening now—anxiety is almost always a "what if" experience, and this is particularly true of agoraphobic panic (what if it gets worse and I embarrass myself); and (c) stopping negative thoughts (thought-stopping techniques were illustrated by one woman who pretended the thoughts came from somebody else whom she named "the old nag"; she would tell the old nag she wasn't listening anymore) (Brehony, 1987).

Obsessive-Compulsive Disorder (OCD)

Definition

The diagnostic criteria for OCD include obsessions—recurrent and persistent thoughts experienced as intrusive and inappropriate—and/or compulsions—repetitive, excessive behaviors that the person feels driven to perform and that are designed to prevent discomfort (APA, 1994).

Incidence

The ECA study identified OCD as the fourth most common diagnosis in women (Robins et al., 1984). In a survey of more than 5,000 high school students, researchers encountered 20 severe cases of OCD, or approximately 1 case for every 250 students. Estimating that for every child with OCD there are three adults, it is projected that there are four million cases of OCD in the United States (Rapoport, 1990).

Etiology

OCD has been identified by psychodynamic theory as a response to event-related anxiety or personal life experience. Neurobiological research in the 1980s, however, has identified the presence of neurological differences and the influence of brain chemistry abnormalities in contributing to the symptoms of OCD (Simoni, 1991). In addition, research has demonstrated the efficacy of selective reduction of serotonin levels in the restoration of normal function.

Treatment

Two very different types of treatment may be effective in dealing with OCD. Climipramine relieves obsessive-compulsive symptoms (Rapoport, 1989). Behavior therapy, which entails repeated exposure of women to the stimulus that sets off the ritualistic acts, is also effective. For example, if a patient has a compulsion that causes her to wash her hands 20 or 30 times a day, her hands may be deliberately dirtied, after which she is prevented from washing them. Although such treatment may sound cruel, it has proved to be effective in severe cases in which traditional forms of psychotherapy have failed. Behavior therapy is more effective in treating compulsions than in treating obsessions. Climipramine is effective in lessening both obsessions and compulsions.

In addition to climipramine, fluoxetine (Prozac), and fluvoxamine have been shown to have anti-OCD effects (Rapoport, 1989). At first glance, it may seem contradictory to claim simultaneously that OCD has a strong biological basis and that behavioral conditioning is effective in reversing it. But because the brain is both a biological organ and the recipient of sensory and psychological inputs, it is to be expected that strictly psychological causes can have biological effects (Rapoport, 1989).

Nursing Implications. Simoni (1991) suggests that, "teaching that presents the client with an understanding that physiological differences, rather than mismanaged emotions, contribute to the disorder will enable the client to accept OCD as an illness, rather than as evidence of personal failure. Support through nursing's caring presence in the client's daily activities, with a focus on the present, will facilitate cooperation in interventions aimed at reducing symptoms through medication or, at the least, increasing client ability to control them through behavior therapy" (p. 22).

Post-Traumatic Stress Disorder (PTSD)

Rape

Rape is a crime of violence, and violence causes symptoms of PTSD in women victims (Schrader, 1990). (See Chapter 18, "Violence Against Women," for further discussion of this subject.) The specific form of PTSD seen in rape victims is called the *rape trauma syndrome*. The essential feature of this disorder is the development of characteristics that follow an event outside the range of usual human experience, an event that would be markedly distressing to almost anyone. The three symptoms of rape trauma syndrome are (a) reexperiencing the traumatic event—recurrent and intrusive distressing recollections of the event, recurrent distressing dreams of the event, sudden acting or feeling as if the traumatic event were recurring, or intense psychological distress at exposure to events that symbolize the traumatic event; (b) persistent avoidance of stimuli associated with the trauma or numbing of general responsiveness—efforts to avoid thoughts or feelings associated with the trauma, efforts to avoid activities or situations that arouse recollections of the trauma, inability to recall an important aspect of the trauma, markedly diminished interest in significant activities, feelings of detachment or estrangement from others, restricted range of affect, or sense of a foreshortened future; and (c) persistent symptoms of increased arousal—difficulty falling or staying asleep, irritability or outbursts of anger, difficulty concentrating, hypervigilance, exaggerated startle response, or physiological reactivity on exposure to events that resemble an aspect of the traumatic event (APA, 1994).

Nursing Implications. Crisis intervention provides the model for initial intervention, which, in addition to addressing emotional and psychological issues, also may require interfacing with legal and medical systems. The long-term effects require a feminist model of psychotherapy that continues to address both societal and psychological issues related to the trauma.

Factors that aid rape recovery are positive self-esteem, a good support system, and an ability to use coping or defense mechanisms effectively. Factors that delay recovery include chronic life stresses, low self-esteem, style of attack (women who are attacked in their own home take longer to recover), victim's acquaintance with the assailant, interracial rape, multiple assailants, and subsequent victimization (Schrader, 1990).

Volunteers have been very effective in rape trauma syndrome because the victim is considered normal—one who was managing adequately in her life prior to the crisis. Telephone counseling programs are also an effective intervention tool (Burgess, 1985). The telephone is effective because it provides quick access to the victim, it places the burden on the counselor to seek out the victim rather than on the victim to seek help, it allows the victim considerable power in the situation, it encourages the victim to resume a normal lifestyle as quickly as possible, it is cost-effective, and it provides a way to discuss difficult issues other than face to face.

Because a significant proportion of women still do not report a rape, nurses should be alert to a syndrome called *silent rape trauma.* As a part of any assessment, ask, "Have you ever been pressured or forced to have sexual activity of any kind?" A diagnosis of silent reaction to rape trauma should be considered when a nurse observes any of the following symptoms during an evaluation interview: (a) increasing signs of anxiety as the interview progresses, such as long periods of silence, blocking of associations, minor stuttering, and physical distress; (b) patient reports of sudden marked irritability or actual avoidance of relationships with men, or marked change in patient sexual behavior; (c) a history of sudden onset of phobic reactions; and (d) persistent loss of self-confidence and self-esteem and attitude of self-blame.

Establishing an alliance with a rape victim is difficult but very important. The goal of the counseling interview is to discuss the victim's emotional reactions and her thoughts and feelings about what happened. This cannot happen without a trusting relationship. During the working phase, the therapist should try to get as complete a picture of the event and its aftermath as possible (Burgess, 1985). The assault must be described in terms of when and where was the victim approached? Who did it? Was he known to the victim? What kind of conversation occurred between the victim and assailant prior to the rape? Did the assailant try to charm her? Did he threaten her or make humiliating comments? What did she say to him?

The actual sexual details may be the most difficult for the victim to discuss. It is generally the topic the victim wishes to forget. However, the sexual details are apt to be the ones that will keep recurring in the victim's mind. Until the victim is able to talk about the details and is somewhat settled within herself when talking about the incident, the details will continue to haunt her and will influence her relationships with other men. It is important to ask about threats and violence. Did the assailant have a weapon? What type of violence was inflicted? It is important to find out how she feels about her struggle or lack thereof. At the time of a rape, many victims decide not to struggle in hopes of saving their lives. The therapist can confirm this universal strategy and help to alleviate guilt. What does the sexual assault mean to her? Was this a first sexual experience? What are her feelings about sex now? Has she been raped before?

A crucial factor in the treatment of sexual trauma is the nurse's own attitude toward the victim. If the nurse finds herself or himself judging the victim rather than trying to understand the situation the victim has experienced, all therapeutic leverage will be lost. Nurses have to come to grips with their own self-identity and prejudices regarding sexuality and violence if they are to be effective in treating a victim of sexual assault (Burgess, 1985).

McArthur (1990) writes about the effectiveness of using reality therapy in a group context with rape victims. Members have an opportunity to learn how others with similar experiences have been able to recover from similar problems. The peer support from members gives an individual a sense of hope. Rape has an effect on the sense of self, effecting a loss of self-esteem, creation of guilt and shame, mistrust in interpersonal relationships, and distorted perceptions of self-worth. Because of the massive injury to the self, rape victims may very quickly become isolated and lonely.

Reality therapy treats the sense of self by offering the victim opportunities to regain self-esteem and resolves guilt and shame by changing the point at which value judgments are made. When the victim develops a passive lifestyle because of chronic feelings of helplessness and powerlessness, the group confronts this in a warm, supportive manner. The group does not

Table 15.2 Functions Performed by Therapeutic Self-Help Groups

Providing hope. Because the members are at different stages, as women enter for their first session they hear success stories.

Requiring women to take responsibility for themselves. They are given a choice about joining the group after hearing what the group is about. They must request group time, if they want it, at each session.

Accepting/building on women's strengths/experiences. Women are encouraged to make attachments in the self-help model. Each woman's personal experience is supported. Intuition is encouraged and trusted.

Fostering interdependence. Women are joined to each other through their common background, issues, and womanhood. Through the simultaneous focus on differences and similarities, the women feel both separate and part of a whole. They develop a sense of interdependence. Participants learn there is strength in asking for help and in joining together.

Mobilizing anger. Given the group rules of no abuse in the group, members gradually feel free to be in touch with their own anger. Members are encouraged to express their anger within the group. They are guided in working out conflicts through assertive communication and problem solving.

Providing a healthy system. The group provides positive self-worth, open communication, clear rules, and a link to society. Women discover flexibility and consistency. The group rules provide limits, which in turn offer the members a sense of structure and protection. Limits are set in a nurturing rather than a punitive way.

Providing knowledge and skills. Women learn about the abuse cycle, how to make a protection plan, how to have healthy sexuality, and how to work with the legal system. They learn communication skills.

Being holistic. Women deal with all the issues that feed into and result from their life situation—finances, child care, housing.

Changing self-image from victim to survivor. The women are helped to see themselves as women in abusive relationships rather than as battered women.

allow excuses for acting out or isolative behavior. The responsibility for the victim's behavior is not with a family who does not understand or with her assailant. The opportunity for making a success of her life, for becoming a survivor instead of a victim, is hers. Members of a rape group form a common bond around their experience and realize that they are able to help others because they understand each other's problems. In helping others, they find a sense of purpose and belonging that restores their own self-esteem.

Victims of Interpersonal Violence

A battered woman is one who stays in a relationship after being repeatedly subjected to coerced, forceful physical, sexual, or psychological behavior. Battering also may include breaking property, severe verbal harassment and criticism, bizarre types of sexuality, and threats to harm other family members (Schrader, 1990).

Nursing Implications. It is critical that battered women learn about the phases in the battering cycle. Therapy is usually necessary. Domestic violence treatment programs, which may be court mandated, have been fairly successful (Rynerson & Fishel, 1993). No type of therapy can take place as long as the woman lives in fear of her partner and a power imbalance exists between them. The batterer must stop his battering. Initial treatment follows a crisis intervention model. Battered women often need to leave their homes and temporarily stay in a safe house or battered women's shelter that provides the initial safety that can allow healing to begin.

Hartman (1987) has found the therapeutic self-help model effective in working with women in abusive relationships. The therapeutic self-help group departs from the traditional group by its use of a professional and a group member as coleaders. The goal of the group is to empower members and foster change. The group acts in a healing manner by performing important functions (see Table 15.2).

Mood Disorders

Definitions

Major depression is a highly prevalent disorder that occurs in both adults and children, most of whom are untreated. For major depression to be diagnosed, at least five of the following symptoms must be present nearly every day: depressed mood, markedly diminished interest in all activities, significant weight loss or weight gain, insomnia or hypersomnia, psychomotor agitation or retardation, fatigue or loss of energy, feelings of worthlessness or inappropriate guilt, diminished ability to concentrate, and/or suicidal ideation with or without a suicidal plan (APA, 1994). The essential feature of bipolar disorders is the presence of one or more manic episodes, usually with a history of a major depression (APA, 1994). Dysthymia is characterized by a chronic mild depressive syndrome for more days than not for at least 2 years (in adolescents, mood can be irritable and duration must be at least 1 year) and that evidences at least two of the following: poor appetite or overeating, insomnia or hypersomnia, fatigue, low self-esteem, poor concentration or difficulty making decisions, and feelings of hopelessness (APA, 1994).

Seasonal pattern specifier for mood disorder (formerly, seasonal affective disorder or SAD) is differentiated by its cyclical seasonality and its atypical depressive symptoms. Current diagnostic criteria include (a) a regular temporal relationship between onset of the mood disturbance and a particular time of the year (e.g., fall or winter), not including cases of seasonality related to psychosocial stresses such as regular winter unemployment; (b) a full remission or change to hypomania/mania, also occurring within a particular time of the year (usually, spring); (c) two episodes in the past 2 years with seasonal relationship; and (d) seasonal episodes substantially outnumber nonseasonal episodes (APA, 1994).

The effects of pattern specifier for mood disorder can be debilitating in the winter, leaving the victim unable to carry out usual activities. Patients subsequently come alive in the spring. In the winter, patients lose their zeal for life, sleep longer but do not feel rested, consume more calories and gain weight, and lose their sex drive and their desire for social interaction (Rosenthal, 1989). Women are frequently unable to maintain a relationship during the winter, causing tension in marriage.

Incidence

In the United States, white, black, and Hispanic women are more than twice as likely as men to suffer from depression (McGrath, Keita, Strickland, & Russo, 1990; Weissman, 1987). This finding persists when income level, education, and occupation are controlled (McGrath et al., 1990). Gender differences in depression have also been reported in at least 10 other countries (McGrath et al., 1990) .

The U.S. Department of Health and Human Services (U.S. DHHS, 1988) reported that, compared with other American women, the death rate for Native American women is six times higher for alcoholism, three times higher for accidental death, three times higher for motor vehicle accidents, and two times higher for suicide—all of which may be associated with depression.

Women ages 18 to 44 have the highest rates of depression (Weissman, 1987). Epidemiological research to date is not definitive about the prevalence of depression among the elderly. Estimates of depression in older women range from less than 2% to more than 50% (McGrath et al., 1990). Several community-based studies indicate that the rates of depression for older men and women are approximately the same (Lewinsohn, Fenn, Stanton, & Franklin, 1986; Smallegan, 1989).

Using ECA data, Weissman (1987) found that in unhappy marriages, women were three times as likely as men to be depressed, and almost half of all women in unhappy marriages were depressed. In happy marriages, the incidence of depression was much lower, but women were almost five times as likely as men in such marriages to experience depression. Tennant, Bebbington, and Hurry (1982) reported that women with children less than 15 years of age had significantly higher rates of psychiatric disorder. However, having children was associated with less psychiatric disorder in men.

Major depression affects approximately 4.5% of women and less than 2% of men (6-month prevalence rate) for a ratio of 2 or 3 to 1. Rates are increasing most rapidly among young adults. Persons at risk for major depression include those who are female, young (born after World War II), separated, divorced or in an unhappy marriage, and who have a family history of major depression (Weissman, 1987).

Dysthmia affects approximately 3% of the adult population and is most common in women under the age of 65, unmarried persons, and young persons with low income. In Weissman's 1988 study, the ratio of women with dysthymia to men ranged from 1.5:1 in the New Haven catchment area to 3:1 in the Durham area. The difference between the rates of lifetime dysthymia for men and for women was greatest in the group that was 45 to 64 years old. There was no association between dysthymia and race, education, or full-time employment.

Bipolar disorder occurs about equally in men and women and has a prevalence in the population of about 0.7% (Taube & Barrett, 1985). Although not very prevalent in society, bipolar disorders are the most serious and socially disruptive forms of depression, carrying a significant risk of death by suicide.

Studies indicate that 5.4% of the population could be labeled as having SAD and 7.6% as having subsyndromal disorder (Rosen et al., 1989). Women are affected four times more often than men (Jacobsen, Wehr, Sack, James, & Rosenthal, 1987). These clients come from all ethnic groups, races, and occupations. In a convenience survey of 65 undergraduate nursing students, using the Seasonal Pattern Assessment Questionnaire, 28% could be classified as having seasonal pattern mood disorder; another 38% scored within subsyndromal levels (Lefler, 1991). These percentages are higher than normed data. Nurses are at a particular risk because of the large number of women in the nursing profession.

Influencing Factors

Age

Major causes for depression in older women are the loss of physical health, the loss of a spouse from death or divorce (McGrath et al., 1990), and financial problems (Fopma-Loy, 1988). In a yearlong study, Bornstein, Clayton, Halikas, Maurice, and Robins (1973) found that 35% of recent widows met the criteria for depression at 1 month and at 4 months after the loss of the spouse, and 17% at 1 year. Factors related to depression in older women may include increasing poverty, isolation as adult children move away and friends and family die, changes in biochemistry as aging occurs, role changes with retirement, and moving to new locations (McGrath et al., 1990). The effects of retirement on women are inadequately researched, but the postretirement period may be a time of major upheaval for them (Formanek, 1987). Certain aspects of socialization may aid older women in resisting depression. Women with close relationships to family and friends may find those supports will prevent depression when they are 65 and over.

Ethnicity

Black women face a number of mental-health-related issues based on their experience with racism and on the historical, cultural, and structural position of black people in American society (McGrath et al., 1990). Although statistics are not readily available for Hispanics/Latinas, Hernandez (McGrath et al., 1990) theorized that traditional cultural male-female role expectations, such as women being passive, manipulated and seduced by men, and obligated to men, may predispose these women to depression. Asian Americans, although a culturally diverse group, must contend with racial and ethnic discrimination. Loo and Ong (1982) reported that Asian American women had lower self-esteem than did Asian American men. Snipp (1990) notes that Native American women are among the least visible and least researched sectors in the U.S. society. Native American women are at risk for many factors associated with depression, including poverty, lack of education, and large numbers of children.

Reproductive-Related Risk Factors

Events related to reproduction—including menstruation, pregnancy, childbirth, infertility, and abortion—are unique experiences for women and have been hypothesized to be related to women's depression, although these events alone do not explain the overall gender difference in depression rates (McGrath et al., 1990).

Between 50% and 80% of women experience "baby blues"—a period of sadness and uncontrollable crying after the birth of a baby. In a study by Freeman, O'Neil, and Lance (McGrath et al., 1990), of 200 infertile couples seeking assistance at a fertility clinic, 40% reported that infertility was the most upsetting experience of their lives.

Abortion does not appear to be a significant risk factor for depression; the predominant response is relief (McGrath et al., 1990). McGrath et al. (1990) note a number of studies reporting that feelings of depression, regret, and guilt may be experienced after an abortion, but they are typically mild and transitory and do not affect general functioning. For the 1% to 2% of women who had serious psychiatric responses following abortion, they typically had a previous psychiatric history and/or felt pressured to have an abortion (against own judgment or religious beliefs) (McGrath et al., 1990).

Personality Traits

Low self-esteem is clearly an important factor in depression. Theoretical explanations for the role of low self-esteem in depression vary. It may be that the reality of women's socialized dependence on others and the external expectations that women respond to the needs of others (with concomitant rewards and punishments) are the key factors in understanding the association between women's relationships and depression (McGrath et al., 1990). Alternatively, more than 200 published studies have examined the role of "explanatory" style in depression, which suggests that people who typically explain negative events as being caused by unchanging, global (or vague), and internal factors have more depression. If women receive more "learned helplessness training" than do men, they may be more likely to develop pessimistic explanatory styles.

Ross and Mirowsky (1989) reported that persons who feel in control of their lives are more likely to attempt to solve problems. Perceived control and ability to solve problems decrease depression. Lerner (1987) hypothesizes that depression is one form of emotional reactivity associated with the loss that occurs when women betray or sacrifice the self in order to preserve relationship harmony. In attempting to navigate the delicate balance between the "I" and "we," women frequently sacrifice the "I" in the service of "togetherness," thus assuming a selfless position in relationships. Jack (1991) linked the silencing of the self to women's subsequent depressions, proposing that socialization as a "good woman" precluded expression of oneself, producing a silent, compliant outer self with an inner angry self.

Nolan-Hoeksema (McGrath et al., 1990) proposed a response style theory to explain gender differences in depression. She suggested that in response to dysphoria (sense of disquiet or restlessness), men engage in physical activities (i.e., have an active response set) to distract them from their mood. Women, in contrast, are less active and ruminate about the causes of their mood. A ruminative response set, as compared with an active response set, may amplify depressive episodes.

Women's Roles

Higher levels of distress among women may be partially a function of their nurturant roles (Turner & Avison, 1989). Gender-role-related differences in exposure and/or responsiveness to events occurring to network members are hypothesized to represent a "cost of caring" for women that translates into elevated levels of depression. Turner and Avison (1989) reported that men and women are equally exposed and equally vulnerable to life events occurring to themselves. However, women were found to be both more aware of and more responsive to events occurring to others. The women studied were more responsive to the negative experiences of others, and this differential responsiveness has significant mental health implications. Women were also found to be at least as capable as men of adjusting to, or resolving, negative personal experiences (Turner & Avison, 1989).

Intimate Relationships

Much of the earlier research on marital status and mental health was reported by Gove (1972) and Nathanson (1975). Gove examined data on mortality, suicide, and mental illness, by marital status and sex, and found that married women generally had noticeably higher rates of mental illness than did married men. He concluded that marriage had a protective effect on men but was detrimental for women because it restricted role possibilities, and housekeeping was a low-prestige activity. Jessie Bernard (1973) reached the same conclusion. Tennant et al. (1982) also reported that within marriage, need for a close and confiding or intimate relationship may affect men and women differently. For women, low intimacy bore a significant relationship to psychiatric disorder but did not do so in men.

Cartwright (1989) found that among a community sample of women undergoing marital separation/divorce, more of the traditional women appeared to be clinically depressed. Early results suggested that nondepressed men and women were strongly identified as assuming the roles of both genders.

Societal homophobia and discrimination pose additional stresses for gay women (Fishel, 1983). Lesbians are 2.5 times more likely to report an attempted suicide sometime in the past than are heterosexual women (McGrath et al., 1990).

Children

Whether homemakers or employed wives, women with young children experience high levels of stress (Gove & Geeken, 1977; McBride, 1988; Nathanson, 1975; Thoits, 1983). In striking contrast to the traditional belief that women require marriage and children for psychological fulfillment, the child-raising period is equated with less life satisfaction, more stress, and more overt mental illness than other periods (Seiden, 1976).

The divorce rate in the United States is the world's highest, and children are spending increasing amounts of time with an overburdened single parent. Although the divorce rate has been steadily dropping since 1980 (U.S. DHHS, 1990), more women are having children outside of marriage. The economic and psychological stresses inherent in raising a child without a live-in partner are great (Fishel, 1986). Today, one family in six is headed by a single mother (Naisbitt & Aburdene, 1990). Tennant et al. (1982) hypothesized that the presence of young children was not directly associated with disorder; rather its effects are mediated through nonemployment. Having young children may keep married women from being employed or make employment more stressful.

Employment

Of any variable investigated, employment has perhaps the most significant bearing on women's health (Nathanson, 1975; Stevens, 1978; Tennant et al., 1982; Turner & Avison 1989). (See Chapter 1, "Women and Their Health.") Married women who are employed typically face much greater time and energy demands than do their unemployed counterparts, but an overload of tasks is not the primary cause of poorer mental health among women. Instead, it is the type of tasks associated with the home and with children that produce the feeling of incessant demands. Turner and Avison (1989) report that employed women tend to be less depressed than do unemployed women, despite the increased burden of depression-relevant stress associated with employment. This finding suggests that overall, the paid worker role must have especially powerful benefits for women.

It is clear that work is an additional source of satisfaction and self-esteem for most women. However, type of employment has specific consequences for women's mental health. Professional women have a higher incidence of depression and suicide than do women in the general population (McGrath et al., 1990). In contrast, Meleis, Norbeck, Laffrey, Solomon, and Miller (1989) reported that the most stressful work situations are unskilled blue-collar and clerical work. At the top of their list of stresses were overload, symptoms such as eye strain and headaches, problems with work space, strained office relationships, and frequent interruptions.

Victimization

Victimization in interpersonal relationships is a significant risk factor in the development of depressive symptomatology in women (McGrath et al., 1990). Carmen, Reiker, and Mills (1984) conducted a chart review of 188 male and female psychiatric inpatients and found that histories of interpersonal victimization were mentioned in the charts of 80 (43%) of the patients. Of those 80, 65 were female. Head injuries from battering could lead to neurological damage, which in turn could lead to persistent depression or other changes in cognition, motivation, and behavior that mirror the symptoms of depression. In a study of 60 battered women, Hilberman and Munson (1977-1978) found that depressive illness was the most frequent diagnostic category. In a series of structured interviews with adult survivors of incest and rape, Roth and Leibowitz (1988) found that the most recurrent themes in these women's self descriptions—helplessness, rage, and self-blame—suggest high rates of depression in that group.

Income

High levels of depressive symptoms are particularly common among individuals with economic problems (McGrath et al., 1990). A longitudinal study that assessed depressive symptoms in the community found that inadequate income was associated with more depressive symptoms (Kaplan, Roberts, Camacho, & Coyne, 1987). Even though the ECA study did not find significant socioeconomic correlates of major depression (Weissman, 1987), dysthymia was more prevalent among young persons with low income (Weissman, Leaf, Bruce, & Florio, 1988).

Table 15.3 Theories of Depression

Psychological models focus on negative thinking or devaluation of oneself, the role of helplessness and negative expectations, loss of self-esteem derived from a sense of helplessness or lack of control in attaining one's desires, object loss derived from separation or disruption of an attachment, and aggressive impulses turned against the self (McGrath et al., 1990).
Behavioral theorists focus on the acquisition of depression-related behaviors such as competence and learned helplessness.
Sociological theorists focus on role deprivation and conflict, as well as lack of control over one's outcomes.
Existential theory focuses on a loss of meaning and purpose to one's existence.
Biological theorists believe the roots of depression to be found in a genetically vulnerable nervous system, depletion of biogenic amines, and hyperarousal.

Demographic Trends

Demographic trends that are placing women at higher risk for depression are increasing numbers of separated, divorced, and widowed women; rising numbers of single parents; the increasing number of people in lower socioeconomic groups; declining employment opportunities in face of increasing demand; and widening differences in income level between women and men (Franks & Rothblum, 1983). There are, however, demographic trends that may have a protective effect. For example, the number of never-married women is increasing, women are marrying later and postponing children and therefore will have fewer children, and more women are working outside the home.

Theories of Etiology of Depression

The dominant theories of depression are psychological, behavioral, sociological, existential, and biological (see Table 15.3). Most researchers and clinicians consider depression to be a complex interaction of many factors (McBride, 1990b; McGrath et al., 1990).

Simmons-Alling (1990) reports that, on average, about one quarter of the first-degree relatives of bipolar patients will have bipolar illness at some point in their lives. The risk to offspring of one parent with affective illness is 27%. However, this risk increases to 75% if both parents have some form of affective disorder. The data suggest that there are genetic and nongenetic forms of depression. Simmons-Alling advises that genetic counseling by responsible clinicians should provide the most direct application of the biological psychiatric findings for the patient and his or her family.

Although genetic and biochemical factors are related to depression (and particularly bipolar mood disorder), the preponderance of major depression and dysthymia in women suggests that psychosocial factors are also significant. Weissman (1987) delineated three of these psychosocial factors as social status, learned helplessness, and marriage. As victims of legal and economic discrimination, women are not able to take care of themselves; they have to depend on men. This dependency on others leads to low self-esteem and depression.

Assessment of Depression

Standardized Tests

The MMPI-Depression Scale is perhaps the best known self-report measure of depression (Hickey & Baer, 1988). It is also used as an outcome measure in the evaluation of treatments of depressive disorders. The most widely used self-report measurement designed explicitly for depression is the Beck Depression Inventory (Beck, 1978). The 21-item scale can be completed and scored quickly and easily, with or without the aid of an interviewer. A similar approach is taken in the Zung Self-Rating Depression Scale (Zung, 1965). The Center for Epidemiological Studies Depression Scale is a self-report scale with 20 items selected from previously validated scales (Radloff, 1977). Its advantages include simple, clear language and the availability of general population norms. The recently developed Inventory to Diagnose Depression, a 22-item self-report scale, is also intended for epidemiological application. It may gain clinical acceptance because of its superior

Table 15.4 Decision-Making Tree for Suicidal Assessment

Nurse: "Are you thinking about Suicide?"

Patient: "Yes."

Nurse assesses suicidal risk (motivation, plan, availability of means, and time frame).

If the patient is at immediate risk, a family member, friend, responsible adult, or health care provider takes the client to an appropriate mental health professional or an emergency resource.

If the person is deemed to be at moderate risk, the nurse generalist can make an appointment with a mental health professional, use a no-suicide contract, give community resource information, identify sources of support, identify reasons not to take self-destructive action, and educate the client.

SOURCE: Adapted from Badger, Cardea, Biocca, and Mishel (1990).

coverage of the DSM-III-R diagnostic criteria. The Hamilton Rating Scale for Depression (Hamilton, 1960) has frequently been used as a measure of severity once depression has been identified. It must be completed by a trained rater or professional, and the interview may require 30 minutes.

Gender Role Assessment

A gender role analysis is an important part of assessment. One should ask, "Which of these symptoms are primarily exaggerations of this woman's feminine gender role? Has this woman had experiences of interpersonal victimization? Are role strains and poverty contributing to her distress? Is she overwhelmed by parenting responsibilities?"

Suicidal Assessment

An ability to assess whether a client is experiencing mild depressive symptoms or a more severe major depression is essential. The generalist-prepared nurse should be held accountable in providing care for mildly depressed women, but a mental health specialist (nursing or other) and/or hospitalization may be necessary for the seriously depressed client. Knowing when to refer depressed clients to mental health professionals is critical in nursing judgment. Severe depression is usually recognized by the "vegetative signs" and by suicidal ideation and/or plan. The vegetative signs include (a) an unexplained weight loss or gain of more than 5% of body weight in one month, (b) the person's inability to handle the activities of daily living, and (c) insomnia (she is unable to sleep more than 3 to 4 hours a night for a week) or hypersomnia (she naps whenever possible in addition to 8 to 10 hours sleep nightly). Severely depressed people may also evidence delusional thinking and/or difficulty concentrating.

Suicidal thoughts or attempts are one of the most serious symptoms of depression and require immediate assessment and intervention. Hospitalization may be indicated to provide a safe environment for the woman. All depressed clients are potentially suicidal and deserve the nurse's attention. A decision-making tree for assessment of suicide risk is a helpful tool (Badger, Cardea, Biocca, & Mishel, 1990) (see Table 15.4).

There are four criteria to measure in assessing the seriousness of a suicidal plan: method, availability, specificity, and lethality (Hatton & Valente, 1984). Has the client specified a method? Is the method of choice available to the attempter? How specific is the plan? If the method is concrete and detailed, with access to it right at hand, the suicide risk increases. How lethal is the method? The most lethal method is shooting, with hanging a close second. The least lethal is slashing one's wrists. Although women formerly relied on pills (lethality dependent on type and amount), they are increasingly more apt to use highly lethal methods.

Some characteristics place people at high risk for suicide. These include multiple high-lethality suicide attempts, rampant hostility toward self or others, alcohol abuse, isolation ("No one cares"), and disorientation (Hatton & Valente, 1984). The more resources available to the client, the more likely that the crisis can be managed. Even with these guidelines, the nurse is often in a position of trying to predict what the combination of signs says about the actual suicide risk now and in the future. She has to make a decision about whether to work with the woman herself, use family and community resources, refer for mental health counseling, or hospitalize the woman immediately. Clinical nurse specialists are frequently faced with such decisions.

Treatment of Depression

Psychotherapy, phototherapy, pharmacotherapy, and electroconvulsive therapy are used, singly or in combination, in treatment of various depressions. The choice of treatment depends on the nature and severity of the depressive symptoms. Psychotherapeutic approaches include a range of psychodynamic, psychoanalytic, behavioral, supportive, cognitive, feminist, family, and group therapies.

Self-Help Strategies to Alleviate Depression

Regular exercise appears to be particularly helpful for depression (Simons, Epstein, McGowan, & Kupfer, 1988). In fact, some claim it is more effective than psychotherapy or medication. In a study by Weiss and Jamieson (1989), nearly one fourth of the women participants of a water exercise program reported feeling depressed at the time of enrollment. All the depressed women reported improvement after 8 weeks or more in the program. For many of the depressed women, the exercise program also provided a support group.

Full-time mothers are particularly vulnerable. DeRosis and Pellegrino (1976) give several suggestions: Arrange at least half a day or evening each week for yourself, maintain at least one personal interest, plan one evening a month to be out alone with your significant other, get information on free or low-cost entertainment (especially the type offering free child care), deepen friendships with other women, and remember that vacations are for mothers as well.

Self-help groups appear to be particularly helpful for persons experiencing grief reactions, such as to divorce, becoming widowed, or being parents of babies who were victims of the sudden infant death syndrome. Other self-help groups for widows have stressed coping skills, such as auto mechanics, how to travel alone, how to manage as a single parent, how to do taxes, and how to get a job, in addition to providing support for loneliness—the major identified problem among widows (Miles & Hays, 1975). (See additional discussion of this topic on page 101.)

Drug Treatment of Depression

An in-depth discussion of drug therapy for depression is beyond the scope of this chapter. General information is presented here; the reader is referred to research by Harris (1988, 1989) and current pharmacology and psychiatric texts.

Antidepressant drugs fall into three major categories: the tricyclics, the atypical antidepressants, and the monoamine oxidase inhibitors (MAOIs). There is no clear, rational, and useful basis for choosing one specific medication over the other in a drug-free depressed patient meeting DSM-IV-R criteria for major depressive disorder (Cole, 1988). Given the risk of hypertensive crisis with MAOIs, it seems sensible to treat a patient initially with a tricyclic antidepressant. If this initial tricyclic antidepressant is poorly tolerated (as it is in about 25% of all patients), another tricyclic with a different pattern of side effects can be tried. Atypical antidepressants such as trazodone (Desyrel), fluoxetine (Prozac), or bupropion (Wellbutrin) sometimes produce a good response in patients who have failed on a tricyclic (Cole, 1988). Atypical antidepressants have distinct side effects (Harris, 1988); the recent alarm about Prozac causing intense suicidal thoughts necessitates educating the clients about this and monitoring them very closely.

If the patient has responded well to a specific antidepressant in the past, that should be the initial medication (Harris, 1988). Because antidepressant response seems to run in families, it can be helpful to find out if a close family member has had any experience with antidepressants.

The patient usually is begun on a low or modest dose of a tricyclic antidepressant; gradually the dosage is increased until undesirable side effects appear or until clinical improvement (Cole, 1988). Orthostatic hypotension usually can be avoided if the dosage is increased slowly. If no improvement is noted in 4 to 6 weeks, the nurse should check the patient's blood level of the drug (Harris, 1988). The client may be metabolizing the drug too rapidly or absorbing it poorly. If so, the dosage can be increased, or another antidepressant drug may be tried. (Whenever there is a change from MAOI drugs to tricyclic drugs, at least 2 weeks should elapse before beginning tricyclics.) In unusual situations, both MAOI and tricyclic drugs are given simultaneously, but very close monitoring is

Table 15.5 Foods Containing Tyramine

Matured cheeses	Pizza
Sour cream	Beef and chicken liver
Bologna and pepperoni	Pickled herring
Italian green beans	Canned figs, raisins, bananas
Snow pea pods	Avocado
Ice cream	Chocolate
Soy sauce	Brewer's yeast
Meats prepared with tenderizers	
Sherry, Chianti wine, beer, vermouth	
Salad dressings containing cheese or monosodium glutamate	

necessary. An adjuvant such as lithium or triiodothyronine may be added (Cole, 1988).

Most tricyclic antidepressants are given at bedtime because they tend to have a sedative effect. Alternately, desipramine and protriptyline are generally less sedative drugs and therefore are better administered during the daytime (Cole, 1988). When higher dosages are being administered, an electrocardiogram is usually obtained to ensure that the drug is not interfering with cardiac conduction.

Other common side effects of tricyclic and other non-MAOI antidepressants include weight gain, tremors, grand mal seizures, nightmares, agitation or mania, and extrapyramidal side effects (Harris, 1988). Anticholinergic side effects include dry mouth, blurred vision (usually temporary), difficulty voiding, constipation, sweating, erection/orgasm difficulty, precipitation of glaucoma, and anticholinergic delirium.

Weight gain is a common complaint of patients on tricyclic antidepressants and the MAOIs; amitriptyline and doxepin are most likely to cause weight gain and many women thus refuse to take them. The atypical antidepressants such as trazadone do not cause weight gain, and fluoxetine can produce weight loss (Harris, 1988). Additional information about management of these side effects, as well as usual daily dosages and interactions with other medications, is covered in Harris's (1988) article.

Hypertensive crisis is the main reason that MAOIs are not prescribed more frequently. The patient should be taught to watch for signs of hypertensive crisis—throbbing occipital headache, stiff neck, chills, nausea, flushing, retroorbital pain, apprehension, pallor, sweating, chest pain, and palpitations (Harris, 1988). This crisis is brought on by the patient eating foods that contain tyramine, a sympathomimetic pressor amine, which normally is broken down by the enzyme, monoamine oxidase. Because antidepressant drugs inhibit monoamine oxidase, patients who take MAOIs without limiting their intake of tyramine can rapidly develop hypertensive crisis (Jackson & Haynes-Johnson, 1988). Tyramine restriction begins the day the patient takes her first dose and continues for 2 weeks after her last dose. Usually the nurse gives the patient a complete list of the foods to avoid as well as emphasizing why they should not be eaten (see Table 15.5). Beverages containing caffeine should be used only in small amounts.

Another drug, lithium, stabilizes mood and is the treatment of choice for bipolar disorder. It has a success rate of 70% to 80% (Harris, 1989). Lithium has a narrow therapeutic window; a slightly low blood level may cause relapse, and a slightly high level may cause an uncomfortable bout of toxicity. An even higher level can be life threatening. When initiating lithium treatment, blood levels are checked every 3 to 5 days. The therapeutic level is 0.8 to 1.2 mEq/L. Once stabilized, blood lithium levels should be checked at least every 3 months, and the therapeutic level can be achieved with serum levels between 0.6 and 0.8 mEq/L. Renal and thyroid functions should be checked at least once or twice a year (Harris, 1989).

Patient education is of utmost importance to ensure medication compliance in the use of lithium (Tirrell & DeForest, 1987). Nurses should inform the patient and family of symptoms of lithium toxicity. Treatment with thiazide diuretics and low-salt diets can reduce the urine output and cause toxic reactions; thus adequate hydration of at least one liter of fluid per day is necessary to maintain sodium and fluid balance. Alcohol intake is discouraged among lithium users. For patients who cannot tolerate lithium, carbamazepine may be used. (See Table 15.6.)

In long-term treatment with antidepressants or lithium, nutritional management is a concern

Table 15.6 Lithium Side Effects and Toxic Effects

Side effects	polyuria, weight gain, fine hand tremor. Memory and cognitive disturbances may interfere with daily functioning. Gastrointestinal side effects may be minimized by taking lithium with meals. Edema is a frequent side effect and probably is caused by lithium's role in stimulating sodium retention in the body (Jackson & Haynes-Johnson, 1988).
Early signs of toxicity	increased output of dilute urine and persistent thirst (Tirrell & DeForest, 1987).
Toxicity	coarse tremors, drowsiness, confusion, diarrhea, vomiting, and ataxia.
Major long-term risks of lithium therapy	hypothyroidism and impairment of the kidneys' ability to concentrate urine. These and other side effects are usually reversible or treatable (Harris, 1989).

of nursing. With patients taking lithium, polydipsia and polyuria are often indirectly responsible for weight gain. To satisfy the need to drink large amounts of fluids, patients may choose sweet drinks (Jackson & Haynes-Johnson, 1988). To minimize weight gain, however, patients should be instructed to drink water or sugar-free drinks instead of sweetened drinks. Fluid intake should be adequate at about 2,500 to 3,000 ml per day, and the patient should be advised of the importance of a normal diet. Light exercise is also an important part of maintaining weight control. Lithium is secreted into the maternal milk and produces severe abnormalities in the hearts of nursing infants, thus lithium is contraindicated not only in pregnancy but also during breastfeeding (Jackson & Haynes-Johnson, 1988).

Another nursing concern for patients on antidepressants is constipation. Constipation can be corrected in most cases by use of a bulking agent such as Dulcolax. Consumption of foods high in fiber (such as Fiber One cereal), increased water intake (about 10 glasses per day), and increased exercise are useful measures to alleviate constipation. Reducing the amount of sweets ingested and substituting no- or low-calorie drinks is usually necessary to help contain weight gain. Dry mouth can be managed by chewing sugar-free gum and sucking on sugar-free candy (Jackson & Haynes-Johnson, 1988).

Psychological Approaches

Female therapists working with women are more likely to achieve therapist-client empathy because they incorporate into their therapeutic role some sense of their core self as a relational being and some internalized experience of being in a subordinate position (McGrath et al., 1990). Existing outcome research does not yet answer the question of whether there is an optimal treatment for women's depression. Clinical practice suggests that cognitive-behavioral therapy (CBT), social skills training, and self-management programs may be effective for depressed women because of their focus on action, mastery, and distraction from depressed rumination (McGrath et al., 1990). Interpersonal therapy (IPT) may be especially helpful for women because it focuses on issues currently viewed as central to the psychology of women—that is, that relationships are the core of a woman's self-esteem. For women, more so than for men, social isolation, relationship loss, and dysfunctional family relationships may precipitate, contribute to, or prolong depression (McGrath et al., 1990). Drugs and psychotherapy are frequently combined in the treatment of depression.

Interpersonal Therapy. IPT is a brief treatment designed to reduce symptoms and improve social functioning in depressed patients (McGrath et al., 1990). The focus is on current interpersonal problems that are secondary to unresolved grief, difficult role transitions, interpersonal role disputes, and social skill deficits (Karasu, 1990). Nurses will recognize this approach as the basis for relationship therapy formulated by Peplau (Field, 1985b) and based on Sullivan's (1953) interpersonal theories. IPT is intense and uses the relationship between the client and therapist as a variable. There is no analysis of transference (patient's unconscious feelings about the therapist, which are triggered by earlier relationships with significant others), and no attention is paid to early life factors that might have been precursors to the current depressed state of the client. The focus is on relationships in the "here and now" and on facilitating the client to develop more effective ways of relating. The goal is not insight but symptomatic relief—relief that may be used in conjunction with antidepressant medication (McGrath et al., 1990).

Often, the client is instructed to read recommended literature written in lay language (Karasu, 1990).

Results from the National Institute of Mental Health Collaborative Study of the Treatment of Depression indicated that 57% to 69% of patients who completed a 16-week course of IPT were symptom free. Treatment effectiveness of IPT did not differ from results obtained with imipramine therapy or CBT, however (Karasu, 1990).

Cognitive Therapy. Cognitive therapy is often helpful with depressed women and can be practiced by generalist-prepared nurses. Cognitive therapy is standardized and brief (15 to 20 sessions) and is characterized by highly specific learning experiences; each session consists of a review of reactions to and results of the previous session, planning specific tasks, and assignment of homework (Karasu, 1990). The therapist is continually active and deliberately interacting with the woman. The therapy is based on the maladaptive cognitions theory that people (especially women) behave on the basis of misconceptions and unrealistic thought patterns. The therapist allies herself with the client against the depressive symptoms that afflict the client. Beck and Greenberg (1974) note three approaches, described below.

The nurse helps the client learn to recognize idiosyncratic thoughts, and this process may help regulate the depression. The client must learn to distance herself emotionally from her thoughts (that is, to view them objectively) with the critical perspective that will enable her to judge whether the thoughts are realistic or justified. A homemaker who sought help because of global feelings of depression, apathy, and inertia was instructed to pay close attention to her thoughts from the time she woke in the morning and throughout the day. After a day or so, she realized that when she began her household chores she would think, "I'm an incompetent housekeeper; I'll never be able to get this done." This is an example of reacting to a single, isolated failure by overgeneralization. The homemaker in the example was directed to look objectively at what she was a failure at (she did not wash her husband's favorite shirt by the time he wanted it); she came to recognize that one mistake did not constitute total failure. Another woman assumed that her friends no longer cared about her because no one telephoned for a day or two. She was helped to weigh the evidence on which her spontaneous conclusions were based and to consider alternative explanations. Actually, of her two best friends, Mary was sick and Joan was out of town. Another client was overly absorbed in the negative aspect of her life. When she was required to write down and report back positive experiences, she recognized her selective attention to the negative (Beck & Greenberg, 1974).

The nurse calls attention to the client's stereotyped themes that influence thinking. The automatic thoughts that constitute the woman's immediate reaction to an event may be a cognitive shorthand for elaborate ideas deeply rooted in past experiences that are no longer relevant. A woman who reported that she made a "fool of herself" in a job interview recognized that this assessment reflected not her actual performance but her tendency to see herself as a subject of humiliation. In reviewing her actual behavior, the nurse was able to shed doubt on the client's perception. In continuing to evaluate new experiences, the woman not only got a more realistic perspective of herself but also learned new skills to cope with confirmed areas of difficulty (Beck & Greenberg, 1974).

The nurse observes that the client holds misconceptions, prejudices, and even superstitions that need to be exposed and evaluated. One female university faculty member experienced intense depression when her promotion to full professor was denied. She was helped to see that she held a set of interlocking premises, such as "If I don't become a full professor, my work and life are meaningless." The faculty member was helped to discover other areas of her academic role and was reminded of the family and friends who were rich sources of gratification. Subjecting her basic premises to a process of validation helped her to stop worrying about recognition and to get more enjoyment out of her work. Meanwhile, she looked at the criteria for promotion and readjusted her priorities to do more publishing. Sometimes, idiosyncratic cognitions take a pictorial rather than a verbal form. A woman who felt depressed following a dinner party told the nurse that she had a spontaneous fantasy during the evening on which her husband left the party with another woman. This woman felt inferior and believed her husband would leave her. With help, she was able to recognize that she was, in fact, unusually accomplished and attractive, and her husband was exceptionally devoted; with this recognition, her depression lifted. Clients can also learn to substitute pleasant fantasies for unpleasant ones. One woman who was depressed because her child required a minor operation was somewhat relieved when she pictured him in a year, playful and happy and without disability (Beck & Greenberg, 1974).

Behavioral Therapy. Behavioral therapy treatments of depression encompass a broad spectrum of strategies and techniques derived from behavioral principles (McGrath et al., 1990). Some of the treatments include training in social skills, assertiveness, relaxation, and increasing the number of pleasant activities in one's life. Graded task assignments also may be used. A depressed homemaker, for instance, may be given a series of tasks starting with simple jobs at which she has a good chance of succeeding and progressing to more complicated tasks. At first, she may be asked only to make beds. In several days she also can cook breakfast. When she has clearly succeeded at a task, however simple, her lethargy decreases and she is motivated to try more.

When a woman's failure to act assertively makes her feel powerless and subsequently depressed, assertion training can be a useful treatment for the depression. Women who know they can handle a situation feel in control of themselves (less helpless); therefore, assertion training can prevent depression. The effectiveness of assertiveness training was researched in the 1970s and has been well documented (Butler, 1976; Galassi & Galassi, 1978; Jakubowski, 1977; Percell, Bermick, & Beigel, 1974; Tregeman & Kassinone, 1977). Assertiveness training is a behavior therapy procedure (Wolpe, 1958) aimed at reducing maladaptive anxiety that prevents a person from expressing herself directly, honestly, and spontaneously. The training involves replacing irrational belief systems with belief systems that support individual rights, the internalization of truthful statements, and the practice of assertive responses.

Models for assertiveness training are described in the literature (Alberti & Emmons, 1974; Bloom, Coburn, & Pearlman, 1975; Galassi & Galassi, 1977). Many schools of nursing offer assertiveness training courses through their continuing education programs. Every nurse should have beginning familiarity with this intervention strategy, for its applicability in professional practice and in working with clients.

Fishel and Jefferson (1983) did assertiveness training with hospitalized emotionally disturbed women and reported that the assertively trained patients had significantly higher change scores than did the comparison subjects. Those diagnosed with depression had more success than did patients with other diagnoses. In a replication of the study with adolescents, the assertively trained group was significantly less depressed than the control group (Jones, 1986). The training lasted 1.5 hours per day for 5 consecutive weekdays. Assertiveness training, role playing, and cognitive rehearsal enable the patient to master specific scenarios that serve as models for real-life achievement.

Cognitive-Behavioral Therapy. Behavioral techniques are often used in combination with cognitive interventions. Gordon and Gordon (1987) designed short-term group intervention to help depressed women reduce their depression, increase their self-esteem, and learn to cope more effectively with daily stress. Examples of topics are self-worth, relationship with self, relationship with others, assertiveness skills, grief, conflict management, and relaxation. During each session, a topic is discussed and activities are conducted to reinforce learning (Gordon & Gordon, 1987). This nursing intervention was evaluated for its effectiveness in relieving symptoms of depression, hopelessness, loneliness, and anxiety in 20 depressed women in Great Britain (Gordon & Gordon, 1987). Significant improvement in women's self-esteem and reduction in expressed feelings of depression and hopelessness were found for those women in the treatment group compared with those in the control group; little change was demonstrated in the treatment group's feelings of loneliness or anxiety, however, or in their level of social adjustment. A 3-year follow-up of the intervention reported that the treatment group was found to have significantly lower levels of depression and hopelessness and significantly higher levels of self-esteem than the no-treatment control group (Gordon, Matwychuk, Sachs, & Canedy, 1988).

Rational-Emotive Therapy (RET). RET, developed over 30 years ago by Albert Ellis (see Ellis & Harper, 1975), is classified as another cognitive-behavioral therapy. Group members are taught Ellis's cognitive analysis system; they keep records of key problem situations that occurred during the week and of the internal dialogues and self-talk that mediated their upset reactions (Wolfe, 1987). The bulk of the session time is spent in helping members identify irrational beliefs and teaching them to challenge or dispute their beliefs and replace them with more rational self-messages. Members are encouraged to take risks and push themselves into previously avoided situations and behaviors, beginning with less anxiety-evoking ones first and working their way up to more difficult ones. Examples are asking questions of your gynecologist or your car mechanic. Other behavioral techniques used regularly include (a) making a contract with the group (e.g., making three positive comments about yourself during each group meeting), (b) allowing yourself to do something you enjoy doing only after you have completed the assignment, (c) doing some nonnormative social behavior to desensitize yourself to your fears of social disapproval, (d) keeping track of the number of times in a day you put yourself down, and (e) practicing RET on a friend to strengthen your own rational thinking (Wolfe, 1987).

Psychodynamic Therapy. The most prevalent forms of therapy in clinical use are derived from psychodynamic theories (McGrath et al., 1990). Karasu (1990) notes that Jacobson has established loss of self-esteem as the central psychological problem among depressed women and exaggerated dependency as a specific weakness. Insight is the primary mechanism of change. The therapeutic relationship is used to examine the transference. The psychodynamic model has several successive goals for the depressed patient: (a) to provide symptom relief through cathartic expression of suppressed aggressive feelings, (b) to lower superego demands and perfectionistic standards so as to reduce feelings of guilt and inadequacy thus allowing self-esteem to be raised, (c) to make clear how current narcissistic wishes for love and excessive expectations in significant relationships are unrealistic, and (d) to uncover and recreate the earlier conflicts from which the current disorder derives (Karasu, 1990).

Phototherapy and Other Interventions for Seasonal Pattern Mood Disorder. Phototherapy has proved to be an effective, noninvasive treatment modality (Rosenthal, Sack, Skwerer, Jacobsen, & Wehr, 1988). Eighty percent benefit from light therapy. An antidepressant effect generally is observed within a few days of starting the phototherapy, and relapse generally occurs within a week of stopping the treatment. Full-spectrum light is superior to other types of light, and 2,500 lux are necessary for an antidepressant effect (Terman, Quitkin, Terman, Steward, & McGrath, 1987). Light therapy clients are instructed to sit no further than 3 feet away from the light and glance at it frequently.

A person who receives a high seasonality score and declares that the seasonal changes are a problem for him or her should be referred to a mental health care professional. A person who receives a reasonably low seasonality score and declares that the changes are only somewhat problematic can be educated by the nurse about subsyndromal type and given the following tips for self-treatment (Lefler, 1991):

- Take walks outside, at noon, without sunglasses, in the winter to receive maximum amounts of sunlight.
- Do extra work in the spring and summer to take some pressure off in the winter.
- Maintain an appropriate diet and exercise program in the winter to help offset weight gain.
- If possible, a trip to a sunnier climate in the winter can be extremely helpful.

Special Female Populations Who Are Depressed

Women in Poverty

Low-income black and white women are likely to receive only drug therapy when they want a chance to discuss their problems with a therapist (Belle, 1984). They experience themselves as blamed by the therapists for their children's problems without receiving any help in solving these problems. In many instances, therapist and client hold such disparate worldviews about the causes of the client's emotional distress that no rapport can be established. Belle (1984) notes that only 7.7% of the white psychologists interviewed by Boyd believed that socioeconomic or system problems were problems experienced by black families.

Mental health services for low-income and minority women will improve as clinicians overcome their classism, racism, and tendency to blame the victim and understand the context of their patients' lives and options (Belle, 1984). If environmental realities are ignored, the patient will become more passive, guilty, and depressed. Because social and economic stresses are often the root cause of emotional disorders, alleviating such stresses often can alleviate the mental health problems as well. Advocacy helps women resolve legal problems, gain the welfare benefits to which they are entitled, and secure job training that can be therapy in itself.

Visits to clients' neighborhoods and homes can be important learning experiences for clinicians and can help them understand their clients' stresses and struggle to cope. Home visits give a powerful message that tells a low-income client she is valued (Belle, 1990). Self-help groups can also be supportive in bringing about social change.

Low-income rural women are especially vulnerable to depression because of lack of social and educational opportunities, inadequate resources in child care, transportation difficulties, isolation, and traditional family role demands regardless of the woman's employment (Haussman & Halseth, 1987). Many mental health centers are not yet designed to facilitate education and prevention; instead, they are often structured according to the medical model, with little consideration for larger community barriers to health. Haussman suggests assertiveness training, cognitive approaches, consciousness-raising groups, feminist therapy, and vocational training. She emphasizes the need for support groups for women who are reentering school, training programs, or employment so they can deal with problems of low self-confidence, role conflict and resulting guilt, and time management.

Women From Underrepresented Ethnic Groups

The occurrence and linking of minority status and role contradiction place black women at risk for depression (Warren, 1994). These women may perceive themselves as being devalued within American society and may have fewer support systems to buffer stressful life circumstances (Carrington, 1980). Furthermore, other health hazards, such as hypertension, alcohol and other substance abuse, and suicide attempts may be related to depression in black women (McGrath et al., 1990; Taylor, 1992). Violence is another risk factor for depression in black women (Barbee, 1992), with both criminal and intimate violence disproportional in black women. Homicide is one of the 10 leading causes of death for black women; reported rape is almost three times that of white women; and aggravated assault is three times that of white women (U.S. Department of Justice, 1991).

Although behavioral, cognitive-behavioral, dynamically oriented, interpersonal, and feminist psychotherapies have been used successfully with some ethnic minority women, they need to be culturally grounded to be effective (McGrath et al., 1990). In general, counseling protocols and interventions have been developed to meet the needs of white males and then generalized to female and ethnic minority populations (Warren, 1994). Thus nurses must develop interventions that are culturally appropriate and address the contextual needs of each woman. Because community support and relationships are important for black women, they should be incorporated into nursing strategies. For example, screening for depression could take place in community settings, such as churches, recreation centers, and health centers. If referral is necessary, community resources and persons with whom black women are comfortable should be used; family, friends, ministers, healers, and social clubs can be included when developing individualized interventions.

Trotman and Gallagher (1987) support the idea that black women experience a safer environment in a group with other black women, where black language allows the full expression of their depth of feelings. The black women's group can provide a safe setting in which the black woman can begin to reexperience some of the painful and damaging incidents of childhood that are indirect results of racism. Also, there appears to be little need to discuss racism in a black women's group, which frees the black woman to go on to the task of taking responsibility for her own life and developing coping strategies that deal with the effects of discrimination and oppression (Trotman & Gallagher, 1987).

Specific suggestions for increasing the effectiveness and relevance of group process for black female clients (Trotman & Gallagher, 1987) include the following: The nurse should be aware of her own race, social class, sex, and age bias; she should be flexible in the design and implementation of group services and be prepared to adopt nontraditional roles; the therapist should not exploit a black client's strengths but, rather, help her get in touch with her needs; the therapist should always consider the social ecology of the black client; and the therapist should anticipate that the period of testing the group leader may last longer with the black member than with the white member.

Older Women

Accurate diagnosis of depression in older women is critical. Nurses are often in the best position to identify potential health problems, to monitor existing problems, and to help the older woman adapt to the aging process (Lum, 1988). Pseudodementia is one of the characteristics of depression in the older adult. A geriatric depression scale has been developed to provide a reliable screening test for depression specifically for the elderly population (Yesavage et al., 1983). Of even greater importance is the evaluation of how medication is affecting the mental health of the elderly woman. Many medicines that treat physical illness, such as antihypertensives and tranquilizers, cause depression in older women and must be carefully monitored (Lum, 1988). Antidepressants can cause as many problems as they resolve unless they are properly regulated and monitored (Lum, 1988).

Countless numbers of organic illness mimic psychiatric episodes (Coyle, 1987), and there are many physical causes of depression (Field, 1985a). Thus, before treating an older woman for depression, physical cause should be ruled out. Diseases that may start with depression as a primary symptom include endocrine (especially thyroid) problems, neurological disorders, heart failure or chronic lung disorders that prevent full oxygenation of the blood, nutritional deficiencies (particularly vitamin B_{12} or folic acid), kidney failure, and chronic infections (Lum, 1988).

Nurses, and clinical specialists in particular, have much to offer related to mental health of the elderly. They have the skills needed to assess both the psychological and physiological functioning of older persons in a variety of treatment settings. Advocacy on behalf of the elderly is another important nursing role. One group of psychiatric nurses in an elderly outreach project planned a series of educational programs to address care planning and management of bizarre and disruptive behaviors by the mentally ill elderly residents, clients, or family members (Smith, Buckwalter, & Albanese, 1990). They provided 28 programs on 16 topics reaching a total of 741 nurses, nursing assistants, and allied health care providers in long-term-care facilities. Such types of educational programs by psychiatric nurse clinical specialists could make a tremendous impact on the well-being of older women in long-term-care settings.

Another role for clinical specialists was reported by Forker and Billings (1989). When asked to speak to a group of black elderly adults in a community day care setting, the therapist transformed them into a social group that talked together about depression and about people being bio-psychosocial-cultural-spiritual beings. From a noncommunicative, disoriented collection of people, the therapist created a feeling of unity and group spirit that began to energize itself and ended in a most creative activity—singing in harmony the song, "This Little Light of Mine, I'm Gonna Let it Shine."

Research has shown that religion is a protective barrier against depression and that black elderly individuals are more intrinsically oriented to religion than are whites (Nelson, 1989). Thus the nurse may wish to encourage elderly clients to participate in religious activities and services.

Elderly widows are frequently documented as at risk for depression. Older women need to grieve, and, frequently, family members, in their concern and love for the elderly individual, may try to speed up the grief process, shutting off communication prematurely (Lum, 1988). Life review and reminiscence help the older woman recognize and value her own personal strengths and get in touch with her personal resources. The depression the older woman experiences can be "reframed" as a normal, necessary, and helpful part of grieving, to be indulged in until the individual no longer needs it (Lum, 1988). Reframing is a technique used to identify the positive aspect of the situation. It inspires hope and empowers the individual. Bereavement groups can be very helpful. After the initial bereavement phase, the nurse can help the widow to discuss how to manage her new lifestyle. Coping strategies such as keeping busy by learning new behaviors and skills, pursuing volunteer work, exercising, and rekindling old relationships as well as initiating new ones increase an elderly client's self-esteem (Poncar, 1989). A difficult decision for the widow is whether to live alone or move near a relative or into a retirement facility (Poncar, 1989). In spite of the expense of remaining in the old family home, the attachment is so great that many widows refuse to move. Living alone also increases their sense of isolation. For those who can afford it, a full-services retirement complex can be a reassuring arrangement. A less expensive option is to rent a room in a home with other older women. Utilities and cleaning are provided, and all the women have access to kitchen and living room space. Meals on Wheels can provide a hot meal daily for those unable to prepare meals. If the home is located near public transportation, it eliminates the need of a car. Other services can be supplemented as needed, and the older woman can maintain some degree of independence while living in a safe environment with other women her age. (See Chapter 6, "Older Women," for discussion of related topics.)

Retirement can pose additional problems for the older woman (Formanek, 1987). Many feel that they cannot retire as long as they are expected to clean the house and cook the meals. Those who have been employed may feel useless and lonely, missing their social contacts and the satisfactions derived from work. Women also worry more about their financial state after retirement. Thus women must begin to plan for their retirement at a young age, especially if they are to ensure having retirement income. Depending on the husband's income could be a grave mistake if they become divorced; also, if he dies first, his retirement plan may not continue to pay the widow.

Many older women are the primary caregivers for husbands who have irreversible memory impairments or debilitating physical illness. Robinson (1989) reported that depression among wife caregivers was related to caregiver health and attitude toward asking for help. Caregivers with a positive attitude reported significantly less depression. Wives generally believed caregiving was their own responsibility, and that they should be able to do it without assistance. This belief seemed to give rise to feelings of failure and dependency when they had to ask for help. Such a negative attitude toward help may be a result of their viewing caregiving as part of their marital responsibility. With more older women caring for dependent family members in the home, nurses need to be doing family work in the home. Meeting with family members to do assessment, plan care, and solve problems related to family needs and resources is an important role for nurses. If older family members are homebound, nurses need to visit them. The caregiver must be encouraged to accept help and be taught survival skills (Wilson, 1989). Survival skills include taking time for self, not taking family members' complaints personally, and setting up realistic expectations for self and family members. The availability of volunteer respite services in the community could make sharing the burden easier for older caregiving women. By having respite services available, the community legitimizes respite as an important resource for caregivers.

Sleep pattern disturbance affects many older women. Recent research (Morin & Azrin, 1988) suggests that geriatric insomnia can be treated with psychological interventions, and that behavioral procedures are more beneficial than cognitive procedures. Behavioral interventions such as going to bed only when sleepy at night, using the bed only for sleep and sex, getting out of bed and going in another room whenever they are unable to fall asleep or return to sleep, repeating this last procedure as often as necessary, rising in the morning at the same time regardless of the amount of sleep obtained during the night, and not napping during the day were found to be effective.

Imagery training, such as imagining a sequence of six neutral objects (candle, hourglass, kite, stairway, palm tree, lightbulb), was also successful but not as successful as the behavioral technique. With their eyes closed, participants concentrated on the image of each object for about 2 minutes. They were instructed to practice the visual-imagery exercises once during the day and whenever they were unable to fall asleep or return to sleep at night.

For the more dependent elderly woman, it is important to see that a balanced diet, hydration, exercise, self-care, and diversional activities are maintained. Warner (1988) found that by simply walking, the elderly produced physical and emotional gains.

Eating Disorders

The most common types of eating disorders found in adolescents and adults are obesity, anorexia nervosa, and bulimia nervosa (Williamson, 1990). Williamson (1990) has proposed a conceptual model based on a preponderance of research that has shown that obesity is a primary antecedent condition of the eating disorders (see Figure 15.1). He also theorizes that when weight gain occurs in a sociocultural climate that emphasizes thinness, especially in women, many young women will develop rigid rules of dietary restraint. When dietary restraint is broken, the person is likely to overeat or binge. If this

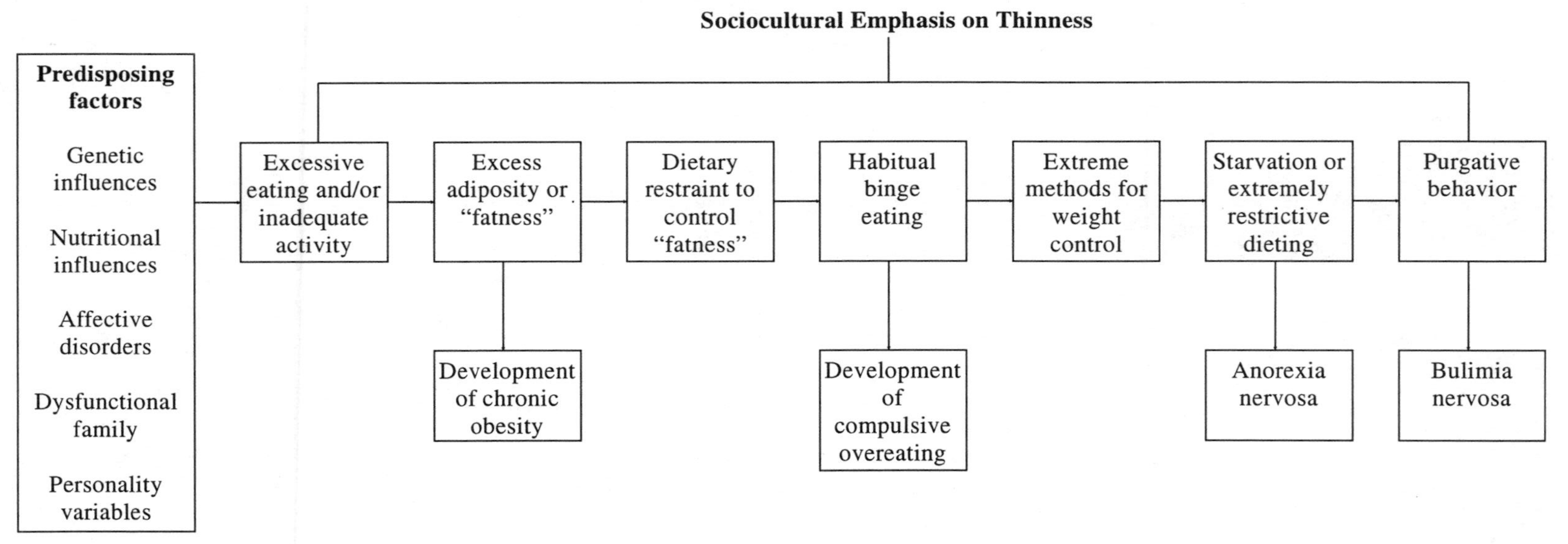

Figure 15.1. Etiologic Model for Eating Disorders
SOURCE: From *Assessment of Eating Disorders* (p. 15), by D. Williamson, 1990, Simon & Schuster International.

dietary restraint becomes habitual, then bingeing is also likely to become habitual. Each binge reinforces the idea that additional rigidity of dietary restraint is required to prevent weight gain.

Definitions

Obesity is not included in the DSM-IV. Tentative diagnostic criteria proposed for the compulsive overeater include recurrent episodes of binge eating (rapid consumption of a large amount of food in a discrete period of time, usually less than 2 hours) at least twice per week for 3 months. Criteria for diagnosis also includes at least three of the following: consumption of high-caloric, easily ingested food during a binge; inconspicuous eating during a binge; repeated attempts at dieting in an effort to lose weight; negative affect often sets the occasion for binge eating; frequent weight fluctuations greater than 10 pounds due to alternating bingeing and dieting; no use of extreme methods to lose weight, such as self-induced vomiting, starvation, or laxatives; awareness that the eating pattern is abnormal; depressed mood following eating binges; and no body image disturbances (Williamson, 1990).

The essential features of anorexia nervosa are refusal to maintain minimally normal body weight; intense fear of gaining weight or becoming fat, even though underweight; a distorted body image; and amenorrhea (APA, 1994).

Essential features of bulimia are recurrent episodes of binge eating characterized by eating a larger amount of food than most people would eat in a discrete period (e.g., 2 hours) and a feeling of lack of control over eating behavior during the episodes, in addition to self-induced vomiting; misuse of laxatives, diuretics, or enemas; fasting; or vigorous exercise to prevent weight gain (APA, 1994). To be diagnosed with bulimia nervosa, a person must have had an average of two binge eating episodes per week for at least 3 months.

Incidence

Prevalence of obesity is hard to document; however, recent research suggests that 20% to 40% of obese patients have significant problems with compulsive binge eating (Williamson, 1990). Of all patients diagnosed with anorexia nervosa, 95% are women. (See Chapter 12, "Nutrition," for additional discussion.)

The prevalence rate for bulimia nervosa among adolescent and young adult women is about 1% (Fairburn & Beglin, 1990). A recent study of college freshmen indicated that 4.5% of the females and 0.4% of the males had a history of bulimia (APA, 1987).

Etiology of Anorexia and Bulimia Nervosa

The Slade model (Heilbrun & Worobow, 1990) for the development of anorexia nervosa proposes that the female may seek success and control in her life by pursuing a thin body through dieting when faced with serious personal problems. Several studies have affirmed the importance of thinness for women in our society. In a group of 33 male and 57 female college students, men were satisfied with their figures, but women desired to be thinner than they thought they were. Women with abnormal eating behaviors desired to be even thinner than what they thought men would find attractive (Zellner, Harner, & Adler, 1989). In a study that evaluated body image distortion and ideal body size preferences in 423 nonbulimic women and 108 bulimics (Williamson, Davis, Goreczny, & Blouin, 1989), bulimics chose current body sizes that were significantly larger than those picked by nonbulimics regardless of actual body size. Bulimics also chose thinner ideal body sizes than did nonbulimics, regardless of actual body size. These results suggest that body image distortion and extreme preference for thinness are fundamental characteristics of bulimia nervosa.

Stuart, Laraia, Ballenger, and Lydiard (1990) investigated the early family experiences of 30 women with bulimia nervosa and 15 women with major depression and compared them with 100 women controls. Bulimics felt rejected by both parents, emotionally distanced from their mothers, and overly controlled by their fathers. The depressives also perceived their parents to be more rejecting than did the normal controls, but it was the fathers who were felt to be less warm emotionally. Bulimics were raised in households with significantly more tension, threats, and physically coercive behavior than the controls, although there was no more actual physical violence. Families of depressives used significantly less rational discussion when compared with the controls. Both patient groups reported more childhood behavioral indicators of unhappiness than the controls. Explanations of eating disorders encompass culture, the social construction of gender, intrapsychic dynamics, and family systems. Physiological features are thought to be consequences rather than causes (Travis, 1988).

Sociocultural Context

Anorexic and bulimic women not only have aberrant eating habits but also engage in rigid and extreme patterns of thinking, feeling, and interacting with others (Schwartz & Barrett, 1988). These patterns are established within the individual's familial and sociocultural contexts. Consequently, these eating disorders cannot be understood or treated effectively without examining such sociocultural contexts. The sociocultural factors that serve to create eating disorders in women are (a) the subordinate position of women in society, (b) the role of nurturer and caretaker occupied by women, and (c) the pressure placed on women to be physically attractive and thin (Schwartz & Barrett, 1988). Bulimia and anorexia nervosa help women satisfy the societal mandate of subordination. Being anorectic or bulimic makes one feel and appear inadequate. Sufferers of both disorders often find themselves in need of physical care. Yet being bulimic or anorectic is very powerful. No one can control their eating or their purging. The disorders are a very indirect method of gaining power and control over one's life. Consequently, eating disorders maintain both the position of the dependent person in need of constant care and attention and the position of a powerful and overcontrolling demagogue. This indirect method of gaining power and control, while remaining subordinate, is congruent with the societal message that women are taught. A woman can perform overly responsible and sacrificial tasks and reward herself only sparingly. The physical numbing effect that results from both self-starvation and purging creates a denial system that helps a person deny hunger, feelings, and needs. Consequently, she can take care of others' needs and deny her own.

The abhorrence of fat and worship of thinness has several consequences for women with eating disorders. One is the struggle it creates between body and will: the will to be thin and the body's need for sustenance. The woman must dissociate from her body's hunger and satiation signals. Because this dissociation is often futile, her low sense of control in the world is accentuated. In cases where the "will" wins, a woman may cling to her new power and become anorectic. If the deprived dieter launches into a binge, she hates herself for the transgression and purges as a way to punish herself and reach her goal of perfect thinness (Schwartz & Barrett, 1988).

In a review of the literature exploring psychodynamic antecedents to anorexia nervosa and bulimia, Jacobson (1988) concludes that abnormal eating patterns suggest the presence of severe psychopathology, the roots of which can be found in an undependable and conflicted parent-infant relationship. The disturbed relationship resurfaces during adolescence when issues of separation and individuation recur. Jacobson suggests viewing the disturbed eating patterns as transitional objects that enable the therapists to focus more on the interpersonal dynamics contributing to the disorder rather than on the symptoms of the disorder. For instance, gorging food and vomiting reflects both the love and hate, and the acceptance and rejection felt toward the significant parent.

Familial Factors

In both "ethnic" and "Americanized" families, there is a sense that men are or should be more valuable, powerful, or competent than women and that a woman's value or competence comes only through her association with a man. In anorectic and bulimic families, the approval of men is stressed as one of the daughter's goals. In both ethnic and Americanized families there is a high degree of conflict, with no perceived method of conflict resolution. Families with an anorectic daughter keep their conflict extremely covert, whereas families with a bulimic member have extreme overt conflict that often lasts for years. In either case, the covert or overt conflicts are never resolved (Schwartz & Barrett, 1988).

The two families differ in some areas. In the Americanized families, there is a great emphasis on achievement, success, and perfection according to male standards. They have an extreme concern about vogue appearance, including dress and pressure to be thin: "The pressure of being perfect for your father through achievement, combined with the desire to please mother through nurturing skills, and attending to the messages of denial, and nonaggressive selflessness, in order to satisfy societal norms creates intense conflicts that the daughter believes she must resolve" (Schwartz & Barrett, 1988, p. 134).

In the more ethnic families, vogue appearance and high achievement are downplayed, whereas values of loyalty to the family and the maintenance of traditional woman's roles are stressed. The values include serving others, perfecting domestic skills, raising children, and staying close to home: "Food often becomes a symbolic language for defining relationships. Anger or rebellion can be expressed by either not eating or vomiting the parent's food—rejecting the mother by rejecting her food and simultaneously rejecting the father in his role of 'bread winner' " (Schwartz & Barrett, 1988, p. 135). The daughters are often intensely worried about the well-being of their parents or their parents' relationship whether married, separated, or divorced. The daughter either becomes involved in the marital issues directly or attempts to satisfy one or both parents because they are not receiving satisfaction from their spouse.

One research study that compared the early family experiences of 30 bulimic women with 100 controls confirms much of the theory just presented (Stuart et al., 1990):

> Women with bulimia described a family characterized by problems, tension, threats, and physical coercion. They perceived themselves as rejected by both parents, with their mother as lacking in warmth and caring and father as overly controlling. They also experienced significant childhood separation anxiety, although they did not experience more actual losses or separations than the control group. They did, however, display many problematic behaviors while growing up, including drug abuse, suicide attempt, alcohol abuse, truancy, and more general emotional problems. The profile that emerges is one of a child in a conflictual family environment that is not demonstrably supportive or self-enhancing, and who expresses her anxiety and unhappiness in a range of maladaptive behaviors throughout her adolescence. (p. 50)

Treatment

Because anorexia and bulimia typically have long periods of development, treatment is especially problematic with periods of relapse. No single therapy has emerged as the treatment of choice, and most hospitalized patients receive a combination of pharmacological interventions, behavior management, and individual, group, and family therapy. Feminist values usually permeate the treatment (Travis, 1988).

Behavioral Treatment

The behavioral treatment plan is based on Williamson's (1990) etiological model for eating disorders discussed earlier in the chapter (see Figure 15.1). He proposed that obesity is a primary antecedent condition of the eating disorders. When weight gain occurs, many women will develop rigid rules of dietary restraint. When such restraint is broken, the woman overeats or binges. If this dietary restraint becomes habitual, then bingeing also is likely to become habitual. The bingeing reinforces the additional rigidity of dietary restraint.

The extent of the overweight or underweight status of a client will determine both the immediacy and the direction of treatment. Seriously underweight patients will need hospitalization. Making a decision about hospitalization is based on weight status, the extent of the problem eating behaviors, the extent of secondary psychopathology, and the success of ongoing outpatient treatment. Severely overweight individuals will require long-term outpatient treatment for weight loss (Williamson, 1990). As an alternative to medical treatment, self-help groups such as Weight Watchers and Tops have been successful in helping overweight women lose weight.

Specific treatment planning for bingeing is essential if it is determined that such bingeing is a problem eating behavior. Nutritional counseling is valuable for virtually all eating disorder clients. Counseling may include helping the obese patient make wise food choices or seeking to correct the misbeliefs regarding both food and weight gain that are typical in anorexia and bulimia (Williamson, 1990).

In behavioral programs for obesity, techniques such as reducing the speed of eating, drinking fluids before meals, leaving food on the plate, and limiting the number of food cues in one's environment have been developed by watching normal and obese people eat. One research study gave people the opportunity to eat as much ice cream as they desired, but they had to remain in the research room afterward. The compulsive overeaters "binged" but the bulimics did not (Duchmann, Williamson, & Stricker, 1989), which suggests that binge eating in bulimia is most likely to occur when environmental circumstances allow purging (Williamson, 1990). Without access to a private place to vomit, bulimics refrain from binge eating. One of the first restrictions on most bulimics in the hospital is to require them to remain in the group setting for 1 hour past meals and to be accompanied to the bathroom.

In addition to learning to eat more regularly and nutritiously, it is also important for eating disorder patients to learn to eat forbidden or feared foods (foods that taste good and or are high in caloric content) without bingeing or purging. Food functions as a phobic stimulus for anorexia and bulimia, and purging serves the function of undoing the act and reducing the anxiety. The behavioral treatment requires patients to eat their feared foods but prevents them from engaging in an escape response such as purging or dietary restriction (Williamson, 1990). In the effort to reduce urges to binge and purge associated with forbidden foods, patients are asked to establish a hierarchy of foods ranging from least forbidden to most forbidden. These foods are entered onto a record sheet so that the patient and the therapist can monitor the patient's progress in learning to eat forbidden foods properly. Early in treatment, the patient is required to eat foods that are low on the list. As treatment progresses, the patient incorporates more and more fearful foods until all foods on the list can be eaten with relative comfort (Williamson, 1990).

Standardized test meals are used to assess progress over the course of treatment (Williamson, 1990). At the pretreatment stage, a meal consisting of standard servings from each of the food groups is served, and the percentage consumed from each food group as well as overall caloric consumption is recorded. In addition, self-rating scales are employed to assess pre- and post-meal anxiety and postmeal urges to binge and/or purge. This assessment serves as the basis for the ongoing evaluation of progress in eating a balanced meal.

Self-monitoring is one of the most widely used procedures in behavioral management of eating disorders (Williamson, 1990). The patient is instructed to record type and amount of foods consumed, mood before and after eating, hunger before and after eating, and environmental circumstances prior to and during eating. This information is used to analyze functional and caloric aspects of eating episodes, which then can be used in treatment. A common finding is that negative affect is often an antecedent to binge eating and often precedes both bingeing and purging in bulimia. In general, obese and bulimic individuals are most likely to overeat or binge when they have skipped one or more meals during the day and are hungry; often, they have recently encountered a distressing or boring situation and overeat when they are alone.

On a daily basis, patients are asked to write down in a notebook each individual eating episode and what they were feeling at the time. Usually, patients are asked to do this self-monitoring for 2 weeks before entering therapy (Williamson, 1990); these data assist in making a diagnosis and case formulation, providing baseline data for assessing treatment outcome, and allowing the patient time to receive feedback about performance in self-monitoring before treatment begins.

Williamson (1990) suggests that eating disorder patients be screened for secondary psychopathology. Anorexics generally have the highest levels of secondary psychopathology, followed by bulimics, who are followed by the compulsive overeater and obese groups.

Family Therapy

A treatment model designed to address sociocultural, familial, and individual factors is family therapy. The primary concepts are influenced by both the structural (Minuchin, Rosman, & Baker, 1978) and the strategic frameworks (Fisch, Weakland, & Segal, 1982). (*Structural* has to do with family roles, and *strategic* has to do with family process.) Because the eating disorders are reinforced by all three factors and help women maintain their sense of self, disorders are very difficult symptoms to treat. The model is composed of three stages: (a) creating a context for change, (b) challenging patterns and expanding alternatives, and (c) consolidation. The interventions of each stage are aimed at restructuring the woman's dysfunctional interactions with food, self, and others so that she is no longer continuing patterns that maintain anorexia or bulimia (Schwartz & Barrett, 1988).

Stage 1 is creating a context for change. The patient and her family are told that as long as her weight and electrolytes do not fall, she will not be hospitalized and she is in charge of what she eats. The patient is seen once a week, and the family is seen once a month. To help the anorexic client to understand the meaning of her illness, she is asked to keep a journal in which she logs the times she thought about food, when she prepared food for others, when she denied herself food, and the times she allowed herself to eat. For each occasion, she records where she was, who she was with, what was happening at that point, and what she was feeling and thinking. She is told at this point not to alter her eating in any way. Keeping a journal makes the client face the extreme nature of her relationship to food without the therapist having to confront her directly (Schwartz & Barrett, 1988). The therapist also explores with the client potentially negative consequences of change in eating habits and what she or her family might have to give up or acknowledge if the client were to eat normally.

Stage 2 is challenging patterns and expanding alternatives. In this stage of treatment, the client and her family are challenged to address the areas of dysfunction directly and to change the way they interact with each other in the process—for example, if both mom and dad use the adolescent as their confidant instead of talking with each other. The last stage of consolidation begins when the client no longer uses therapy to process her life with her friends, family, and work; instead, she talks about the changes she is making, the risks she is taking, and how she is viewing life differently (Schwartz & Barrett, 1988).

Group Therapy

During hospitalization, group psychotherapy can be particularly useful for the patient with an eating disorder and the problems of distortion of body image (Oehler & Burns, 1987). Some argue that group therapy should be the treatment of choice. In one report, adolescent girls discussed issues such as feminine identity and heterosexual issues. Oedipal themes were addressed often, because many of the girls were being treated within a psychoanalytic framework. They used the group to discover that others had similar sexual feelings (Oehler & Burns, 1987).

Pharmacotherapy

In 1988, research accumulated suggesting that eating disorders are related to depression. In fact, some bulimic women respond well to antidepressants (McGrath et al., 1990).

Dissociative Identity Disorder

The essential feature of dissociative identity disorder (DID) is the presence within the person of two or more distinct personalities or personality states (each with its own relatively enduring pattern of perceiving, relating to, and thinking about the environment and self). At least two of these identities or personality states recurrently take full control of the person's behavior (APA, 1994). Informal diagnostic signs include reports of periods of amnesia, sometimes lasting for days, and behavior that is often hysterical, suggestible, and easily hypnotizable. If electroencephalograms (EEGs) are performed on different alternative personalities, each EEG reading will be different (Lego, 1988).

Recent reports suggest that this disorder is not nearly as rare as has commonly been thought. However, there continues to be polarization of the mental health care community on the frequency of the disorder (Drew, 1988). DID occurs from three to nine times more frequently in females than males.

Etiology

DID develops in childhood and is a result of the defensive process of dissociation. A child splits off or blocks out feelings, memories, and events that are too painful to deal with by any other means as a way to survive (Anderson & Ross, 1988). An extremely dysfunctional, abusive family life can precipitate dissociative process. Putnam, Guroff, Silberman, Barban, and Post (1986) studied 100 MPD patients and found that 97% of the patients had experienced extreme childhood trauma, 83% were sexually abused, 75% were physically abused, and 68% were both physically and sexually abused.

Treatment

The most common treatment is extended psychotherapy with hypnosis. Over time the patient is encouraged to abreact all the traumas of childhood (which are nearly always severe) and to understand intellectually what has happened (Lego, 1988). The goal of this treatment is fusion of the many personalities into one whole person.

A second treatment is extended psychoanalysis without hypnosis. The patient is encouraged over time to bring dissociated aspects of the past life into conscious awareness. Again, the goal is fusion into one person (Lego, 1988).

Although nurses do not usually do psychotherapy with clients having DID, knowing how the illness manifests itself and recognizing the high risk of DID in clients who have been sexually abused is critical for nurses working in any setting. Nurses should be alert to patients who act differently at subsequent appointments or times of the day or who allude to periods of memory loss. More often, nurses care for DID patients when they come into the hospital. Nursing issues during hospitalization include a fear of fostering dissociation in the patient and how to foster integration (Lego, 1988). Nurses should have a chart of all the personalities and what they represent, so that they will be recognized when they appear. The nurse treats the alter (other personality) with kindness and respect, remembering that each alter is a stratum of the total self.

If the alter is a child, the nurse relates to whatever age the alter presents. Child alters usually hold memories of the abuse and feelings such as hurt, pain, and fear. Expression of these feelings and memories may be difficult. Age-appropriate activities are implemented with the child alters to help form a trusting relationship. Such activities may include drawing, playing, or walks in the snow (Anderson & Ross, 1988). Lego (1988) recommends that the alter be reminded that she is part of the host personality. The nurse emphasizes safety. Hospitalization is recommended so that all the personalities can appear and experiences can be abreacted. DID patients present a tremendous drain on staff and arouse many feelings that must be processed.

Policy Implications for Improving Mental Health of Women

The mental health of women is profoundly affected by the social, economic, and psychological consequences of inequality in our society today, for gender inequality increases women's vulnerability to stress and the potential for mental disorders. Policy changes directed toward eliminating sex role stereotyping, decreasing poverty through work opportunities, assuring adequate child care, promoting neighborhood helping services, improving self-esteem, and fostering self-help groups have been recommended by professional and lay groups alike.

Eliminating Sex Role Stereotyping

The price society pays for maintaining sex role stereotyping is very high. According to the President's Commission on Mental Health Report (1978a), the most extensive and most recent government study on mental health (much of which has not been implemented),

> Intervention in the social system has potential for effecting a far greater change than does individual or group psychotherapy. For example, implementation of affirmative action plans and a reduction in the extent to which jobs are segregated by sex would raise the earning potential of millions of women. The resultant increase in income would reduce the impact of life stress and raise the self-concept of women on a scale not possible through remedial psychotherapies. The development of a network of day-care systems in the community would free more welfare mothers to work and would relieve the stress of many mothers already working. Appointment of a representative number of women to policymaking positions in Federal, State, and Local agencies would permit the concerns of women to be expressed in the decisions that impact on the lives of all American women. . . . Legal enforcement of court-mandated child support payments would raise the living standard of millions of American women and children. Federal laws covering the kidnapping of children by the noncustodial parent would eliminate crisis situations for many parents and children. Such interventions in the social system are preventive measures and ultimately will reduce the need and the cost of remedial services. (p. 1065)

Women have made little headway on the Capitol Hill leadership ladder. For appropriate policy development on their behalf, whether at federal, state, or local levels, women must participate at all levels of the decision-making process (Russo, 1984). Women constitute more than half of the population and more than half of all voters; thus women are tremendously underrepresented in the group that determines the laws of this country. However, policy development alone is insufficient—policies must be implemented. The reader is referred to the President's Commission on Mental Health (1978a) for a discussion on recommendations to change the social status of women and thereby lessen their need for mental health services.

In addition to policy changes, Weinraub and Brown (1983) suggest four child-rearing techniques that parents and other adults can use to combat the negative effects of sex role stereotypes on children's interests and aspirations: (a) Parents can call children's attention to sex role reversals when they occur and model such behaviors themselves; (b) parents can distinguish between sex role stereotypes and personal conformity to them; (c) children can be helped to put sex role stereotypic models of men and women in a sociohistorical framework; and (d) children can be helped to develop skills so that they can transcend stereotypes.

Decreasing Poverty Through Work

A second policy for improving women's mental health is through promoting work opportunities. Work is a crucial source of satisfaction and self-esteem for most women (California Task Force, 1990; Sales & Frieze, 1984) and provides women opportunities to increase income and thus remove themselves from poverty.

According to Sales and Frieze (1984), changes in the formal policies of work settings, including more equitable hiring practices for desirable jobs, reduced pay differentials, and greater possibilities for on-the-job training and promotions would increase the attractiveness of employment for women. Employers are encouraged to accommodate their workers' status as new parents by offering parental leaves, flexible work schedules, or worksite child care services. In addition, government policies could encourage child care use through tax benefits, subsidizing programs, and setting quality standards. Women also need more realistic preparation for the demands of the marketplace, including more experiences for adolescent girls with independence, competition, and teamwork in home, school, and community. Policies that enhance the conditions of female employment would also enhance the mental health of women.

Meleis et al. (1989) have offered similar recommendations to management to reduce work stress for clerical women, including providing training programs to enhance a sense of personal growth; teaching strategies to decrease strained relationships between supervisors and coworkers; providing child care, particularly during school vacations and child illness; increasing worker participation in decision making; and offering stress reduction and health promotion programs.

A woman's sense of self is intimately related to her connections to others. Within the workplace, programs could be developed that build on a recognition of women's shared concerns and their capacity for mutual support and facilitation. Low-income women in particular need programs offering sharing, support, and affirmation (Kaplan & Surrey, 1984). In addition, corporations could recognize and support the total demands placed on these women's lives, including their responsibilities at home—allowing some choice in selecting the hours and days to work (flextime) is a useful beginning. Time away from work required to tend to a sick child could be considered as valid as sick leave. "Cafeteria" benefit programs could be instituted so that corporate contributions to the cost of child care would be an option. Most important, women should be solicited by corporations for requests as to what additional options would facilitate their daily lives and hence their capacity to function more effectively.

Prevention efforts must aim to halt the feminization of poverty and to increase women's opportunities. Enforcement of existing laws that promise equality of opportunity to women and members of minority groups must be a high priority (Belle, 1984). Helping girls and young women develop marketable skills will enhance their employability as adults. Female students are not now sufficiently encouraged to study mathematics and science, to pursue technical skills, or to enroll in government-sponsored apprenticeship programs that will lead to well-paying jobs. Training programs that help women enter nontraditional employment areas are essential. Pay scales for traditional women's jobs must also be upgraded so that women can actually support their families. The lack of high-quality affordable child care prevents many women from entering the labor force and prevents many more from holding well-paying full-time jobs. Without a job, many poor women survive by receiving welfare benefits.

The majority of individuals receiving financial aid from the government from the Aid to Families With Dependent Children (AFDC) are mothers with young children. The California Task Force (1990) reported that being a welfare recipient can be destructive to self-esteem, encourages a "learned helplessness," and undermines one's efforts to be personally and socially responsible. Many painful questions about the impact of welfare on individuals, families, and the nation have been posed. Does welfare destroy the incentive to work? Promote teenage pregnancy? Discourage marriage and a stable family life? Does it encourage a cycle of dependency on government assistance that is passed from one generation to another? The California Task Force emphasizes that all aid programs need to help people move toward high self-esteem and financial self-sufficiency. Often, welfare recipients need training in vocational and educational opportunities, independent living skills, and interpersonal communications. The Task Force recommends that inservice self-esteem training be given to staff who work with welfare recipients and that welfare reform programs be implemented to alter attitudes and enhance motivation.

There is currently a nationwide movement toward getting people off welfare and into private sector jobs (Naisbitt & Aburdene, 1990). Some 39 states have enacted workfare programs, designed to get women off welfare (Naisbitt & Aburdene, 1990). Congress has mandated that all states must have workfare programs. Two successful welfare programs are the Massachusetts program that has saved taxpayers more than $281 million (Naisbitt & Aburdene, 1990) and the Michigan Opportunity and Skills Training.

Belle (1990) argues that recent efforts to force poor women into the labor force as the price they must pay for continuing to receive their meager welfare benefits are extremely dangerous. She postulates that with all its stigma and frustrations, welfare dependency is a highly undesirable option, and women who choose it do so out of great need. Coercing women into humiliating job searches will not improve the mental health of women.

Child Care

An equal division of child care responsibilities for both parents would help decrease the overload felt by women. The school system could also share the responsibility for child care. Far too many children are staying at home unsupervised because school ends so early in the afternoon. The school could provide after-school programs with scheduled activities and supervised play until the usual workday ends (Fishel, 1981). For middle-school-aged children, perhaps a study hall in the school library after the regular school day would be helpful to both parents and children.

The necessity of government or private sector support for child care for poor women has already been discussed as a necessary prerequisite for women to work. Minimum wage earnings minus the expenses of child care leaves many poor women in debt.

Naisbitt and Aburdene (1990) agree that day care is a necessary service in the next decade, but they propose that it should be available as an employee benefit. Currently, in companies providing day care, most do not have on-site facilities but offer some financial help or referral services. Some companies issue vouchers or pay a portion of costs. One company reported a 31% drop in absenteeism among parents who used day care centers and a 10% drop in the turnover rate (Naisbitt & Aburdene, 1990). Another company, whose employees were 85% women, had a 57% turnover rate before implementation of a day care center. After the company spent $250,000 on the day care center, the turnover immediately dropped to 31% and fell to only 3% 10 years later.

Neighborhood Helping Networks

Health professionals do not and cannot provide help for most individuals. Of the mental health problems with which people must cope, 80% are solved through help from the person's social network (President's Commission, 1978a). The natural helping network includes spouses, neighbors, coworkers, friends, and acquaintances from church and civic groups. The self-help groups discussed in the section on depression are also examples of the social system acting to reduce isolation and stressful life situations. These resources can and do provide major preventive and crisis help for women; those who have social supports may escape the potentially negative effects of crises and changes. Every new mother, for example, needs another mother with whom she can discuss the many concerns of parenting. The concept of social support is so important in promoting women's mental health that an entire section of the President's Commission on Mental Health (1978a) was devoted to exploring ways to expand the model of community support systems.

Improving Self-Esteem

The Task Force to Promote Self-Esteem and Personal Social Responsibility (California Task Force, 1990) reported that self-esteem is the most likely candidate for a "social vaccine"—something that empowers women to live responsibly and that inoculates them against the lures of crime, violence, substance abuse, teen pregnancy, child abuse, chronic welfare dependency, and educational failure.

The California Task Force (1990) identified two critical forces in improving and promoting self-esteem: parents and schools. High self-esteem is vital to a parent's ability to provide a healthy environment for the child. Nurses need to assist parents to develop their own self-esteem and to become more knowledgeable, capable, and effective in nurturing their children's positive self-esteem and personal responsibility.

Because children spend so much of their time in school, the environment of the school also plays a major role in the development of self-esteem. Young people who have high self-esteem are less likely to become pregnant as teenagers. People with high self-esteem themselves are less likely to engage in destructive and self-destructive behavior, including child abuse, substance abuse, violence, and crime.

Self-Help Groups

Part of the feminist therapy effort has been to promote alternatives to therapy, such as consciousness-raising (CR) groups and self-counseling. As opposed to therapeutic groups and group psychotherapy, self-help groups are for the most part organized and operated by group members (Marram, 1984). In addition, self-help groups often become social advocacy groups.

The processes involved in self-help groups are social affiliation, indoctrination in self-control, modeling of methods of coping with stress, and provision of an agenda of actions that change the social environment. The cognitive processes identified by Levy (1976) involve the following actions: Remove mystification by providing a rationale for problems; give information and advice; expand perceptions of problems and actions to cope with problems; provide support for change; decrease social isolation; and develop a new subculture for identification. The power of the self-help group, according to Riessman (1976), enables members to feel and use their own strengths to control their own lives. In self-help groups, the persons who have already lived through difficult experiences are critical in helping others with similar experiences. Not only do these persons know what the experience is like, but they also have learned how to play the required new role (e.g., a mother who has recently returned to paid employment).

Effectiveness of self-help groups has not been well researched or documented because they are run by the lay public. Certainly most are familiar with the success of self-help groups such as Alcoholics Anonymous, Weight Watchers, and TOPS. A number of groups for women who have been sexually abused and/or battered have also been reported in recent years to be very effective.

One of the goals of many self-help groups for women is CR—the key focus being that problems experienced by women are social rather than individual in origin (Travis, 1988). Indeed, one of the first things women discover in these groups is that personal problems are political. Individual experiences of shame, dependency, and anger are common to others. These experiences rest on shared conditions characterized by issues of dominance and power. Therefore, the sharing and analyzing of personal experiences becomes a means of raising women's consciousness of their joint status as a class, revealing that their future hopes and destinies are shared by women in general (Travis, 1988). Rape crisis centers, abortion counseling services, and shelters for battered women around the country often started as ideas in CR groups.

The first women's CR groups appeared in scattered locations across the United States in 1967 and 1968, as women began to focus attention on their own devalued status as females in male-defined movements. CR groups also served the function of educating the community at large about sexism and discrimination, particularly in the early 1970s when society did not generally believe women were subjected to prejudice or discrimination (Travis, 1988).

CR groups are deliberately small, generally with 4 to 12 members so that each person gets adequate amounts of time to speak at each meeting. The group members usually sit in a circle, allowing face-to-face communication. Meetings are held at regular intervals, usually in members' homes.

The 1970s and 1980s gave rise to multiple sources for CR for women, including the large, national women's rights organizations; women's caucuses within academe, business, labor, and the professions; women's studies courses; feminist service agencies; lesbian political groups; feminist music, theater, art, literature, and scholarship; and CR groups. Therefore, many CR groups have been the result of, rather than the source of, women's feminist identity (Kirsh, 1987). "The ideology may be less frequently verbalized as 'the personal is political,' yet the essence of this slogan remains the foundation of the groups, as women see each other through personal change in the context of problems generated by society" (Kirsh, 1987, p. 52).

Feminist Therapy

Contemporary views on the psychology of women need to be built into the core curricula and inservice education programs for mental health professionals. Among today's nurses, disagreement with the principles of feminist philosophy is rare. As Sampselle (1990) has noted,

> Because nurses often provide care to women at critical developmental points, it is important that the practice of nursing reflect the principles of feminism. By challenging traditional attitudes and values, nurses can have a beneficial effect on women's self-concept and sense of self-ownership. Incorporating feminist philosophy into practice can make it more likely for women to become full partners in sexual, social and economic relationships and to be valued for a wide range of contributions to society. (p. 246)

Techniques that are most compatible with feminist therapy are bibliotherapy (recommending books for clients to read), cognitive reprogramming, CR groups, RET, sex role analysis, women's studies, bioenergetics, gestalt exercises, psychodrama, systemic desensitization, assertion training, behavioral rehearsal, contracts and homework assignments, communications training, and physical fitness.

In feminist therapy, clients are encouraged to identify the effects of sexism on their own lives and the lives of other women. Working toward social change is seen as an important contributor to personal empowerment. The concept of empowerment reflects a general goal to not only improve self-esteem but to change the nature of relationships, both personal and political (Travis, 1988).

Two principles have prevailed as cornerstones of feminist therapy: the theoretical orientation that the personal is political and the egalitarian nature of client-therapist relationships. Travis (1988) also argues that women therapists should conduct therapy with women clients. Unfortunately, standard training does not focus on the process of building affective connectedness and empathic relations between client and therapist; therefore, male therapists enter professional practice somewhat less prepared than female therapists and need more supervision on entry into practice (Brody, 1984; Sturdivant, 1980; Travis, 1988; Walker, 1984).

Four concepts identified by Travis (1988) are fundamental to feminist therapy: dominance relations, dependency, anger, and power. In dominance relations, the idea is that women mostly occupy subordinate positions and that this is a social condition with psychological consequences—it is not brought about by the psychological traits of women. Dominance continues to be played out between intimate partners, manifesting itself not only in violence but in more subtle ways that influence decisions about how the couple spends their money and their time and raises their children.

Dependent acts include expressions of helplessness, weeping, frailty, and clumsiness. Dependent acts are expected elements of traditional femininity, and these acts are learned and are continually reinforced. By acting dependent, females retain the approval of others and avoid censure for rule violation. Persistent reliance on dependency can have long-term costs. Women become very frightened that they will not be able to survive without the dominant male. Men who support this pattern do so because it ensures that they are competent and that their wives will not leave.

Homicide is often the only way a pathologically dependent family member can psychically separate from the engulfing family. One may speculate that battering is based on a male pathological fear of abandonment and the subsequent need to dominate the woman completely.

Feminist theorists have developed new perspectives on dependency, in which dependency does not reflect lack of individuation but instead reflects a desire to be in relationship to others or to have a relational identity. Women are more likely to view interpersonal events as opportunities for growth than are men. Men have more difficulty attending to relationships. Sexual gratification, presented as a need for physical release, is one area in which men frequently also seek gratification of their needs for closeness and connection. Men's expression of rage toward infidelity by their partners not only represents a confrontation with the separateness of the other but also contains threats to the satisfaction of dependency needs. The fact that women want more relational connection than men desire contributes to much conflict.

Relational work cannot be pursued effectively unless all parties have a firm sense of self as unique and independent from others. Women need to develop a sense of identity separate from the roles they hold as parents and spouses.

In a dyadic relationship, the less "needy" partner is in a more powerful position because that person can always exert influence by a threat of withdrawal or indifference. Because women are more likely to perceive a threat to the relational commitment, they will make compromises to retain a relationship. Men frequently do not realize the extent of their own need for relationship until they have lost it. This has been especially evident in divorce research, which shows that women initiate separation much more frequently than men because they want more from a relationship. Divorced men frequently did not know anything was wrong and are very surprised at how much they miss their family (Fishel & Samsa, 1993).

Women often say they are hurt when they are angry. Men say they are angry when they are hurt. Compared to men, women risk paying a higher social cost when they express anger. The apparent lack of anger among women who have been mistreated may stem from the belief that they don't deserve anything better. Oftentimes, women may contribute substantially to the financial security of the family, manage the physical comforts of home and hearth, and provide emotional support and nurturing for their male partners who maintain a single role, that of the "good provider." It is generally agreed that men do not nurture their wives to the extent that women nurture their husbands.

As subordinates, women should want to gain control of their lives, to ensure more responsive attention to their own needs, and to establish new social structures. However, women consistently deny that they want power or often deny that they even need it. Fear that the man will leave prevents women from exerting power in the relationship. Feminists view power as empowerment—the ability to acknowledge one's own strengths and capabilities; they do not see it as producing conflicts with others. As women acquire a sense of their own authenticity, their expressions of power should be less conflicted.

Women's Mental Health Agenda

After a decade of reports underscoring the inadequacy of existing scientific knowledge for understanding gender differences in mental disorder and its treatment, the National Institute of Mental Health (Russo, 1990) developed a women's mental health research agenda with five priority areas for research: poverty, multiple roles for women, mental health issues of older women, violence against women, and diagnosis and treatment of mental disorders in women. Data that supports the need for research in these critical areas affecting mental health of women have been presented in this chapter and can be found in Chapters 1, 6, 7 ("Women and Health Care"), and 18. Much work needs to be done to improve the sociopolitical context of women's lives that negatively influences women's mental health.

References

Alberti, R., & Emmons, M. (1974). *Your perfect right.* San Luis Obispo, CA: Prometheus.

American Psychiatric Association. (1987). *Diagnostic and statistical manual of mental disorders* (3rd ed., rev.). Washington, DC: Author.

American Psychiatric Association. (1994). *Diagnostic and statistical manual of mental disorders* (4th ed.). Washington, DC: Author.

Anderson, G., & Ross, C. (1988). Strategies for working with a patient who has multiple personality disorder. *Archives of Psychiatric Nursing, 2*(4), 236-243.

Badger, T., Cardea, J., Biocca, L., & Mishel, M. (1990). Assessment and management of depression: An imperative for community-based practice. *Archives of Psychiatric Nursing, 4*(4), 235-241.

Barbee, E. L. (1992). African-American women and depression: A review and critique of the literature. *Archives of Psychiatric Nursing, 4*(5), 257-265.

Beck, A. T. (1978). *Beck depression inventory* (rev. ed.). Philadelphia: Center for Cognitive Therapy.

Beck, A. T., & Greenberg, R. (1974). Cognitive therapy with depressed women. In V. Franks & V. Burtle (Eds.), *Women in therapy* (pp. 113-131). New York: Brunner/Mazel.

Belle, D. (1984). Inequality and mental health: Low income and minority women. In L. Walker (Ed.), *Women and mental health policy* (Vol. 9, pp. 135-150). Beverly Hills, CA: Sage.

Belle, D. (1990). Poverty and women's mental health. *American Psychologist, 45*(3), 385-389.

Bernard, J. (1973). *The future of marriage.* New York: World.

Bloom, L. Z., Coburn, K., & Pearlman, J. (1975). *The new assertive woman.* New York: Dell.

Bornstein, P. E., Clayton, T. J., Halikas, J. A., Maurice, W. L., & Robins, E. (1973). The depression of widowhood after 13 months. *British Journal of Psychiatry, 122,* 561-566.

Brehony, K. (1987). Self-help groups with agoraphobic women. In C. Brody (Ed.), *Women's therapy groups* (pp. 82-94). New York: Springer.

Brody, C. (1984). Authenticity in feminist therapy. In C. Brody (Ed.), *Women therapists working with women* (Vol. 7, pp. 11-21). New York: Springer.

Burgess, A. (1985). *Psychiatric nursing in the hospital and the community* (4th ed.). Englewood Cliffs, NJ: Prentice Hall.

Butler, P. (1976). Techniques of assertive training in groups. *International Journal of Group Psychotherapy, 26,* 361-371.

California Task Force. (1990). *Toward a state of esteem: The final report of the California Task Force to Promote Self-Esteem and Personal and Social Responsibility.* Sacramento: California State Department of Education, Bureau of Publications.

Carmen, B., Reiker, P. B., & Mills, T. (1984). Victims of violence and psychiatric illness. *American Journal of Psychiatry, 141*(3), 378-382.

Carrington, C. H. (1980). Depression in black women: A theoretical appraisal. In L. F. Rogers-Rose (Ed.), *The black woman* (pp. 265-271). Beverly Hills, CA: Sage.

Cartwright, R. D. (1989, August). *Sleep and dreams in depressed men and women undergoing divorce.* Paper presented at the annual meeting of the American Psychological Association, New Orleans.

Childs-Clarke, A., Whitfield, W., Cadbury, S., & Sandu, S. (1989). Anxiety management groups in clinical practice. *Nursing Times, 85*(30), 49-52.

Cole, J. (1988). The drug treatment of anxiety and depression. *Medical Clinics of North America, 72*(4), 815-830.

Coyle, M. (1987). Organic illness mimicking psychiatric episodes. *Journal of Gerontological Nursing, 13*(1), 31-35.

DeRosis, H., & Pellegrino, V. (1976). *The book of hope: How women can overcome depression.* New York: Bantam.

Dilsance, S. (1989). Generalized anxiety disorder. *American Family Physician, 39*(2), 137-144.

Drew, B. (1988). Multiple personality disorder: An historical perspective. *Archives of Psychiatric Nursing, 2*(4), 227-230.

Duchmann, E. G., Williamson, D. A., & Stricker, P. M. (1989). Bulimia, dietary restraint, and concern for dieting. *Journal of Psychopathology and Behavioral Assessment, 11*(1), 1-13.

Ellis, A., & Harper, R. (1975). *A guide to rational living.* North Hollywood, CA: Wilshire.

Fairburn, C., & Beglin, S. (1990). Studies of the epidemiology of bulimia nervosa. *American Journal of Psychiatry, 147*(4), 401-408.

Field, W. (1985a). Physical causes of depression. *Journal of Psychosocial Nursing, 23*(10), 6-11.

Field, W. (1985b). *The psychotherapy of Hildegard E. Peplau.* Austin, TX: University of Texas Press.

Fisch, R., Weakland, J., & Segal, L. (1982). *The tactics of change.* San Francisco: Jossey-Bass.

Fishel, A. (1981). Mental health. In C. Fogel & N. Woods (Eds.), *Health care of women: A nursing perspective* (pp. 582-627). St. Louis: C. V. Mosby.

Fishel, A. (1983). Gay parents. *Issues in Health Care of Women, 4*(2/3), 139-164.

Fishel, A. (1986). Separation and divorce. In J. Griffith-Kenney (Ed.), *Contemporary women's health: A nursing advocacy approach* (pp. 339-358). Menlo Park, CA: Addison-Wesley.

Fishel, A., & Jefferson, C. (1983). Impact of assertiveness training on hospitalized emotionally disturbed women. *Journal of Psychosocial Nursing, 21*(1), 22-27.

Fishel, A., & Samsa, G. (1993). Role perceptions of divorcing parents. *Health Care for Women International, 14*(1), 87-98.

Fodor, I. G. (1974). The phobic syndrome in women: Implications for treatment. In V. Franks & V. Burtle (Eds.), *Women in therapy* (pp. 132-168). New York: Brunner/Mazel.

Fopma-Loy, J. (1988). The prevalence and phenomenology of depression in elderly women: A review of the literature. *Archives of Psychiatric Nursing, 2*(2), 74-80.

Forker, J., & Billings, C. (1989). Nursing therapeutics in a group encounter. *Archives of Psychiatric Nursing, 3*(2), 108-112.

Formanek, R. (1987). Depression and older women. In R. Formanek & A. Gurian (Eds.), *Women and depression* (pp. 272-281). New York: Springer.

Franks, V., & Rothblum, E. (1983). Concluding comments, criticism, and caution: Consistent conservatism or constructive change? In V. Franks & E. Rothblum (Eds.), *The stereotyping of women* (pp. 259-270). New York: Springer.

Galassi, M. D., & Galassi, J. P. (1977). *Assert yourself: How to be your own person.* New York: Human Sciences Press.

Galassi, M. D., & Galassi, J. P. (1978). Assertion: A critical review. *Psychotherapy: Theory, Research and Practice, 15*(1), 16-29.

Gordon, V., & Gordon, E. (1987). Short-term group treatment of depressed women: A replication study in Great Britain. *Archives of Psychiatric Nursing, 1*(2), 111-124.

Gordon, V., Matwychuk, A., Sachs, E., & Canedy, B. (1988). A 3-year follow up of a cognitive-behavioral therapy intervention. *Archives of Psychiatric Nursing, 2*(4), 218-226.

Gove, W. R. (1972). The relationship between sex roles, marital status, and mental illness. *Social Forces, 51*(1), 34-44.

Gove, W. R., & Geeken, M. R. (1977). The effect of children and employment on the mental health of married men and women. *Social Forces, 56*(1), 66-76.

Hamilton, M. A. (1960). A rating scale for depression. *Journal of Neurology and Neurosurgery Psychiatry, 23*(1), 56-61.

Harris, E. (1988). The antidepressants. *American Journal of Nursing, 88,* 1512-1518.

Harris, E. (1989). Lithium. *American Journal of Nursing, 89,* 190-194.

Hartman, S. (1987). Therapeutic self-help group: A process of empowerment for women in abusive relationships. In C. Brody (Ed.), *Women's therapy groups* (pp. 67-81). New York: Springer.

Hatton, C., & Valente, S. (1984). *Suicide assessment and intervention.* Norwalk, CT: Appleton-Century-Crofts.

Haussman, M., & Halseth, J. (1987). Reexamining women's roles: A feminist approach to decreasing depression in women. In C. Brody (Ed.), *Women's therapy groups* (pp. 217-226). New York: Springer.

Heilbrun, A., & Worobow, A. (1990). Attention and disordered eating behavior: II. Disattention to turbulent inner sensations as a risk factor in the development of anorexia nervosa. *Psychological Reports, 66,* 467-478.

Hickey, J., & Baer, P. (1988). Psychological approaches to the assessment and treatment of anxiety and depression. *Medical Clinics of North America, 72*(4), 911-923.

Hilberman, E., & Munson, K. (1977-1978). Sixty battered women. *Victimology: An International Journal, 2,* 460-470.

Jack, D. C. (1991). *Silencing the self: Women and depression.* Cambridge, MA: Harvard University Press.

Jackson, R., & Haynes-Johnson, V. (1988). Nutritional management of patients undergoing long-term antipsychotic and antidepressant therapies. *Archives of Psychiatric Nursing, 2*(3), 146-152.

Jacobsen, F. M., Wehr, T. A., Sack, D. A., James, S. P., & Rosenthal, W. E. (1987). SAD: A review of the syndrome and public health implications. *American Journal of Public Health, 77,* 57-60.

Jacobson, J. (1988). Speculations on the role of transitional objects in eating disorders. *Archives of Psychiatric Nursing, 2*(2), 110-114.

Jakubowski, P. A. (1977). Self-assertive training procedures for women. In E. Rawlings & D. Carter (Eds.), *Psychotherapy for women* (pp. 168-190). Springfield, IL: Charles C Thomas.

Jones, J. (1986). *Assertiveness training with hospitalized emotionally disturbed adolescents.* Unpublished masters thesis, University of North Carolina, Chapel Hill.

Kaplan, G., Roberts, R., Camacho, T., & Coyne, J. (1987). Psychosocial predictors of depression: Prospective evidence from the Human Population Laboratory Studies. *American Journal of Epidemiology, 125,* 206-220.

Kaplan, A., & Surrey, J. (1984). The relational self in women: Developmental theory and public policy. In L. Walker (Ed.), *Women and mental health policy* (Vol. 9, pp. 79-94). Beverly Hills, CA: Sage.

Karasu, T. (1990). Toward a clinical model of psychotherapy for depression: II. An integrative and selective treatment approach. *American Journal of Psychiatry, 147*(3), 269-278.

Kirsh, B. (1987). Evolution of consciousness-raising groups. In C. Brody (Ed.), *Women's therapy groups* (pp. 43-54). New York: Springer.

Knowles, R. (1981, January). Dealing with feelings: Managing anxiety. *American Journal of Nursing,* pp. 110-111.

Laraia, M., Stuart, G., & Best, C. (1989). Behavioral treatment of panic-related disorders: A review. *Archives of Psychiatric Nursing, 3*(3), 125-133.

Lefler, A. (1991). *A winter's tale.* Paper presented for honors credit, North Carolina Collection, Davis Library, University of North Carolina, Chapel Hill.

Lego, S. (1988). Multiple personality disorder: An interpersonal approach to etiology, treatment, and nursing care. *Archives of Psychiatric Nursing, 2*(4), 231-235.

Lerner, H. G. (1987). Female depression: Self-sacrifice and self betrayal in relationships. In R. Formanek & G. Gurian (Eds.), *Women and depression* (Vol. 11, pp. 200-221). New York: Springer.

Levy, L. (1976). Self-help groups: Types and psychological processes. *Journal of Applied Behavioral Science, 12,* 310-322.

Lewinsohn, P. M., Fenn, D. S., Stanton, A. R., & Franklin, J. (1986). Relation of age at onset to duration of episode in unipolar depression. *Psychology and Aging, 1*(1), 63-68.

Loo, C., & Ong, P. (1982). Slaying demons with a sewing needle: Feminist issues for Chinatown's women. *Berkeley Journal of Sociology, 27,* 77-88.

Lum, T. (1988). An integrated approach to aging and depression. *Archives of Psychiatric Nursing, 2*(4), 211-217.

Marram, G. (1984). *Group and family therapy.* St. Louis: C. V. Mosby.

Maser, J., & Woods, S. (1990). Biological basis of panic: Psychological interactions. *Psychiatric Medicine, 8*(3), 121-141.

McArthur, M. (1990). Reality therapy with rape victims. *Archives of Psychiatric Nursing, 4*(6), 360-365.

McBride, A. (1988). Mental health effects of women's multiple roles. *Image: Journal of Nursing Scholarship, 20*(1), 41-47.

McBride, A. (1990). Psychiatric nursing in the 1990s. *Archives of Psychiatric Nursing, 4*(1), 21-28.

McGrath, E., Keita, G., Strickland, B., & Russo, N. (1990). *Women and depression: Risk factors and treatment issues* (Final report of the APA National Task Force on Women and Depression). Washington, DC: American Psychological Association.

Meleis, A., Norbeck, F., Laffrey, S., Solomon, M., & Miller, L. (1989). Stress, satisfaction, and coping: A study of women clerical workers. *Health Care of Women International, 10*(4), 319-334.

Miles, H., & Hays, D. (1975). Widowhood. *American Journal of Nursing, 75,* 280-282.

Miller, J. (1973). Phobias after marriage. In J. Smeller (Ed.), *Psychoanalysis and women* (pp. 287-300). New York: Penguin.

Minuchin, S., Rosman, B., & Baker, L. (1978). *Psychosomatic families: Anorexia nervosa in context.* Cambridge, MA: Harvard University Press.

Morin, C. M., & Azrin, N. H. (1988). Behavioral and cognitive treatments of geriatric insomnia. *Journal of Consulting and Clinical Psychology, 56*(5), 748-753.

Naisbitt, J., & Aburdene, P. (1990). *Megatrends 2000.* New York: Avon.

Nathanson, C. A. (1975). Illness and the feminine role: A theoretical review. *Social Science Medicine, 9,* 57-62.

Nelson, P. (1989). Ethnic differences in intrinsic/extrinsic religious orientation and depression in the elderly. *Archives of Psychiatric Nursing, 3*(4), 199-204.

Oehler, J., & Burns, M. (1987). Anorexia, bulimia, and sexuality: Case study of an adolescent inpatient group. *Archives of Psychiatric Nursing, 1*(3), 163-171.

Peplau, H. (1963). A working definition of anxiety. In S. Burd & M. Marshall (Eds.), *Some clinical approaches to psychiatric nursing* (pp. 333-338). New York: Macmillan.

Percell, L., Bermick, P., & Beigel, A. (1974). The effects of assertive training on self-concept and anxiety. *Archives of General Psychiatry, 31,* 502-504.

Poncar, P. (1989). The elderly widow: Easing her role transition. *Journal of Psychosocial Nursing, 27*(2), 611.

President's Commission on Mental Health. (1978a). *Mental health of women: Task panel reports* (Vol. III). Washington, DC: Government Printing Office.

President's Commission on Mental Health. (1978b). *Research and public attitudes and use of media for promotion of mental health: Task panel reports* (Vol. IV). Washington, DC: Government Printing Office.

Putnam, F. W., Guroff, J. J., Silberman, E., Barban, K., & Post, R. M. (1986). The clinical phenomenology of MPD: Review of 100 recent cases. *Journal of Clinical Psychiatry, 47*(6), 285-293.

Radloff, L. S. (1977). The CES-D scale: A self-report depression scale for research in the general population. *Applied Psychological Measurement, 1,* 385-401.

Rapoport, J. (1989, March). The biology of obsessions and compulsions. *Scientific American,* pp. 83-89.

Rapoport, J. (1990). *The boy who couldn't stop washing.* New York: Plume.

Riessman, F. (1976). How does self-help work? *Social Policy, 7,* 41-45.

Robins, L. N., Helzer, J. E., Weissman, M., Orvaschel, H., Gruenberg, E., Burke, J., & Regier, D. (1984). Lifetime prevalence of specific psychiatric disorders in three sites. *Archives of General Psychiatry, 41,* 949-958.

Robinson, R. (1989). Predictors of depression among wife caregivers. *Nursing Research, 38*(6), 359-363.

Rosen, L., Targum, S., Terman, M., Bryant, M., Hoffman, H., Raspar, S., Hamovit, J., Docherty, J., Welch, B., & Rosenthal, N. (1989). Prevalence of seasonal affective disorder at four latitudes. *Psychiatry Research, 31*(2), 131-144.

Rosenthal, N. E. (1989). *Seasons of the mind.* New York: Bantam.

Rosenthal, N. E., Sack, D. A., Skwerer, R. G., Jacobsen, F. M., & Wehr, T. A. (1988). Phototherapy for seasonal affective disorder. *Journal of Biological Rhythms, 3*(2), 101-120.

Ross, C. E., & Mirowsky, J. (1989). Explaining the social patterns of depression: Control and problem solving—or support and talking? *Journal of Health and Social Behavior, 30*(2), 206-219.

Roth, S., & Leibowitz, L. (1988). The experiences of sexual trauma. *Journal of Traumatic Stress, 1,* 79-108.

Russo, N. (1984). Women in the mental health delivery system: Implications for research and public policy. In L. Walker (Ed.), *Women and mental health policy* (Vol. 9, pp. 21-42). Beverly Hills, CA: Sage.

Russo, N. (1990). Overview: Forging research priorities for women's health. *American Psychologist, 45*(3), 368-373.

Rynerson, B., & Fishel, A. (1993). Domestic violence treatment programs. *Journal of Family Violence, 8*(3), 253-266.

Sales, E., & Frieze, I. (1984). Women and work: Implications for mental health. In L. Walker (Ed.), *Women and mental health policy* (Vol. 9, pp. 229-246). Beverly Hills, CA: Sage.

Sampselle, C. (1990). The influence of feminist philosophy on nursing practice. *Image, 22*(4), 243-247.

Schrader, S. (1990). Ending the violence. *Insight, 11*(2), 11-15.

Schwartz, R., & Barrett, M. J. (1988). Women and eating disorders. In L. Braverman (Ed.), *Women, feminism and family therapy* (pp. 131-144). New York: Harrington Park.

Seiden, A. (1976). Overview: Research on the psychology of women: II. Women in families, work and psychotherapy. *American Journal of Psychiatry, 133,* 1111-1123.

Simmons-Alling, S. (1990). Genetic implications for major affective disorders. *Archives of Psychiatric Nursing, 4*(1), 67-71.

Simoni, P. (1991). Obsessive-compulsive disorder: The effect of research on nursing care. *Journal of Psychosocial Nursing, 29*(4), 19-23.

Simons, A. D., Epstein, L. H., McGowan, C. R., & Kupfer, D. J. (1988). Exercise as a treatment for depression: An update. *Clinical Psychology Review, 5,* 553-568.

Smallegan, M. (1989). Level of depressive symptoms and life stresses for culturally diverse older adults. *The Gerontologist, 29*(1), 45-50.

Smith, M., Buckwalter, R., & Albanese, M. (1990). Geropsychiatric education programs: Providing skills and understanding. *Journal of Psychosocial Nursing, 28*(12), 8-12.

Snipp, C. M. (1990). A portrait of American Indian women and their labor force experiences. In S. E. Rix (Ed.), *The American woman, 1990-1991: A status report* (pp. 265-272). New York: Norton.

Stevens, S. (1978). The mad housewife syndrome. In C. Kneisl & H. Wilson (Eds.), *Current perspectives in psychiatric nursing: Issues and trends* (pp. 83-93). St. Louis: C. V. Mosby.

Stuart, G., Laraia, M., Ballenger, J., & Lydiard, R. B. (1990). Early family experiences of women with bulimia and depression. *Archives of Psychiatric Nursing, 4*(1), 43-52.

Sturdivant, S. (1980). *Therapy with women: A feminist philosophy of treatment.* New York: Springer.

Sullivan, H. (1953). *The interpersonal theory of psychiatry.* New York: Norton.

Taube, C., & Barrett, S. (1985). *Mental health, U.S. 1985* (DHHS Publication No. 86-1378, ADM). Rockville, MD: National Institutes of Mental Health.

Taylor, S. E. (1992). The mental health status of black Americans: An overview. In R. L. Braithwaite & S. E. Taylor (Eds.), *Health issues in the black community* (pp. 20-34). San Francisco: Jossey-Bass.

Telch, M., Lucas, J., & Nelson, P. (1989). Nonclinical panic in college students: An investigation of prevalence and symptomatology. *Journal of Abnormal Psychology, 98*(3), 300-306.

Tennant, C., Bebbington, P., & Hurry, J. (1982). Female vulnerability to neurosis: The influence of social roles. *Australian & New Zealand Journal of Psychiatry, 16*(3), 135-140.

Terman, M., Quitkin, F. M., Terman, J. S., Steward, J. W., & McGrath, P. J. (1987). A comparison of normal, bipolar, and seasonal affective disorder subjects using the Seasonal Pattern Assessment Questionnaire. *Journal of Affective Disorders, 14,* 257-264.

Thoits, P. A. (1983). Multiple identities and psychological well-being. *American Sociological Review, 48*(2), 174-187.

Tirrell, C., & DeForest, D. (1987). Neuroendocrine factors in affective disorder. *Archives of Psychiatric Nursing, I*(4), 225-229.

Travis, C. (1988). *Women and health psychology.* Hillsdale, NJ: Lawrence Erlbaum.

Tregeman, S., & Kassinone, H. (1977). Effects of assertive training and cognitive components of rational therapy on assertive behaviors and interpersonal anxiety. *Psychological Reports, 49,* 535-542.

Trotman, F., & Gallagher, A. (1987). Group therapy with black women. In C. Brody (Ed.), *Women's therapy groups* (pp. 118-131). New York: Springer.

Turner, R. J., & Avison, W. R. (1989). Gender and depression: Assessing exposure and vulnerability to life events in a chronically strained population. *Journal of Nervous and Mental Disorders, 177*(8), 443-455.

U.S. Department of Health and Human Services. (1988). *Chart series book.* Washington, DC: Government Printing Office.

U.S. Department of Health and Human Services. (1990). *Monthly vital statistics report* (Vol. 38, No. 12, Suppl. 2). Washington, DC: National Center for Health Statistics, U.S. Government Printing Office.

U.S. Department of Justice. (1991). *Criminal victimization in the United States: 1973-88 trends.* Washington, DC: Government Printing Office.

Walker, L. (1984). *Women and mental health policy* (Vol. 9). Beverly Hills, CA: Sage.

Warner, D. R. (1988, January). Walking to better health. *American Journal of Nursing,* pp. 64-66.

Warren, B. J. (1994). Depression and African-American women. *Journal of Psychosocial Nursing, 32*(3), 29-33.

Weinraub, N., & Brown, L. (1983). The development of sexrole stereotypes in children: Crushing realities. In V. Franks & E. Rothblum (Eds.), *The stereotyping of women* (pp. 30-58). New York: Springer.

Weiss, C., & Jamieson, N. (1989). Women, subjective depression, and water exercise. *Health Care for Women International, 10*(1), 75-88.

Weissman, M. (1987). Advances in psychiatric epidemiology: Rates and risks for major depression. *American Journal of Public Health, 77*(4), 445-451.

Weissman, M. (1990). Epidemiology of panic disorder and agoraphobia. *Psychiatric Medicine, 8*(2), 3-14.

Weissman, M., Leaf, P., Bruce, M., & Florio, L. (1988). The epidemiology of dysthymia in five communities: Rates, risks, comorbidity, and treatment. *American Journal of Psychiatry, 145*(7), 815-819.

Whitley, G. (1989). Anxiety: Defining the diagnosis. *Journal of Psychosocial Nursing, 27*(10), 7-12.

Williamson, D. (1990). *Assessment of eating disorders.* New York: Pergamon.

Williamson, D., Davis, C., Goreczny, A., & Blouin, D. (1989). Body-image disturbances in bulimia nervosa: Influences of actual body size. *Journal of Abnormal Psychology, 98*(1), 97-99.

Wilson, H. (1989). Family caregiving for a relative with Alzheimer's dementia: Coping with negative choices. *Nursing Research, 38*(2), 94-98.

Wolfe, J. (1987). Cognitive-behavioral group therapy for women. In C. Brody (Ed.), *Women's therapy groups* (pp. 163-173). New York: Springer.

Wolpe, J. (1958). *Psychotherapy by reciprocal inhibition.* Stanford, CA: Stanford University Press.

Wood, W. (1990). The diagnosis and management of panic disorder. *Psychiatric Medicine, 8*(3), 197-209.

Yesavage, J., Brink, T. L., Rose, T. L., Lum, O., Huang, V., Adley, M., & Leirer, V. O. (1983). Development and validation of a geriatric depression screening scale: A preliminary report. *Journal of Psychiatric Research, 17*(1), 37-49.

Zellner, D., Harner, D., & Adler, R. (1989). Effects of eating abnormalities and gender on perceptions of desirable body shape. *Journal of Abnormal Psychology, 98*(1), 93-96.

Zung, W. (1965). A self-rating depression scale. *Archives of General Psychiatry, 12*(1), 63-70.

Supplemental Readings

Blazer, D., & Williams, C. (1980). Epidemiology of depression and dysphoria in an elderly population. *American Journal of Psychiatry, 137,* 439-443.

Brown, G., Bhrolchain, M., & Harris, T. (1975). Social class and psychiatric disturbance among women in an urban population. *Sociology, 9*(2), 225-254.

Chesler, P. (1972). *Women and madness.* Garden City, NY: Doubleday.

Chodorow, N. (1978). *The reproduction of mothering: Psychoanalysis and the sociology of gender.* Berkeley: University of California Press.

Dinnerstein, D. (1976). *The mermaid and the minotaur: Sexual arrangements and human malaise.* New York: Harper & Row.

Dohrenwend, B. P., & Dohrenwend, B. S. (1965). The problem of validity in field studies of psychological disorders. *Journal of Abnormal Psychology, 70,* 52-69.

Elkin, I., Shea, T., Watkins, J., Imber, S., Sotsky, S., Collins, J. F., Glass, D. R., Pilkonis, P. A., Leber, W. R., Docherty, J. P., Fiester, S. J., & Perloft, M. (1989). National Institute of Mental Health treatment of depression collaborative research program: General effectiveness of treatments. *Archives of General Psychiatry, 46,* 971-982.

Fopma-Loy, J. (1989). Geropsychiatric nursing: Focus and setting. *Archives of Psychiatric Nursing, 3*(4), 183-190.

Gilbert, L. (1979). Feminist therapy. In A. Brodsky & R. Hare-Mustin (Eds.), *Women in psychotherapy* (pp. 245-265). New York: Guilford.

Gilligan, C. (1982). *In a different voice: Psychological theory and women's development.* Cambridge, MA: Harvard University Press.

Gordon, V. (1982). Themes and cohesiveness observed in a depressed women's support group. *Issues in Mental Health Nursing, 4,* 115-125.

Gulesserian, B., & Warren, C. (1987). Coping resources of depressed patients. *Archives of Psychiatric Nursing, 1*(6), 392-398.

Halleck, S. (1978). Therapy is the handmaiden of the status quo. In B. Backer, P. Dubbert, & E. Eisenman (Eds.), *Psychiatric/mental health nursing* (pp. 434-444). New York: Van Nostrand.

Jahoda, M. (1958). *Current concepts of positive mental health.* New York: Basic Books.

Joyce, T., & Mocan, N. (1990). The impact of legalized abortion on adolescent childbearing in New York City. *American Journal of Public Health, 80*(3), 273-278.

Koss, M. P. (1990). The women's mental health research agenda: Violence against women. *American Psychologist, 45*(3), 374-380.

Lerner, H. G. (1988). *Women in therapy.* Northvale, NJ: Jason Aronson.

Levine, S. (1974). Sexism and psychiatry. *American Journal of Orthopsychiatry, 44,* 327-336.

Lewinsohn, P. M. (1974). Clinical and theoretical aspects of depression. In R. S. Calhoun, H. E. Adams, & R. M. Metchell (Eds.), *Innovative treatment methods in psychopathology* (pp. 63-120). New York: John Wiley.

Miller, J. B. (1976). *Toward a new psychology of women.* Boston: Beacon.

Moss, M., & Frieze, I. (1984). *College students' perceptions of career success strategies for male and female occupations.* Unpublished manuscript, University of Pittsburgh.

Murray, C. (1984). *Losing ground.* New York: Basic Books.

Parmelee, P., Ratz, I., & Lawton, M. (1989). Depression among institutionalized aged: Assessment and prevalence estimation. *Journal of Gerontology, 44*(1), 22-29.

Pearlin, R., & Schooler, C. (1978). The structure of coping. *Journal of Health and Social Behavior, 19*(1), 221.

Preston, D., & Dellasega, C. (1990). Elderly women and stress: Does marriage make a difference? *Journal of Gerontological Nursing, 16*(4), 26-32.

Russo, N., & Olmedo, E. (1983). Women's utilization of outpatient psychiatric services: Some emerging priorities for rehabilitation psychology. *Rehabilitation Psychology, 28*(3), 141-155.

Sanchez, V., Lewinsohn, P., & Larson, D. W. (1980). Assertion training: Effectiveness in the treatment of depression. *Journal of Clinical Psychology, 36,* 526-529.

Seligman, M. (1975). *Helplessness: On depression, development and death.* San Francisco: Freeman.

Spar, J., & Larue, A. (1990). *Geriatric psychiatry.* Washington, DC: American Psychiatry Press.

Tavris, C., & Wade, C. (1984). *Longest war.* San Diego, CA: Harcourt Brace Jovanovich.

Verbrugge, L. (1983, March). Multiple roles and physical health of women and men. *Journal of Health and Social Behavior,* pp. 16-30.

Yalom, I. (1985). *Theory and practice of group psychotherapy* (2nd ed.). New York: Basic Books.

Zimmerman, M., & Coryell, W. (1987). The inventory to diagnose depression (IDD): A self-report scale to diagnose major depressive disorder. *Journal of Consulting and Clinical Psychology, 55*(1), 55-59.

16

Women in the Workplace

BONNIE ROGERS

This chapter explores trends in women's work, the effects of employment on women's roles, and common health hazards for women in the workplace. It also describes actions that women, nurses, other health care professionals, employers, and government leaders can take to promote health for women in the workplace.

Trends in Women's Work

In the past three decades, the number of women in the workforce has more than doubled (National Center for Health Statistics, 1989). During this period, such factors as economics, women's changing roles, increased job opportunities, and laws against sex discrimination have influenced job availability and advancement opportunities.

During the 17th and 18th centuries in preindustrial America, women's work was linked to the home and family. Men performed primarily agricultural work; women maintained the home and manufactured nearly all materials used in daily life, including clothing, soap, candles, and shoes (Flexner, 1959). With the advent of industrialization in the 19th and 20th centuries, factories began to produce many of these products, and women then began to devote more time to maintaining a nurturing home environment. However, many women—particularly unmarried women—began to work for mills, trades, and railroads, usually in sales, accounting, and bookkeeping positions (Baker, 1964).

In the early 20th century, more women became involved in social reforms, such as improving sanitary and environmental conditions. They also entered professions such as teaching, social work, and nursing. Few married women worked outside the home because they remained heavily involved in child rearing and domestic work (Fox & Heise-Biber, 1984). Industrialized work was difficult and hazardous, required long hours, and offered few opportunities for advancement, thus providing little incentive for women to pursue this type of work.

As men went off to war during World War II, however, more women entered the workforce and assumed jobs traditionally held by men.

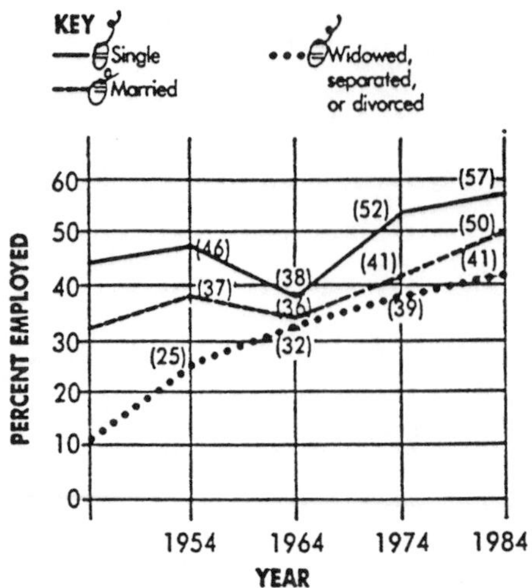

Figure 16.1. Recent Trends in Employment of Women
SOURCE: National Center for Health Statistics (1989).

After the war, many women remained in the labor force. Since that time, the number of women working outside the home has increased steadily, regardless of marital status. (For a graphic representation, see Figure 16.1.) In 1950, women made up 34% of the civilian labor force; by 1984, they accounted for 53% of the civilian force and 48% of the total employed population (Bureau of Labor Statistics [BLS], 1985).

Many factors have contributed to the increased number of women in the workforce, including the following:

- Economic necessity to provide or supplement family income, especially in households headed by single women
- A decrease in births and child rearing, resulting in more time for work activities
- A change in women's attitudes toward work that has favored full-time careers rather than part-time jobs
- A change in family and societal attitudes toward women's roles and work contributions
- The influence of political forces, such as the women's rights movement, that have increased social awareness and asserted women's rights

Even though more women work outside the home, most work in traditionally "female" occupations, such as nursing, teaching, and service and secretarial positions (for details, see Table 16.1). Many women also continue to perform most or all of the work within the home. Although women are represented in all occupations, they remain overrepresented in clerical, service, and sales positions and underrepresented in managerial, executive, and skilled-labor positions. Women are also underrepresented in nontraditional jobs for women, those in which women make up 25% or less of the total number of workers, such as construction and skilled trade work (U.S. Department of Labor [USDOL], 1986).

Work and Women's Multiple Roles

In the past 20 years, increased education, equal opportunity laws, and delayed childbearing have increased employment opportunities for women (LaRosa, 1988). At the same time, the role of the working mother has become more widely accepted, and technological advances have made home-related chores less time-consuming. These changes and advances have simplified women's entry into the workforce.

Many women who hold full-time jobs also retain other roles and responsibilities; that is, many are also wives, mothers, heads of households, and students. Not surprisingly, employed women who continue to bear the responsibility for managing the home and family risk role overload, conflicting role demands, role differentiation problems, and emotional stress (Baruch & Barnett, 1986). For some women, these conflicts can lead to frustration, anger, and anxiety.

Work responsibilities usually require a significant commitment of time and energy and may disrupt family and personal life and create guilt feelings, especially when the needs of family members are not met. This is particularly true for women who cannot separate multiple roles easily or restructure household responsibilities (McGovern & Matter, 1992). Although many employed people can manage household affairs, the amount of time available to spend with children is reduced. (Some researchers assert that this is not harmful to children even though parents may feel guilty [Fox & Heise-Biber, 1984].) Some parents compensate for the reduced time through supportive child care and restructuring of household tasks and other activities. Because most working women do not

Table 16.1 Occupations of Men and Women (age 18 or older) Employed in the United States, 1983 to 1985 (in percentages)

Occupation	*Male*	*Female*
Executive, administrative, and managerial	13.3	8.8
Professional specialty	11.0	13.5
Technicians and related support	2.6	3.3
Sales	9.7	11.2
Administrative support, including clerical	5.2	26.3
Private household	0.1	1.6
Protective service	2.2	0.5
Service, except protective and household	5.6	13.9
Farming, forestry, and fishing	4.3	1.0
Precision production, craft, and repair	18.9	2.3
Machine operators, assemblers, and inspectors	7.4	6.6
Transportation and material moving	6.6	0.8
Handlers, equipment cleaners, helpers, and laborers	4.8	1.3
Unknown occupation and military	1.6	1.7

SOURCE: National Center for Health Statistics (1989).

relinquish their household work, they maintain two jobs. Typically, the division of household tasks between partners is unequal because most men dedicate themselves to their employment, not to household tasks (Fox & Heise-Biber, 1984).

Working women who live with partners must manage not only the home but also interpersonal and work relationships. Pressure and stress may be high among couples in which both partners have comparable occupational success or in which the woman's success exceeds that of her partner. If the partner is supportive, conflict probably will be minimal. However, if both partners are work-driven high achievers, the relationship may suffer. Major changes, such as job relocations, may tax the relationship. Compromise and adjustments are necessary for the couple to continue living together. They may have to alternate employment opportunities or remap their plans in considering each major change. Time management of both the job and household responsibilities is especially important in nurturing the relationship.

Multiple roles and responsibilities require adaptation to minimize conflict and stress. Partners can use several approaches, such as limiting other obligations, learning to say no, delegating responsibilities, sharing more household responsibilities, and maintaining some separation of work and home life. They may need to manage stress related to work roles, especially when the job includes competition, role ambiguity, and role conflict. Unmanaged stress at work can cause psychological strain, job dissatisfaction, and overall frustration and may increase stress at home.

Some researchers believe that women with multiple roles may experience role conflict and role overload, causing adverse effects on health and well-being (Baruch & Barnett, 1986). However, Froberg, Gjerdingen, and Preston (1986) purport that when women perform multiple roles, they receive certain benefits from each role, such as increased social contact and satisfaction, which contribute to better health and to mental well-being. Social support at work from supervisors and peers can reduce job-related and other forms of stress. These benefits may be enhanced by employers who offer work support groups, counseling and referral services, and job restructuring through task reevaluation and reassignment (Cronin-Stubbs & Rocks, 1985; Norbeck, 1985; Norbeck & Resnick, 1986).

In discussing social support related to well-being in working women, Pugliesi (1988) indicated that employment-related experiences are important in enhancing self-esteem. Autonomy in one's work, work complexity, and variability in work challenge represent important components of self-esteem and self-confidence. From interviews with 534 employed women, Pugliesi concluded that social support and self-esteem had positive effects on their well-being. Marriage had a negative effect on self-esteem, which was attributed to role conflict. However, role multiplicity (for example, wife, mother, and employee) did not negatively affect well-being. The findings suggest that multiple roles affect self-esteem and well-being in complex—sometimes conflicting—ways, thus requiring further research.

McBride (1988) reported role strain (subjective response to external role stress) in relation to somatization (symptoms caused by psychological effects), depression, anxiety, mental illness, discomfort, anger, hostility, and dissatisfaction. Waldron and Jacobs (1989) examined the effects of multiple roles on health through a 10-year longitudinal study of 3,252 women who were between the ages of 30 and 44 at the beginning of the study. Using a 22-item health questionnaire, they found that women with multiple roles had significantly better health. However, the effects of specific roles and role combinations differed according to race. Unmarried white women in the workforce and married white women not in the workforce experienced relatively good health. Black women who had children and were in the workforce had better health than those who were not in the workforce. For whites, parental status did not affect health; for blacks, marital status did not affect it. The positive effects of employment were attributed to providing a buffer against the stresses of child rearing, time away from children's demands, and social support on the job. Waldron and Jacobs concluded that multiple roles had beneficial health effects for mothers and did not contribute to role overload or conflict for women with children.

McEntee and Rankin (1983) surveyed 103 self-identified professional and business women to examine the relationships between multiple roles and mind-body distress disorders and work absenteeism. Their findings indicated that women with multiple roles did not have a higher incidence of illness or work absenteeism than those who had only a single role.

Woods (1985) pointed out that women with traditional beliefs about sex roles may approach role conflict in ways that do not serve their best interests. In fact, they may not be able to resolve the conflict, and their mental health may be compromised through internalization of the conflict. Women with nontraditional beliefs about sex roles are less likely to have mental health problems because they can express their feelings, deal with conflict, and negotiate support.

Using the Cornell Medical Index MR Scale, a 195-item instrument that measures such factors as behavior, feelings, moods, and symptoms, Woods (1985) examined women's mental health in relation to multiple roles. She studied 140 randomly selected married women who were clients at a family health clinic and reported the following findings:

- The number of roles the women performed was not related directly to mental health problems.
- Traditional beliefs about sex roles had a negative influence on mental health.
- The parenting role had a minimal influence on mental health.
- Sharing and confiding with the partner and others had a positive influence on mental health.

Woods concluded that nontraditional beliefs about sex roles were important in protecting the mental health of women with multiple roles, such as spouse, employee, and parent. This conclusion may reflect the ability of women with less traditional views to deal with role conflicts, especially because partner task sharing and confiding had a positive influence on mental health.

Clark (1988) studied 44 working and nonworking mothers to identify attitudinal differences toward career orientation, maternal-infant relationship, and satisfaction with mothering. No significant differences were noted between the groups on maternal separation anxiety, effects of separation on the child, and work orientation. Working mothers expressed more adaptive attitudes to child rearing and more satisfaction with their mother role than did nonworking mothers. The home-oriented, nonworking mothers were more anxious about leaving the child at home even though they believed separation was beneficial.

In addition to the traditional multiple roles that women have assumed, the role of caregiver for elderly parents is becoming increasingly common. Those who assume this role need emotional support as well as knowledge about elder care. Because women provide most elder care—usually in the home—this adds to their role burden (Brody & Schoonover, 1986). Institutions that provide child care facilities and allow flextime, job sharing, and working at home (when appropriate) may help women manage the demands of multiple roles.

Workplace Hazards

Women constitute the largest group of workers in offices, schools, and hospitals and other health care environments. They are also well represented in other occupations, such as housekeeping, manufacturing, and assembly line work. Because each occupation poses different health

Table 16.2 Health Hazards and Effects in Some Occupations That Employ Women

Occupation	*Common Hazards*	*Potential Health Effects*
Arts	Solvent and paint exposure	• Central nervous system (CNS) depression • Dermatitis • Blood dyscrasia
Battery manufacturing	Lead	• Hematologic disorders • Neuromuscular disorders • Adverse reproductive effects
Clerical	Exposure to video display terminals	• Musculoskeletal disorders, especially those caused by cumulative trauma • Eyestrain
	Poor workstation design	• Musculoskeletal fatigue • Headache
Construction	Lifting	• Lower back strain
	Noise	• Hearing loss • High blood pressure
	Chemical exposure	• Asbestosis • Skin and respiratory disorders
	Hazardous positions or equipment	• Falls • Injuries • Electrocution • Death
Cosmetology	Chemical exposure (for example, to hair dyes, sprays, and solvents)	• Respiratory irritation • Dermatitis
Dentistry	Mercury	• Pneumonitis • Neuropsychiatric disorders
	Biological agent exposure	• Infectious diseases
	Anesthetic gas exposure	• Hepatic and reproductive toxicity
Farming[a]	Pesticide exposure	• Blood dyscrasia • Cholinergic symptoms, such as headache, sweating, seizures, and gastrointestinal (GI) disturbances
	Heat	• Heat stress • Exhaustion • Stroke
	Heavy lifting	• Musculoskeletal injury
	Hazardous equipment	• Amputation • Lacerations and contusions
Housekeeping	Solvent exposure (for example, to benzene, toluene, xylene, or dioxane)	• Hematologic disorders • CNS depression • Dermatitis • Respiratory irritation
	Lifting	• Lower back strain • Falls • Lacerations and contusions
Laboratory	Biological agent exposure	• Infectious diseases, such as hepatitis
	Solvent exposure	• Neurological disorders
	Anesthetic gas exposure	• Hepatic and reproductive disorders

(continued)

hazards, a list of all health hazards encountered by women in all occupations would be impractical. (For an overview of the hazards associated with some common occupations, see Table 16.2.) Instead, this section focuses on health hazards for the largest single group of female workers—health care employees—and briefly relates these hazards to other occupations. Then it highlights reproductive hazards, which are of concern to many working women.

Professional and technical workers represent the largest sector of the hospital workforce. Registered nurses are the largest group (989,000), followed by technologists (404,000), managers (199,000), physicians (165,000), and therapists (125,000). Nonprofessionals represent the second

Table 16.2 Continued

Occupation	*Common Hazards*	*Potential Health Effects*
Laundry or dry cleaning	Chemical exposure (for example, to detergents or solvents)	• Dermatitis • Respiratory irritation • Neurological disorders • Hematologic disorders
	Lifting	• Back injury
	Heat	• Heat stress • Dehydration • Fatigue
Nursing	Lifting	• Lower back strain
	Falls and slips	• Lacerations and contusions • Fractures
	Radiation	• Cancer • Sterility
Nursing, medicine, and pharmacy	Biological agent exposure	• Infectious diseases, such as hepatitis, cytomegalovirus infection, and acquired immunodeficiency syndrome (AIDS)
	Anesthetic gas or chemotherapeutic or sterilizing agent exposure	• Chromosomal aberrations • Adverse reproductive effects • Dermatitis • Cancer
	Stress	• GI disorders • Fatigue • Headache
Sales	Stress	• GI disorders • Headache • Fatigue
	Prolonged standing	• Lower back pain • Varicose veins
Semiconductor manufacturing	Chemical exposure (for example, to arsenic)	• Blood dyscrasia • Burns • Cancer • Dermatitis • Neurological disorders • GI disturbances
	Repetitive motion	• Cumulative trauma disorders • Back injury
Textiles	Noise	• Hearing loss • High blood pressure • Headache
	Chemical exposure (for example, to dyes and cleaning agents)	• Dermatitis • Renal or hepatic damage • Respiratory irritation
	Heat	• Dehydration • Exhaustion
	Inadequate equipment	• Injuries • Lacerations • Amputations

a. Farming is included because most farms are family operated.

largest sector of the hospital workforce. Most of them are clerical workers (743,000), nurse's aides (484,000), and employees in food, laundry, and housekeeping services (388,000). Data suggest that women make up 75% of the total hospital workforce and more than 90% of several hospital occupations, such as 97% of nurses, 93% of medical records management personnel, and 91% of dietary service employees (Zoloth & Stellman, 1987).

According to Rogers and Travers (1991), major hazards for health care workers can be classified as biological, chemical, environmental/mechanical, physical, and psychosocial (see Table

Table 16.3 Summary of Major Occupational Hazards for Health Care Occupations

Biological

These hazards include biological or infectious agents, such as bacteria, viruses, fungi, or parasites. They may be transmitted via contact with infected clients or contaminated body secretions or fluids.

Chemical

These hazards include various chemicals, such as medications, solutions, and gases, that are potentially toxic or irritating to body systems.

Environmental/mechanical

These hazards are factors in the work environment that cause or increase the risk of accidents, injuries, strain, or discomfort. They include poorly designed equipment, inadequate lifting devices, and slippery floors.

Physical

These hazards include physical agents in the work environment that can cause tissue trauma, such as noise, radiation, electricity, and extreme temperatures.

Psychosocial

These hazards are factors and situations associated with the job or work environment, such as shift work and sexual harassment, that create or increase stress, emotional strain, or interpersonal problems.

16.3). Many of these hazards are also present in other occupations.

Biological Hazards

Nurses, dental and laboratory personnel, and other health care professionals are commonly exposed to biological agents. Those who work directly with infectious clients or come into contact with infected body fluids or tissues are at highest risk for illness from blood-borne pathogens. Infections can be transmitted from the client to the health care worker by various routes, such as direct contact, needlestick, and inhalation of droplets, and include varicella, rubella, staphylococcus, streptococcus, herpes simplex virus, cytomegalovirus, human immunodeficiency virus (HIV), and hepatitis B virus infections (for details, see Table 16.4).

Hepatitis B virus is the most serious infectious agent that health care workers face (Triolo, 1989b). The Centers for Disease Control (CDC, 1988) estimates that more than 300,000 cases of hepatitis B infection occur annually and that 12,000 health care workers are exposed occupationally, resulting in 600 hospitalizations and 200 deaths per year. Needlestick injuries are a common mode of transmission of this infection (Jackson, Dechario, & Gardner, 1986; Jacobson, Burke, & Conti, 1983; Neuberger, Harris, Kundin, Bischone, & Chin, 1984). To reduce this hazard, employers should offer hepatitis B vaccine to high-risk employees, including nurses, laboratory personnel, phlebotomists, and dental personnel.

Recently, concern has grown about exposure to HIV, the agent that causes acquired immunodeficiency syndrome (AIDS). Current data suggest that the risk of acquiring HIV through occupational exposure is less than 1% (CDC, 1988). However, potentially exposed workers consistently should take blood and body fluid precautions as recommended by the CDC (Lewy, 1991). These precautions include, but are not limited to, the following procedures:

- Wash hands before and after contact with clients, even when gloves have been used. If hands come into contact with blood, body fluids, or human tissue, wash them immediately with soap and water.
- Wear gloves when contact with blood, body fluids, or contaminated surfaces is anticipated.
- Wear a gown or plastic apron if blood splattering is likely.
- Wear a mask and protective goggles if aerosolization or splattering is likely, as in certain dental and surgical procedures, wound irrigation, postmortem examinations, and bronchoscopy.
- Keep mouthpieces, resuscitation bags, or other ventilation devices readily available in areas where the need for resuscitation is predictable. This minimizes the need for emergency mouth-to-mouth resuscitation.
- Handle sharp objects in a manner that prevents accidental cuts or punctures. Do not break or unnecessarily handle used needles or reinsert them into the original sheaths. Immediately after use, discard them intact in a puncture-resistant, needle disposal container.
- Report to the employee health service any accidental needlestick, mucosal splash, or contamination of an open wound with blood or body fluids.

Table 16.4 Common Biological Exposures of Health Care Workers

Agent	*Mode of Transmission*
Cytomegalovirus	Direct contact with contaminated secretions
Hepatitis A virus	Ingestion of contaminated food, water, or milk (fecal-oral route)
Hepatitis B virus	Contact with contaminated blood or body fluids
Herpes simplex virus	Direct contact with contaminated secretions
Human immunodeficiency virus (HIV)	Direct contact with contaminated blood or body fluids
Influenza virus	Inhalation of droplet respiratory secretions or direct contact with the virus
Meningococcal bacteria	Inhalation of droplet respiratory secretions
Rubella virus	Contact with respiratory secretions
Sarcoptes scabies (itch mite)	Direct contact with mite from an infected client
Staphylococcus bacteria	Direct contact with an infected lesion
Streptococcus bacteria	Direct contact with large-droplet respiratory secretions
Mycobacterium tuberculosis bacillus	Direct contact with bacillus or inhalation or ingestion of airborne droplets
Varicella-zoster virus	Direct contact with virus or inhalation of airborne droplets

- Clean up blood spills promptly with a disinfectant solution, such as 1:10 to 1:100 bleach solution.
- Consider all client specimens biohazardous and bag them for transport to laboratories.

Teachers, child care workers, and social workers may also face biological hazards on the job. However, their risk of exposure is considerably less than that of health care professionals.

Chemical Hazards

In the health care industry, women are exposed to numerous chemical agents, such as anesthetic gases, antineoplastic agents, solvents, sterilizing agents, and germicides. Such exposure can harm many organ systems, such as the reproductive, gastrointestinal (GI), endocrine, and immune systems (Brodsky & Cohen, 1985; Landrigan, Meinhardt, & Gordon, 1984; National Institute for Occupational Safety and Health, 1977; Nikula, Kivinitty, & Leist, 1984; Rogers, 1986; Rogers & Emmett, 1987; Seleven, Lindbohm, Polsci, Hornung, & Hemminski, 1985).

Typically, chemicals enter the body through inhalation, absorption, or ingestion. The consequence of the exposure is determined largely by the body's ability to detoxify and excrete these substances. It may also depend on the type of chemical hazard.

Types of Hazards

The American National Standards Institute (1977) has classified dusts, fumes, gases, mists, and vapors as chemical hazards in the workplace.

Dusts. These solid particles are generated by handling, crushing, grinding, detonating, or applying rapid impact to organic or inorganic materials, such as rock, ore, metal, coal, wood, and grain. They do not tend to flocculate (form loose masses), except under electrostatic force. They do not diffuse in air because of their weight.

Fumes. These solid particles are generated by condensation of a gas, usually after volatilization (passage into vapor form) of molten metal, such as zinc, copper, or magnesium, or after a chemical reaction, such as oxidation. Fumes flocculate and sometimes coalesce (fuse or blend).

Gases. These invisible substances, such as hydrogen fluoride, ammonia, sulfuric acid, and phosgene, diffuse through an enclosed space; they can be changed to a liquid or solid state by increasing pressure and decreasing temperature.

Mists. These suspended liquid droplets result from condensation of a gas or from dispersion of a liquid by splashing, foaming, or atomizing.

Vapors. These gaseous forms of substances that normally are solid or liquid result from increased pressure or decreased temperature. Vapors diffuse.

Effects of Hazards

The effects of chemical hazards are determined by the type of chemical as well as by the dose, concentration, and duration of exposure and the individual's genetic inheritance and health history. Not all chemicals are harmful. However, several may have serious health effects when workers are exposed to them for long periods, especially in hospitals (Zoloth & Stellman, 1987). Because chemicals are ubiquitous, measures should be taken to reduce health risks. For example, workers and workplaces should be monitored carefully and protective devices used consistently.

The effects of chemical hazards may be acute or chronic and systemic or localized. They can range from overt clinical manifestations to alterations that are noticeable only at the cellular level. These effects include cancer, reproductive problems, and genetic and clinical effects.

Cancer. Some environmental substances can induce target-organ-specific cancer in human beings. For example, asbestos has been linked to mesothelioma.

Reproductive Problems. Some substances, such as lead, mercury, and benzene, can have adverse reproductive effects, including infertility, spontaneous abortion, and fetotoxicity. (For more information, see the "Reproductive Hazards" section of this chapter.)

Genetic Effects. Alkylating agents and other substances can change deoxyribonucleic acid (DNA), although the significance of the change is unclear. Debate continues on whether the toxic effects on genetic material lead to cancer and reproductive problems.

Clinical Effects. Target tissue damage may occur in several organs and body systems, such as the lungs, heart, liver, or skin. For example, vinyl chloride directly affects the liver, and phosgene produces lower respiratory tract irritation.

Occupations at Risk. In addition to health care workers, women in housekeeping trades, manufacturing, office work, assembly lines, and construction trades may be exposed to chemical hazards.

Many people consider household work to be "women's work"; some do not even view it as work. Paradoxically, more than 1 million household women workers are employed in such paid positions as housekeepers, cleaners, and janitors (USDOL, 1986), and this number is probably underreported. While performing this work, women are exposed to various solvents, cleaning agents, and pesticides, which can be health hazards, especially when used in confined spaces.

Women who work in manufacturing facilities and offices may be exposed to organic solvents, such as toluene, which are used for degreasing and cleaning machinery. Assembly line workers, especially those in the electronics industry, also commonly face exposure to chemical cleaning and degreasing agents. Exposure to these agents may result in adverse effects that range from skin rashes, headaches, and dizziness to such long-term effects as bone marrow depression.

Women in construction trades face other hazards, including exposure to asbestos during demolition work, lime and silica in cement, fumes from welding, diesel exhaust, organic solvents, wood dust, fiberglass, and chemical wastes in the soil.

Environmental/Mechanical Hazards

Environmental/mechanical hazards create unsafe or inadequate working conditions that may result in accident or injury. Currently, the most common work-related injuries for women are musculoskeletal disorders—particularly back injuries and carpal tunnel syndrome—and the effects of electromagnetic exposure to or prolonged use of video display terminals (VDTs—a computerized combination of video monitor and typewriter keyboard designed to speed information storage and retrieval).

Back Injuries

In 1984, Troup reported a high incidence of back pain (159 cases per 1,000 nurses) related to lifting techniques performed without assistance. These lifts were bulky and asymmetrical and required awkward positions. More recently, Agnew (1987) found that although back injuries were the third most common injury, they accounted for the most lost work days and were the most prevalent injury in nursing. According to McAbee (1988), the major factors that contribute to back injury are heavy, repeated lifting, use of improper lifting techniques, and previous back injury. Other contributing factors include age, sex, length of time in employment, posture, and physical activity.

Carpal Tunnel Syndrome

Compression of the median nerve in the carpal canal usually results from tasks associated with repetitive motion, vibration, and forced gripping (Schenck, 1989). It affects three times as many women as men, probably because women commonly hold the jobs that require repetitive tasks (such as typing, supermarket checking, assembly line processing) and tight handgripping of tools.

Effects of Video Display Terminals

Women occupy most jobs in offices, including those in health care facilities. Throughout the country, the office environment has been reshaped by VDTs. Electrons beamed from a cathode ray tube onto the display screen interact with phosphorus in the screen to produce light in the form of letters and numbers.

Problems with machine design and maintenance, work area layout and lighting, and job design (such as lack of control over job tasks and work pacing) combine to produce physical and psychological health problems for VDT users. Although VDTs have made work easier and more convenient, they also have had major adverse effects on the health of users. VDT users have reported the following health complaints:

- Eyestrain and other vision problems resulting from extended screen viewing
- Headaches and musculoskeletal strain, particularly of the neck, back, arms, and wrists, caused by prolonged sitting without breaks at workstations that, typically, are designed improperly
- Increased stress from work reorganization, changes in responsibilities, isolation from coworkers, and requirements for increased work output (Farbach & Chapman, 1990)

To minimize these adverse effects, VDT users should take the following precautions:

- Take at least one 15-minute break every hour or one 30-minute break every 2 hours, depending on the workload.
- Take breaks away from the VDT in an open area, where the eyes can focus at greater distances.
- Alternate 1 hour of work on the VDT with 1 hour of work that requires viewing at greater distances and more body movement (McGowan, 1985).
- Use a radiation and glare guard over the VDT screen.
- Work at least one arm's length from the VDT screen.
- Reduce the screen brightness to a comfortable level.
- Adjust the body position to decrease stress on the lower back (e.g., adjust the height of the chair back or use a slanted footrest).

Occupations at Risk

Besides affecting those in the health care industry, environmental or mechanical hazards may be a threat to housekeepers, assembly line workers and others in manufacturing facilities, clerical workers, and construction workers.

Like nursing, housekeeping and cleaning services usually require heavy lifting, which may cause back and other musculoskeletal injuries. Women on assembly lines or in certain manufacturing facilities commonly face similar problems.

Similar musculoskeletal problems are associated with several jobs held primarily by women, such as cashiers, food checkers, typists, and keyboard operators. Jobs that require rapid, repetitive motion of the fingers, hands, wrists, and arms commonly cause cumulative trauma disorders, such as tenosynovitis (tendon sheath inflammation) and carpal tunnel syndrome. Such disorders are becoming more common among assembly line workers, garment workers, maids, poultry processors, cashiers, and clerical workers. Fortunately, most musculoskeletal injuries can be reduced by enhancing the ergonomics—that is, human engineering in the workplace—for example, by improving tool and workstation design (Knave, Wibom, Voss, Hedstrom, & Bergqvist, 1985).

The United States has more than 18 million clerical workers, and approximately 75% of them are women (BLS, 1986). Although commonly considered safe and clean, office work poses various environmental hazards that are typically unrecognized or ignored. For example, the widespread use of computers in offices has raised concern about exposure to low levels of radiation. Although the risks of low-level radiation exposure are unclear and unsubstantiated, the risks of VDT use include the following:

- Long periods of standing or sitting—sometimes in awkward positions. Prolonged sitting may cause blood pooling and edema in the lower legs. Poor sitting postures or prolonged standing can create postural imbalance, which may lead to back pain, muscle stress, and overall fatigue.
- Repetitive movements, which may cause or aggravate musculoskeletal problems, such as carpal tunnel syndrome or other repetitive motion disorders (Burt, 1991).

For women in construction, the most common environmental hazards involve falls from scaffolds, ladders, and roofs; falls on the ground; being struck by objects; and injuries from hand tools (BLS, 1986).

Physical Hazards

Usually, these hazards involve heat, cold, noise, or radiation. In the workplace, women primarily hold jobs that expose them to noise and radiation.

Noise

Noise is excessive or undesirable sound. Noise exposure can occur in any environment with an excessive sound level, causing hearing loss and psychological stress. For example, critical care nurses often complain about noise from medical equipment.

Hearing loss results from acoustic trauma. It may occur instantly from a sharp, loud noise, such as an explosion, or it may occur progressively from long-term exposure to excessive noise (McCandless & Butler, 1983). Progressive hearing loss is more common, and its severity depends on the intensity, frequency, and duration of noise exposure. It produces no pain even though sensory cells are damaged. However, it may cause tinnitus and slightly diminished hearing. The absence of pain makes progressive noise-induced hearing loss particularly insidious because it usually is noticed only after considerable permanent damage has occurred.

Sound is measured by frequency, or pitch, in hertz (Hz) and by magnitude of pressure in decibels (dB). Industrial noise usually impairs hearing at relatively high frequencies and causes maximum hearing loss at around 4,000 Hz. When measured with audiometric instruments, the threshold of hearing (the level at which audiometric tones first can be heard) normally occurs at roughly 0 dB (Berger & Royster, 1988). An overall estimate of hearing loss is calculated by averaging thresholds of hearing from 500 to 2,000 Hz. For normal hearing, the threshold ranges from 0 to 25 dB; for slight hearing loss, from 25 to 40 dB; for mild loss, from 40 to 55 dB; for moderate loss, from 55 to 70 dB; for severe loss, from 70 to 90 dB; and for profound loss, greater than 90 dB (see Figure 16.2). However, loss of hearing of higher frequencies may produce greater functional impairment because the person cannot clearly hear high-pitched sounds, such as children's and some adult's voices, rustling leaves, and some musical instruments (Berger & Royster, 1988) (for more information, see Table 16.5).

Since the early 1980s, the Occupational Safety and Health Administration (OSHA, 1983) has required that sound levels be measured on an 8-hour, time-weighted average (TWA), which is the exposure level averaged over time. It also has required that the TWA does not exceed 90 dB. OSHA has limited exposure to 115 dB to no more than 15 minutes. It has also limited exposure to impulsive or impact noise to no more than 100 impulses with a peak sound level of 140 dB. Employee exposure to noise above the permissible exposure level (PEL) must be reduced to within permissible limits by engineering or administrative controls. When these controls cannot reduce employee exposure to within the PEL, they must be supplemented with personal protective equipment.

The OSHA hearing conservation program indicates that when employee noise exposure equals or exceeds a TWA of 85 dB, protective and monitoring measures must be implemented. Although the 8-hour, TWA PEL is 90 dB, 85 dB is the trigger level for a formal OSHA-defined hearing conservation program. The intent of this program is to prevent hearing impairment in additional workers.

In environments where noise is potentially damaging, employees should wear a personal protective device: earplugs, which are inserted

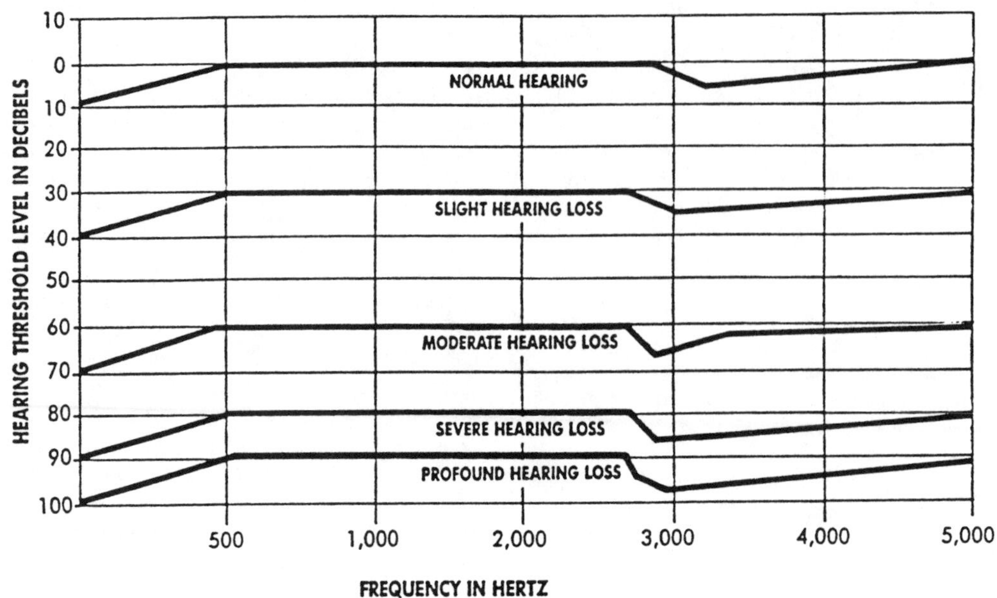

Figure 16.2. Degrees of Hearing Loss
SOURCE: Adapted from Berger and Royster (1988).

Table 16.5 Common Sounds[a] and Their Effects

Sound	*Decibels*	*Effects*
	140	Pain threshold
Jet takeoff	130	
	120	
Large stamping press	110	Short exposure can cause permanent hearing loss.
Chain saw	100	Prolonged exposure can cause moderate to severe hearing loss. Hearing protectors may help prevent some loss.
Concrete drilling	90	Prolonged exposure can cause mild to moderate hearing loss. Hearing protectors are required.
Vacuum cleaner	80	Prolonged exposure can cause slight hearing loss. Hearing protectors are recommended.
	70	
Conversation	60	No effect on hearing
	50	
Soft whisper	40	No effect on hearing
Crunchy breakfast cereal	30	No effect on hearing
	20	
	10	
	0	Threshold of hearing

SOURCE: Adapted from Berger and Royster (1988).
a. Measured in decibels from the threshold of hearing to the threshold of pain.

into the ear, or earmuffs, which cover the external ear. For maximum protection, employees can use both devices simultaneously (Hamernik & Davis, 1988).

Radiation

Ubiquitous in the environment, radiation can be categorized as ionizing (able to ionize or split electrons off atoms) or nonionizing (unable to ionize atoms).

Ionizing Radiation. When ionizing radiation strikes living tissue cells, it can kill them directly (for example, by causing burns or hair loss) or it can alter their genetic material (for example, by causing cancer or reproductive damage) (Upton, 1982). The risks of exposure to low levels of ionizing radiation are not fully known because of the lack of information about low-level exposure and the need for enormous samples to study this association (Land, 1980).

The radiation dose depends on time, distance, and shielding. The greatest dangers to workers are from scatter exposure (small amounts of radiation deflected or reflected from the beam into the immediate vicinity) and accidental exposure by inadvertently entering an area not marked as a radiation area or by equipment that is not maintained properly. Workers at relatively high risk for exposure include those in diagnostic radiology (including radiography, fluoroscopy, and angiography; dental radiography; and computed tomography), in nuclear medicine (such as centers that use radioisotope implants), and in radiopharmaceutical laboratories. They should be monitored carefully by occupational health personnel for exposure at their workstations, which also should be assessed for radiation safety.

Different sources of radiation produce different amounts of radiation. General background radiation in the environment from rocks, building materials, radon, and the human body accounts for about 100 to 150 millirems (mrems) per year. The average chest X ray produces approximately 30 mrems of radiation exposure. The Nuclear Regulatory Commission has set maximum exposure limits of 500 mrems per year for occupational exposure to ionizing radiation and 125 mrem per quarter for nonoccupational exposure (Upton, 1982).

For employees who may be exposed to ionizing radiation from X rays and radioisotopes, Lewy (1991) strongly recommends the following protective measures:

- Ensure that rooms with radiation sources are marked properly and entered only by authorized personnel.
- Have the client or family member hold X-ray films in place. If the client must be held, ask a family member to do so. If a staff member must hold the film or client, plan to rotate this task to minimize the dose per individual staff member.
- Allow only the client and trained personnel in any room where portable X-ray units and radioisotopes are used.
- Give adequate warning to nearby workers when a portable X-ray unit is to be used.
- Ensure that X-ray controls are located so that inadvertent activation of the unit cannot occur.
- Keep X-ray room doors closed when equipment is in use.
- Check the X-ray machine before each use to ensure that the secondary radiation cones and filters are in place.
- Clearly identify clients who have received radioactive implants or other radiological treatments. Also label bedding, dressings, wastes, and similar material from such clients.
- Wear a lead apron, gloves, and goggles when working in the direct field or when scatter radiation levels are high. Expect all such protective equipment to be checked annually for cracks in the lead.
- Wear a dosimeter badge (instrument that measures radiation exposure) when working with or near sources of ionizing radiation. Dosimeter badges should be analyzed regularly by a laboratory with good quality control. These results should be recorded along with each employee's personal radiation exposure and the receipt and disposition of all radioisotopes (Lewy, 1991).

Nonionizing Radiation. This type of radiation is the electromagnetic emission of photons, which generally have insufficient energy to produce atom ionization (Levy & Wegman, 1988). Forms of nonionizing radiation include ultraviolet light, microwaves, laser beams, radio waves, and television waves, which have lower frequencies than ionizing radiation and contain less energy. Nonionizing radiation may be absorbed by individuals and cause changes in tissue molecules, leading to energy dissipation in the form of heat.

Health care workers who are exposed to germicidal lights receive nonionizing radiation from ultraviolet light; other occupations may be exposed to other forms of nonionizing radiation. The source of radiation determines which occupations are at risk, the monitoring techniques that can be used, and the precautions (such as the use of shields or goggles) that may be taken.

Occupations at Risk. Exposure to excessive noise commonly occurs in heavy industrial settings, such as textile and paper mills, furniture factories, aircraft hangars, manufacturing facilities, or stamping operations. Excessive noise also can occur in offices and other workplaces, such as hospitals, increasing the workers' risk of noise-induced hearing loss.

Health care workers commonly are exposed to ionizing radiation from certain diagnostic tests, nuclear medicine treatments, and radiopharmaceutical laboratory work. Many other workers are at risk for exposure to at least low doses of ionizing radiation, such as atomic energy plant workers, electron microscopists, television repair people, nuclear submarine workers, and uranium miners. However, relatively few women hold such positions.

The source of nonionizing radiation determines which occupations are at risk. For example, ultraviolet light exposure results from welding arcs, germicidal lights, and sunlight. Therefore, it is associated with welding, certain health care occupations, and outdoor jobs. Microwave exposure can result from radar, satellite communications, and microwave ovens, so it is associated with the operation of radar or satellite communication equipment and cooking.

Psychosocial Hazards

Stress and sexual harassment are two common psychosocial hazards that working women must face. Both can produce a variety of adverse effects and are common in the health care field and such diverse occupations as manufacturing and office work.

Stress

Stress is any external or internal demand that exceeds the individual's ability to cope or adapt. Rogers and Travers (1991) state that stress from the work environment can be influenced by personal, situational, organizational, technological, and environmental factors (for details, see Table 16.6).

Table 16.6 Factors Affecting Worker Stress

Personal
These factors include demographics (such as age and gender), motivation, health status, personality type (such as passive or aggressive), coping and communication skills, and multiple roles.
Situational
These factors are related to job conditions, such as a burdensome workload, conflicts with managers or coworkers, job dissatisfaction, unreasonable expectations, and tight schedules.
Organizational
These factors are related to business policies and operational controls, such as lack of shared decision making, role ambiguity, ineffective leadership, inadequate resources, lack of opportunity for challenge or growth, inadequate job safety, and poor economic and professional incentives.
Technological
These factors are related to technological advances that cause such concerns as rapid changes in work processes or equipment without adequate training, increased interaction with computers, work depersonalization, and lack of knowledge about handling sophisticated technology.
Environmental
These factors are related to the characteristics of the workplace, such as poor workstation design, shift work, clutter, passive smoking, noise, and inadequate ventilation, lighting, and hygiene.

Work-related stress can be ubiquitous and insidious, producing physical effects (such as headaches, backaches, GI upset, and increased susceptibility to infections and accidents) and psychological effects (such as anxiety, guilt, sleep disturbances, apathy, cynicism, and exhaustion). These effects may culminate in burnout, a syndrome in which the worker experiences emotional exhaustion, withdrawal from work situations, and feelings of failure (Jacobson & McGrath, 1983; Lewy, 1991). Persistent, unrelieved stress can reduce productivity, increase accidents and absenteeism, and lead to maladaptive behaviors, such as substance abuse.

Shift work, a common job-related stressor, occurs in various occupations, including factory work, airline work, waitressing, police work, and fire fighting. However, shift work is particularly common in hospitals because staffing must be provided 24 hours a day. Studies have shown that shift work, especially night and rotating shift work, has a negative effect on health care workers' general well-being and performance. This effect is attributed to the regular disruption of the individual's circadian rhythms, which results in insomnia, altered eating patterns, elimination disturbances, tiredness, anxiety, and depression (Moore-Ede & Richardson, 1985; Siebander & McGovern, 1991). Dunham (1977) also has reported that shift workers tend to have lower rates of participation in social organizations and higher rates of family problems, sexual problems, and divorce.

The same factors that affect stress are thought to contribute to substance abuse. Throughout the United States, substance abuse has become a major occupational problem. Thompson (1990) summarizes substance abuse in U.S. industries:

- Between 10% and 23% of all U.S. workers use dangerous drugs on the job.
- As many as one in five workers in the United States has a drug or alcohol problem.
- About 65% of young people entering the workforce have used illegal drugs.
- About 14.7 million Americans suffer from alcoholism or problem drinking—an estimated 7% of all adults and 19% of adolescents between ages 14 and 17.
- One of three Americans aged 12 or older has used marijuana, hallucinogens, cocaine, heroin, or psychotherapeutic drugs; one of five has done so within the past year.
- Alcohol and drug abuse cost the U.S. economy more than $100 billion annually.

Data suggest that health care professionals are at unusually high risk for substance abuse. For example, scientists believe that chemical dependence among nurses and physicians is 30 to 100 times greater than that of the general population (Cronin-Stubbs & Schaeffner, 1985). Nearly 20% of nurses and physicians are impaired by alcohol or drug abuse, and 67% of cases reviewed by state boards of nursing are drug related (Triolo, 1989a).

Employers may be able to reduce stress and substance abuse in the workplace by developing strategies to deal with these psychosocial problems and by providing employee assistance programs that offer counseling and rehabilitation. (For more information, see Chapter 15, "Mental Health," and Chapter 22, "Drug Abuse Among Women.")

Sexual Harassment

Sexual harassment (any unwanted verbal or physical sexual advance) includes sexual comments and suggestions, pressure for sexual favors accompanied by outright or subtle threats concerning one's job, physical assault, and rape. In the workplace, sexual harassment is a problem for many women (Horgan, 1986). Studies indicate that 42% to 88% of working women report having been sexually harassed on the job (Levy & Wegman, 1988).

In some occupations, sexual harassment may be particularly prevalent. For example, women recently have pursued construction jobs. Yet they still account for only 1.6% of the construction workforce (BLS, 1985). In this traditionally male-dominated trade, women may face isolation, hostility, and sexual harassment, which may be significant sources of stress.

Psychological trauma and stress-related physical symptoms can result from sexual harassment. Both effects are compounded if the woman's job is in jeopardy, if she is forced to resign, or if she is fired as a result of the harassment situation. In one study of 500 women who were sexually harassed on the job, 46% stated that the harassment interfered with their work performance, and 36% reported that it led to physical illness, such as GI disturbances, depression, and headaches (Chavkin, 1986).

Sexual harassment is illegal. It is a violation of rights under Title VII of the Civil Rights Act of 1964 and of the fair employment practice laws in many states. A woman who is fired or resigns because of harassment may be entitled to unemployment compensation. Organized protest against managers for sexual harassment is a protected activity under the National Labor Relations Act. In many instances, however, a woman may need to seek legal help, contact a local or state agency that deals with fair employment practices, or contact the federal Equal Employment Opportunity Commission. Employee assistance programs that offer counseling also may help a woman who has been sexually harassed on the job.

Reproductive Hazards

An increasing number of pregnant women work outside the home, and about 75% of all working women are in their childbearing years (BLS, 1985). During these years, women face various reproductive hazards in the workplace. Some of these hazards can not only affect women before, during, and after conception but also affect their fetuses and children (for details, see

Table 16.7). In addition, some employers may use these hazards to discriminate against women employees.

The effect of work on reproductive health is complex because various work-related exposures can occur. For example, exposure to many chemicals and other substances, such as drugs, anesthetic gases, heavy metals, pesticides, and organic solvents, can disrupt the menstrual cycle or affect pregnancy or embryonic or fetal development (Barnard-Radford, 1987). Another factor that adds complexity is the fact that, initially, many women do not realize they are pregnant and therefore remain at risk for continued exposure to toxic agents in the workplace. Public policies must be developed to safeguard the health of the working pregnant woman and her fetus and to recognize the social contribution of childbearing (Chavkin, 1986).

Table 16.7 Chronology[a] of Adverse Effects on Reproductive and Children's Health

Before conception
Menstrual disorders in women
Sexual dysfunction in men
Reduced fertility in women and men
Genetic damage to male and female germ cells, which can be passed on to children (causing disease or birth defects) or cause spontaneous abortion or stillbirth
At conception
Difficulty in conceiving, for example, interference with the sperm's ability to fertilize the egg
During pregnancy
Spontaneous abortion, stillbirth, cancer, disease, or birth defects caused by substances (such as certain drugs, chemicals, and viruses) crossing the placenta and reaching the fetus or by direct action, as in radiation exposure
During the neonatal period
Toxic effects on the neonate's development as a result of chemicals being excreted into breast milk
During childhood
Toxic effects on the child's development as a result of exposure to substances inadvertently brought home on the parents' work clothes.

SOURCE: Adapted from Hricko and Brunt (1976).
a. The timing of the workplace exposure helps determine the specific effects.

Types of Hazards and Their Effects

Most current knowledge about reproductive hazards comes from laboratory animal studies. Although the study of reproductive hazards is relatively new and measurement of toxicity is still evolving, several biological, chemical, and physical agents in the workplace represent clear hazards to reproductive health.

Transmission of biological (infectious) agents to pregnant women is a serious concern, especially for those working in health care, laboratory, and child care settings. For example, rubella and cytomegalovirus infection are known to cause congenital malformations (Adler, 1986; Brady, 1986; Miller, Cradock-Watson, & Pollock, 1982; Nelson & Sullivan-Bolyai, 1987). Primary herpes simplex virus (HSV) infection can cause reproductive problems for the mother, such as spontaneous abortion. If HSV is contracted in the third trimester, it can cause problems for the neonate during birth (see Chapter 24, "Sexually Transmitted Diseases") (Lewy, 1991).

The adverse reproductive effects of some chemicals and other substances have been known for a long time (for some examples, see Table 16.8). Centuries ago, the Ancient Romans recognized lead as a hazard. More than 100 years ago, European women exposed to lead in the pottery industry were found to be at increased risk for sterility, spontaneous abortion, stillbirth, and neonatal death. At the turn of the century, studies of women exposed to lead on the job prompted several European governments to prohibit them from working with the metal. Numerous other agents such as mercury also came under scrutiny during the 19th and early 20th centuries. Now, the cumulative effects of such environmental agents as organic solvents, ethylene oxide, antineoplastic agents, lead, arsenic, and other metals are suspected of germ-cell chromosomal damage. If conception occurs, such damage is generally embryolethal because more than 90% of chromosomally abnormal fetuses spontaneously abort (Rudolph & Forest, 1990).

Concern exists not only for the pregnant woman and birth outcome but also for exposures occurring around the time of conception. Female hospital workers have provided most of the evidence related to adverse reproductive effects of exposure to environmental agents. Several studies have reported adverse reproductive effects

Table 16.8 Adverse Reproductive Effects of Selected Substances

	Adverse Reproductive Effects								
Chemical	*Infertility*	*Fecundity*	*Mental Disorders*	*Prematurity/Low Birth Weight*	*Spontaneous Abortion*	*Stillbirths*	*Birth Defects*	*Contaminated Breast Milk*	*Animal Studies*
Anesthetic agents	•				•			•	
Anilene			•						
Antineoplastic agents					•	•	•	•	
Arsenic, ethylene oxide					•			•	
Benzene			•				•	•	•
Boron		M							•
Cadmium	•	M		•				•	•
Carbon disulfide		M	•		•				•
Carbon monoxide				•					
Chlordecone,* ethylene dibromide, manganese	•	M							•
Chloroprene	•	M	•	•					
Chromium, copper, nickel									•
DDT								•	•
Dieldrin								•	
Formaldehyde			•	•					
Lead	•	M	•		•	•	•	•	•
Mercury		F		•				•	•
Polychlorinated biphenyl (PCB)*			•	•			•	•	•
Toluene		M	•	•					
Vinyl chloride				•	•	•			•

SOURCE: Office of Technology Assessment (1986).
KEY: • = presence of adverse effect; M = male; F = female; * = no longer manufactured.

for women exposed to anesthetic gases, antineoplastic agents, or sterilizing agents. Substances can affect the germ cell or act as teratogens, affecting the developing fetus. Although environmental agents can affect the fetus at any stage, they are most likely to affect fetal development during the first trimester. Known teratogens include antineoplastic agents, lead, and ionizing radiation. Exposure to organic mercury or lead in the second or third trimester is less likely to cause birth defects but may cause intrauterine growth delay (LaDou, 1990).

To assess reproductive risks, the nurse needs to obtain a complete and detailed health history and to characterize the extent of the exposure through workplace and biological monitoring and observation of workplace practices. To manage the risk, the employer and employee should minimize harmful exposure, primarily through engineering controls and also through use of personal protective devices, such as gloves and clothing.

Discrimination Based on Reproductive Capacity

In an effort to equalize job opportunities for women, Title VII of the 1964 Civil Rights Act prohibits discrimination on the basis of sex. Furthermore, the Pregnancy Discrimination Act of 1978 requires that employers treat women affected by pregnancy, childbirth, or related conditions the same as any other temporarily disabled worker. This law protects a woman from being fired, rejected for a job, or denied promotion because she is pregnant. It also entitles a woman who cannot work at her usual job because of pregnancy or a related condition to the same disability benefits as any temporarily disabled worker. For example, if a man with a broken leg is entitled to job modification, light duty, job transfer, sick leave, disability leave, or health insurance, a pregnant woman must be granted the same. The law does not require employers to provide benefits to disabled workers, but it does prohibit reducing benefits, such as maternity leave (Rudolph & Forest, 1990).

As women have assumed jobs traditionally held by men, more emphasis has been focused on reproductive health issues and fetal hazards. Some industries have developed fetal protection policies that deny employment to women of reproductive capacity and in at least one case required sterility as a condition of women's employment (Murphy, 1990). These conditions of employment appear incompatible with Title VII, which prohibits discrimination based on "pregnancy, childbirth, or related conditions." Although the problem is complex, women are supposed to be protected by law.

In considering these policies, three appellate courts arrived at basically the same conclusion: Policies that target fertile or pregnant women are sex discriminatory, even if the purported justification is a benign one related to health protection (Bertin, 1987). The courts also agreed that restrictive policies can be justified only under limited circumstances and that employers must demonstrate the following facts:

- The chemical or condition poses a significant or unreasonable threat to the fetus, not just a speculative or hypothetical risk.
- Exposure at levels hazardous to the fetus is likely to occur.
- The risk is confined to female exposure. In other words, the male reproductive system is not similarly susceptible to injury.
- A substantial body of expert opinion supports these conclusions to the extent that "an informed employer could not responsibly fail to act."

Workplace Health Promotion

The Occupational Safety and Health Act of 1970 entitles every working man and woman to a safe and healthful workplace. The goal of the act is to protect workers from adverse health effects related to work. Regardless of the workplace, the employer must provide a safe and healthful work environment and prevent situations that contribute to work-related injury and illness. Employers can implement health promotion strategies that help educate workers about risks on the job and methods to minimize or eliminate risks. They can offer preplacement examinations to applicants to obtain baseline health data and make appropriate recommendations for job assignments. They can also use periodic examinations to monitor women who may be at greater risk, such as those who are pregnant.

Education is an extremely important part of a worker health and safety program. The more employees know about specific workplace hazards, the more effectively they can help minimize workplace health risks. All employees should know the general hazards of the workplace, the specific hazards related to their particular job (such as exposure to toxic substances), implications for reproductive health, and protective measures. Preconception and prenatal education and counseling should be offered at the worksite.

Recognizing that many jobs women hold are quite stressful, employers should provide employee assistance and counseling programs for workers at risk. Programs should specify signs and symptoms of stress, stress management techniques, crisis intervention, and referrals for long-term counseling. Health programs should be designed to meet the needs of the target work group while containing costs for the employee and employer.

Although occupational health nurses are ideally suited to influence worker health, fewer than 25,000 occupational health nurses are available at worksites (American Nurses Association, 1989). Employers need to recognize that health promotion services are needed at work and that occupational health nursing is a cost-effective way to meet this need. Nurses in work settings are uniquely prepared to assess the work environment, identify potential and actual workplace hazards, and design and implement health supervision, counseling, education, and related programs (Collins, 1990). Commonly, this is done within a multidisciplinary framework to identify hazards accurately and develop effective risk reduction programs.

Occupational health nurses can use materials that guide effective health care delivery at the workplace, paying particular attention to preventive health care strategies (American Association of Critical-Care Nurses, 1989; American Association of Occupational Health Nurses, 1987). They can consider all aspects of women's health when promoting and protecting the health of the U.S. workforce.

In summary, occupational health hazards to women are ubiquitous and can cause serious problems for them and their families. To improve their health and that of the United States' entire workforce, legislators, policy makers, program planners, health care providers, and the workers themselves must work together to develop and implement strategies to promote and protect workplace health.

The occupational health nurse is pivotal in this movement. The nurse can serve as a catalyst to make the workplace safer and healthier for all employees and can develop and implement specific strategies designed to protect women's health in the workplace.

References

TRENDS IN WOMEN'S WORK

Baker, J. (1964). *Technology and women's work.* New York: Columbia University Press.

Bureau of Labor Statistics. (1985). *U.S. Department of Labor handbook of labor statistics* (Bulletin 2217). Washington, DC: Government Printing Office.

Flexner, E. (1959). *Century of struggle: The women's rights movement in the U.S.* Cambridge, MA: Belkings.

Fox, M., & Heise-Biber, S. (1984). *Women at work.* Boston: Mayfield.

National Center for Health Statistics. (1989). Health characteristics of workers by occupation and sex: U.S., 1983-85. *Advanced data from vital and health statistics* (Publication No. 89-1250). Hyattsville, MD: Public Health Service.

U.S. Department of Labor. (1986). *Facts of U.S. working women.* Washington, DC: Government Printing Office.

WORK AND WOMEN'S MULTIPLE ROLES

Baruch, G., & Barnett, R. (1986). Role quality, multiple role involvement, and psychological well-being in midlife women. *Journal of Personality and Social Psychology, 51*(3), 578-585.

Brody, E., & Schoonover, C. (1986). Patterns of parent-care when adult daughters work and when they do not. *The Gerontologist, 26*(4), 372-381.

Clark, M. C. (1988). Working and non-working mothers' perceptions of their careers, their infants' needs, and satisfaction with mothering. *Health Visit, 61*(4), 103-106.

Cronin-Stubbs, D., & Rocks, C. (1985). Stress, social support, and burnout of critical care nurses: The results of research. *Heart and Lung, 14*(1), 31-39.

Fox, M., & Heise-Biber, S. (1984). *Women at work.* Boston: Mayfield.

Froberg, D., Gjerdingen, D., & Preston, M. (1986). Multiple roles and women's mental and physical health: What have we learned. *Women and Health, 11*(2), 79-96.

LaRosa, J. (1988). Women, work, and health: Employment as a risk factor for coronary heart disease. *American Journal of Obstetrics and Gynecology, 158*(6), 1597-1602.

McBride, A. B. (1988). Mental health effects of women's multiple roles. *Image: Journal of Nursing Scholarship, 20*(1), 41-47.

McEntee, M. A., & Rankin, E. (1983). Multiple role demands, mind-body distress disorders, and illness-related absenteeism among business and professional women. *Issues in Health Care of Women, 4*(2/3), 117-190.

McGovern, P., & Matter, D. (1992). Work and family: Competing demands affecting worker well-being. *AAOHN Journal, 40*(1), 24-25.

Norbeck, J. (1985). Types and sources of social support for managing job stress in critical care nursing. *Nursing Research, 34*(4), 225-230.

Norbeck, J., & Resnick, B. (1986). Balancing career and home: How the OHN can relieve stress to improve employee health. *AAOHN Journal, 34*(1), 20-25.

Pugliesi, K. (1988). Employment characteristics, social support, and the well-being of women. *Women's Health, 14*(1), 35-58.

Waldron, I., & Jacobs, J. A. (1989). Effects of multiple roles on women's health: Evidence from a national longitudinal study. *Women and Health, 15*(1), 3-19.

Woods, N. (1985). Employment, family roles, and mental ill health in young married women. *Nursing Research, 34*(1), 4-10.

WORKPLACE HAZARDS

Adler, S. (1986). Nosocomial transmission of cytomegalovirus. *Pediatric Infectious Disease, 5*(2), 239-246.

Agnew, J. (1987). Back pain in hospital workers. *Occupational Medicine: State-of-the-Art Reviews, 2*(3), 609-616.

American National Standards Institute. (1977). New York.

Barnard-Radford, J. (1987). Women and chemicals. *Occupational Health, 39,* 316-325.

Berger, E., & Royster, J. (1988). *EAR.* Indianapolis, IN: Cabot Corporation.

Bertin, J. (1987). Reproduction, women, and the workplace: Legal issues. *Occupational Medicine: State-of-the-Art Reviews, 1*(3), 497-507.

Brady, M. T. (1986). Cytomegalovirus infections: Occupational risk for health professionals. *American Journal of Infection Control, 14*(5), 197-203.

Brodsky, J., & Cohen, E. (1985). Health experiences of operating room personnel. *Anesthesiology, 63*(4), 461-463.

Bureau of Labor Statistics. (1985). *U.S. Department of Labor handbook of labor statistics* (Bulletin 2217). Washington, DC: Government Printing Office.

Bureau of Labor Statistics. (1986). *Injuries to construction workers.* Washington, DC: Government Printing Office.

Burt, S. (1991). Carpal tunnel syndrome among employees at a window hardware manufacturing plant. *AAOHN, 39*(12), 576-577.

Centers for Disease Control. (1988). Update: Universal precautions for prevention of transmission of human immunodeficiency virus, hepatitis B virus, and other bloodborne pathogens in health care settings. *Morbidity and Mortality Weekly Report, 37,* 377-388.

Chavkin, W. (1986). Work and pregnancy. *Obstetrics and Gynecological Survey, 41*(8), 467-472.

Cronin-Stubbs, D., & Schaeffner, J. (1985). Professional impairment: Strategies for managing the troubled nurse. *Nursing Administration Quarterly, 9*(3), 44-54.

Farbach, P., & Chapman, L. (1990). VDT work duration and musculo-skeletal discomfort. *AAOHN Journal, 38*(1), 32-36.

Hamernik, R. P., & Davis, R. I. (1988). Noise and hearing impairment. In B. S. Levy & D. H. Wegman (Eds.), *Occupational health: Recognizing and preventing work-related disease* (pp. 247-261). Boston: Little, Brown.

Horgan, D. (1986). Sexual harassment. *AAOHN Journal, 34*(2), 83-86.

Hricko, A., & Brunt, M. (1976). *Working for your life: A women's guide to job health hazards.* Berkeley: University of California, Labor Occupational Health Program, Health Research Group.

Jackson, M., Dechario, D., & Gardner, D. (1986). Perceptions and beliefs of nursing and medical personnel about needle handling practices and needlestick injuries. *American Journal of Infection Control, 14*(1), 1-10.

Jacobson, J., Burke, J., & Conti, M. (1983). Injuries of hospital employees from needles and sharp objects. *Infection Control, 4*(2), 100-102.

Jacobson, S., & McGrath, H. M. (1983). *Nurses under stress.* New York: John Wiley.

Knave, B., Wibom, R. I., Voss, M., Hedstrom, L. D., & Bergqvist, U. (1985). Work with video display terminals among office employees. *Scandinavian Journal of Work Environment & Health, 11,* 457-466.

LaDou, J. (1990). *Occupational medicine.* Norwalk, CT: Appleton & Lange.

Land, C. E. (1980). Estimating cancer risks from low doses of ionizing radiation. *Science, 209*(12), 1197-1203.

Landrigan, P. J., Meinhardt, T. S., & Gordon, J. (1984). Ethylene oxide: An overview of toxicologic and epidemiologic research. *American Journal Industrial Medicine, 6*(2), 103-115.

Levy, B., & Wegman, D. (1988). *Occupational health: Recognizing and preventing work-related disease.* Boston: Little, Brown.

Lewy, R. (1991). *Employees at risk.* New York: Van Nostrand Reinhold.

McAbee, R. (1988). Nurses and back injuries: A literature review. *AAOHN Journal, 36*(5), 200-209.

McCandless, G., & Butler, G. (1983). Noise. In W. Rom (Ed.), *Environmental and occupational medicine* (pp. 707-718). Boston: Little, Brown.

McGowan, T. (1985). What we've learned about lighting for office VDUs. *The Office,* 124-125.

Miller, E., Cradock-Watson, J. E., & Pollock, T. M. (1982). Consequences of confirmed maternal rubella at successive stages of pregnancy. *Lancet, 2,* 781-784.

Moore-Ede, M. C., & Richardson, G. S. (1985). Medical implications of shift work. *Annual Review of Medicine, 36,* 607-617.

Murphy, J. (1990). Fetal protection v. women's jobs: Case is before the Supreme Court. *Nation's Health,* pp. 1-4.

National Institute for Occupational Safety and Health. (1977). *Occupational exposure to waste anesthetic gases and vapors* (DHEW Publication No. 77-140). Cincinnati, OH: National Institute for Occupational Safety and Health.

Nelson, K. E., & Sullivan-Bolyai, J. Z. (1987). Preventing teratogenic viral infections in hospital employees: The cases of rubella, cytomegalovirus, and varicella-zoster virus. *Occupational Medicine: State of the Art Reviews, 2*(3), 471-498.

Neuberger, J. S., Harris, J., Kundin, N. D., Bischone, A., & Chin, T. (1984). Incidence of needlestick injuries in hospital personnel: Implications for prevention. *American Journal Infection Control, 12*(3), 171-176.

Nikula, E., Kivinitty, K., & Leist, J. (1984). Chromosome aberrations in lymphocytes of nurses handling cytostatic agents. *Scandinavian Journal of Work and Environmental Health, 10*(2), 71-74.

Occupational Safety and Health Administration. (1983). *Occupational exposure to noise: Final standard* (29 CFR 1910.95. U.S. Department of Labor). Washington, DC: Government Printing Office.

Office of Technology Assessment. (1986). *Reproductive health hazards in the workplace.* Washington, DC: Government Printing Office.

Rogers, B. (1986). Exposure to waste anesthetic gases. *AAOHN Journal, 34*(11), 574-579.

Rogers, B., & Emmett, E. (1987). Handling antineoplastic agents: Urine mutagenicity in nurses. *Image: Journal of Nursing Scholarship, 19*(3), 108-113.

Rogers, B., & Travers, P. (1991). An overview of work-related hazards in nursing: Health and safety issues. *Heart and Lung, 20*(5), 486-499.

Rudolph, L., & Forest, C. (1990). Female reproductive toxicology. In J. LaDou (Ed.), *Occupational medicine* (pp. 275-287). Norwalk, CT: Appleton & Lange.

Schenck, R. (1989). Carpal tunnel syndrome: The new industrial epidemic. *AAOHN Journal, 37*(6), 226-231.

Seleven, S., Lindbohm, M., Polsci, C., Hornung, R., & Hemminski, K. (1985). A study of occupational exposure to antineoplastic drugs and fetal loss in nurses. *New England Journal of Medicine, 313*(19), 1173-1178.

Siebander, M. J., & McGovern, P. (1991). Shiftwork: Consequences and considerations. *AAOHN Journal, 39*(2), 558-567.

Thompson, B. (1990). *Substance abuse and employee rehabilitation.* Washington, DC: Bureau of National Affairs.

Triolo, P. (1989a). Occupational health hazards of hospital staff nurses: Part I. Overview and psychosocial stressors. *AAOHN Journal, 37*(6), 232-237.

Triolo, P. (1989b). Occupational health hazards of hospital staff nurses: Part II. Physical, chemical, and biological stressors. *AAOHN Journal, 37*(1), 274-279.

Upton, A. C. (1982). The biological effects of low-level ionizing radiation. *Scientific American, 246*(2), 41-49.

U.S. Department of Labor. (1986). *Facts of U.S. working women.* Washington, DC: Government Printing Office.

Zoloth, S., & Stellman, J. (1987). Hazards of healing: Occupational health and safety in hospitals. In A. H. Stromber, L. Larwood, & B. A. Gutek (Eds.), *Women at work: An annual review* (pp. 45-68). Newbury Park, CA: Sage.

WORKPLACE HEALTH PROMOTION

American Association of Critical-Care Nurses. (1989). *AACN handbook on occupational hazards for critical care nurses.* Newport Beach, CA: Author.

American Association of Occupational Health Nurses. (1987). *Comprehensive guide to establishing an occupational health service.* Atlanta, GA: Author.

American Nurses Association. (1989). *Facts about nursing, 1988-1989.* Kansas City, MO: Author.

Collins, J. (1990). Health care of women in the workplace. *Health Care of Women International, 11*(1), 21-32.

17

Choices in Childbearing

KATHRYN RHODES ALDEN
BETTY GLENN HARRIS

Contemporary women are faced with a variety of choices when they consider childbearing. Technological advances have made it possible for a majority of women to choose whether to have children, how many to bear, and when to have them. For each pregnancy conceived, a number of other options can be considered: Expectant parents must choose a health care provider, select a place for birth, and decide whether to attend preparation for childbirth classes. In anticipation of the birth, they will need to make decisions about breast-feeding. Those with a history of cesarean birth may consider whether to attempt a vaginal birth.

Nurses who work with women increase their ability for self-care when they sensitize women to the choices in childbearing that are available to them. Nurses are often called on to consult about issues, resources, and potential outcomes for options under consideration. This chapter explores some of the options women contemplating motherhood might face and some factors that should be considered in making decisions.

Preconception Health Care

Traditionally, women have entered pregnancy without specific preconception planning with a health care professional. Indeed, a large proportion of pregnancies continue to occur without specific planning by the parents. Unless there is a history of reproductive problems or a chronic medical problem, preconception assistance is sought primarily for fertility impairments. As information accumulates, however, health professionals and, often, their women clients are putting increasing emphasis on planning conception and on the importance of preconception health care. Such care has the potential to increase maternal health during pregnancy and the probability for birth of a normal healthy infant.

Reasons cited by health professionals for preconception care are to (a) increase the chance of a healthy embryo and fetus, (b) decrease the possibility of maternal illness or complications of pregnancy, (c) adjust ongoing medical treatment of chronic illnesses in anticipation of pregnancy, (d) allay anxiety about potential outcomes, (e) permit needed educational/instructional activities, (f) permit planning for early assessment or intervention for fetus or woman at high risk, (g) foster general good health of the woman and her family, (h) permit desired timing of conception (optimum sperm maturation time or length of time between pregnancies), (i) ensure that needed immunizations or tests are completed prior to initiation of pregnancy, and (j) make lifestyle or environmental changes that are needed.

Prepregnancy health care begins with a comprehensive review of the woman's medical and health history. Information should be sought on family health history with special attention to any report of relatives with conditions such as "slowness," "large head," or "seizures" that suggest a potential for genetic defects. This is followed by the health history of the prospective parents. Special attention is given to previous illnesses, childhood diseases, and immunization history. Attention should also be paid to any history of exposure to radiation or environmental toxins that could adversely affect ovum or sperm, so questions about previous medical treatments, work environments, and living conditions should be included. Finally, current health status should be assessed. Nutritional status, current therapies, and working conditions are all important indicators of physical readiness for pregnancy. Testing should include hemoglobin and hematocrit levels, hepatitis B and rubella antibody titers, possibly human immunodeficiency virus (HIV) antibodies, and urinalysis. With this information available, the nurse can assess potential threats to fetal or maternal health status and plans made, with the client, to deal with identified risk factors.

Preconception care should be part of routine primary care. It may be provided by all health professionals who provide care to couples of childbearing age. Because many individuals who could profit from prepregnancy care are unaware of resources and unfamiliar with the need for planning prior to pregnancy, primary health care providers should be aware of the need and offer care when appropriate. Family planning services should include a brief discussion of preconception services as part of contraception services, and physicians and nurse practitioners should mention the possibility as part of general care. Because many of the individuals who could profit most from planning pregnancy may not have access to or participate in routine primary care, health education classes in the school system could be used to introduce the idea to potential parents.

Partner Involvement

Once pregnancy begins, health care tends to focus almost entirely on the pregnant woman and developing fetus. Therefore, whenever possible, inclusion of both potential parents in preconception assessment is highly desirable. Involving both emphasizes that conception and parenthood are a shared responsibility and fosters joint involvement in planning for a healthy pregnancy. In addition, having both persons present permits each to raise relevant questions and to receive answers directly.

Pregnancy Timing

Timing of conception is important. Congenital malformations have been found to be higher in infants of both very young (under 15 years) and much older women (over 40 years). (See Chapter 19, "High-Risk Childbearing," for a discussion of age as a pregnancy risk factor.) Review of a woman's typical menstrual cycle permits identification of the most likely time of ovulation and thus allows the couple to plan intercourse. Use of commercially available ovulation predictor kits can further help to pinpoint the most fertile period. This increases both the likelihood of conception and that the fetus will be normal. Paternal genetic history, radiation exposure, and environmental toxins are known to have consequences for the quality of sperm, and pregnancy timing may be altered to provide for maturation of the healthiest possible sperm.

Another timing issue relates to the time between conceptions. Very short interconceptional periods are associated with an increased fetal and infant mortality and decreased mental ability in the children produced. This is especially true for birth intervals under one year, when conception would have occurred within 3 months of a prior birth, but the effect is present when subsequent conception occurs within 2 years after a prior delivery. The mechanism is thought to be lack of hormonal regulation, leading to (a) release of "aged" gametes or (b) suboptimal physical or hormonal environment for the developing embryo. Birth intervals of 2 years or more permit complete recovery of the mother and complete hormonal restabilization, enhancing the chance for a healthy conception. Although long birth intervals may be problematic for some women, particularly women approaching the end of their fertile years, very short interconceptual periods increase the potential for fetal loss or infant abnormality.

Nutrition

Preconception health care also provides information about nutrition and permits counseling about needed changes prior to conception. Dimperio (1990) noted that nutritional issues should be addressed because some problems require resolution before conception, and because changes in eating habits is a long-term effort, intervention should begin well before pregnancy is contemplated. Among the issues with potentially negative effects are significant under- or overweight, certain disease states with metabolic or nutritional components, and the levels of vitamins and trace minerals consumed. (See Chapter 12, "Nutrition," for a discussion of these topics.)

Medical conditions such as gastrointestinal disorders, maternal phenylketonuria, or kidney disease, which affect nutritional status, either directly or via the therapy required for their control, should be carefully evaluated and the women's condition stabilized prior to conception. The physiology of metabolic conditions and the pharmacology of any medications should be considered in assisting individuals to plan for a healthy pregnancy. For example, sodium, a mineral necessary for the health of pregnant women, may be restricted in women with heart disease or essential hypertension.

Previous Reproductive Experience

Women and their partners may also seek preconceptional health care because of concerns arising from previous reproductive experiences. Past difficulty conceiving, miscarriage, fetal or perinatal death, or a child with structural or functional abnormalities may cause anxiety about future childbearing. Answering their questions requires a reliable history of the previous episode, review of any relevant records, and perhaps tests that identify potential chromosomal, hormonal, or structural problems.

Having a previous spontaneous abortion (SAB) is the most common reason for seeking genetic counseling. Most spontaneous abortions occur in the first trimester, and approximately half of the aborted embryos have chromosomal abnormalities (Cefalo & Moos, 1988). The potential for a successful pregnancy following SAB is good, however. In a classic study, Warburton and Fraser (1964) found that the risk for recurrent SAB increased very slowly. Specifically, the probability of not miscarrying was about 88% with a first pregnancy as opposed to 76% following one spontaneous abortion. These figures pertain only to aggregates; in any specific instance, if an identified reason for pregnancy loss exists and that cause is continuing, the possibility for carrying a healthy pregnancy may be much different.

Because, in most instances, a chromosomal analysis is not made for a first SAB, little can be planned other than early, careful surveillance of subsequent pregnancies. If chromosomal abnormalities are known to have existed in an embryo, karyotyping or determination of the total morphological characteristics of the chromosomal makeup of the parents is possible. Because there is little therapy designed to change chromosomal abnormalities available, however, couples may enter another pregnancy with plans for early surveillance, and perhaps chorionic villus sampling or amniocentesis, to assess the health of a developing fetus. (See Chapter 19 for a discussion of these procedures.)

For recurrent spontaneous abortions, abnormalities of the mother's genital tract should be considered. If X ray of the uterus and fallopian tubes (hysterosalpingogram) detects abnormalities, surgical correction may be possible prior to attempting another pregnancy. Finally, for second trimester abortions, cervical incompetence should be considered. Careful assessment of a subsequent pregnancy with early, repeated examination of the cervix is indicated. If effacement begins, surgical closure of the cervix (cervical cerclage) may be effective.

Medical Disorders

Preconception counseling is crucial for many women with chronic disease. This is particularly true when the organ system affected will be further stressed by pregnancy, as in women with heart disease or cystic fibrosis, or when the disease is treated with medications that are dangerous to an embryo. A full consideration of all disease states that increase pregnancy risks is beyond the scope of this chapter; this topic is discussed in depth in Chapter 19.

Disease states that compromise maternal function in ways that are likely to be exaggerated by pregnancy are not particularly common. Pregnancy affects all systems, typically increasing adaptive demands on the maternal organism. Cardiac, respiratory, and renal systems are greatly affected, and women with disease of these systems should be carefully assessed. The stress of pregnancy is different at various stages of pregnancy. Prepregnancy counseling permits assessment of maternal physiological status, counseling about the risk to both mother and fetus, and planning for careful monitoring.

Probably the most common chronic disease where preconception care can make a major difference is diabetes mellitus. It has long been known that glycemic control is related to the incidence of malformations in infants born to diabetic women. In an excellent prospective study, Kitzmiller et al. (1991) demonstrated the impact of preconceptional care. Offspring of 84 diabetic women who entered care a median of 17 weeks before conception were compared with 110 infants born to diabetic women entering care after conception. Only 1 of the 84 infants (1.2%) had a congenital malformation, a bilateral inguinal hernia. In comparison, 12 of the 110 (10.9%) born to women without preconceptional glycemic control had malformations; seven of those malformations affected the heart and two of which were lethal. This compares with a 2% to 4% malformation rate in the population at large. The authors concluded that all diabetic women of childbearing age should be made aware of preconceptional services whether or not pregnancy is being contemplated at present.

Environmental Conditions

Environmental toxins in the workplace may affect the reproductive potential of both men and women. There are over 55,000 chemicals in commercial use; many have known associations with sterility, miscarriage, and birth defects. Among the reproductive consequences of workplace hazards are sterility, impaired sexual functioning, miscarriage, birth defects, and an increased incidence of childhood cancer. In addition to chemicals, infectious agents, stress, and radiation are potential problems in the workplace. Health care providers have a responsibility to inform men and women contemplating future childbearing of the risks and assist them in taking steps to protect themselves appropriately. (See Chapter 16, "Women in the Workplace," for a thorough discussion of this topic.)

Care Provider and Birthplace Options

Perhaps no choice is more important for a woman during pregnancy than that of health care provider, because that provider influences all other components of the childbearing experience. Typically, the setting for birth and philosophy of care is defined by choice of provider, and often, so are many specifics of the birth experience. Examples of factors heavily influenced by choice of caregiver are ability to choose types of pain relief, type of fluid replacement during labor, position for delivery, and probability of an episiotomy. Some women, especially those pregnant for the first time, appear to assume that caregivers are much alike and select one with little thought or information.

Although this chapter focuses on women's choices, it is important to recognize that few choices may be available for women without independent financial resources or adequate insurance. Although countries with a national health care system, such as Canada, may have care available, for American women with minimal resources, it may be difficult to find a source of accessible, competent care. Local health departments or medical schools may offer public clinics. The care offered may range from adequate to excellent, but the same individual may not deliver both prenatal care and care during delivery and recovery. Nurses in health departments or other public clinics may provide prenatal care, with physician consultation available, and delivery care may be provided by someone else. Medical school clinic personnel may change frequently as medical students and residents move through their rotations. Physicians in private practice may accept Medicaid reimbursement for maternity care, but because of the low level of compensation and the paperwork involved, many physicians either refuse to accept Medicaid patients at all or limit the number for whom they will provide care. Health care providers helping women to consider childbirth options need to be aware of the limitations that exist and be able to help women assess opportunities for care that are available and learn how to access that care. Arranging for care involves knowing whom to contact, the circumstances and cost of care delivery, and how to negotiate with providers for care that comes closest to meeting women's preferences and needs. Providing such information to women will help them to make the best choices available to them. Even for the middle-class woman with adequate resources, childbirth options are frequently limited by the unavailability of a full range of services within reasonable distance. Caregiver and birthplace options will be discussed as though they were separate, although in fact there is much overlap in provider/place options. The following discussion presents some of the options in care provider and birthplace that may be considered. Much of the data available on women's responses to caregiver and to place of birth are from studies of patient satisfaction. It has been recognized that there are some specific pitfalls to these studies (Drew, Salmon, & Webb, 1989; Lumley, 1985; Seguin, Therrien, Champaign, & Larouche, 1989). Among the more obvious are whether the questions are asked by someone perceived to be reporting to the caregiver, and the time after birth when questions are asked. For most women, there is a "honeymoon" period after the birth of a healthy infant, when women express a more positive attitude about the care received. As that recedes and a more realistic picture emerges, women typically express higher levels of criticism. Each expectant woman and her family will need to consider what is reasonably available to her and make choices within that framework.

Care Providers

In general, three categories of personnel may attend and manage births. These are physicians (obstetricians and family practice physicians), nurse-midwives, and independent (or lay) midwives. Physicians dominate in the management of pregnancy and birth. At present, less than 2% of births are managed by nurse-midwives (Aaronson, 1987) and about 1% or less by independent midwives (Butter & Kay, 1988). This leaves approximately 97% of births supervised by physicians. The Canadian experience is similar; in 1986, 99% of births were physician supervised (*Report of the Task Force,* 1987, p. 11). A comparison of the three types of care providers in terms of training, interventions, approach, clients, and client satisfaction is found in Table 17.1.

Physicians, especially obstetricians, have intensive postgraduate training in the management of pregnancy and birth. In general, a great deal of emphasis is placed on reproduction as a high-risk function and on the more sophisticated biomedical approaches to dealing with biomedical problems. Their approach is typified by vigilance about complications, pharmacological management of problems, a directitorial approach in dealing with women, and a less personal approach than that of other maternity health care providers (Baruffi, Strobino, & Paine, 1990; Dewees, 1991; Sakala, 1988).

Women have emphasized the importance of physician communication skills (Seguin et al., 1989; Zweig, Kruse, & LeFevre, 1986). For women wishing to have their obstetric care provided by a physician, choosing one may be difficult. A common source of information is friends and family who typically have little basis for comparison. Independent childbirth educators have information but may be constrained by political considerations from ranking physicians. Women's groups may keep information on members' satisfaction with physicians, and it is worth asking whether they have such a service. In the end, a woman may have to schedule a "first prenatal visit" and make an assessment at that time. She should be prepared to ask questions about those elements of the management of pregnancy and birth that are important to her. For example, if she prefers an unmedicated birth, she might ask the physician about support for prepared childbirth and whether medication will be ordered without careful consultation with the expectant mother. If support is expressed by the physician, a follow-up question should be asked about the proportion of the clientele who deliver without medication. Furthermore, in a group practice, she might ask whether other physicians' results are similar and, if not, what choice would she have about caregiver during labor and birth. Similar questions could be constructed about other elements of the reproductive experience, and these questions should be asked of other partners in the practice as she sees them. If considering a family practice physician, she might ask which obstetricians provide backup if referral to a specialist is needed. If the answers received are not satisfactory, an expectant mother needs to feel free to change caregivers until she finds someone with

Table 17.1 Comparison of Birth Attendants

	Physician	*Nurse-Midwife*	*Independent Midwife*
Training	M.D.—Extensive postgraduate education with emphasis on high risks of reproduction	Registered nurse with additional training in care of normal obstetric clients	Varies widely from formal training to self-taught
Intervention	Pharmacological management Medical management more often than nurse-midwives Increased number of procedures	Noninterventionist	Prevention, supportive Natural preparations
Approach	Directive, often impersonal May be paternalistic High-risk	Encourage active participation Collaborative	Collaborative
Clients	Low- and high-risk obstetric clients	Low-risk and uncomplicated clients Referral to M.D. for complications	Desiring homebirth Alternative health care
View of client	Wanted improved communication Wanted more involvement in own care Wanted more information	Client satisfaction high	Not known

SOURCES: Adapted from Aaronson (1987); Chute (1985); Dewees (1991); Seguin, Therrien, Champagne, and Larouche (1989); and Zweig, Kruse, and LeFevre (1986).

whom she feels comfortable. Such discussion should occur early in pregnancy so that there is time for any desired changes to occur.

Nurse-midwives, although numerically few, offer an alternative childbearing experience. Nurse-midwife care typically encourages active participation of the woman and her family during the reproductive process, including birth. For women experiencing an uncomplicated pregnancy, nurse-midwifery may be a desirable alternative.

Independent midwives, sometimes called "lay midwives," are a third potential source of care. Independent midwives vary widely in background and training. Women desiring homebirth may find that only an independent midwife will provide care at home. The number of practicing independent midwives is small, and they are concentrated in certain geographic areas, such as Utah (Sakala, 1988), Michigan (Kay, Butter, Chang, & Houlihan, 1988), and California (Mills, 1976).

Health care professionals may be approached about the option of independent midwives or homebirth. If such care is available, it is incumbent on physicians and nurses to be aware of the quality of care provided and to evaluate that care realistically rather than emotionally.

The Place of Birth

For some women, the issue of birthplace is equally as important as the question of health care provider. There are three primary options: hospital, alternative birth center, and home. Because there is a tendency for health care providers to gravitate to a particular worksite, some of the issues involved in this choice have been touched on earlier. Each option will be discussed briefly.

Hospitals are the site for the majority of births. The range of services provided by hospitals, however, varies tremendously. Some small hospitals provide maternity care, but if complications arise and an operative delivery becomes necessary, these hospitals must either transfer the mother or call in personnel to provide anesthesia and operating room services. At the other end of the spectrum, large medical centers are equipped and staffed with specialists to handle any emergent problem on a 24-hour basis, including intensive care facilities for the small or ill neonate. Factors that may affect expectant parents' decisions include geographic accessibility, provision of admitting privileges to the physician of choice, anticipated cost, hospital policies regarding family participation in birth and immediate care of the newborn, visiting policies, and the availability of special services, such as parent classes or lactation consultants.

Many hospitals, in an attempt to respond to consumer demand for a more homelike birthing experience, have developed in-hospital birthing centers. This shift in focus by physicians to a near-total concentration on the fetus as the object of care, with the accompanying routine use of multiple technologies, has become the source of much conflict between health care providers who believe that the provider is in a better, more knowledgeable position to determine what the consumer's childbearing experience will be and consumers who believe that they have the right to determine what their childbearing experience will be. The effect of this attitude was to create a rather widespread climate of criticism and distrust of hospitals and obstetricians (Arms, 1975; Arney, 1982; Ehrenreich & English, 1978; Inch, 1984; Wertz & Wertz, 1977). Many care providers became much more responsive to consumers, seeking alternatives that were both judged safe by the physician and acceptable to consumers. For hospitals, these included in-hospital home-style birthing rooms and a variety of policy changes. Wertz and Wertz (1977) note that the decline in births (which occurred in the 1970s and 1980s) was responsible for much of this change, as hospitals competed for the maternity patients that were available. For example, Pridham and Schutz (1983) recount the experience of one midwestern university hospital where, in an evaluation of patient satisfaction with care, respondents wanted more opportunities to be with the infant and other family members throughout the hospitalization. Policy changes were implemented to respond to those desires. It is also probable that the malpractice crisis of the 1980s, with the frequent assertion that lack of communication was the most common cause for bringing suit, further increased the willingness of hospitals to respond to consumer desires.

Consumers should be aware that there is wide variation in the care available between birthplaces within the same category and even between that given by different practitioners within a particular birthplace. It is not uncommon to find traditional, physician-dominated medical practice occurring in a hospital-based "birthplace." The concerned consumer of maternity care must be prepared to ask questions and do some real research; general reassurances or global promises are inadequate evidence on which to make decisions.

In a hospital with flexible policies, responsive to the desires of consumers, and with physicians, nurse-midwives, and obstetric nurses committed to helping expectant women and their families have an optimal birthing experience, both physical safety and emotional satisfaction are possible. The birthing in-house center can provide a homelike place for delivery, with family participation encouraged and support for each woman's individual efforts provided. Technological resources are available if necessary but kept out of sight and used only with true medical indications. At the same time, all the facilities of the traditional delivery room are available if complications occur, and surgical facilities are available if operative delivery becomes necessary. For the woman at risk or with complications, the hospital remains the birthplace of choice.

Alternative birth centers (ABCs) are another possible choice. Falling midway between the hospital and a home delivery, these centers provide a place for prenatal care, birth, and immediate aftercare of the normal patient. Commonly, midwives practice in these ABCs, with physician backup either on site or easily accessible, or there may be joint midwife/physician practice arrangements. In an attempt to look at the outcome of participation in freestanding birth centers, Rooks et al. (1989) studied 11,814 women admitted to 84 freestanding birth centers. They found an intrapartum and neonatal mortality rate of 1.3 per 1,000 births, a 4.4% cesarean delivery rate, and a rate of 7.9% of the women who developed serious complications. One woman in six (15.8%) was transferred to a hospital. They concluded that the care provided at these centers was safe and effective and provided a reasonable alternative for low-risk women.

Patients often choose an ABC experience because they desire to have more influence over their childbirth experience. Annandale (1987) found that women choosing an ABC often did so in reaction to hospital environments, practices, and the perceived lack of personal control patients would have there. Furthermore, many women specifically preferred a nonphysician provider and, often, a female nonphysician provider. Induction, fetal monitoring, and medication administration were all elements that women choosing ABC care wanted to be able to influence. Patient anxiety often became quite high when the possibility of transfer to hospital arose; uncertainty and ambivalence were common. Klee (1986) compared women choosing ABCs, homebirth, and conventional labor and delivery. She found that those choosing ABCs and homebirth shared critical views of conventional hospital care, but in different ways. ABC choosers wanted the greater comfort and fewer interventions associated with birth there but still wanted the technological apparatus and hospital environment available if needed. Fewer than half of the women initially choosing ABC care actually delivered there. Most, however, were satisfied with their care, having been convinced that the transfer to conventional care was necessary because of risk to themselves or their infant. Women expressed similar reasons for choosing an ABC to Mackey (1990)—a better atmosphere, avoidance of transfer for delivery, extended baby contact, an alternative to homebirth, and fewer interventions and caregivers. Among her respondents, 74% delivered in the birthing center and expressed satisfaction with their care.

Homebirth is chosen by a small proportion of women. The development of ABCs or home-style delivery rooms, providing many of the experiences that originally led women and their families to choose homebirth, has blunted that movement. Homebirth advocates frequently have had negative experiences with hospitals and choose homebirth in an attempt to exercise more control or to avoid repeating those painful experiences. McClain (1983) found that women who chose homebirth viewed medical interventions such as pain medication, oxytocin augmentation, electronic fetal monitoring, and episiotomy as primarily negative. They tended, as did women choosing other birthplaces, to discount the risks and exaggerate the benefits of the birth setting they had chosen. Other research (Arms, 1975; Ehrenreich & English, 1978; Inch, 1984) has shown how difficult it is to avoid medical interventions in hospital settings and the extent to which medical care has become an instrument of social control (Waitzkin, 1984). Homebirth choosers may judge that the risks of homebirth are limited and unlikely, whereas the negative experiences associated with hospitals are certain to occur.

Because of medical control, few physicians or certified nurse-midwives will provide care for homebirth. Frequently, independent midwives can practice only in the home setting. These midwives often provide prenatal care (Sakala, 1988), and homebirth under those circumstances has been found to be quite safe (Mehl, 1976). Some women choose to be attended only by their family or friends and may make extensive preparations for homebirth. When considering statistics for homebirths, it is important to know the basis for assignment to a category. Many states report all out-of-hospital births together, thus lumping together the planned homebirth, often preceded by months of careful preparation, with the unexpected, precipitant labor. Complications are much more likely to accompany the unplanned and unexpected birth at home (Mehl, 1976). Although certainly not supported by the medical establishment, homebirths have provided a satisfactory alternative for some women.

Education for Pregnancy and Birth

The American educational system does not prepare individuals for pregnancy, childbirth, or parenthood, and informal preparation, through family discussions or participation in caring for young siblings or relatives, is increasingly rare for many young people. As a result, individuals contemplating parenthood often lack information about what will be happening to them and how they can best deal with the physiological and emotional phenomena of reproduction.

Nurses, because of their knowledge, communication skills, acceptability to couples, and position in the health care system, are responsible for a large part of the education that is provided to couples concerning the reproductive experience. Indeed, education of expectant and new parents now consumes large portions of nurses' time, either in the provision of didactic courses or in on-the-spot teaching. All professional nurses are prepared by their education and practice to participate in such teaching, particularly the immediate, situation-based teaching needed in clinic and hospital settings. Advanced preparation for prenatal teaching is also available and is especially useful for the nurse teaching in group situations or when a more sophisticated psychological approach, with exploration of feelings and adjustment of expectations, is involved.

A variety of options are available to couples desiring to learn more about the pregnancy, birth, and early parenting experience. Among the potential resources are self-instructional approaches, such as reading, discussion with others, and viewing of films or listening to audiotapes. It is helpful for the nurse to be aware of

Table 17.2 Goals for Prenatal Teaching

- Provide information on processes of pregnancy, birth, and parenting to enhance self-care and informed decision making.
- Create an atmosphere that promotes discussion of feelings and concerns and encourages questions about the women's experiences of pregnancy.
- Foster communication between the expectant mother and her family, partner if present, and health care providers to enhance trust.
- Provide information on health promotion and maintenance skills during the maternity cycle.
- Teach skills needed to deal with stresses of labor, delivery, and puerperium.
- Teach skills needed to care for newborn.

NOTE: Reflecting the client-centered approach to childbirth education, specific goals and objectives are based on the identified and validated needs of our clients. However, the general goals listed above are appropriate to most prenatal teaching.

Table 17.3 Topics for Childbirth Classes

- Overview of conception, fetal development, pregnancy
- Nutrition, including assistance with planning for special needs
- Management of common discomforts of pregnancy
- Information on hospital or birth center—what to expect, precedences, policies
- Discussion of breast-feeding or bottle-feeding, circumcision of male infants, and rooming-in or central nursery care
- Overview of labor processes with description of changes specific to each stage/phase of labor
- Specific tips for mother and coach on handling sensations of labor
- Information on medical management, including medication, fetal monitoring, forceps and/or vacuum extraction procedures, cesarean delivery, induction/augmentation of labor, episiotomy
- Roles of mother, coach, and health care providers during labor
- Overview of immediate postpartum period, including hospital care, baby changes
- Characteristics and behaviors of newborn
- Care of the newborn
- Adjustment to parenthood

NOTE: Although the specific information offered in childbirth classes may differ with the method of preparation for childbirth, a common core of content is generally discussed in all classes, including the topics listed here.

a variety of materials that may be helpful to expectant couples. In addition, childbirth education (CBE) classes are commonly attended by some subpopulations of expectant parents. Effectively helping women and their partners select among the many options available requires that the nurse know the types of classes available and information about each. Because expectant parents are, in general, adult learners, classes that emphasize adult education teaching strategies, such as focusing on learner-defined goals, providing for discussion instead of giving primarily lecture content, and finding new ways to use material learned in other contexts, should be selected.

Common Aspects of Preparation for Birth Classes

There is very little difference in the results achieved by different methods of preparation for childbirth. This may be due to the fact that all methods include similar activities. Although the specific information offered may differ from one "method" of preparation to another, the activities involved show marked parallels. All provide information on the reproductive experience, body-toning exercises, breathing techniques to enhance coping during labor, and information about potential medical interventions. Goals for prenatal teaching and topics generally included in childbirth classes are given in Tables 17.2 and 17.3.

Education About Pregnancy and Birth

A large proportion of all class time is spent in teaching expectant parents about the phenomena of pregnancy, labor, birth, and the immediate postpartal period. Many persons approach reproduction with profound ignorance of what constitutes a normal reproductive sequence and therefore have no basis from which to evaluate the sensations they experience. Lack of information, coupled with the inexorable approach of the time of birth, tends to make expectant parents anxious about labor and their ability to cope. At the same time, general ignorance is often made more distressing by whispers and hints from friends and relatives about obstetric complications and disasters. A straightforward, normal birth seems to cause little comment, whereas a complicated or mismanaged birth is discussed in detail. It is difficult for young women and their partners who are uneducated about the process of pregnancy and birth to ignore the frightening ideas and remember only the normality and excitement of birth.

Childbirth educators attempt to replace ignorance with knowledge and erroneous conceptions with accurate detail. Reassured by the normalcy of what she is experiencing, the parturient woman and her partner can then learn what sensations are to be expected, how these sensations are to be interpreted, and what responses on their part will be useful in dealing with them.

Exercises

This more physical portion of class typically includes exercises that are designed to promote comfort during pregnancy and to prepare for the work of labor. Information on posture and body mechanics is included, largely for the comfort provided during late pregnancy. Typically, information is given on walking, sitting, and lifting objects in ways that preserve optimum appearance, avoid maternal injury, and promote fetal health. Although walking is the optimum exercise for support of circulation in the lower extremities, other exercises can be useful adjuncts, especially for working mothers or those who because of climate or home responsibilities cannot walk enough. A variety of activities for the lower extremities, such as ankle circling or heel pointing, are appropriate. Frequently, information is also given on the cause and management of leg cramps. For example, women may be taught to dorsiflex the foot to relieve cramps rather than massage the cramping muscle. A variety of muscle toning exercises may be taught, including at least one exercise such as bent leg lifts, partial sit-ups, or the pelvic rock, which has the goal of increasing abdominal muscle tone. Other exercises may be included that stretch and tone leg and pelvic muscles (tailor sitting, squatting), expand respiratory capacity ("climbing a rope"), or exercise other muscle groups. Probably the most comprehensive book on exercises for expectant mothers is that by Elizabeth Noble (1982).

The CBE teacher should select all activities carefully. Information about the effect of exercise during pregnancy is accumulating, but there are no general medical guidelines available (Artal-Mittelmark, Wiswell, Drinkwater, & St. Jones-Repovich, 1991). Guidelines for assessing the ability of a woman to engage in exercise are available (American College of Obstetrics and Gynecologists [ACOG], 1985; Artal-Mittelmark et al., 1991). In general, women who were active before pregnancy can continue activities during pregnancy, provided that their temperature does not exceed 38.9° C (102° F) (Drinkwater & Artal-Mittelmark, 1991) and they avoid bouncy movements and deep flexion or extension of the joints. These limits are necessary because higher temperatures have been associated with fetal damage and because the joint changes that accompany pregnancy make them vulnerable to damage when under increased pressure. Exercises may require adaptation as pregnancy advances, and the woman should be instructed to avoid high-intensity exercises during the final trimester.

Preparation of the Breasts for Breast-Feeding

This section should include information about the added support needed by the enlarging breast for both breast-feeding and bottle-feeding women and, for those considering breast-feeding, instruction in nipple and skin care.

Techniques for Coping With Labor

Although education about the phenomena of reproduction and what to expect during the different phases of the experience may do much to diminish anxiety, practice of specific techniques provides skill in those activities that will be useful during labor. It is certainly possible to coach an unprepared woman through labor effectively. However, the possibility of success is heightened for those individuals who approach labor possessing skills that can be used in an essentially automatic fashion. The following skills are an integral part of all preparation for childbirth approaches.

Relaxation. In an early review of the literature, Humenick (1981) concluded that the concept of relaxation is a state of low arousal that is the antithesis of the "fight-or-flight" response and the decrease of somatic and autonomic responses, such as muscle tension, breathing rate, and metabolism. Relaxation is taught in all CBE classes, with a very common form being the progressive relaxation. Training in progressive relaxation is often supplemented by some form of neuromuscular dissociation technique, in which the student is taught to contract certain muscle groups while keeping others relaxed. More recently, to promote options and expand learning possibilities for parents, some childbirth educators have begun to include biofeedback approaches and yoga or transcendental meditation techniques. The parturient is taught to practice these techniques under a variety of conditions, preferably with the person who will accompany her during labor. The expectation is that she will gain skill in relaxation and that during labor she will use relaxation during her contractions to promote comfort, conserve energy, and avoid eliciting the autonomic responses, with accompanying catecholamine release, that can serve to lengthen labor by contributing to uncoordinated uterine contractions (Fox, 1979; Lederman, Lederman, Work, & McCann, 1978; Levinson & Shnider, 1974). Practicing relaxation skills with the individual who will be the woman's companion during labor permits both to learn the skills. It also permits them to learn together which techniques are more effective and to develop ways of communicating about the techniques that will be useful during the stress of labor.

Breathing Techniques. For many couples, preparation for birth is synonymous with learning "the breathing." However, regardless of what breathing technique is advocated, there are a number of basic objectives for training breathing in prenatal care classes. Hilbers (1982) suggests that the method selected should accomplish the following: (a) eliminate inefficient use of muscles so that the oxygen cost of breathing is decreased, (b) include relaxed patterns that enhance opening of airways, (c) maintain adequate oxygenation for mother and baby, (d) augment physical and mental relaxation, (e) decrease or increase neural input from muscle and joint receptors in the thorax according to the need of the mother at a given time (this relates to the concept that alterations in stimulus affect the gate control mechanism and may diminish pain), (f) provide a means of attention focusing, (g) provide confidence building, (h) strengthen respiratory muscles for use in expulsion, and (i) control for hyperventilation or other inadequate ventilation patterns.

If the technique used accomplishes these goals, it does not appear to make a great deal of difference which type of breathing method is practiced. Specific patterns adapted largely from the Lamaze, Dick-Read, and Bradley methods may be taught. It is useful for the labor nurse to be familiar with the methods being used in a specific geographic area so that she can assist the couple with the method they have learned and to which they are often very committed. Attempting to teach an alternative method to a trained couple during labor is rarely effective and is generally very distressing to the laboring family.

Types of Preparation for Childbirth Classes

A discussion of the philosophy and practice of the different types of preparation for childbirth is beyond the scope of this chapter. Classes may be offered that include Lamaze classes, Bradley method classes, or classes that are eclectic in approach.

Although most classes offered to expectant parents involve preparation for coping with pregnancy and planning for delivery, classes and discussion groups are also provided to meet special needs. Among these are early pregnancy classes, review classes for repeat parents, sibling classes, and classes to prepare for cesarean birth. These special classes are outlined in Table 17.4.

Effectiveness of Childbirth Classes

Information about the effectiveness of CBE is often contradictory (Broome & Koehler, 1986; Geden, Beck, Brouder, & O'Connell, 1983; Green, Coupland, & Kitzinger, 1990; Jones, 1986; Leventhal, Shacham, & Easterling, 1989; Stevens, 1977). Precise identification of CBE effects is difficult because attenders at CBE classes are self-selected and tend to be older and more educated. Furthermore, the practices of health care professionals have a profound effect on the ability of couples to use their learned techniques effectively (Shearer, 1990).

CBE classes are continuing to evolve. Geden et al. (1983) reviewed the literature and concluded that breathing patterns, effleurage, and timing of contractions were of limited or inconsistent

Table 17.4 Special Classes for Expectant Women

Early pregnancy classes

- Provide information about the first trimester of pregnancy and preparation for rest of pregnancy
- Emphasis on normalcy of pregnancy, reactions to diagnosis of pregnancy
- Content on nutrition, exercise, lifestyle changes, safe working conditions
- May vary from a single class to a series of four to six
- Peer support

Classes for repeat parents

- Review of content on labor and delivery and practice in relaxation, breathing, comfort measures
- Discussion of issues involved in parenting two or more children
- Discussion of prior birth experiences
- Usually three to four classes

Sibling classes

- Prepares children to attend birth and/or understand hospital experiences
- Discussion of newborn
- Orienting children to the hospital environment
- Must determine what child knows and what child wants to do
- Goal is to decrease sense of separation children may feel when sibling is born

Grandparent classes

- Focus on changes in maternity and pediatric changes
- Goal is to sensitize grandparents to contemporary experiences so that they can be understanding and supportive

Preparation for cesarean birth

- Goal is to assist women to view birth as more salient than surgery
- Content includes reasons for cesarean birth; decision-making process in trial of labor, emergency, and elective surgery; procedures to expect prior to and during surgery; how they may participate; expectations of immediate recovery period, hospitalization; long-range recovery; participation in infant care
- Peer support and discussion of their experiences
- Organization for parents and professionals: C/SEC, Inc., 23 Cedar St., Cambridge, MA 02140

SOURCES: Adapted from Maloni, McIndoe, and Rubenstein (1987) and Spadt, Martin, and Thomas (1990).

benefit and could be de-emphasized in classes. Other techniques that are more effective, including relaxation, husband/partner presence, and sensory transformation, should be emphasized. Lindell (1988) suggested that a woman may cope better if she spends some time becoming aware of her response to contractions "rather than immediately starting a prescribed pattern of breathing"; thus finding her own way to work during labor. Such suggestions, although reasonable, do not seem likely to meet everyone's needs. At present, given the incomplete state of knowledge about the effectiveness of various techniques and how their usefulness is affected by the expectations of the woman and her significant others, the characteristics of her labor, and the behavior of health care providers, a broad flexible program of preparation for childbirth seems desirable. For now, clients might seek classes with the following characteristics: (a) information sufficient to meet their educational needs, (b) a variety of breathing techniques with general guidelines for use, (c) concentrated practice of relaxation in a variety of positions and using a variety of approaches, and (d) instruction in guided imagery (cognitive rehearsal and/or fantasy) and sensory transformation. At the same time, an attitude of confidence and trust should be conveyed. Finally, suggestions for assessing the contractions of labor (their strength, pattern, and the sensations they cause) can be offered. Optimally, at the end of CBE classes, women and their partners will possess information about birth, confidence in their abilities, and a variety of breathing, relaxation, and other comfort techniques to use as needed during labor. Although childbirth should not be viewed as a test, the experience of coping adequately with a stressful situation can provide the woman with a good foundation from which to begin mothering her newborn child (Humenick, 1981; Humenick & Bugen, 1981; Seiden, 1978). CBE classes provide tools to assist the woman to cope with labor to the full extent of her ability.

Health care professionals who work with pregnant women and their families will, of necessity, do a great deal of teaching. They may also offer group classes at times. It is desirable, however, that they be aware of their limitations and be ready to assist prospective parents to find needed information in a congenial setting and in a format that is appropriate for them. Frequently, this will require referral to others for instruction. The health care professional has a responsibility to be aware of community resources, to inform clients about appropriate learning opportunities, and to be conversant with the cost, approach, and information offered in local classes. Women and their families can discuss the content and approach with individual teachers before deciding whether to attend classes, and if so, which to attend.

In conclusion, for women experiencing an uncomplicated pregnancy, nurse-midwifery care is a reasonable alternative. Especially for those who desire an alternative to hospital birth, care by a certified nurse midwife (CNM) in an alternative birthing center may be a desirable approach. Women who wish to participate maximally in their pregnancy and birth may find midwifery care especially suitable for them. Before making a final decision, expectant mothers may also wish to find out about the physicians who provide consultation and to whom she may be referred if complications arise and about the policies and procedures regarding transfer to physician or hospital care.

Vaginal Birth After Cesarean

During pregnancy, parents are faced with an array of decisions, many of which are related to the birthing experience. For those individuals who have delivered a previous infant by cesarean section, there are two available birthing methods for the anticipated delivery: repeat cesarean section or a vaginal birth after cesarean (VBAC).

Incidence of Cesarean and VBAC

During the last two decades, cesarean rates have escalated at an alarming rate, from 5.5% in 1970 to 22.7% in 1985. One third of these were elective repeat cesareans (Placek & Taffel, 1988). Statistics from 1986 to 1988 have demonstrated a less dramatic increase in the overall cesarean rate, from 24.1% to 24.7%. Although the rate of VBAC has increased steadily from 3.4% in 1980 to 12.6% in 1988, the incidence of repeat cesareans has also risen, nearly doubling since 1980 to a current rate of 9.0%. Thus repeat cesareans continue to account for approximately one third of all cesarean births and remain the single most common reason for cesarean section (Myers & Gleighen, 1990; Placek & Taffel, 1988; Taffel, Placek, & Moien, 1990).

Standard of Practice

Until recent years, the common standard of obstetric practice has been to perform elective repeat cesarean section on any woman with a history of previous cesarean delivery. However, in recent years, rising cesarean rates prompted the medical community and consumers to question the necessity of routine repeat cesareans. The safety of vaginal birth after cesarean has been well documented (Eriksen & Buttino, 1989; Martin, Morrison, & Wiser, 1988) and has provided an impetus for the medical profession to reexamine and redefine the former standards, making VBAC the recommended alternative to repeat cesarean.

In 1988, the ACOG published *Guidelines for Vaginal Delivery After a Previous Cesarean Birth,* recommending VBAC as the standard of care unless there were specific indications for cesarean delivery in the current pregnancy. These guidelines reflected changes from the 1982 and 1985 guidelines and extended VBAC to women with more than one previous cesarean. In addition, prohibition of VBAC for any woman with multiple gestation or a macrosomic infant and a recommendation for continuous electronic fetal monitoring were removed from previous guidelines (ACOG, 1988).

When compared with repeat cesarean, VBAC is associated with decreased maternal and perinatal morbidity and mortality (ACOG, 1988). There are definite advantages for both the mother and the infant when the delivery method is vaginal instead of surgical birth by cesarean. There are also specific risks associated with this procedure. Risks and benefits are outlined in Table 17.5.

Table 17.5 Benefits and Risks of Vaginal Birth After Cesarean (VBAC)

	Mother	*Infant*
Benefits	• Mortality rate half of cesarean section	• Mortality and morbidity comparable to vaginal birth without previous cesarean section
	• Morbidity (infection, blood loss, thromboembolic) rate lower than that of cesarean section	• Respiratory complications fewer than with cesarean section
	• Decreased risk of injury to uterus, urinary tract, bowel	• Labor thought to facilitate infant's adaptation to extra-uterine life
	• Less postpartum pain than with cesarean section	
	• Shorter (1-3 day) hospitalization	
	• Cost approximately half that of cesarean section	
	• Psychological benefit of increased sense of control and participation in birth process	
Risks	• Complete uterine rupture: rare, occurs almost exclusively in vertical uterine incisions; associated with shock, major blood loss	• With complete uterine rupture, rapid fetal death may occur

SOURCES: Adapted from Clark (1988); Dahll, Mittal, Grover, and Dahll (1987); Eriksen and Buttino (1989); Haq (1988); Lagercrantz and Slotkin (1986); Laufer et al. (1987); Lavin, Stephens, Miodovnik, and Barden (1982); Martin, Morrison, and Wiser (1988); Miller (1988); Phelan, Clark, Diaz, and Paul (1987); Placek and Taffel (1988); and Stedman and Kline (1990).

Success Rates for VBAC

Reports since 1985 indicate that, of those women selected for a trial of labor, 80% to 81% can deliver vaginally and avoid cesarean delivery (Martin et al., 1988). Women with the highest VBAC success rates (87%-93%) are those who have given birth vaginally before, whether before or after the cesarean, and those whose prior cesarean was due to a breech presentation. Lower success rates are reported for women whose previous cesarean was for failure to progress or cephalopelvic disproportion (CPD). However, studies have indicated that one third to one half the women whose primary cesarean was for CPD are able to deliver an even larger infant by VBAC (Dahll, Mittal, Grover, & Dahll, 1987; Flamm, Dunnett, Fischermann, & Quilligan, 1984; Silver & Gibbs, 1987; Stovall, Shaver, Solomon, & Anderson, 1987).

In those instances when VBAC is unsuccessful and the trial of labor results in repeat cesarean, it is most commonly due to CPD, failure to progress, or fetal distress. Patient request has been cited as the next most common reason for repeat cesarean after a trial of labor (Dahll et al., 1987; Eglinton et al., 1984; Haq, 1988; Jarrell, Ashmead & Mann, 1985).

Eligibility Criteria for VBAC

To be a candidate for a trial of labor, the woman must have a transverse lower segment uterine incision. A classical vertical uterine incision is an absolute contraindication to VBAC, due to the increased risk of uterine rupture. The previous cesarean must have been done for a nonrecurring problem, such as breech presentation, fetal distress, failure to progress, and so on. In other words, the indications that necessitated the original cesarean should no longer exist. A true contracted pelvis, although rare, is an absolute contraindication for a trial of labor. An active case of genital herpes at the time of labor is also a contraindication to VBAC.

In the past, a trial of labor was limited to those women with one previous cesarean delivery and a single fetus in vertex position. ACOG guidelines now extend eligibility for a trial of labor to women with a history of two or more previous cesareans, provided there are no contraindications. Multiple gestation is evaluated on an individual basis to determine whether a trial of labor is appropriate.

Another contraindication is patient refusal after full discussion of the risks and benefits. The physician should discuss the option of VBAC with the woman early in the prenatal period. The woman must consent to a trial of labor; the physician cannot force the issue when the patient is opposed.

The choice of a physician and hospital also affects eligibility for a trial of labor. ACOG (1988) recommends that there must be professional and institutional resources capable of performing a cesarean within 30 minutes from the time the decision is made that a cesarean is necessary. This is an expectation of all hospitals with obstetric service and therefore does not limit VBAC to larger institutions (ACOG, 1988; Martin et al., 1988).

Other Considerations

In past years, there has been controversy concerning the use of oxytocin for augmentation of VBAC labor. More recent studies indicate that there is no increased risk associated with administration of oxytocin for labor augmentation in the VBAC patient with a transverse lower segment incision than in the general population (ACOG, 1988; Flamm et al., 1987; Horenstein & Phelan, 1985). Likewise, the use of epidural anesthesia during a trial of labor has been controversial. However, there is no longer any evidence that epidural anesthesia is contraindicated in a trial of labor (ACOG, 1988; Flamm, Lim, Jones, Newman, & Mantis, 1988; Phelan, Clark, Diaz, & Paul, 1987).

Decision Making

In their 1989 study, "Choice of a Childbirth Method After Cesarean," Murphy and Harvey found that the majority of women perceived themselves to be the primary decision makers for a birth method. Those individuals most influential in the decision-making process were the woman's husband/partner and the health care provider (McClain, 1985; Murphy & Harvey, 1989). The attitude of the physician and the manner in which information is given are extremely important in influencing the woman to opt for VBAC or repeat cesarean (Lipson, 1984).

The choice of a childbirth method is based, in large part, on previous birth experience and anticipated consequences of the selected birthing method. Those women who choose a trial of labor are more likely to view their initial cesarean birth experience negatively and place a high value on experiencing a vaginal birth. Often, their main reason for selecting VBAC is to experience a vaginal birth to participate in the birthing process and because they perceive the experience as a personal, feminine accomplishment. They also wish to avoid the pain, recovery time, and risks associated with cesarean section (Foster, Jacobson, & Valenzuela, 1988; Lipson, 1984; McClain, 1985; Murphy & Harvey, 1989).

The most common reason for choosing a repeat cesarean is to avoid an unsuccessful labor. These women often experienced long, debilitating labors and felt rescued by the cesarean from which they recovered quickly. They are often fearful of the uncertainty of VBAC and prefer the predictability of a repeat cesarean. A repeat cesarean is perceived as more convenient because it can be scheduled to accommodate employment, child care, or other needs. Women who desire sterilization often decide on repeat cesarean so that tubal ligation can be performed concurrently with the cesarean (Foster et al., 1988; Lipson, 1984; McClain, 1985; Murphy & Harvey, 1989).

Women also base their decision on their beliefs about the safety of each birthing method. Murphy and Harvey (1989) found that the majority of mothers who chose VBAC believed that vaginal birth was safer for both mother and infant. Those women who chose a repeat cesarean believed in greater safety of the infant with cesarean birth but greater safety of the mother with vaginal birth.

Implications for Nursing

VBAC is a safe and sensible option for the majority of women who previously experienced cesarean section. It is the responsibility of health care professionals to provide accurate and current information to women and their partners regarding the risks and benefits of vaginal birth compared with repeat cesarean. Education of parents should begin early in the prenatal period and should continue throughout pregnancy. The individuals who choose a trial of labor should be encouraged to participate in childbirth classes and to seek support from other VBAC parents. It is important that the parents understand and accept that a trial of labor may result in cesarean delivery. When parents are well prepared and well informed, they are more likely to experience a successful VBAC, and at the same time are more capable of accepting disappointment should another cesarean be necessary.

The Infant Feeding Decision: Breast-Feeding or Bottle-Feeding

The selection of an infant feeding method is one of the most emotion-laden decisions for parents of a newborn infant, especially for the mother who ultimately makes the decision. Parents view feeding as the focus of an intimate relationship with the new family member. Because feeding is one of the few measurable outcomes of early parenting, perceived success fosters parents' self-images as nurturers and providers. Nurses caring for childbearing women must be informed regarding the advantages and disadvantages of breast-feeding and bottle-feeding (see Table 17.6). As health professionals, nurses are instrumental in assisting childbearing women with infant feeding issues and decisions. Nursing roles include education, counseling, and client advocacy.

Through preconceptional and prenatal education, nurses provide information to women about breast-feeding and bottle-feeding as they foster informed decision making. It is essential that nurses be knowledgeable with regard to both methods and consider the cultural and psychosocial factors known to influence the infant feeding decision as they teach and counsel childbearing women. In working with expectant parents, the nurse should include the father or partner in discussions of feeding methods, realizing that the woman's final decision will be influenced to a great extent by this person.

Whether the mother chooses to breast-feed or bottle-feed, the nurse should support the decision and provide further education as needed. For example, the woman who elects to breast-feed can be directed to breast-feeding classes. When the infant is born, the mother will require assistance from nursing staff as she begins to breast-feed her infant. Support and encouragement from nurses and other health care professionals are factors known to influence breast-feeding positively. Lactation specialists, now employed by many health care facilities, are an invaluable resource for breast-feeding mothers throughout the period of lactation. Organizations such as La Leche League provide education, support, and counseling for breast-feeding mothers.

The mother who chooses bottle-feeding will need instruction in equipment and formula preparation; she may also need assistance with actual feeding methods once the infant is born. As a client advocate, the nurse can direct the lower income mother to the Women, Infants, and Children (WIC) program and assist her in applying for the program.

Conclusion

Health care providers will be consulted about a wide variety of birth-related options. To function effectively in this role, it is essential for the provider to have a wide knowledge about the resources available to the expectant mother and to be able to assist the woman in assessing those options in light of her own resources and desires. When chosen by a woman as provider for care during pregnancy, professionals have a responsibility to clients about their practice routines as well as a continuing responsibility to inform women and their families about options throughout the childbearing process. As Trandel-Korenchuk (1982) notes, many providers assume that informed consent is needed only for high-risk procedures. That assumption is incorrect; consent is needed for a procedure that involves any form of touch. Consent is an irrelevant concept if that consent is not informed. Informed consent, in turn, requires that the individual be informed about the specifics of any contemplated procedure, potential risks, possible benefits, and reasonable alternatives.

Options for families during the childbearing experience are expanding. Although geography, resources, and knowledge may continue to limit the ability of some women to achieve their desired childbearing experience, the options are increasing. Health care professionals can assist by continuing to expand the choices available to women and by informing their clients about the possibilities available to them.

Table 17.6 Comparison of Breast-Feeding and Bottle-Feeding

	Breast-Feeding	*Bottle-Feeding*
Maternal advantages	• Increases maternal uterine tone and uterine involution • Decreased risk of postpartum hemorrhage • Return to prepregnancy weight more quickly • Provides bonding experience • When successful, increases maternal role attainment • Convenient • Less expensive • Encourages relaxation	• Convenience • Opportunity for father and other family members to feed infant • Sharing of feeding allows mother more free time • Easier to determine amount infant receives • Requires less frequent feedings
Infant advantages	• Considered optimal food for first six months • Provides immunologic protection against infection • Nonallergenic • Nutritionally adequate, complete • Less likely to overfeed • Tactile stimulation can foster sense of security • Fosters social interaction between mother and infant	• Maternal-infant closeness can be obtained • Commercial formulas are safe, satisfactory means of meeting nutritional needs
Disadvantages	• Initially can be physically and emotionally draining for mother • If unsuccessful, women may feel guilt, grief, failure • Initial physical discomfort of lactation (e.g., sore nipples, engorgement) • Some mothers have inadequate milk supply • Exhausting initially • Requires large time commitment • More difficult to be separated from infant	• Infants tend to gain weight faster • Cost of formula • Potentially less opportunity for social interaction between mother and infant • Lack of anti-infective and anti-allergenic properties of breast milk
Contraindications	• Chronic, debilitating maternal illness such as myasthenia gravis, lupus erythematoses, neoplastic disease • Treatment regimens such as chemotherapy • Infant condition such as congenital lip or mouth and esophageal defect, both of which interfere with sucking • Galactosemia in infant	

SOURCES: Adapted from American Academy of Pediatrics (1982); Anholm (1986); Arango (1984); Gonzales (1990); Gulick (1986); Hanson et al. (1985); Howie, Forsyth, Ogston, Clark, and Florey (1990); Lawrence (1989); Maclean (1990); and Poskitt (1988).

NOTE: As with any health care decision, to make an informed choice, the mother needs adequate information related to the advantages and disadvantages of breast-feeding and bottle-feeding. Whichever method the mother chooses, she needs support and reassurance that she can adequately satisfy the needs of her growing infant. The success or failure of the infant feeding method depends, in large part, on support the mother receives from her family, including the father of the infant, friends, and health care providers.

References

PRECONCEPTION HEALTH CARE

Cefalo, R. D., & Moos, M. (1988). *Preconceptional health promotion: A practical guide.* Rockville, MD: Aspen.

Dimperio, D. (1990). Preconceptional nutrition. *Journal of Pediatric and Perinatal Nutrition, 2*(2), 65-78.

Kitzmiller, J. L., Gavia, L. A., Gin, G. A., Jovanovic-Peterson, L., Main, E., & Zigrant, W. O. (1991). Preconception care of diabetes: Glycemic control prevents congenital anomalies. *JAMA, 265*(6), 731-736.

Warburton, D., & Fraser, F. C. (1964). Spontaneous abortion risks in man: Data from reproductive histories collected in medical genetics unit. *American Journal of Human Genetics, 16*(1), 1-22.

CARE PROVIDER AND BIRTHPLACE OPTIONS

Aaronson, L. S. (1987). Nurse-midwives and obstetricians: Alternative models of care and client "fit." *Research in Nursing and Health, 10,* 217-226.

Annandale, E. C. (1987). Dimensions of patient control in a free-standing birth center. *Social Science and Medicine, 25*(11), 1235-1248.

Arms, S. (1975). *Immaculate deception: A new look at women and childbirth in America.* Boston: Houghton Mifflin.

Arney, W. R. (1982). *Power and the profession of obstetrics.* Chicago: University of Chicago Press.

Baruffi, G., Strobino, D. M., & Paine, L. L. (1990). Investigation of institutional differences in primary cesarean birth rates. *Journal of Nurse-Midwifery, 35*(5), 274-281.

Butter, I. H., & Kay, B. J. (1988). State laws and the practice of lay midwifery. *American Journal of Public Health, 9,* 1161-1169.

Chute, G. E. (1985). Expectation and experience in alternative and conventional birth. *JOGNN, 14*(1), 61-67.

Dewees, C. B. (1991). *A study of maternity care provider models and neonatal hypoglycemia.* Unpublished doctoral dissertation, University of North Carolina at Chapel Hill.

Drew, N. C., Salmon, P., & Webb, L. (1989). Mothers', midwives' and obstetricians' views on the features of obstetric care which influence satisfaction with childbirth. *British Journal of Obstetrics and Gynaecology, 96*(9), 1084-1088.

Ehrenreich, G., & English, D. (1978). *For her own good: 150 years of the expert's advice to women.* Garden City, NY: Anchor.

Inch, S. (1984). *Birthrights: What every parent should know about childbirth in hospitals.* New York: Pantheon.

Kay, B. J., Butter, I. H., Chang, D., & Houlihan, K. (1988). Women's health and social change: The case of lay midwives. *International Journal of Health Services, 18*(2), 223-236.

Klee, L. (1986). Home away from home: The alternative birth center. *Social Science and Medicine, 21*(1), 9-16.

Lumley, J. (1985). Assessing satisfaction with childbirth. *Birth, 12*(3), 141-145.

Mackey, M. C. (1990). Women's choice of childbirth setting. *Health Care for Women International, 11*(2), 175-189.

McClain, C. S. (1983). Perceived risk and choice of childbirth service. *Social Science and Medicine, 17*(23), 1857-1865.

Mehl, L. E. (1976). Statistical outcomes of homebirths in the U.S.: Current status. In D. Stewart & L. Stewart (Eds.), *Safe alternatives in childbirth* (pp. 127-139). Chapel Hill, NC: National Association of Parents and Professionals for Safe Alternatives in Childbirth (NAPSAC).

Mills, N. (1976). The lay midwife. In D. Stewart & L. Stewart (Eds.), *Safe alternatives in childbirth* (pp. 127-139). Chapel Hill, NC: NAPSAC.

Pridham, K. F., & Schutz, M. E. (1983). Parental goals and the birthing experience. *JOGNN, 12*(1), 50-55.

Report of the Task Force on the Implementation of Midwifery in Ontario. (1987). Toronto: Province of Ontario.

Rooks, J. P., Weatherby, N. L., Ernst, R. K. M., Stapleton, S., Rosen, D., & Rosenfield, A. (1989). Outcomes of care in birth centers: The national birth center study. *New England Journal of Medicine, 321,* 1804-1811.

Sakala, C. (1988). Content of care by independent midwives: Assistance with pain in labor and birth. *Social Science and Medicine, 26*(11), 1141-1158.

Seguin, L., Therrien, R., Champagne, F., & Larouche, D. (1989). The components of women's satisfaction with maternity care. *Birth, 16*(3), 109-113.

Waitzkin, H. (1984). The micropolitics of medicine: A contextual analysis. *International Journal of Health Services, 14*(3), 339-378.

Wertz, R. W., & Wertz, D. C. (1977). *Lying-in: A history of childbirth in America.* New York: Free Press.

Zweig, S., Kruse, J., & LeFevre, M. (1986). Patient satisfaction with obstetric care. *Journal of Family Practice, 23*(2), 131-136.

EDUCATION FOR PREGNANCY AND BIRTH

American College of Obstetrics and Gynecology. (1985). *Exercise during pregnancy and the postnatal period* (ACOG home exercise programs). Washington, DC: Author.

Artal-Mittelmark, R., Wiswell, R. A., Drinkwater, B. L., & St. Jones-Repovich, W. E. (1991). Exercise guidelines for pregnancy. In R. Artal-Mittelmark, R. A. Wiswell, & B. L. Drinkwater (Eds.), *Exercise in pregnancy* (pp. 299-312). Baltimore: Williams & Wilkins.

Broome, M. E., & Koehler, C. (1986). Childbirth education: A review of effects on the woman and her family. *Family and Community Health, 9*(1), 33-44.

Drinkwater, B. L., & Artal-Mittelmark, R. (1991). Heat stress and pregnancy. In R. Artal-Mittelmark, R. A. Wiswell, & B. L. Drinkwater (Eds.), *Exercise in pregnancy* (pp. 261-269). Baltimore: Williams & Wilkins.

Fox, H. A. (1979). The effects of catecholamines and drug treatment on the fetus and newborn. *Birth and the Family Journal, 6*(3), 157-165.

Geden, E., Beck, N., Brouder, G., & O'Connell, E. (1983). Identifying procedural components for analogue research of labor pain. *Nursing Research, 32*(2), 80-83.

Green, J. M., Coupland, V. A., & Kitzinger, J. V. (1990). Expectations, experiences, and psychological outcomes of childbirth: A prospective study of 825 women. *Birth, 17*(1), 15-24.

Hilbers, S. M. (1982). A look at breathing patterns and the behavioral brain. In S. S. Humenick (Ed.), *Expanding horizons in childbirth education* (Vol. 2, pp. 43-54). Washington, DC: American Society for Psychoprophylaxis in Obstetrics (ASPO)/Lamaze.

Humenick, S. S. (1981). Mastery: The key to childbirth satisfaction? A review. *Birth and the Family Journal, 8*(2), 79-83.

Humenick, S. S., & Bugen, L. A. (1981). Mastery: The key to childbirth satisfaction? A study. *Birth and the Family Journal, 8*(2), 4-90.

Jones, L. C. (1986). A meta-analytic study of the effects of childbirth education on the parent-infant relationship. *Health Care for Women International, 7,* 357-370.

Lederman, R. P., Lederman, E., Work, B. A., & McCann, D. S. (1978). The relationship of maternal anxiety, plasma catecholamines, and plasma cortisol to progress in labor. *American Journal of Obstetrics and Gynecology, 132,* 495-500.

Leventhal, H., Shacham, S., & Easterling, D. V. (1989). Active coping reduces reports of pain from childbirth. *Journal of Consulting and Clinical Psychology, 57*(3), 365-371.

Levinson, G., & Shnider, S. M. (1974). Catecholamines: The effects of maternal fear and its treatment on uterine function and circulation. *Birth and the Family Journal, 6*(13), 167-174.

Lindell, S. G. (1988). Education for childbirth: A time for change. *JOGNN, 17*(2), 108-112.

Maloni, J. A., McIndoe, J. E., & Rubenstein, G. (1987). Expectant grandparents class. *JOGNN, 16*(1), 26-29.

Noble, E. (1982). *Essential exercises for the childbearing years.* Boston: Houghton-Mifflin.

Seiden, A. M. (1978). The sense of mastery in the childbirth experience. In M. T. Notman & C. C. Nadelson (Eds.), *The woman patient* (Vol. I, pp. 87-105). New York: Plenum.

Shearer, M. H. (1990). Effects of prenatal education depend on the attitudes and practices of obstetric caregivers. *Birth, 17*(2), 73-74.

Stevens, R. J. (1977). Psychological strategies for management of pain in prepared childbirth: I. A review of the research. *Birth and the Family Journal, 3*(4), 157-164.

VAGINAL BIRTH AFTER CESAREAN

American College of Obstetricians and Gynecologists. Committee on Obstetrics. (1988). *Guidelines for vaginal delivery after a previous cesarean birth.* Washington, DC: American College of Obstetricians and Gynecologists.

Clark, S. L. (1988). Rupture of the scarred uterus. *Obstetrics and Gynecology Clinics of North America, 15*(4), 737-744.

Dahll, K., Mittal, S., Grover, V., & Dahll, G. (1987). Childbirth following primary cesarean section: Evaluation of a scoring system. *International Journal of Gynaecology and Obstetrics, 25,* 199-205.

Eglinton, G., Phelan, S., Yeh, S., Diaz, F., Wallace, T., & Paul, R. (1984). Outcome of a trial of labor after prior cesarean section. *Journal of Reproductive Medicine, 29*(1), 3-8.

Eriksen, N. L., & Buttino, L. (1989). VBAC: A comparison of maternal and fetal morbidity to elective repeat cesarean section. *American Journal of Perinatology, 6*(4), 375-379.

Flamm, B., Dunnett, C., Fischermann, E., & Quilligan, E. (1984). Vaginal delivery following cesarean section: Use of oxytocin augmentation and epidural anesthesia with internal tocodynamic and internal fetal monitoring. *American Journal of Obstetrics and Gynecology, 148*(6), 759-763.

Flamm, B., Goings, J., Fuelberth, N., Fischermann, E., Jones, C., & Hersh, E. (1987). Oxytocin during labor with previous cesarean section: Results of a multicenter study. *Obstetrics and Gynecology, 70*(5), 709-712.

Flamm, B., Lim, O., Jones, C., Newman, L., & Mantis, J. (1988). Vaginal birth after cesarean section: Results of a multi-center study. *American Journal of Obstetrics and Gynecology, 158*(5), 1079-1084.

Foster, T., Jacobson, J., & Valenzuela, G. (1988). *Choice of trial of labor after cesarean section* (Abstract). Las Vegas: Society of Perinatal Obstetricians.

Haq, C. (1988). Vaginal birth after cesarean delivery. *American Family Physician, 37*(6), 167-171.

Horenstein, J., & Phelan, J. (1985). Previous cesarean section: The risks and benefits of oxytocin usage. *American Journal of Obstetrics and Gynecology, 151*(5), 564-569.

Jarrell, M., Ashmead, G., & Mann, L. (1985). Vaginal delivery after cesarean section: A five year study. *Obstetrics and Gynecology, 65*(5), 628-632.

Lagercrantz, H., & Slotkin, T. (1986). The stress of being born. *Scientific American, 254,* 100-107.

Laufer, A., Hodenius, V., Friedman, L., Duncan, N., Gay, C., MacPherson, S., & Barrows, N. (1987). Vaginal birth after cesarean section: Nurse midwifery management. *Journal of Nurse-Midwifery, 32*(1), 41-47.

Lavin, J., Stephens, R., Miodovnik, M., & Barden, T. (1982). Vaginal delivery in patients with a prior cesarean section. *Obstetrics and Gynecology, 59*(2), 135-148.

Lipson, J. (1984). Repeat cesarean births: Social and psychological issues. *Journal of Obstetric, Gynecologic, and Neonatal Nursing, 13*(3), 157-162.

Martin, J., Morrison, J., & Wiser, W. (1988). Vaginal birth after cesarean section: The demise of routine abdominal delivery. *Obstetrics and Gynecology Clinics of North America, 15*(4), 719-736.

McClain, C. (1985). Why women choose trial of labor or repeat cesarean section. *Journal of Family Practice, 21*(2), 210-216.

Miller, J. (1988). Maternal and neonatal morbidity and mortality in cesarean section. *Obstetrics and Gynecology Clinics of North America, 15*(4), 629-638.

Myers, S., & Gleighen, N. (1990). 1988 U.S. cesarean section rate: Good news or bad? *New England Journal of Medicine, 323*(3), 200.

Murphy, M., & Harvey, S. (1989). Choice of a childbirth method after cesarean. *Women and Health, 15*(2), 67-85.

Phelan, J., Clark, S., Diaz, F., & Paul, R. (1987). Vaginal birth after cesarean section. *American Journal of Obstetrics and Gynecology, 157*(6), 1510-1515.

Placek, P., & Taffel, S. (1988). Recent patterns in cesarean delivery in the United States. *Obstetrics and Gynecology Clinics of North America, 15*(4), 607-627.

Silver, R., & Gibbs, R. (1987). Predictors of vaginal delivery in patients with a previous cesarean section who require oxytocin. *American Journal of Obstetrics and Gynecology, 156*(1), 57-60.

Stedman, C. M., & Kline, R. C. (1990). Intraoperative complications and unexpected pathology at the time of cesarean section. *Obstetrics and Gynecology Clinics of North America, 15*(4), 745-769.

Stovall, R., Shaver, D., Solomon, S., & Anderson, G. (1987). Trial of labor in previous cesarean section patients, excluding classical cesarean sections. *Obstetrics and Gynecology, 70*(5), 713-717.

Taffel, S., Placek, P., & Moien, M. (1990). 1988 U.S. cesarean section rate at 24.7 per 100 births: A plateau? *New England Journal of Medicine, 323*(3), 199-200.

THE INFANT FEEDING DECISION: BREAST-FEEDING OR BOTTLE-FEEDING

American Academy of Pediatrics. (1982). Policy statement based on task force report: The promotion of breast feeding. *Pediatrics, 69*(5), 654-661.

Anholm, P. (1986). Breastfeeding: A preventive approach to health care in infancy. *Issues in Comprehensive Pediatric Nursing, 9*(1), 1-10.

Arango, J. O. (1984). Promoting breastfeeding: A national perspective. *Public Health Reports, 99*(6), 559-565.

Gonzales, R. B. (1990). A large scale rooming-in program in a developing country: The Jose Fabella Memorial Hospital. *International Journal of Gynecology and Obstetrics, 31*(Suppl. 1), 31-34.

Gulick, E. E. (1986). The effects of breast feeding on toddler health. *Pediatric Nursing, 12*(1), 51-54.

Hanson, L. A., Andersson, B., Carlsson, B., Fallstrom, S., Mellander, L., Porras, O., Soderstrom, T., & Eden, C. S. (1985). Protective factors in milk and the development of the immune system. *Pediatrics Supplement, 75*(1), 172-176.

Howie, P. W., Forsyth, J. S., Ogston, S. A., Clark, A., & Florey, C. D. (1990). Protective effect of breastfeeding against infection. *British Medical Journal, 300,* 11-16.

Lawrence, R. A. (1989). *Breastfeeding: A guide for the medical profession* (3rd ed.). St. Louis: C. V. Mosby.

Poskitt, E. M. E. (1988). *Practical paedetric nutrition.* London: Butterworths.

CONCLUSION

Trandel-Korenchuk, D. M. (1982). Informed consent: Client participation in childbirth decisions. *JOGNN, 11*(5), 379-381.

SUPPLEMENTAL READINGS

American Academy of Pediatrics. (1984). Task force on infant feeding practices: Executive summary. *Pediatrics Supplement, 71,* 579-585.

American Academy of Pediatrics Committee on Nutrition. (1981). Nutrition and lactation. *Pediatrics, 68*(3), 435-443.

American Dietetic Association. (1986). Position of the American Dietetic Association: Promotion of breast feeding. *Journal of the American Dietetic Association, 86*(11), 1580-1585.

American Medical Association. (1979). Concepts of nutrition and health. *JAMA, 242*(21), 2335-2338.

American Public Health Association. (1981). Policy statements, 8022 (PP): Infant feeding in the United States. *American Journal of Public Health, 71*(2), 207-211.

Auerbach, K. G. (1990). Assisting the employed breastfeeding mother. *Journal of Nurse-Midwifery, 35*(1), 26-34.

Baranowski, T., Bee, D. E., Rassin, D. K., Richardson, C. J., Brown, J. P., Guenther, N., & Nadar, P. R. (1983). Social support, social influence, ethnicity, and the breastfeeding decision. *Social Science Medicine, 17*(21), 1599-1611.

Bevan, M., Mosley, D., Labach, K., & Solimaro, G. (1984). Factors influencing breastfeeding in an urban WIC program. *Journal of the American Dietetic Association, 84*(5), 563-567.

Black, R. F., Blair, J. P., Jones, V. N., & DuRant, R. H. (1990). Infant feeding decisions among pregnant women from a WIC population in Georgia. *Journal of the American Dietetic Association, 90*(2), 255-259.

Bloom, M. (1981). The romance and power of breastfeeding. *Birth and the Family Journal, 8*(4), 259-269.

Chamberlain, G., & Lumley, J. (1986). *Prepregnancy care: A manual for practice.* New York: John Wiley.

Eckhardt, K. W., & Hendershot, G. E. (1984). Analysis of the reversal in breastfeeding trends in the early 1970's. *Public Health Reports, 99*(4), 410-415.

Ford, K., & Labbok, M. (1990). Who is breastfeeding? Implications of associated social and biomedical variables for research on the consequences of method of infant feeding. *American Journal of Clinical Nutrition, 52*(3), 451-456.

Gabriel, A., Gabriel, K. R., & Lawrence, R. A. (1986). Cultural values and biomedical knowledge: Choices in infant feeding. *Social Science Medicine, 23*(5), 501-509.

Grossman, L. K., Fitzsimmons, S. M., Larson-Alexander, J. B., Sachs, L., & Harter, C. (1990). The infant feeding decision in low and upper income women. *Clinical Pediatrics, 29*(1), 30-37.

Heritage, C., & Cunningham, M. (1985). Persistent pulmonary hypertension associated with elective cesarean deliveries. *American Journal of Obstetrics and Gynecology, 152*(6), 627-629.

Hill, P. D., & Humenick, S. S. (1989). Insufficient milk supply. *Image, 21*(3), 145-148.

Humenick, S. S. (1982). The many modes of relaxation. In S. S. Humenick (Ed.), Expanding horizons in childbirth education (Vol. 2, pp. 3-8). Washington, DC: ASPO/Lamaze.

Institute of Medicine. (1990). *Nutrition during pregnancy.* Washington, DC: National Academy Press.

Jones, R. (1990). The politics of reproductive biology: Exclusionary policies in the United States. In W. P. Handwerker (Ed.), *Births and power: Social change and the politics of reproduction* (pp. 39-51). Boulder, CO: Westview.

Maclean, H. (1990). *Women's experience of breastfeeding.* Toronto: University of Toronto Press.

Martinez, G. A. (1984). Ross Laboratories National Mothers Survey: Reports for 1981, 1982, 1983. Columbus, OH: Ross Laboratories Marketing Research Department.

Martinez, G. A., & Krieger, F. W. (1985). Milk-feeding patterns in the United States. *Pediatrics, 76*(6), 1004-1008.

Morse, J. M., Harrison, M. J., & Prowse, M. (1986). Minimal breastfeeding. *JOGNN, 15*(4), 333-338.

Pipes, P. (1985). *Nutrition in infancy and childhood* (3rd ed.). St. Louis: C. V. Mosby.

Public Health Service. (1989). *Caring for our future: The content of prenatal care.* Washington, DC: Public Health Service, Department of Health and Human Services.

Rassin, D. K., Richardson, C. J., Baranowski, T., Nader, P. R., Guenther, N., Bee, D. E., & Brown, J. P. (1984). Incidence of breastfeeding in a low socioeconomic group of mothers in the U.S.: Ethnic patterns. *Pediatrics, 73*(2), 132-137.

Sarett, H. P., Bain, K. R., & O'Leary, J. C. (1983). Decisions on breastfeeding or formula feeding and trends in infant feeding practices. *American Journal of Diseases in Children, 137,* 719-725.

Simoupoulos, A. P., & Grave, G. D. (1984). Factors associated with the choice of infant feeding practice. *Pediatrics Supplement, 74*(2), 603-614.

Spadt, S. K., Martin, K. R., & Thomas, A. M. (1990). Experiential classes for siblings-to-be. *MCN, 15*(3), 184-186.

Stahl, M., & Guida, D. (1984). Slow weight gain in the breastfed infant: Management options. *Pediatric Nursing, 10*(2), 117-120.

PART IV

18

Violence Against Women

JACQUELYN C. CAMPBELL
KÄREN LANDENBURGER

Scope of the Problem

Violence against women is pervasive in our society, occurring in all socioeconomic and ethnic groups. The causes, consequences, and remedies of violence must be seen within the context of a society that permits violence and/or fails to punish adequately those individuals who perpetrate crimes against women—a society that permits treating women as a commodity or an object that must be dominated. Violence against women can be conceptualized as an issue of control of women; each of the forms in which it is seen serves to keep individual women within the control of individual men (Breines & Gordon, 1983). Collectively, the sum total of acts of violence against women can be viewed as one of many forms of patriarchal social control (Hanmer & Maynard, 1987). There are many levels of complexity between the individual act of violence and patriarchal society, and the answer to violence against women is not simply equal status for women (Counts, Brown, & Campbell, 1992; Hoff, 1990). However, this overall conceptual framework of violence against women as a form of social control provides the background for understanding the various forms of violence as part of one continuum, ranging from sexual harassment to homicide. All have health care implications and opportunities for nursing interventions.

Forms of Violence Against Women: Definitions and Incidence

Homicide

Approximately 90% of adult female homicide victims in the United States are killed by men (Campbell, 1992; Mercy & Saltzman, 1989). More than three fourths of these women are killed by a family member, most often an intimate partner (husband, lover) or ex-intimate partner. In the majority of the murders by male partners, the homicide was preceded by abuse of the female (Campbell, 1992). The leading cause of death for young (15-35 years old) African American women is homicide, and it is the 11th leading cause of premature death for women in the general population (U.S. Department of Health and Human Services [DHHS], 1990).

Abuse of Female Partners

Abuse is a multifaceted phenomenon. Abuse of a female partner can be defined as repeated physical, sexual, and/or emotional assault within a context of coercive control by an intimate partner (or ex-partner). A context of coercive control refers to the environment of isolation; denial of economic resources; forced sex; and threats against children, family, and personal property that abusers impose on their female partners. According to the latest national random survey, one of every six, or 16% of, American couples experience at least one incident of physical assault each year (Straus & Gelles, 1990).

Although women also assault their male partners, such violence is far more frequently in self-defense, less likely to cause injury, and less often accompanied by coercive control in other spheres of life (Saunders, 1989). Because abuse of female partners tends to escalate in severity and frequency over time, the minor violence can be expected to increase to serious battering if not recognized as a serious problem and interrupted by health care professionals. Given the magnitude of the problem, woman abuse constitutes a major national health problem.

Dating Violence

Dating violence or courtship violence is of endemic proportions in our society. The phenomenon of physical abuse in dating relationships has become a focus of research in the past 10 years. Dating violence, similar to other forms of violence, crosses socioeconomic status and ethnic groups. Sigelman, Berry, and Wiles (1984) found in a study of dating relationships that one half of the college students studied reported having been victims of dating violence. Although Makepeace (1981) found that more females than males engaged in violent behavior, he found that females suffered more severe violence in terms of injury and tactics used against them. Females reported sustaining three times as much mild injury (slapping) and twice as much moderate injury (hitting, punching) as males and were the only ones to report severe injury (beating up or use of a weapon). In marital abuse it was found that the acts of violence by women were most often in response to violence by male partners. In addition, men claimed to use violent behaviors as a means of intimidating their partners, whereas women claimed the use of violence as a means of self-defense.

Societal and individual factors are at the core of violence in dating relationships. Societal roles that frame males as aggressors and women as passive recipients and the belief that women wish to be controlled are factors that support the use of aggressive behavior in dating relationships. Because of the inclination of women to either ignore violence or label incidence of violence as a product of some other dynamic (e.g., alcohol or stress) during dating relationships and to romanticize courtship, partners marry and abuse continues in the marital relationship (Landenburger, 1989; Lloyd, 1991).

Female Partners

At least 1.8 million women per year in the United States are battered by their male partners (Straus & Gelles, 1990). The exact incidence and prevalence of wife abuse is difficult to determine. In a study of violence in the home, Gelles (1972) found that 56% of husbands hit their wives at least once within the year preceding the study, whereas 20% hit their wives from six times a year to daily. In a study administered to women admitted to the hospital for emergency room treatment (excluding rape), Appleton (1980) reported that 35% of the women stated they had been struck by their abusers with the intent of causing harm. Divorce statistics, police records, and emergency room statistics alone cannot be used to determine a reliable frequency of wife abuse (Martin, 1976). In divorce cases, the incidence of abuse is often negotiated off the record. Often, police records do not include an official category for wife abuse; it is listed under domestic violence, which can include any assaults occurring in the home. Emergency room statistics are often inaccurate because of the hesitancy of some women to state that they have been victims of abuse and the failure of health care professionals to ask and document appropriately (Drake, 1982; Goldberg & Tomlanovich, 1984: Stark & Flitcraft, 1979; Tilden, 1989; Tilden & Shepherd, 1987). Taking into account the aforementioned factors and the fact that most investigators looked only at physical abuse, it is surmised that the physical and psychological abuse of women involved in male-female relationships takes place in a large proportion of all relationships between spouses and those individuals who are cohabiting.

Characteristics of Abuse

The characteristics of abuse vary and are often contradictory. Abuse of female partners is found in all economic, social, and cultural categories. Walker (1979) pointed out that battering is more common at higher socioeconomic levels than cited evidence indicates because few of these victims are seen in emergency departments or hospitals due to social pressures and alternative resources. However, most studies have found higher levels of abuse in relationships in which the male's income, occupation, and stability of employment is low (Hotaling & Sugarman, 1986; Petersen, 1980; Straus & Gelles, 1990). There is also research support for abuse being related to "status inconsistency" between the partners, such as the husband's having less education and/or less occupational prestige than his wife (Gelles, 1972; Straus & Gelles, 1990). In addition, it is clear that men who feel they should have the final say in household decisions (whether they do or not) and/or otherwise feel their male role is threatened are likely to compensate with aggression toward their female partners (Campbell & Humphreys, 1984; Straus & Gelles, 1990; Tolman & Bennett, 1990).

Abuse is also more likely to occur in couples in which there is a great deal of stress from outside occurrences (e.g., job loss, death in family) as well as discord, argument, and verbal aggression between the partners (Hotaling & Sugarman, 1986; Straus & Gelles, 1990). There is also recent evidence that abuse is more frequent in couples cohabiting, separated, or divorced than in those currently married (Hotaling & Sugarman, 1990). The majority of studies indicate that men who were exposed to violence in childhood (child abuse or abuse of their mothers) are more likely to assault their wives, but the evidence is mixed as to whether or not childhood violence increases the risk for women to become abused partners. In fact there are very few personal or demographic characteristics of women consistently indicated by research to be predictive of their becoming victims of adult abuse.

An important component of the violent situation is whether or not alcohol is involved. Evidence suggests that alcohol consumption is related to violent acts between family members. From both research reviews and the most recent national random survey, it appears that chronic alcohol problems in the male are more predictive of female battering than acute intoxication prior to an incident (Straus & Gelles, 1990; Tolman & Bennett, 1990). However, only approximately half of batterers have problems with alcohol, and although most experts consider alcohol a factor in abuse, it is not seen as causative (Goodstein & Page, 1981; Hilberman, 1980; Tolman & Bennett, 1990). Walker (1979) drew on over 120 interviews with battered women and concluded that men beat the women whether or not alcohol consumption had occurred. Curing alcohol problems does not necessarily help abuse problems, and both must be treated as separate problems with specific interventions.

Sexual Violence

Sexual violence against women includes rape (date or acquaintance, stranger, and marital), incest, and prostitution.

Rape

Rape, the act of forced sexual intercourse, is both a social and political issue (Barry, 1984). At least 120 per 100,000 women over the age of 12 report rape or attempted rape each year in the United States, and the incidence is increasing (U.S. DHHS, 1990). Although major strides have taken place in the United States in the treatment of rape victims and in the prosecution of rape, women are still often seen as being responsible for the occurrence of the rape. If a woman's appearance is deemed sensual or she is walking the streets at night or otherwise placing herself in a potentially vulnerable situation, she is seen as complicit in the assault. Generally, society views women as responsible for men's behavior.

Rape outside of marriage can be divided into two categories: date or acquaintance rape and stranger rape. Although both forms are sexual assault, differences can be seen in how others attribute blame to the victims of rape. Until recently, it was generally believed that if women followed normative social behaviors they would not be raped. In a sense, women were viewed as the perpetrators of the assault and had to prove that they did not cause the assault. Although women who are raped by a stranger are now more frequently viewed as unwilling victims, women experiencing date rape are often seen either as willing victims or as responsible for the assault.

Date rape among young people only recently gained attention as a threat to women. Women are at high risk for various forms and levels of physical and sexual violence in their dating relationships (Bird, Stith, & Schladale, 1991). Lloyd (1991) claims that half of all dating relationships include some form of physical aggression, including date rape. Sigelman et al. (1984) found only rare reports of female-committed sexual violence, whereas more women reported having been victims of sexual aggression than did men. Makepeace (1986), querying the perceived motivation for violence, found that eight times as many females as males felt that forced sex has been attempted. Because of the tendency to remain silent about experiences including physical aggression and the difficulty of labeling what constitutes this form of behavior, the exact incidence remains ambiguous.

Kanin (1985) reported that peer pressure influenced the desire of males to be sexually active, contributing to the rape of intimate partners, whether or not they had been sexually involved. In addition, submissiveness may be construed by the aggressor as acceptance of force. Women may feel obligated to respond to sexual demands in established relationships, and men may think that they have a right to make these demands. Lloyd (1991) hypothesizes that the greater the proclivity to rely on social norms in the formulation of behavior, the greater the likelihood of a power differential between the male and the female, which may and often does lead to violence. Because social norms ascribe to women the role of maintaining relationships, blame is placed on women for the abuse that takes place. Subsequently, the role of the male and his responsibility as the perpetrator of violence becomes a secondary issue. The opposing roles of initiator and gatekeeper set up an adversarial relationship in courtship.

"Marital" Rape

Approximately 10% to 14% of American women have been raped within marriage or within a long-term cohabiting relationship (Russell, 1982). This form of sexual abuse can happen in a marriage that is otherwise nonviolent, but it most often occurs along with physical battering. In fact, 40% to 45% of battered women are also being raped on an ongoing basis by their partners (Campbell, 1989b). This sexual trauma has specific emotional and physical sequelae that are separate from those of physical abuse. Women have reported such chronic difficulties as urinary, vaginal, and anal trauma, pain, and infections (Campbell & Alford, 1989). Physically abused women who are also sexually abused have even lower self-esteem, especially in the area of body image, than do those who are only physically beaten (Campbell, 1989b). The male partner who sexually abuses his wife as well as physically abuses her is a particularly violent and dangerous batterer in terms of homicide potential.

The sexual assault laws of the United States were based on traditional English law that stated that a man had the right to force his wife into sex and that her marriage vow constituted perpetual and irrevocable consent to sex at his desire. As recently as 1980, 47 states recognized this "right" of men by adding marital rape exemptions to sexual misconduct laws. In other words, the sexual assault laws of almost all states applied to all men except husbands. By 1990, only 10 states still retained that exception, but the fact that in the United States it is legal for a man to rape his wife is indicative of the vestiges of attitudes that condone violence against women.

Incest

Incest, a matter of common concern in our society, is a sexual act whereby a parent or a significant person who a child trusts abuses that trust and exerts control over a child. The traditional legal definition of incest is usually limited to sexual intercourse between blood relatives. Finkelhor (1980) has broadened that definition to include explicit sexual contact.

The incidence of incest is difficult to determine. According to Russell, Schurman, and Trocki (1988), in a study of African American and white American women, 16% and 17%, respectively, were incestuously abused during childhood. Difficulties in obtaining the incidence of incest in our society are a result of societal avoidance of the topic or disbelief that it truly takes place. Children often block from their memories the assaults to cope psychologically with an untenable situation. Usually, children are hesitant to speak of the abuse. They may have been threatened not to speak of the incidents, and often children do not possess the vocabulary to describe what is happening to them. These causes are even more profound in cases of incest in which the perpetrator is someone whom the child trusts and depends on.

A child's age, the degree of molestation, a child's interpretation of the experience, and the duration of the sexual relationship influence the psychological, sexual, and interpersonal impact of childhood sexual assault (Finkelhor, 1986). Some behavioral manifestations of sexual abuse include precocious sexual activity, including the use of sex-specific language beyond a child's developmental years; aggressive sexual behaviors; a change in a child's normal patterns of behavior; and an increased level of sexual behavior, such as the preoccupation with fondling his or her genitals or those of others or promiscuity (Browne & Finkelhor, 1986; Cornman, 1989; Deyoung, 1982). Long-term effects of childhood sexual abuse include depression; social isolation; difficulties in future intimate relationships, especially with men; guilt; and low self-esteem (Alexander, Neimeyer, Follette, Moore, & Harter, 1989; Draucker, 1989; Rew, 1989). The child's search for some way to make sense of the incest along with the above symptoms persist into adulthood. The adult's understanding of the experiences and constructing some meaning of the past childhood experiences are essential in recovering from childhood trauma (Draucker, 1989; Silver, Boon, & Stones, 1983).

Other Forms of Violence Against Women

Barry (1984) and other theorists (e.g., Daly, 1990; Spratlen, 1988) consider prostitution and sexual harassment to be forms of sexual oppression against women. Prostitution is an institution that economically exploits women. Although economic exploitation is an important factor, sexual domination of women can be viewed as the foundation that supports prostitution in the United States. The majority of prostitutes have been sexually assaulted in childhood and adolescence and are often forced into prostitution by violence or threats of such from individual men or by drug addiction first imposed by male partners (Hartman, Burgess, & McCormack, 1987).

The incidence of sexual harassment is difficult to determine. Some researchers claim it is as high as 25% (Fitzgerald, Shullman, et al., 1988). Usually, sexual harassment is perpetrated by men against women. Sexual harassment is an interaction between two or more people in which one person is the recipient of unwanted sexual behavior by another person (Spratlen, 1988). Sexual harassment includes gender-specific verbal and nonverbal harassment; inappropriate and offensive sexual advances; and sexual bribery, coercion, and assault (Fitzgerald, Weitzman, Gold, & Ormerod, 1988). In most cases of sexual harassment, there is a power differential between the victim and the perpetrator. The power one individual has over another can lead to a fear in reporting the events, with the harassment continuing and psychological healing prohibited.

Health Care Costs

It is believed that most women victimized by violence first enter the health care system through prenatal clinics and/or emergency rooms (Tilden, 1989). Generally, these women are seeking assistance for injuries sustained during physically abusive episodes (Appleton, 1980; Goldberg & Tomlanovich, 1984; Rounsaville, 1978; Tilden & Shepherd, 1987). If the high incidence of abuse between intimate partners is taken into account, it is likely that battering could be cost-effectively assessed at routine health exams and/or at times when women seek treatment for depression, fatigue, parenting problems, and marital difficulties.

Because of the stigma involved, women and health care providers are often reluctant to initiate discussion about abuse. However, the majority of battered women say they would have talked about the issue with a health care professional if they were asked (Drake, 1982; Goldberg & Tomlanovich, 1984). Because abuse is often insidious, starting with minor psychological abuse and building to more severe physical incidents, it often remains unrecognized by victims and health care providers alike until a severe episode forces attention on the situation. Stigma and inadequate assessment lead to women continually seeking health care for a variety of complaints with the underlying problem being virtually unmentioned.

Within emergency room departments alone, at least 18% of women presenting with trauma have been abused (Tilden, 1989). Care in the emergency room is often fragmented and necessarily oriented toward life and death situations. Therefore, women are not adequately assessed for prior physical or sexual abuse and so receive little or no emotional support or intervention specific to their needs (Campbell, 1991). It can be surmised that the cost to the health care system is phenomenal, with little or no positive outcome. A cycle persists in which women seek care and receive either no intervention or interventions that are grossly ineffective (Campbell & Sheridan, 1989). This cycle perpetuates feelings of anger and inadequacy within health care providers, resulting in blame placed on women for their lack of compliance with remedies offered.

History and Culture

Evidence of violence against women precedes written history and can be found in the earliest recorded documents. Traditionally, rape has been used by invading armies to subjugate conquered peoples; various forms of violence (e.g., stoning to death, "gang" rape) were recorded as punishments for women who engaged in adultery and/or premarital sex; abuse of female partners is referred to in the Bible and condoned in the Koran. There also is some evidence of early societal forms where apparently totally nonviolent societies were based on gender and class equality, partnership rather than domination of one group over another (Eisler, 1988). This type of community was conquered and eventually replaced by more dominating forms of societal organizations. Since then, history is replete with accounts of various forms of violence against women, such as witch burnings, foot binding, and suttee, the Indian practice of widows throwing themselves (or being coerced) onto their dead husbands' funeral pyres because their existence as single women would be so destitute. Some analyses of recorded historical evidence suggest that periods and cultures of relatively greater gender equality (e.g., precolonial Ojibwa Native Americans; Minoan Crete circa 2,000 BCE; contemporary Wape of Papua, New Guinea) were accompanied by less violence against women or at least more societal outcry against violent practices (Counts et al., 1992; Eisler, 1988). However, relative gender equality is difficult to measure, because there are many different arenas in a society in which female and male status or power can be contrasted. By any measure, all of recorded history reflects societal control by males and accompanying violence against women.

Various other forms of violence against women are found in cultures different from our own (Campbell, 1985; Stern, 1992). Young women found not to be virgins customarily can be (and still occasionally are) stoned to death in Saudi Arabia. Infanticide of female infants is more common than that committed against male infants, especially in cultures in which there is a strong gender preference for males. Female infants are also fed after male children and therefore may starve to death in countries such as India. Hindu India is also the site of dowry murders or bride burnings in which wives are killed for inadequate dowries or when they threaten to obtain a divorce because the dowry would then have to be returned. Sexual trafficking (selling into prostitution) of young girls is a serious problem in Thailand. The killing of wives accused of adultery by their husbands was condoned by law in Brazil until the early 1990s, when feminist groups were finally successful in initiating legal reform. Gang rape is used in some areas of New Guinea to chastise young women who do not conform to their prescribed subservient roles.

The most pervasive form of violence against women in other cultures is genital mutilation or female circumcision, which has been performed on more than 90 million African women and girls (Stern, 1992). Genital mutilation involves clitoral circumcision, clitoridectomy, labial excision, or infibulation (sewing of the labia majora after excision of the labia minora and clitoris) (Levinson, 1989). The purposes of these practices are to control women's sexuality by preventing any female sexual pleasure and ensuring virginity before marriage and fidelity afterward. Because the practice is often conducted without anesthesia and in unsterile conditions, it frequently results in severe infections and death. Although it takes place primarily in the Middle East and Africa, immigrants to the United States are often affected and may continue the practice. Genital mutilation of girls has been compared to circumcision of the male in terms of both being cultural sex-related practices. However, the major differences are not only degree of physical harm but also inequality between the sexes and the sexual control of women.

There is debate over whether genital modification can be considered abuse or if it is a ritualistic form of entry into womanhood. Similarly, in an emic view (from within a culture) the other practices mentioned earlier can be said to be part of cultural norms and therefore not subject to international censure. Yet these practices contribute to male control over women in all of these societies, and individual women have little choice about whether to be victimized. An etic (external) view of violent practices is that certain standards should apply across cultures, despite culturally specific norms. In support of this more etic view, the United Nations has taken the stand that genital mutilation and the other forms of violence against women are subject to international censure.

Correlates of Violence Against Women

Cross-cultural and historical research efforts are beginning to identify societal correlates of violence against women that either enhance or deter such practices. These factors are important in both understanding the societal context for such violence and identifying useful prevention and public policy measures.

In a quantitative cross-cultural analysis of family violence using aggregate anthropological data, Levinson (1989) found that the most important predictors of wife beating around the world were economic inequality between genders, violent conflict resolution, male domestic authority, and divorce restrictions for women. Using more in-depth descriptions from 14 diverse societies with a variety of levels of violence against women, Counts et al. (1992) found that community-level sanctions against battering and sanctuary for beaten wives was important in preventing occasional wife beating from escalating to ongoing abuse. An examination of ethnographies from a variety of cultures written by women led Campbell (1985) to suggest that cultural norms of relatively low autonomy of wives (including restricted divorce), definitions of manhood that include an emphasis on toughness and control of women, and strong importance of the wife/mother role were predictive of wife abuse. When cultures define the wife/mother role as the sole or primary role for women, women who are hit by their husbands often find it difficult to escape, the same mechanism that occurs where divorce is restricted.

Strong cultural gender preference for males is associated with forms of violence against women other than wife beating, as is general low status of women, especially in terms of political power and economic autonomy. Generally, where there are other forms of violence against women, wife beating is also prevalent. As cultural norms regarding women change along with political upheaval, the degree and frequency of violence against women can be expected to change also. For instance, the early 1990s have seen a severe curtailment of women's autonomy in Algeria, whereas the status of women has been increasing steadily in Zimbabwe since the 1980s revolution. Although it is difficult to ascertain exact rates, women in both of these countries feel that the incidence of violent practices against them increases as autonomy decreases and vice versa. However, it may be that in cultures in which women have remained strictly controlled by law and tradition, to keep female autonomy circumscribed, violence against women only needs to be permitted rather than frequently committed (Campbell, 1985).

Theoretical Frameworks for Understanding Violence Against Women

As well as general theories explaining violence against women, specific theories have been posited attempting to explain the causes and nature of wife abuse. Understanding the environmental, interpersonal, and interactional dynamics that occur during a woman's experiences of abuse assists in determining why women remain in or leave an abusive relationship. The experience of being abused within the context of a significant relationship can be understood by clarifying the views women have of themselves as individual persons and the meaning they attach to their interactions with others and the environment. Because abuse is a multicontextual problem, no one theory can totally explain the dynamics of abusive relationships. The different theories viewed as a whole are helpful in identifying the societal, familial, and individual components that contribute to the existence and continuation of violence against women within our culture.

Theories About Wife Abuse

Intraindividual Theories

Gelles and Straus (1988) have categorized theories about violence among intimates into three groups: intraindividual theories, sociopsychological theories, and sociocultural theories. Intraindividual theories focus on individual characteristics. Personality traits inherent in individuals, such as low self-esteem, poor impulse control, and psychopathology, can lead to violent behavior. The difficulty with this approach is that social context is ignored, and perpetrators are relieved from responsibility for their malbehavior. In addition, the majority of abusers cannot be diagnosed with major psychopathology.

Within the intraindividual view, alcohol and drug abuse are viewed as mechanisms that break down natural inhibitions against deviant behavior. Walker (1984) claims that alcohol and drug abuse are not causal factors for abuse but are excuses used to relieve individuals from responsibility for abusive behaviors. Although abuse is prevalent in relationships in which one or both individuals misuse alcohol and drugs, it is also present when these chemicals are not used.

Sociopsychological Theories

In sociopsychological theories, such as exchange theory, social learning theory, learned helplessness, symbolic interactionism, and attribution theory, the source of violence and the explanations for the behavior of those victimized are located within interpersonal interactions.

Exchange Theory

Exchange theory examines abuse within a costs-rewards framework. Abuse is the result of interactions in which benefits and rewards are exchanged. If rewards are not acquired, the exchange is ended. Rewards for the abuser include increased power and instant gratification of demands. This approach is based on the premise that the exchange is mutual, and there is consent between the players in the interaction. Within exchange theory, an abused woman's efforts to stop the abuse often remain unheeded. Blame for the abuse and responsibility for the abuse are placed on the woman as well as on her perpetrator. This supports the myth that women ask for abuse and could end the unwanted behavior if they wished to do so.

Social Learning Theory

Social learning theory claims that abusive behavior is learned from exposure to violence. Within this framework, abuse is learned to be a normative means of control that is passed down within the family. Research supports the theory that violence can be learned. Of men who are abusive toward their female partners, 80% were either abused as children or were witnesses to violence between parents (Herrenkohl, Herrenkohl, & Toedler, 1983). Although this theory links violence in the family of origin with men who batter, it does not explain why some men who were either indirect or direct victims become abusive, whereas the majority do not. Research evidence less clearly supports women "learning" to be victims of abuse from childhood experience than men learning to be perpetrators (Hotaling & Sugarman, 1986).

Learned Helplessness

Seligman and Garber (1980) have advanced the view that in conditions wherein individuals find that specific outcomes are not related to (noncontingent with) their behavior, they exhibit signs of learned helplessness. There are three basic components of this syndrome: (a) passivity or lack of motivation toward controlling one's environment, (b) a negative stance, according to which one believes that actions taken will result in failure, and (c) a belief that outcomes are uncontrollable. Thus, if a person does not believe that he or she has control over outcomes but instead believes such control is not possible, then the person responds accordingly with learned helplessness. Clinically, the syndrome is seen as apathy, depression, low self-esteem, and an inability to see ways out of the situation. These symptoms are more chronic and severe depending on the degree to which the person blames himself or herself for the situation, feels alone in the situation, and feels the situation is unchangeable (Abramson, Seligman, & Teasdale, 1978). According to Walker (1977-1978), learned helplessness can be used as a framework for examining the behavior of battered women. Women involved in relationships in which they are physically, sexually, and/or psychologically abused by their partners progress through a cycle of violence. As efforts to stop the violence are unsuccessful, women's feelings of helplessness are supported. This cycle of abuse contains three stages: (a) the preincident tension stage; (b) the acute incident stage; and (c) the forgiving, calm, loving stage. This cycle is repeated until the relationship ends with either divorce or the death of one of the parties involved in the abuse. The cycle of abuse, contrition, and forgiveness becomes a pattern of interaction between the couple that is expected. Over time, contrition and forgiveness attenuate as the bonds of trust between the couple are diminished, resulting in a distancing from and a false presentation of self to other family members (Denzin, 1984a, 1984b; Dutton & Painter, 1981).

Symbolic Interactionism

According to Denzin (1984b) the exploration of abuse as an experience within the family conforms well to a symbolic interactionist approach. Symbolic interactionism is focused on how people socially construct meaning. Situations shape the nature of individual's responses, and roles implicit in situations give a person reason to act in a certain manner (Blumer, 1967; Denzin, 1985). Within this framework, abuse is viewed as a process that occurs intermittently over time and involves a continuing relationship with a high likelihood of recurrence (Denzin, 1984b; Frieze, 1979; Walker, 1984). As the abuse continues, it becomes embedded in a context of inauthentic attachment, the expectancy of future violence, and patterns of emotionality. In patterns of emotionality, individuals try to regain through violent means that which has been lost through previous violent interactions (Denzin, 1984a; Ferraro & Johnson, 1983; Frieze, 1983). Within inauthentic attachment, a couple seeks to regain the feelings of attachment they once had for one another. The tendency to review past interactions and apportion blame is a process that draws attention away from essential aspects of the relationship. The couple tries to atone for past behaviors. The ongoing cycle of abuse, contrition, and forgiveness results in an internal conflict over the true nature of the relationship versus a mythical view of relationships. The desire for the actual relationship to compare favorably with the mythical relationship results in the woman blaming herself for the abuse that has occurred. The abuse is minimized, and the behavior of the woman becomes the focal area of concern. As the abuse continues, a woman's self-esteem diminishes, resulting in the belief that she has no option but to stay in the relationship (Frieze, 1983; Miller & Porter, 1983).

The problem with both the learned helplessness and symbolic interactionist frameworks is that they do not explain how the majority of abused women eventually leave the relationship or otherwise make the violence end (Campbell, 1989a, 1991). They also do not explain the research finding that women become more active over time in seeking help (Gondolf, 1988). Women also tend to blame themselves less for abuse over time (Frieze, 1979).

Attribution Theory

Often, a woman who is abused is stigmatized not for the abuse itself but for the role others attribute to her for causing or, more often, not ending the abuse. The responsibility for the abusive situation is often attributed to the woman, offering evidence to her that aspects of her personality or behavior are to blame (Frieze, 1979; Miller & Porter, 1983). A woman is influenced by attributions of cause and blame for the abuse she sustains. When a woman is labeled by others as being abused, expectations and judgments about her behavior are formulated by others. The internalization of the labels designated by others influences a woman's view of herself and becomes a potentially important part of her subsequent behavior (Cooley, 1967; Strauss, 1959). She also searches for explanations as to why this is happening to her. These explanations take the form of a woman questioning her ability to perform the roles of wife and mother regardless of her achievements. She may blame herself for the problems of other family members even though she may not be responsible for these problems. As she continues in the abusive relationship, the sum of the past events and the meaning she makes of the events influence her current view of herself and her life.

Research on women who have experienced rape by a stranger suggests that if she blames her own behavior (as opposed to a personality characteristic) for the attack and subsequently changes that behavior, she may feel less vulnerable to another attack and thereby recover from the rape trauma more quickly (Burgess & Holmstrom, 1974; Janoff-Bulman & Frieze, 1983). In addition, Campbell (1989a) found that for her sample of battered women, those who blamed themselves along with their partners (interaction blame) were less depressed and had higher self-esteem than those who blamed their husband or partner alone. However, those who blamed themselves solely were the most depressed. Although these findings suggest that some self-blame can be useful in assisting women to believe they can control outcomes, these attributions also place most of the blame and responsibility of negative outcomes on women and can be harmful (Janoff-Bulman & Frieze, 1983). More research is needed to understand these issues.

Sociocultural Theories

Current evidence suggests that pressures or social conditions in the external environment lead to abuse and that a combination of external pressures and individual experiences and meaning that contribute to the ongoing nature of abuse (Breines & Gordon, 1983; Dutton & Painter, 1981; Ferraro & Johnson, 1983; Frieze, 1983; Rouse, 1984). The most salient factor that leads to abuse is the overall acceptance and practice in American society of violence as a means of maintaining, demonstrating, or regaining control. The news media and television are filled with incidents of "acceptable" violence. Men are socialized in a manner that holds in esteem acts of aggression and control. Most children grow up with fairy tales, nursery rhymes, and television shows that depict violence as appropriate behavior. If a child learns that abuse is an acceptable form of behavior through stories and is confronted with actual abuse of self or acts of parental violence, there is a greater likelihood of abuse being a normal mode of behavior for that child in the future (Dobash & Dobash, 1979). As long as there are positive social sanctions on using physical force to control others, there is a high probability that many individuals will extend this use beyond that which is considered acceptable.

Systems theory has been used to explain family violence, including wife abuse, by Straus and Gelles (1990). Although this theoretical framework includes the issues of both societal gender inequality and the domestic control of wives as predictors of wife abuse, its emphasis on stressors and considering all forms of family violence together makes it less explanatory for violence against women.

Certain family conflicts seem to trigger violent outbursts. The demands a woman may make on her husband to attain a better job, to be a better father, or to stop drinking are often seen as criticisms of his role as head of the household and may lower an already shaky self-esteem (Goodstein & Page, 1981). In the United States, a woman's role in the family, generally, is subordinate to the male. Acts of violence are often precipitated by what is seen as a violation of this role. In many incidents, a woman's suggesting that she find a job to help support the family has been met with abuse by her partner. A woman's planning to work outside of the home is still responded to with jealousy or feelings of inadequacy by many men (Faludi, 1992). Conflicts over how children should be raised and the timing of pregnancy have also been named as precipitating factors for abuse (Steinmetz, 1977).

Pearlin (1975) first described the relationship between status equality and stress in marriage. He stated that when there are norms of inequality existing in society and these norms are considered important within the marriage relationship, there is likely to be conflict between the couple. This view is supported by Martin (1976), who found that conflict in many of the middle-income couples stemmed from the inferiority feelings of the husband when the woman was successful professionally.

Status inconsistency as a precursor of wife abuse is one of the research findings that supports a feminist framework explanation for violence against women (see Chapter 8, "Frameworks for Nursing Practice With Women"). The findings from historical and cultural analyses also generally support the premises that violence against women in all its forms is fundamentally related to the patriarchal structures and attitudes that permeate almost all cultures historically and currently (Dobash & Dobash, 1979; Hanmer & Maynard, 1987; Levinson, 1989; Smith, 1990).

Recent feminist analyses of the behavior of victimized women also contribute to our understanding. Rather than emphasizing the pathology of women who have experienced violence, such analyses are stressing women's strengths (Gondolf, 1988; Hoff, 1990). Without minimizing the potential and actual health care problems of these women, such an approach can be incor-

Table 18.1 Rape Trauma Syndrome

Acute Phase (disorganization)

Immediate effect: shock and disbelief, expressed emotional response (anger, fear, anxiety, crying) or controlled style (feelings masked or hidden, calmness, subdued affect)

Physical reactions: sleep disturbances, eating disturbances, injury at sites of forced sexual activity

Emotional reactions: fear of death, humiliation, guilt, shame, embarrassment, self-blame, anger, desire for revenge, mood swings, irritation, and caution with others

Cognitive reactions: trying to block thoughts of assault, trying to think how to undo what has happened, trying to think how she could have escaped

Long-term process (reorganization)

Physical reactions: stress-related symptoms, menstrual problems, chronic vaginal symptoms

Traumatic stress syndrome: hypervigilance (anxiety, sleep disturbances, impaired concentration), reexperiencing trauma (flashbacks, nightmares), numbness and avoidance

Other emotional responses: self-blame, low self-esteem, phobias, fear of AIDS

Relationship problems: sexual problems, including lack of desire and inability to reach orgasm; other social contacts constrained; lack of trust in men; disruption of family relationships

SOURCE: Adapted from Burgess and Holmstrom (1979) and Baker, Burgess, Brickman, and Davis (1990).
NOTE: The rape trauma syndrome includes an acute phase of disorganization lasting a few days to a few weeks and is followed by a long-term process (up to 2 years postassault) of lifestyle reorganization. The characteristics of or responses to each phase are shown here. Nurses can use this information when assessing clients who have experienced rape.

porated into nursing research and practice to their advantage.

Nursing Theories

Several of the broad nursing conceptual frameworks have been applied to the issues of violence against women. Limandri (1986) applied Roy's (1976) framework to help in understanding the nursing role in increasing women's effective adaptation to abuse. Campbell (1986) illustrated the use of a homicide assessment instrument as a means of increasing abused women's self-care agency (ability to care for one's own health) from Orem's (1990) theory of nursing. Stuart (Stuart & Campbell, 1989) used Rogers's (1970, 1986) framework for research to further identify homicide risk factors in abusive relationships. Parse's (1985) theory was used by Butler and Snodgrass (1991) to direct nursing care of an abusive couple so that they learned to coexist together.

Midrange nursing theories have also been introduced (i.e., theories that include a limited number of variables and focus on a limited aspect of reality). The early nursing research of Ann Burgess (Burgess & Holmstrom, 1974, 1979) established the notion of a rape trauma syndrome and has been elaborated by researchers in many different disciplines (see Table 18.1). Her current work has established a midrange theory of trauma encapsulation that explains the variety of behaviors seen in victims of childhood sexual abuse (Hartman & Burgess, 1988). Children are unable to process the trauma and therefore "encapsulate" it, some almost totally. They may experience indirect effects, such as physical symptoms, but may not fully recall the trauma until adulthood. However, this defense prevents the memory from being processed, depletes psychic energy, and interferes with normal development. Ongoing intervention is needed for these children.

Landenburger (1989) developed a midrange theory of the process of entrapment in and recovery from an abusive relationship. Her research indicated that a woman passes progressively through a process including four phases: binding, enduring, disengaging, and recovering. The binding phase incorporates a description of the initial development of the relationship and the beginnings of abuse within the relationship. The positive aspects of the relationship are the primary focus for the woman and dominate the negative aspects of the relationship. During the second phase, enduring, a woman sees herself as putting up with the abuse. Whereas in the first phase, a woman subconsciously tended to overlook the bad, she now consciously blocks out the negative aspects of the relationship. She focuses on a solution to the abuse and in doing so places partial or total responsibility for the abuse on herself. During the disengaging phase, an identity with other women in her situation begins to form. During this phase a woman tends to place a conscious label on what is happening to her. She takes more risks to seek help and tries to find people who will support her instead of seeking support from those who blame or question her. The love she thought her partner had for her is recognized as an obsession. She becomes angry with herself and her partner. This anger mobilizes her to leave the relationship. The recovering phase contains the period of initial readjustment after a woman has left her abusive partner until she regains a "balance" in her life. The woman has to grieve the loss of her relationship and the loss of her partner. This period can take years, and many women are unable fully to pass through this phase. A woman works at understanding the meaning of her past experiences so that she can obtain a balance in her life. Further development and application of theory specific to nursing roles include the assessment and identification of the needs specific to this population of women. Nurses must become actively involved in identifying women who are at risk for abuse. Nurses should make it a routine practice to assess all women for signs and symptoms of abuse. Women should be offered information from which they can learn more about abusive relationships and resources available to them. Efforts must center not only on helping a woman but on conveying to her the effects of an abusive environment on children.

Nursing Research

The majority of nursing research on violence against women has been on wife abuse, with only some research on sexual abuse. Nursing research has added a unique perspective to knowledge development about violence against women because of its holistic perspective. The literature in most other disciplines tends to concentrate on documenting emotional effects and sociological and psychological contextual factors. Medical research on violence against women has only recently begun to be published and has tended to concentrate on determining the prevalence of abuse and/or sexual abuse in various medical settings and diagnostic groups. The nursing research to date has been more concerned with responses to and characteristics of the various forms of victimization rather than on causation and medical issues. Nursing research has generally avoided the victim-blaming approaches of much of the other discipline research, especially the early studies. There have also been connections with grassroots movements against wife abuse and sexual assault by most nursing researchers that has strengthened use of research results for advocacy on behalf of battered women. Two of the early studies that are considered "classic" examples of groundbreaking quality research in the area of violence against women were conducted by nurses on rape and wife abuse respectively (Burgess & Holmstrom, 1974; Parker & Schumacher, 1977). Nursing research has provided much of the impetus for the recent official health care system concern with abuse during pregnancy (Helton, McFarlane, & Anderson, 1987).

The findings from nursing research that have been supported by other research and that can be considered trustworthy have made significant contributions to the knowledge base about violence against women. Nursing research has established that at least 8% of women in prenatal and primary care settings are abused by a male partner and approximately 20% of women in emergency departments have a history of abuse (Bullock, McFarlane, Bateman, & Miller, 1989; Goldberg & Tomlanovich, 1984; Helton et al., 1987; Stark et al., 1981). Other nursing studies indicated that such violence is usually not documented correctly in medical records so that they could be used in court and that abused women do not feel they have been appropriately assessed and treated (Brendtro & Bowker, 1989; Drake, 1982). However, Tilden and Shepherd (1987) demonstrated that training of emergency room personnel about abuse can significantly increase the accurate identification of abused women.

Nursing research has also established some of the detrimental physical and emotional effects of wife abuse, abuse during pregnancy, marital rape, incest, and stranger rape (Brunngraber, 1986; Bullock & McFarlane, 1989; Burgess & Holmstrom, 1974; Campbell, 1989a; Campbell & Alford, 1989). Studies conducted by nurses have also helped explain why women remain in abusive relationships in terms of lack of resources, concern for children, realistic fear of being killed by the abuser, and loss of a sense of self (Campbell, 1986; Landenburger, 1989; Lichtenstein, 1981; Ulrich, 1991). As well as the harmful outcomes, nursing research has identified significant strengths of battered women, such as taking care of themselves and their children in most aspects of their lives, indica-

Table 18.2 Female Responses to Battering

Strengths
Awareness and concern for children
Developing survival strategies
Developing support systems
Developing resistance strategies
Appropriate help seeking
Developing stronger ties with other women
Determination to avoid future exploitation
Changing from blaming self to blaming the batterer over time
Developing self-awareness
Developing independence
Making sense of the situation
Physical problems
Injury (facial, head, trunk, proximal rather than distal)
Stress-related physical symptoms (e.g., choking sensations, hyperactive gastrointestinal system)
Injury-related physical symptoms (e.g., arthritis, chronic pain, neurological symptoms)
Physical sequelae of forced sex: pelvic inflammatory disease, sexually transmitted diseases, urinary tract infections, being inorgasmic, anal and vaginal tearing, unwanted pregnancies, AIDS, painful intercourse
Physical sequelae of abuse during pregnancy: spontaneous abortions, placenta previa, low-birth-weight infant
Psychological (emotional and cognitive) problems
Depression (ranging from transient to suicidal)
Low self-esteem
Self-blame
Fear
Traumatic stress syndrome: hypervigilance (anxiety, sleep disturbances, impaired concentration), reexperiencing trauma (flashbacks, nightmares), numbness and avoidance
Learned helplessness: depression, low self-esteem, apathy, problem-solving difficulties, feelings of loss of control, inability to escape
Substance abuse

NOTE: Nursing research has established physical and emotional effects of violence against women. Study findings have also identified significant strengths of battered women. This knowledge can be used in the assessment and development of interventions when working with women clients who have experienced violence in their lives.

tions of normal processes of grieving and recovering, and cultural and social support influences on responses to battering (Campbell, 1989b; Hoff, 1990; Torres, 1987) (see Table 18.2). Taken cumulatively, these findings are beginning to indicate data-based nursing interventions that will in many cases support the clinical suggestions already in the literature.

Despite the many positive aspects of nursing research, there are many gaps and improvements to be made. There are many opportunities to use larger, more culturally diverse samples of women and to document the prevalence of violence against women in each type of health care setting. More important, there is a need for nursing research to begin to test theories explaining the responses of women to abuse and nursing interventions designed to be helpful to them.

Nursing Care

Assessment

Assessment for all forms of violence against women should take place—ideally, by nurses—for *all* women entering the health care system (see Table 18.3). The assessment should be ongoing and stress confidentiality. A thorough assessment gathers information on physical, emotional, and sexual trauma from violence; risk for future abuse; cultural background and beliefs; perceptions of the woman's relationships with others; and the woman's stated needs. The assessment should be conducted in private. Other adults who are present could be an abuser and should be directed toward the waiting area and told that it is policy that, initially, women are

Table 18.3 Assessment for Abuse

Physical safety
Legal needs
Support needs and options
Economic status
Feelings of blame, isolation, fear, and responsibility
Resources available to women
Immediate and future
Community shelters
Support groups and counseling
Legal options
Safety plan
Economic assistance

NOTE: Assessment for violence against women should be a part of every health history done by nurses for all women regardless of their point of entry to the health care system. At each contact, nurses should assess their clients on the points listed here. Assessment must take place in a private, confidential setting.

seen alone. Women should be asked directly if they have been or are currently in an abusive relationship either as a child or as an adult. They should also be asked if they have ever been forced into sex that they did not wish to participate in. Shame and fear often make disclosure difficult. Verbal acknowledgment of the seriousness of the situation and emotional and physical support assist women in talking about past or current circumstances.

Women can be categorized into three groups in terms of abuse: no risk, low risk, or moderate to high risk. Women with no signs of current or past abuse are considered at no risk. At the initial assessment, a woman may be hesitant to speak of concerns she may have. Future visits should include questioning a woman about whether there have been any changes in her life or whether she has additional information or questions about topics discussed at previous visits.

Women at low risk show no evidence of recent or current abuse. Education that helps a woman gain perspective on her situation and her needs should be discussed. Resource materials including group and individual formats can be suggested. It is important that the nurse is identified as a supportive and knowledgeable person. The risk level should be recorded, and preventive measures and teaching should be documented.

Assessment of moderate to high risk includes evaluation of a woman's fear for both psychological and physical abuse. Lethality potential should be assessed (Campbell, 1986). Risk factors for lethality include behaviors such as stalking or frequent harassment, threats or an escalation of threats, use of weapons or threat with weapons, excessive control and jealousy, and public use of violence (see Table 18.4). Statements from an abuser such as "If I can't have you, no one can" should be taken seriously. In all cases, a history of abuse and alcohol and drug use should be collected on both partners and carefully documented. The determined risk level should also be documented, and any past or present physical evidence of abuse from prior or current assault should be either photographed or shown on a body map as well as described narratively. It is important that the assailant be identified in the record, which can be accomplished by the use of quotes from the woman or subjective information. These records can be very important for women in future assault and/or child custody cases, even if she is not ready to make a police report at the present time (see Table 18.5).

Nursing Interventions

Immediate care for a woman in a potentially harmful or present abusive situation involves the development of a safety plan. Questions that are important to ask include the following: "How can we help you be safe? Do you have a place to go?" A woman can be assisted to look at the options available to her. Shelter information, access to counseling, and legal resources should be discussed. If a woman wants to return to her partner, she can be helped in the development of plans that can be carried out if the abuse continues or becomes more serious.

Table 18.4 Risk Factors for Homicide in Abusive Relationships

Physical abuse increasing in frequency and/or severity
Abuser has used a weapon (gun, knife, baseball bat) against her
Abuser has threatened to kill her
Abuser chokes or attempts to choke her
Gun in the home
She is forced into sex
Children abused
Abuse during pregnancy
Abuser is violent outside of the home
Abuser uses crack, amphetamines, "ice," or combination drugs
Abuser is drunk every day or almost every day or is a "binge" drinker
Abuser is violently and constantly jealous
Abuser makes statements such as "If I can't have you, no one can."
Abuser controls most or all of her daily activities, money, and so on
Either partner has threatened or tried to commit suicide

NOTE: Potential for lethality must be assessed when a woman is in a violent relationship. The factors listed here are indicators of lethality.

Table 18.5 Elements of Appropriate Documentation of Battered Women

History
Description of past and present injuries
Photographs of visible injuries
Body map with notation of past and present injury
Record of her description of incident, including name of her assailant
Specific notation as to occurrence and nature of any forced sex
Physical
Notation of complete physical exam, including neurological exam
Notation of pelvic exam if history of forced sex
Notation of X ray of past and present bone injuries

NOTE: It is important that the nurse document risk for abuse, level of risk, past or present abuse, and information regarding the assailant. Both historical information and physical findings are included in documentation. This information may be essential for women involved in assault or child custody cases.

Whenever there is evidence of sexual assault within the past 24 to 48 hours, whether by father or father figure, husband, boyfriend, acquaintance, or stranger, a rape kit examination should be performed. In many settings, nurses are conducting these exams with accuracy equal to that of physicians and better results in terms of rapport with female victims, willingness to spend sufficient time to do a thorough and empathetic exam, and willingness to testify in court when necessary (DiNitto, Martin, Norton, & Maxwell, 1986). Advocacy for female victims of violence includes ascertaining who is conducting rape kit exams in hospitals in the nurse's community and working to change policy if necessary so that nurses are conducting the exams.

Women who are survivors of past psychological, physical, and sexual abuse can benefit from survivor groups or individual counseling. Lists of resources such as rape crises clinics and support groups for survivors of incest or physical and emotional abuse should be made available.

Prevention

Prevention, public policy, and social attitudes are intertwined. Our society has taken a major step toward the secondary prevention of abuse and sexual assault through the establishment of programs that encourage women and children to speak about their experiences. We need to support these programs further by trusting the women who confide in us. In the development of laws that punish child and woman abuse, we have given support to the victims of abuse, but often they are again victimized by our disbelief of their experiences, the devaluing of the effects of these assaults on their persons, and our focus on assisting the perpetrators of the crimes.

Primary prevention would encompass a total attitudinal change within the values of our society. Both girls and boys would be taught human values of interdependence, respect for human life, and a commitment to empathy and strength in the development of the human species regardless of sex, race, or socioeconomic status. Continued progress would be made toward eliminating the feminization of poverty and ensuring gender parity in the sharing of economic resources. In addition, local communities would make it clear that violence against women is not to be tolerated by eliminating pornography, mandating arrest of wife abusers, and creating a general climate of nonviolence.

Women victimized by violence are in need of assistance in making decisions and taking control of their lives. Nurses are involved with women at key times when they can be screened for the presence or absence of all forms of abuse. Mechanisms for screening women who are either abused or at risk for abuse from male partners and other intimates are available (Campbell & Humphreys, 1984; Helton et al., 1987). To intervene effectively, nurses must understand abuse as a cumulative process that must be examined as a continuum (Landenburger, 1989; Mills, 1985). During this process, the abuse, the relationship, and a woman's view of self change, requiring time-specific interventions. Research indicates that blame and responsibility for the victimization that is inflicted on the woman by the male is attributed by society to women (Drake, 1982; Landenburger, 1989). Subsequently, either women are assisted in a manner that discounts their feelings and further devalues them or the abuse is ignored. Through understanding the societal contexts that perpetuate violence and shape a woman's responses to experiencing violence, nursing is in a key position to intervene with individual women. Nurses can also work toward changing public policy in general and specific health care policies so that violence toward women decreases in our society.

References

Abramson, L. Y., Seligman, E. P., & Teasdale, J. D. (1978). Learned helplessness in humans: Critique and reformulation. *Journal of Abnormal Psychology, 87*(1), 49-74.

Alexander, P. C., Neimeyer, R. A., Follette, V., Moore, M. K., & Harter, S. (1989). A comparison of group treatments of women sexually abused as children. *Journal of Consulting and Clinical Psychology, 57*(4), 479-483.

Appleton, W. (1980). The battered woman syndrome. *Annals of Emergency Medicine, 9*(2), 45-63.

Baker, T. C., Burgess, A. W., Brickman, E., & Davis, R. C. (1990). Rape victims' concerns about possible exposure to HIV infection. *Journal of Interpersonal Violence, 5*(1), 49-60.

Barry, K. (1984). *Female sexual slavery.* New York: New York University Press.

Bird, G. W., Stith, S. M., & Schladale, J. (1991). Psychological resources, coping strategies, and negotiation styles as discriminators of violence in dating relationships. *Family Relations, 40*(1), 45-50.

Blumer, H. (1967). Society as symbolic interaction. In J. G. Manis & B. N. Meltzer (Eds.), *Symbolic interaction: A reader in social psychology* (pp. 139-148). Boston: Allyn & Bacon.

Breines, W., & Gordon, L. (1983). The new scholarship on family violence. *Signs: Journal of Women in Culture and Society, 8,* 490-531.

Brendtro, M., & Bowker, L. H. (1989). Battered women: How can nurses help. *Issues in Mental Health Nursing, 10,* 169-180.

Browne, A., & Finkelhor, D. (1986). Impact of child sexual abuse: A review of the research. *Psychological Bulletin, 99*(1), 66-77.

Brunngraber, L. S. (1986). Father-daughter incest: Immediate and long-term effects of sexual abuse. *Advances in Nursing Science, 8*(4), 15-35.

Bullock, L., & McFarlane, J. (1989). Battering/low birth-weight connection. *American Journal of Nursing, 89,* 1153-1155.

Bullock, L., McFarlane, J., Bateman, L., & Miller, V. (1989). Characteristics of battered women in a primary care setting. *Nurse Practitioner, 14*(6), 47-55.

Burgess, A. W., & Holmstrom, L. L. (1974). The rape trauma syndrome. *American Journal of Psychiatry, 131,* 981-986.

Burgess, A. W., & Holmstrom, L. L. (1979). *Rape: Crisis and recovery.* Bowie, MD: Brady.

Butler, M. J., & Snodgrass, F. G. (1991). Beyond abuse: Parse's theory in practice. *Nursing Science Quarterly, 4*(1), 76-82.

Campbell, J. C. (1985). Beating of wives: A cross-cultural perspective. *Victimology: An International Journal, 10*(14), 174-185.

Campbell, J. C. (1986). Nursing assessment for risk of homicide with battered women. *Advances in Nursing Science, 8*(4), 36-51.

Campbell, J. C. (1989a). A test of two explanatory models of women's responses to battering. *Nursing Research, 38*(1), 18-24.

Campbell, J. C. (1989b). Women's responses to sexual abuse in intimate relationships. *Health Care for Women International, 8,* 335-347.

Campbell, J. C. (1991). Public health conceptions of family abuse. In D. Knudson & J. Miller (Eds.), *Abused and battered* (pp. 35-48). New York: Aldine de Gruyter.

Campbell, J. C. (1992). "If I can't have you, no one can": Power and control in homicide of female partners. In J. Radford & D. E. H. Russell (Eds.), *Femicide: The politics of woman killing* (pp. 99-113). Boston: Twayne.

Campbell, J., & Alford, P. (1989). The dark side of marital rape. *American Journal of Nursing, 89,* 946-949.

Campbell, J., & Humphreys, J. (1984). *Nursing care of victims of family violence.* Reston, VA: Reston.

Campbell, J. C., & Sheridan, D. (1989). Emergency nursing with battered women. *Journal of Emergency Nursing, 15*(1), 12-17.

Cooley, C. H. (1967). Looking-glass self. In J. G. Manis & B. N. Meltzer (Eds.), *Symbolic interaction: A reader in social psychology* (pp. 139-148). Boston: Allyn & Bacon.

Cornman, B. J. (1989). Group treatment for female adolescent sexual abuse victims. *Issues in Mental Health Nursing, 10,* 261-271.

Counts, D., Brown, J., & Campbell, J. (1992). *Sanctions and sanctuary: Cultural perspectives on the beating of wives.* Boulder, CO: Westview.

Daly, M. (1990). *Gyn ecology: The metaethics of radical feminism.* Boston: Beacon.

Denzin, N. K. (1984a). *On understanding emotion.* San Francisco: Jossey-Bass.

Denzin, N. K. (1984b). Toward a phenomenology of domestic family violence. *American Journal of Sociology, 90*(3), 483-513.

Denzin, N. K. (1985). Emotion as lived experience. *Symbolic Interaction, 8*(2), 223-240.

Deyoung, M. (1982). *The sexual victimization of children.* Jefferson, NC: McFarland.

DiNitto, D., Martin, P. Y., Norton, D. B., & Maxwell, M. S. (1986). After rape: Who should examine survivors. *American Journal of Nursing, 86,* 538-540.

Dobash, R. E., & Dobash, R. (1979). *Violence against wives.* New York: Free Press.

Drake, V. K. (1982). Battered women: A health care problem. *Image, 19*(2), 40-47.

Draucker, C. B. (1989). Cognitive adaptation of female incest survivors. *Journal of Consulting and Clinical Psychology, 57*(5), 668-670.

Dutton, D., & Painter, S. L. (1981). Traumatic bonding: The development of emotional attachments in battered women and other relationships of intermittent abuse. *Victimology: An International Journal, 6*(2), 139-155.

Eisler, R. (1988). *The chalice and the blade.* San Francisco: Harper & Row.

Faludi, S. (1992). *Backlash.* New York: Crown.

Ferraro, K. J., & Johnson, J. M. (1983). How women experience battering: The process of victimization. *Social Problems, 30,* 325-339.

Finkelhor, D. (1980). Risk factors in the sexual victimization of children. *Child Abuse and Neglect, 4,* 265-273.

Finkelhor, D. (1986). *A sourcebook on child sexual abuse.* Beverly Hills, CA: Sage.

Fitzgerald, L. F., Shullman, S. L., Bailey, N., Gold, Y., Ormerod, M., Richards, M., Swecker, J., & Weitzman, L. (1988). The incidence and dimensions of sexual harassment in academia and the work place. *Journal of Vocational Behavior, 32,* 152-175.

Fitzgerald, L. F., Weitzman, L. M., Gold, Y., & Ormerod, M. (1988). Academic harassment: Sex and denial in scholarly garb. *Psychology of Women Quarterly, 12*(4), 329-340.

Frieze, I. H. (1979). Perceptions of battered wives. In I. H. Frieze, D. Bar-Tal, & J. S. Carroll (Eds.), New approaches to social problems (pp. 79-108). San Francisco: Jossey-Bass.

Frieze, I. H. (1983). Investigating the causes and consequences of marital rape. *Signs: Journal of Women in Culture and Society 8*(3), 325-339.

Gelles, R. J. (1972). *The violent home.* Beverly Hills, CA: Sage.

Gelles, R. J., & Straus, M. A. (1988). Determinants of violence in the family: Toward a theoretical integration. In W. R. Burr, R. Hill, F. I. Nye, & I. L. Reiss (Eds.), *Contemporary theories about the family* (Vol. 1, pp. 549-581). New York: Free Press.

Goldberg, W. G., & Tomlanovich, M. C. (1984). Domestic violence victims in the emergency department. *Journal of the American Medical Association, 251,* 3259-3264.

Gondolf, E. W. (1988). *Battered women as survivors: An alternative to treating learned helplessness.* Lexington, MA: Lexington Books.

Goodstein, R. K., & Page, A. W. (1981). Battered wife syndrome: Overview of dynamics and treatment. *American Journal of Psychiatry, 138*(8), 1036-1044.

Hanmer, J., & Maynard, M. (1987). *Women, violence and social control.* Atlantic Highlands, NJ: Humanities Press.

Hartman, C. R., & Burgess, A. W. (1988). Information processing of trauma. *Journal of Interpersonal Violence, 3,* 443-457.

Hartman, C. R., Burgess, A. W., & McCormack, A. (1987). Pathways and cycles of runaways: A model for understanding repetitive runaway behavior. *Hospital and Community Psychiatry, 38*(3), 292-299.

Helton, A., McFarlane, J., & Anderson, E. (1987). Prevention of battering during pregnancy: Focus on behavioral change. *Public Health Nursing, 4*(3), 166-174.

Herrenkohl, K. C., Herrenkohl, R. C., & Toedler, L. J. (1983). Perspectives on the intergenerational transmission of abuse. In D. Finkelhor, R. Gelles, G. Hotaling, & M. Straus (Eds.), *The dark side of families: Current family violence research* (pp. 305-316). Beverly Hills, CA: Sage.

Hilberman, E. (1980). The "wife beater's wife" reconsidered. *American Journal of Psychiatry, 137*(11), 1336-1347.

Hoff, L. A. (1990). *Battered women as survivors.* London: Routledge.

Hotaling, G. T., & Sugarman, D. B. (1986). An analysis of risk markers in husband to wife violence: The current state of knowledge. *Violence and victims, 1*(2), 101-124.

Hotaling, G. T., & Sugarman, D. B. (1990). A risk marker analysis of assaulted wives. *Journal of Family Violence, 5*(1), 1-14.

Janoff-Bulman, R., & Frieze, I. H. (1983). A theoretical perspective for understanding reactions to victimization. *Journal of Social Issues, 39*(2), 1-17.

Kanin, E. J. (1985). Date rapists: Differential sexual socialization and relative depravation. *Archives of Sexual Behavior, 6*(1), 67-76.

Landenburger, K. L. (1989). The process of entrapment in and recovery from an abusive relationship. *Issues in Mental Health Nursing, 10*(3), 165-183.

Levinson, D. (1989). *Family violence in cross-cultural perspective.* Newbury Park, CA: Sage.

Lichtenstein, V. R. (1981). The battered woman: Guidelines for effective nursing intervention. *Issues in Mental Health Nursing, 3,* 237-250.

Limandri, B. J. (1986). Research and practice with abused women: Use of the Roy adaptation model as an explanatory framework. *Advances in Nursing Science, 8*(4), 52-61.

Lloyd, S. A. (1991). The dark side of courtship: Violence and sexual exploitation. *Family Relations, 40*(1), 14-20.

Makepeace, J. M. (1981). Courtship violence among college students. *Family Relations, 30*(2), 97-102.

Makepeace, J. M. (1986). Gender differences in courtship violence victimization. *Family Relations, 35,* 383-388.

Martin, D. (1976). *Battered wives.* New York: Pocket Books.

Mercy, J. A., & Saltzman, L. E. (1989). Fatal violence among spouses in the United States, 1976-85. *American Journal of Public Health, 79,* 595-599.

Miller, D. T., & Porter, C. A. (1983). Self-blame in victims of violence. *Journal of Social Issues, 39*(2), 139-152.

Mills, T. (1985). The assault on the self: Stages in coping with battering husbands. *Qualitative Sociology, 8*(2), 103-123.

Orem, D. E. (1990). *Nursing: Concepts of practice.* New York: McGraw-Hill.

Parker, B., & Schumacher, D. (1977). The battered wife syndrome and violence in the nuclear family of origin: A controlled pilot study. *American Journal of Public Health, 67,* 760-761.

Parse, R. (1985). *Man, living and health: A theory of nursing.* New York: John Wiley.

Pearlin, L. I. (1975). Status inequality and stress in marriage. *American Sociological Review, 40,* 344-357.

Petersen, R. (1980). Social class, social learning, and wife abuse. *Social Service Review, 40,* 390-406.

Rew, L. (1989). Long-term effects of childhood sexual exploitation. *Issues in Mental Nursing, 10,* 229-244.

Rogers, M. E. (1970). *An introduction to a theoretical base for nursing.* Philadelphia: F. A. Davis.

Rogers, M. E. (1986). Science of unitary human beings. In B. M. Malinski (Ed.), *Explorations in Martha Rogers' science of unitary human beings* (pp. 3-8). Norwalk, CT: Appleton-Century-Crofts.

Rounsaville, B. J. (1978). Battered wives: Barriers to identification and treatment. *American Journal of Orthopsychiatry, 48,* 487-494.

Rouse, L. P. (1984). Models, self-esteem, and locus of control as factors contributing to spouse abuse. *Victimology: An International Journal, 9*(1), 130-141.

Roy, C. (1976). *An introduction to nursing: An adaptation model.* Englewood Cliffs, NJ: Prentice Hall.

Russell, D. E. H. (1982). *Marital rape.* New York: Macmillan.

Russell, D. E. H., Schurman, R. A., & Trocki, K. (1988). The long-term effects of incestuous abuse: A comparison of Afro-American and white American victims. In G. E. Wyatt & G. J. Powell (Eds.), *Lasting effects of child sexual abuse* (pp. 119-134). Newbury Park, CA: Sage.

Saunders, D. (1989). Wife abuse, husband abuse, or mutual combat: A feminist perspective on the empirical findings. In K. Yllö & M. Bograd (Eds.), *Feminist perspectives on wife abuse* (pp. 90-113). Newbury Park, CA: Sage.

Seligman, M., & Garber, J. (1980). *Human helplessness: Theory and applications.* New York: Academic Press.

Sigelman, C. K., Berry, C. J., & Wiles, K. A. (1984). Violence in college students' dating relationships. *Journal of Applied Social Psychology, 5/6,* 530-548.

Silver, R. L., Boon, C., & Stones, M. H. (1983). Searching for meaning in misfortune: Making sense of incest. *Journal of Social Issues, 39*(2), 81-102.

Smith, M. (1990). Patriarchal ideology and wife beating: A test of a feminist hypothesis. *Violence and Victims, 5*(4), 257-273.

Spratlen, L. P. (1988). Sexual harassment counseling. *Journal of Psychosocial Nursing, 26*(2), 28-33.

Stark, E., & Flitcraft, A. (1979). Medicine and patriarchal violence: The case against the patriarchy. *Social Problems, 9,* 461-493.

Stark, E., Flitcraft, A., Zuckerman, D., Grey, A., Robison, J., & Frazier, W. (1981). *Wife abuse in the medical setting* (Domestic Violence Monograph No. 7). Rockville, MD: National Clearinghouse on Domestic Violence.

Steinmetz, S. K. (1977). *The cycle of violence: Assertive, aggressive, and abusive family interaction.* New York: Praeger.

Stern, P. N. (1992). Woman abuse and practice implications within an international context. In C. M. Sampselle (Ed.), *Violence against women* (pp. 143-152). New York: Hemisphere.

Straus, M. A., & Gelles, R. (1990). *Physical violence in American families.* New Brunswick: Transaction.

Strauss, A. (1959). *Mirrors and masks: The search for identity.* Glencoe, IL: Free Press.

Stuart, E., & Campbell, J. C. (1989). Assessment of patterns of dangerousness with battered women. *Issues in Mental Health Nursing, 10,* 245-260.

Tilden, V. P. (1989). Response of the health care delivery system to battered women. *Issues in Mental Health Nursing, 10,* 309-320.

Tilden, V. P., & Shepherd, P. (1987). Increasing the rate of identification of battered women in an emergency department: Use of a nursing protocol. *Research in Nursing and Health, 10,* 209-215.

Tolman, R. M., & Bennett, L. W. (1990). A review of quantitative research on men who batter. *Journal of Interpersonal Violence, 5,* 87-118.

Torres, S. (1987). Hispanic-American battered women: Why consider cultural differences? *Response, 10*(3), 20-21.

Ulrich, Y. (1991). Women's reasons for leaving abusive spouses. *Women's Health Care International, 12,* 465-473.

U.S. Department of Health and Human Services. (1990). *Healthy people 2000: National health promotion and disease prevention objectives (DHHS Publication No. PHS 91-50213). Washington, DC: Government Printing Office.*

Walker, L. E. (1977-1978). Battered women and learned helplessness. *Victimology: An International Journal, 2*(3-4), 525-534.

Walker, L. (1979). *The battered woman.* New York: Harper & Row.

Walker, L. (1984). *The battered woman syndrome.* New York: Springer.

19

High-Risk Childbearing

CATHERINE INGRAM FOGEL
LYNNE PORTER LEWALLEN

Most expectant mothers will have an uneventful pregnancy with a favorable outcome. Pregnancy itself is not an illness but a normal life cycle event. However, of the approximately 3.9 million women giving birth in the United States each year, at least 500,000 will be designated as being at high risk (Cohen, Kenner, & Hollingsworth, 1991). When a high-risk pregnancy occurs, the challenge to nursing is great. This chapter will provide knowledge needed by the nurse providing care to the client experiencing the biological, emotional, and social crises of high-risk pregnancy by (a) defining the concept of high-risk pregnancy; (b) exploring the scope of the problem; (c) presenting information about specific risk factors; (d) discussing identification of the high-risk client, including diagnostic procedures for determining the client at risk; and (e) analyzing appropriate nursing interventions.

Definition and Scope of the Problem

Traditionally, a high-risk pregnancy has been defined as one in which the mother or infant (or fetus) has a significantly increased chance of mortality or morbidity when compared with a "low-risk" pregnancy, in which an optimal outcome is expected for both, either before, during, or after birth. A broader definition is needed to allow for consideration of morbidity or mortality resulting from a variety of causative agents—physical, psychological, or sociocultural—that place the mother, fetus, or both at risk at any time during the childbearing cycle. Childbearing carries with it the potential for risk because of the numerous factors involved, many of which are impossible to predict or control. These risks exist on a continuum ranging from little or no risk to the woman and her family to the risk of death for the mother and/or fetus.

An understanding of the extent and seriousness of high-risk childbearing may be gained by examining the statistical data available on maternal mortality and morbidity, infant mortality, and perinatal mortality. Maternal mortality rates have declined sharply in the United States over the past half century from 376.0 deaths per 100,000 live births in 1940 to 8 per 100,000 in 1989 (Horton, 1992). This represents a decrease of over 98%. Over the years, the majority of maternal deaths have been caused by hemorrhage, pregnancy-induced hypertension (PIH), and infection. Although this triad still accounts for most maternal deaths, medical management of these complications has improved tremendously, accounting for the vast improvement in mortality figures. Despite this, women of color have a maternal mortality rate more than twice as high as the rate of white women—16.6 deaths per 100,000 live births in 1986 (Atrash, Koonin, Lawson, Franks, & Smith, 1990). Effects of coagulation disorders, such as embolism, have emerged as a significant cause of maternal morbidity and mortality. African American women generally have had a higher incidence of complications of pregnancy that are associated with clotting problems, such as PIH (Saftlas, Olson, Franks, Atrash, & Pokras, 1990).

It could be argued that childbirth is much safer today if only maternal mortality rates are considered; however, maternal morbidity rates must also be considered, and these are not available. Although, occasionally, statistics surface indicating, for example, that 2.6% of all pregnant women in the United States experienced preeclampsia during the years 1979 to 1986 (Saftlas et al., 1990), there is no uniform system of reporting maternal morbidity and therefore no way of knowing what is the true incidence of maternal morbidity. Furthermore, our definition of high risk is not limited to, or measured in, medical complications or deaths alone. There are many other social, psychological, and economic factors to be considered. These are discussed later in the section on specific risk factors.

In considering the scope of high-risk pregnancy, the infant mortality rate should also be considered. Compared with other countries having comparable populations and technologies, the United States ranks 21st in infant mortality (Wegman, 1991). Infant mortality rates have shown improvement over the years, decreasing from 10 in 1,000 live births in 1970 to 9.8 in 1,000 live births in 1991, the lowest ever recorded in the United States. However, in that year, black infants died at more than twice the rate of white infants (18.6/1,000 live births versus 8.1 per 1,000 live births) (Horton, 1992). The incidence of low birth weight (less than 2,500 gm [5 lb. 8 oz.]) also has relevance to the magnitude of the problem, because these infants are more apt to be the product of a high-risk pregnancy, contribute significantly to infant mortality, and have more physical problems in life.

The United States' low birth weight rate has not changed significantly in more than 30 years. In 1950, 7.6% of all live births were considered to be low birth weight. Today, 7% of all live births in the United States produce infants who weigh less than 2,500 gm. When race is considered, wide discrepancies in levels are seen—5.7% for whites and 12.7% for blacks (U.S. Bureau of the Census, 1990). Deaths for low birth weight infants in the neonatal period are 30 times more frequent than for infants of average or normal birth weight. It is now widely believed that if birth weight could be improved, infant mortality would be substantially reduced.

Risk Factors

Obstetrics has long recognized that some women are more likely to experience poor outcomes of pregnancy than others. Hippocrates recognized that the outcomes of pregnancy were influenced by intrinsic, extrinsic, and environmental factors. Traditionally, risk factors have been viewed only in the medical model framework; that is, only medical, obstetric, or physiological risk factors were considered. In recent years, health professionals have recognized that a more comprehensive approach to high-risk pregnancy is necessary, and risk assessment has developed into a valuable tool for evaluating risk status in pregnancy. The pregnant woman does not exist in a vacuum, and factors such as age, parity, environmental influences, and emotional disturbances are equally as important to consider as specific disease entities, such as hypertension or diabetes.

It is possible to group the factors associated with at-risk childbearing into broad categories based on threats to health and pregnancy outcome. Categories of risk include biophysical, psychosocial, sociodemographic, and environmental. Those risks considered to be biophysical in nature include factors that originate within the mother or fetus and affect the development or functioning of either. Sociodemographic risks arise from characteristics of the mother and her family that place the childbearing unit at increased risk. Psychosocial risks involve those maternal behaviors and adverse lifestyles that have a negative impact on the health of the mother and her unborn fetus. Internal conflicts, emotional distress, and disturbed interpersonal relationships also are considered to be risk factors, as are inadequate social support and unsafe cultural practices. Environmental factors arise from circumstances outside of the woman and her family and include hazards of the workplace and her general environment.

Risk factors are interrelated and cumulative in their effects. Rarely is serious risk incurred with the presence of a single factor. Usually, high-risk status occurs because several factors are identified simultaneously. It is important to remember that risk is incurred by a unit; a threat to the health and well-being of the mother will most often have an adverse effect, direct or indirect, on the fetus. In addition, some threats that arise within the fetus itself can threaten the mother. At times, the mother will be at greater risk, whereas in other instances the fetus will be. However, whenever the mother is seriously threatened, the fetus will also be in jeopardy. Extending this concept further, pregnancy exists within the context of a family unit; and, therefore, whenever the woman and her fetus are threatened, there is likely to be a negative impact on the rest of the family. Conversely, risk to the pregnant woman can be intensified by a poor family situation and lack of social support.

Biophysical Risk Factors

Genetic

Genetic factors may interfere with normal fetal/neonatal development, result in congenital anomalies, and/or create difficulties for the pregnant woman. Defective maternal or paternal genes as well as transmittable inherited disorders can cause genetic disease or defects. Deviations in fetal development place the fetus and, at times, the mother at risk. The most obvious risks are those resulting from chromosomal abnormalities; however, other less aberrant deviations create risk. Multiple pregnancies carry an increased risk for low-birth-weight infants as well as create excessive stress on a woman. Large fetal size can create dystocia (abnormal labor) and cephalopelvic disproportion (fetal head is too large or mother's pelvis is too small to permit vaginal birth). Certain genetically determined maternal or paternal characteristics can be risk factors in childbearing. ABO incompatibility (incompatibility of blood types) and Rh incompatibility with its attendant anemia and hyperbilirubinemia are examples of such characteristics. The degree of severity in this instance is related to the degree of antibody sensitization incurred by the mother.

Nutritional Status

Nutritional status is an important, if not the most important, determinant of pregnancy outcome. Fetal growth and development cannot progress normally without adequate nutrition. Studies indicate that height of the mother and her weight during pregnancy can affect fetal growth and subsequent birth weight and that these effects are independent and cumulative (DeBruyne & Rolfes, 1989). It is thought that maternal size may be a factor affecting the ultimate size of the placenta. There is also an interrelationship between infant birth weight and the amount of weight gained during pregnancy (see Chapter 12, "Nutrition"). In the first trimester, severe limitation of the supply or transport of nutrients may cause restriction of the materials and energy needed by cell synthesis and cell differentiation and thus produce malformations or death of the embryo. After the first trimester, malnutrition would not have teratogenic effects but could limit fetal growth. Nutrient requirements are greatest in the last trimester of pregnancy, when the cells are increasing in size and number. Even small nutritional restrictions could be serious at this time, resulting in low-birth-weight offspring and compromised maternal wellbeing (DeBruyne & Rolfes, 1989).

Nutritional risk factors present at the beginning of pregnancy include very young age (< 15 years); previous poor pregnancy outcomes or three pregnancies in the past 2 years; tobacco, alcohol, or drug use; inadequate diet due to chronic illness or food fads; and weight less than 85% or greater than 120% of standard weight for height. Inadequate or excessive weight gain and hematocrit less than 33% during pregnancy are also indicators of nutritional risk.

Table 19.1 Major Physiological Causes of Maternal Morbidity

Medical complications/obstetric illnesses
- Anemias, particularly sickling disorders and persistent anemia
- Diabetes (including glucose intolerance of pregnancy)
- Epilepsy
- Heart disease
- Hypertensive conditions (for example, pregnancy-induced hypertension or chronic hypertension)
- Infections, especially those that are sexually transmitted (i.e., gonorrhea, herpes, and AIDS), and urinary tract infections
- Kidney disease
- Pelvic surgery
- Deep venous thrombophlebitis
- Malignant neoplasms, including breast and cervical
- Rh incompatibility

Medical and Obstetric Complications

Medical complications of previous and current pregnancies (e.g., insulin-dependent diabetes, cardiac illness), obstetric illnesses (e.g., PIH or placenta previa), and pregnancy losses have long been identified as risk factors and are discussed in every standard obstetric textbook. The more common causes of maternal mortality are given in Table 19.1.

It has been recognized for many years that obstetric complications tend to recur in subsequent pregnancies. Furthermore, it has been clearly documented that a woman with a history of a prior pregnancy loss is at increased risk for future losses. The etiology of this risk factor varies depending on when in the pregnancy it occurs. In early pregnancy, the major risk factors are genetic abnormalities and structural anomalies of the reproductive tract. As pregnancy progresses, obstetric complications and chronic medical diseases of the mother become the major risk factors.

Sociodemographic Risk Factors

Although it is sometimes possible to ascribe childbearing risk to biophysical factors alone, in most instances it is not. Sociodemographic factors seem to be associated with increased risk in many instances. Sociodemographic factors are defined as factors that dictate lifestyle and influence participation in social behaviors such as substance abuse. They are interdependent and determined by where an individual lives, her access to services, and her family's values and attitudes. It is possible to identify sociodemographic factors that indicate high risk; however, it is not possible to determine the specific ways in which these factors will create problems for a given women. Sociodemographic risk factors include low income, lack of prenatal care, age, parity, residence, and race.

Low Income

For over half a century, it has been noted that the population most at risk during childbearing is among the most underprivileged socioeconomically. Poverty seems to underlie many other risk factors. Inadequate financial resources are highly correlated with low birth weight and increased infant mortality rates.

The poor experience increased risk because of poor general health prior to and during pregnancy and poor or nonexistent prenatal care. Low-income mothers often do not seek prenatal care at all or they do so late in pregnancy (Institute of Medicine, 1988). Low-income women are more likely to have medical complications of pregnancy, which predispose them to perinatal mortality; experience increased prenatal morbidity with increased risk of mortality; and more often report a history of prior prenatal loss, which places them at greater risk for fetal loss with a current pregnancy. Also, they are considerably more predisposed to illnesses and obstetric complications during pregnancy.

Poverty also has an indirect effect on high-risk pregnancy in that other significant risk factors, such as nutritional status, emotional disturbances, and environmental influences, are affected by socioeconomic status.

Lack of Prenatal Care

Lack of prenatal care is a major factor in placing the pregnant woman at risk because the opportunity is lost for early diagnosis and treatment of obstetric complications. It is possible to identify many women at risk for preterm birth or a low-birth-weight infant early in pregnancy when corrective measures could be begun. Women with no prenatal care are three times more likely to deliver a low-birth-weight infant than women with adequate prenatal care (Lia-Hoagberg et al., 1990). The number of infants born to women with either no prenatal care, or prenatal care that started in the third trimester or later, has increased from 5.1% in 1980 to 6.9% in 1988 (U.S. Bureau of the Census, 1990). Many of the women who receive inadequate prenatal care are poor or members of ethnic minorities (Ahmed, McRae, & Ahmed, 1990).

The Institute of Medicine (1988) has identified four major categories of barriers to prenatal care: (a) financial barriers, (b) inadequacy of the system, (c) organization and atmosphere of prenatal care services, and (d) cultural and personal barriers. Financial barriers are some of the most frequently described in the literature. In a study done in Washington, D.C., Ahmed et al. (1990) found that the poorest women were the most likely to receive the least adequate prenatal care. Transportation is also a barrier to prenatal care for poor women and can be especially severe for women in rural areas, who live far from the nearest health care provider (Kalmuss & Fennelly, 1990; McDonald & Coburn, 1988).

Prenatal clinics, which may be the only available site for care for poor women, are often unpleasant (Institute of Medicine, 1988). Many women complain about the depersonalization of care, and there is little incentive to return for care or initiate it in subsequent pregnancies. In too many cases, the visit is brief and routinized with little or no time for asking questions, discussing the client's concerns, or for client education. The waiting time is often measured in hours for a visit that takes minutes, in which it appears nothing has been done. If the preventive and maintenance measures are not explained to the client, the whole experience may be seen as valueless, time-consuming, expensive, and irrelevant. Women may rarely see the same health care provider on a regular basis, thus receiving little continuity of care (Institute of Medicine, 1988; Lia-Hoagberg et al., 1990).

Many women do not understand the need for early and continued prenatal care. Their orientation to health care is one of treatment, not prevention and maintenance. Pregnant women, regardless of income, may not know what type of care is available, how to make an appointment, when to go for the first visit, or how to get this information. Others may feel they already know how to care for themselves and believe that as long as the baby moves and they feel healthy, routine prenatal care is unnecessary. Weeks or months may elapse between the time a woman first suspects pregnancy and the time when she first sees a health care provider. At times, the fact of pregnancy is denied until it is evident to others. Others may be so frightened of or uncomfortable with health care providers and the health care system that they delay or avoid seeking prenatal care (Miller, Margolis, Schwethelm, & Smith, 1989; Poland, Ager, & Olson, 1987).

Age

Age has long been considered a crucial variable in determining high-risk pregnancy. Traditionally, women at either end of the childbearing continuum have been considered to be at high risk during pregnancy, because the incidence of poor outcomes is increased in each. An examination of statistics reveals that risk and poor outcomes are high in the very young (aged 15 and under), drop to minimal levels during the 20s, and then rise continually until the end of the childbearing years. However, research findings support the theory that age is related to poor outcomes in some instances but not in others. The conclusion should not automatically be drawn that it is dangerous for women outside the optimal age range to bear children. Both physiological and psychological variables should be considered in assigning risk.

Adolescent Mothers. The percentage of births to teenagers has been declining in the past decade, primarily due to the relatively small numbers of children born after the baby boom. Recent statistics, however, demonstrate that the fertility rate for adolescents under the age of 15 is increasing (U.S. Bureau of the Census, 1990). Data on the physiological risks of adolescent childbearing are conflicting. Some research has indicated that early childbearing has a biological advantage, whereas others have found that it is associated with increased complications. Frequently cited pregnancy complications in adolescents include anemia, PIH, prolonged labor, contracted pelvis, and cephalopelvic disproportion (Cefalo & Moos, 1988). The latter two are generally more common in deliveries at less than age 15. Although childbearing in the later teen years does not seem to carry risk significantly higher than childbearing in the 20s, it is generally thought that biological risks are significant for perinatal outcomes when the pregnancy occurs less than 3 years after menarche (Cefalo & Moos, 1988). Mothers under the age of 15 have a 60% higher maternal mortality rate than do mothers over 20, and the infant mortality in their offspring is two to four times greater (Cefalo & Moos, 1988). Researchers and clinicians have long agreed that adolescent childbearing is associated with long-term social and economic problems, including lower educational achievement, lower incomes, increased dependence on governmental support programs, higher rates of divorce, and higher parity. Furthermore, it has been assumed that early childbearing occurred in generation after generation. However, results from a longitudinal study of adolescent pregnancy and its outcomes conducted over 20 years in urban Baltimore indicate that this is not always the case (Furstenberg, Levine, & Brooks-Gunn, 1990). Nearly two thirds of the daughters of adolescent mothers delayed their first birth until age 19 or later; however, those who did have an adolescent birth appeared to be even more vulnerable than their mothers to economic dependence and poverty.

Mature Mother. Although childbearing after the age of 35 is far less common than between the ages of 18 and 34, the birthrate of women 35 years or older has steadily increased since 1979 (U.S. Bureau of the Census, 1990). Two phenomena may help to explain this trend. First, the number of women over the age of 35 is the largest it has ever been due to the maturing of individuals born during the post-World War II baby boom. Second, many women are delaying childbearing because of desires to continue their education, career priorities, financial concerns, late and second marriages, and infertility (Mansfield & McCool, 1989). Older pregnant women are often referred to in negative terms such as the *elderly primigravidas, obstetrically senescent,* and *postmature,* and as participating in childbearing in the "twilight" of their reproductive years. As more and more women elect to defer their childbearing to their 30s and 40s, it is essential that less offensive terms be used. For example, the term *mature primigravida* has been recommended as a suitable replacement for the pejorative elderly primigravida (Kirz, Dorchester, & Freeman, 1985).

It is traditional for clinicians to view women over the age of 35, especially first-time mothers, as high-risk patients. Risks associated with childbearing at an advanced age do not arise from age alone but rather are affected by numerous lifestyle, historical, social, and demographic factors as well—the number and spacing of previous pregnancies; genetic disposition of the parents; and the medical history, lifestyle, nutrition, and prenatal care of the mother. Socioeconomic factors influencing later childbearing include income, education, housing, and social networks.

After comprehensively reviewing existing data on pregnancy outcomes for women of advanced maternal age, Hansen (1986) concluded that the ability to conceive decreases and the incidence of problems for those who do conceive is greater than that of the general population. Problems the mature mother may experience include hypertension (including PIH) diabetes, extended labor, cesarean delivery, placenta previa, abruptio placentae, spontaneous abortion, and maternal mortality. Her offspring is at greater risk for low birth weight, macrosomia (increased body weight and size), chromosomal abnormalities, congenital malformations, and neonatal mortality.

Although maternal mortality rates for women of all ages have decreased dramatically in the past 5 decades, women 35 years and older are at increased risk for mortality from pregnancy-related causes (Horton, 1992). The leading causes of death in the older woman are obstetric hemorrhage followed by embolism and hypertensive conditions. Although maternal mortality rates are adversely affected by increasing age, ethnicity and socioeconomic status tend to be more crucial indicators of maternal risk than do adolescent or mature childbearing.

An increased incidence of chromosomal abnormalities is indisputably linked to increased age. And certain congenital malformations are positively associated with maternal age. It appears that an increase in chromosomal nondisjunction occurs in the aging oocyte. Prolonged exposure to pollutants, pesticides, radiation, and other environmental and occupational hazards may also play a role. The correlation between age and Down's syndrome (trisomy 21) is well known; however, the age-related risks of other chromosomal abnormalities are not as well known. Chromosomal abnormalities such as trisomy 18 (Edward's syndrome), trisomy 13 (Patau's syndrome), and XX genotype (Klinefelter's syndrome) are more frequent with advancing maternal age.

Gravidity affects optimum childbearing age; as birth order increases so does the optimum childbearing age. For example, risk for fetal mortality is lowest at maternal age 18 in primigravidas and at age 26 for women having their fourth pregnancy.

Having a child in one's 30s or 40s can have considerable psychological impact. Some women may experience strong conflict regarding the effect of childbearing on their career, lifestyles, and relationships. They may experience a sense of displacement, feeling neither in step with their peers nor in step with those women having babies in their teens and 20s. Some women may feel embarrassed or even ashamed at a pregnancy that occurs so late in their reproductive lives. Until recently, it was a learned cultural role that a woman did not become pregnant in middle life. Motherhood was considered a task to be completed before the age of 40. Other women are delighted at beginning a delayed family and may have the additional satisfaction of achieving a long-desired and long-deferred goal. If they have experienced infertility problems, there may be a sense of relief and additional accomplishment. For some women, fear is present—fear of a high-risk pregnancy, of increased risks to self and offspring, and fear of death for self and child.

Although childbearing is perhaps more problematic for women in their late 30s and 40s, there is no specific age at which the risks suddenly escalate; rather, increase in risk is gradual. Furthermore, recent research findings suggest that the higher perinatal mortality rates associated with advanced maternal age may be ameliorated by intensive, high-risk prenatal and intrapartal care (Kirz et al., 1985) and that present-day older women are healthier than older women in the past, so pregnancy in this otherwise healthy group would pose few risks (Mansfield & McCool, 1989). On the basis of an analysis of the research on the risks of childbearing at an advanced maternal age, Mansfield and McCool (1989) concluded that life circumstances surrounding the pregnancy and childbirth experiences of younger and older women account for a considerable portion of the risks ascribed to reproductive age. They identified three factors associated with increased risks: (a) the older woman's increasing likelihood of chronic diseases that adversely affect pregnancy outcomes, (b) more invasive medical management of middle-aged women's pregnancies and labors with resulting iatrogenically caused complications, and (c) demographic characteristics suggesting that in the past midlife pregnancy was associated with poverty or subfertility, and that today it is associated with healthy middle-class women who postponed their childbearing.

Parity

The number of previous pregnancies a woman has had can be a high-risk factor and is closely associated with age. Some authorities consider first pregnancies to be potentially high risk, no matter what the age of the mother. However, more risk is incurred when the first pregnancy is at either end of the childbearing-age spectrum. The incidence of PIH and dystocia is higher in first births; and firstborns have higher rates of morbidity and mortality. Infants born to unmarried mothers, who are disproportionately represented in first pregnancies, are known to have higher mortality rates. High parity, especially more than five closely spaced pregnancies, also brings increased risk.

Marital Status

Marital status can be considered a high-risk factor because mortality and morbidity rates are higher for nonmarital than marital births (U.S. Bureau of the Census, 1990). For example, unmarried women have a significantly greater risk of developing PIH (Saftlas et al., 1990). Nonmarried women are more likely to have inadequate prenatal care than are married women (13.2% vs. 3.7%). Nonmarital pregnancies more often occur in the youngest age group (15 years and under), which is at extremely high risk for medical problems.

Residence

Where a woman lives can be associated with an increase in childbearing risk. There are large variations in prenatal care, depending on place of residence. In general, women in metropolitan areas have more prenatal visits than do those in nonmetropolitan areas. Women who live in rural areas have fewer opportunities for specialized health care. The incidence of maternal mortality is slightly higher for both white and nonwhite women living in rural areas. This is likely related to low socioeconomic level, increased age (women continue childbearing longer in rural areas), higher fertility levels and parities, and less availability of health care. Women living in the inner city also experience increased risks. These women are often poor and begin childbearing earlier and continue it longer, having greater numbers of children. Health care in the inner city may be of a poorer quality than that offered in more affluent sections of the city.

Ethnicity

Ethnicity alone is not a major contributing factor in childbearing risk. Although a small number of genetic disorders are racially transmitted, they are not a large component of genetic risk conditions. Race, as an indicator of other sociodemographic factors, presents another picture, however. Nonwhite women are more than three times as likely as white women to die of pregnancy-related causes, and the risk for black women is the highest of all racial groups (Horton, 1992). Infant mortality rates among blacks are more than twice as high as those of whites (Witwer, 1990). Babies of black women have the highest rates of prematurity (18.3%) in the United States (Witwer, 1990). Furthermore, the percentage of nonwhite, low-birth-weight infants is twice that of whites. Prenatal care has been shown to be more beneficial for blacks than for whites even in a population of women at low risk for giving birth to a low-birth-weight infant (Murray & Bernfield, 1988).

Psychosocial Risk Factors

Certain lifestyle patterns and maternal behaviors can have an adverse impact on pregnancy outcomes. Use of alcohol and tobacco is widely accepted in our society, despite widespread health education efforts to inform the public about the dangers of their use. Many women view use of tobacco, alcohol, and drugs as merely habitual and/or medicinal in nature and do not realize that they are consuming biologically active substances that cross the placental barrier. Nicotine, caffeine, alcohol, and drugs can influence reproduction either through direct action on the embryo or fetus or indirectly when maternal equilibrium is disturbed.

Smoking

There is a strong, consistent, causal relationship between maternal smoking during pregnancy and reduced birth weight. Infants of mothers who smoke weigh less than do infants of nonsmokers at all gestational ages. On the average, smokers' babies weigh from 150 to 250 gm less than nonsmokers' babies, and twice as many weigh less than 2,500 gm. Neonatal mortality rates for single live births of low-birth-weight infants are significantly higher for infants of smoking mothers. Studies have also documented a direct increase in mortality risk as smoking level increases. There is an increase in spontaneous abortion rates but no significant increase in stillbirth or major fetal anomalies among women who smoke. Wen et al. (1990) found that women over the age of 35 who smoked had an increased incidence of both low-birth-weight infants and preterm delivery as compared to younger women who smoked. It would seem that age increases the detrimental effect of cigarette smoking during pregnancy.

There is some suggestion that there is an increased incidence of premature rupture of the membranes in smokers. There may also be an increased risk for women smokers who are anemic, are of low socioeconomic status, or have prior poor obstetric histories and who aggravate poor nutritional status by smoking (Coste, Job-Sprira, & Fernandez, 1991; DeBruyne & Rolfes, 1989). Olsen, Pereira, and Olsen (1991) found that women who drank 2 ounces of alcohol per week and smoked more than 15 cigarettes per day averaged a 459 gm lower birthweight in their infants than did women who drank the same amount of alcohol but did not smoke.

Caffeine

Caffeine, although shown to be a teratogen in mice, has not been shown to cause birth defects in humans (Narod, de Sanjose, & Victora, 1991). Heavy consumption of caffeine (equivalent to 3 or more cups of percolated coffee per day), however, has been related to a slight decrease in birthweight (Caan & Goldhaber, 1989; Narod et al., 1991). (See Chapter 22, "Drug Abuse Problems Among Women.")

Alcohol

Although the precise effects of maternal alcohol use in pregnancy have not been quantified and the mode of action is unexplained, there is sufficient evidence to conclude that maternal alcohol consumption has a number of varied negative reproductive effects (see Chapter 22). Because of the magnitude and risk of mental deficiency in infants of alcoholic women, a woman who is a chronic alcoholic should be counseled regarding effective birth control measures. If she becomes pregnant, she should be informed of the risks of alcohol exposure to the fetus and offered the option of abortion. New data have shown that women who are "social drinkers" may have children with fetal alcohol effects (FAE), which can include learning disabilities and hyperactivity. It is recommended that a woman consume no alcohol during pregnancy (Barbour, 1990).

Drugs

Drugs taken during pregnancy may adversely affect the developing fetus; these drugs may include those prescribed by a health care provider, those bought over the counter, or those commonly abused. Drugs can be teratogenic (cause congenital malformations), cause metabolic disturbances, produce chemical effects, or cause depression and/or alteration of the central nervous system function. When any medication is administered during pregnancy, the benefits must be weighed against the risk inherent in its use. Table 19.2 summarizes the potential effects of many drugs on the mother and her fetus.

Drug abuse during pregnancy is a major problem in the United States. Often, women who abuse drugs have inadequate or no prenatal care (Ahmed et al., 1990; Kalmuss & Fennelly, 1990), and the incidence of maternal complications is markedly higher, especially prematurity and precipitate labor. In addition, the incidence of sexually transmitted diseases (STDs) is increased in drug addicts. (See Chapter 24, "Sexually Transmitted Diseases," for a discussion of perinatal effects of STDs.) All addictive drugs affect the fetus, and the infant will demonstrate withdrawal symptoms shortly after delivery. The risks involved in multiple drug abuse are more complicated and not yet clearly understood; furthermore, the long-term effects of intrauterine drug exposure, neonatal withdrawal syndrome, and any subsequent treatment are not known. Chapter 22 explores the problem of drug abuse in women in depth.

Intravenous drug users (IVDUs) often engage in high-risk activities, such as sharing needles and unprotected sexual intercourse with a variety of partners. Often, female heroin users have irregular menstrual cycles and are infertile, but pregnancy can occur. The longer the addiction, the greater the severity of the withdrawal symptoms in the infant. When a woman is addicted to heroin, abrupt abstinence ("cold turkey") is not recommended, because it can cause damage to the fetus, such as intrauterine convulsions and possible stillbirth (Cefalo & Moos, 1988). There are two alternate approaches available: detoxification and methadone maintenance. In the detoxification program, complications for the mother and child are low birth weight, meconium-stained amniotic fluid (indicating fetal distress), and increased likelihood of breech presentation. The methadone program appears to have better results in that pregnancy complications are similar to the average obstetric population; however, low birth weight at term is frequent. The infant will also go through drug withdrawal after birth if the mother is on methadone, and the withdrawal may be severe and prolonged.

Cocaine is one of the most dangerous of the illicit drugs used in pregnancy. Ingested by sniffing, injection, or smoking ("crack" cocaine), it causes severe vasoconstriction, followed by rebound vasodilation. Cocaine can cause vaginal bleeding, preterm labor, and abruptio placentae during pregnancy. Dangers to the fetus include asphyxia, meconium-stained amniotic fluid, prematurity, and drug withdrawal after birth, leading to long-term irritability and altered responsivity to caretakers (Abel & Sokol, 1988; "Caring for Cocaine's Mothers & Babies," 1989; Lynch & McKeon, 1990; Mastrogiannis, Decavalas, Verma, & Tejani, 1990). Genitourinary tract abnormalities, such as hypospadias and hydronephrosis, have also been reported in infants exposed to cocaine in utero (Chasnoff, 1989).

Approximately 14% of women use marijuana at some point during their pregnancies (Abel & Sokol, 1988). Most studies show no increase in congenital malformations in babies exposed to marijuana in utero, but dysmorphic facial features

Table 19.2 Direct and Indirect Effects of Maternal Drug Abuse

Class of Drugs	*Direct Effect (fetal risk)*	*Indirect Effect (maternal behavior)*[a]
Amphetamine and related substances[b]	Congenital defects (i.e., cardiac abnormalities, bifid encephaly, biliary atresia, eye, and central nervous system defects) Withdrawal syndrome (i.e., poor state control, lability, poor consolability) Growth retardation past neonatal stage Decreased birth weight, length, head circumference Increased incidence of preterm delivery Increased perinatal mortality rate	Intoxication, seizures, cardiac arrhythmias, respiratory paralysis Withdrawal with paranoid and suicidal ideation; suicide a major complication Violent and aggressive behavior, may harm self or others while reacting to delusions Are stimulants and thus share traits and risks with cocaine
Cannabis	May retard placental development and result in reduced blood flow to fetus Abnormalities of nervous system, immaturity, and disruption of fetal sleep patterns Decreased birth weight, length, head circumference Increased stillbirth and neonatal mortality Meconium staining Withdrawal symptoms at birth Use near delivery can prolong or shorten labor due to effects on infant behavior	Accidents, particularly auto, due to impaired motor coordination May harm self or others while reacting to delusions
Cocaine	Hyperactivity of fetus Abruptio placentae with onset of uterine contractions and labor with subsequent increased incidence of prematurity Intrauterine growth retardation Intrauterine cerebral infarctions Meconium staining Withdrawal symptoms Congenital anomalies (i.e., cardiac, genitourinary, limb) Neonatal neurobehavioral dysfunction Sudden infant death syndrome (SIDS) Increased incidence of spontaneous abortion Necrotizing enterocolitis Visual and auditory dysfunction Seizures Long-term developmental neurobehavioral disabilities	Seizures after large doses Cardiac arrhythmias, respiratory paralysis, death Paranoid and suicidal ideation, suicide Violent or aggressive behavior May harm self or others while reacting to delusions
Hallucinogens	Congenital malformations, particularly ocular Increased incidence of spontaneous abortion	In rare cases may act irrationally and harm self or others Suicidal behavior, suicide, major depression, panic disorder
Inhalants	No information available	Impaired motor coordination Central nervous system depression Cardiac arrhythmia, sensitization of heart to epinephrine, ventricular fibrillation, sudden death
Opioids		Opioid depression with coma, shock pinpoint pupils, depressed respiration, death due to intoxication Withdrawal occurs rarely unless woman has severe physical disorder

Table 19.2 Continued

Class of Drugs	*Direct Effect (fetal risk)*	*Indirect Effect (maternal behavior)*[a]
Codeine	Musculoskeletal defects, cleft lip and palate, cardiac and circulatory system defects Neonatal withdrawal with respiratory depression	No studies available
Meperidine	Decelerated fetal heart rate Drug-induced respiratory depression Hypotension Impaired behavioral responsibility	No studies available
Methadone	Growth retardation Smaller head circumference Depression of interactive behavior, state controls Elevated systolic blood pressure Low birth weight (< 30%) Increased incidence of breech presentation Chromosome damage Neonatal narcotic withdrawal Increased morbidity and mortality Increased incidence of SIDS Increased incidence of stillbirth	Maternal withdrawal produces marked fetal response that contraindicates detoxification during pregnancy
Morphine Heroin Opium	Increased pre- and postnatal growth deficiency Mental and neurological deficiencies High morbidity, mortality Chromosomal breakage, mitosis depression, chromosomal aberration Drug-induced respiratory depression Vascular change Meconium staining Hypoxic episodes Narcotic withdrawal syndrome (85%)	
Pentazocine	Neonatal respiratory depression	
Phencyclidine (PCP)	Withdrawal with tremors, irritability hypertonia Sudden agitation, change in level of consciousness, sleeplessness, bizarre eye movements Vomiting and diarrhea Meconium staining Respiratory distress Spasticity Cerebellar malformation Dysmorphology Microcephaly Increased risk of prematurity, low birth weight	Death from respiratory depression, suicide May harm self or others Violence, self-abuse, mutilation
Sedative Hypnotic Anxiolytic	Congenital defects Central nervous system depression	
Diazepam	Hypotonia, lethargy, sucking difficulties Intrauterine growth retardation, tremors, irritability, hypertonaia, diarrhea/vomiting Disturbances in neonatal thermogenesis and regulation	

(continued)

Table 19.2 Continued

Class of Drugs	*Direct Effect (fetal risk)*	*Indirect Effect (maternal behavior)*[a]
	Loss of beat-to-beat variability in fetal rate Decreased fetal movements Respiratory depression, apneic spells if drug overdose Congenital malformations (e.g., cleft lip and/or palate, craniofacial asymmetry, cardiac defects)	
Barbiturates	Withdrawal symptoms	Accidental overdose and death Seizures with withdrawal Injuries associated with hallucinations Memory impairment may place women at risk

SOURCE: Adapted from Jones and Lopez (1990).
NOTE: To effectively counsel women regarding drug use and abuse, the nurse must have comprehensive knowledge of the potential effects of many drugs on the mother and her fetus. The effects of the major categories of drugs are described in this table.
a. Effects listed are in addition to those associated with the effects of the lifestyle often seen among women who abuse drugs, such as poor nutrition; increased infections, particularly STD; injuries; and inadequate prenatal care.
b. Risks associated with abuse of substances.

have been reported (Cefalo & Moos, 1988). Significant increases in preterm delivery and meconium-stained amniotic fluid have been found, and animal studies have also shown an increased incidence of intrauterine growth retardation with cannabinoid exposure. Infants born to marijuana users may show tremors and a diminished startle response during the first 1 to 3 weeks of life, suggesting delayed nervous system development (Abel & Sokol, 1988).

Psychological Status

Childbearing is one of the most critical periods in the life of an individual or family. Even under optimal circumstances, pregnancy, birth, and the postpartum period trigger profound and complex physiological, psychological, and social changes. For the individual, it is a period of increased ego vulnerability, whereas for the family it is a time of change. It has long been suggested that there is a relationship between emotional distress and obstetric complications. Results of earlier studies (McDonald, 1968; Nuckolls, Cassel, & Kaplan, 1972) supported the existence of such a relationship; however, at present, the literature does not provide conclusive evidence of a causal relationship between emotional factors and pregnancy complications (Rutter & Quine, 1990).

Anxiety and stress during pregnancy are associated with antepartum complications, prematurity, and intrapartum complications but not low birth weight (Levin & DeFrank, 1988). Depression has also been associated with prematurity (Molfese, Bricker, et al., 1987). Work-related psychosocial stress is related to preterm, low-birth-weight delivery in those women who did not want to work (Homer, James, & Seigel, 1990). The woman who has experienced severe emotional disturbances prior to conception may be unable to handle the additional stress of pregnancy. Severe emotional disturbances in which there is incapacitating depression and/or loss of touch with reality can have a significant negative impact on maternal-fetal attachment and on family equilibrium.

In addition to specific intrapsychic disturbances and dysfunctional behavioral lifestyles, such as addiction, there are other psychosocial factors that may place the mother or infant at risk, including the following:

- Maternal, paternal, or familial history of child or spouse abuse
- Insufficient support systems (e.g., inadequate family support systems, families prone to crisis, families unable to fulfill usual functions of a family)
- Family disruption or dissolution (e.g., divorce, death, military service, abandonment)

- Maternal role changes/conflicts (e.g., alterations in lifestyle, career, self, responsibilities, or conflict about role expectations)
- Noncompliance with cultural norms (e.g., nonmarital pregnancy)
- Unsafe cultural, ethnic, or religious practices (e.g., refusal to have blood transfusions or seek medical care)
- Situational crises (e.g., unintended or unwanted pregnancy)

Environmental Risk Factors

Pregnant women are exposed to a variety of substances that can have an impact on fertility and fetal development, the chance of a live birth, and their children's subsequent mental and physical development. Furthermore, evidence derived from numerous studies suggests that environmental factors are significantly associated with reproductive risk. Factors involved include infections, radiation, chemicals such as pesticides, therapeutic drugs, illicit drugs, industrial pollutants, cigarette smoke, stress, and diet. Furthermore, paternal exposure to mutagenic agents (ethylene oxide, solvents used in refineries, and solvents and chemicals used in the manufacturing of rubber products) in the workplace was associated with an increased relative risk of spontaneous abortions in a recent study in Finland (Lindbohm et al., 1991). (See Chapter 16, "Women in the Workplace," and Table 16.3 for additional information regarding some of the known environmental agents associated with congenital defects.) Exposure at different trimesters can result in a number of different outcomes, and any one outcome can be the effect of a variety of actions occurring at a number of different stages.

The majority of pregnant women work during their pregnancy (Culpepper & Thompson, 1990). Decisions regarding the degree of risk that pregnant women incur in the workplace depend on a number of factors: potential risk of exposure to mutagenic and teratogenic agents, increased risk resulting from the interaction of physiological alterations of pregnancy and the demands of a particular occupation, and the general physical condition of the mother. Decisions regarding pregnant women and work should be based on a determination of the degree of risk present, the mother's need and/or desire to work, and her access to prenatal care. Chapter 16 provides an in-depth discussion of this topic.

Identification of High-Risk Status

Identification of pregnancies that are at greater than average risk is a basic tenet of prenatal care. It is essential that nurses identify the high-risk client(s) if the hazards of childbearing are to be reduced and nursing strategies aimed at risk reduction developed. The earlier the client is identified, the greater are the chances for a favorable outcome. Ideally, potential risk is determined during well-woman examinations, premarital examinations, or preconceptional evaluations so that diagnosis, specific treatment, appropriate family planning, and other preventive measures can be instituted prior to conception. This is rarely the case, however, and if a woman has not received consultation prior to conception, risk screening should begin with the initial prenatal visit.

Identification of risk status has been approached in various ways, ranging from reiterating the importance of listening carefully to what every woman says about her past and current obstetric, medical, and social circumstances to formal risk assessment. Risk assessment systems differ widely in complexity, ranging from a simple, six-question approach (Scurletis, Turnbull, & Corkley, 1973) to complex multifactorial analyses (Aubrey & Pennington, 1973; Hobel, Youkeles, & Forsythe, 1979; Molfese, Thomson, Beadnell, Bricker, & Manion, 1987). They may be specific to a particular outcome, as in those designed to identify women at high risk for preterm labor (Herron, Katz, & Creasy, 1982), or general (Hobel et al., 1979).

Many high-risk factors can be established by asking each pregnant woman the following questions:

- How old are you?
- How many pregnancies have you had?
- How far did you go in school?
- Have you had a previous fetal death?
- Have you had a child born alive who is now dead?
- What is your marital status?

Questions that could be added to this list to elicit additional information include the following:

- Have you had a child that weighed less than 5 pounds at birth?
- What did you weigh when you got pregnant?

- When did you begin prenatal care?
- How often have you come for prenatal care during this pregnancy?

Using these questions, the nurse can do a rough screening of pregnant women and alert the health care team to potential risk factors. Many of these questions are among the first asked a woman at her initial prenatal visit; yet few nurses put the answers into the perspective of high risk. A variety of more comprehensive and/or more complex screening tools are available to the nurse as guidelines for identifying clients at high risk for poor pregnancy outcomes. Variables commonly used in these tools tend to cluster in the following categories: demographic, socioeconomic status, obstetric history, medical history, course of the current pregnancy, and, most recently, electronic fetal monitoring data (Marshall, 1989). Two purposes are met by the use of screening tools such as these: (a) identification of problems that pose threats to health during the childbearing cycle and (b) collection of research data for prospective studies identifying high-risk clients among the childbearing populations.

Recently, questions have been raised as to the effectiveness of any one screening tool (Molfese, Thomson, et al., 1987) and of formal risk scoring in general (Alexander & Keirse, 1989). After evaluating the tools currently in use, Alexander and Keirse (1989) concluded that formal risk screening appeared to be a mixed blessing for the individual woman and her baby. Although such systems are instrumental in providing a minimum level of care and attention in areas in which pregnancy itself is not considered to be a sufficient reason to provide these, in other health care systems in which a minimum level of prenatal care is already provided, risk scoring can result in a "profusion of interventions," such as ultrasounds, amniocentesis, and biophysical profiles (Alexander & Keirse, 1989, p. 361). Main and associates (Main & Gabbe, 1987; Main, Richardson, Gabbe, Shong, & Weller, 1987) have also emphasized the lack of evidence in favor of formal risk scoring as a means of reducing adverse pregnancy outcomes. When risk scoring is applied in clinical practice, there is a very real danger that a potential risk of an adverse outcome may be replaced by the certain risk of treatments and interventions whose benefits have not been demonstrated and whose hazards are largely unknown. It is essential that the nurse in prenatal settings using formal risk scoring systems be knowledgeable of the benefits and risks associated with these instruments. For example, the nurse should realize that identification of low risk could change over the course of a woman's pregnancy or that a designation of high-risk status should not automatically mean that a battery of tests should be ordered; rather, the usefulness of each should be evaluated.

Assessment of Risk Status

It is important that assessment of risk status be done throughout the maternity cycle. Checkpoints for assessment include the initial prenatal visit, each subsequent prenatal visit, admission to labor and delivery, during labor, immediately postpartum, and termination of postnatal care following the postpartum checkup.

Maternal Physical Risk Status

Clinical assessment is an essential component of risk status in addition to any formal risk scoring systems that are employed. Clinical assessment of at-risk status is the gathering of data from physical examination and measurement. These data are obtained through abdominal examination, including fundal height measurement and determination of fetal position; assessment of maternal and fetal vital signs; and measurement of maternal weight. A review of systems for characteristic indicators of complications (e.g., periorbital edema as an indicator of PIH) should be done. (See Chapter 9, "Well-Woman Assessment," for specific information on this topic.)

Laboratory and diagnostic tests provide additional important information regarding risk status and are useful adjuncts in evaluating pregnant clients. Tests such as clean-catch urines for asymptomatic bactiuria can be used to screen the total obstetric population to detect women at risk for increased perinatal loss prior to their developing clinical symptoms associated with pathological processes. Additional information on this subject can be found in Chapter 9.

Maternal Psychological Risk Status

High-risk childbearing women and their families must cope with two distinct crises—the normal developmental crisis of childbearing and the crisis of high-risk status and resulting uncertainty as to the eventual outcome. Pregnancy and illness are uncommon experiences; the usual coping mechanisms may not work, coping abilities may be severely stressed, and new ways of behaving may need to be developed.

In the past decade, health care professionals have recognized that medically and obstetrically healthy women who have unmet psychosocial needs might become "at risk" when these needs are unattended. Women with known medical and obstetric problems that increase risk in pregnancy or women who give evidence of severe social-emotional dysfunction receive the majority of attention, time, interest, money, and effort from health teams. The normal patient, the woman who is physically healthy and emotionally and socially stable, receives much less attention. This group can be divided into three types: (a) clients in good physical, social, and emotional equilibrium whose pregnancy progresses normally, clients having adequate social support, and clients experiencing no undue stress. These women will probably remain healthy and assume the parental role with minimal support and counseling. (b) Some are physically healthy but have emotional or social problems that are not identified by the health care practitioner. These clients' needs may not be identified or met. (c) Others are not currently stressed, but their background places them at risk for potential problems. It is important to identify the latter two groups of clients and offer supportive and preventive services to them. Table 19.3 provides criteria by which these clients may be identified. Obstetrically normal and abnormal pregnant clients who are determined to be at psychosocial risk have a good potential for positive change. It is important that they receive the energy, time, caring, and expertise of nursing.

It is important to accurately assess the woman's ability to proceed through the developmental tasks of pregnancy. Inability to do so, or pregnancy maladaptation, is strongly correlated with inadequate identification with the fetus, lack of compliance with therapeutic regimens, difficulties in developing a real perception of the infant, and problems regarding the development of lasting attachment to the child. The mother's mood (sense of well-being versus depression, anxiety) and maternal reactions to discomfort and body changes should be evaluated. Women must make major alterations in their self-concept and their role definitions as they move through pregnancy. High-risk status may impede the successful completion of the maternal developmental tasks of confirming and accepting pregnancy, ensuring safe passage, acceptance of the child by significant others, attachment, and giving of oneself (Rubin, 1984).

All pregnant women must come to believe that their pregnancies are real. The pregnant woman who is at high risk or who has had past reproductive failures may experience difficulty with this task. Anxiety over the outcome may be expressed by intensified physical symptoms or asking for repeated physical examinations in an effort to prove the pregnancy is real. Others may delay seeking prenatal care. Ambivalence is extremely common for all women during the time in which pregnancy becomes a reality to them and their families; resolution usually occurs by the end of the first trimester or when fetal movement is perceived. These feelings are accentuated when negative physical signs indicate problems or when unanticipated complications disrupt the parents' daily lives. Both parents may experience alternating feelings of love and concern, fear and anger, toward the fetus and each other. Although hoping for a positive outcome, the parents may experience negative feelings if the mother's health is endangered. For women who had difficulty getting pregnant or have lost several pregnancies, these feelings may be particularly disturbing. Ambivalence often makes it difficult for the couple to communicate with each other. If each is afraid to express dissatisfaction, anger, fear, or resentment, communication becomes strained. The partners may not be able to provide each other with the emotional support needed to cope with a high-risk pregnancy. Ambivalence is assessed in terms of how honestly it is expressed and whether it continues past the second trimester.

Another essential psychological task for a pregnant woman is incorporating the fetus into her body image. This may be hard for those with a history of infertility or previous poor pregnancy outcomes. Fear of loss may prevent attachment to the developing fetus. Helping women to hear fetal heart tones, identifying signs of the progressing pregnancy to them, and pointing out fetal movement can assist them in seeing the pregnancy as reality and as part of their body image.

Later in the pregnancy, women should begin to see the fetus as a separate entity. They will begin to plan for their babies; dreams and fantasies intensify at this time. Women experiencing a high-risk pregnancy may be unable to plan and

Table 19.3 Criteria for Identifying Clients at Risk for Psychosocial Dysfunction

Criteria	*Behavioral Clues*
Significant ambivalence or negative feeling toward pregnancy evidenced after 20 weeks gestation	1. No questions asked regarding pregnancy, labor and delivery, or infant care 2. Vague plans regarding delivery or postpartum period 3. No questions asked about fetal growth or heart beat 4. Unrealistic expectations regarding labor (i.e., painless labor, labor lasts 3 days) and delivery or postpartum adjustment (i.e., will be able to return to work in 1 week) 5. Negative perception of past deliveries, denies pregnancy, body changes, or fetal movement 6. Expresses persistent feeling of wanting to escape or get it over with—prior to last month or in greater intensity than is customarily expressed by pregnant women 7. Noncompliance with medical suggestions; carries out lifestyle activities (i.e., smoking, not eating, drinking alcohol) that are potentially harmful 8. Persistent physical complaints 9. Views pregnancy as grèatly interfering with lifestyle or self-image
Insecurity or negative feelings regarding mothering skills	1. Limited child care experience 2. Client is youngest child—extended dependent role herself, possibly incompatible with needs of infant 3. Limited experience with nurturing or setting limits 4. No positive parenting role model 5. History of abuse or neglect of client or in her family 6. Adolescent with conflicting developmental needs 7. Difficulty in previous childbearing adjustments 8. Current parent-child interaction problem

SOURCE: Allen, E., & Mentz, M. L. (1981). Are normal patients at risk during pregnancy? *JOGNN,10,* 348-353. Copyright by J. B. Lippincott, adapted with permission.
NOTE: Pregnant women who are medically and obstetrically at low risk who have unmet psychosocial needs may be at risk for problems during the childbearing cycle. This table lists criteria by which these women may be identified by nurses.

may postpone all preparations for the upcoming baby. Women who are concerned about premature labor are apt to be especially cautious. As labor and delivery become imminent, any doubts the couple may have had about their ability to parent will increase. The woman who delivers early may not complete her psychological preparation for transition to parenthood. Those couples who have remained unconvinced that the pregnancy would end in a live, healthy infant may also be unprepared for their roles as parents.

Additional indications of pregnancy maladaptation include persistent denial of the pregnancy past quickening, inability to develop an emotional attachment to the fetus, and inability to see the fetus as a separate individual. Indications of denial of the pregnancy include denial of change in body function or appearance, delaying prenatal care until late in the pregnancy, and not keeping appointments or noncompliance with suggested health practices, such as weight gain or vitamin supplementation. When faced with a diagnosis of high-risk status, parents may express denial as a defense against attachment to an infant who may not survive. Denial is often present when other pregnancies have proceeded normally or if the mother feels well. Preoccupation with vague emotional or physical complications may be noted. Late in pregnancy, the woman might dress and act as though she is not pregnant. Lack of attachment can be seen when there is little or no response to quickening or disturbing responses such as, "She never stops kicking. I can't get any sleep. I wish she'd leave me alone." Absence of nesting behavior in the third trimester, particularly in primigravidas, as evidenced by not choosing names or preparing a room, may indicate lack of attachment; however, lack of nesting is common when fetal viability is borderline throughout pregnancy. When evaluating a couple's ability to work through the crisis of a high-risk pregnancy, it is useful to ask, Are internal strength and social support present or absent? Are anxiety and tension at an unbearable level, or are escape mechanisms available to decrease anxiety?

Assessment of potential parenting ability is an essential component of maternal psychological risk status assessment. The factors that influence parenting abilities are laid down long before pregnancy actually begins. How the client and partner were parented, the role models available to them, their beliefs about appropriate methods of childbearing, and their individual personalities all affect their parenting styles. Assessment of parental role preparation determines how much the couple want to be parents, how much preparation they have made, if and how the couple see themselves in the parenting role, and how much life change they have anticipated. The couple relationship should be evaluated to determine the degree of mutuality and interdependency present and what support the expectant mother has experienced in the past. The question "What kind of mother do you want to be?" should be asked. Answers to the effect of "like my own mother" are a positive sign.

Women at psychosocial high risk may evidence excessive concern over the sex of the unborn infant, suggesting that the mother expects her baby to fulfill her own needs, or that she wishes to please her partner by giving him a child of the sex he desires. When an infant or child is expected to meet the needs of a parent and fails, as he or she invariably must, neglect and abuse may result. Sleep disturbances, lack of affect, and withdrawal or isolation from support persons can signal depression. Noting that symptoms have developed after pregnancy occurred helps to determine the etiology of the depression. Although suicide is less likely during pregnancy, it does occur, particularly when a woman feels desperate or overwhelmed. Mothers may feel overwhelmed with too many children or children born too close together. It is important to determine whether a woman who has considered abortion or placing the child for adoption and then decided against those options freely made her decision.

Family isolation is a frequent cause of psychosocial high risk. The following questions should be routinely included in prenatal assessment: "How long have you lived in this area? Where do you live now? Where does most of your family live? How often do you see your mother or other close relatives?" Observing who accompanies a woman on her prenatal visits may provide additional clues to poor social support or isolation.

Becker (1982) has developed a tool to assess three themes: (a) the way in which the woman is adapting to pregnancy, (b) the supports and resources available to the woman, and (c) the lifestyle and personal belief system ascribed to by the woman and her family (see Table 19.4). When these categories are assessed, comprehensive nursing diagnoses can be formulated and individualized quality health care provided. Ideally, such care will result in improved childbearing experiences for the woman and healthier outcomes for the woman, her baby, and her family.

Women with high-risk pregnancies often experience a period of self-doubt, blame, and guilt. They may feel guilty if their health is the cause of the risk situation. If the pregnancy was planned, a woman may wonder if she was doing the right thing in attempting the pregnancy; if it was unplanned, she may feel she is being punished. Often women will attribute the problem to something they did or did not do. A diabetic mother may feel she ate too many sweets, and a mother who is hypertensive may feel guilty because she did not follow her medication schedule. Women who feel guilty and view their situation as punishment present a special challenge to nurses. If they expect punishment, they may be unwilling to take actions to improve their condition or to cooperate with health care professionals.

Many high-risk mothers experience considerable anger. Women who have planned their pregnancy, taken meticulous care of themselves, and still are at serious risk may be bitter. Anger may be expressed toward health care providers who were expected to have prevented or solved the problem. Feelings of failure may be experienced by both the woman and her partner if successful childbearing is equated with success

Table 19.4 Guidelines for Identification of Prenatal Risk

Aspects of physical and psychosocial adaptation

- Age
- Initial response to this pregnancy
- Planned or unplanned pregnancy
- Feelings about this pregnancy
- Desired family size
- Perception of pregnancy affecting present activities and responsibilities
- Perception of parenthood affecting future activities and plans
- Current developmental task of pregnancy: coping skills; fantasies about pregnancy; changes in mood and effect on others
- Sexual functioning during pregnancy: changes in sexual functioning; feelings about and/or problems with sexual functioning
- Nature of verbal interest expressed about self and fetus
- Preparations for prenatal classes (type, when completed?), place of delivery, other children in mother's absence, and new sibling
- Menstrual history: problems with menstruation; last normal menstrual period; expected date of confinement
- Height and prepregnancy weight
- Past obstetric history: dates, course, outcomes
- Present obstetric status: course, abdominal assessment, quickening, fetal heart beat, blood pressure, urinalysis, weight and pattern of gain, signs of any major complications of pregnancy
- Past medical history: illness, date, treatment, outcome, surgery; childhood diseases; current immunization status; allergies; venereal disease; emotional problems
- Family medical history: illnesses, emotional problems, genetic defects (both sides of family)
- Loss of significant other in past year
- Food intolerances (lactose, nausea/vomiting), food cravings, and pica
- Iron-vitamin-mineral dietary supplements used
- Elimination patterns: changes and/or problems with remedies used
- Pattern of rest, sleep: difficulties with, remedies used

Aspects of personal belief system and lifestyle

- Date first sought prenatal care for this pregnancy and in prior pregnancies
- Reasons for seeking and receiving prenatal care
- Beliefs about pregnancy and childbirth: cultural beliefs subscribed to regarding childbearing (antepartum, intrapartum, postpartum)
- Racial-ethnic group
- Beliefs about role of the father during pregnancy and labor and father's role in child care
- Perception of needs of fetus
- Perception of needs of infant and proposed methods to meet these needs
- Contraceptive history: methods used, failures and/or problems with, knowledge of alternate methods, willingness to use
- Patterns of use of tobacco, alcohol, prescription and nonprescription drugs, illegal drugs; perception of effects on health of self and fetus
- Patterns of nutrient intake: food dislikes, history of/method of dieting—when
- Planned method of infant feeding: why chosen
- Occupation: present, former, how long, work requirements, hazards, amenities, plans regarding current occupation
- Recreational activities: plans to continue with, use of seat belt in car, pets in home
- Community activities
- Perception of health care personnel and agencies, prior experiences with
- Date of last physical examination, including breast examination, Pap smear, chest X-ray, and dental checkup
- Breast self-examination done regularly; if not, interest in learning about

Table 19.4 Continued

Aspects of support and resources
- Address: how long there, housing accommodations, phone, plans to move—when, where, why
- Level of education and future plans for education
- Religious preference; nominal or active involvement
- Marital status: years
- Father of baby: age, occupation, educational level, racial-ethnic group, religious preference
- Family composition: household members
- Communication patterns with significant others
- Communication patterns with health personnel
- Perception of support system (mate, family, friends, community agencies) available and willingness to use
- Type of prenatal service receiving and perception of its adequacy
- Available transportation
- Social service/community agencies involved with: how long and contact person
- Self-concept and perceived ability to cope with life situations
- Body-image concept: prepregnancy, currently; response to physiological changes of pregnancy
- Mate's response to body changes in pregnancy
- Feelings about parenting that woman received as a child; history of separation from mother—what age?
- Prior experiences with infants; knowledge of infant care
- Feelings about previous pregnancies, labor, puerperium, and mothering skills
- Knowledge of reproduction, labor and delivery, and puerperium

SOURCE: Becker, C. H. (1982). Comprehensive assessment of the healthy gravida. *JOGNN, 11*(6), 375-378. Copyright by J. B. Lippincott, adapted with permission.
NOTE: The categories described here are used to assess adaptation to pregnancy, formulate nursing diagnoses, and develop individualized nursing interventions.

as a man or woman. Any threat to a woman's sense of adequacy during pregnancy may affect the next developmental period. For example, if she feels that she has performed unsatisfactorily in the task of producing a healthy baby, she may feel inadequate in the role of mother. In a study of high-risk and low-risk women and their partners, Mercer, Ferketich, DeJoseph, May, and Sollid (1988) found that high-risk women reported significantly less optimal functioning as mothers than did low-risk women.

In a high-risk pregnancy, the usual fears and fantasies of pregnancy are intensified as a woman fears for herself and her infant. Her fears of mutilation, death, and deformity, commonly repeated by many pregnant women, may be intense and concern may be expressed about what the infant will be like and how the infant will be accepted by family and community.

Pregnant women use family and friends as role models. Particularly important is a woman's relationship with her own mother, a major determinant in how she herself will act in the maternal role. Attitudes, beliefs, and practices of her peer group and ethnic group also significantly affect how she defines and implements her concept of the maternal role. Behavior of persons in a woman's peer group is determined largely by their expectations of childbearing. Usually, this is in terms of normalcy with a happy ending of healthy mother and baby. If a healthy outcome is in doubt, friends and family may be uncomfortable. Some health care professionals may display withdrawal behaviors and avoid contact with the high-risk mother. Every culture has a complexity of rituals and beliefs that support the childbearing experience. These are the values with which women and their families define and evaluate their childbearing experiences. "Be fruitful and multiply" is still representative of the dominant childbearing ethic of American culture today.

Women do not experience childbearing in a vacuum but, rather, within a social support system and community in a cultural framework. The structure of the family system and dynamics of interpersonal relationships are profoundly influenced by high-risk childbearing. A careful evaluation of the family and social system is essential. The social support systems, particularly partner and family, are highly significant in assessing stressors, coping abilities, and planning nursing care. Specific areas of assessment that determine the adequacy and influence of partner, family, and social support systems include family composition, support system, and financial situation.

Table 19.5 Amniotic Fluid Studies[a]

Color	The presence of meconium (a black to greenish appearance) may indicate fetal distress and possible fetal death. At times, the amniotic fluid will appear whitish or opaque due to cell sloughing. This is not necessarily a cause for alarm.
Bilirubinoid pigments	Peak levels are obtained between 16 and 30 weeks gestation, and a steady decline occurs thereafter with disappearance occurring by 36 weeks. Levels of less than .015 indicate a gestational age of greater than 36 weeks and a normal pregnancy.
Creatinine concentration	Levels of creatinine in the amniotic fluid increase with gestational age and therefore are useful in determining fetal maturity. A creatinine level of 2.0 or greater indicates probable fetal maturity.
Lecithin/sphingomyelin (L/S) ratio	This ratio has proved to be of considerable value in determining fetal pulmonary maturity, indicating surface-active phospholipids. When the L/S ratio is 2:1, fetal lungs are assumed to be mature. The presence of phosphatidylglycerol (PGL) also indicates fetal lung maturity.

a. Studies most commonly done on amniotic fluid to determine fetal maturity and well-being.

Additional information regarding psychosocial assessment of pregnant clients is found in Chapter 9.

Fetal Testing in High-Risk Pregnancy

When women have been identified as at risk, laboratory data and diagnostic tests can provide information on the intrauterine well-being of the fetus.

Chorionic Villus Sampling

Chorionic villus sampling is a new procedure and can be used as an alternative to amniocentesis for prenatal diagnosis of chromosomal abnormalities. It has the advantage of being done in the first trimester, so that fetal treatment, if applicable, could begin earlier or so that a first-trimester abortion, which is safer and easier to perform than a second-trimester abortion, could be performed. With chorionic villus sampling, a small portion of the chorion frondosum (small projections from the egg sac that later develop into the placenta) is taken and analyzed. New uses for chorionic villus sampling include DNA analyses for diagnosing diseases such as hemophilia, muscular dystrophy, and cystic fibrosis.

Complications of chorionic villus sampling include spontaneous abortion, infection, and possible Rh sensitization in Rh negative mothers. Some physicians administer Rh immunoglobulin prophylactically to all Rh negative women undergoing this procedure.

A study conducted in Great Britain found that clients who had chorionic villus sampling were generally pleased with the procedure, primarily because of the earlier diagnosis it allowed. The main aftereffects of the procedure were reported as pelvic pain, usually lasting less than 24 hours, and vaginal bleeding (McCormack, Rylance, MacKenzie, & Newton, 1990).

Amniocentesis

Amniocentesis is done at approximately 16 weeks gestation to detect genetic disorders and diagnose fetal defects, including chromosomal anomalies, skeletal disorders, and central nervous system disorders; amniocentesis is performed at 30 weeks gestation or later to assess fetal maturity and well-being. The structural chemical components and activity of fetal cells in amniotic fluid can provide valuable information regarding fetal well-being and maturity (see Table 19.5).

Amniocentesis is the transabdominal aspiration of amniotic fluid from within the uterine cavity. It may be done in the outpatient clinic. Although it is a relatively simple and safe procedure, there are risks associated with it: trauma, bleeding, initiation of labor, and infection (Kappy, McTigue, & Guzman, 1993).

Ultrasound or Echo Sounding

Ultrasound or echo sounding has added to the health professional's repertoire of diagnostic techniques that assess fetal growth and determine maternal problems. The technique consists of sending very short pulses of low-intensity, high-frequency soundwaves into the mother's uterus. The returning echo signals are transmitted onto a screen that builds up a two-dimensional picture of the intrauterine contents, which can then be photographed for a permanent record. Ultrasound provides a useful technique for assessing gestational age. The crown-rump length (CRL), biparietal diameter (BPD), and femur length measurements are obtained and the ratios between them calculated. These are then compared to those expected at various gestational ages. It should be noted that (a) accuracy in determining fetal gestational age is expressed as plus or minus 2 weeks; (b) accuracy is decreased when the technique is used late in pregnancy; and (c) estimates of gestational age based on ultrasonography obtained after 24 weeks gestation to term may vary from 2 to 4 weeks (Kurtz & Needleman, 1988). Ultrasound is a valuable tool for "dating" pregnancies and determining estimated date of delivery (EDD) in clients who are uncertain about when their last menstrual period occurred; this is especially critical when early delivery is a concern, as with the client who is at risk for preterm delivery or the client with insulin-dependent diabetes. Ultrasound is most reliable in estimating weeks of gestation when done in the second trimester.

Ultrasound is also used to document intrauterine growth retardation. By doing a series of ultrasound readings over time (usually at 2-week intervals), it is possible to demonstrate growth or lack of growth in utero. Location of placental site and cord insertion may also be determined with ultrasound. Locating the site of implantation is valuable in the diagnosis of placenta previa and when deciding where to do amniocentesis or cesarean section. Multiple pregnancy may be confirmed through ultrasound. Certain anomalies, such as hydrocephaly, anencephaly, hydatidiform mole, or conjoined twins, can be diagnosed through ultrasound. There is no evidence to date that ultrasonography in human pregnancy has any harmful biological or physical effects (Neilson & Grant, 1989).

When a woman is to have an ultrasound, she should be encouraged to drink four to six glasses of fluid—but not to void before testing—to increase bladder fullness. Ultrasound waves will not traverse air; the fluid-filled bladder displaces the small bowel and provides a medium that can be easily penetrated by sound waves.

Fetal Movement Count

Maternal monitoring of fetal movements is a simple and inexpensive test of fetal well-being that can be performed daily. It should be used as a screening test that suggests other diagnostic tests rather than obstetric intervention. In the fetal movement count, or "kick" count, the woman identifies the presence and frequency of fetal movements. In normal circumstances, fetal movements average 200 per day at 20 weeks gestation, 575 per day at 32 weeks gestation, and 282 per day at term (Sandovsky, 1985). Usually normal counts suggest a healthy fetus, whereas decreased counts suggest possible fetal difficulty. Kick counts can be instituted at 27 weeks gestation and afterward.

Clients are taught to record the number of fetal movements during a period of time from 30 minutes to 1 hour and are instructed to do this from one to three times daily. The woman is advised to choose a time when she can relax and also when she knows her baby is active. She can stimulate fetal movement by lying on her left side, eating a light snack, drinking orange juice, touching or moving her abdomen, or making a sudden noise by clapping her hands. The client stops counting when she records four to six movements in a 30-minute period. She should continue to count for an additional hour or more if she does not note three movements in 30 minutes. The woman is advised to contact her health care provider if she notes fewer than 10 movements in two 1-hour periods spaced 12 hours apart, no movements on awakening, fewer than three movements in 8 hours, or if she is worried for any reason (Chez & Sandovsky, 1984). Changes in fetal activity should be further evaluated. At the same time, it is important to remind the client that wide variations in fetal movements exist in each woman and each pregnancy.

Nonstress Test

The nonstress test (NST) is designed to evaluate the health of the fetus by assessing the response of the fetal heart rate to fetal movement. It is used whenever the health care provider is concerned about fetal well-being. Although an NST may be performed at any point in the second or third trimester, it is most commonly used in the third trimester. Healthy fetuses will have heart rate accelerations during and after movement. NSTs are often used in women who might be expected to have a fetus with decreased well-being, such as those with preterm labor, hypertensive disorders such as PIH, diabetes mellitus, intrauterine growth retardation, and prolonged gestation.

An NST is best conducted in the morning to early afternoon hours, about 2 hours after a meal, and when a woman is not under the influence of any stimulant or depressant drugs. Women can be advised to eat a snack before the test to help ensure there are recordable fetal movements. The client is placed in the left-lateral or semi-Fowler's position to avoid compression of the aorta or the vena cava, which can reduce uterine blood flow and result in temporary fetal hypoxemia and an abnormal test. Blood pressure is monitored initially and every 10 to 15 minutes during testing to identify any maternal hypotension. If this occurs, it should be corrected by changing the mother's position (Huddleston, Williams, & Fabbri, 1993). An external fetal monitoring device similar to that used in labor is then attached to her abdomen. The fetus is monitored for 20 to 90 minutes. An NST is considered "reactive" or favorable if at least two fetal heart rate accelerations of at least 15 beats over the baseline heart rate, lasting at least 15 seconds, occur during a 20-minute period in response to fetal movement (Huddleston et al., 1993). If minimal fetal movement is present during the NST, the client can touch or rock her abdomen to move the fetus or drink orange juice, the sugar content of which will stimulate the fetus.

If the test is abnormal, or "nonreactive," further investigation should be done, possibly including a contraction stress test (see following section). NSTs have a very high false-positive rate (approaching 75%), meaning that many healthy fetuses are judged as possibly unhealthy by this test (Gaffney, Salinger, & Vintzileos, 1990). The time intervals between each NST are individually determined and commonly vary between daily and biweekly (Devoe, 1990; McCaul & Morrison, 1990).

Contraction Stress Test

The adequacy of placental respiratory capabilities can be evaluated by the contraction stress test (CST), also sometimes called the oxytocin challenge test (OCT). This test is based on the premise that late decelerations of the fetal heart rate (decrease in fetal heart rate that begins about 30 seconds after the contraction begins, with the lowest point occurring after the peak of the contraction) indicate fetal hypoxia and distress. Uterine contractions decrease blood flow, and, therefore, oxygen is not transferred to the placenta. If the placenta has adequate oxygen stores, then transient decreases will not cause changes in the fetal heart rate; however, if the fetus does not have adequate reserves and placental insufficiency is present, the fetal heart rate decreases at or slightly after the peak of the contraction. Late deceleration of the fetal heart indicates that the fetus cannot tolerate stress—that there is uteroplacental insufficiency and the fetus is in jeopardy.

CST is done in the last trimester if there is a question of fetal distress or in presence of maternal high risk or disease. As with the NST, women are positioned in the left-lateral or semi-Fowler's position. External fetal monitoring equipment is then applied. Oxytocin is administered intravenously continuously in increasing amounts until mild uterine contractions are produced. This constitutes a "stress situation" for the fetus. Oxytocin administration is continued until three palpable contractions, lasting 40 to 60 seconds, are observed in a 10-minute period. Alternatively, the woman is asked to stimulate her nipples by gently pulling or twisting them until uterine contractions that meet the above criteria result (nipple stimulation contraction stress test, or NSCST). A test is considered positive when late decelerations occur with 50% or more of contractions during a period of adequate uterine contractions. At this point, delivery is considered advisable and fetal maturity studies (ultrasound, amniocentesis) are done. When a CST is not interpretable as either negative or positive, it should be repeated within 24 hours. A suspicious test result is one in which occasional late decelerations occur. In a negative result, there are no late decelerations when adequate contractions are present. In this case, CST should be repeated every 7 days until delivery (Huddleston et al., 1993). A slight risk of CST is that preterm labor may ensue. Thus the CST is usually avoided in women with threatened preterm labor, incompetent cervix, or multiple gestation. Other relative contraindications to CST are placenta previa, previous uterine rupture, previous vertical cesarean section, and premature rupture of the membranes.

Table 19.6 Biophysical Profile[a]

Fetal muscle tone	Evaluated by ultrasonography. Fetal muscle tone develops earlier than any of the other indicators measured, so it is less sensitive to hypoxia. Therefore, the fetus would be quite stressed before fetal muscle tone would be affected.
Fetal movements	Evaluated by ultrasonography. Normally, one would expect to see at least three fetal movements in 30 minutes. Consideration must be taken, however, of the fetus's sleep/wake states. It is normal for the fetus to have sleep states and, consequently, not move for a time.
Fetal breathing movements	Begin after 20 weeks gestation. Absence of fetal breathing movements may mean that a portion of the brain is depressed due to hypoxia.
Fetal reactivity	A nonstress test is considered part of the biophysical profile. A reactive nonstress test is considered normal and evaluates the reactivity of the fetal heart to fetal movement. This reactivity does not develop until about the beginning of the third trimester, so it may be missing if a very immature fetus is evaluated. Reactivity is very sensitive to hypoxia, so it may be the first indicator to be depressed in beginning hypoxia.
Qualitative amniotic fluid volume	Amniotic fluid volume is assessed by ultrasonography. Normally, one would expect to see amniotic fluid present throughout the uterine cavity or at least large pockets of fluid.

SOURCES: Adapted from Gaffney, Salinger, and Vintzileos (1990); Huddleston, Williams, and Fabbri (1993); and McCaul and Morrison (1990).
NOTE: In some instances, a sixth parameter is evaluated and the placenta is "graded." A placenta may receive a grade of 0, signifying an immature placenta; 1 or 2, which signifies a normal mature placenta; or 3, which signifies a placenta that has significantly aged. A placenta with a grade of 3 may contribute to uteroplacental insufficiency, with resultant fetal hypoxia.
a. This test can assess fetal hypoxia by examining five indicators, each with a differing sensitivity to hypoxia.

Biophysical Profile

The biophysical profile (BPP) is a noninvasive test that evaluates fetal behavior, and it may be more reliable than either NSTs or CSTs alone. This test is done at 28 weeks gestation or later and is used for women who are at high risk of fetal hypoxia, such as those with PIH. An external fetal monitor and ultrasound machine are used to perform this test. The components of this assessment procedure are given in Table 19.6.

The maximum score that can be obtained on a BPP is 10 (12 if the placenta grading is included); the minimum score is 0. Each variable receives 2 points for a normal response, 1 point for an abnormal response, and 0 for no response or a very abnormal response. These scores must be evaluated individually, but a score of 6 or less is generally seen as worrisome. Not all centers measure all indicators, so the maximum possible score may vary from institution to institution, and this must be taken into consideration when interpreting the BPP. The BPP has a 72% false-positive rate (McCaul & Morrison, 1990).

The BPP seems to offer the advantage of determining varying degrees of fetal compromise; however, it is possible that the profile may not be as predictive of uteroplacental reserve as tests requiring fetal stress, such as CST. A major advantage of the biophysical profile is that with ultrasound, additional information about the fetus also may be gathered (Huddleston et al., 1993). A note of reservation regarding the use of these tests has been sounded by Mohide and Keirse (1989), who caution that the use of these tests has not been demonstrated to confer benefits in the care of an individual woman. For this reason, they believe that biophysical tests of fetal well-being should be considered of experimental value only, rather than as validated clinical tools, and urge that carefully conducted research trials that evaluate their usefulness be carried out.

Nursing Management

Even before conception, nursing can be instrumental in preventing high-risk childbearing. The importance of preconceptional care in preventing the negative outcomes of a high-risk pregnancy cannot be overemphasized. (See Chapter 17, "Choices in Childbearing," for a discussion of this topic.) Although the information presented in this chapter about risk factors, tools that detect high risk, and an understanding of the meaning of high risk suggests possible areas of assessment, it is crucial that nurses listen to what their clients say about their needs, concerns, and stressors.

Optimum care is achieved when the same person sees the parent(s) at each visit. Development of a helping relationship is essential; trust and continuity of care greatly facilitate nursing care. Once a relationship is established, identification of new problems, management of existing ones, and assessment of client understanding are made easier. Continuity of care facilitates better communication of information, better coordination of procedures, and more accurate evaluation of the client's ability to follow recommendations.

A growing role for the nurse is that of caring for and assisting the high-risk pregnant woman in her home. New technologies have enabled some women with such conditions as preterm labor, PIH, or bleeding to remain at home and to become an active participant in their care. In this era of skyrocketing health care costs, home care for the high-risk pregnant woman has been shown to be very cost-effective. For instance, in the case of a pregnant woman at 27 weeks gestation with preterm labor, hospitalization until term would cost, at minimum, $25,400. If the woman's preterm labor was not treated, and she delivered at 27 weeks, the costs of neonatal intensive care for her infant would exceed $154,000. Home care for this same woman from 27 weeks gestation until term would cost approximately $2,100 (Dahlberg, Parker, & Knox, 1989). Careful assessment by a community health nurse of the physical environment of the home and available support systems will help determine if home care is an appropriate alternative for a high-risk pregnant woman.

Some nursing care activities can be managed by the client herself at home, such as fetal movement counts, blood glucose monitoring, and blood pressure monitoring. Other activities require nursing interventions in the home, such as electronic fetal monitoring, administration of tocolytics either by mouth or by subcutaneous pump, and performance of NSTs (Harmon & Barry, 1989; Zuspan & Rayburn, 1991). The nurse has a major role as client educator in all of these activities.

Nursing roles include teaching and explanation, for it is important that the client have a thorough understanding of her condition and treatment regimen. Without this, she will not be able to participate fully in her care. She should understand the precautions involved in her care, her particular risk factors, and any hospitalization anticipated. Furthermore, parameters of normal pregnancy—expected body change, diet, exercise, emotional changes, routine care during pregnancy, infant care, progress of labor and delivery—should be explained. The problem-solving method of teaching is most successful. The client, with the nurse's assistance, is involved in gathering the necessary facts and determining solutions. This encourages the client's involvement, as opposed to the traditional mode in which the nurse provides ready-made answers that stifle client participation. When the client works out the solution herself, it is more lasting and effective and she is more likely to implement it.

When a woman is diagnosed as being high-risk during her pregnancy, many choices are taken away from her. Women today are encouraged by popular literature and by health care professionals to "take charge" of their childbirth experience. They are encouraged to interview and choose an obstetrician or midwife who shares their philosophy of childbirth and to choose to give birth in a facility that allows things that are important to them, such as early rooming-in, breast-feeding, or early discharge. They may consider the option of giving birth in their homes.

Choice about these and many other factors is limited when a woman has a high-risk pregnancy. Some physicians may not be prepared to manage a high-risk pregnancy, and the use of a midwife would probably be out of the question. Community hospitals and family-centered birthing facilities may not be equipped to deal with a known high-risk pregnancy or with a potentially compromised newborn. Prenatal exercise, work, travel, and child care may all be restricted. During labor, fetal monitoring will most likely have to be continuous, limiting freedom of movement. Analgesia or anesthesia during labor will be controlled by the woman's medical condition, not the couple's wishes or plans. The option of a vaginal delivery may not be available for the high-risk pregnant woman, depending on her condition. For the high-risk pregnant woman, pregnancy may be anything but the normal, healthy time often portrayed by the media and her friends.

Nurses must support high-risk mothers as they cope with loss of choice and control over their childbearing experiences. Nurses can assist their clients in identifying the choices they do have and encourage them to take control over these aspects of their care. Women must be helped to understand the rationales behind the treatments and procedures they undergo. A knowledge of the reasons for the treatment and what to expect can provide a sense of control for women and their families and assist them to be more informed consumers of the health care services offered during this time.

Women may also need to grieve the loss of a fantasized normal pregnancy. A woman may have anticipated pregnancy for years, imagining what it would be like and planning how she and her family would like the experience to be. Almost no one plans for a high-risk pregnancy, and a woman must let go of her fantasies before she can fully experience the reality of her actual pregnancy.

Often, hospitalization prior to labor is necessary. Family separation, unfamiliar hospital routines, and discomfort contribute to a reluctance to enter or remain in the hospital. At-risk mothers often assume a dependent role, with loss of control over what they may and may not do. A team approach that involves the client in planning can reduce the stress of hospitalization. This returns a measure of control to the client and helps to reduces the stress of separation and disruption.

High-risk childbearing brings with it physical, emotional, maturational, situational, and social crises. Demands are enormous for women and their families. It requires skilled care from concerned, caring health care practitioners. Nursing care should be individualized and comprehensive so that the client(s) may maximize her (their) strengths and minimize inherent stressors.

References

Abel, E. L., & Sokol, R. J. (1988). Marijuana and cocaine use during pregnancy. In J. R. Neibyl (Ed.), *Drug use in pregnancy* (pp. 223-230). Philadelphia: Lea & Febiger.

Ahmed, F., McRae, J. A., & Ahmed, N. (1990). Factors associated with not receiving adequate prenatal care in an urban black population: Program planning implications. *Social Work in Health Care, 14*(3), 107-123.

Alexander, S., & Keirse, M. J. N. C. (1989). Formal risk scoring during pregnancy. In I. Chalmers, M. Enkin, & M. J. N. C. Keirse (Eds.), *Effective care in pregnancy and childbirth* (Vol. 1, pp. 345-365). Oxford, UK: Oxford University Press.

Allen, E., & Mentz, M. L. (1981). Are normal patients at risk during pregnancy? *JOGNN, 10,* 348-353.

Atrash, H. K., Koonin, L. M., Lawson, H. W., Franks, A. L., & Smith J. C. (1990). Maternal mortality in the United States, 1979-1986. *Obstetrics and Gynecology, 76*(6), 1055-1060.

Aubrey, R. H., & Pennington, J. C. (1973). Identification and evaluation of the high risk pregnancy: The perinatal concept. *Clinics in Obstetrics and Gynecology, 16*(1), 3-29.

Barbour, B. G. (1990). Alcohol and pregnancy. *Journal of Nurse-Midwifery, 35*(2), 78-85.

Becker, C. H. (1982). Comprehensive assessment of the healthy gravida. *JOGNN, 11*(6), 375-378.

Caan, B. J., & Goldhaber, M. K. (1989). Caffeinated beverages and low birthweight: A case-control study. *American Journal of Public Health, 79*(9), 1299-1300.

Caring for cocaine's mothers and babies. (1989). *NAACOG Newsletter, 16*(10), 1, 406.

Cefalo, R. C., & Moos, M.-K. (1988). *Preconceptional health promotion.* Rockville, MD: Aspen.

Chasnoff, I. J. (1989). Cocaine, pregnancy, and the neonate. *Women and Health, 15*(3), 23-35.

Chez, R., & Sandovsky, E. (1984). Teaching patients how to record fetal movements. *Contemporary OB/GYN, 24*(4), 85-86.

Cohen, S. M., Kenner, C. A., & Hollingsworth, A. O. (1991). *Maternal, neonatal, and women's health nursing.* Springhouse, PA: Springhouse Corporation.

Coste, J., Job-Sprira, N., & Fernandez, H. (1991). Increased risk of ectopic pregnancy with maternal cigarette smoking. *American Journal of Public Health, 81*(2), 199-201.

Culpepper, L., & Thompson, J. E. (1990). Work during pregnancy. In I. R. Merkatz & J. E. Thompson (Eds.), *New perspectives on prenatal care* (pp. 211-234). New York: Elsevier.

Dahlberg, N. L. F., Parker, L., & Knox, G. E. (1989). A new home care challenge: The high risk antepartal client. *Caring, 8*(10), 24-26, 28, 30.

DeBruyne, L. K., & Rolfes, S. R. (1989). *Life cycle nutrition.* New York: West.

Devoe, L. D. (1990). The nonstress test. *Obstetrics and Gynecology Clinics of North America, 17*(1), 111-128.

Furstenberg, F. F., Levine, J. A., & Brooks-Gunn, J. (1990). The children of teenage mothers: Patterns of early childbearing in two generations. *Family Planning Perspectives, 22*(2), 54-61.

Gaffney, S. E., Salinger, L., & Vintzileos, A. M. (1990). The biophysical profile for fetal surveillance. *MCN, 15*(6), 356-360.

Hansen, J. P. (1986). Older maternal age and pregnancy outcome: A review of the literature. *Obstetrics & Gynecology Survey, 41S,* 726-742.

Harmon, J. S., & Barry, M. (1989). Antenatal testing, mobile outpatient monitoring service. *JOGNN, 18*(1), 21-24.

Herron, M. H., Katz, M., & Creasy, R. K. (1982). Evaluation of a preterm birth prevention program: Preliminary report. *Obstetrics and Gynecology, 59,* 452-456.

Hobel, C. J., Youkeles, L., & Forsythe, A. (1979). Prenatal and intrapartum high-risk screening: II. Risk factors reassessed. *American Journal of Obstetrics and Gynecology, 135,* 1051-1056.

Homer, C. J., James, S. A., & Seigel, E. (1990). Work-related psychosocial stress and risk of preterm, low birthweight delivery. *American Journal of Public Health, 80*(2), 173-177.

Horton, J. A. (1992). *The women's health data book.* Washington, DC: Jacobs Institute of Women's Health.

Huddleston, J. F., Williams, G. S., & Fabbri, E. L. (1993). Antepartum assessment of the fetus. In R. A. Knuppel & J. E. Drukker (Eds.), *High-risk pregnancy: A team approach* (pp. 62-77). Philadelphia: W. B. Saunders.

Institute of Medicine. (1988). *Prenatal care: Reaching mothers, reaching infants.* Washington, DC: National Academy Press.

Jones, C. L., & Lopez, R. E. (1990). Drug abuse in pregnancy. In I. R. Merbatz & J. E. Thompson (Eds.), *New perspectives on prenatal care* (pp. 273-318). New York: Elsevier.

Kalmuss, D., & Fennelly, K. (1990). Barriers to prenatal care among low-income women in New York City. *Family Planning Perspectives, 22*(5), 215-231.

Kappy, K. A., McTigue, M., & Guzman, E. R. (1993). Premature rupture of the membranes. In R. A. Knuppel & J. E. Drukker (Eds.), *High-risk pregnancy: A team approach* (pp. 378-395). Philadelphia: W. B. Saunders.

Kirz, D. S., Dorchester, W., & Freeman, R. K. (1985). Advanced maternal age: The mature gravida. *American Journal of Obstetrics and Gynecology, 152,* 7-12.

Kurtz, A., & Needleman, L. (1988). Ultrasound assessment of fetal age. In P. Callen (Ed.), *Ultrasonography in obstetrics and gynecology* (2nd ed., pp. 47-64). Philadelphia: W. B. Saunders.

Levin, J. S., & DeFrank, R. S. (1988). Maternal stress and pregnancy outcomes: A review of the psychosocial literature. *Journal of Psychosomatic Obstetrics and Gynecology, 9,* 3-16.

Lia-Hoagberg, B., Rode, P., Skovholt, C. J., Oberg, C. N., Berg, C., Mullett, S., & Choi, T. (1990). Barriers and motivators to prenatal care among low-income women. *Social Science and Medicine, 30*(4), 487-495.

Lindbohm, M.-L., Hemminki, K., Bonhomme, M. G., Anttila, A., Rantala, K., Heikkila, P., & Rosenberg, M. J. (1991). Effects of paternal occupational exposure on spontaneous abortions. *American Journal of Public Health, 81*(8), 1029-1033.

Lynch, M., & McKeon, V. A. (1990). Cocaine use during pregnancy. *JOGNN, 19*(4), 285-292.

Main, D. M., & Gabbe, S. G. (1987). Risk scoring for preterm labor: Where do we go from here? *American Journal of Obstetrics and Gynecology, 157,* 789-793.

Main, D. M., Richardson, D., Gabbe, S. G., Shong, J., & Weller, S. C. (1987). Prospective evaluation of a risk scoring system for predicting preterm delivery in black inner city women. *Obstetrics and Gynecology, 69,* 61-66.

Mansfield, P. K., & McCool, W. (1989). The "advanced maternal age" factor. *Health Care for Women International, 10,* 395-415.

Marshall, V. A. (1989). A comparison of two obstetric risk assessment tools. *Journal of Nurse-Midwifery, 34*(1), 3-7.

Mastrogiannis, D. S., Decavalas, G. O., Verma, U., & Tejani, N. (1990). Perinatal outcome after recent cocaine usage. *Obstetrics and Gynecology, 76*(1), 8-11.

McCaul, J. F., & Morrison, J. C. (1990). Antenatal fetal assessment. *Obstetrics and Gynecology Clinics of North America, 17*(1), 1-16.

McCormack, M. J., Rylance, M. E., MacKenzie, W. E., & Newton, J. (1990). Patients' attitudes following chorionic villus sampling. *Prenatal Diagnosis, 10*(4), 253-255.

McDonald, R. L. (1968). The role of emotional factors in obstetrical complications: A review. *Psychosomatic Medicine, 30*(2), 222-237.

McDonald, T. P., & Coburn, A. F. (1988). Predictors of prenatal care utilization. *Social Science and Medicine, 27*(2), 167-172.

Mercer, R. T., Ferketich, S. L., DeJoseph, J., May, K. A., & Sollid, D. (1988). Effect of stress on family functioning during pregnancy. *Nursing Research, 37,* 268-275.

Miller, C. L., Margolis, L. H., Schwethelm, B., & Smith, S. (1989). Barriers to implementation of a prenatal care program for low income women. *American Journal of Public Health, 79,* 62-64.

Mohide, P., & Keirse, M. J. N. C. (1989). Biophysical assessment of fetal well-being. In I. Chalmers, M. Enkin, & M. J. N. C. Keirse (Eds.), *Effective care in pregnancy and childbirth* (Vol. 1, pp. 477-492). Oxford, UK: Oxford University Press.

Molfese, V. J., Bricker, M. C., Manion, L. G., Beadnell, B., Yaple, K., & Moires, K. A. (1987). Anxiety, depression, and stress in pregnancy: A multivariate model of intrapartum risks and pregnancy outcomes. *Journal of Psychosomatic Obstetrics and Gynecology, 7,* 77-92.

Molfese, V. J., Thomson, B. K., Beadnell, B., Bricker, M. C., & Manion, L. G. (1987). Perinatal risk screening and infant outcome. Can predictions be improved with composite scales? *Journal of Reproductive Medicine, 32,* 569-576.

Murray, J. L., & Bernfield, M. (1988). The differential effect of prenatal care on the incidence of low birth weight among blacks and whites in a prepaid health care plan. *New England Journal of Medicine, 319,* 1385-1391.

Narod, S. A., de Sanjose, S., & Victora, C. (1991). Coffee during pregnancy: A reproductive hazard? *American Journal of Obstetrics and Gynecology, 164*(4), 1109-1114.

Neilson, J., & Grant, A. (1989). Ultrasound in pregnancy. In I. Chalmers, M. Enkin, & M. J. N. C. Keirse (Eds.), *Effective care in pregnancy and childbirth* (Vol. 1, pp. 419-439). Oxford, UK: Oxford University Press.

Nuckolls, K., Cassel, V., & Kaplan, B. (1972). Psychosocial assets, life crises and the prognosis of pregnancy. *American Journal of Epidemiology, 95*(5), 431-441.

Olsen, J., Pereira, A. C., & Olsen, S. F. (1991). Does maternal tobacco smoking modify the effect of alcohol on fetal growth? *American Journal of Public Health, 81*(1), 69-73.

Poland, M. L., Ager, J. W., & Olson, J. M. (1987). Barriers to receiving adequate prenatal care. *American Journal of Obstetrics and Gynecology, 157,* 297-303.

Rubin, R. (1984). *Maternal identity and the maternal experience.* New York: Springer.

Rutter, D. R., & Quine, L. (1990). Inequalities in pregnancy outcome: A review of psychosocial and behavioral mediators. *Social Science and Medicine, 39*(5), 553-568.

Saftlas, A. F., Olson, D. R., Franks, A. L., Atrash, H. K., & Pokras, R. (1990). Epidemiology of preeclampsia and eclampsia in the United States, 1979-1986. *American Journal of Obstetrics & Gynecology, 16*(2), 460-465.

Sandovsky, E. (1985). Fetal movements. In J. Queenan (Ed.), *Management of high-risk pregnancy* (2nd ed., pp. 183-193). Oradell, NJ: Medical Economics.

Scurletis, T., Turnbull, C. D., & Corkley, D. C. (1973). High risk indicators of fetal, neonatal and postnatal mortalities. *North Carolina Medical Journal, 34*(3), 183-192.

U.S. Bureau of the Census. (1990). *Statistical abstract of the United States* (110th ed.). Washington, DC: Government Printing Office.

Wegman, M. E. (1991). Annual summary of vital statistics—1990. *Pediatrics, 88*(6), 1081-1092.

Wen, S. W., Goldenberg, R. L., Cutter, G. R., Hoffman, H. J., Cliver, S. P., Davis, R. D., & Du Bard, M. B. (1990). Smoking, maternal age, fetal growth, and gestational age at delivery. *American Journal of Obstetrics and Gynecology, 162,* 53-58.

Witwer, M. B. (1990). Prenatal care in the United States: Reports call for improvements in quality and accessibility. *Family Planning Perspectives, 22*(1), 31-35.

Zuspan, F. P., & Rayburn, W. F. (1991). Blood pressure self-monitoring during pregnancy: Practical considerations. *American Journal of Obstetrics and Gynecology, 164,* 2-6.

20

Unwanted Pregnancy

DONA J. LETHBRIDGE

The occurrence of an unwanted pregnancy is a difficult situation for a woman. She may consider terminating the pregnancy, a complex decision in itself, or she may carry the pregnancy to term, deciding whether or not she will keep and raise the child or relinquish it for adoption. Any course taken when an unwanted pregnancy occurs involves decision making that includes consideration of biological, emotional, social, familial, and ethical/moral factors. Nurses working with women with unwanted pregnancies encourage and help with the consideration of all pertinent factors; assess available social support, including that of partners and families; refer women to supportive agencies as appropriate; support them as they carry out their decision; and act as advocates for the women's rights to make their own decisions. This chapter will include a discussion of the concept of unwanted pregnancy as well as the outcomes of unwanted pregnancies: carrying an unwanted pregnancy to term and keeping the infant, relinquishing the infant for adoption, and undergoing an induced abortion.

Why Might Unwanted Pregnancies Occur?

Unwanted pregnancies may occur for many reasons. These include cultural norms about women's roles and the meaning of childbearing, difficulties choosing and using contraception, and psychological issues.

Cultural Norms

In some cultures, within and outside the United States, childbearing is an expected role and function for women. Childbearing may represent entry into womanhood. The nurturing of children may be considered the most noble of callings for women. These ideals, however, may clash with modern roles for women that include occupational goals and independence. They may also conflict with personal inclinations and interests. A woman may conform to social or cultural ideals that are at odds with personal interests and goals and end up conceiving an unwanted pregnancy.

Difficulties Choosing and Using Contraception

Unwanted pregnancies occur because of a failure to use contraception effectively. There are relatively few contraceptive methods available, and if a woman is kept from using one or more methods by physiological or medical constraints or personal preference she has even fewer methods from which to choose (Lethbridge, 1991). Contraceptive failures occur through user failure or method failure. User failures include failure to use a barrier method during an episode of intercourse, forgetting to take some birth control pills during a cycle such that ovulation occurs, not checking an IUD string and not noticing that it has fallen out, and misuse of coitus interruptus. Method failures would include such events as condom breakage, dislodgement of a diaphragm, or repatency of a ligated vas deferens after a vasectomy.

Some unwanted pregnancies occur because of failure to initiate contraceptive use or because of the use of less effective methods. Mosher and Bachrach (1987), for instance, report that young women wait an average of 1 year to initiate an effective contraceptive method, such as the birth control pill or the diaphragm, after becoming sexually active.

Psychological Issues

A pregnancy may occur to meet needs other than the desire to bear and raise a child. Luker (1975), in a classic study of women who had chosen abortion, described women's estimation of the costs of using contraception and the benefits of becoming pregnant during an episode of intercourse. In some cases, pregnancy, if it occurred, was seen as an acceptable outcome because it might mean marriage or a closer relationship with the partner. When a pregnancy occurred, however, and its benefits did not materialize, it was not wanted in and of itself.

The occurrence of an unwanted pregnancy might result from less conscious processes as well, wherein the woman desires to be pregnant or to have a child while being unable to accommodate a child into her life.

Prevalence of Unwanted Pregnancy

Unwanted pregnancies are difficult to categorize. Whether or not a pregnancy is wanted may change throughout the antepartum course. Unwanted pregnancies must also be distinguished from those that are unplanned or unintended. Finally, there is a difference between a pregnancy unwanted by the woman or couple and a pregnancy that is socially considered undesirable, such as the pregnancy of an unmarried adolescent.

It is important to note that feelings about how much a pregnancy is wanted may change throughout the course of the pregnancy. In a classic theoretical paper, Pohlman (1965) discussed the concept of unwanted pregnancy. At conception, a pregnancy might have been unplanned and undesired but later, as the pregnancy progressed, it is accepted and wanted. The first trimester of pregnancy may be a period of ambivalence when, regardless of whether the conception was planned and wanted, feelings of happiness are accompanied by feelings of regret and even panic.

In the National Survey of Family Growth (NSFG), most recently taken in 1988, 8,460 women, randomly sampled, were interviewed regarding their contraceptive use (Williams & Pratt, 1990). The survey included data on wanted and unwanted pregnancies, as perceived at the time of conception, that were carried to term. It does not include data on pregnancies that were aborted. It shows that 10.3% of all children born in the previous 5 years were described as unwanted at the time of conception by the mother (Williams & Pratt, 1990). The percentage of unwanted conceptions for black women was 22.8%, higher than for the general population of women.

Furthermore, the proportion of unwanted births rose between 1982 and 1988, from 7.7% to 10.3%. This is most pronounced among women living in poverty, in whom the proportion of unwanted births rose by almost 75%, from 10.2% to 17.4%. In 1988, the percentage of unwanted pregnancies among poor black women (35%) was more than double that of poor white women (17%).

It is also important to distinguish pregnancies that are perceived as unwanted by the women carrying them from those perceived as undesirable by society, because a pregnancy considered socially undesirable or unwanted may, in fact, be wanted by the individual woman. For instance, of those births to never-married women aged 15 to 19 years, 76.8% were reported as wanted (planned or mistimed) at conception (Williams & Pratt, 1990). Yet many people would consider these conceptions as undesirable and unwanted by the larger society. Over 837,000 teenage pregnancies were estimated for the year 1988, 23,000 to those aged 14 and younger (Trussell, 1988). Of these pregnancies, only 16% are intended—that is, purposefully conceived.

Women's Choices When Pregnancies Are Unwanted

An unwanted pregnancy may be carried to term with the child kept and raised by the birth mother or a family member, carried to term with the child relinquished for adoption, or terminated by abortion. In 1987, a ratio of 28.9 abortions to 100 pregnancies was estimated for women ages 15 to 45 (Henshaw, Koonin, & Smith, 1991). For women under 20 years of age, the ratio was 41.6 abortions to 100 pregnancies; for women over 40, it was 44.3. Few infants are relinquished for adoption at birth. The 1982 and 1988 NSFG data showed only 62 reports in each survey of infants relinquished for adoption (Bachrach, Stolley, & London, 1992).

Unwanted Pregnancies Carried to Term With the Infant Kept and Reared

More studies have been made of adolescents' than of adult women's decisions to carry the pregnancy to term and keep the child or to relinquish it for adoption. In a study of over 13,000 adolescents' willingness to bear and rear a child outside of marriage, it was found that 41% of blacks, 29% of Hispanics, and 23% of non-Hispanic whites said they either would have or would consider having a child outside of marriage (Abrahamse, Morrison, & Waite, 1988). Those adolescents who reported problem behavior in school, such as absenteeism and cutting classes, were more likely to indicate willingness to have a child outside of marriage, when variables such as socioeconomic status or ethnicity were controlled. The higher the educational aspirations, the less the willingness to consider rearing a child outside of marriage.

There has been little or no study of the effect on women of bearing children from unwanted conceptions, except for the large body of literature on the effects of pregnancy on adolescent girls, a population in which pregnancy is considered socially unwanted. Studies of the outcome of unwanted pregnancy on women generally tend to focus on the effect on the infant, although these studies are also relatively few.

In a study of women denied abortions in Czechoslovakia, it was found that there was no difference in neonatal birth weights and lengths from those infants from wanted pregnancies, but that women with unwanted pregnancies were less likely to breast-feed or did so for a shorter period (David & Matejcek, 1981). Data taken from the National Longitudinal Survey of Labor Market Experience of Youth showed no difference in neonatal birth weights or breast-feeding (Marsiglio & Mott, 1988). These studies suggest that there may not be major behavioral differences, at least those that would seriously jeopardize the neonate, during the prenatal period when a pregnancy is unwanted. However, the National Natality Survey data were analyzed to determine a relationship between how much a pregnancy was wanted and smoking behavior (Weller, Eberstein, & Bailey, 1987). A 23% increase in the probability that a woman would stop smoking was found when a pregnancy was classified as wanted.

In a study of women in their 30s who became pregnant while adolescents and chose to rear their child, it was found that a substantial majority completed high school, found regular employment and, although some spent some time on welfare, did escape dependence on public assistance (Furstenberg, Brooks-Gunn, & Morgan, 1987). Most ended up having fewer births than they originally expected at the time they first became pregnant. However, many seemed to have not fared as well as they might have if they had postponed childbearing. Having borne and reared children while adolescents decreased the likelihood of economic success. However, those women who bore children during their adolescent years who were from more economically secure and better educated families were more likely to succeed. Educational aspirations were also found to relate to later economic success. Women who had more children within 5 years after their first had less economic success later in life.

Nursing Implications for Unwanted Pregnancies Carried to Term With the Infant Kept and Reared

There is little in the literature that guides nursing care for the woman who is bearing and keeping a child from an unwanted pregnancy. General nursing principles would suggest, however, that it would be important for such women to be helped to understand their feelings about the pregnancy and the subsequent child. Women may be referred for counseling and ongoing support as they work through their feelings and work to care for an infant that they had not wanted.

Women carrying unwanted pregnancies may be in difficult social situations, either unmarried or in financial difficulty. They may become estranged from parents or significant others because of their choice to continue the pregnancy and keep the infant. Such women may need help in obtaining financial support and referral to programs such as Women, Infants and Children (WIC) for nutritional support. They may need help, especially if they are young, in continuing with their education or following through on occupational goals. Child care may be an especially difficult problem, and women may need help in finding appropriate child care or financial support for it. They may need help in finding new sources of social support, such as peer groups for single parents or resources for parents under stress.

Pregnancies Relinquished for Adoption

There is little research available on the effect on birth mothers of relinquishing infants for adoption. In the literature on adoption, emphasis is placed on the impact of children being raised in adoptive homes and on the needs of adoptive parents. This orientation may be rooted in the social belief that a woman giving up her child is doing the best thing and does not desire to keep the child. Historically, in Western industrialized cultures, adoptions occurred to help the child escape the stigma of illegitimacy (Stroud, 1987). Hence adoptions came to be shrouded in secrecy. Today, adoptions may still be handled by public agencies or conducted privately, with restriction of information and contact between the birth parents and adoptive parents. However, more adoptions are now being conducted more openly, with some form of a continued relationship between the birth and adoptive parents. Adoption is receiving more official recognition in that the U.S. Office of Adolescent Pregnancy Programs promotes adoption as an option for pregnant adolescents (Klerman, 1983).

Generally, the studies that have been conducted on the experiences of mothers who have relinquished infants are limited by small samples but provide some directions for clinical practice and future research. For example, one study of 20 patients in psychotherapy who were white, middle-class women who before they were 20 years old had relinquished infants, reported that this was a painful and difficult event with long-lasting consequences (Rynearson, 1982). They perceived the relinquishment as externally forced by their parents, social norms, and the needs of the infant. Similarly, Pannor, Baran, and Sorosky (1978) reported that women continued to have problems resolving the adoption and experienced continued emotional pain, incomplete grieving, and difficulties relating to or making the decision to have subsequent children. Deykin, Campbell, and Patti (1984) suggested that the loss resulting from relinquishment is incomplete. Although the mother initiated the separation, the child, albeit lost to her, continues to exist.

Devaney and Lavery (1980) interviewed 50 women who had relinquished infants and found that the firmness of women's decision to relinquish and their ability to live with that decision rested on the availability of the opportunity to talk about their feelings regarding the event with concerned family, friends, or health care professionals. Women reported that seeing the infant helped them confirm their decision in that they had a face to remember. Women reported difficulty with health care personnel, feeling avoided by them and, in some cases, feeling the object of their hostility. They also described wanting their birthing experience to be as rewarding and emotionally fulfilling as that of any other woman. The last time they saw the infant was described as a time of great sorrow.

Finally, McLaughlin, Manninen, and Winges (1988) studied 269 adolescents who had either relinquished a child at birth or chosen to rear their child. They found that members of both groups were as likely to complete high school, but relinquishers were more likely to complete vocational training or have aspirations for higher education. Those who relinquished were more likely to delay marriage, to be employed within a year after the birth, and to live in higher income households. Those who chose to rear their infants were more likely to become pregnant again and to choose to terminate subsequent pregnancies. In this study, it was found that both groups indicated very high levels of satisfaction with their decision.

Nursing Implications for the Woman Relinquishing Her Infant for Adoption

Nurses are in an optimal position to provide care and support for the woman relinquishing her child. Nurses providing prenatal care are positioned to help the woman as she begins and progresses through the decision-making process. Nurses in the maternity setting provide care for the woman laboring and delivering a child she will relinquish. Nurses delivering mother-baby care provide the opportunity for the mother to be with and know her infant. They are frequently with her as she implements her decision, relinquishing the infant before discharge from the maternity unit. Finally, nurses in all aspects of practice meet women who have relinquished infants in the past and may need help resolving feelings about their loss.

The available research on the situation of the woman relinquishing her child suggests specific implications for nursing care. First, the woman must be supported to make her own decision, considering all the alternatives. Denial of the pregnancy may lessen the time for decision making. The nurse may help her to acknowledge the pregnancy so that she may begin to think about the choices available to her.

The decision may be very difficult and she may waver in her belief in the correctness of it. The nurse should help her to see that this is a natural part of decision making when the choice is difficult. The nurse may help the woman to seek a delay in making the decision if she is not sure that it is what she wants to do. Others, such as the woman's family or partner, may seek to influence the woman either to relinquish the infant or to keep it. The nurse may need to be an advocate for the woman if others seem to be pushing her to make a decision one way or another or more rapidly than she is ready to.

Although state legislation differs, generally, a signed release of custody of the infant will take place more than 72 hours after birth (Rhodes, 1988). After a waiting period, a petition for termination of parental rights is filed in court. Thus, before termination of parental rights is granted, there is a time when the decision may be revoked.

Studies of relinquishment suggest that many women do not have the opportunity to grieve the loss of their infant. Health care workers, family, and friends may deny the extent of the loss to the woman, believing that it is best to "forget" the infant as soon as possible to lessen her grief and sadness. There is no formal ritual, such as a funeral, to mark the loss of the infant and to permit formal expression of her grief (Weinreb & Murphy, 1988). The nurse may encourage the mother to take mementos and pictures of the child as remembrances. The nurse sharing the experience as the mother relinquishes the child may also be one the mother can talk openly with about her grief.

The nurse may help women to reveal their history as a birth mother, to remove the secrecy from this part of their lives, to own the experience of having had an infant and the ongoing impact of having relinquished it. This task may be especially difficult because, although women are expected to give up an "illegitimate" child for adoption, relinquishing an infant is not sanctioned by society, and the nurse may have to support the woman and help her deal with her feelings of shame.

In addition, because the time women are hospitalized for the delivery is short and they are removed from the health care system after they have delivered and been discharged, the nurse may help women, while still hospitalized, to anticipate grief. The nurse may help women to predict how it will be to return to their previous lifestyle and those situations that will be painful, such as seeing other babies, birthdays, and so on.

During the time of decision making, the nurse may help women to consider their own needs, because it is easier for women to consider first the needs of the infant and those of others, such as their partners, other children, or families (Rynearson, 1982). If they relinquish the infant, they may never see their child again but may return to their previous lifestyle (Devaney & Lavery, 1980). If they keep the child, they will not have the pain of relinquishment but may need to end their education and find employment and a home.

Women report needing to have as fulfilling a birth experience as possible and to see and care for their infants. Although planning to relinquish the child for adoption, many still report anxiety that their infant will be healthy and normally developed. Nurses should point out positive characteristics of the infant. Furthermore, the father of the infant, grandparents, and significant others may also be grieving the relinquishment of the infant. If the woman is unmarried, however, the decision to relinquish is solely hers (Rhodes, 1988). Women who have relinquished a child may need help in exploring whether or not they will search for the child or see the child if the child searches for them (Weinreb & Murphy, 1988).

Nurses will need to work out their own feelings about the relinquishment of children by mothers. Feelings may range from disapproval of nonmarital sexual activity, where responsibility for the outcome of that activity—childbearing—is being shirked, to extreme identification with the pain of the loss of the infant.

Ending an Unwanted Pregnancy With Induced Abortion

Abortion remains a common approach to handling an unwanted pregnancy, with almost 30% of all pregnancies, or 1.6 million per year, being terminated in the first or second trimester (Henshaw et al., 1991). On the basis of national data collected in 1986 and 1987 mainly by the Alan Guttmacher Institute, Henshaw et al. (1991) report that women having abortions are predominantly white (65%), younger than 25 (59%), and unmarried (82%). A majority had no previous live births (53%) and no previous abortions (58%). Approximately half of abortions were performed before 9 weeks gestation, and 97% were curettage procedures. Since 1980, the rate of abortions per 1,000 women has increased for women of minority status and those younger than the age of 15.

Reasons for Undergoing Abortion

Relatively few reasons are commonly given for undergoing abortion. The Alan Guttmacher Institute found that 75% of women reported having a baby would interfere with work, school, or other responsibilities (Torres & Forrest, 1988). About 66% said they could not afford to have a child, and approximately half said they did not want to be a single parent or they had relationship problems. Unmarried women were more likely than currently married women to undergo abortion to prevent others from knowing they had had sex or become pregnant.

Early Abortion

Early or first trimester abortions are carried out using vacuum curettage, whereby the cervix is dilated and uterine contents are removed using suction. An alternative method is dilatation and curettage (D & C), whereby uterine contents are removed through scraping of the endometrial wall. Less commonly used methods include menstrual extraction, postcoital contraception, and RU 486, a method currently not available in the United States.

Vacuum Curettage

The most common form of first trimester abortion in the United States is the vacuum curettage, where the products of conception are evacuated using a suction pump. The uterine lining is then scraped with a sharp curette to remove any remaining conceptus and to confirm that the abortion is complete. Vacuum curettage is often performed under local anesthesia and is usually performed between 6 and 12 weeks gestation. If performed before 6 weeks, there is a greater risk of missed or retained products of conception. After 12 weeks, there is a greater risk of uterine perforation and uterine atony and bleeding.

Sometimes, a dried seaweed of laminaria may be used to initiate cervical dilation. It is inserted approximately 24 hours before the procedure, into the external and internal cervical ossi, and as it swells, it dilates the cervical canal. If laminaria is not used, the cervix will be dilated using progressively larger cervical dilators. Although paracervical block lessens pain in the lower uterine segment, painful uterine cramping may occur during cervical D & C.

Physical recovery time following first trimester abortion is short with most women discharged from the clinic within an hour or two. Mild cramping may continue for several days. Postprocedure bleeding is similar to a menstrual period. Possible complications include endometrial infection, postprocedure bleeding because of retained products of conception, or, rarely, uterine perforation.

RU 486 (Mifepristone)

RU 486 is an abortion-causing agent that was discovered accidentally in France in 1975 by researchers studying glucocorticoid steroids (Ulmann, Teutsch, & Philibert, 1990). RU 486 has been found to be an effective means of inducing abortion in early pregnancy and has been approved for use in many countries. It has not been approved, but it is presently being tested for use in the United States.

RU 486, a progesterone antagonist, is able to bind to progesterone receptors in the uterus more readily than progesterone itself. The action of RU 486 induces menstrual bleeding and the sloughing off of the endometrium (the decidua in the pregnant uterus) and reverses progesterone's calming influence on the myometrium, stimulating uterine contractions that help to dislodge the embryo (Klitsch, 1989). The increased level of prostaglandins occurring with the drop in progesterone levels also softens the cervix, promoting effacement and dilation.

In studies, RU 486 has been found to be most effectively used up to 6 weeks after the last menstrual period. In the first 6 weeks, approximately 10% of pregnancies are not successfully aborted, possibly because prostaglandin levels are too low to stimulate uterine contractions. After 6 weeks gestation, it is thought that the placental production of progesterone is high enough to overwhelm the effects of RU 486.

Side effects reported include bleeding as well as nausea and cramping (Grimes, 1988; Ulmann, Dubois, & Philibert, 1987). In France where RU 486 has been approved as an abortifacient, it is currently used in conjunction with prostaglandins and is administered vaginally or by injection. In these cases, for early pregnancy, 95% of terminations are successfully achieved within a day or two (Klitsch, 1989). If RU 486 is taken alone, it may take 7 to 10 days for the abortion to be complete because prostaglandin levels will need to rise sufficiently to stimulate uterine contractions.

Dilatation and Curettage (D & C)

With D & C, a sharp curette is used to scrape the uterine lining to remove uterine contents. It requires greater cervical dilation, takes longer to empty the uterus, causes more blood loss, and is more painful than vacuum curettage. It is more likely to result in retained products of conception because some may be missed by the curette.

Other Methods of Early Abortion

Other methods of early abortion include postcoital contraception, also called the "morning-after pill," which contains estrogen or estrogen-progesterone combinations; a procedure termed menstrual extraction; and RU 486. Postcoital contraception includes either a combination of ethinyl estradiol and norgestrel (marketed as Ovral) or high-dose estrogen ethinyl estradiol (for example, Estinyl) (Hatcher et al., 1990). Combination pills are thought to act by disrupting luteal phase function, endometrial development, and tubal transport of the fertilized ovum. High-dose estrogens are thought to prevent implantation of the blastocyst through disruption of the endometrium or decreased production of progesterone by the corpus luteum. Preparations are administered within 12 to 24 hours after unprotected intercourse and should result in a menstrual period within 2 to 3 weeks.

Menstrual extraction is a method of abortion that may be used up to 2 weeks after the missed menstrual period, even before a pregnancy has been diagnosed. A 4- to 5-millimeter catheter is inserted through the cervical canal and the uterine contents are extracted using suction. No anesthesia or cervical dilation is necessary, and it may be performed in an outpatient facility. In past decades, menstrual extraction was performed by women themselves, or by women for each other, outside of health care facilities. If the availability of abortion continues to be limited by the U.S. Supreme Court's reversal of the 1973 *Roe vs. Wade* decision and by restrictive legislation passed by state governments, the use of illegal

Legal Status of Abortion in the United States

Abortion was a relatively common and accepted practice in the United States during much of the 19th century and was performed by lay abortionists as well as by midwives and others (Mohr, 1978). The first attempt to regulate abortion was enacted by Connecticut in 1821, when abortions were permitted before quickening (perceived fetal movement) but were illegal thereafter. In the mid-1800s, however, physicians and the American Medical Association pushed to make abortion illegal in the United States. Mohr (1978) suggests that part of the motivation was to restrict the practice of lay abortionists and midwives. Nineteenth-century feminists also supported the anti-abortion movement in an effort to discourage promiscuity on the part of men (Ginsburg, 1989). Between 1840 and 1860, 40 states enacted legislation making abortion at any stage of gestation a crime unless performed by a physician. Physicians had the right to determine the need for an abortion, especially to protect the life of the mother (Luker, 1984).

In the first half of the 20th century, women obtained abortions if a physician agreed that her life was endangered (Ginsburg, 1989). Other women used illegal abortionists. Ginsburg (1989) suggests that the American public became aware of inconsistencies in how endangerment to the life of the mother was interpreted. The public became more aware of and sympathetic to the abortion issue with the celebrated Sherri Finkbine case, in which a mother of four and the host of a children's television program tried to obtain an abortion because she had taken thalidomide during her fifth pregnancy (Luker, 1984). Between 1967 and 1972, 14 states passed reform legislation permitting legalized abortion (Ginsburg, 1989). By 1970, abortion laws were challenged in the courts as constitutionally vague and violating the civil rights of women.

On January 22, 1973, the Supreme Court handed down the decisions known as *Roe vs. Wade* and *Doe vs. Bolton* (see Hatcher et al., 1990). The Court set forth the following guidelines:

1. In the first trimester, the abortion decision and its performance must be left to the judgment of the pregnant woman and her physician.
2. In the second trimester, the state, in promoting its interest in the health of the pregnant woman, may choose to regulate the abortion procedure in ways that are reasonably related to her health.
3. For the state of pregnancy subsequent to viability, the state, in promoting its interest in the potentiality of human life, may, if it chooses, regulate and even forbid abortion except when necessary, according to appropriate medical judgment, for the preservation of the life or health of the pregnant woman.

Definitions of viability vary state by state, but they generally range from 20 to 24 weeks gestation.

Since 1973, there have been attempts to make abortion laws more restrictive. On July 3, 1989, in the decision known as *Webster vs. Reproductive Health Services,* the Supreme Court supported the Missouri abortion law, which included the statement that "the life of each human being begins at conception" (Supreme Court decision cited in Hatcher et al., 1990). The Court further ruled that states could place restrictions on abortion, such as waiting periods, informed consent requirements, parental/spouse notification, and hospitalization requirements, such as requiring all abortions to be performed in hospitals rather than permitting the use of clinics.

In 1988, Title X funds, provided to clinics by the federal government for family planning purposes, were restricted, in that clinics supported by these funds were prohibited from providing any information about abortion, including neutral information and information when it was requested. This became known as the "Gag Rule." In 1990 and 1991, various states considered or passed very restrictive abortion laws that are expected to be brought to the Supreme Court. Other states have passed constitutional amendments through referenda putting the rights of *Roe vs. Wade* into state law before they may be further eroded by the Supreme Court (Donovan, 1989). In 1993, shortly after his inauguration, President Clinton repealed the Gag Rule.

abortion and home-based menstrual extraction procedures may increase.

RU 486 is a progesterone antagonist that is taken orally in one 600-mg dose (Klitsch, 1989). Used in conjunction with prostaglandin administration, it is being tested in Great Britain, Sweden, and China and marketed in France to induce abortion up to 7 weeks gestation (Ullman, Teutsch, & Philibert, 1990). It is not currently available in the United States.

Late Termination of Pregnancy

Late or second-trimester abortions are performed through the use of prostaglandin injection or vaginal suppositories, or instillation of prostaglandin, hypertonic saline, or hypertonic urea into the amniotic sac in the uterine cavity. Although occasionally performed as early as 14 weeks, uterine instillation is most common between 16 and 20 weeks or up to whatever the state defines as the age of viability. During this period, the uterus is adequately enlarged and palpable over the suprapubic arch to allow access to the uterus through the abdominal wall without risking penetration of the bladder or bowel.

Second-trimester abortions may also be performed through dilatation and evacuation (D & E), used at 13 to 16 and possibly to 20 weeks gestation, whereby uterine contents are removed through vacuum, scraping, and forceps. Other second-trimester abortions may be performed through hysterotomy (i.e., through an incision in the uterus) or with hysterectomy (i.e., removal of the uterus). With a late abortion, regardless of the method, a woman will experience breast changes and lactation and may experience other postpartum changes, such as cramping and emotional lability. Physiological recovery time is approximately 2 weeks.

Prostaglandin Administration

Prostaglandins may be administered intramuscularly, as vaginal suppositories, or through uterine instillation. They stimulate uterine contractions and eventual expulsion of the fetus.

Prostaglandin E2 is available in 20-mg suppositories that may be inserted into the posterior vaginal fornix (Mueller, 1991). After cervical dilation through the use of laminaria sticks, prostaglandin suppositories are inserted every 3 to 5 hours until delivery. The mean abortion time is 15 to 17 hours, with 80% of patients delivering within 24 hours. Another mode, prostaglandin F2, may be administered intramuscularly and is given every 1 to 2 hours until labor is induced.

For uterine instillation, approximately 20 to 40 mg or 8 ml of prostaglandin F2 is injected into the uterine cavity. Laminaria sticks may also be used to aid in dilation of the cervix, thus shortening the length of labor. Uterine contractions will be initiated in approximately 6 to 12 hours, and expulsion of uterine contents will take place in approximately 24 hours.

Once contractions have begun, oxytocin may be administered intravenously to maintain or increase contractions, as well as to inhibit postabortion bleeding. Side effects due to smooth muscle stimulation, such as nausea and vomiting, abdominal cramps, and diarrhea, may occur. In addition, bronchospasms, convulsions, or transient blood pressure elevations may occasionally occur. Because this procedure may be performed up to 24 weeks in some states and the prostaglandin is not a feticide, a live fetus may be expelled. In these cases, hospitals and health care professionals must determine whether such neonates will be given life-sustaining treatment.

Hypertonic saline is now less commonly used because of dangerous side effects and delay in the onset of labor, but it is a feticidal agent. Approximately 200 ml of amniotic fluid is withdrawn through the uterine wall and the same amount of 20% to 25% hypertonic saline is instilled. Contractions will begin within 8 to 40 hours, and oxytocin will be used to augment contractions. Risks with this procedure include failure to abort, incomplete placental separation, bleeding, disseminated intravascular coagulation, and hypernatremia with convulsions and coma if the saline is infused directly into the circulatory system.

Hypertonic urea is another agent instilled into the amniotic cavity. It is also a feticide. Approximately 200 ml of amniotic fluid is removed and 200 ml of water containing 80 gm of urea is slowly instilled. It has a high failure rate when used alone and is usually used in combination with prostaglandins or oxytocin.

During these methods of late abortion, the woman will experience the process of labor with associated pain. Analgesia will not be used until contractions are well established. After the abortion is complete, bleeding will be scanty, not unlike that during a menstrual period.

Dilatation and Evacuation (D & E)

D & E is performed in the second trimester, between 13 and 16 weeks, although it may be performed up to 20 weeks. It is a combination of first-trimester vacuum curettage and D & C procedures, but greater cervical dilation is necessary because of the larger fetal size. A combination of vacuum, curettage, and crushing forcep may be used to remove the products of conception. There is greater risk of uterine bleeding, uterine perforation, and cervical damage than with early abortions. Oxytocin to induce uterine involution or vasopressin to constrict uterine blood vessels may be used to reduce uterine bleeding.

Hysterotomy and Hysterectomy

A hysterotomy may be performed to remove a second-trimester fetus if tubal sterilization is also being done or if there are other indications, such as the need for a myomectomy to remove fibroids. The period of recovery is similar to that for a cesarean section. A first- or second-trimester abortion may also be performed in conjunction with a hysterectomy, if a hysterectomy was planned for other reasons.

Mortality and Morbidity

It is difficult to estimate maternal mortality from induced abortion, because deaths after abortion may be attributed to other causes, such as sepsis or hemorrhage, and for some women, the procedure will have taken place in secrecy. In developing countries, estimates of maternal mortality from abortion include 7% of maternal deaths in Indonesia, 17% in Argentina, and 29% in Ethiopia (Zahr & Royston, 1991). In the United States, it is estimated that there is one death per 100,000 abortion procedures, and that women are seven to 25 times more likely to die from childbirth than from legal abortion (Rosenberg & Rosenthal, 1987).

The long-term physical risks of abortion are unclear. The surgeon general's report on the medical and psychological impact of abortion concluded that infertility, miscarriage, low birth weight, and other reproductive problems are no more frequent among women who experienced abortion than they are among the general population of women ("More on Koop's Study," 1990).

Short-term complications of abortion, however, include infections, retained products of conception, continued pregnancy, cervical or uterine trauma, and bleeding. These may be minimized, however, with diligent assessment for risk factors. Hatcher et al. (1990) recommend that risks are lessened if (a) the abortion is performed early in pregnancy, (b) the woman is in good health, and the practitioner is experienced, (c) there are no abnormalities of the uterus, (d) local anesthesia is used, (e) the woman knows how to care for herself after the abortion and understands the symptoms of complications, (f) follow-up care is available, (g) the evacuated contents of the uterus are carefully inspected to detect signs of ectopic or molar pregnancy, (h) Rh-negative women receive Rh immunoglogulin (Rho[D]Ig), and (i) there are no preexistent infections.

Emotional Sequelae of Abortion

There have been myriad studies on sequelae to abortion. Many of them have been weakened through presenting an ideological stance, particularly against abortion (Adler, 1992; Shusterman, 1976; Wilmoth, deAlteriiss, & Bussell, 1992). There has been, for instance, the call for identification of a new clinical disease called "postabortion syndrome," presumably suffered by most women who have had abortions (Wilmoth et al., 1992). The actual incidence of negative sequelae depends on how it is defined, from "troubled" feelings to severe psychiatric illness. Studies have focused on women in the immediate postabortion period, but there are fewer studies of women's experiences after abortion over the long term. Nevertheless, many women predominantly describe feelings of relief after abortion, combined with other feelings, such as guilt or sadness (Illsley & Hall, 1976; Osofsky, Osofsky, & Rajan, 1971; Wilmoth et al., 1992).

Adler (1975) studied the postabortion responses of 95 women and identified three categories of responses. One was described as positive emotions of happiness and relief. Another was described as socially based emotions, such as shame, guilt, and fear of disapproval, related to the social stigma of abortion. The third was internally based negative emotions, such as regret, anxiety, depression, doubt, and anger, related to the meaning of pregnancy for the woman. Adler described most women as experiencing ambivalence, with some level of negative feelings accompanying positive ones.

Lemkau (1988) has presented four areas of inquiry that would enable identification of women that might be troubled by unresolved negative effects of an abortion. These are (a) the characteristics of the woman prior to and around the time of the abortion, (b) the nature of social support and prevailing cultural attitudes about abortion, (c) characteristics of the medical environment and abortion procedure, and (d) events subsequent to the abortion that may have aroused postdecisional conflict.

Questions that relate to the characteristics of the woman around the time of the abortion help to determine the meaning of the pregnancy and the abortion to the woman. One important consideration is the age of the woman at the time of the abortion. It has been suggested that adolescent and unmarried women have more difficulty with postabortion emotional sequelae (Adler, 1975). Marecek (1987) found that young women had fears about their future fertility if they underwent abortion. Younger women may also have fantasies about parenting as a way of obtaining unconditional love and through abortion, losing that opportunity (Hatcher, 1976).

Women who had difficulty making the decision to undergo abortion may have greater difficulty adjusting afterward (Lemkau, 1988). Women's attitudes toward abortion and beliefs about conception and childbearing may determine their adjustment postabortion. Those with strong beliefs against abortion may suffer guilt and remorse afterward (Adler, 1975; Payne, Kravitz, Notman, & Anderson, 1976). However, women who are strongly in favor of the right to abortion may also suffer postabortion negative sequelae but be less able to acknowledge those feelings (Lemkau, 1988).

Questions about the use of contraception may be used to determine if the pregnancy was intended to meet goals for the woman that went beyond childbearing per se, such as attempting to keep a relationship together through becoming pregnant (Luker, 1975).

Women's ability to cope or adjust after abortion may influence their emotional recovery from the procedure. Major, Mueller, and Hildebrandt (1985) found that women who expected that they would cope well after their abortion did in fact do so. A study that was aimed at raising women's expectations that they would cope well after their abortion found that the treated group adjusted better and had decreased depression in the immediate postabortion period and 3 weeks later (Mueller & Major, 1989).

Some studies have found that social support is related to women's adjustment to having undergone abortion. Women were more likely to feel positive after abortion if their partner or significant other was supportive (Llewelyn & Pytches, 1988; Moseley, Follingstad, Harley, & Heckel, 1981). Others have found that those women most distressed postabortion were those whose relationship had deteriorated or broken up (David, Rasmussen, & Holst, 1981; Freeman, 1978). Being coerced into an abortion by a parent or partner has been related to more pronounced negative emotional sequelae (Friedman, Greenspan, & Mittleman, 1974).

The context in which the abortion occurred and the event itself may also influence women's feelings later. Adler and Dolcini (1986) found that later abortions were related to a more difficult adjustment. When an abortion is delayed, the woman may have experienced fetal movement, causing her to fantasize about the potential infant. A delay in seeking the abortion may indicate ambivalence. However, it may also indicate difficulty in arranging the abortion and having to overcome social and financial obstacles (Lee, 1969). Perceived negative attitudes of abortion staff and perceived physician incompetence may also be related to more negative feelings after the procedure (Bracken, 1978).

A late abortion may also take place because of the discovery of fetal abnormality. If the pregnancy was wanted, the abortion may be especially difficult for the woman. Because fetal abnormalities are often not discovered until the second trimester, after amniocentesis or ultrasound, a woman may have become attached to the developing fetus. In these cases, women may be especially sensitive to the conditions under which the abortion takes place as well as grieve for the loss of their infant (Friedman et al., 1974; Neidhardt, 1986).

Finally, women reconstruct events in their past on the basis of subsequent experiences (Lemkau, 1988). If women have abortions when they are young and then go on to bear and rear children, they may have renewed or belated feelings of grief or regret, remembering or fantasizing about the child they did not bear. If they have subsequent difficulties with conceiving or carrying a pregnancy to term, they may attribute them to a previous abortion, as either physical damage or moral retribution. Finally, any other significant loss may reawaken feelings of loss of a terminated pregnancy.

Nursing Implications

Nursing Care for the Woman Undergoing Abortion

Nurses may be involved with women during the time an unwanted pregnancy has been diagnosed and they are deciding whether or not to undergo abortion. Nurses also have a role during abortions, assessing and counseling women before the procedure, providing care and support during the procedure, and teaching and counseling for postabortion self-care. Nurse practitioners may perform abortions. Nurses in all aspects of practice may meet women who have had abortions in the past and continue to have difficulty resolving feelings about terminating their pregnancies.

During the preabortion period, when the decision to undergo abortion is still being made, the nurse can help the woman to gain insight into her feelings about the pregnancy and to explore how she feels about the prospect of abortion versus the alternatives of bearing and relinquishing or rearing the child. When a woman is considering abortion, nurses can help her to explore how she feels about abortion. An abortion is both a termination of a pregnancy as well as a surgical procedure, and both aspects will have meaning and implications for the woman. The nurse should help her to consider her feelings about the physiological, emotional, and moral aspects, as well as her familial, social, and cultural beliefs about abortion. A questionnaire such as that presented in Table 20.1 may help a woman explore her moral beliefs about abortion (Parsons, Richards, & Kanter, 1990). It was developed to reveal those who have extreme moral views about abortion, whether strongly against or strongly pro-choice. Midrange scores on the questionnaire identify those who are ambivalent.

Nurses can help the woman to objectively weigh the factors supporting and opposing the alternatives for resolving the pregnancy (see Table 20.2). Nurses must ascertain that a choice of abortion is solely the woman's decision and that she has not been unduly influenced by others' wishes. The relationship with the partner should also be explored, whether or not he is available to support the woman emotionally and financially and what she thinks will be their future relationship. The woman should be helped to reflect on how she became pregnant, whether it was a contraceptive failure, a conscious decision that changed after conception, or possibly an unconscious act that influenced the nonuse of contraception. The nurse should also explore with the woman her knowledge and feelings about the pregnancy and abortion—how she perceives the fetus and what she knows about the abortion procedure. Women may have limited information about what the procedure will entail, especially young women planning a second-trimester abortion. Finally, the nurse should ascertain what support is available to the woman as she goes through the abortion and for the period after the procedure.

Nurses are also responsible for teaching women about the procedure. Depending on the woman's level of knowledge, this may entail providing information about reproductive anatomy and physiology; the abortion procedure; postabortion physiological and emotional responses; postabortion self-care information, including signs of complications; and contraception. Because many women are highly anxious preceding the abortion, repetition may be necessary. A variety of teaching strategies, such as pamphlets, visual aids, and models, should be used to present the information. Sharing the information that most women have a variety of emotional responses after an abortion may help to lessen women's concern after the abortion if they, too, have a similar range of feelings. In some cases, members of the woman's support system may also be given the information so that they may augment the woman's information if necessary. It may also be helpful to share the belief with women that they will be able to cope after the abortion. Although it has been tested only on a short-term basis, expectations that women would adjust well related to women's better adjustment postabortion (Major et al., 1985).

A complete history and physical assessment are also necessary. Pregnancy dating that includes a pregnancy test, menstrual history, history of when coitus occurred, and bimanual exam to ascertain uterine size is essential to ensure that the abortion procedure planned is the one appropriate to the gestational age. An obstetric history should also be taken, including previous pregnancies, abortions, and deliveries, as well as

Table 20.1 Reasoning About Abortion Questionnaire

		1	*2*	*3*	*4*	*5*
P	Abortion is a matter of personal choice.	SDA	DA	MF	A	SA
M	Abortion is a threat to our society.	SDA	DA	MF	A	SA
P	A woman should have control over what is happening to her own body by having the option to choose abortion.	SDA	DA	MF	A	SA
M	Only God, not people, can decide if a fetus should live.	SDA	DA	MF	A	SA
M	Even if one believes that there may be some exceptions, abortion is still basically wrong.	SDA	DA	MF	A	SA
M	Abortion violates an unborn person's fundamental right to life.	SDA	DA	MF	A	SA
P	A woman should be able to exercise her rights to self-determination by choosing to have an abortion.	SDA	DA	MF	A	SA
P	Outlawing abortion could take away a woman's sense of self and personal autonomy.	SDA	DA	MF	A	SA
P	Outlawing abortion violates a woman's civil rights.	SDA	DA	MF	A	SA
M	Abortion is morally unacceptable and unjustified.	SDA	DA	MF	A	SA
P	In my reasoning, the notion that an unborn fetus may be a human life is not a deciding issue in considering abortion.	SDA	DA	MF	A	SA
M	Abortion can be described as taking a life unjustly.	SDA	DA	MF	A	SA
P	A woman should have the right to decide to have an abortion on the basis of her own life circumstances.	SDA	DA	MF	A	SA
P	If a woman feels that having a child might ruin her life, she should consider an abortion.	SDA	DA	MF	A	SA
M	Abortion could destroy the sanctity of motherhood.	SDA	DA	MF	A	SA
M	An unborn fetus is a viable human being with rights.	SDA	DA	MF	A	SA
P	If a woman feels she can't care for a baby, she should be able to have an abortion.	SDA	DA	MF	A	SA
M	Abortion is the destruction of one life for the convenience of another.	SDA	DA	MF	A	SA
M	Abortion is the same as murder.	SDA	DA	MF	A	SA
P	Even if one believes that there are times when abortion is immoral, it is still basically the woman's own choice.	SDA	DA	MF	A	SA

SOURCE: From Parsons, N. K., Richards, H. C., & Kanter, G. D. P. (1990). Validation of a scale to measure reasoning about abortion. *Journal of Counseling Psychology, 37,* 107-112. Copyright 1990 by the American Psychological Association. Adapted by permission.
NOTE: This instrument is scored by summing the personal reasoning (P) items and subtracting them from the moral reasoning (M) items. The total sum represents how polarized a woman is about abortion. Scores range from 40—very strongly in favor of abortion to –40—very strongly against abortion. A midrange score indicates mixed feelings.
SDA = strongly disagree; DA = disagree; MF = mixed feelings; A = agree; SA = strongly agree.

previous reproductive surgeries that might have altered the genitourinary system or might influence the abortion procedure. A general medical history should be taken to identify possible risk factors, especially those that indicate that the abortion should take place in a hospital. Examples

Table 20.2 Factors Weighing Toward and Against Abortion, Bearing and Relinquishing the Child, and Bearing and Rearing the Child When a Pregnancy Is Unwanted

	Abortion	*Adoption*	*Rearing*
Biological:			
Toward	Pregnancy and childbearing contraindicated Fetal anomalies	Child is born	Child is born
Against	Pain of abortion Possible complications	Challenge of pregnancy Pain of childbirth	Challenge of pregnancy Pain of childbirth
Emotional:			
Toward	Desire not to have a child	Child has potential for good life Pleasure of giving birth Genetic continuation	Able to nurture one's own child Pleasure of giving birth Genetic continuation
Against	Attachment to fetus/potential child	Pain of loss	Dislike of partner Not wanting child
Social/Familial:			
Toward	Educational and occupational goals Economically stressed No partner or family support Other family responsibilities	Educational and occupational goals Economically stressed No partner or family support Other family responsibilities	Provide new family member
Against	Strong social and cultural prohibitions	Social and cultural prohibitions	Should not stress children already born Should not have more children than one can support
Moral:			
Toward	Desire not to overpopulate world	Every child deserves opportunity for successful life	Should take responsibility for own children
Against	Belief in the sanctity of life Belief that women should bear consequences of sexual choices	Belief that women should bear consequences of sexual choices	Should not keep a child if it cannot be well supported

are sickle cell anemia, cardiac or kidney disease, diabetes, and epilepsy. Lab work to ensure an adequate hematocrit and blood typing should also be done in case a blood transfusion should be necessary. Those women who are Rh-negative will need Rho(D)Ig after the procedure. A Pap smear and culture for gonorrhea to decrease the risk of postabortion infection should also be done. Many practitioners give antibiotics prophylactically to prevent postabortion infection. (See Table 20.3 for information on nursing care for women undergoing vacuum curettage or D & C.)

Nursing Care for the Woman Undergoing a Second-Trimester Abortion

Second-trimester abortions are generally conducted in hospitals. Commonly, the woman will see the health care practitioner 24 hours before the procedure for the insertion of laminaria. She may also enter the hospital the night before the abortion and have laminaria inserted at that time as well as at the time of the abortion. Laminaria might continue to be inserted until labor ensues.

Table 20.3 Nursing Care of the Woman Undergoing Vacuum Curettage and/or D & C

Preprocedure assessment

- Assess women's feelings about terminating the pregnancy.
- Review the process she used as she made her decision to undergo abortion.
- Assess support available to her from her partner, family, and social network.
- Review plans she has made to care for herself after the abortion.
- Do a physical assessment and history, with attention to pregnancy dating, current health status, drugs currently used, Rh determination, factors that might increase risks (such as postabortion bleeding and low hematocrit).

Nursing care during the abortion

- Assess and support woman's companion(s) and help them to provide support to the woman.
- Assist woman to empty her bowel and bladder.
- Cleanse vaginal area with antiseptic solution such as Betadine or Phisohex.
- Help the woman to know what to expect throughout the procedure: Warn her of the feeling of the cold antiseptic on the vaginal walls, the speculum, the injection of local anesthetic, the sound of the vacuum machine, the cramping feeling that accompanies the suction.
- Sit with the woman and offer a hand for her to hold.
- Assess her response throughout the procedure.

Postabortion nursing care

- Observe for a vagal response, such as diaphoresis, pallor, tachycardia, or fainting, which may result from cervical dilatation or uterine wall manipulation.
- Assess uterine bleeding and cramping.
- Provide teaching for postabortion self-care, including
  - signs of postabortion bleeding—bleeding beyond 1 week, although light vaginal flow or spotting may continue for several weeks
  - signs of postabortion sepsis—foul odor to vaginal discharge, more than light cramping beyond 2 days after the abortion, temperature over 100°F
  - no use of tampons for one week
  - no vaginal intercourse until bleeding stops
  - no douching until bleeding stops
  - resume normal eating habits and activities, avoiding strenuous exercise for 2 to 3 days
  - use of birth control even if next menstrual period has not occurred, because ovulation can occur
  - a telephone number to be used for signs of postabortion complications or if she has questions
- Provide birth control counseling.
- Make a 2-week follow-up appointment to ensure recovery is on course.

With hypertonic saline and urea, 200 ml of amniotic fluid will be withdrawn. The solution, or 200 ml of hypertonic saline or urea, will then be injected—20 ml of prostaglandins. With hypertonic urea, the solution will be injected very slowly, sometimes using a drip device.

With hypertonic saline and urea, labor will not ensue for 12 to 24 hours. With prostaglandins, contractions may begin soon after the injection, with labor in progress up to 12 hours later. Prostaglandins frequently cause nausea and vomiting and antiemetics should be given. Pain medication may be used, but it is often withheld until labor is well established in order not to slow progress. The pain of a second-trimester abortion may be exacerbated by the woman's anxiety or feelings about the abortion. Unlike normal labor, when the woman has the birth of her infant to anticipate, the labor of an abortion results only in the end of the pregnancy. A woman undergoing second-trimester abortion is most helped by the presence of a supportive person. The nurse should stay with the woman in labor and support the woman's partner or support persons as well. (See Table 20.4 for information about nursing care for the woman undergoing prostaglandin instillation.)

The nurse should monitor the course of labor so that it may be anticipated when the fetus will be expelled. The umbilical cord should be clamped and passage of the placenta monitored. This is the time of greatest risk of bleeding.

The woman may desire to see the fetus and the nurse should support her in doing so if that

Table 20.4 Nursing Care for the Woman Undergoing Prostaglandin Instillation

Instillation procedure
Assist woman to empty her bowel and bladder, especially necessary because of the danger of injection into a full bladder or intruding bowel.
Cleanse abdominal wall with antiseptic.
Prepare woman for steps of the instillation procedure:
Injection of local anesthesia
Use of ultrasound to guide needle to amniotic sac
Feeling of pressure as needle passes through abdominal musculature and uterine wall
Labor and passage of the fetus
Assess and support woman's companion(s) and help them to provide support to the woman.
Assess beginning of labor.
Monitor contractions and progress of labor.
Provide pain medication after labor is established and administer antiemetic as necessary.
Teach psychoprophylactic breathing, such as is usually used during labor.
Help woman to see the fetus after the abortion if she desires.
Monitor expulsion of the placenta.
Postabortion care
Monitor vaginal bleeding and fundal involution.
Teach postabortion self-care, including signs of physiological recovery and complications; postabortion processes, such as lactation and hormonally based emotional lability; contraceptive use; and resumption of normal activities and sexual intercourse.

is her wish. She may wish to know the sex, although this is often not apparent before 18 or 20 weeks of gestation.

Postabortion Discharge Instructions

Before discharge, information about self-care and signs of complications should be reinforced. Women should be taught that vaginal bleeding will be similar to that during a menstrual period and will last up to a week. Bleeding should not continue beyond 7 days or resume before 4 weeks after the procedure. If her menstrual period has not returned by 8 weeks after the procedure, she should notify her health care practitioner. There may be light cramping for a day or two. She should take her temperature twice a day; if it rises above 100°F, she should suspect an infection and contact her health care provider. Additional signs of infection include continued bleeding, passage of clots, a foul odor to the vaginal discharge, continued cramping, and passage of light-colored tissue, possibly indicating retained products of conception.

In addition, she should not resume normal activities for a day or two and should especially avoid strenuous activities during that time. She should not use tampons or douche and should avoid vaginal intercourse until bleeding stops. She should return for a postabortion checkup after 2 weeks, at which time a repeat pregnancy test should be done.

Nurses' Feelings About Abortion

Many nurses believe abortion is wrong or they have personal feelings about childbearing and abortion that make it difficult for them to work with women undergoing abortions. Although such nursing organizations as the Association of Women's Health, Obstetric and Neonatal Nurses (AWHONN, formerly NAACOG) have positions supporting women's right to choose abortion, no nurse should have to care for a woman undergoing abortion unless no other nurse is available or the woman's life is in danger.

A nurse with negative feelings and beliefs about abortion will be unable to deliver supportive and nonjudgmental nursing care. It is important that nurses be aware of their feelings about the issue of abortion. Even the nurse who is in favor of women's right to abortion may find caring for some situations difficult. Being aware of their own feelings will enable nurses to find the support and emotional outlets they need so that they may continue to deliver competent and sensitive care.

Decision Making for Unwanted Pregnancy

When an unwanted pregnancy is conceived, a woman's choices as to how to proceed are time limited. She must decide whether she will terminate the pregnancy or carry it to term. Ideally, this decision should be made during the first trimester, when an abortion is less traumatic, but must be made before 20 to 24 weeks, whichever the state defines as the age of viability. If abortion is not chosen and the pregnancy is carried to term, then the woman must decide whether to relinquish the infant for adoption or to rear the child.

In making a decision that relates to one's life situation and well-being, all alternative options should be considered. Both short-term and long-term costs and benefits for each course of action should be evaluated. The nurse may assist in providing the information that women will need to consider all the alternatives and their ramifications.

Women's initial decision making about whether to terminate a pregnancy will necessarily follow their recognition that they may be pregnant, and that decision may be delayed if indicators of pregnancy are not identified (Patterson, Freese, & Goldenberg, 1986). Because decision making may be taking place in a context of crisis or panic, it may be difficult for women to make reasoned, well-thought-out choices. Janis and Mann (1979) describe decision making during times of crises as often including denial of the urgency of the situation as well as grasping at an immediate solution that will defuse the situation but that may not be the best course of action. In cases of unwanted pregnancy, women may deny that they are pregnant until an abortion is not possible or must take place in the second trimester. Women may also immediately undergo abortion to resolve the difficulty of the pregnancy without considering the alternatives. Women may need help in distinguishing between negative feelings that are part of the ambivalence of the first trimester of pregnancy and objective aspects of their lives that would make a pregnancy difficult and unwanted.

It may be said that the decision to abort is always a difficult one. Even if the woman does not feel an emotional attachment to the fetus or the thought of childbearing, does not disapprove of abortion, and is relatively immune to social attitudes about termination of pregnancy, abortion is still a physically painful and difficult procedure (Wells, 1989). And, in reality, many women will feel conflict about terminating a pregnancy.

Women may want to terminate their pregnancies but not have the knowledge or resources to obtain an abortion. Torres and Forrest (1988) report that of those having a late abortion, 71% reported not having realized they were pregnant or the actual gestation of their pregnancy. Almost half reported difficulty arranging the abortion, especially raising the money for it. Approximately one third, and 63% of those who were less than 18 years of age, were afraid to tell their partner or parents that they were pregnant.

Similarly, abortion facilities may not be available. In 1985, 82% of all U.S. counties lacked health care practitioners who provide abortion (Henshaw, Forrest, & Van Vort, 1987). In 1985, abortion clinics constituted only 15% of providers but performed 60% of all procedures. During 1986, charges for a first-trimester, nonhospital abortion ranged from $75 to $900, with the average being $213. Only 39% of nonhospital abortion facilities accepted state reimbursement, and only 55% offered some reduction in charges. In most cases, women need to pay for their abortions before the procedure. Thus pregnancies may be carried to term because of the nonavailability of funds for abortion.

A woman considering abortion or relinquishment should make the decision for herself, without pressure or coercion by others (see Table 20.2 for factors a woman must consider). As noted by Lemkau (1988), it may be difficult for women to make a decision that is self-serving and based on their own needs, because women are socialized to put others' needs before their own. Part of women's needs may include the desire to be pregnant, to be a mother, or to nurture. They will need to consider how they will cope with the pain of loss of the child and the opportunity to be a mother in relation to the benefits of continuing life without adding new child-rearing responsibilities. In many cases, the costs of choosing to rear the child may be high, with changes in educational and occupational plans, a constricted social life, financial stress, and the hard work of child care. Nevertheless, the pain of relinquishing a child is often severe and long lasting, and many women choose abortion rather than carrying a pregnancy to term and then giving up the child.

Summary

This chapter has included a discussion of unwanted pregnancy, including the categorization of pregnancies as wanted or unwanted, some reasons for the occurrence of an unwanted pregnancy, and data on prevalence. The alternative courses for resolving an unwanted pregnancy, including bearing and relinquishing the child, rearing the child, or aborting the pregnancy are discussed in terms of decision making; biological, emotional and social effects; and nursing implications.

References

Abrahamse, A. F., Morrison, P. A., & Waite, L. J. (1988). Teenagers willing to consider single parenthood: Who is at greatest risk? *Family Planning Perspectives, 20,* 13-23.

Adler, N. (1975). Emotional responses of women following therapeutic abortion. *American Journal of Orthopsychiatry, 45,* 446-454.

Adler, N. (1992). Abortion: A social-psychological perspective. *Journal of Social Issues, 35,* 100-119.

Adler, N., & Dolcini, P. (1986). Psychological issues in abortion for adolescents. In G. B. Melton (Ed.), *Adolescent abortion: Psychological and legal issues* (pp. 74-95). Lincoln: University of Nebraska Press.

Bachrach, C. A., Stolley, K. S., & London, K. A. (1992). Relinquishment of premarital births: Evidence from national survey data. *Family Planning Perspectives, 24,* 27-32.

Bracken, M. (1978). A causal model of psychosomatic reactions to vacuum aspiration abortion. *Social Psychiatry, 13,* 135-145.

David, H. P., & Matejcek, Z. (1981). Children born to women denied abortion: An update. *Family Planning Perspectives, 13,* 32-34.

David, H., Rasmussen, N., & Holst, E. (1981). Postpartum and postabortion psychotic reactions. *Family Planning Perspectives, 13,* 88-92.

Devaney, S. W., & Lavery, S. F. (1980). Nursing care for the relinquishing mother. *JOGNN, 9,* 375-378.

Deykin, E., Campbell, L., & Patti, P. (1984). The post-adoption experience of surrendering parents. *American Journal of Orthopsychiatry, 54,* 271-280.

Donovan, P. (1989). The 1988 abortion referenda: Lessons for the future. *Family Planning Perspectives, 21,* 218-223.

Freeman, E. W. (1978). Abortion: Subjective attitudes and feelings. *Family Planning Perspectives, 10,* 150-155.

Friedman, C., Greenspan, R., & Mittleman, F. (1974). The decision-making process and the outcome of therapeutic abortion. *American Journal of Psychiatry, 131,* 1332-1337.

Furstenberg, F. F., Brooks-Gunn, J., & Morgan, S. P. (1987). Adolescent mothers and their children in later life. *Family Planning Perspectives, 19,* 142-151.

Ginsburg, F. D. (1989). *Contested lives: The abortion debate in an American community.* Berkeley, CA: University of California Press.

Grimes, D. A. (1988). Early abortion with a single dose of the antiprogestin RU-486. *American Journal of Obstetrics and Gynecology, 158,* 1307.

Hatcher, R. A., Stewart, F., Trussell, J., Kowal, D., Guest, F., Stewart, G. K., & Cates, W. (1990). *Contraceptive technology, 1990-1992.* New York: Irvington.

Hatcher, S. (1976). Understanding adolescent pregnancy and abortion. *Primary Care, 3,* 407-425.

Henshaw, S. K., Forrest, J. D., & Van Vort, J. (1987). Abortion services in the United States, 1984 and 1985. *Family Planning Perspectives, 19,* 63-70.

Henshaw, S. K., Koonin, L. M., & Smith, J. C. (1991). Characteristics of U.S. women having abortions, 1987. *Family Planning Perspectives, 23,* 75-81.

Illsley, R., & Hall, M. H. (1976). Psychosocial aspects of abortion: A review of issues and needed research. *Bulletin of the World Health Organization, 53,* 83-103.

Janis, I. L., & Mann, L. (1979). *Decision making: A psychological analysis of conflict, choice, and commitment.* New York: Free Press.

Klerman, L. V. (1983). Adoption: A public health perspective. *American Journal of Public Health, 73,* 1158-1160.

Klitsch, M. (1989). *RU 486: The science and the politics.* New York: Alan Guttmacher Institute.

Lee, N. H. (1969). *The searchfor an abortionist.* Chicago: University of Chicago Press.

Lemkau, J. P. (1988). Emotional sequelae of abortion. *Psychology of Women Quarterly, 12,* 461-472.

Lethbridge, D. J. (1991). Women's experience with contraception: Towards a theory of contraceptive self-care. *Nursing Research, 40,* 276-280.

Llewelyn, S. P., & Pytches, R. (1988). An investigation of anxiety following termination of pregnancy. *Journal of Advanced Nursing, 13,* 468-471.

Luker, K. (1975). *Taking chances: Abortion and the decision not to contracept.* Berkeley: University of California Press.

Luker, K. (1984). *Abortion and the politics of motherhood.* Berkeley: University of California Press.

Major, B., Mueller, P., & Hildebrandt, K. (1985). Attributions, expectations, and coping with abortion. *Journal of Personality and Social Psychology, 48,* 485-599.

Marecek, J. (1987). Counseling adolescents with problem pregnancies. *American Psychologist, 42,* 89-93.

Marsiglio, W., & Mott, F. L. (1988). Does wanting to become pregnant with a first child affect subsequent maternal behaviors and infant birth weight? *Journal of Marriage and Family, 50,* 1023-1036.

McLaughlin, S. D., Manninen, D. L., & Winges, L. D. (1988). Do adolescents who relinquish their children fare better or worse than those who raise them? *Family Planning Perspectives, 20,* 25-32.

Mohr, J. (1978). *Abortion in America: The origins and evolution of national policy.* New York: Oxford University Press.

More on Koop's study of abortion. (1990). *Family Planning Perspectives, 22,* 36-39.

Moseley, D. T., Follingstad, D. R., Harley, H., & Heckel, R. (1981). Psychological factors that predict reaction to abortion. *Journal of Clinical Psychology, 37,* 276-279.

Mosher, W. D., & Bachrach, C. A. (1987). First premarital contraceptive use: United States, 1960-82. *Studies in Family Planning, 18,* 83-95.

Mueller, L. (1991). Second-trimester termination of pregnancy: Nursing care. *JOGNN, 20,* 284-289.

Mueller, P., & Major, B. (1989). Self-blame, self-efficacy, and adjustment to abortion. *Journal of Personality and Social Psychology, 57,* 1059-1068.

Neidhardt, A. (1986). Why me? Second trimester abortion. *American Journal of Nursing, 86,* 1133-1135.

Osofsky, J. D., Osofsky, H. J., & Rajan, R. (1971). Psychological effects of legalized abortion. *American Journal of Orthopsychiatry, 42,* 215-234.

Pannor, R., Baran, A., & Sorosky, A. D. (1978). Birth parents who relinquished babies for adoption revisited. *Family Process, 17,* 329-337.

Parsons, N. K., Richards, H. C., & Kanter, G. D. P. (1990). Validation of a scale to measure reasoning about abortion. *Journal of Counseling Psychology, 37,* 107-112.

Patterson, E. T., Freese, M. P., & Goldenberg, R. L. (1986). Reducing uncertainty: Self-diagnosis of pregnancy. *Image, 18,* 105-109.

Payne, E., Kravitz, A., Notman, M., & Anderson, J. (1976). Outcome following therapeutic abortion. *Archives of General Psychiatry, 33,* 725-733.

Pohlman, E. (1965). Unwanted conception: Research on undesirable consequences. *Eugenics Quarterly, 14*(2), 143-154.

Rhodes, A. M. (1988). Options and issues for pregnant adolescents. *Maternal-Child Nursing, 13,* 427.

Rosenberg, M. J., & Rosenthal, S. M. (1987). Reproductive mortality in the United States: Recent trends and methodologic considerations. *American Journal of Public Health, 77,* 833-838.

Rynearson, E. K. (1982). Relinquishment and its maternal complications: A preliminary study. *American Journal of Psychiatry, 139,* 338-340.

Shusterman, L. R. (1976). The psychosocial factors of the abortion experience: A critical review. *Psychology of Women Quarterly, 1*(1), 79-106.

Stroud, J. (1987). Social history of adoption. *Midwife, Health Visitor and Community Nurse, 23,* 434-437.

Torres, A., & Forrest, J. D. (1988). Why do women have abortions? *Family Planning Perspectives, 20,* 169-176.

Trussell, J. (1988). Teenage pregnancy in the United States. *Family Planning Perspectives, 20,* 262-272.

Ullman, A., Dubois, C., & Philibert, D. (1987). Fertility control with RU 486. *Hormone Research, 28,* 274-278.

Ullman, A., Teutsch, G., & Philibert, D. (1990). Are you 486? *Scientific American, 262*(6), 274-278.

Weinreb, M. L., & Murphy, B. C. (1988). The birth mother: A feminist perspective for the helping professional. *Women and Therapy, 7,* 23-36.

Weller, R. H., Eberstein, I. W., & Bailey, M. (1987). Pregnancy wantedness and maternal behavior during pregnancy. *Demography, 24,* 407-412.

Wells, N. (1989). Management of pain during abortion. *Journal of Advanced Nursing, 14,* 56-62.

Williams, L. B., & Pratt, W. F. (1990). Wanted and unwanted childbearing in the United States: 1973-1988. *Advance data from vital and health statistics* (No. 189). Hyattsville, MD: National Center for Health Statistics.

Wilmoth, G. H., deAlteriiss, M., & Bussell, D. (1992). Prevalence of psychological risks following legal abortion in the U.S.: Limits of the evidence. *Journal of Social Issues, 48*(3), 37-66.

Zahr, C. A., & Royston, E. (1991). *Maternal mortality: A global factbook.* Geneva: World Health Organization.

21

Sexuality in Women's Lives

LINDA A. BERNHARD

Sexuality is an integral part of life, an important aspect of women's health, and a complex—yet fascinating—topic of study.

Men and women experience sexuality differently. Unlike most men, who view sexuality primarily as genital activity, most women view it as a total body experience that cannot be separated from the context of life. Men commonly think of sexuality quantitatively, for example, in terms of the number of times one has engaged in a particular behavior. In contrast, women tend to take a qualitative approach, focusing on the meaning of sexual activity and the depth of feelings involved.

No two women experience sexuality in exactly the same way. Nor does a woman's sexuality remain static. It is dynamic, changing throughout her life. It includes a wide range of experiences expressed in different ways at different times. These experiences include everything from dressing or kissing to masturbation or intercourse. Throughout her life, a woman can have a variety of sexual experiences with different partners, with the same partner, or by herself.

To familiarize nurses with the many facets of women's sexuality, Chapter 21 begins with an introduction to sexual terms, myths, and identity. Next it presents the anatomy and physiology of female sexuality, followed by a discussion of sociocultural influences on sexuality and sexual lifestyles. It continues by describing developmental and other considerations in sexuality and then investigating common sexual problems, including various types of sexual dysfunction. The chapter concludes with an exploration of sexual health promotion, highlighting the nurse's role in assessment and intervention.

Introduction

Female sexuality is a multidimensional, biopsychosocial phenomenon that consists of at least four components: sexual desire, sexual response, view of oneself as female, and presentation of oneself as woman (Bernhard, 1988).

Sexual desire (also called sexual drive or libido) refers to the innate urge for sexual activity, which is produced by activation of a specific system in the brain and experienced as a specific sensation that moves a person to seek out or be receptive to sexual experience (Kaplan, 1979). Sexual desire can vary in intensity across the life span. It is learned through sexual experiences and feelings of pleasure, enjoyment, or dissatisfaction during sexual activity. This component of sexuality also includes a woman's interest in and desired frequency of sexual activity as well as her preference for a sexual partner of the opposite, same, or either sex.

Sexual response refers primarily to the biological aspects of sexuality. It includes the physical ability to engage in sexual activity and experience orgasm. Because all body systems are involved in sex, impairment of any system may alter an individual's sexual response. This component of sexuality may be subdivided into capacity (ability to engage in sexual experiences) and activity (actual sexual experiences).

The view of oneself as female is a self-perception that includes gender identity (identification of oneself as female); a sense of having characteristics traditionally considered feminine, masculine, or both; and body image—classically defined by Schilder (1950) as the view of one's body and its relationship to the environment. A woman's view of her body and how realistic is her idea of her appearance to others influences her confidence in social and sexual situations.

The final component of sexuality is the way a woman presents herself to society as a woman. Commonly called gender (or sex) role behavior, this component includes all the behaviors that a woman uses to disclose herself as a woman to other people, such as style of dress, hairstyle, walk, speech patterns, and use of cosmetics. Presentation primarily involves a woman's internalization of social and cultural stereotypes and expectations of women's behavior in that culture (Heilbrun, 1981).

Every part of the body is important to a woman's sexual expression and presentation of self to society, and body language is especially important in sexual communication. Body language is the expression of feelings, desires, conflicts, and attitudes through facial expression, posture, gestures, and movement (Kahn & Holt, 1990).

Language of Sexuality

The language used to refer to sexuality can add to the complexity of the topic in several ways. For instance, terms that women use to refer to sexuality frequently do not appear in indexes or other information databases, so when women seek information, they may not be able to find it. The term *sexuality,* for example, does not appear in many databases, but the terms *sex* and *sexual behavior* do. This fact may reflect a bias toward tangible evidence, rather than abstract concepts, which frequently are the concepts women use.

The perceived meanings of certain terms also can add complexity to sexuality. This occurs because individuals may have different interpretations and connotations of words such as *sex, sexuality, sexual dysfunction,* and *orgasm.*

Furthermore, much of the language of sexuality is outdated because the meanings and societal expectations related to terms have changed. For example, the term *premarital sex* formerly referred to sexual intercourse between adolescents, which was socially taboo. Today, over half of all adolescents engage in intercourse and other sexual behaviors, which have become more socially acceptable. These changes have reduced the importance of the term *premarital sex* to almost nothing. Also, the terms *premarital, extramarital,* and *nonmarital* reflect the social standards that marriage is the desired goal and that sexuality should be reserved for marriage. Yet considerable sexual activity occurs outside marriage and is widely condoned, except by some individuals and religions. Thus these terms no longer have clear meanings, although they are still used in many places.

Another language problem that affects women's sexuality are the terms *virgin* and *virginity.* Traditionally, the term *virgin* referred to a woman who had not engaged in intercourse. Society valued virginity and expected a woman to lose her virginity only by engaging in penile-vaginal intercourse with her husband on their wedding night. By this outdated definition, a sexually abused girl has lost her virginity and a lesbian who never engages in sexual intercourse with a man is a virgin forever (even though she regularly may practice many other sexual activities).

The term *defloration* is related to virginity. Technically, defloration refers to rupture of the hymen. Historically, it implied the woman's loss of the "flower" of virginity (Kahn & Holt, 1990) and was expected to occur during the first sexual intercourse. This rarely happens now because a young girl's hymen may rupture during various physical activities, such as bicycle riding.

Because of these language difficulties, terms related to sexuality must be clarified and differentiated. *Sex* refers to one's biological assignment based on anatomy. This term also can describe various forms of sexual expression but usually refers to genital sexual activity. *Sexual behavior* means all activities—genital and other—that a woman uses to express her sexuality. *Sexual functioning* implies an assessment of the level or quality of one's sexual activities.

Today, women are redefining their sexuality. Women's definitions of sexuality differ from traditional definitions; they suggest that sexuality is something individuals create, not something that is imposed on them.

Women define sexuality on the basis of what they have discovered and created for themselves through relevant feelings, experience, and politics. Frequently, sensuality, closeness, mutuality, love, and relationships are included in women's definitions of sexuality.

Sexual Myths

Traditionally, society has mythologized women's sexuality in two ways: as Eve (or whore) or as Mary (or madonna). The Eve myth views a woman's sexuality as uncontrolled and her eroticism so great that she is dangerous to men. The Mary myth trivializes or denies a woman's sexuality. In fact, it views her as nonsexual, except for sexuality directly related to childbearing. Yet most of society expects women to fit this sexual image. Although both views are unhealthy images of women's sexuality, they frequently appear today in advertising, films, and social institutions (Muff, 1982).

Another harmful myth is that certain women, such as nuns and elderly, disabled, or obese women, are asexual because of their differences. Similar to the Mary myth, this view assumes that such women have no sexual needs, feelings, or actions. Of course, no person is asexual.

Alternatively, society has also defined certain women, such as black women, stewardesses, and nurses, as supersexual. As in the Eve myth, society may believe these women to be sexually dangerous. In reality, they experience sexuality as individuals within the context of their lives.

Other myths about sexuality exist. The two most pervasive are that sexuality refers only to heterosexual activities and that the highest form of sexuality is heterosexual coitus. In reality, no sexual lifestyle or activity is better than any other, and women experience all varieties.

Sexual Identity

A part of self-identity, sexual identity is a woman's awareness of herself as heterosexual, lesbian, or bisexual. Sexual identity develops through conscious and unconscious awareness of others and through learning from them how to be and act. One observes the roles and behaviors of others like oneself and then views oneself similarly. For example, a woman whose roles and behaviors are like those of most other women is likely to be heterosexual.

Difficulties with a woman's sexual identity can occur when the behaviors she observes do not match those that she enacts or wishes to enact. For example, a female adolescent who feels sexually attracted to women but does not know that lesbians exist and who observes only heterosexual behaviors is likely to believe that something is wrong with her.

Traditionally, sexual identity development has meant that people are sexually attracted to persons of the opposite sex or the same sex, act on the attraction, and come to accept the identity congruent with their actions. This implies that people are heterosexual or homosexual. Yet sexual identity development is much more complex. Research suggests that some women may have incongruence between their sexual identity and sexual behaviors—for example, when a woman feels she is a male and continues to behave as a woman (Silber, 1990). Furthermore, sexual identity is not static; it can and does change throughout life. For example, a heterosexual woman may redefine her sexual identity as bisexual or lesbian after engaging in sexual exploration with a woman.

Acknowledging one's sexual identity involves placing oneself in a category created by society (such as heterosexual, lesbian, or bisexual) or invented by oneself (sexual being). Acknowledging one's sexual identity is also a component of taking responsibility for one's sexuality (Trebilcott, 1984). For a woman, taking responsibility also involves acknowledging and understanding her experiences and feelings about sexuality. It requires considering different sexualities and consciously choosing a sexual identity, which can raise the woman's consciousness and ultimately make her stronger and more independent in this and other areas of life.

Cassell (1984) believes the central fault in many women's sexuality is a failure to take responsibility for their sexuality. She asserts that this causes women to fear their sexuality, become dependent, and desire only to be "swept away" by a man.

Anatomy and Physiology of Female Sexuality

Every part of a woman's body is a potential sexual organ and may play a role in the sexual response cycle.

Sexual Organs

Unlike the cardiovascular or other body systems, a sexual system does not exist. This may explain the lack of study about sexuality and its expression. Although some textbooks (Pernoll, 1991) describe the reproductive system as the "sexual system," this is misleading because every part of a woman's body is a potential sexual organ. Furthermore, the clitoris (the primary organ of female sexuality) is not part of the reproductive system. Yet it is the only organ that has sexual pleasure as its only purpose.

The clitoris is located at the top of the labia where the tissue folds come together. Filled with nerve endings, it is exquisitely sensitive to tactile stimulation, especially its tip (the glans). Usually, direct clitoral stimulation is pleasing, but overstimulation can cause pain. For most women, some clitoral stimulation must occur for them to achieve orgasm.

The female breasts also are sexual organs that are not part of the reproductive system. Although their only function is to produce milk, they are highly valued by women and men in this culture as sexual organs. Therefore, loss of a breast may be extremely distressing to a woman because she no longer may feel completely female.

Breasts vary greatly in size from woman to woman. A woman may increase her breast size through augmentation to enhance her sexuality. One with extremely large breasts may decrease their size through reduction to enhance her physical health, comfort, and sexuality. After mastectomy, a woman may undergo breast reconstruction surgery so that she can feel like a "whole" woman again.

Reproductive organs that double as sexual organs are the external genitalia (including the labia majora, labia minora, and mons pubis) and the internal genitalia (including the vagina, uterus, and ovaries).

Another sexual organ is the sensitive area around the urethra and on the anterior vaginal wall. Known as the Graefenberg spot, G spot, or urethral sponge, this area swells when stimulated and can lead to orgasm (Federation of Feminist Women's Health Centers, 1981; Ladas, Whipple, & Perry, 1982). In a large national survey, 84% of the women believed that a sensitive area exists in the vagina and produces pleasurable feelings when stimulated; 66% reported that they have such an area. Of the latter group, 73% said they experienced orgasms when the area was stimulated (Davidson, Darling, & Conway-Welch, 1989).

Sexual Response Cycle

Although physiology is only a small part of women's sexuality, the nurse must understand it to provide appropriate care. In the 1960s, Masters and Johnson (1966) first identified the sexual response cycle—a highly orderly sequence of physiological responses to sexual stimuli. Chapter 3, "Women's Bodies," provides in-depth information on their research.

In the 1970s, Kaplan (1979) reinterpreted the sexual response cycle, identifying three phases: desire, excitement, and orgasmic. Although Kaplan's excitement and orgasmic phases resemble those of Masters and Johnson, the desire phase is unique. According to Kaplan (1979), desire is a subjective state of excitement accompanied by sexual arousal that is physiologically produced by activating a specific neural system in the brain and is mediated by testosterone. Kaplan's cycle does not include a plateau or resolution phase.

The American Psychiatric Association (APA, 1994) describes a sexual response cycle in its *Diagnostic and Statistical Manual of Mental Disorders* (*DSM-IV*). This cycle combined those of Masters and Johnson and Kaplan to form four phases: appetitive, excitement, orgasm, and resolution. Its appetitive phase is similar to Kaplan's desire phase; the other three phases resemble those of Masters and Johnson, except that the plateau and excitement phases are combined. (For a summary, see Figure 21.1.)

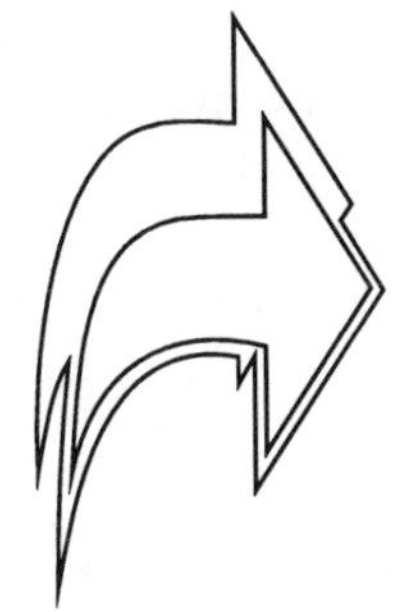

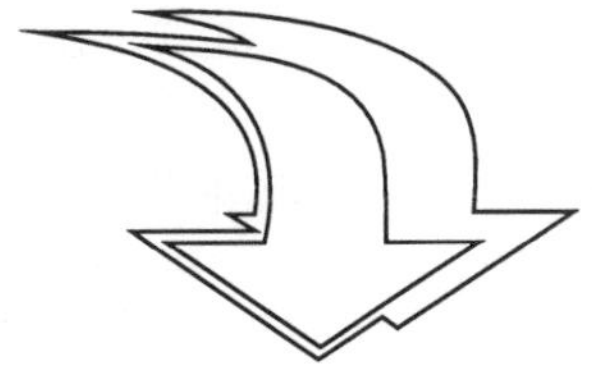

Appetitive Phase
In this primarily psychological phase, sexual fantasies and desire for sexual activity lead to sexual arousal.

Excitement Phase
Pelvic vasocongestion and vaginal lubrication are the hallmarks of this phase, which also produces myotonia, external genital swelling, and breast tumescence.

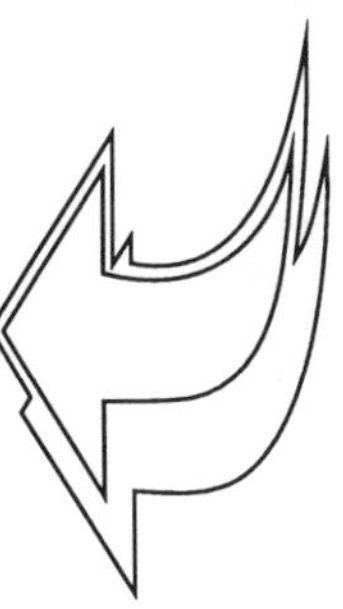

Orgasm Phase
Orgasm marks the peak of sexual pleasure followed by the sudden release of muscle tension in rhythmic contractions throughout the pelvis.

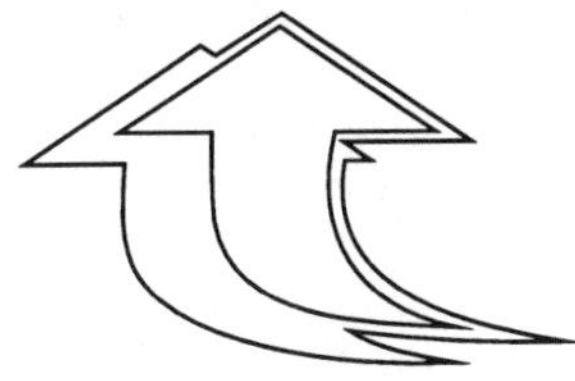

Resolution Phase
The body returns to a state of physical and mental relaxation, and the individual experiences a general sense of well-being. With continued stimulation, the woman can immediately repeat the sexual response cycle.[a]

Figure 21.1. *DSM-IV* Sexual Response Cycle
SOURCE: Adapted from American Psychiatric Association (1994).
NOTE: a. Women may repeat the cycle more quickly than men because women do not experience a refractory period (time after an orgasm when restimulation and orgasm are not possible for a man).

Although orgasms achieved by various sexual behaviors show no physiological differences, women report subjective differences. They state that orgasms achieved through masturbation are more intense and physically satisfying than orgasms achieved during sexual intercourse, which are more satisfying psychologically (Davidson & Darling, 1989).

Many people believe orgasm is the goal of sexual activity. However, focusing on orgasm may be antithetical to sensuality and relaxed sexual activity. Some women are well satisfied with tender sexual activities that include sharing of good feelings but do not necessarily include orgasm.

Some women do not experience orgasms. Others experience orgasms with some sexual activities, but not with sexual intercourse. Although these women may enjoy intercourse, they may pretend to have an orgasm because they feel that their partner expects it, believe it demonstrates their sexual adequacy, or wish to signal that sex is "done."

No obvious action lets a woman know that she has had an orgasm. Consequently, some women do not know that they experience orgasms. Investigating this, Warner (1984) asked women about their "peak of physical response," or the point of the most intense physical feelings during sexual activity. Of the women studied, 80% identified their peak as orgasm, but only 47% described it as "throbbing" sensations or other physical sensations most likely related to orgasm. If the woman did not have an orgasm, vasocongestion may not return completely to normal. If she has sexual activity many times without orgasm, she may develop pelvic congestion (Charles & Glover, 1985), which can result in severe pelvic discomfort.

Sociocultural Influences on Women's Sexuality

The world into which a woman is born determines her culture. Culture determines the meanings of sexual events and behaviors and gives the woman ways to understand and judge aspects of sexuality.

Family training and socialization into gender roles begins at birth—or even before, if fetal sex is known. Family attitudes and behaviors related to such things as affection, nudity, and masturbation teach a woman how to deal with aspects of sexuality. For example, a woman from a family that treated sex as a taboo subject learns that sex is bad.

Most of the literature about women's sexuality is based on white, middle-class women. Although little is known about the sexuality of women from other cultures, the existing information clearly shows that culture strongly influences a woman's experience of her sexuality (Smith, 1990).

Some information about black women and sexuality exists. Some people have viewed black women as extremely sexual. However, this view may stem from the sexual use and abuse of slave women (Staples, 1972). Data suggest that black women have sexual intercourse at a younger age, engage in extramarital intercourse more frequently, and have more liberal attitudes about sex than do white women (Weinberg & Williams, 1988). However, House, Faulk, and Kubovchik (1990) report that black women have lower sexual desire than do white women: Black women desired sex an average of twice per week, whereas white women desired it three times per week.

General discussions of sex and sexuality are common in the black community, yet private discussions about sex between a woman and her partner may be limited by fear of the man's response and distrust of the partner (Fullilove, Fullilove, Haynes, & Gross, 1990). Furthermore, lack of sexual communication is associated with imbalances in gender-based power.

When poor and working-class black women were asked about sexual roles for women, they identified two: good girl and bad girl (Fullilove et al., 1990). The good girl is most likely to engage in serial monogamy, whereas the bad girl is likely to have multiple sexual relationships simultaneously. The bad girl also is more likely to initiate sexual activity with a man, engage in sexual acts considered taboo, and be considered sexually aggressive. The black women strongly viewed sex as the consummation of a relationship rather than as an isolated pleasure-giving act.

Women's Sexual Lifestyles

A sexual lifestyle is the pattern and context of one's sexuality (Laws & Schwartz, 1977). The most commonly accepted sexual lifestyle for a woman is marriage to a monogamous partner. During the sexual revolution of the 1960s and 1970s, this lifestyle lost some of its traditional status as the best one for women and men. Since the advent of acquired immunodeficiency syndrome (AIDS) and neoconservatism, however, it has regained its former status.

For those who are not married, society dictates that coupling or partnership is the most desirable lifestyle. It assumes that single individuals (including divorced and widowed women and lesbians) are in transition until they find a partner.

Some women choose nonmonogamous marriage as their sexual lifestyle. They may participate with their husband in sexual activities with other individuals or couples (swinging). Other heterosexual women may choose to live with a man without being married; they may be sexually monogamous or nonmonogamous.

Other sexual lifestyles include lesbianism and bisexuality. Women in these lifestyles may be single or have a partner. They may have many sexual partners or only one. The most typical pattern for lesbians is serial monogamy. (For more information, see Chapter 10, "Lesbian Health Care.")

The bisexual lifestyle is poorly understood. Bisexual women experience sexual desire for persons of either sex. They may have sexual partners of both sexes simultaneously or serially. Many are married but maintain lesbian relationships. Some married women become bisexual after being introduced to lesbianism through swinging. Some bisexual women have committed lesbian relationships yet also have sexual relationships with men.

Celibacy (abstinence from sexual activity) is another sexual lifestyle. When consciously chosen, celibacy can allow a woman to devote her time and full attention to other activities without putting energy into sex (Kitzinger, 1983). However, some women hesitate to admit to this lifestyle because they think society expects them to want to be sexually active. Celibacy can also be involuntary—for example, when an individual is between relationships.

Sexual Behaviors

Almost every woman needs to express her sexuality, yet individuals vary greatly in their expression of it. Sexual behavior refers to the actions women use in sexual expression, including genital and nongenital activities. However, this section focuses on genital activities because nongenital activities can include everything from women's style of dress or gestures to their interactions with others.

For years, women's motivation for sexual behavior was thought to be the expression of love or commitment to their sexual partners. Recent studies have investigated this assumption. Leigh (1989) studied heterosexual men and women, gay men, and lesbians to determine their reasons for having—and not having—sex. Although small numerical differences in scores existed among groups, all women were more likely than men to engage in sex to express emotional closeness. They were also more likely than men to avoid sex because they were not interested or did not enjoy sex. Hatfield, Sprecher, Pillemer, Greenberger, and Wexler (1988) showed that most women desire love and intimacy from a sexual encounter.

When asked what they most desired from a sexual relationship, women reported that they would like their sexual partners to talk more lovingly and be more seductive, complimentary, warm, and involved. Married and single women also desired more directions from their partners during sexual encounters, and married women desired their partners to be more experimental (Hatfield et al., 1988).

Like men, women participate in all types of sexual behaviors. Unlike men, they typically view each activity (such as kissing, caressing, or manual genital stimulation) as an end in itself, rather than as foreplay for intercourse (Denney, Field, & Quadagno, 1984). However, almost no literature describes the meaning of various sexual activities to women.

A common issue that can arise between a woman and her sexual partner is different levels of sexual desires. For example, one may want sex frequently, whereas the other wants it rarely. To minimize tension, the couple may need to compromise on the frequency and nature of sexual activities. They also may need to learn how to communicate their desires without making judgments about the partner.

Intercourse

For many women, penile-vaginal intercourse is the preferred sexual activity. However, they are sensitive to the situation or environment in which intercourse occurs. Situational factors, such as fear of discovery, worry about a sick child, anxiety that a child might enter the room, or fear of being heard, may interfere with a woman's full expression of her sexuality.

After intercourse, many women experience afterglow (a time of emotional and physical relaxation). They view afterglow as an important time of closeness and communication, in which they enjoy caressing or talking with their partner.

Women usually engage in sexual intercourse for sexual pleasure but may engage in it for other reasons as well. For example, they may want to release tension, reconcile after a disagreement, conceive, or simply be touched or held.

The frequency of intercourse has been a topic of much social interest. According to a national study, sex is a regular part of life for most married couples: About two thirds have sex at least once a week, even after more than 10 years of marriage. Also, more than 75% of nonmarried heterosexual couples (cohabitors) have sex at least once a week (Blumstein & Schwartz, 1983).

For both types of couples, however, the frequency of sex decreases as the duration of the relationship increases (Blumstein & Schwartz, 1983). Decreased frequency of intercourse may result from a reduction in the woman's or her partner's health and sexual desire. It also can be caused by a decrease in partner availability—for example, if a job requires overnight travel. For older heterosexual women (married and widowed), lack of availability of a satisfactory partner commonly results in cessation of intercourse.

Oral intercourse (oral sex) refers to sexual contact between one partner's mouth and the other's genitals. Oral contact with a man's genitals is known as *fellatio*; oral contact with a woman's genitals is known as *cunnilingus.* Oral sex is a common sexual practice among women. According to Blumstein and Schwartz (1983), 90% of heterosexual couples engage in fellatio and 93%

engage in cunnilingus; 96% of lesbians engage in cunnilingus.

Although many women find cunnilingus stimulating, a woman may hesitate to let her partner perform it unless she feels totally clean. This is because society has taught men and women that the vagina is dirty and smelly. Women seem to have less ambivalence about performing fellatio because the penis is assumed to be clean and exciting.

Anal intercourse (anorectal sex) refers to insertion of a penis, dildo, or other object into the rectum as a part of sexual activity. This form of intercourse is different from digital or oral stimulation of the anus only because penetration occurs. A woman may receive or give anal intercourse with a male or female partner.

Many people find anal intercourse unappealing or repugnant. Some think it is dirty, others worry that it will damage rectal tissue, and many associate it with AIDS or gay men and thus are unwilling to engage in it. Nevertheless, some women find rectal penetration extremely satisfying sexually. Recent research suggests that up to 10% of women engage in anal intercourse frequently (Voeller, 1991).

Masturbation

Also known as *autoeroticism,* masturbation is an important sexual behavior. Kinsey (1953) reported that 62% of the women in his sample had masturbated, Hite (1976) reported that 82% of the women in her sample had masturbated, and today it is generally believed that most women do. However, a recent study of low-income, inner-city women showed that only 31% had ever masturbated, that 25% currently masturbated, and that only half of that group masturbated to orgasm (House, Faulk, & Kubovchik, 1990).

Dodson (1987) calls masturbation a primary form of sexual expression because it usually is the first form of sexual activity. As self-sexuality, it is valid as one's total sex life.

Unfortunately, many women were taught that masturbation is unacceptable and could cause harm. They learned that their genitals were ugly and that they should not look at or touch them. In reality, masturbation is normal; its only harm is the anxiety and guilt it may trigger in women who were socialized to believe that masturbation is taboo.

Masturbation is a way for adolescents to learn about their physical responses and pleasurable sensations, to explore the body, and to discover erotic feelings. Moreover, masturbation is a safe sexual outlet for an adolescent who does not wish to engage in other sexual activities. By learning how to masturbate, a woman can become orgasmic. This learned sexual skill also may help a woman teach her partner how to please her.

Although women may use many techniques for masturbation, most employ direct, manual stimulation of the clitoris. Other techniques include manipulating the genitals manually, rubbing the clitoris and vulva against an object, tensing the vaginal muscles, inserting a finger or object into the vagina, running water over the genitals, or wearing tight clothing. The methods are limited only by the woman's creativity. For many women, mutual masturbation with a partner is an alternative to intercourse or a pleasant addition to the sexual repertoire.

Kegel exercises (isometric exercises used to strengthen the pubococcygeal muscle by contracting it) also are a form of self-stimulation that may be used in masturbation (Kuhns-Hastings, 1988). Health care providers commonly recommend Kegel exercises to women to help prevent stress incontinence or to strengthen the muscles after childbirth. However, these exercises can be done anywhere at any time, and doing them can be sexually pleasurable. During intercourse, Kegel exercises can increase a woman's awareness of her genitals and may enhance enjoyment for both partners.

Sexual devices such as dildos, ben wa balls, and candy panties add variety and fun to some women's sexual experiences. Perhaps the most commonly used women's sex toy is a vibrator. Electric and battery-operated vibrators come in many different shapes, sizes, and colors. Their chief advantage during masturbation is that they do not experience fatigue as a person may, so they can provide stimulation for as long as desired. Today, many women also use condoms and dental dams (rubber devices that cover the teeth and oral cavity) as sex toys as well as protection against AIDS.

Fantasy

Another form of women's sexual expression, fantasy (creation of mental images that develop as the woman desires) has become recognized as a legitimate sexual behavior (Dodson, 1987). It certainly is the most common sexual behavior: In one study, 97% of single college women reported having sexual fantasies (Pelletier & Herold, 1988). However, research has shown that fantasies are associated negatively with age. In other words, older women have fewer fantasies than do younger women (Pelletier & Herold, 1988).

During a fantasy, the woman is in control and can think about anything—even something that might displease her if it were real. She may use fantasy by itself as a sexual behavior or combine it with other behaviors to enhance the experience.

A woman may have been taught that fantasies are unhealthy or that they represent what she really wants. Consequently, if she fantasizes about rape or bestiality (sex with an animal), for example, she may feel guilty. If a lesbian has heterosexual fantasies, she may question her sexual identity. These concerns are unnecessary, however, because fantasies are normal and cannot be wrong (Gordon & Snyder, 1989).

Some women use erotica (explicit descriptions or representations of sexual activity) to enhance sexual pleasure during fantasy or other sexual activities. However, many women accept erotica only if it represents women positively, has aesthetic value, or was created by women (Califia, 1983). Some women do not accept any erotica: They consider it pornography, which is demeaning and degrading to women.

Touch

Touching is an extremely important sexual activity for most women. According to the Hite Report (Hite, 1976), women want physical closeness, cuddling, and caressing more than they want intercourse. Lesbians also report a desire for more touching and caressing than genital activity (Blumstein & Schwartz, 1983).

Massage is a form of touch that can be performed using various techniques on specific parts of the body, such as the face, hands, or feet, or on the entire body. Usually, oil or lotion is used during massage to prevent unpleasant heat or friction. Massage also is a form of communication and an act of physical caring and healing that can be channeled into a form of sexual expression. Having a massage requires surrender of control and total acceptance of receiving rather than giving, which is what most women are used to doing. It is relaxing, therapeutic, and sensual and can be sexual when performed by a woman's partner. Self-massage also can be combined with masturbation for added pleasure (Dodson, 1987).

Sadomasochism

Sadomasochism, sometimes called S/M, is a form of erotic ritual that involves acting out sexual fantasies in which one partner is dominant (top) and the other partner is submissive (bottom). In sadomasochism, individuals derive sexual arousal, pleasure, and gratification from inflicting pain or humiliation (sadism) or experiencing pain or humiliation (masochism).

Heterosexual and bisexual women and men, lesbians, and gay men may engage in sadomasochism. However, this sexual behavior is controversial because many people—especially feminists—think it is dangerous and acts out in sexual behavior the violence of patriarchal society. These views have helped make sadomasochism a hidden behavior and a sexual subculture by stigmatizing sadomasochism and those who engage in it.

The sadomasochistic ritual, or scene, is preceded by negotiation of the role each partner will play, and identification of specific activities that will occur and the limits of those activities—including a cue word or action for the submissive partner to stop the scene. The dynamic is eroticized consensual exchange of power (Califia, 1983).

Little is known about the women and men who participate in sadomasochism. One study based on questionnaires placed in publications for sadomasochists had only 52 (28%) female respondents. Most of these women were heterosexual, a third were bisexual, and only one was lesbian. Less than 25% of the women were prostitutes. Most were introduced to the subculture by another person and most made their contacts through advertisements. Women reported an average of 8.6 partners and 53 sadomasochistic sexual encounters in the past year: Men had 3.4 partners and 25 encounters (Breslow, Evans, & Langley, 1985).

Developmental and Other Considerations

Most of the literature about female sexuality is based on typical young adult and midlife women who are white, middle-class, and healthy. Therefore, the previous sections of the chapter have focused primarily on their sexuality. This section presents the variations in sexual expression in women at different developmental stages and in those who otherwise are not considered typical for social or other reasons.

Adolescence

Adolescence marks a time of awareness of and changes in sexual feelings. During this time, young women and men experiment with their sexuality and engage in a wide variety of behaviors, including kissing, petting, and genital stimulation without penile penetration. These activities may result in orgasm for one or both partners. Many adolescents also participate in sexual intercourse. Research reports that the average age of first voluntary intercourse is 17.2 for white women and 16.7 for black women (Wyatt, 1989).

On the basis of interviews with a large number of adolescent women, Thompson (1990) reported that they began sexual activity in one of two scenarios: (a) Intercourse "just happened." The women were unprepared, uninformed, and often unwilling. Many of them thought the experience was "nice"; others found it to be disappointing, boring, or painful. (b) Intercourse was planned. These young women satisfied their own curiosity by initiating sex. They used contraception and were sexually informed. Many of them had prior masturbation and petting experiences.

Lesbian adolescents began sexual activity in either scenario. Their first heterosexual experiences resembled those of the heterosexual adolescents. However, they were more likely to experience the second scenario when they engaged in lesbian sexual activity. Most were orgasmic the first time and reported the experience of lesbian sexual activity as highly positive and emotionally rewarding.

Pregnancy

Sexuality during pregnancy is a concern for many women and their partners. Although women vary greatly in their sexuality during pregnancy, research and anecdotal reports suggest that women's sexual activity tends to decline throughout the pregnancy. Also, they commonly experience decreased sexual desire, sexual satisfaction, and frequency of intercourse (Bogren, 1991).

During the first trimester, most women feel less sexual because of the physical discomforts associated with early pregnancy, such as nausea, vomiting, and fatigue. In the second trimester, some women become more sexual because they feel better physically and are happy with the pregnancy. However, they may need to try new sexual positions to accommodate their enlarging abdomens. During the third trimester, women's sexual feelings typically wane, especially as the delivery date nears. They may feel tired and uncomfortable; some women may experience painful spastic (rather than rhythmic) uterine contractions during orgasm (Masters & Johnson, 1966).

Throughout pregnancy, women and their partners may worry about the effects of intercourse on the fetus. Early in the pregnancy they may fear spontaneous abortion; later, they may be concerned about damaging the fetus. Although controversy exists, most experts believe that intercourse in healthy women does not endanger the fetus (Mueller, 1985).

However, sexual activity late in pregnancy can trigger labor in several ways. Cervical stimulation, orgasm, prostaglandins in semen, and breast stimulation all can produce uterine contractions that lead to labor (Kahn & Holt, 1990). In fact, women may engage in intercourse near term in an attempt to start labor.

Lactation

Although women vary greatly in their sexuality, many experience decreased sexual desire during lactation. This can cause depression and guilt, particularly if they do not understand the cause of this change. Decreased desire primarily results from low estrogen levels. It may be exacerbated by decreased vaginal secretions (also caused by low estrogen levels), which can lead to dyspareunia (painful intercourse) unless a lubricant is used.

Old Age

Older women commonly are believed by society and themselves to be asexual. Unfortunately, women who accept this belief may give up a very important part of themselves. If they think that to be old is to be sexless, they may be trapped in a self-fulfilling prophecy and begin to withdraw from—rather than engage with—the important people in their lives (Rice, 1989). Yet sexual activity may contribute to serenity and happiness in old age (Fogel & Lauver, 1990; Rice, 1989).

Research into the sexuality of older people concludes that, although sexual interest and behaviors may decrease somewhat, most older people maintain sexual relationships if they have a partner. For women especially, the availability of a willing and able partner is the key to maintaining sexual activity (Malatesta, 1989).

Sexual behavior patterns in old age resemble those in midlife. In one study, past sexual behaviors correlated strongly with present behaviors in healthy women and men from the ages of 80 to 102 (Bretschneider & McCoy, 1988).

In women, the effects of aging include decreased estrogen levels and tissue elasticity. This can cause vaginal tissue thinning, which can result in vaginal irritation or discomfort with penetration. If the irritation leads to inflammation, atrophic vaginitis can occur. Other factors that predispose older women to atrophic vaginitis may include increased time to achieve complete arousal and lubrication as well as diminished lubrication.

With age, women lose fatty tissue in the labia and mons pubis, resulting in tenderness and easily damaged skin or abrasions in that area. Orgasms may decrease in intensity or become painful. The women's breasts may sag and decrease in size. Although these breast changes may alter a woman's view of herself sexually, they do not affect her capacity for sexual response.

Physical changes may require a woman to alter her sexual activity. For example, she may need to use a water-soluble lubricant to increase vaginal comfort, or she may take a hormone replacement to minimize such changes as vaginal tissue thinning. She can be encouraged to enjoy—rather than worry about—the increased time to achieve full arousal. If sexual activity is unsatisfying or uncomfortable, a woman may try different sexual positions. If she is fatigued in the evening, she may benefit from engaging in sexual activities in the morning or afternoon, instead of the evening.

Older women reportedly need touch and closeness more than genital activity. Kissing may be a satisfactory expression of sexuality. Although the primary motivation for most women to engage in sexual activity is to gain a sense of connection, mutuality, or love, a recent study showed that the physical motivation increases and love motivation decreases with age (Sprague & Quadagno, 1989).

Approximately 5% of older women live in nursing homes and other institutions, and most are forced into celibacy. The staff may frown on or strictly forbid sexual activity, even masturbation, in subtle ways (for example, by not providing privacy) and obvious ways (for example, by shaming or publicly embarrassing women who act on their sexual needs). This forced lack of sexual expression can lead to depression (Rice, 1989).

Widowhood

Generally, the death of a woman's husband is an extremely stressful event that can affect her sexuality. Typically, a woman's identity is defined through her relationships, especially her relationship with her husband. Therefore, when she loses her husband, she also may lose her sense of self. At the same time, she may develop a new identity as a widow—a stereotyped sad woman.

Little is known about the sexuality of widows. However, numerous factors can affect a widow's sexuality, including the suddenness of the husband's death and her extramarital sexual experience, age, and sexual satisfaction in the marriage. These factors were associated with sexual desire and the resumption of sexual intercourse in a group of widows during the first 14 months of bereavement: Younger widows whose husband's death was expected and who had extramarital sexual experience and were less sexually satisfied in the marriage experienced sexual desire and resumed intercourse earlier than did other widows (Kansky, 1986).

Malatesta, Chambless, Pollack, and Cantor (1988) conducted a study of 118 white widows between the ages of 40 and 89. They found that the loss that caused unhappiness was more likely to be the loss of heterosocial activities, such as going places with or confiding in a man, rather than the loss of specific sexual activities. Unhappiness related to sexual activity loss, such as intercourse and hugging, was associated with the widow's age: The younger the widow, the more she missed sexual activities. Regardless of age, personal appearance and attractive clothes were meeting sexual needs.

Remarriage after widowhood is correlated with age. Women who become widows before the age of 35 are likely to remarry, but the likelihood of marriage diminishes with increasing age. Less than 5% of women widowed after the age of 55 ever remarry (Cleveland & Gianturco, 1976).

Disability

Disabilities may range from blindness, deafness, or paralysis to mental illness or cancer. They may be congenital or acquired. A woman's experience of her disability and its effects on her sexuality may be related to the time of its onset. DeHaan and Wallander (1988) reported that women with early-onset physical disabilities (congenital disabilities or those acquired before the age of 3) were less likely to engage in sexual activities than were women who had late-onset disabilities (those acquired after age 18) or women with no disabilities (women between the ages of 3 and 18 were not included in the study sample). Like older women, disabled women typically are perceived by society as asexual. Although they may become friends or confidantes, they may be considered (by themselves and others) unfit to be sexual partners or mothers. Therefore, many heterosexual and lesbian women with disabilities remain single (Fine & Asch, 1981).

Health care providers also may perceive disabled women as asexual. In a study of gynecologic care, only 26% of disabled women (average age 43) reported being asked about their sexual history. About half would have liked information about sexuality or wanted to discuss feelings about sexuality. However, only 19% were offered sexual information by their gynecologist, and only 6% requested such information (Beckmann, Gittler, Barzansky, & Beckmann, 1989). In another study, women who were totally blind before the age of 10 had lower sex knowledge scores, reported receiving less sex information, and received that information at a later age than did sighted women (Welbourne, Lifschitz, Selvin, & Green, 1983).

Body image is an important aspect of sexuality for many women with disabilities. If the disability has caused a body alteration, such as limb amputation or paralysis, or if it requires the use of an assistive device, such as a cane or wheelchair, the woman may view her body as a problem and as a source of anxiety rather than pleasure. Her acceptance of societal beliefs may cause her to feel that she cannot be sexual and is not sexually appealing. Such acceptance may limit her to masturbation and other self-expressions of sexuality and may prevent her from seeking sexual partners. Some women will choose others with disabilities as sexual partners because they share feelings and experiences.

Prostitution

Although prostitution is called the oldest profession, many people do not consider it to be legitimate employment. In this country, in fact, society views prostitution as a criminal offense and condemns women who are prostitutes. This is a classic example of a sexual double standard: Selling sex is a serious crime, but buying sex is not.

The sexuality of prostitutes has rarely been studied. However, the AIDS crisis has begun to focus attention on prostitutes. Although they are blamed for the spread of AIDS, little attention is paid to their personal risks. Yet because of the number of sexual encounters prostitutes have, they and their clients and private sexual partners are at high risk for HIV infection.

Two studies recently examined the sexuality of prostitutes. Freund, Leonard, and Lee (1989) identified the types of sexual activities in which prostitutes engaged and described their sexual partners. The most frequently performed sexual activity was fellatio (62%) and the second (23%) penile-vaginal intercourse with their clients, 49% of whom were seeing them at least once a week.

Savitz and Rosen (1988) concluded that prostitutes derive pleasure or enjoyment from their sexual activities. In understanding this conclusion, one must consider the context of these women's lives. Being labeled a prostitute may give them greater freedom to enjoy sex and admit that they do.

Sexual Problems

Because sexuality is multidimensional, many situations and factors can cause sexual problems or difficulties for women. This section discusses two common causes: illness and sexual dysfunction.

To determine how a particular situation or factor affects a woman's sexuality, the nurse must consider all of the components of sexuality and must keep in mind that individuals respond to events differently: Something that affects one woman may not affect another.

Illness

Little empirical research exists about the effects of various physical and mental disorders on women's sexuality. The existing literature suggests that women's sexuality can be affected by the following:

- Chronic illness, such as diabetes, asthma, arthritis, cancer, or heart or kidney disease
- Acute illness, such as a sexually transmitted disease (STD)
- Surgery, such as cholecystectomy, hysterectomy, mastectomy, or an orthopedic procedure, and other procedures
- Trauma, such as spinal cord injury

The nurse should keep in mind that illness and treatment of illness do not alter sexuality in all cases. One study demonstrated no significant differences in sexual desire, function, and performance between women with nonalcoholic liver disease and the general female population (Bach, Schaffner, & Kapelman, 1989).

Although the effects of acute illness on sexuality may be brief in time, the impact can be considerable. Fatigue and pain, symptoms commonly associated with acute illness, may require postponement of sexual activity. STDs often necessitate refraining from sexual activity until a cure is obtained (see Chapter 24, "Sexually Transmitted Diseases") or altering one's sexual practices, as when use of a condom is needed or oral-genital contact must be avoided.

The effects of trauma on sexuality are often devastating and lifelong. Spinal cord injuries most often occur to young adults who experience instantaneous, profound, and complex insults to their total well-being, including their sexual self (Sackett, 1990). A discussion of the myriad effects of trauma on sexual functioning and sexuality is beyond the scope of this text. Furthermore, little is known about the effect of spinal cord injuries on female sexuality.

However, chronic illness is more likely to produce difficulties with sexual desire and arousal than with orgasm (Schover, 1989). General symptoms of chronic illness, such as fatigue, stress, and pain, may diminish a woman's energy, especially her energy for sexual expression. If so, the woman and her partner may need to participate in sexual activity at a time of day when they feel most able. They may also need to experiment with various positions to enhance comfort and pleasure and to avoid excess fatigue or stress. Good communication between partners is essential in maintaining satisfactory sexual activities.

Changes in physical appearance, such as those caused by arthritis, weight loss, or surgery, may reduce self-esteem and alter body image, directly or indirectly influencing a woman's sexuality. In a study of end-stage renal disease, women reported extreme changes in body image, self-concept, and femininity caused by weight gain and surgical scars that had a negative effect on their sexuality (Rickus, 1987).

Most studies of women with diabetes suggest that they are likely to have multiple sexual difficulties, especially orgasmic dysfunction and inadequate lubrication. One study found that Type I diabetes was not associated with sexual difficulties, but Type II diabetes had many negative effects on sexual desire, orgasmic capacity, lubrication, and sexual satisfaction (Schreiner-Engel, Schiavi, Vietorisz, & Smith, 1987). A study of women with Type I diabetes demonstrated negative effects on sexual desire, lubrication, and orgasmic ability, which increased with the women's age and the duration of diabetes (Bahen-Auger, Wilson, & Assalian, 1988). Even when researchers have conducted multiple studies of the effects of an illness on women's sexuality, inconsistencies and differences among studies point to the need for further study.

Women with gynecologic cancer usually have severe sexual difficulties after diagnosis and treatment. Studies consistently have shown that women experience decreased frequency of intercourse and decreased sexual excitement or arousal (Andersen, Anderson, & deProsse, 1989; Schover, Fife, & Gershenson, 1989).

Hysterectomy frequently is performed as a part of gynecologic cancer treatment but may also be done to treat many other disorders. Although researchers have studied the effects of hysterectomy on women's sexuality, their results vary considerably. Older studies, such as the one by Dennerstein, Wood, and Burrows (1977), reported negative effects, including increased dyspareunia and decreased sexual desire, enjoyment, orgasm, and lubrication. More recent studies demonstrated positive outcomes, such as increased frequency of and satisfaction with intercourse (Gath, Cooper, & Day, 1982). Some studies also have shown an association between women's expectations about the effects of hysterectomy and its actual effects on sexuality (Bernhard, 1986; Dennerstein et al., 1977).

Breast cancer threatens the sexuality of most women. In a society that views women's breasts as sexual organs, a woman and her partner may feel that the loss of a breast is devastating to their sexuality. Even if a woman undergoes breast reconstruction, she may worry about her sexuality. Although death is the primary concern of most women with breast cancer, altered sexuality frequently becomes a major concern when she learns that she is expected to survive.

Some women may have greater sexuality problems when faced with breast cancer. These include women who dislike their breasts, have a negative self-image, have a history of unpleasant sexual experiences, have been abused sexually, worry about finding a sexual partner, lack a support system, are uncomfortable discussing personal and sexual concerns, or sustain severe adverse effects from treatment (Schain, 1985). Lesbians have rarely been acknowledged in breast cancer research, but Arbogast (1985) found that the effects of mastectomy on lesbian sexuality were similar to those on the sexuality of heterosexual women and their partners.

Sexual difficulties may arise from treatments other than surgery. For example, diazepam (Valium) is the drug most commonly prescribed for women (Riley & Riley, 1986). Yet research has shown that diazepam causes a dose-related impairment of sexual response in women, producing decreased arousability, lubrication, speed and sensation of orgasm, and general satisfaction.

On the other hand, treatments can improve some women's sexuality. For example, women with ulcerative colitis who underwent proctocolectomy that preserved continence experienced enhanced sexual functioning, increased frequency of intercourse, and reduced dyspareunia, primarily because of improved health (Metcalf, Dozois, & Kelly, 1986).

Sexual Dysfunction

Sexual dysfunction refers to impaired, incomplete, or lack of expression of normal human sexual desires and responses. However, these concerns become dysfunctions only when they cause subjective discomfort (Renshaw, 1983). Masters and Johnson (1970) reported that half of married couples experience sexual dysfunctions at some time during their marriage. Renshaw (1983) indicated that partner dissatisfaction may precipitate acknowledgment of a dysfunction.

Sexual dysfunctions may result from various causes. In the past, most were thought to derive from psychological factors. Today, however, many are known to result from physical or organic factors such as chronic disease (diabetes), medications (antihypertensive agents), and surgery. Traumatic sexual experiences, such as incest and rape, can lead to sexual dysfunction in women. Relationship difficulties also may trigger dysfunction. For example, if a woman discovers that her partner has been sexually unfaithful, she may become dysfunctional with that partner.

Numerous factors tend to maintain sexual dysfunction, such as inadequate or incorrect sexual knowledge or lack of effective communication between partners. Anxiety or depression about the inability to deal with the dysfunction may make it worse. Sexual difficulties also can escalate if both partners experience dysfunction.

Sexologists and sex therapists define three principal sexual dysfunctions in women: inhibited sexual desire (lack of interest in sexual activity), anorgasmia (inability to achieve orgasm), and vaginismus (vaginal muscle spasms that interfere with intercourse). Some also include dyspareunia (Masters & Johnson, 1970). They treat these and other sexual dysfunctions with sex therapy, including education and counseling (for more information, see Table 21.1).

Psychiatrists (APA, 1994) acknowledge these four dysfunctions as well as sexual aversion disorder (extreme repulsion by and avoidance of almost all genital sexual contact) and female sexual arousal disorder (partial or complete failure to attain or maintain vaginal lubrication and swelling or sexual excitement). However, these dysfunctions go beyond the scope of nursing and must be treated by a health care practitioner with extensive training in sex counseling and therapy.

Sex Addiction

Although some health care professionals doubt the validity of sexual addiction, women of all sexual orientations identify themselves as sex addicts. Formerly, these women may have been called nymphomaniacs.

In women, sex addiction is the inability to stop sexual behavior despite serious consequences, such as disease, unwanted pregnancy, violence, sexual dysfunction, or job or financial loss (Carnes, 1986). Kasl (1989) distinguishes between addictive sex and sex addiction. Addictive sex

Table 21.1 Common Sexual Dysfunctions

Description	*Cause*	*Treatment*
Inhibited sexual desire		
Lack of interest in sexual activity is the most common sexual dysfunction for which women seek help (Stuart, Hammond, & Pett, 1987). Women with the dysfunction are less likely than other women to express romantic love feelings for their partners and to be satisfied with their ability to listen to their partners (Stuart et al., 1987).	Unknown, but may be caused by biological, psychological, and relationship factors and associated with high stress levels.	• Sensate focus therapy (deliberate form of touching as a communication method). Both partners participate in sensate focus therapy and must communicate feelings to their partner through touch. The therapist directs the couple to touch certain parts of their partner's body and avoid others. This therapy progresses until the partners touch all parts of each other's bodies and become sexually aroused. • Psychotherapy. • Communication skills training.
Anorgasmia		
The inability to experience orgasm can be primary (preorgasmia), in which the woman has never experienced orgasm, or secondary (situational anorgasmia), in which she has experienced orgasms but does not experience them with this partner, at this time, or during a particular sexual activity. Primary anorgasmia is more common than secondary orgasmia.	Primary anorgasmia: previous sexual trauma, current relationship issues, lack of education and information about sexual matters, sociocultural stigma, or interpersonal concerns (Heiman & Grafton-Becker, 1989). Secondary anorgasmia: use of psychoactive drug (Segraves, 1988), episiotomy scars, or oophorectomy is commonly reported (e.g., see Dennerstein, Wood, & Burrows, 1977) but the mechanism of action is not known (i.e., we don't know how or why).	• Directed masturbation. In this behavioral therapy that relies on desensitization, the woman is taught to examine her genitals, touch them without expecting arousal, then touch them to produce pleasurable feelings, and finally masturbate by touching those areas with increasing duration and intensity. When taught to masturbate, most anorgasmic women experience orgasms relatively easily and quickly (Barbach, 1980). The chief obstacle in this therapy may be a woman's reluctance to touch herself and receive pleasure from doing so.
Vaginismus		
This dysfunction is characterized by involuntary, spasmodic, sometimes painful contractions of the pubococcygeal and other muscles of the vaginal introitus (Leiblum, Pervin, & Campbell, 1989). Although some health care professionals consider vaginismus rare, sex therapists think it may be more common but that women do not seek help for the problem unless they desire to have children.	Rape or other sexual trauma, strong conservative religious values in the family of origin, dyspareunia, or hostile feelings toward the sexual partner (Leiblum et al., 1989).	• Desensitization through insertion of progressively larger dilators into the vagina by the woman or her partner. • Psychotherapy if the woman needs to overcome a particular trauma.

(continued)

is the mistaken use of sex as a form of power or love. Sex addiction occurs when addictive sex escalates and the woman cannot control it, resulting in harmful consequences, obsessions, and a decreased ability to perform normal daily functions. In women, sex addiction reflects an

Table 21.1 Continued

Description	*Cause*	*Treatment*
Dyspareunia		
This dysfunction causes pain in the labia, vagina, or pelvis during or after sexual intercourse (Glatt, Zinner, & McCormack, 1990). Its incidence is unknown, but may affect up to 60% of women (Glatt et al., 1990).	Organic disorders, such as vaginal or urinary tract infection, endometriosis, and anatomic or structural variations; decreased estrogen supply; mechanical irritation from such things as excess douching or use of deodorant soaps; developmental factors, such as family religious taboos or teachings that the vagina should not be touched; sexual trauma, such as rape or incest; and relational concerns, such as hostile feelings toward the partner, lack of complete arousal, or personal problems (Lazarus, 1989).	• Treatment related to underlying physical cause. For example, if a urinary tract infection was present, antibiotic treatment should relieve the infection—and the dyspareunia. • Psychotherapy related to underlying psychological or relational problems.

NOTE: The four most common sexual dysfunctions in women are inhibited sexual desire, anorgasmia, vaginismus, and dyspareunia. To help a client with one of these dysfunctions, the nurse should be familiar with their characteristics, causes, and treatments.

internalization of traditional (male) norms of sexuality, including power, aggressiveness, and control.

Women may experience sex addiction in many ways, but the underlying themes of pain, fear, loneliness, and desperation are the same as in other addictions. Many female sex addicts were abused as children (Kasl, 1989). Some seek many partners, some have few, and others simply masturbate. Some sex addicts engage in prostitution; others participate in sadomasochistic relationships. These women share one common feature: Their goal is the "high" of orgasm, which allows a momentary escape from the pain in their lives.

Sources of help exist for sex-addicted women. The most common are 12-step programs that focus on the recovery process. These programs are based on the Alcoholics Anonymous model, which has helped many people recover from alcoholism addiction.

Sexual Health Promotion

All women's health care providers should offer sexual health promotion as a part of care. In the 1970s, interest in sexuality ran high: Many medical and nursing schools incorporated sexual content into their curricula and addressed sexual health concerns. Unfortunately, that interest was not sustained. Today, these schools devote little attention to sexuality-related topics, except for AIDS. Although AIDS is a crucial topic, so are all the other actual and potential sexual health problems that women experience. The need for sexual health promotion continues.

Nursing Care

To provide effective sexual counseling and client care, nurses first must be comfortable with their own sexuality. Acceptance of one's own sexuality and awareness of one's sexual biases is paramount in assisting a client.

To help achieve this acceptance and awareness, Brash (1990) suggests that the nurse use a "Model of Sexual Health for Nurses." As the first step in providing sexual health care, she suggests that the nurse focus on these five statements or assertions:

- I know and accept my sexual self and my body as OK.
- I choose a sexual lifestyle that fits and satisfies me.
- I am sexually assertive.
- I am free to express masculine and feminine sides of myself.
- I am sexually competent and sexually responsible.

Of course, these assertions do not apply only to nurses: They could be used by any health care provider or client to promote sexual health.

The second requirement for nurses is current, accurate knowledge about sexual health and the effects of various illnesses and treatments on sexuality. The nurse's knowledge base should also include strategies for managing problems as well as resources, such as sex therapists and books, pamphlets, films, and other educational materials.

The third requirement for a nurse who wants to provide sexual counseling is an appropriate attitude. In one study, women preferred these qualities in a provider with whom they would discuss sexual concerns: empathy and comfort in talking with the woman, good training, confidentiality, and lack of embarrassment (Metz & Seifert, 1988). The nurse not only should be comfortable discussing sexuality but should also have a genuine desire to help. Research has shown that healthy women and women with medical or surgical problems desire more sexual counseling, especially from female nurses (Baggs & Karch, 1987; Krueger et al., 1979).

Frequently, the health care provider and client assume that the other will introduce the topic of sexual health problems, and when neither does, sexual problems are overlooked. To prevent this, the nurse should initiate a discussion of sexual health and problems. In one gynecologic office practice, the use of these two simple questions elicited sexual concerns that the female clients had not mentioned earlier: "Are you sexually active? Are you having any sexual difficulties or problems at this time?" (Bachmann, Leiblum, & Grill, 1989).

When promoting a client's sexual health, the nurse must remember never to make assumptions about her sexual behavior, feelings, or attitudes. By keeping an open mind, the nurse will be able to understand the client better. The nurse should establish a mutual understanding of sexual terms to ensure effective communication with the client.

Assessment

A sexual health assessment is essential for sexual health promotion. First, the nurse should make the client comfortable and put her at ease. The assessment should take place in a private environment, and the client must understand that her information will be kept strictly confidential. These steps help promote trust and encourage the client to share her feelings and concerns. The nurse should allow adequate time for the assessment so that the client does not feel rushed.

The information to be collected depends on the client's problem and its potential to cause sexual difficulties. The nurse should not uncover sexual information and needs without a reason and a plan for dealing with it.

The nurse may use one of many guides for sexual assessment. (For an example, see Chapter 9, "Well-Woman Assessment.") Alternatively, the nurse can take an individualized approach tailored to the work setting. For example, a clinic nurse may take a complete sexual history; a hospital staff nurse may obtain only information relevant to the problem being treated in the hospital. Of course, the client may not reveal some relevant information, such as a history of incest or an illegal abortion. The nurse should be available when the client decides to disclose such information. (See Chapter 9, for suggestions regarding encouraging disclosure of sensitive information.)

The nurse should use data collected from the complete assessment—including the sexual assessment—to formulate the appropriate nursing diagnoses as well as the expected outcomes and nursing interventions.

Intervention

The most common approach to sexual counseling is the PLISSIT model (Annon, 1976). In this classic model, the acronym PLISSIT stands for four levels of sex counseling: permission, limited information, specific suggestions, and intensive therapy (see Table 21.2).

Conclusion

Sexuality is a vital aspect of women's lives that can provide great enjoyment—as well as numerous health problems. Some health care providers interact daily with women but never address their sexual health concerns. To help correct this oversight and promote sexual health, this chapter has given readers a breadth of information about women's sexuality.

Table 21.2 The PLISSIT Model

Permission (P)
At this level, the nurse encourages the client to talk about her sexual concerns and gives the client professional permission to function sexually, as she typically does. (However, the nurse should withhold permission for sexual behaviors that may harm the client or her partner. Although few behaviors are regularly harmful, some may be harmful for a time—for example, having intercourse following pelvic surgery). Giving permission meets most clients' needs, allowing them to continue their current behaviors and relieving anxiety about normality. All nurses should be able to give permission to clients. For example, women may be given permission to be sexually aroused by normal feelings or to engage in safe activities that arouse sexual feelings, such as masturbation or fantasizing.
Limited information (LI)
By providing limited information, the nurse answers the client's spoken—and unspoken—questions on the basis of clinical knowledge and an understanding of what other clients have asked and what a client needs to know about a particular problem or concern. For example, the nurse might give an older client information that dispels myths about sexuality and aging. The purpose of intervention at this level is to provide facts directly related to the client's concerns or to relieve a specific concern or anxiety. All nurses can provide limited information.
Specific suggestions (SS)
Many staff nurses and all advanced nurse practitioners should be able to make specific suggestions. At this level, the nurse focuses on the client and her unique concerns. For example, the nurse might help a client with chronic obstructive pulmonary disease and her partner by suggesting specific sexual positions that require the least amount of energy. The nurse could assist a diabetic client who experiences hypoglycemia after intercourse by pointing out ways to alter her timing of intercourse or diet plan so that intercourse remains a pleasant activity.
Intensive therapy (IT)
Intervention at this level requires the skill of a nurse with special preparation in sexuality or sex therapy or referral to a specially trained practitioner. Intensive therapy is recommended for a client with a sexual dysfunction or one who needs more counseling than the nurse can provide. The nurse must be aware of the limits of personal knowledge and skill and should make appropriate referrals when these limits are reached. Intensive therapy may be an appropriate intervention when a woman experiences sexual aversion disorder or vaginismus.

NOTE: Adapted from Annon (1976) who developed the PLISSIT model as an intervention tool for clients with sexual problems. The model defines four levels of sex counseling: permission, limited information, specific suggestions, and intensive therapy. It takes a behavioral approach to treating sexual problems and requires increasing knowledge and clinical skills as interventions increase in complexity.

The successful women's health nurse should keep two goals in mind: (a) to promote women's sexual health through thorough assessment and appropriate interventions and (b) to conduct and read research on women's sexuality and sexual health care. This will help nurses and their clients achieve their main goal: to be comfortable with their bodies and their sexuality.

References

INTRODUCTION

Bernhard, L. A. (1988). Women's sexuality. In C. J. Leppa & C. Miller (Eds.), *Women's health perspectives: An annual review* (pp. 71-89). Phoenix, AZ: Oryx.

Cassell, C. (1984). *Swept away: Why women fear their own sexuality.* New York: Simon & Schuster.

Heilbrun, A. B., Jr. (1981). *Human sex-role behavior.* New York: Pergamon.

Kahn, A. P., & Holt, L. H. (1990). *The A-Z of women's sexuality.* New York: Facts on File.

Kaplan, H. S. (1979). *Disorders of sexual desire.* New York: Brunner/Mazel.

Muff, J. (1982). Hand-maiden, battle-ax, whore. In J. Muff (Ed.), *Socialization, sexism, and stereotyping* (pp. 113-156). St. Louis: C. V. Mosby.

Schilder, P. (1950). *The image and appearance of the human body.* New York: International Universities Press.

Silber, L. (1990). Research note negotiating sexual identity: Non-lesbians in a lesbian feminist community. *Journal of Sex Research, 27*(1), 131-140.

Trebilcott, J. (1984). Taking responsibility for sexuality. In R. Baker & F. Elliston (Eds.), *Philosophy and sex* (pp. 421-430). Buffalo, NY: Prometheus.

ANATOMY AND PHYSIOLOGY OF FEMALE SEXUALITY

American Psychiatric Association. (1994). *Diagnostic and statistical manual of mental disorders* (4th ed.). Washington, DC: Author.

Charles, D., & Glover, D. D. (1985). Psychosexual problems related to pelvic pain. In M. Farver (Ed.), *Human sexuality: Psychosexual effects of disease* (pp. 159-168). New York: Macmillan.

Davidson, J. K., Sr., & Darling, C. A. (1989). Self-perceived differences in the female orgasmic response. *Family Practice Research Journal, 8*(2), 75-84.

Davidson, J. K., Sr., Darling, C. A., & Conway-Welch, C. (1989). The role of the Grafenberg spot and female ejaculation in the female orgasmic response: An empirical analysis. *Journal of Sex and Marital Therapy, 15*(2), 102-120.

Federation of Feminist Women's Health Centers. (1981). *A new view of a woman's body.* New York: Touchstone.

Ladas, A. K., Whipple, B., & Perry, J. D. (1982). *The G spot and other recent discoveries about human sexuality.* New York: Holt, Rinehart & Winston.

Masters, W. H., & Johnson, V. E. (1966). *Human sexual response.* Boston: Little, Brown.

Pernoll, M. L. (Ed.). (1991). *Current obstetric and gynecologic diagnosis and treatment.* Norwalk, CT: Appleton & Lange.

Warner, J. (1984). Physical and affective dimensions of peak of female sexual response and the relationships to self-reported orgasm. In H. I. Lief & Z. Hoch (Eds.), *International research in sexology* (pp. 91-96). New York: Praeger.

SOCIOCULTURAL INFLUENCES ON WOMEN'S SEXUALITY

Fullilove, M. T., Fullilove, R. E., Haynes, K., & Gross, S. (1990). Black women and AIDS prevention: A view towards understanding the gender rules. *Journal of Sex Research, 27*(1), 47-64.

House, W. C., Faulk, A., & Kubovchik, M. (1990). Sexual behavior of inner-city women. *Journal of Sex Education and Therapy, 16*(3), 172-184.

Smith, L. S. (1990). Human sexuality from a cultural perspective. In C. I. Fogel & D. Lauver (Eds.), *Sexual health promotion* (pp. 87-96). Philadelphia: W. B. Saunders.

Staples, R. (1972). The sexuality of black women. *Sexual Behavior, 2*(6), 4-15.

Weinberg, M. S., & Williams, C. J. (1988). Black sexuality: A test of two theories. *Journal of Sex Research, 25*(2), 197-218.

WOMEN'S SEXUAL LIFESTYLES

Kitzinger, S. (1983). *Women's experience of sex.* New York: G. P. Putnam.

Laws, J. L., & Schwartz, P. (1977). *Sexual scripts: The social construction of female sexuality.* Hinsdale, IL: Dryden.

SEXUAL BEHAVIORS

Blumstein, P., & Schwartz, P. (1983). *American couples.* New York: Morrow.

Breslow, N., Evans, L., & Langley, J. (1985). On the prevalence and roles of females in the sadomasochistic subculture: Report of an empirical study. *Archives of Sexual Behavior, 14*(4), 303-317.

Califia, P. (1983). *Sapphistry: The book of lesbian sexuality.* Tallahassee, FL: Naiad.

Denney, N. W., Field, J. K., & Quadagno, D. (1984). Sex differences in sexual needs and desires. *Archives of Sexual Behavior, 13*(3), 233-245.

Dodson, B. (1987). *Sex for one: The joy of self-loving.* New York: Harmony.

Gordon, S., & Snyder, C. W. (1989). *Personal issues in human sexuality.* Boston: Allyn & Bacon.

Hatfield, E., Sprecher, S., Pillemer, J. T., Greenberger, D., & Wexler, P. (1988). Gender differences in what is desired in the sexual relationship. *Journal of Psychology and Human Sexuality, 1*(2), 39-52.

Hite, S. (1976). *The Hite report.* New York: Macmillan.

Kinsey, A. C. (1953). *Sexual behavior in the human female.* Philadelphia: W. B. Saunders.

Kuhns-Hastings, J. (1988). Management of female incontinence with Kegel exercises. *American Association of Occupational Health Journal, 36*(2), 78-83.

Leigh, B. C. (1989). Reasons for having and avoiding sex: Gender, sexual orientation, and relationship to sexual behavior. *Journal of Sex Research, 26*(2), 199-209.

Pelletier, L. A., & Herold, E. S. (1988). The relationship of age, sex guilt, and sexual experience with female sexual fantasies. *Journal of Sex Research, 24*(2), 250-256.

Voeller, B. (1991). AIDS and heterosexual anal intercourse. *Archives of Sexual Behavior, 20*(3), 233-276.

DEVELOPMENTAL AND OTHER CONSIDERATIONS

Beckmann, C. R. B., Gittler, M., Barzansky, B. M., & Beckmann, C. A. (1989). Gynecologic health care of women with disabilities. *Obstetrics and Gynecology, 74*(1), 75-79.

Bogren, L. Y. (1991). Changes in sexuality in women and men during pregnancy. *Archives of Sexual Behavior, 20*(1), 35-45.

Bretschneider, J. G., & McCoy, N. L. (1988). Sexual interest and behavior in healthy 80- to 102-year-olds. *Archives of Sexual Behavior, 17*(2), 109-129.

Cleveland, W. P., & Gianturco, D. T. (1976). Remarriage probability after widowhood: A retrospective method. *Journal of Gerontology, 31*(1), 99-103.

DeHaan, C. B., & Wallander, J. L. (1988). Self-concept, sexual knowledge and attitudes, and parental support in the sexual adjustment of women with early- and late-onset physical disability. *Archives of Sexual Behavior, 17*(2), 145-161.

Fine, M., & Asch, A. (1981). Disabled women: Sexism without the pedestal. *Journal of Sociology and Social Welfare, 8*(2), 233-248.

Fogel, C. I., & Lauver, D. (1990). *Sexual health promotion.* Philadelphia: W. B. Saunders.

Freund, M., Leonard, T. L., & Lee, N. (1989). Sexual behavior of resident street prostitutes with their clients in Camden, New Jersey. *Journal of Sex Research, 26*(4), 460-478.

Kansky, J. (1986). Sexuality of widows: A study of the sexual practices of widows during the first fourteen months of bereavement. *Journal of Sex and Marital Therapy, 12*(4), 307-321.

Malatesta, V. J. (1989). Sexuality and the older adult: An overview with guidelines for the health care professional. *Journal of Women and Aging, 1*(4), 93-118.

Malatesta, V. J., Chambless, D. L., Pollack, M., & Cantor, A. (1988). Widowhood, sexuality and aging: A life span analysis. *Journal of Sex and Marital Therapy, 14*(1), 49-62.

Mueller, L. S. (1985). Pregnancy and sexuality. *JOGNN, 14*(4), 289-294.

Rice, S. (1989). Sexuality and intimacy for aging women: A changing perspective. *Journal of Women and Aging, 1*(1-3), 245-264.

Savitz, L., & Rosen, L. (1988). The sexuality of prostitutes: Sexual enjoyment reported by "street walkers." *Journal of Sex Research, 24,* 200-208.

Sprague, J., & Quadagno, D. (1989). Gender and sexual motivation: An exploration of two assumptions. *Journal of Psychology and Human Sexuality, 2*(1), 57-76.

Thompson, S. (1990). Putting a big thing into a little hole: Teenage girl's accounts of sexual initiation. *Journal of Sex Research, 27*(3), 341-361.

Welbourne, A., Lifschitz, S., Selvin, H., & Green, R. (1983). A comparison of the sexual learning experiences of visually impaired and sighted women. *Journal of Visual Impairment and Blindness, 77*(6), 256-259.

Wyatt, G. E. (1989). Reexamining factors predicting Afro-American and white American women's age at first coitus. *Archives of Sexual Behavior, 18*(4), 271-298.

SEXUAL PROBLEMS

Andersen, B. L., Anderson, B., & deProsse, C. (1989). Controlled prospective longitudinal study of women with cancer: I. Sexual functioning outcomes. *Journal of Consulting and Clinical Psychology, 57*(6), 683-691.

Arbogast, C. Q. (1985, August). Mastectomy: How does it affect women's sexual behavior? *Sexual Well-Being,* pp. 5-6.

Bach, N., Schaffner, F., & Kapelman, B. (1989). Sexual behavior in women with nonalcoholic liver disease. *Hepatology, 9*(5), 698-703.

Bahen-Auger, N., Wilson, M., & Assalian, P. (1988). Sexual response of the type I diabetic woman. *Medical Aspects of Human Sexuality, 22*(10), 94-100.

Barbach, L. (1980). *Women discover orgasm.* New York: Free Press.

Bernhard, L. A. (1986). *Sexuality expectations and outcomes in women having hysterectomies.* Unpublished doctoral dissertation, University of Illinois at Chicago.

Carnes, P. J. (1986). Progress in sexual addiction: An addiction perspective. *SIECUS Report, 14*(6), 4-6.

Dennerstein, L., Wood, C., & Burrows, G. D. (1977). Sexual response following hysterectomy and oophorectomy. *Obstetrics and Gynecology, 49*(1), 92-96.

Gath, D., Cooper, P., & Day, A. (1982). Hysterectomy and psychiatric disorder: I. Levels of psychiatric morbidity before and after hysterectomy. *British Journal of Psychiatry, 140,* 335-350.

Glatt, A. E., Zinner, S. H., & McCormack, W. M. (1990). The prevalence of dyspareunia. *Obstetrics and Gynecology, 75*(3, pt. 1), 433-436.

Heiman, J. R., & Grafton-Becker, V. (1989). Orgasmic disorders in women. In S. R. Leiblum & R. C. Rosen (Eds.), *Principles and practice of sex therapy* (2nd ed., pp. 51-88). New York: Guilford.

Kasl, C. D. (1989). *Women, sex, and addiction.* New York: Ticknor & Fields.

Lazarus, A. A. (1989). Dyspareunia: A multimodal psychotherapeutic perspective. In S. R. Leiblum & R. C. Rosen (Eds.), *Principles and practice of sex therapy* (2nd ed., pp. 89-112). New York: Guilford.

Leiblum, S. R., Pervin, L. A., & Campbell, E. H. (1989). The treatment of vaginismus: Success and failure. In S. R. Leiblum & R. C. Rosen (Eds.), *Principles and practice of sex therapy* (2nd ed., pp. 113-138). New York: Guilford.

Masters, W. H., & Johnson, V. E. (1970). *Human sexual inadequacy.* Boston: Little, Brown.

Metcalf, A. M., Dozois, R. R., & Kelly, K. A. (1986). Sexual function in women after proctocolectomy. *Annals of Surgery, 204*(6), 624-627.

Renshaw, D. C. (1983). Recognition and treatment of sexual disorders. *Pennsylvania Medicine, 86*(12), 64-67.

Rickus, M. A. (1987). Sexual concerns of the female patient: Research study and analysis. *ANNA Journal, 14*(3), 192-195.

Riley, A. J., & Riley, E. J. (1986). The effect of single dose diazepam on female sexual response induced by masturbation. *Sexual and Marital Therapy, 1*(1), 49-53.

Sackett, C. (1990). Spinal cord conditions and sexuality. In C. I. Fogel & D. Lauver (Eds.), *Sexual health promotion* (pp. 384-406). Philadelphia: W. B. Saunders.

Schain, W. S. (1985). Breast cancer surgeries and psychosexual sequelae: Implications for remediation. *Seminars in Oncology Nursing, 1*(3), 200-205.

Schover, L. R. (1989). Sexual problems in chronic illness. In S. R. Leiblum & R. C. Rosen (Eds.), *Principles and practice of sex therapy* (2nd ed., pp. 319-351). New York: Guilford.

Schover, L. R., Fife, M., & Gershenson, D. M. (1989). Sexual dysfunction and treatment for early stage cervical cancer. *Cancer, 63*(1), 204-212.

Schreiner-Engel, P., Schiavi, R. C., Vietorisz, D., & Smith, H. (1987). The differential impact of diabetes type on female sexuality. *Journal of Psychosomatic Research, 31*(1), 23-33.

Stuart, F. M., Hammond, D. C., & Pett, M. A. (1987). Inhibited sexual desire in women. *Archives of Sexual Behavior, 16*(2), 91-106.

SEXUAL HEALTH PROMOTION

Annon, J. (1976). *Behavior treatment of sexual problems.* San Francisco: Harper & Row.

Bachmann, G. A., Leiblum, S. R., & Grill, J. (1989). Brief sexual inquiry in gynecologic practice. *Obstetrics and Gynecology, 73*(3, pt. 1), 425-427.

Baggs, J. G., & Karch, A. M. (1987). Sexual counseling of women with coronary heart disease. *Heart and Lung, 16*(2), 154-159.

Brash, K. C. (1990). Toward a model of sexual health for nurses. *Holistic Nursing Practice, 4*(4), 62-69.

Krueger, J. C., Hassell, J., Goggins, D. B., Ishimatsu, T., Pablico, M. R., & Tuttle, E. J. (1979). Relationship between nurse counseling and sexual adjustment after hysterectomy. *Nursing Research, 28*(3), 145-150.

Metz, M. E., & Seifert, M. H. (1988). Women's expectations of physicians in sexual health concerns. *Family Practice Research Journal, 7*(3), 141-152.

Supplemental Readings

Fann, V. (1990, Fall). Touching women. *Woman of Power,* p. 74.

Jackson, M. (1984). Sex research and the construction of sexuality: A tool of male supremacy? *Women's Studies International Forum, 7*(1), 43-51.

Lamb, M. A. (1990). Psychosexual issues: The woman with gynecologic cancer. *Seminars in Oncology Nursing, 6*(3), 237-243.

Lott, B. (1987). Sexuality: A feminist perspective. In K. Kelley (Ed.), *Females, males, and sexuality* (pp. 175-211). Albany: State University of New York Press.

McFarland, G. K., & McFarlane, E. A. (1989). *Nursing diagnosis and intervention: Planning for patient care.* St. Louis: C. V. Mosby.

Schwarz-Applebaum, J., Dedrick, J., Jusenius, K., & Kirchner, C. W. (1984). Nursing care plans: Sexuality and treatment of breast cancer. *Oncology Nursing Forum, 11*(6), 16-24.

Segraves, R. T. (1988). Psychiatric drugs and inhibited female orgasm. *Journal of Sex and Marital Therapy, 15*(3), 202-207.

Wyatt, G. E., Peters, S. D., & Guthrie, D. (1988a). Kinsey revisited, Part I: Comparisons of the sexual socialization and sexual behavior of white women over 33 years. *Archives of Sexual Behavior, 17*(3), 201-239.

Wyatt, G. E., Peters, S. D., & Guthrie, D. (1988b). Kinsey revisited, Part II: Comparisons of the sexual socialization and sexual behavior of black women over 33 years. *Archives of Sexual Behavior, 17*(4), 289-332.

22

Drug Abuse Problems Among Women

CHRISTINE VOURAKIS

Alcohol consumption and other drug use was a regular part of life in colonial America. Men's drinking, however, was much more open and was the focus of temperance societies and groups attempting to stamp out excessive drinking and drunkenness. For example, during the latter half of the 19th century, groups such as the Woman's Christian Temperance Union (WCTU) focused their efforts on drunkenness in men. Historically, women's drug use was not openly acknowledged, and the existence of drug problems in women was generally denied.

In contrast to past centuries, the 20th century has shown a gradual decline in the concealment of drug use and dependency among women. In fact, since the 1960s, there has been a growing interest in women's drug problems and treatment separate from those of men. Until this time, programs were primarily established for men, and women needing treatment were often admitted to these existing programs. In the 1970s, women-only groups in mixed-sex treatment settings were becoming more widespread and programs specifically for women were established. These programs operated for several years with minimal research evaluating which aspects were helpful and how programs could be made more effective. Eventually, by the early 1980s, researchers began to identify program factors important for women and subgroups of women (Beckman & Amaro, 1986; Beckman & Kocel, 1982; Boyd & Mast, 1983; Marsh, 1982; Vourakis, 1983, 1989).

This chapter will focus on women in the United States and will cover the following topics: (a) a definition of selected terms used in this chapter; (b) a history of women and drug use; (c) a rationale for current emphasis on women's drug consumption; (d) a discussion of the prevalence of drug use and abuse/dependency among women (selected data on Canadian women will be included in this section); (e) identification of the predictors of drug abuse and dependency in women; (f) the problem of drug use during pregnancy; (g) an overview of selected issues for intervention; and (h) a discussion of treatment, prevention, and suggested areas for future investigation. For an in-depth discussion of drug abuse, including theories of causation and treatment (including types of treatment) and the pharmacology of the drugs of abuse and their biopsychosocial manifestations, the reader is encouraged to see the published materials cited here: Dimijian (1976), Estes and Heinemann (1986), Jack (1989, 1990a, 1990b), Jaffe (1985), and Ray and Ksir (1987).

Definition of Terms

Drug Use. Drug use refers to the nontherapeutic consumption of any psychoactive chemical, excluding food substances, that is known to have potential for abuse. For the purposes of this chapter the term does not refer to potential consequences of drug consumption but is used in a scientific sense to assist in the understanding of the types and/or degree of drug consumption by segments of the population at any point in time. Selective prescription medications, alcohol, and other licit drugs such as caffeine and nicotine are included in this category.

Drug Abuse. Drug abuse refers to the use of any psychoactive chemical that poses significant consequences to biological, psychological, and/or social health. Drugs or chemicals may be abused for a brief period of time, episodically, or on a continuing basis. Although patterns of abuse normally persist for a month or more, a single episode of abuse may include, for example, the consumption of alcohol above safe limits immediately before operating a motor vehicle. Problems as a result of abusing drugs may occur in people who are not necessarily chemically dependent and include, for example, car accidents, divorce, and arrest for drunken driving.

Chemical Dependency or Addiction. Chemical dependency or addiction is characterized by compulsion, loss of control over the circumstances of drug use, continued use despite adverse consequences, frequent relapses after periods of abstinence, and the inability to decrease use voluntarily. With many drugs, these characteristics are frequently accompanied by a psychological and/or a physical withdrawal syndrome after cessation of use. Alcohol dependency and heroin addiction are examples of chemical dependency.

Historical Perspective

Although not clearly documented, American women were most likely drinking alcoholic beverages prior to the 18th century. There is evidence that in addition to heavy alcohol use (Lender & Martin, 1982) women were consuming opiates and cocaine from the late 18th century to the period just prior to World War II (Musto, 1987).

Middle-class women were most affected by cultural norms for appropriate behavior in the 18th and 19th centuries. For example, the temperance movement throughout the 19th century had a profound effect on the form and context of women's drug use. To avoid ostracism or derision, women learned to "hide" their drug use by using patent medicines under the respectable cloak of treatment for "female health conditions." In general, female conditions referred to such problems as discomfort around pregnancy and premenstrual difficulties. Whether women's drug consumption was for female conditions or for other purposes, it was made "respectable" by the preparation and presentation of many popular drugs—for example, opiates, sedatives, cocaine, and alcohol as patent medicines. In fact, during the period 1850 to 1880, women were twice as likely as men to be addicted to legal patent medicines (Terry & Pellens, 1928). Patent medicine use became increasingly popular and flourished from the late 18th century until the early part of the 20th century, when restrictions on the sale and use of these drugs began to dampen their rampant use (Musto, 1977).

Women from all social classes used alcohol and other drugs, differing only in form or type, depending on sanctions, preference, cost, and availability. Lower- and upper-class women used patent medicines as well, but to a lesser extent than middle-class women. Lower-class women were heavy gin users, whereas middle- and upper-class women combined whiskey and opiates (Morgan, 1974).

Although at this point it is clear that American women from all social classes have been consumers of a variety of drugs for well over two centuries, this behavior, until fairly recently, has largely remained hidden from public scrutiny. The hidden nature of women's drug use and abuse can best be explained by the social mores governing female behavior during the late 18th and early 19th centuries. Women were expected to portray an image of purity and goodness in the limited but esteemed roles of wife and mother. These inflexible expectations exemplified the repression of women and their concomitant powerlessness over their life circumstances. Within the narrow parameters of women's roles, "deviant" behavior such as drug use required the establishment of mechanisms to mask the activity. To be noticeably drunk or to be labeled an addict was highly stigmatizing for women and still is to a large extent today.

By the time of World War II, the number of government regulations had increased to the point of severely limiting the availability of patent medicines containing psychoactive drugs. For the most part, middle- and upper-class women continued to obtain mood-altering drugs through their physicians, and indigent women were forced to seek their drugs (other than alcohol) through illegal channels.

It is interesting to note that during times of social upheaval drug use among American women escalated. Worth (1991), in her literature review, identifies three major periods in U.S. history when a significant increase in women's drug abuse was documented. The first period was from 1840 to 1880. During this time the Civil War was fought, a significant number of people immigrated into the United States, there was migration from the eastern part of the United States to the West, large numbers of both men and women moved from the farm to the city in search of work, and it was a period of massive, rapid industrialization.

The second period of major social, economic, and political upheaval was from 1890 to 1930 during World War I and the economic depression following the stock market crash. The escalated pattern of drug use established by women during the war and depression years continued into the 1930s. Although remaining hidden, middle-class women were combining alcohol with prescribed drugs, especially sleeping medications, during the 1930s. Women in the upper and lower classes continued their use of illicit drugs (e.g., heroin, cocaine, morphine, and opium) during this time. Historical documents such as pharmacy and medical records were helpful in revealing the extent of women's drug use during this period. Mexican American women living in the southwestern United States increased their use of marijuana. This group, like middle-class white women, remained hidden (S. Sorrell, cited in Worth, 1991).

Although social structures were altered during both the first and second periods of social upheaval, women's roles, for the most part, changed much more slowly. Women had few legal and individual rights and remained greatly oppressed. Some of the ways women were oppressed included the perpetuation of the belief that they were intellectually and physically inferior to men, the exercise of little, if any, control over economic resources, and the lack of a voice in the political structure, in part because they were not allowed to vote. This oppression, along with female role restrictions, posed considerable stress for women lacking the skills and options to cope effectively during times of major social tumult.

Although women's roles have become more flexible since World War II, especially with the help of the civil rights and women's movements, economic and political oppression remains. Women are still fighting for equal pay for equal work and for the same rights and opportunities in the social environment as those afforded to men.

The period from 1960 to 1980 was also characterized by an increase in women's abuse of a variety of drugs. The rapid social changes during this period have had a considerable effect on American families and, subsequently, on women's roles. Women have had to function within a milieu of increasing strain and fragmentation. More women than ever are in the workforce, and the divorce rate has increased dramatically as has the number of single-parent families headed by women (Worth, 1991). Within this context, it is not surprising that women have continued and at times escalated their patterns of drug use to cope with anxiety; the pressures of dwindling supports, both familial and economic; and the increasing role demands.

Although there was no noticeable increase in alcohol consumption during this period, use of other drugs was on the rise. For example, both Canadian and American women exceeded men in their use of prescribed drugs (Abelson, Fishburne, & Cisin, 1977; Cooperstock, 1971). Antianxiety agents (e.g., Valium and Librium) emerged in the 1960s and were immediately popular with women. In one cross-sectional study of households (Parry, Balter, Mellinger, Cisin, & Manheimer, 1973), women were more than twice as likely as men to use sedatives; minor tranquilizers, including the antianxiety agents; and stimulants. In their review of the literature, Prather and Fidell (1978) found an increase in women's use of heroin, marijuana, and other psychoactive drugs. Men were using more illicit drug substances than were women, but women were beginning to move closer to the level of male consumption in their use of cocaine; and this trend has continued into the 1980s (Clayton, Voss, Robbins, & Skinner, 1986).

Rationale for Current Concern

There is some speculation that the recent surge of interest in women's drug use and drug dependency is related to the concern for the fetus in pregnant women, especially since the emergence of the crack cocaine epidemic. This is certainly an important public health concern; however, a number of other factors interacting over the last 3 decades have sparked increased openness and growing public interest. A few of these factors are mentioned here; however, this list is by no means exhaustive. One of these is the evolving flexibility in women's roles, bringing about their participation in a variety of occupations in increasing numbers and their growing visibility in all areas of public life. Furthermore, women themselves, particularly feminists influenced by the civil rights and women's movements, have been advocating for women with health problems, such as drug dependency, and have been bringing attention to their neglected needs. Finally, the emergence of the "disease concept of alcoholism," starting in the 1960s, had a major effect on both men and women who were alcohol dependent. It helped to move alcoholism away from a moral problem to an illness that was treatable. This concept of a disease has broadened to include other drugs.

Prevalence

Determining the prevalence of drug abuse and dependence among women continues to be a challenge. Prevalence is a treatment concern because program planners need to justify the extent of the problem and its distribution to develop programs for intervention. In addition, subgroups need to be identified to target prevention programs. The confusion and lack of clarity over the years in determining how many women are drug dependent is, in part, related to cultural and social factors.

There has been an evolving broad acceptance of social consumption of alcohol and other drugs by women in the U.S. culture over the past few decades. The media may have assisted in this trend in that women have been portrayed, alone or with men, in flattering contexts by alcohol and tobacco advertisers. Advertisers, using the print media, have been relentless in their promotion of smoking among women, particularly young women. Women are also often the target of advertisers promoting over-the-counter drugs (e.g., cold and cough products, sedatives, and appetite suppressants).

Although somewhat lessened and certainly less hidden, drunkenness and addiction are still less acceptable in women than in men. Although men still drink and use illicit drugs to a much greater extent than do women, young women are drinking in increasing numbers and are rapidly approaching males in numbers of new drinkers. One survey revealed regular heavy drinking by a significant proportion of high school girls. Of the sample of girls in the 12th grade, 30% had consumed five or more drinks at least once in the past 2 weeks (Thompson & Wilsnack, 1984).

Women who abuse drugs are frequently polydrug abusers—that is, they use more than one psychoactive drug simultaneously or sequentially. Patterns of drug use may be influenced by socioeconomic status (SES), age, and ethnicity. For instance, subgroups of young women may develop patterns of marijuana use or combine marijuana use with alcohol, whereas women over the age of 60 are more likely to use minor tranquilizers alone or with alcohol. Although many women have a drug of choice, when that drug is not available they may temporarily shift drugs. Others use different drugs to combat the prolonged effects of a particular drug or to ward off the symptoms of withdrawal when they cease taking their drug of choice, or they may use drugs in combination to achieve certain effects. For example, in one study of women in which alcohol was the drug of choice, those who were over the age of 30 frequently combined alcohol with minor tranquilizers. Those women who were under 30 more often combined alcohol with marijuana and stimulants (i.e., cocaine and amphetamines) (Harrison & Belille, 1987).

Alcohol

Past national surveys of American drinking indicate that at least two thirds of women over 18 years old drank low to moderate levels of alcohol without personal, social, or environmental consequences (Cahalan, Cisin, & Crossley, 1969; Clark & Midanik, 1982). This stability has been confirmed in more recent surveys by both Fillmore (1984) and Hilton (1987, 1988) except for an increase in the proportion of heavy drinkers among younger women. Employed women in their 20s had higher rates of frequent heavy drinking than did previous cohorts measured at the same age (Hilton, 1987). Although Canada tends to be a more conservative nation than the United States, a 1988 national survey estimated that 7 million (69.8%) Canadian women used alcohol in the past year (Staff, 1991), similar to the proportion of American women who drink.

From a national survey, Hilton (1987) has determined that the proportion of female drinkers from the ages of 18 to 49 with dependence symptoms is between 5% and 6%. After this age, the proportion drops to 1%. The proportion is much higher for drinking-related problems (e.g., arrest, divorce, or traffic accidents). Twelve percent of women in the 18 to 29 age range and 6% of women in the 30 to 40 age range reported drinking-related problems. Scarcely any women over 60 years old reported drinking-related problems. Compared to white women, black women have higher rates of abstention and lower rates of heavy drinking (Herd, 1988). Of those black women who drink heavily, they tend to become alcohol dependent and suffer alcohol-related biopsychosocial consequences more rapidly than do white women (Amaro, Beckman, & Mays, 1987). For instance, alcohol-dependent black women are at higher risk for health problems such as cirrhosis of the liver and esophageal cancer (Herd, 1988).

Asian (Kitano & Chi, 1986-1987) and Hispanic (Caetano, 1989) women have high rates of abstention and lower rates of heavy drinking compared to white women. In her review of the literature, Sun (1991) determined that the low rate of alcohol and drug problems in Asian American women is related to culturally restrictive roles of Asian women, Confucianism and Taoism belief systems stressing moderation, and the fact that Asia is traditionally a nondrinking society. As younger Asian American women become increasingly integrated into American society, alcohol and other drug use may begin to reflect patterns similar to those in the dominant culture. Although patterns of drinking among younger Mexican American women are changing, traditional Mexican society, which is known for definite cultural sanctions against women's drinking, contributes to a lower rate of alcohol and other drug problems among this population.

One way to approximate the extent of the alcohol problem in women is to identify the number of women who seek help. Women make up approximately 20% of the alcohol problem treatment population (National Institute on Drug Abuse, 1980), and 34% of Alcoholics Anonymous (AA) members are women (AA, 1987). These indicators, although helpful, are not definitive, because for a variety of reasons women may not seek treatment or attend AA.

Other Drugs

Women use the same variety of drugs that men use; however, they tend to use certain drugs in greater amounts than do men. Men are twice as likely to use opiates, sedatives, inhalants, phencyclidine (PCP), hallucinogens, and nitrites, whereas women, particularly young women, abuse stimulants (e.g., cocaine, amphetamine and amphetamine-like drugs) to a slightly greater extent than do men (quite possibly due to the popularity of "diet pills"). High school females are also smoking tobacco cigarettes (which contain the highly addictive stimulant nicotine) more than are males (Johnston, O'Malley, & Bachman, 1987). A 1990 Gallup survey revealed that 3.6 million (36%) of Canadian women aged 18 years or older had smoked cigarettes in the past week, compared to 3.2 million males (34%). In the 1988 national survey, 54.2% of adult Canadian women said that they had ever smoked in their lives (Staff, 1991). Considering the severe health consequences from tobacco use, there is growing alarm related to women's attraction to smoking.

Women tend to use more prescribed psychoactive drugs than men. One national survey indicated that 29% of the women and 13% of the men reported using mood-altering prescription drugs during the past year (Parry et al., 1973). It is difficult to determine how many women are heroin addicts; however, it is estimated that they compose approximately 20% to 25% of that population, or about 100,000 women. Cocaine use is hard to determine; however, there was a major increase in use for both sexes during the 1970s. It was estimated that by 1980,

28% of young people between the ages of 18 and 25 had at least tried cocaine, and one third of this group had used the drug in the past month (Smith, 1984).

Drug Problem Predictors and Risk Factors

It should be pointed out that most of the predictors of problems have been identified from research on women in treatment; however, the identified predictors offer some criteria for classifying subgroups of women on which to focus prevention programs and to monitor for early intervention. Women at risk for developing drug abuse problems cross age, ethnic, and SES groupings. Women in crisis or experiencing one or more stressful life events (e.g., marital discord or divorce, death of a loved one, severe financial stress, or life circumstances that bring about rapid change in their lives) and who have one or more of the following risk factors are at risk for drug dependency problems.

Women at risk have the following characteristics: (a) They have a history of trauma in their lives (e.g., physical abuse and sexual victimization) (Covington, 1986; Miller, Downs, Gondoli, & Keil, 1987; National Institute on Alcohol Abuse and Alcoholism, 1981). (b) They suffer from low self-esteem and feelings of inadequacy, incompetence, and great anxiety (McLachlan, Walderman, Birchmore, & Marsden, 1979). (c) They feel chronically lonely, bored, and depressed and have difficulty coping with marital conflict and life transitions (e.g., menopause) (Marsh, Colten, & Tucker, 1982). (d) They have first-degree relatives with alcohol-dependency problems (Knupfer, 1982). In her review of the literature, Knupfer (1982) noted that there was a higher incidence of depressive diagnoses in alcohol-dependent women and sociopathic diagnoses in alcohol-dependent men. On the basis of her findings she proposed that

> family histories of women alcoholics show far greater incidence of affective disorders in first degree relatives and of alcoholism in all relatives. These findings have led to the postulation of a "broad spectrum" disease process presumably consisting of some sort of vulnerability which in men is more likely to result in alcoholism or sociopathy and in women more likely to result in depressive illness. (p. 15)

(e) They must cope with the strain of alterations in role due to changes in the social structure and the concomitant changes in many families with fixed or limited incomes. Included here are women who, although reluctant, are forced to enter the workforce, women who are divorced, and women who are single parents (Gomberg, 1982). (f) They have chronic problems specific to women's health (e.g., dysmenorrhea or other pelvic pain, emotional difficulties related to infertility problems, or reproductive problems) and tend to gravitate toward mood-altering chemicals as the primary form of coping with these problems (Busch, McBride, & Benaventura, 1986; Wilsnack, 1973a, 1973b). (g) They may be lesbians and having difficulty coping with feelings of dependency and a lack of a sense of personal power in their lives (Diamond & Wilsnack, 1978). (h) They use drugs as a form of escapism from painful feelings or stress and have a spouse or significant other who is a drug abuser (Beckman & Amaro, 1986; National Institute on Alcohol Abuse and Alcoholism, 1981).

The Problem of Drug Use During Pregnancy

Prevalence

The problem of pregnant women who use illicit drugs has become a major public issue in the 1990s. It is estimated that approximately 30,000 pregnant women receive drug treatment each year, although about 105,000 need treatment yearly (Institute of Medicine [IOM], 1990). Although more specific data are needed to evaluate potential fetal harm, it is helpful to have some idea of the scope of illicit drug abuse by pregnant women. A national household survey in 1988 (National Institute on Drug Abuse, 1988) indicated that approximately 9.3 million women in high-fertility age brackets (15 to 35 years) used an illicit drug at least once in the previous year and 4.9 million did so in the previous month. Considering that the annual birthrate is about 9%, it is estimated that there are between 350,000 and 625,000 annual fetal exposures to one or more instances of maternal illicit drug consumption.

In an important study by Chasnoff, Landress, and Barrett (1990), urine was collected for analysis on 100% of all public and 70% of all private first prenatal visits by women in a Florida county. During this first appointment, each of the women submitted a urine sample for a blind toxicological screen. The urine was effectively screened for opiates, cocaine, and marijuana. Positive results were found for one or more of these substances among 16.3% of the public versus 13.1% of the private pregnant women. When separated by race, 14.1% of black women and 15.4% of the white women tested positive for one or more of the drugs.

The initial cluster of symptoms known as fetal alcohol syndrome (FAS) was first described in 1973. The extent of this problem in the United States varies by the study population. In studies of lower SES black and American Indian mothers the estimated rate is 2.6 per 1,000 births compared to 0.6 per 1,000 births in studies of white mothers of middle SES. If only the population of alcohol-dependent women is considered, the estimated incidence is as high as 25 per 1,000 live births. Fetal alcohol effects (FAE), a label recommended when only some of the criteria for FAS are met, are estimated to be three times higher than the estimates given above among the general population and four times higher in the alcohol-dependent population (Abel, 1984).

Effects of Alcohol and Other Drug Use During Pregnancy

Drug effects during pregnancy are variable among women and often depend on the interaction of a number of factors, which include but are not limited to the following: (a) types of drug(s), including over-the-counter and prescription drugs, and amount consumed; (b) route of administration; (c) length of last episode of consumption; (d) stage of pregnancy; (e) body defenses of embryo or fetus; (f) body defenses of mother; (g) genetic factors; (h) general physical health of mother, including nutritional status; and (i) mother's emotional health. Thus, based on the understanding of the variability of embryonic and fetal effects, it is not surprising therefore, in relation to alcohol consumption, that far fewer cases of FAS and FAE have been reported relative to the amount of pregnant alcohol abusers (U.S. Department of Health and Human Services [DHHS], 1990).

Our main concern in this chapter is psychoactive drug use; however, pregnant women may consume a variety of over-the-counter and prescription drugs alone or in combination with psychoactive drugs. Drug use of any type may be harmful during the prenatal period. Continued use of drugs during pregnancy may be due to one of the following reasons: (a) lack of awareness of being in a state of pregnancy, (b) lack of awareness of the potential harmful effects of drugs during pregnancy, or (c) chemical dependency. In addition to an assessment of their drug consumption, women currently pregnant or planning pregnancy need information related to the potential effects of drug use during this period.

In Ancient Greece, newly married couples were instructed to refrain from alcohol consumption on their wedding night because it was believed that alcohol could harm future offspring (Haggard & Jellinek, 1942), demonstrating a long history of concern; however, concern and knowledge about the unsafe use of alcohol and other drugs during pregnancy was somewhat disregarded during most of the first half of the 20th century (Geller, 1991). Since the 1960s, concern has been more consistent. Through various means, women have been cautioned against alcohol and other drug use during pregnancy; and there has also been a growing body of research on the effects of drug use, and in particular alcohol use, during various stages of embryonic and fetal development.

Drug consumption during the period of organ differentiation, which occurs during the first 3 months of pregnancy, can cause major embryonic or fetal physical damage (Tuchmann-Duplessis, 1987). Some organ systems, such as the central nervous system (CNS), can be affected at any time during the pregnancy. FAS, the well-known problem attributed to alcohol consumption during pregnancy, is characterized by pre- and postnatal growth retardation, mental retardation and other CNS dysfunction, distinctive craniofacial features (e.g., small head, wide space between the eyes, thin upper lip and short palpebral fissures), and other major organ malformations (Clarren & Smith, 1978). FAE, lower birth weights, and lower levels of mental development have been attributed to babies born to mothers who drink compared to those of nondrinking mothers. At this time, it is not clear which characteristics make some women's pregnancies more susceptible to the effects of alcohol. Furthermore, although we know that babies with severe cases of FAS have been born to some heavy-drinking mothers, less is known about the subtle effects of low alcohol consumption during pregnancy (U.S. DHHS, 1990). It is recommended that couples planning pregnancy abstain from all alcohol and other drug use before pregnancy unless a prescribed drug is absolutely necessary.

Although the CNS stimulants caffeine and nicotine are the most common "uppers" consumed during pregnancy, cocaine use has grown over the past two decades. All three are presumed to cause problems, but there is clearer evidence of the effects of nicotine and cocaine. The available information on caffeine is deficient, and some of the research reports demonstrate conflicting evidence on caffeine's effects. Caffeine is available in so many products that the amount consumed on a daily basis is difficult to determine. Furthermore, there is some speculation that one reason for conflicting research findings relative to caffeine's effect may be related to a combined effect of caffeine with other substances, such as nicotine—that is, effects attributed to caffeine may actually be related to the combination of caffeine with other substances consumed (Abbott, 1986). There is some evidence that spontaneous abortions are more common in women who are moderate to heavy caffeine users (Srisuphan & Bracken, 1986; Weathersbee, Olsen, & Lodge, 1977).

Pregnant women who use tobacco are at higher risk for spontaneous abortions, premature births, and having low-birth-weight babies (Hogue & Sappenfield, 1987; Koop, 1986). The same fetal complications can occur from using cocaine at any time during pregnancy. Cocaine use has also been known to increase the risk of cerebral infarction in the newborn and to have an effect on cognitive and behavioral development (Chasnoff et al., 1990). Infant withdrawal from cocaine is less dramatic than withdrawal from opiates. Cocaine-exposed infants tend to be somewhat withdrawn and less responsive to caretakers than are normal infants (Chasnoff, Burns, Schnoll, & Burns, 1985).

Pregnant opiate users are prone to deliver infants with low birth weight and low Apgar scores. In addition to withdrawal, these infants are prone to a host of complications, including respiratory distress, jaundice, congenital malformations (Ostrea & Chavez, 1979), and sudden infant death syndrome (Ward et al., 1986). Withdrawal in opiate-exposed infants is characterized by CNS hyperirritability, gastrointestinal problems, and respiratory difficulties.

Criminal Punishment of Pregnant Drug-Dependent Women

Some pregnant women who use drugs during pregnancy or who are drug dependent face criminal punishment if their situation comes to the attention of the local prosecutor. Several states are establishing precedents as an increasing number of women are being arrested and prosecuted for using drugs during pregnancy (Moss, 1991). Although the apparent motivation for incarcerating drug-dependent women is endangerment to the fetus due to drug use, in some circumstances, incarceration of these women may pose additional risks to the fetus.

The fear of prosecution and the lack of trust generated by current trends in the United States are counterproductive to achieving adequate drug abuse prevention and early intervention as well as prenatal care for women who use drugs during pregnancy. These women may avoid sharing drug use information during prenatal and other health care visits because they fear arrest.

Drug-dependent pregnant women have been singled out and punished in ways that are unprecedented. A double standard is currently applied to these women, and they are receiving harsher sentences than those levied on men and nonpregnant women (American Nurses Association, 1991). Although some women are able to enter treatment in lieu of prosecution, others are not; for example, a woman in Florida was convicted of delivering drugs through the umbilical cord and sentenced to 14 years probation (Stone, 1990). Another woman, a 20-year-old in Houston, Texas, was convicted in an unusual case of cocaine possession. During a particular day that she spent in a Houston crack house, she apparently delivered her 3.5 pound (2 months premature) stillborn fetus. It was reported that she smoked crack for several hours while in the crack house and the fetus was found to contain enough cocaine to kill an adult. She was sentenced to 12 years in prison ("Mom Gets 12 Years," 1991).

Health care providers have voiced concern that prosecuting pregnant women will discourage many of them from seeking prenatal care. In a position statement released on April 5, 1991, by the American Nurses Association (ANA), a similar concern was expressed. Another concern is that at this time inadequate treatment is available for drug-dependent women who are pregnant, and existing drug treatment programs, due in part to liability concerns, often refuse to admit women who are pregnant. The ANA's statement supports the development of adequate treatment tailored to the special needs of women of childbearing age and opposes the criminal prosecution of women for use of drugs during pregnancy.

Selected Issues for Intervention

Drug abuse among women is a complex issue frequently inseparable from other women's issues (e.g., poverty, physical vulnerability to selected chemicals; physical and sexual abuse, including incest and battering; sexism; depression; and AIDS). For example, this understanding of the interconnection of drug abuse with other issues that women face is a useful argument to lobby for more efficient use of existing services, increased research, and program funding. This is especially important for subgroups of women with limited resources, including informational resources and access to adequate treatment.

The private sector of the drug abuse treatment industry caters to clients who can afford services or who have insurance that pays a substantial proportion of treatment costs. The public sector of the drug abuse treatment industry has not adequately addressed the needs of the aggregate of women not served by the private sector. Current fiscal constraints on the national, state, and local levels have severely affected community-based accessible treatment and prevention programs offering comprehensive services for these women.

Although it is suggested that all pregnant women be assessed for alcohol and other drug (AOD) abuse (Campinha-Bacote & Bragg, 1993), ideally, every client, including women of childbearing age, should be routinely assessed for AOD abuse by a primary health care provider. The ANA supports professional nurses' systematically assessing clients, in any setting, for AOD abuse and other health problems that frequently accompany AOD abuse (i.e., AIDS/HIV, mental health problems, and tuberculosis). Furthermore, the ANA supports "one-stop shopping"—offering multiple services at the same location (ANA, 1993). For example, AOD abuse treatment services could be available in primary health care facilities and primary health care in drug treatment centers. A benefit for pregnant women is that these women would be assessed and identified earlier for AOD abuse in conjunction with other health problems, increasing the possibility for early detection, intervention, and referral if necessary. In addition, this health care management approach is likely to be more cost-effective than traditional approaches.

Effects of Drug Abuse on Women's Bodies

Until the last 20 years, investigators have been inconsistent in reporting gender differences in drug abuse research. This is especially true in reporting gender differences in the biological effects of drugs on the body. Women were often not even included in samples, and when they were, results were frequently reported without identifying variation by gender.

A review of the current scholarly literature reveals an increased sensitivity to gender differences in theoretical articles and research reports, although the bulk of research on gender differences related to biological effects is most significant for alcohol. There is some evidence that other drugs affect physical health; nonetheless, they do so to a lesser extent than does alcohol and in basically similar ways for both sexes.

Of all the drugs of abuse, alcohol has the most toxic effects on the body. If unattenuated or insufficiently metabolized, significant amounts entering the bloodstream can damage important body organs within a short period of time. It is known that a more rapid progression of physical deterioration after fewer years of heavy consumption differentiates women from men. Women tend to develop symptoms of alcoholic hepatitis and cirrhosis after fewer years of uncontrolled drinking (Galambos, 1972; Lelbach, 1974). A consistent finding is that after ingesting an equivalent amount of alcohol, women tend to maintain higher blood levels of alcohol than men. Although several theories related to body weight, metabolism, and hormonal level differences have been put forth over the years, more recent research has demonstrated significant progress in understanding this phenomenon. A study by Frezza et al. (1990) used both male and female alcoholics and nonalcoholics. Their first-level findings were similar to previous research and showed differences in blood alcohol levels for males and females in both alcoholics and nonalcoholics. For the next phase of their research, they administered equivalent amounts of alcohol intravenously to all subjects and found no differences.

This finding led them to reexplore alcohol metabolism, and they went on to discover gender differences in the stomach's ability to oxidize alcohol. Women in the study had lower amounts of alcohol dehydrogenase (a stomach enzyme), thereby increasing by a third the amount of unmetabolized alcohol entering the bloodstream.

Alcohol-dependent women appear to have a higher prevalence of a number of clinical problems compared to nonalcohol-dependent women. There appears to be a higher prevalence of problems in the postovulation phase of the menstrual cycle, amenorrhea, anovulation, pathological changes in the ovaries (Hughes et al., 1980; Valimaki et al., 1984), and some indication of precipitation of early menopause (Gavaler, 1985).

Physical Abuse and Sexual Victimization

There is a growing interest in the effect of past physical abuse and sexual victimization on long-term recovery in drug-dependent women. There is some indication that women in recovery from drug problems who address the meaning and impact of these abusive experiences on their lives are at lower risk for drug relapse. Investigators identify a substantial number of substance-abusing women as having a history of sexual victimization (Benward & Densen-Gerber, 1975; S. S. Covington, cited in Root, 1989; M. A. Hayek, cited in Evans & Schaefer, 1987; Rohsenow, Corbett, & Devine, 1988). In one study, over half of the women alcoholics in the sample reported a history of at least one incident of rape (Murphy, Coleman, Hoon, & Scott, 1980). Another study demonstrated that alcohol-dependent women are more likely than nonalcohol-dependent women to be subjected to repeated incidents of physical and sexual abuse (Covington, 1986).

Sometimes, it is not until much later in recovery from drug-dependency problems that past issues of abuse emerge. Many women in recovery from drug-dependency problems discover that they have multiple addictions (e.g., overspending, compulsive overeating, bulimia, and/or gambling). Addressing these addictions becomes part of their overall recovery process. Eating disorders (e.g., compulsive overeating and bulimia) in both nondrug-dependent women and recovering drug-dependent women have been linked to issues of past physical and sexual abuse. Thus problems of abuse should be addressed whenever they emerge in the recovery process.

Gender Role and Chemically Dependent Women

The issue of gender role conflict and its relation to chemical dependency in women is complex and unresolved. A major obstacle is the lack of uniformity with regard to the normative standard for gender role behavior in males and females. It is doubtful that with a constantly changing society and with various cultural, social class, and individual perceptions of social roles, a uniform standard can be reached. It is even doubtful that subgroup standards will hold up within relatively homogeneous samples, because, for example, members within a social class may choose from a number of alternative lifestyles that they may find acceptable and yet that may not be considered the norm. What is the norm? As Schuckit and Morrissey (1976) point out, a number of studies take for granted that there exists a clearly delineated role set that distinguishes the role behavior of American women. Knupfer (1982) identifies the muddle around a number of dimensions of social role: "This is the difficulty posed by the confusion about what is normative or deviant, normal or pathological, traditional or modern, about women's roles" (p. 21).

At times subtle, but often not so subtle, is the general attitude that the masculine role is more valued in our society. If the expectation is that the female adhere to the more feminine role, yet she has learned that this role is inferior, she is likely to experience conflict whether she is drug dependent or not. Knupfer (1982) discusses the concept of status inferiority in relation to the female embracing her social role. This concept refers to the actual second-class status label placed on the role of women.

Studies exploring the psychological conformity of chemically dependent women to their gender role have generally suffered from small samples and inappropriate control groups. An assumption has been, for example, that alcohol-dependent women act more masculine than do nonalcohol-dependent women. Researchers refute this assumption and assert that findings indicate an overidentification with the female roles of wife and mother on a conscious level; alcohol-dependent women struggle more both interpersonally and intrapersonally with gender role identity (Gomberg, 1974; Parker, 1972; Wilsnack, 1973b). There is some support for the finding that alcohol-dependent women, although not exemplifying a standard of differences in femininity or masculinity (more or less on either dimension) compared to nonalcohol-dependent women, demonstrate more conflict in their gender role attitudes and behavior (Anderson, 1980). A study by Scida and Vannicelli (1979) compared psychology students and alcohol-dependent women with scales measuring femininity and gender role conflict. This study included a sample of 24 alcohol-dependent women, 68 psychology students, and 9 nonstudent volunteers. Their findings indicated that discrepancies between one's actual view of self and idealized view of self may be a factor in alcohol dependency. Most of the studies on gender role conflict exhibit problems not only in sampling methods but in the reliability of the measurements used to measure gender role conflict.

The confusion concerning the concept of gender role is clearly stated by Knupfer (1982):

> As for gender role research, it appears to this reviewer that, for the time being, it would be desirable to concentrate on what women do, what they feel, and what in their environment promotes intoxication rather than focusing on their identity as females. The gender role concepts are too varied and confused; perhaps we must await further clarification from research devoted to such concepts before we can use them fruitfully in the study of problem drinking. (p. 31)

Beckman (1981) recognized the problems inherent in measuring unconscious gender role identity and suggested that future research concentrate on the personal style of a subject's gender role behavior and the difference between this personal identity and the perceived identity or behavior by society.

Depression and Chemically Dependent Women

Chemically dependent women appear to have more mental health problems in their families of origin than do men. In his literature review, Schuckit (1972) noted more affective disorders in alcohol-dependent women's families. In addition, alcohol-dependent women have a higher incidence of alcohol dependency in their families of origin (Jones, 1972; Winokur & Clayton, 1968).

In the area of mental health problems, women are considered to have a higher incidence of depression (Guttentag, Salasin, & Belle, 1980), and alcohol-dependent women are more likely than alcoholic men to be diagnosed with an affective disorder (Schuckit & Morrissey, 1976). In their extensive review of the mental health literature, Guttentag et al. (1980) determined that low-income mothers of young children were at greatest risk for depression. The stresses imposed on the lives of these depressed women may put them at higher risk for drug abuse problems. In a study by Schuckit, Pitts, Reich, King, and Winokur (1969), women with a primary affective disorder were found to be younger, had fewer years of alcoholic drinking, had a higher incidence of suicide attempts, and seemed to respond better to treatment. Midanik's (1983) data from a 1979 survey concludes that there is a need for clearer operational definitions of conceptual terms used in the fields of chemical dependency and depression. She found that specific criteria for alcohol problems often characterized depression in women. This conclusion was based on one of her findings that, for example, "the more stringent the criteria for defining problem drinking, the more likely that a female problem drinker will also report depressive symptoms (34-57%)" (p. 19).

Corrigan (1980) conducted a longitudinal study seeking some basic descriptive data from a cross section of women in treatment. She interviewed 150 women after their initial entry into a treatment program. Chosen for the study were 14 program settings in the Northeast—inpatient, outpatient, and AA groups. Subjects were chosen from all consecutive admissions during a period beginning in March 1974; follow-up interviews were conducted after a lapse of 13 months from initial treatment. The subjects consisted of a heterogeneous group of urban and suburban women spanning the SES continuum and including 40 professional women. They were primarily white women, with 32 blacks in the sample. In the follow-up interview of the women in her study, Corrigan found a significant improvement in the emotional health scores of the sample. She attributed this decrease in emotional symptomatology largely to a decrease in drinking.

A history of emotional, physical, and sexual abuse, as well as other social factors, needs closer examination when attempting to determine antecedents to depression in women.

AIDS

The issue of AIDS and drug use is an important consideration in drug-dependent women, primarily because of intravenous (IV) drug use and unsafe sexual behavior. Heterosexual women who are drug dependent are more likely than heterosexual drug-dependent males to have partners who are IV drug users. These women are at higher risk for HIV infection, not only because they share needles with their partner and others but because they have unsafe sex with their male partner and others. Women who practice unsafe sex are potentially exposed to HIV infection and a host of other sexually transmitted diseases. It is not uncommon for many female drug abusers who are dependent on illicit drugs to lack the financial resources to support their habit. Women in these situations are often desperate and frequently exchange sex for drugs (Darrow et al., cited in Karan, 1989).

Karan (1989) reported that as of January 2, 1989, 6,983 (8%) of the total AIDS cases reported to the Centers for Disease Control (CDC) were women. Of these women, 52%, or 3,622, were IV drug users. Of female drug users, 90% are heterosexuals. Of the IV drug users, 30% are women, of whom 90% are in their childbearing years (p. 395). Furthermore, the rate of AIDS is 11 to 13 times higher for black and Hispanic women, when adjusted for population size, in comparison to whites (CDC, 1989). Not only do drug-dependent women expose themselves to HIV infection by administering drugs intravenously and/or participating in unsafe sexual practices, but most of these women are in their childbearing years, which poses the potential risk, if they become pregnant, of bearing a child with an HIV infection.

As mentioned earlier, although some treatment is available, it is insufficient for women of childbearing age. Treatment accessibility for pregnant women is a particular problem. In addition to comprehensive programs that address their varied needs (Kendall & Chavkin, 1992), drug-dependent heterosexual women need education and support relative to practicing safer sex to prevent HIV infection in themselves and their offspring. In addition, these women will need to address issues of self-esteem and self-image as well as guilt and shame.

Treatment of Drug-Dependent Women

Although the treatment literature on the needs of drug-dependent women has tended to be drug specific (e.g., focusing on alcohol-, cocaine-, or heroin-dependent women), there is a growing realization that women are often multidrug abusers and/or may shift their drug preference(s) over time. Although some differences do exist among women who prefer different drugs, the differences are more often related to lifestyle, sociodemographic, and economic factors.

Treatment Characteristics of Drug-Dependent Women

The treatment characteristics of drug-dependent women are changing. Although, in general, women in treatment for drug-dependency problems do not fit a specific profile in relation to most sociodemographic characteristics, there has been an overall downward shift in the age of women in treatment. In general, the average age of women entering treatment has been between 40 and 50 years old; however, a growing number of younger women are participating in treatment. One author estimates that women of childbearing age now represent the largest group among drug-dependent women. The author further estimates that the average age of the pregnant addict is 24 and that she is more likely than not to have children (Daghestani, 1989).

These younger women, unlike some of the older married women in treatment, are presenting with a history of job and economic instability and many are not receiving adequate treatment. The IOM, in its 1990 report, expressed concern for these women and suggested the following action:

> The committee recommends that a special study initiative be undertaken by the National Institute on Drug Abuse, in conjunction with other relevant agencies of the Public Health Service, on the treatment of drug abuse and dependence among adolescents and women who are pregnant or rearing young children. (p. 199)

Women in drug treatment complain of more medical problems than do their male counterparts, and often medical problems precipitate entry into treatment (Mondanaro, 1981). Many drug-dependent women have a history of disruption and chaos in their family of origin and considerable stress in their current living situation. In addition to being a result of instability in their lives, stress is exacerbated by multiple interpersonal, family, and social losses. It is not uncommon for a significant proportion of these women to have drug-abusing or abusive partners (Braiker, 1984; Daghestani, 1989).

Treatment Needs

Treatment for women was basically an unaddressed issue until the social movements of the 20th century. In particular, the women's movement, the alcoholism movement, and a boost in federal spending in the mid-1970s for research on heroin-dependent women assisted in elevating concern for and visibility of all chemically dependent women and their treatment needs. Although some progress has been made in women's treatment over the past 20 years, women are still considered a minority group in treatment. This minority group status stems from the fact that the number of men in programs is overwhelmingly greater; most programs are not designed for women; women are underrepresented in treatment; and, as a group, women have a lower status in society (Reed, 1985).

Selected Reports of Treatment Needs and Effectiveness

One review of past research found only 23 studies published between 1950 and 1978 that contained information about gender-related outcomes. Among the hundreds of studies reporting on the treatment outcome of alcoholics, relatively few noted gender differences or even included women in their samples. In about half of the studies, there was no detailed information on sex differences in outcome rates, yet there were enough raw data to allow the reviewer to conduct appropriate statistical analyses. In essence, only 23 studies specifically concentrated statistical tests on gender differences. Of the 23 studies, 15 failed to note any difference in outcome rates for men and women. This finding does not support the frequent assertion that women have poorer outcome rates than do men. More improvement for women was noted in 5 of the studies, and more improvement for men was noted in 3 (Annis, 1980).

In the 1980s, there was a significant increase in the number of published research reports on gender differences in alcohol-dependent men and women. As identified in the report of the IOM (1990), clinical data (Braiker, 1984; Beckman & Amaro, 1986) provide support for the following differences in male and female alcoholics, suggesting differing programming needs:

> Women are more likely than men to have (a) primary affective disorders (as well as depressed/sad mood states); (b) serious liver disease; (c) marital instability; (d) instability of family of origin; (e) spouses with alcohol problems; (f) lower self-esteem; (g) a pattern of drinking in response to major life crises; (h) a history of sexual abuse; (i) opposition to treatment from family and friends; and (j) more child care responsibilities, which is inferred from data indicating that women in treatment are more likely to be divorced and single heads of households than men. (IOM, 1990, p. 357)

These findings as noted earlier have relevance to all drug-dependent women and are important considerations for treatment. Women who are drug dependent are a diverse group with a variety of different needs. Although it is not unusual for women in recovery to have some problems in common (e.g., coping with aspects of withdrawal, sexism, and past physical and sexual abuse), women may be quite dissimilar on several dimensions. It is reported that it would be more helpful for them to be with people more similar to themselves in background and style of daily living, with whom they could discuss a number of concerns (e.g., ongoing life problems, economic matters, and relationship issues) (Vourakis, 1989).

SES is an important dimension in treatment selection. Women who differ in SES often have dissimilar lifestyle, life factors that precipitate stress, and differ in perception of stress (Vourakis, 1989). Middle- and upper-class women with intact marriages may have entirely different needs for and expectations of treatment than do lower-class women and women who are single mothers on welfare. The IOM, in its 1990 report, identifies several dimensions to consider when planning programs for subgroups of alcohol-dependent women:

> It is important to note that there are also many subgroups within the population of women that may have specific needs for differential treatment services in addition to those required by all women. Typologies have been suggested based on personality differences, sexual orientation, age of onset, race/ethnicity, psychopathology, other drug use, childbearing status and socioeconomic factors (Schuckit and Morrissey, 1976; Braiker, 1982; Dawkins and Harper, 1983; Vannicelli, 1984; Lex, 1985; Amaro, Beckman and Mays, 1987; Blume, 1987; Roman, 1988). (p. 357)

In a review of gender differences in the efficacy of various treatment approaches, it was found that group therapy was a positive treatment modality in four of the studies in which women were more improved than men (Annis, 1980). This is in contrast to those reports of the alcoholic woman's preference for individual counseling (Curlee, 1971; Gomberg, 1974). Annis (1980) suggested sensitizing outcome criteria to the individual client in treatment. For example, if employment is not an outcome of success for a specific group of clients, more appropriate measures must be established. She encouraged research in the development and refinement of outcome criteria. Annis's review led her to conclude that the home situation and social ties outside the home were positive variables in outcome success.

In her 1980 study, Corrigan found that 71% of the sample were abstinent for at least 1 month before the follow-up interview. Many of these women had experience with AA as well as inpatient or outpatient treatment. This finding lends credence to the encouragement of a supportive self-help group for the recovering woman. Employment did not prove to be a significant outcome variable for abstinence in the women as a group. The lower-income and black women in Corrigan's sample were significantly less likely to alter drinking patterns even after treatment. She suggested alternative approaches, including programs offering a longer duration of treatment.

It should be kept in mind that qualitative measures were not used in Corrigan's (1980) study, and it was not the purpose of the researcher to do so. One must therefore review the data with some caution and skepticism. For instance, the employment factor poses questions that can be explored by in-depth examination of the women's relationship to their work. Is the job satisfactory? Is this the career of choice? Are there differences among the women in the various SES categories in relation to their values, feelings, and attitudes concerning employment? Because of the heterogeneity of chemically dependent women, qualitative investigation must play an important role in the current emphasis on research.

It is speculated that there is more rapid development of negative symptoms in alcoholic women. Knupfer (1982) raises some issues concerning the shorter interval of alcoholic drinking in women and entry into treatment. The shorter interval for women may not necessarily mean that the disease has advanced to the same degree in both sexes. It may simply mean that the alcoholic has drained all social supports. Knupfer goes on to say that

> it appears that, once men and women are far enough advanced in alcoholic drinking (which might be termed destructive, compulsive, or addictive drinking), their symptoms are much the same. What differs is the effect the frequent intoxication has on the lives of men and women because of the differences between them in social functions and cultural expectations. (p. 6)

The draining of social supports and the rapid downward spiral noted in alcoholic women may be partly explained by a grounded theory study conducted by Hutchinson (1986). Her qualitative study explored the process through which nurses become chemically dependent. Part of her data was obtained from interviews with 20 chemically dependent nurses ranging in age from 21 to 55, 18 of whom were women. Her data analysis revealed that the nurses' basic social psychological problem was perceived pain. Among the subjects, the pain varied from psychological to physical. Personal, work, social, and physical stresses contributed to the pain described by the nurses. This experienced pain had an effect on the rate of the process of their becoming chemically dependent.

The researcher described the process of self-annihilation (which was prompted by the nurses' perceived pain) as a self-destructive process. The self-annihilation process was distinguished by a trajectory toward a downhill course (Hutchinson, 1986). In a later study, Hutchinson (1987) explored the process of recovery in nurses and found a recovery process characterized by movement away from self-annihilation and toward self-integration. Self-integration is marked by the following stages: (a) surrendering, (b) accepting, and (c) committing. It is "a voyage to self-discovery" (Hutchinson, 1987, p. 340).

It is important to realize that almost nothing has been done to define *treatment* and, in particular, what aspects, qualities, or methods are used. Although some progress has been made in bringing attention to gender differences in relation to treatment needs, research is necessary to evaluate a variety of treatment models, techniques, and services currently used and their effects on client outcomes (Reed, 1987; Vannicelli, 1986). In addition, the interaction or enhancement of treatment with outside treatment-stabilizing factors (e.g., job and family or other social support) needs to be considered when evaluating treatment outcome (Marsh & Miller, 1985).

Treatment Referral and Availability

If treatment for various subgroups of drug-dependent women is available in a community, then health professionals must be knowledgeable about program services and how to refer clients needing assistance. Furthermore, health professionals need to learn about the variety of self-help groups for chemically dependent people in their community (Vourakis, 1990). Self-help groups, especially those modeled after the 12-step program of AA, have helped many people lead fruitful drug-free lives. Women should be encouraged to attend many different groups before deciding on which groups to attend on an ongoing basis. If they find groups with people like themselves, with whom they feel comfortable and willing to participate, they are more likely to be successful in these programs (Vourakis, 1989).

In general, to reach long-term abstinence, drug-dependent women must be motivated to accept assistance and follow a program of recovery. Health professionals who are supportive and not punitive may be able to motivate women to seek treatment. Unfortunately, until adequate treatment is available, women of lower SES will continue to suffer the consequences of their addiction. These women are particularly vulnerable to the interaction of a number of problems, which are compounded if they additionally have a drug abuse problem. Primary health care providers and other health professionals frequently have contact with these women in a variety of health care settings. Those who are in desperate need of services—poor, ethnically diverse women—and single mothers, particularly those who are pregnant or pregnant with children, are the least likely to have services accessible to them.

Prevention

Prevention of drug problems is more likely to be successful if a broad community approach is used. The general acceptance of drug use and the pervasiveness of drug abuse and dependency in our society requires an approach that goes beyond the individual user. The public health model offers a broad approach to prevention, and not only the host (user or potential user) is targeted but also the agent (drug) and the environment (community). Lubinski (1991) advocates a public health model as a strategy for the prevention of drug problems. She identifies the environment as "community attitudes, practices and policies which can either nurture or discourage alcohol and other drug problems from manifesting themselves" (p. 180).

Women have a history of leadership in prohibition activities (e.g., WCTU), are involved in such activities in the present (e.g., Mothers Against Drunk Driving [MADD]), and are an excellent resource for leadership in the prevention movement to come. Impetus for women's leadership and participation in prevention activities might stem from their knowledge of the devastating effect of drugs and alcohol on women's bodies after fewer years of excessive use compared to men. Furthermore, women are vulnerable to victimization and brutalization when they are intoxicated with chemicals or when their partner is intoxicated. In addition, Lubinski (1991) notes that "Alcoholism and drug addiction reinforce the second-class status of women in our society by rendering women incapable of self-actualization by undermining women's ability to take concrete steps, individually or collectively, to improve the quality of their own lives or of women generally" (pp. 180-181).

Efforts should be made through the print and broadcast media to portray images using alternative healthy means of relaxing, coping with stress, and have fun. Influencing legislative and other policy-making bodies to change zoning laws (e.g., to eliminate from residential neighborhoods billboards that glamorize smoking and drinking for women and to prevent the sale of alcoholic beverages at corner grocery stores) is another way women could direct their prevention efforts. Policy-making bodies could also be lobbied to increase taxes on legal drug substances (e.g., caffeine, nicotine, and alcohol). Funds raised from these taxes could be used for prevention activities. These are but a sampling of the many strategies and activities that could be used to continue the prevention efforts already underway in the United States and other parts of the world. The threat of drug abuse is continuous; therefore, prevention must be considered an ongoing process requiring vigilant attention and nurturance.

Future Research

Overall, although still in the early stages of development, research on drug use and problems among women is beginning to create a body of knowledge that gives direction to program planners and policy makers and provides direction for new lines of investigation. Current areas of study are becoming more clearly delineated, and many scholars are formulating research questions from a new consciousness unencumbered by past research traditions. A few areas needing attention from researchers, in addition to the growing practice of identifying samples of drug-dependent women separate from men, include (a) the changing female role and associated changes in drug use by women, (b) distinctions between use of psychoactive drugs for legitimate health problems and for abusive use, (c) continued development of a body of knowledge on drugs other than alcohol and their effects on women, (d) continued development of a body of knowledge on the effects of drug use during pregnancy, and (e) continued investigation into effective treatment and prevention programs and strategies for subgroups of high-risk women.

Summary

American women have been using and abusing substances in recent years, similar to patterns established over two centuries ago. If we exclude pregnant women, one major change from historical patterns is the increased acceptance of women's social drug use. Furthermore, there is increased recognition that a significant number of women in all social classes and ethnicities abuse drugs and are drug dependent; and many women seem less reluctant to acknowledge problems publicly and seek help. The exception to this is the pregnant drug-dependent woman, who fears prosecution if the addiction is identified. A need to encourage and make available treatment for these women in lieu of prosecution is advocated.

As noted, women's treatment remains inadequate for those without the resources to afford private services. Continued advocacy and research on women's needs is necessary to bring attention to the plight of underserved women. It will take the efforts of women to spearhead changes in public policy and health care to ensure that drug-dependent women receive adequate services. Women must also continue to increase their efforts in the area of prevention; there is a great deal at stake for women, who are most often the victims of their own and/or others, drug problems.

References

Abbott, P. J. (1986). Caffeine: A toxicological overview. *Medical Journal of Australia, 145*(7), 518-521.

Abel, E. L. (1984). *Fetal alcohol syndrome and fetal alcohol effects.* New York: Plenum.

Abelson, H. I., Fishburne, P. M., & Cisin, I. (1977). *National survey on drug abuse: 1. Main findings.* Rockville, MD: National Institute on Drug Abuse.

Alcoholics Anonymous. (1987). *About AA.* New York: Alcoholics Anonymous World Services.

Amaro, H., Beckman, L., & Mays, V. (1987). A comparison of Black and White women entering alcohol treatment. *Journal of Studies on Alcohol, 48*(3), 220-228.

American Nurses Association. (1991). *Position statement on opposition to criminal prosecution of women for use of drugs while pregnant and support for treatment services for alcohol and drug dependent women of childbearing age.* Kansas City, MO: Author.

American Nurses Association. (1993). *Position statement on the health care service system and linkage of primary care, alcohol and other drug, mental health, and HIV/AIDS related services.* Kansas City, MO: Author.

Anderson, S. C. (1980). Patterns of sex-role identification in alcoholic women. *Sex Roles, 6,* 231-243.

Annis, H. M. (1980). Treatment of alcoholic women. In G. Edwards & M. Grant (Eds.), *Alcoholism treatment in transition* (pp. 128-139). Baltimore: University Park Press.

Beckman, L. J. (1981). The psychosocial characteristics of alcoholic women. In S. Cohen (Ed.), *Drug abuse and alcoholism: Current critical issues* (pp. 14-26). New York: Haworth.

Beckman, L. J., & Amaro, H. (1986). Personal and treatment. *Journal of Studies on Alcohol, 47*(2), 135-145.

Beckman, L. J., & Kocel, K. M. (1982). The treatment-delivery system and alcohol abuse in women: Social policy implications. *Journal of Social Issues, 38*(2), 139-151.

Benward, J., & Densen-Gerber, J. (1975). Incest as a causative factor in antisocial behavior: An exploratory study. *Contemporary Drug Problems, 4,* 323-340.

Boyd, C., & Mast, D. (1983). Addicted women and their relationships with men. *Journal of Psychosocial Nursing and Mental Health Services, 21*(2), 10-13.

Braiker, H. B. (1984). Therapeutic issues in the treatment of alcoholic women. In S. C. Wilsnack & L. J. Beckman (Eds.), *Alcohol problems in women* (pp. 349-368). New York: Guilford.

Busch, D., McBride, A. B., & Benaventura, L. M. (1986). Chemical dependency in women: The link to OB/GYN problems. *Journal of Psychosocial Nursing and Mental Health Services, 24*(4), 26-30.

Caetano, R. (1989). Drinking patterns and alcohol problems in a national sample of U.S. Hispanics (NIAAA

Monograph No. 18, ADM 89-1435). In National Institute on Drug Abuse (Ed.), *The epidemiology of alcohol use and abuse among U.S. minorities* (pp. 147-162). Washington, DC: Government Printing Office.

Cahalan, D., Cisin, I. H., & Crossley, H. M. (1969). *American drinking practices: A national study of drinking behavior and attitudes.* New Haven, CT: College and University Press.

Campinha-Bacote, J., & Bragg, E. J. (1993). Chemical assessment in maternity care. *MCN, 18*(1), 24-28.

Centers for Disease Control. (1989). Update: Acquired immunodeficiency syndrome—United States, 1981-1988. *Morbidity and Mortality Weekly Reports, 38,* 232.

Chasnoff, I., Burns, W., Schnoll, S., & Burns, K. (1985). Cocaine use in pregnancy. *New England Journal of Medicine, 313,* 666-669.

Chasnoff, I. J., Landress, J. J., & Barrett, M. E. (1990). The prevalence of illicit-drug or alcohol use during pregnancy and discrepancies in mandatory reporting in Pinellas County, Florida. *New England Journal of Medicine, 322*(17), 1202-1206.

Clark, W. B., & Midanik, L. (1982). *Alcohol use and alcohol problems among U.S. adults: Results of the 1979 national survey* (Alcohol and Health Monograph No. I, Publication No. ADM 82-1190). Washington, DC: National Institute on Alcohol Abuse and Alcoholism.

Clarren, S., & Smith, D. (1978). The fetal alcohol syndrome. *New England Journal of Medicine, 298,* 163-167.

Clayton, R. R., Voss, H. L., Robbins, C., & Skinner, W. F. (1986). *Gender differences in drug use: An epidemiological perspective* (Research monograph 65). Washington, DC: National Institute on Drug Abuse.

Cooperstock, R. (1971). Sex differences in the use of mood-modifying drugs: An explanatory model. *Journal of Health and Social Behavior, 12,* 238-244.

Corrigan, E. M. (1980). *Alcoholic women in treatment.* New York: Oxford University Press.

Covington, S. S. (1986). Facing the challenges of women alcoholics: Physical, emotional and sexual abuse. *Focus on Family, 9*(3), 10-11, 37, 42-44.

Curlee, J. (1971). Sex differences in patient attitudes toward alcoholism treatment. *Quarterly Journal of Studies on Alcohol, 32,* 643-650.

Daghestani, A. N. (1989). Psychosocial characteristics of pregnant women addicts in treatment. In I. J. Chasnoff (Ed.), *Drugs, alcohol, pregnancy and parenting* (pp. 7-16). Hingham, MA: Kluwer Academic.

Diamond, D. L., & Wilsnack, S. C. (1978). Alcohol abuse among lesbians: A descriptive study. *Journal of Homosexuality, 4*(2), 123-142.

Dimijian, G. C. (1976). Contemporary drug abuse. In A. Goth (Ed.), *Medical pharmacology principles and concepts* (pp. 297-329). St. Louis, MO: C. V. Mosby.

Estes, N. J., & Heinemann, M. E. (1986). *Alcoholism: Development, consequences, and interventions* (3rd ed.). St. Louis, MO: C. V. Mosby.

Evans, S., & Schaefer, S. (1987). Incest and chemically dependent women: Treatment implications. In E. Coleman (Ed.), *Chemical dependency and intimacy dysfunction* (pp. 141-173). New York: Haworth.

Fillmore, K. M. (1984). When angels fall: Women's drinking as cultural preoccupation and as reality. In S. C. Wilsnack & L. J. Beckman (Eds.), *Alcohol problems in women: Antecedents, consequences and interventions* (pp. 7-36). New York: Guilford.

Frezza, M., Di Podova, C., Pozzato, G., Terpin, M., Baraona, E., & Lieber, C. S. (1990). High blood alcohol levels in women. *New England Journal of Medicine, 322*(2), 95-99.

Galambos, J. T. (1972). Alcoholic hepatitis: Its therapy and prognosis. In H. Popper & F. Schaffner (Eds.), *Progress in liver diseases* (Vol. 4, pp. 242-277). New York: Grune & Stratton.

Gavaler, J. S. (1985). Effect of alcohol on endocrine function in post-menopausal women: A review. *Journal of Studies on Alcohol, 46,* 495-516.

Geller, A. (1991). The effects of drug use during pregnancy. In P. Roth (Ed.), *Alcohol and drugs are women's issues: 1. A review of the issues* (pp. 101-106). Metuchen, NJ: Scarecrow.

Gomberg, E. S. (1974). Women and alcoholism. In V. Franks & V. Burtle (Eds.), *Women in therapy* (pp. 169-190). New York: Brunner/Mazel.

Gomberg, E. S. L. (1982). Historical and political perspectives: Women and drug use. *Journal of Social Issues, 38*(1), 9-23.

Guttentag, M., Salasin, S., & Belle, D. (1980). *The mental health of women.* New York: Academic Press.

Haggard, H. W., & Jellinek, E. M. (1942). *Alcohol explored.* New York: Doubleday, Doran.

Harrison, P. A., & Belille, C. A. (1987). Women in treatment: Beyond the stereotype. *Journal of Studies on Alcohol, 48,* 574-578.

Herd, D. (1988). Drinking by black and white women: Results from a national survey. *Social Problems, 35*(5), 493-505.

Hilton, M. E. (1987). Drinking patterns and drinking in 1984: Results from a general population survey. *Alcoholism (NY), 11,* 167-175.

Hilton, M. E. (1988). Trends in U.S. drinking patterns: Further evidence from the past 20 years. *British Journal of Addictions, 83*(1), 269-278.

Hogue, C., & Sappenfield, W. (1987). Smoking and low birth weight: Current concepts. In M. J. Rosenberg (Ed.), *Smoking and reproductive health* (pp. 97-108). Littleton, MA: PSG.

Hughes, J. N., Cofte, T., Perret, G., Jayle, M. S., Sebaoun, J., & Modigliani, E. (1980). Hypothalamo-pituitary ovarian function in 31 women with chronic alcoholism. *Clinical Endocrinology, 12,* 543-551.

Hutchinson, S. (1986). Chemically dependent nurses: The trajectory toward self-annihilation. *Nursing Research, 35*(4), 196-201.

Hutchinson, S. A. (1987). Toward self-integration: The recovery process of chemically dependent nurses. *Nursing Research, 36*(6), 339-343.

Institute of Medicine. (1990). *Treating drug problems* (Vol. 1). Washington, DC: National Academy Press.

Jack, L. (Ed.). (1989). *Nursing care planning with the addicted client* (Vol. I). Skokie, IL: Midwest Education Association.

Jack, L. (Ed.). (1990a). *The core curriculum of addictions nursing.* Skokie, IL: Midwest Education Association.

Jack, L. (Ed.). (1990b). *Nursing care planning with the addicted client* (Vol. I). Skokie, IL: Midwest Education Association.

Jaffe, J. H. (1985). Drug addiction and drug abuse. In A. G. Gilman, L. S. Goodman, T. W. Rall, & F. Murad (Eds.), *Goodman and Gilman's the pharmacological basis of therapeutics* (pp. 532-581). New York: Macmillan.

Johnston, L. D., O'Malley, P. M., & Bachman, J. G. (1987). *National trends in drug use and related factors among American high school students and young adults, 1975-1986* (DHHS Publication No. ADM 87-1535). Washington, DC: Government Printing Office.

Jones, R. W. (1972). Alcoholism among relatives of alcoholic patients. *Quarterly Journal of Studies on Alcohol, 33,* 810-817.

Karan, L. D. (1989). AIDS prevention and chemical dependence treatment needs of women and their children. *Journal of Psychoactive Drugs, 21*(4), 395-399.

Kendall, S. R., & Chavkin, W. (1992). Illicit drugs in America: History, impact on women and infants, and treatment strategies for women. *Hastings Law Journal, 43*(3), 615-643.

Kitano, H. H. L., & Chi, I. (1986-1987). Asian-Americans and alcohol use. *Alcohol Health and Research World, 11*(2), 42-47.

Knupfer, G. (1982). Problems associated with drunkenness in women: Some research issues (DHHS Publication No. ADM 82-1193). In National Institute on Alcohol Abuse and Alcoholism (Ed.), *Special population issues: Alcohol and health* (Monograph No. 4, pp. 3-39). Rockville, MD: Government Printing Office.

Koop, C. E. (1986). Smoking and pregnancy. *American Pharmacy, NS26* (7), 34-35.

Lelbach, W. K. (1974). Organic pathology related to volume and pattern of alcohol use. In R. J. Gibbins, Y. Israel, H. Kalant, R. E. Popham, W. Schmidt, & R. G. Smith (Eds.), *Research advances in alcohol and drug problems* (pp. 327-364). New York: John Wiley.

Lender, M., & Martin, J. (1982). *Drinking in America.* New York: Free Press.

Lubinski, C. (1991). Advocacy: Prevention strategies and treatment services sensitive to women's needs. In P. Roth (Ed.), *Alcohol and drugs are women's issues: 1. A review of the issues* (pp. 178-182). Metuchen, NJ: Scarecrow.

Marsh, J. C. (1982). Public issues and private problems: Women and drug use. *Journal of Social Issues, 38*(2), 153-165.

Marsh, J. C., Colten, M. E., & Tucker, M. B. (1982). Women's use of drugs and alcohol: New perspectives. *Journal of Social Issues, 38*(1), 1-8.

Marsh, J. C., & Miller, N. A. (1985). Female clients in substance abuse treatment. *International Journal of the Addictions, 20*(6/7), 995-1019.

McLachlan, J. F. C., Walderman, R. L., Birchmore, D. F., & Marsden, L. R. (1979). Self-evaluation, role satisfaction and anxiety in the woman alcoholic. *International Journal of the Addictions, 14*(6), 809-832.

Midanik, L. (1983). Alcohol problems and depressive symptoms in a national survey. *Advances in Alcohol and Substance Abuse, 2*(4), 9-28.

Miller, B. A., Downs, W. R., Gondoli, D. M., & Keil, A. (1987). The role of childhood sexual abuse in the development of alcoholism in women. *Violence and Victims, 2*(3), 157-172.

Mom gets 12 years for cocaine in fetus. (1991, July 2). *San Francisco Chronicle,* National Report sec., p. 6.

Mondanaro, J. (1981). Medical services for drug dependent women. In G. M. Beschner, B. G. Reed, & J. Mondanaro (Eds.), *Treatment services for drug dependent women* (Vol. 1, pp. 208-257). Rockville, MD: National Institute on Drug Abuse.

Morgan, W. H. (1974). *Yesterday's addicts, American society and drug abuse 1865-1920.* Norman: University of Oklahoma Press.

Moss, K. L. (1991). Punishing pregnant addicts. In P. Roth (Ed.), *Alcohol and drugs are women's issues: 1. A review of the issues* (pp. 107-113). Metuchen, NJ: Scarecrow.

Murphy, W. D., Coleman, E., Hoon, E., & Scott, C. (1980). Sexual dysfunction and treatment in alcoholic women. *Sexuality and Disability, 3,* 240-255.

Musto, D. (1977). Historical highlights of American drug use 1800-1940. In C. Kryder & S. P. Strickland (Eds.), *Americans and drug abuse* (pp. 3-8). Aspen, CO: Aspen Institute for Humanistic Studies.

Musto, D. (1987). *The American disease, origins of narcotic control.* New York: Oxford University Press.

National Institute on Alcohol Abuse and Alcoholism. (1981). *Spectrum: Alcohol problem prevention for women by women* (DHHS Publication No. ADM 81-1036). Washington, DC: Government Printing Office.

National Institute on Drug Abuse. (1980). *Data from the client-oriented acquisition process (CODAP): State statistics 1978* (Statistical Series E, No. 13). Washington, DC: Government Printing Office.

National Institute on Drug Abuse. (1988). Data from the Drug Abuse Warning Network (DAWN): Annual data, 1987 (Statistical Series I, No. 7, DHHS Publication No. ADM 88-1584). Rockville, MD: National Institute on Drug Abuse.

Ostrea, E., & Chavez, C. (1979). Perinatal problems (excluding neonatal withdrawal) in maternal drug addiction: A study of 830 cases. *Journal of Pediatrics, 94,* 292-295.

Parker, F. B. (1972). Sex role adjustment in women alcoholics. *Quarterly Journal of Studies on Alcohol, 33,* 647-657.

Parry, H. L., Balter, M., Mellinger, G., Cisin, I. H., & Manheimer, D. I. (1973). National patterns of psychotherapeutic drug use. *Archives of General Psychiatry, 71,* 769-783.

Prather, J. E., & Fidell, L. S. (1978). Drug use and abuse among women: An overview. *International Journal of the Addictions, 13,* 863-885.

Ray, O. S., & Ksir, C. (1987). *Drugs, society and human behavior.* St. Louis, MO: Times Mirror/Mosby College.

Reed, B. G. (1985). Drug misuse and dependency in women: The meaning and implications of being considered a special population or minority group. *International Journal of the Addictions, 20*(1), 13-62.

Reed, B. G. (1987). Developing women-sensitive drug dependence treatment services: Why so difficult? *Journal of Psychoactive Drugs, 19*(2), 151-164.

Rohsenow, D. W., Corbett, R., & Devine, D. (1988). Molested as children: A hidden contribution to substance abuse? *Journal of Substance Abuse Treatment, 5*(1), 13-18.

Root, M. P. P. (1989). Treatment failures: The role of sexual victimization in women's addictive behavior. *American Journal of Orthopsychiatry, 59*(4), 542-548.

Schuckit, M. A. (1972). The woman alcoholic. *Psychiatry in Medicine, 3*(1), 31-43.

Schuckit, M. A., & Morrissey, E. R. (1976). Alcoholism in women: Some clinical and social perspectives with an emphasis on possible subtypes. In M. Greenblatt & M. A. Schuckit (Eds.), *Alcoholism problems in women and children* (pp. 5-35). New York: Grune & Stratton.

Schuckit, M. A., Pitts, F. N., Reich, T., King, L. J., & Winokur, G. (1969). Alcoholism I. Two types of alcoholism in women. *Archives of General Psychiatry, 20,* 301-306.

Scida, J., & Vannicelli, M. (1979). Sex role conflict and women's drinking. *Journal of Studies on Alcohol, 40*(1), 28-44.

Smith, D. E. (1984). Diagnostic treatment and aftercare approaches to cocaine abuse. *Journal of Substance Abuse Treatment, 1*(1), 5-9.

Srisuphan, W., & Bracken, M. B. (1986). Caffeine consumption during pregnancy and association with late spontaneous abortion. *American Journal of Obstetrics and Gynecology, 154*(1), 14-20.

Staff. (1991, May). Stats—Facts: Women (Addiction Research Foundation). *The Journal* (an official publication of the Addiction Research Foundation), pp. 13-14.

Stone, A. (1990, April 4). Mother cleared of giving cocaine to child at birth. *USA Today,* Newsmakers sec., p. 2.

Sun, A. P. (1991). Issues for Asian American women. In P. Roth (Ed.), *Alcohol and drugs are women's issues: 1. A review of the issues* (pp. 125-129). Metuchen, NJ: Scarecrow Press.

Terry, C., & Pellens, M. (1928). *The opium problem* (Committee on Drug Addiction). New York: Bureau of Social Hygiene.

Thompson, K., & Wilsnack, R. (1984). Drinking problems among female adolescents: Patterns and influences. In S. Wilsnack & L. Beckman (Eds.), *Alcohol problems in women: Antecedents, consequences and intervention* (pp. 37-65). New York: Guilford.

Tuchmann-Duplessis, H. (1987). Embryonic clinical pharmacology. In T. M. Speight (Ed.), *Avery's drug treatment principles and practice of clinical pharmacology and therapeutics* (3rd ed., pp. 65-78). Auckland, New Zealand: Adis.

U.S. Department of Health and Human Services. (1990). *Seventh special report to the U. S. Congress on alcohol and health* (DHHS Publication No. ADM 90-1656). Washington, DC: Government Printing Office.

Valimaki, M., Pelkonen, R., Salaspuro, M., Harkonen, M., Hirvonene, E., & Ylikahri, R. (1984). Sex hormones in amenorrheic women with alcoholic liver disease. *Journal of Clinical Endocrinological Metabolism, 59*(1), 133-138.

Vannicelli, M. (1986). Treatment considerations. In National Institute on Alcohol Abuse and Alcoholism (Ed.), *Women and alcohol: Health related issues* (Research Monograph No. 16, pp. 130-153). Washington, DC: Government Printing Office.

Vourakis, C. (1983). Women in substance abuse treatment. In G. Bennett, C. Vourakis, & D. S. Woolf (Eds.), *Substance abuse: Pharmacologic, developmental and clinical perspectives* (pp. 383-399). New York: John Wiley.

Vourakis, C. (1989). *The process of recovery for women in Alcoholics Anonymous: Seeking groups "like me"* (Doctoral dissertation, University of San Francisco). Ann Arbor, MI: University Microfilms International. (No. 8917924)

Vourakis, C. (1990). Evolving process of recovery, change, and growth. In L. Jack (Ed.), *The core curriculum of addictions nursing* (pp. 117-139). Skokie, IL: Midwest Education Association.

Ward, S., Schuetz, S., Krishna, V., Bean, X., Wingert, W., Wachsman, L., & Keens, T. (1986). Abnormal sleeping ventilatory pattern in infants of substance-abusing mothers. *American Journal of Diseases of Children, 140,* 1015-1020.

Weathersbee, P., Olsen, L., & Lodge, J. (1977). Caffeine and pregnancy: A retrospective survey. *Postgraduate Medicine, 62*(1), 64-69.

Wilsnack, S. C. (1973a). The effects of social drinking on women's fantasy. *Journal of Abnormal Psychology, 82*(1), 44-63.

Wilsnack, S. C. (1973b). Sex role identity in female alcoholism. *Journal of Abnormal Psychology, 82,* 253-261.

Winokur, R. F., & Clayton, P. J. (1968). Family history studies: IV. Comparison of male and female alcoholics. *Quarterly Journal of Studies on Alcohol, 29,* 885-891.

Worth, D. (1991). American women and polydrug abuse. In P. Roth (Ed.), *Alcohol and drugs are women's issues: 1. A review of the issues* (pp. 1-9). Metuchen, NJ: Scarecrow.

23

Common Symptoms
Bleeding, Pain, and Discharge

CATHERINE INGRAM FOGEL

Throughout her life, the average woman will experience bleeding, pain, or discharge associated with her reproductive organs or functions. Many women will seek out nurses as advisers, counselors, and health care providers for these concerns. To meet their clients' needs, nurses must have accurate, up-to-date information. Nurses must be able to distinguish normal characteristics from pathological alterations, identify pathology when it exists, and understand the meaning of the symptoms or illness for the client. This chapter provides the needed information to meet these objectives. Symptoms are discussed in terms of (a) their normal parameters, (b) common causes, and (c) general assessment. Specific causes of symptoms are addressed in terms of (a) their definition and description, (b) data collection and differential diagnosis, and (c) management. Preventive measures, alternatives to medical management, and self-care strategies are emphasized.

Bleeding

Typically, women menstruate for about 40 years. Once the irregular nature of menses in the first 2 to 3 years following menarche subsides and a cyclic, predictable pattern of monthly bleeding is established, women may worry about any deviation from that pattern or from what they have been told is normal for all menstruating women. Vaginal bleeding that does not conform to expected patterns is a concern shared by most women at some point in their lives. Thus "abnormal" bleeding—too often or too seldom or not at all, too little or too much—is a very common symptom seen by women's health care practitioners.

Bleeding that is perceived as abnormal or unusual evokes fear and anxiety. Throughout the ages, blood has been seen as the life-giving and life-sustaining substance, and its loss therefore is viewed as life threatening. Bleeding provokes a sense of urgency and a need to do something.

Differences in cyclic bleeding patterns or bleeding that is perceived as abnormal may evoke fears regarding reproductive or sexual abilities. Sexual identity and role are closely tied to menstrual functioning for many women; therefore, any occurrence that alters this function may be perceived as a threat.

Normal Parameters

Knowledge of the normal parameters of menstruation is essential in the assessment of abnormal vaginal bleeding in women. Chapter 3, "Women's Bodies," discusses the menstrual cycle in detail. Normal menstrual patterns are averages based on observations and reports from large groups of healthy women. When counseling the individual woman, it is important to remember that these values are averages only. As the Federation of Feminist Women's Health Centers (1981) so aptly stated, the 28-day cycle is a medical myth. Although the majority of women do have approximately monthly cycles, other healthy and fertile women can have cycles more or less frequently. Although no woman's cycle is exactly the same length every month, the typical month-to-month variation in an individual's cycle is usually plus-or-minus 2 days; however, greater normal variations are frequently noted. Abnormal bleeding may occur at any age and for a variety of reasons.

Common Causes

Most women seek care for one of three reasons associated with bleeding: amenorrhea, spotting, and changes in the menstrual cycle that are thought to be abnormal. Abnormal genital bleeding is the most common reason for gynecologic office visits. For approximately 75% of women, the cause of bleeding is benign (e.g., normal variations of the menstrual cycle) (Murata, 1990); however, 25% of abnormal bleeding results from pathology, much of which can be life threatening. The etiology and incidence of a woman's bleeding problems alter significantly throughout her life cycle (see Table 23.1).

Abnormal or unusual bleeding may last only a few hours or persist for several weeks. It can vary from spotting to hemorrhage and may be associated with the passage of clots. Abnormal bleeding is presumed to be uterine in origin until proved otherwise. It may be associated with a range of symptoms varying from severe pain and cramps to no discomfort at all.

Life Cycle Variations

An understanding of the physiological variations present in several age groups is essential in determining whether a bleeding pattern is normal or abnormal. Menstrual cycle length is most irregular in the 2 years after menarche and the 3 to 5 years before menopause, when anovulatory cycles are most common. Irregular bleeding, both in length of cycle and in amount, is the rule rather than the exception in early adolescence. It takes approximately 15 months for completion of the first 10 cycles and an average of 20 cycles before ovulation occurs regularly (Shulman, 1990). Cycle lengths of 22 to 40 days are not unusual, and during the first 2 years postmenarche, intervals of 3 to 6 months between menses can be normal (Simmons, 1988). Additional information on this topic is found in Chapter 3.

Irregular bleeding is also common during the perimenopausal years; the majority of women experience an alteration in interval between menses and character of flow in the 5 years preceding menopause. (See Chapter 3 and Chapter 5, "Midlife Women's Health," for additional discussion of this topic.)

General Assessment

The initial step in the assessment, diagnosis, and management of abnormal gynecologic bleeding is a comprehensive problem-specific history. Also essential to the assessment process is a thorough physical examination. Selected laboratory tests are used to confirm information obtained by history taking and physical examination and to suggest interventions.

History

An important first piece of information is the client's age (Shulman, 1990) because it may suggest possible causes of bleeding. Next in the assessment process is an exploration of why the client sought care (presenting problem or chief concern). Ask first about why she has sought care for the bleeding and why the bleeding is worrying her. Particular attention should be given

Table 23.1 Common Causes of Gynecologic Bleeding Through the Life Cycle

Childhood to Teens	*Childbearing Years*	*Peri- to Postmenopausal Years*
Foreign bodies: cotton, paper, safety pins, sand, sticks Pinworms: excoriation from scratching Trauma: self-inflicted or from sexual abuse Estrogen withdrawal spotting in neonate Vaginitis: commonly STD (e.g., gonorrhea, human papilloma virus) Rectal and urethral bleeding may appear to be vaginal Systemic disease: leukemia Medications: oral contraceptives Malignancy: adenocarcinoma of cervix or vagina Vulvular skin disorders Precocious puberty Alterations in hormones of menstruation: anovulatory cycles Systemic: weight, exercise, psychological	Contraception: oral contraceptive pills, intrauterine device, Norplant Pregnancy: implantation, early loss Infection: sexually transmitted disease (STD), cervicitis, pelvic inflammatory disease Cervical erosion/eversion Benign masses: endometriosis, uterine leiomyomas Malignancy: cervical, uterine, adenocarcinoma associated with diethylstilbestrol Systemic illness: hypothyroidism, hyperthyroidism, thrombocytopenia purpura, blood dyscrasias Systemic: weight, exercise, psychological Medication: marijuana, thiazide, diuretics, anticoagulents, anticholinergics, phenothiazines, corticosteroids Trauma Mittlestaining with ovulation Hormonal imbalance: corpus luteum cyst, anovulatory cycles Cervical stenosis	Malignancy: cervical, endometrial Benign neoplasms: uterine leiomyomas Hormone alterations: anovulatory cycles, sustained endometrial proliferation Hormonal replacement therapy Trauma: coital injury Pregnancy Systemic illness: hypothyroidism, hyperthyroidism, Cushing's disease Medications

NOTE: The cause of gynecologic bleeding varies depending on a woman's age. An understanding of how life cycle affects etiology of gynecologic bleeding is important when gathering a history from women seeking care for this problem.

to her description of the vaginal bleeding itself. Information regarding the severity (onset, duration, frequency, or interval), amount, color, and character of the bleeding is gathered. This information is critical to diagnosis yet frequently difficult to obtain accurately because women often find it difficult to describe their bleeding. Shulman (1990) suggests that an important element of well-woman care is encouraging all women to keep a calendar of the days, amount, and character of her bleeding as a lifelong menstrual habit. Such an activity can sensitize women to their normal cycle variations and help them to determine more easily when to seek care.

The client may be asked, "Is the bleeding enough to use a tampon or pad?" If so, she should be asked which form of sanitary protection she uses (tampons or pads), what type (regular/super or maxi/mini), and the number of tampons or pads used per hour or per day. Because studies have shown little correlation between the number of pads used and the actual volume of menstrual flow, it is important to ask how saturated each pad is when changed. Increase or decrease in the number of pads or tampons used is a good subjective indicator of changes in amount of bleeding or menstrual flow. Included in the assessment should be the woman's personal patterns of changing protection, for this can influence perceptions of blood loss. When collecting information about amount of bleeding, it is useful to ask women to quantify bleeding in terms they are familiar with, using units such as teaspoon, tablespoon, cupfuls. Information about the color of the bleeding—dark brown, bright red, pink—is also gathered. When possible, the nurse should observe the stained pad or tampon to provide additional data regarding color and amount of bleeding.

The nurse next inquires about the presence of associated symptoms: clots; pain and its location, type, duration, and what relieves it or makes it worse; foul odor; vaginal discharge; fever; shaking chills; gastrointestinal symptoms, such as diarrhea, constipation, or nausea and vomiting; and urinary frequency, urgency, and dysuria

Table 23.2 Menstrual History Questions

When was your last period (LMP)? Was this a normal period for you? If not, how was it different?
When was your period before your last period (PMP)? Was this period normal? If not, how was it different?
How many days are there usually between your periods?
How many tampons/pads would you say you use each day? How full or saturated would you say your pad/tampon was when you changed it?
Do you have any bodily signs (e.g., breast tenderness or swelling) that tell you that your period is coming? If yes, what are they? Do any of these changes cause you to change your daily routine? How upsetting are these?
Do you have any bodily changes with your period? If yes, what are they? Do any of these changes cause you to change your daily routine? How upsetting are these?
When did you have your first period? How was that for you?

NOTE: Obtaining a detailed menstrual history is an essential component of assessment of gynecologic bleeding. Information on past patterns is needed to evaluate accurately present bleeding problems. These questions are used to gather comprehensive data on a woman's menstrual history.

(painful urination). Women are asked specifically about the presence of pregnancy symptoms, sexual activity, and trauma. Nurses should inquire as to whether the client had bleeding problems before. Finally, the nurse asks about relationship of the symptoms to the client's menstrual cycle (when in the cycle does bleeding occur?); sudden changes in weight; major recent life events; changes or stresses; extreme diets; and drug use, including marijuana.

After information on the reason the woman sought care is obtained, her complete gynecologic history should be reviewed (Lichtman & Papera, 1990a). Given the variability in biological patterns of menstruation and individual perceptions, it is critical that the nurse obtain a detailed menstrual history. (See Chapter 9, "Well-Woman Assessment," and Table 23.2.) This information is essential in comparing the present concern to past patterns. If this history is not obtained, false assumptions are too easily made and can result in inappropriate interventions. Knowledge of a woman's age at menarche and, when relevant, age at menopause, as well as prior menstrual patterns, can provide significant diagnostic clues. An important additional question to ask is, "How does this bleeding compare to your normal periods?" Menstrual flow characteristics provide important diagnostic data. For example, regular cycles with recent altered menstrual flow may indicate early pregnancy, whereas short cycles or premenstrual spotting may indicate low progesterone levels. Having a menstrual calendar for the previous 6 to 12 months is advantageous. Women are asked about skipping periods. Knowing if a woman's cycles are ovulatory or anovulatory helps to narrow the differential diagnosis. The presence of premenstrual symptoms such as breast tenderness, fluid retention, and cramping with bleeding are progesterone-induced changes suggesting ovulation, whereas heavy, irregular bleeding is associated with anovulatory cycles. Mittelschmerz (pain at ovulation) and dsymenorrhea (pain with menses) are also absent in anovulatory cycles.

Obstetric, contraceptive, and sexual histories are important because they may suggest possible causes of bleeding. The number of pregnancies and the outcome of each should be noted. In addition, specific problems associated with contraception or pregnancy should be recorded. Bleeding with sexual intercourse may indicate infection or a structural abnormality such as a polyp or lesion. Bleeding following a period of amenorrhea in a woman who has had previous spontaneous abortions suggests that she may be miscarrying now. A history of an intrauterine device or hormonal implant in place suggests a cause of intramenstrual bleeding. If the woman is heterosexually active, ask about association of symptoms with coitus, and if dyspareunia is present. Murata (1990) states that all genital bleeding in a premenarcheal child should be viewed as sexual abuse until disproved.

Any information available from previous gynecologic examinations and surgical procedures is noted; however, because clients often are not given sufficient information or explanation regard-

Table 23.3 Common Drugs That May Alter Menstrual Bleeding

Generic Name	*Trade Name*
Amphetamines*	Desoxyn, Obetrol*
Anticoagulants	Coumadin, Heparin
Benzodiazepines*	
Diazepam, oxazepam	Valium, Serax*
Benzomide derivatives	Pronestyl, Matulane
Butyrophenones*	Haldol, Inapsine*
Cannabis	Marijuana
Chlordiazepoxide	Librium
Cimetidine*	Tagamet*
Ethyl alcohol	Whiskey, wine, beer
Isoniazid*	INH*
Methyldopa*	Aldomet*
Monoamine oxidase inhibitors	Eutonyl, Nardil
Opiates*	Morphine, Heroin, Methadone*
Phenothiazines*	Compazine, Thorazine, Phenergan*
Rauwolfia	Raudixin
Prostaglandin inhibitors	Motrin, Indocin
Reserpine*	Serpasil*
Spironolactone*	Aldactone*
Steroids	
Gonadal	
Estrogen*	Premarin,* (also oral contraceptives)
Progesterones*	Provera,* (also oral contraceptives)
Testosterone*	Android*
Thyroid	Synthroid, Cytomel
Thioxanthenes*	Navane*
Tricyclic antidepressants	Elavil*

SOURCE: Murata, J. M. (1990). Abnormal genital bleeding and secondary amenorrhea. *JOGNN, 19*(1), 26-36. Copyright J. B. Lippincott, reprinted with permission.
NOTE: Knowledge of which medication may affect the menstrual cycle is important for nurses obtaining histories from women seeking care for gynecologic bleeding or amenorrhea or for well-woman assessment.
* May also produce galactorrhea.

ing the indications for and results of such procedures, previous health care providers or institutions may need to be contacted. If additional information is obtained from these sources, it should always be shared fully with the woman and explained in terms that she clearly understands.

The menstrual cycle may be affected by chronic illness, acute illness, or medications and drugs (see Table 23.3); thus a client's medical history and her current medical status can suggest previous unsuspected health problems. For example, if a woman reported to her nursing practitioner that she recently had experienced diarrhea, weight loss, and palpitations, she should be evaluated further for hyperthyroidism, a cause of menstrual alterations such as oligomenorrhea. Similarly, indicators of systemic bleeding such as bruising or petechiae also should be investigated. Gaines (1981) suggests that exposure to radiation or toxic chemicals that could damage the ovaries, endometrium, or hypothalamus should be considered when a woman presents with a bleeding problem. A family history may be helpful, because some bleeding problems (e.g., endometriosis and endometrial or ovarian cancer) may have a familial association (Shulman, 1990). A family history of delayed menarche, infertility, or heavy irregular menses may suggest polycystic ovary disease in female relatives, whereas family history of blood dyscrasia may indicate a bleeding disorder in the women.

The menstrual cycle responds to the components of a woman's lifestyle. Therefore, clients are asked about recent changes in weight and exercise patterns, and a nutritional history and 24-hour diet recall are obtained. Given that eating disorders such as anorexia and bulimia are prevalent in women in the United States and may be associated with cycle alterations and amenorrhea, this possibility should be considered and investigated. The nurse should ask about the woman's social situation, social supports, and family life. She should ask how the client has been feeling and assess her for psychological disturbances, such as depression and anxiety.

Physical Examination

A thorough physical examination is indicated when assessing abnormal vaginal bleeding and includes far more than just a pelvic examination. Observation of the woman's general condition and taking her vital signs will provide an immediate estimation of the severity of the problem. For example, if a woman is pale and clammy with a rapid pulse and low blood pressure, hypovolemic shock from a ruptured ectopic pregnancy would be suspect, even if she gives a history of irregular spotting and mild abdominal cramps. A woman who gives a history of heavy bleeding and needing to change her maxi pads every hour, yet has a normal blood pressure and pulse, is able to go about her daily activities without difficulty, and whose mucous membranes and nailbeds are pink, is most likely not hemorrhaging as she describes. If some doubt exists as to the degree of blood loss, the patient can be tested for orthostatic changes in pulse and blood pressure and a hematocrit obtained.

A complete physical exam may uncover endocrine disturbances, coagulation disorders, or nutritional problems. Significant findings include delayed or precocious sexual maturation; galactorrhea; hirsutism; signs of thyroid disease, such as thyroid enlargement or nodules, excessively dry or moist skin, exophthalmos, and palmar erythemia; signs of Cushing's syndrome, such as moon face, buffalo hump, excessive acne, and facial plethora; petechiae and bruising; and obesity or anorexia.

A complete pelvic examination, including speculum and bimanual assessment, should be done. During the speculum examination, the nurse assesses the source, amount, color, character, and odor of any observed bleeding. To assess the possibility of bleeding from sites other than the cervix and uterus, the nurse must carefully inspect the external genitalia, urethra, and rectum for bleeding, redness, hemorrhoids, or lesions. It is important to identify the exact source of bleeding. The nurse locates and swabs the cervix free of any blood present and observes whether the bleeding reoccurs. If the os or cervix is not the source of bleeding, the vagina is cleansed and inspected for bleeding sites. Occasionally, an excoriated lesion such as a venereal wart can cause extensive, bright red genital bleeding (Murata, 1990). During the bimanual examination, the nurse palpates for any abnormal enlargements, masses, tenderness, or fixation of organs in the pelvis, cervix, and vagina. Chandelier's sign, or exquisite tenderness on cervical motion, suggests adnexal inflammation, such as pelvic infection or ectopic pregnancy. The rectal exam can reveal hemorrhoids, which may be mistaken for vaginal bleeding or spotting.

Laboratory Tests

Even though the history and physical examination may suggest a diagnosis, certain laboratory tests should be done. Because pregnancy is a frequent cause of bleeding in women of childbearing age, a pregnancy test is done first. A hematocrit should be obtained, and if the bleeding is significant, a complete blood count with differential count, platelet count, and coagulation survey should be ordered to assess the degree of anemia and assist in the diagnosis (Connell, 1989). When indicated by history or physical examination, the nurse should obtain a Papanicolaou (Pap) smear, wet smears to identify vaginitis, cervical cultures for gonorrhea and chlamydia, and/or cervical mucus for the presence of ferning (see Chapter 9 and Chapter 24, "Sexually Transmitted Diseases"). Ferning of cervical mucus suggests adequate estrogenization (see Chapter 25, "Infertility"). Assessment of cervical mucus is possible when bleeding is light. In a suspected early pregnancy loss, a more sensitive pregnancy test, such as one that tests for the B subunit of human chorionic gonadotropin (B-HCG), would be appropriate. In addition, a variety of diagnostic procedures may be indicated and necessitate referral to a gynecologist or other specialist for evaluation. Such procedures may include endometrial biopsy, biopsy of a visible lesion, or colposcopy (an examination of cervical epithelium using a colposcope, which provides increased magnification). Ultrasound and X-ray studies may be needed to arrive at an accurate diagnosis. At times, surgery such as dilatation and curettage (D & C) or laparoscopy may be necessary to determine the cause of the bleeding problem.

Shulman (1990) suggests that for the woman with a chronic bleeding problem in which the diagnosis is not clear, having her record her bleeding and chart her basal body temperature

Table 23.4 Causes of Amenorrhea

Level of Alteration	*Condition/Cause*
Hypothalamus	Generalized hypothalamic disorder
	Isolated gonadotropin deficiency
	Functional: exercise, weight alterations, environmental stress, anxiety, grief
	Functional pseudocyesis, emotional shock
	Exposure to toxins
Pituitary	Tumors (adenomas, cysts) of gland, stalk, suprasellar space
	Insufficiency or failure: Sheehan's syndrome, Simmonds's disease
	Chiari-Frommel syndrome and other amenorrhea-galactorrhea disease
Ovarian	Stein-Leventhal syndrome
	Neoplasms, cysts
	Ovarian failure (premature menopause)
	Infection: severe pelvic inflammatory disease, mumps oophoritis
	Primary gonadal disorder
	Hypogonodotropic hypogonadism
Thyroid	Hyperthyroidism
	Hypothyroidism
Anatomical	Congenital absence of ovaries
	Congenital anomalies: absent or hypoplastic uterus, imperforate hymen, transverse vaginal system, congenital absence of vagina
Physiological	Pregnancy
	Postpartum: Sheehan's syndrome, Chiari-Frommel syndrome
	Menopause
Chronic Disease	Tuberculosis, nephritis, rheumatoid arthritis, cirrhosis, alcohol abuse, Type I diabetes mellitus, adrenal disorders
	Obesity (polycystic ovaries)
Medication	Oral contraceptives
	Phenothiazines
	Dilantin, digitalis, reserpine, cytoxic drugs

NOTE: Amenorrhea is a symptom of many different conditions and pathologies. A knowledge of multiple etiologies of amenorrhea guides an assessment of these symptoms.

(BBT) and cervical mucus may provide very useful information. If normal hypothalamic-pituitary-ovarian function can be shown by a biphasic temperature chart with ovulatory mucus patterns (see Chapters 3 and Chapter 25), she may be able to avoid part of a lengthy, costly diagnostic workup.

Amenorrhea

Defined as the absence or cessation of menstrual flow, amenorrhea is the clinical manifestation of a variety of disorders. The criteria used to determine when the clinical problem of amenorrhea exists are not uniform. In general, the absence of both menarche and secondary sexual characteristics in a woman by age 14, or the absence of menarche by age 16 regardless of the presence of normal growth and development, should be evaluated (Speroff, Glass, & Kase, 1989). When a previously normally menstruating woman ceases to do so for three cycle lengths or 6 months, it also is considered abnormal and should be investigated. Although it is an artificial distinction that is not usually helpful for the evaluation of amenorrheic women (Clarke-Pearson & Dawood, 1990), amenorrhea has been traditionally classified as primary (no previous menstruation) or secondary (cessation of menses after a period of menstruation). Amenorrhea is a symptom and may result from any defect or interruption in the hypothalamic-pituitary-ovarian-uterine axis. Amenorrhea also may result from anatomical abnormalities, other endocrine disorders, chronic disease, medications, and emotional reasons (see Table 23.4).

Assessment

Assessment begins with a thorough history and physical examination. Shulman (1990) recommends that the first step, at times overlooked, is to be sure that the woman is not pregnant.

The extent to which nurses are involved in the diagnosis of amenorrhea for women of any age depends on their level of educational preparation, clinic or practice protocols, and consultation agreements. All nurses working with women should be prepared to collect the historical information outlined and should be skilled in physical examination procedures. Many nurses will be able to order basic laboratory studies; however, ordering special X rays, computerized axial tomography (CAT scan), or magnetic resonance imaging (MRI) should be done only after consultation and referral.

Adolescent Client. For adolescents presenting with amenorrhea, areas to explore during history taking include (a) stages and ages of pubertal developmental changes, if any; (b) onset of concern regarding amenorrhea; (c) whose concern it is (parent or client); and (d) the meaning this symptom has for the client and her family. A past medical history is taken, focusing on past illness, hospitalizations, operations, and allergies. Because chronic systemic disease (renal, pulmonary, cardiovascular) may also cause pubertal and menstrual delay (Shulman, 1990), the presence of such conditions is noted. A family history of the onset of puberty and menarche for the client's mother, sisters, and maternal aunts is also pertinent. Girls tend to menstruate at about the same time as their mothers and grandmothers (Ouellette, MacVicar, & Harlan, 1986), and a family history of late menarche can be significant. Information about the girl's school and home situation and her habits is gathered. Additional information about lifestyle and habits to be gathered include diet; exercise patterns; and substance use, including cigarettes, prescription and over-the-counter medications, illicit drugs, and alcohol. In addition, the adolescent is asked about her sexual activity and contraceptive use.

During the physical exam, the patient's age, absolute weight and height, and percentile weight and height are obtained. The presence or absence of normal female secondary sexual characteristics (e.g., pubic hair, axillary hair, fat distribution on hips and thighs) and presence of female secondary virilization (e.g., increase in body or facial hair) are recorded. Breast development indicates a strong likelihood of adequate endogenous estrogen, reflecting probably adequate ovarian estrogen output, whereas no breast development suggests low endogenous estrogen output because of failure or dysfunction of the hypothalamic-pituitary-ovarian axis at any level (Clarke-Pearson & Dawood, 1990). A pelvic examination will help establish if an adolescent has a normal vagina, cervix, and uterus and can assist in excluding pregnancy as a possible cause of amenorrhea. A vaginal smear can also be obtained at this time to determine the presence of superficial cells in the vaginal epithelium, which would suggest that the woman is eugonadal (Shulman, 1990).

Adult Woman. When the woman is postpubertal and has been menstruating for some time before becoming amenorrheic, a similar diagnostic process is undertaken. The underlying causes, however, are somewhat different from those considered when menses has never occurred. With amenorrhea that occurs after menstruation has been established, a functioning hypothalamic-pituitary-ovarian-uterine axis has been established. Again the first step is to rule out pregnancy, because it is the most probable cause of secondary amenorrhea. The nurse asks about any symptoms associated with pregnancy such as breast tenderness, nausea and vomiting, or fatigue. A thorough contraceptive history is obtained because amenorrhea may occur with progestin-only contraceptives or with progesterone-containing injectable contraceptives. Amenorrhea may occur temporarily when a woman stops taking birth control pills: If this lasts more than 6 months, however, other causes are investigated.

In assessing the adult amenorrheic woman, in addition to a careful menstrual and contraceptive history, data are obtained regarding medications; sources of stress such as marital discord, chronic anxiety, recent travel, and changes in work or school; symptoms of past and present illness; present weight; weight 1 year ago; and amount of daily exercise. Any recent uterine infections, abortions, and D & C procedures are noted.

The physical examination includes observation of both breasts for discharge. When present, the character of the discharge—milky, clear, dark, light, bloody, thick, thin—is noted. During the vaginal exam, the nurse observes for presence of cervical mucus and atrophy. The bimanual examination provides information on the size of the uterus and adnexa. Laboratory tests often performed are Pap smear, evaluation of cervical mucus, and cytological evaluation of vaginal smear (maturation index). A maturation index is obtained by studying the type of vaginal cells present in a smear of the lateral midvagina. Three types of cells are identified—parabasal, intermediate, and superficial. The percentage of superficial cells can be used as a rough gauge of estrogen effect. If the percentage of superficial cells present is 10% or less, the estrogen effect is assumed to be slight, whereas more than 30% indicates a marked estrogen effect. In addition, if 50% or more of the cells are basal cells, low estrogen effect is also indicated. If inflammation (e.g., chronic cervicitis or vaginitis) is present, the maturation index is not a reliable index of estrogen effect (Clarke-Pearson & Dawood, 1990). In addition, tests for thyroid-stimulating hormone (TSH) levels, follicle-stimulating hormone (FSH) and leuteinizing hormone (LH) levels, HCG levels, and prolactin levels may be ordered.

Perimenopausal Women. Amenorrhea is a cardinal signal of menopause, usually after a time (up to 8 or 10 years) of menstrual changes in flow and frequency (see Chapters 3 and 5). Menopause is suggested by the presence of elevated LH and FSH levels. At times a woman in her mid-40s may have a short period of amenorrhea followed by a positive pregnancy test. Because some pregnancy tests that measure HCG, and not just the beta subunit of HCG, also measure FSH and LH, it is possible to obtain a false-positive result, resulting in considerable confusion and possible distress for the woman. Therefore, it is essential that pregnancy testing in this age group should be done with a specific assay for the beta subunit of HCG (Shulman, 1990).

Nursing Management

Regardless of the etiology, what amenorrhea means to an individual woman is varied and often negative. She may feel she is not really a woman, that her "marriage-ability" is compromised and her ability to conceive and bear children threatened. She may worry about her appearance or about peer acceptance or approval. It can be a source of much distress and concern as the woman wonders, "What is wrong with me?" Although her health is usually not seriously endangered, it may compromise a woman's biological ability to reproduce. Nurses can help the client to acknowledge negative feelings and work through the feelings. Comments such as, "I'm wondering if this makes you feel different from others" or "It must be really hard to think you may never have children" can stimulate discussion. Some fears may be reality based; the client may indeed be infertile. In such instances the client will need to gain some acceptance of this fact and develop a self-concept not rooted in childbearing functions. The nurse might ask her client to think of all the things that she does well or feels good about. Sexual issues often surface and must be examined. Nurses will need a thorough understanding of how they view female roles and what constitutes "female identity" before they can assist their clients in exploring and resolving these issues.

Once pregnancy has been ruled out, a course of progestin is used to evaluate estrogen status. The client is most commonly given 5 to 10 mg of the oral progestin medroxyprogesterone acetate twice a day for 5 days (Doody & Carr, 1990). Withdrawal bleeding within 7 days demonstrates she has adequate estrogen and also confirms that she has a normal outflow tract (vagina, patent cervix, uterus). In these instances, the cause of amenorrhea is believed to be anovulation.

If withdrawal bleeding does not occur in the eugonadal adolescent after a course of progestin, an anatomical defect in the uterus or vagina is likely and indeed may have been suspected or found during the pelvic exam. Such defects may be the result of an imperforate hymen or an absent vagina and, perhaps, uterus (Mayer-Rokitansky-Küster-Hauser syndrome) or testicular feminization (androgen insensitivity syndrome).

When amenorrhea is due to hypothalamic disturbances or occurs in the absence of anatomical defect, system illness, pituitary lesions, or other organic causes, the nurse is an ideal health professional to assist women, for many of the causes are potentially reversible (e.g., stress, weight loss for nonorganic reasons), and counseling and education are primary interventions and appropriate nursing roles.

Often the primary medical management approach to hypothalamic amenorrhea is to "wait and see." Given that other diagnostic entities have been ruled out, the "cure" for hypothalamic amenorrhea is the production of the gonadotropin-releasing factor by the hypothalamus, which may take months to occur. It is not necessarily physiologically harmful for a woman not to menstruate for several months. On the other hand, the chronic persistence of amenorrhea associated with estrogen stimulation to the endometrium without adequate progesterone may result in endometrial hyperplasia. When the management plan is to observe and reevaluate, the nurse has an important role in education and support of the client. Women can be taught to make symptothermal observations using menstrual calendars, temperature charts, and cervical mucus characteristics (see Chapter 14, "Fertility Control," for information regarding these techniques). These observations can aid in documenting ovulation.

When a stressor known to predispose a client to hypothalamic amenorrhea is identified, initial management involves addressing the stressor. Together the woman and nurse plan how to decrease or discontinue medications known to affect menstruation; correct weight loss; deal more effectively with psychological stress; and eliminate substance abuse, including alcohol and marijuana.

Current research on the interaction between nervous system or neurotransmitter functions and hormonal regulation throughout the body has demonstrated a biological basis for the relation of stress to physiological processes. The nurse and client working together can identify, cope with, and possibly resolve sources of stress in the client's life. Teaching the client deep-breathing exercises and relaxation techniques are simple yet effective stress reduction measures. Referral for biofeedback or massage therapy may also be useful. In some instances, referrals for psychological therapy may be indicated.

Amenorrhea has been associated with strenuous exercise in some women athletes (see Chapter 13, "Exercise"). What is not clear is whether the amenorrhea results from exercise alone, amount of body fat, or dietary changes (e.g., decrease in red meat consumption). If a woman's exercise program is thought to contribute to her amenorrhea, several options exist for management. She may decide to decrease the intensity or duration of her exercise program or to gain some weight and see if the problem resolves itself. Coming to accept this alternative may be difficult for one who is committed to a strenuous exercise regimen, and the nurse and client may meet in several sessions before the woman elects to try exercise reduction. The nurse and client also should investigate other factors that may be contributing to the amenorrhea and develop plans for altering lifestyle and decreasing stress. If amenorrhea continues after decreasing exercise level and/or gaining weight and altering lifestyle, hormonal therapy may be indicated to prevent additional problems.

The perimenopausal woman should be counseled to note and possibly record her changing patterns of bleeding as well as any other changes that may occur, such as hot flushes, headaches, and insomnia. These can then be reviewed with the woman, and she can be reassured that although these symptoms may be disturbing, all are normal effects of changing ovarian function.

Spotting

Spotting, or small amounts of bloody vaginal discharge, is usually intermenstrual and varies in color from pink to dark brown. It may be a symptom of a relatively innocuous or benign condition, or it can be an indication of a serious, possibly life-threatening situation. Typical examples of problems that are often first indicated by spotting are spontaneous abortion, various gynecologic infections, and malignancy. Spotting is also often experienced in conditions more characteristically associated with pain, such as ectopic pregnancy (see the section on pain in this chapter). In addition, conditions such as trichomoniasis, Chlamydia, gonorrhea, and venereal warts and cervicitis may cause spotting (see the discussion on vaginal discharge in this chapter and in Chapter 24).

Spotting may be associated with oral contraceptive usage. Some women report midcycle spotting—known as *mittelstaining*—which occurs because of hormonal fluctuations during ovulation. Some women may experience "implantation bleeding" or spotting that occurs at the time of implantation of a pregnancy. In addition, spotting may occur in the perimenopausal years as ovarian function changes.

Spontaneous Abortion

Spontaneous abortion is the natural termination of a pregnancy before the fetus is considered to be viable (approximately 20-24 weeks after the last menstrual period or a fetal weight of 500 grams or less). Although *abortion* is correct medical terminology, many women may associate this term with the voluntary termination of a pregnancy and thus may view it as criminal or believe it is sinful or wrong. *Miscarriage* for the lay public indicates spontaneous or involuntary loss of a pregnancy. An awareness of this distinction that many women make is useful in obtaining an accurate history.

At least 15% of clinically recognized pregnancies abort spontaneously. Recent research suggests that the spontaneous abortion rate may be much higher, and researchers speculate that if women were monitored continuously, the rate might be as high as 50% (Keye, 1987; Scott, Disaia, Hammond, & Spellacy, 1994). Almost 80% of all spontaneous abortions occur before the 12th week of gestation; of these, the majority occur before the 8th week (Scott, 1986) and, perhaps, before the woman is aware that she is pregnant. She may notice that her period is somewhat delayed and that when it begins the flow is heavier than usual, but she does not identify this as an early spontaneous abortion, an important point to remember when taking a history.

Spontaneous abortions can occur for many reasons. Nearly 80% are attributed to abnormal genetic or chromosomal makeup; the remaining result from maternal factors (Beischer & MacKay, 1986). When a cause can be identified, it is in one of three categories: abnormalities of the ovum; abnormalities of the female reproductive tract, such as uterine anomalies or incompetent cervix; or maternal host factors (e.g., chronic disease or infection).

The characteristic symptoms of spontaneous abortion are persistent uterine bleeding and cramping. The process of abortion is often progressive, with the symptoms increasing in severity with each subsequent stage.

Assessment. When any woman of childbearing age seeks care with a concern of vaginal spotting, the possibility of spontaneous abortion must be investigated. Information focusing on a description of the present vaginal bleeding, menstrual history, and prior obstetric and pertinent medical history should be gathered. It is particularly important to ask the woman for a description of any tissue she may have passed. She also should be asked whether she has had a pregnancy test and, if so, what type, when, and what the results were. The time frame in which the woman's symptoms have developed is useful as well and can be compared to her usual menstrual patterns and the date of her last menstrual period.

Abdominal palpation is done to determine uterine size (suggestive of week of gestation of pregnancy) and tenderness (may indicate infection). When indicated by the week of gestation, presence or absence of fetal heart tone should be determined. A gentle speculum exam may suggest the source of the bleeding and help rule out other possible causes. Inspection of the cervix and vagina for bleeding and aborted tissue should also be done. A bimanual examination provides information of uterine size and consistency and helps determine whether cervical effacement and dilatation are present.

Certain laboratory studies may provide additional information on the woman's condition. A pregnancy test is done to establish a baseline, even though results are often equivocal. Frequently, the woman experiencing a spontaneous abortion will have a negative or weakly positive urine pregnancy test, and results may remain positive for as long as 2 weeks after fetal death. A complete blood count with differential white blood cell count and blood type is done. With persistent or considerable blood loss or in a woman already compromised by low iron stores or low hemoglobin levels, anemia may be present. Sepsis, more likely with incomplete or missed abortions, should be suspected when the white blood cell count is elevated. Serum HCG level measurements and serial sonography may help establish a diagnosis in cases of threatened or possible missed abortion. With sonography, the presence or absence of gestational sac growth in very early pregnancy and fetal movement and heart palpation after the 8th or 9th week of pregnancy can be established.

Nursing Management. Management of a woman with a threatened abortion (slight spotting, mild cramps, internal cervical os closed, no tissue passed) is noninterventionist. She is advised to rest and refrain from sexual intercourse for 2 weeks after the bleeding stops. No treatment has been shown with certainty to affect the outcome, and the number of women who have a threatened abortion and who continue the pregnancy is small. Clarke-Pearson and Dawood (1990) estimate that less than 30% of these patients have viable fetuses when first seen and that 80% will progress to abortion regardless of medical management. Refraining from intercourse will prevent additional uterine stimulation and decrease the potential introduction of infectious agents into the vagina, cervix, and uterus. Any woman with symptoms of a spontaneous abortion should be told of the possible progression of her condition and contact her health care provider promptly if the symptoms progress. She should also be instructed to save any tissue that she passes so that it can be examined. Because of the emotionally charged nature of the situation, it is best to have written information available for her to take home to supplement what she has been told during her health care visit. Her anxiety level may prevent her from hearing or understanding what is said to her. Frequent prenatal visits should be scheduled to assess uterine growth to observe for signs of missed abortion. Hematocrit levels are checked frequently to detect the development of anemia.

When increased bleeding and pain and dilatation of the internal cervical os indicate that abortion is inevitable or that an incomplete abortion has occurred, prompt evacuation of the uterus is done. Uterine size and amount of bleeding will determine the method chosen. In a complete abortion, when the uterus is well contracted, the cervix closed, and the bleeding minimal, curettage may or may not be done. RhoGam is given to all nonsensitized Rh negative women within 72 hours after abortion.

When a woman has experienced a missed abortion, she most always expels the products of conception within 3 weeks of fetal demise (Hayashi & Castillo, 1986). Current medical management is to wait 4 weeks for spontaneous resolution and then evacuate the contents of the uterus if needed. Throughout this waiting period, it is essential that maternal fibrinogen and platelet levels be followed and coagulation levels obtained, because prolonged retention of the conceptus may lead to coagulation abnormalities. Many women will not want to wait once they know that they have suffered a missed abortion; in these cases, evacuation of the uterus should be done then without waiting.

A spontaneous abortion is a crisis situation for women and their families. Unexpected vaginal bleeding always causes anxiety, and fears about reproductive capacity may surface. Feelings of guilt are common as women attempt to identify possible causes for the pregnancy loss; clients should be informed of the probable cause (when known) and any possible available treatment. If no discernible reason can be identified, they can be reassured that in the majority of cases, abortion eliminates a fetus that was defective. Reassurance can be offered that most women who experience spontaneous abortion subsequently have normal pregnancies and that women who have experienced early pregnancy losses are often highly fertile in their subsequent menstrual cycles (Wilcox et al., 1988). Based on an assumption that pregnancies conceived in the first cycle after an early pregnancy loss were at particularly high risk, current clinical practice has often been to advise women to use birth control after a spontaneous abortion. Wilcox and associates (1988) suggest that this practice should be reconsidered on the basis of their findings that pregnancies conceived in the first cycle after a pregnancy loss were not at particularly high risk. This is particularly important for older women, whose ability to conceive and maintain a pregnancy may decline with time.

The nurse assesses the client's physical status and psychological functioning. Monitoring of vital signs; assessment of amount and type of bleeding; determination of the character, type, and location of pain; and identification of potential complications are specific areas of nursing responsibility. Women are taught about the normal course of recovery for spontaneous abortion and what the danger signs are. They are instructed to report any fever, excessive or prolonged bleeding, foul-smelling discharge, or persistent back or abdominal pain. Appropriate contraceptive counseling should be provided.

Women's feelings about their pregnancy loss, their coping behaviors, the amount of anxiety or depression experienced, and where they are in the mourning process are explored with them. Each will need time to mourn, to express what she is feeling (including anger), and to talk about what has happened to her. Any feelings of grief, anger, or guilt must be worked through at her own pace. This is not a time to focus on possible future pregnancies with happier outcomes; women may feel that this is insensitive or is an attempt to minimize their grief.

Malignancy

Spotting may be a signal of cancer of the reproductive tract and the first symptom of gynecologic cancer that the woman notes. Unfortunately, spotting usually does not occur until metastasis has begun and thus is a symptom of potentially life-threatening magnitude. Screening for reproductive malignancies is discussed in Chapter 9. Chapter 27, "Chronic Illnesses and Women," discusses reproductive cancers, and Chapter 26, "Reproductive Surgery," outlines many of the surgical interventions commonly used when a woman has reproductive cancer.

Alterations in Cyclic Bleeding

Women may seek health care for a variety of alterations in their normal cyclic patterns of bleeding. These concerns are usually associated with amount, duration, interval, or irregularity.

Oligomenorrhea/Hypomenorrhea

The term *oligomenorrhea* often is used to describe decreased menstruation, either in amount or time, or both. However, oligomenorrhea more correctly refers to infrequent menstrual periods characterized by intervals of 40 to 45 days or longer, whereas hypomenorrhea refers to scanty bleeding at normal intervals. The etiology of oligomenorrhea includes many of the causes of amenorrhea in that the difference in menstrual function may be only a matter of degree.

The assessment and diagnostic approach is similar to that for amenorrhea except that tests for intactness of the vagina are not necessary. Diagnosis focuses on abnormalities of hypothalamic, pituitary, or ovarian function. Oligomenorrhea can also be physiological or part of a woman's normal pattern for the first few years after menarche or for several years before menopause (Shulman, 1990). The periods of oligomenorrhea may be interspersed with episodes of very heavy bleeding (dysfunctional uterine bleeding, discussed elsewhere in this chapter).

Treatment is aimed at reversing, if possible, the underlying cause. Alternatively, hormonal replacement therapy using progestins, with or without estrogens, is begun promptly to avoid the complications of unopposed estrogen production (endometrial hyperplasia) or of lowered estrogen (vaginal dryness, hot flashes/flushes, osteoporosis).

Important components of the nursing role when working with women experiencing menstruation characterized by prolonged intervals between cycles are education and counseling. The cause of the problem and the rationale for a specific therapeutic regimen should be discussed with the client. She can be taught how to use a BBT chart to ascertain her menstrual patterns. The preventive value and disadvantages of hormonal replacement therapy should be thoroughly discussed with the client. If a client chooses medical intervention, she should be taught how to take the medications, made aware of side effects of any drugs, and provided written instructions. (See Chapter 5 for further discussion of menopausal hormonal therapy.) Teaching and counseling emphasize the importance of the woman's keeping careful records of her vaginal bleeding.

One of the most common causes of scanty menstrual flow or hypomenorrhea is oral contraceptives (OCs). Because approximately 13.8 million women in the United States and about 60 million worldwide (Hatcher et al., 1994) are currently taking OCs, it is important that the nurse explain in advance that the use of OCs decreases menstrual flow by as much as two thirds. This effect is caused by the continuous action of the progestin component, which produces a decidualized endometrium with atrophic glands. It should be noted that implantation bleeding, or spotting that occurs about the time of implantation of a pregnancy, occurs about the time of an expected period and may be mistaken for a period of short duration. A few women continue to have menses after conception, and these are lighter and shorter than usual. Hypomenorrhea may also be caused by structural abnormalities of the endometrium or uterus that result in partial destruction of the endometrium, such as Asherman's syndrome, in which adhesions resulting from curettage or infection obliterate the endometrial cavity, or caused by congenital partial obstruction of the outflow tract.

Metrorrhagia

In the broadest sense, metrorrhagia, or intermenstrual bleeding, refers to any episode of bleeding, whether spotting, menses, or hemorrhage, that occurs at a time other than the normal menses. Mittelstaining, a small amount of bleeding or spotting that occurs at the time of ovulation (14 days prior to onset of next menses), is considered normal. The cause of mittelstaining is not known; however, it is a common occurrence that can be documented by its repetition in the menstrual cycle.

Often, intermenstrual bleeding is directly related to the contraceptive a woman uses. Women taking OCs may experience midcycle bleeding or spotting. If the contraceptive pill does not sufficiently maintain a hypoplastic endometrium, it will begin to shed, usually in small amounts at a time, a process called "breakthrough bleeding." Breakthrough bleeding is most common in the first three cycles of OCs. The lowered potency of OCs (thus enhancing their safety) has decreased the amount of available hormones, making it more important that blood levels be kept constant. Thus the suggestion that a woman take her pill at exactly the same time each day may alleviate the problem. She may establish a routine in which she takes her pill when she does some never-omitted activity, perhaps brushing her teeth. Suggesting that she double up on pills for a day or two if breakthrough bleeding occurs may also be helpful (Clark-Coller, 1991). If the spotting continues, a different formulation of OC that increases either the estrogen or progestin component can be tried (see Chapter 14 for information on oral contraception formulation). Increasing the estrogenic potency of the pill is helpful in treating spotting early in the cycle, whereas increasing the progestational potency may be useful in late cycle spotting.

Contraceptive implants, such as Norplant, which are filled with synthetic progestin, may also cause midcycle bleeding, especially in the first several cycles after implantation. Women should be advised of this and counseled to report continuation of breakthrough bleeding after the first three to six cycles to their health care provider.

Although intrauterine devices (IUDs) are not used as commonly as they have been in the past, a prevalent side effect of their use is intermenstrual bleeding. Women with an IUD may experience spotting between their periods and heavier menstrual flow. The mechanism of action of the IUD is thought to be that of a foreign body that sets up a local inflammatory process in the uterine cavity. This creates a hostile environment to the fertilized ovum, preventing implantation. An unintended side effect of this process is an endometrium that tends to become hypertrophied every month and breaks down about midcycle. Because many other conditions (e.g., infection, pregnancy, myomas) may cause midcycle bleeding, it is important to rule these out when making a decision about continued use of the IUD for contraception. If these are ruled out, the IUD can be left in place. However, because of the possibility of anemia, iron supplementation by diet or pills or both should be considered (Hatcher et al., 1994).

When a woman seeks care for intermenstrual bleeding, the nurse must always consider the possibility that the woman is, or recently has been, pregnant. Bleeding between periods can be a sign of spontaneous abortion, ectopic pregnancy, molar pregnancy, retained products of conception, or postpartum or postabortion endometritis. Other possible causes of intermenstrual bleeding include trauma, foreign objects, endocervical or uterine polyps, benign functional ovarian cysts, benign neoplasms, cervical erosion, infection, and malignancies of the reproductive tract.

A complete bleeding history as previously described in this chapter should be obtained. The nurse should ask if the woman has noticed that the bleeding is associated with any other event, such as douching or intercourse. Women are asked if they are sure the bleeding is vaginal rather than rectal.

During the physical exam, the practitioner should note carefully the quality, quantity, and source of any observed bleeding. Often, however, there is no obvious bleeding or source for the bleeding when the woman seeks care. If a diagnosis cannot be made, women are asked to return during the next episode of intermenstrual bleeding. Because many women prefer not to have a pelvic exam when they are bleeding and because they may have been told that they should not have their well-woman exam and Pap smear during their period, the nurse should emphasize the importance of their return. Even if the woman is bleeding, wet smears to examine vaginal discharge, Pap smear, and cervical cultures can be done. Biopsy of any visible lesions, ultrasound for any palpated pelvic mass, D & C, or laporascopy may also be indicated.

Treatment of intermenstrual bleeding depends on the cause and may include reassurance and education concerning mittelstaining, observation of three menstrual cycles for presumed functional ovarian cyst, adjustment of an oral contraceptive, removal of foreign bodies, or treatment for vaginal infections. More complex treatment may consist of removal of polyps; evaluation and treatment of abnormal Pap smear, including colposcopy, biopsy, cautery, cryosurgery, and/or conization and, finally, surgery; chemotherapy; and radiation treatment for malignancy. The primary roles for the nurse include education, counseling, consultation, and referral.

Menorrhagia (Hypermenorrhea)

Excessive menstrual bleeding, either in duration of flow or amount (> 80 ml) occurring at regular intervals, can cause grave distress and inconvenience. It is one of the most common of gynecologic conditions and is the reason many women visit their health care provider each year. A single episode of heavy bleeding may occur, or a woman may experience regular flooding as a pattern in which she changes tampons or pads every few hours for several days. A precise definition of menorrhagia is difficult to establish because of the wide variations of normal patterns already described. Shulman (1990) suggests that if the woman herself considers the amount or duration of bleeding to be excessive, the problem should be investigated. Hemoglobin and hematocrit provide objective indicators of actual blood loss. If bleeding necessitates changing a pad every hour for 7 days, hospitalization should be considered.

The causes of heavy menstrual bleeding are many, including hormonal disturbances, systemic disease, benign and malignant neoplasms, infection, and contraception. Often, the woman using an IUD for contraception may have heavier and longer periods because of excessive endometrial buildup and subsequent sloughing. Women with IUDs should be advised that increased bleeding is likely. This side effect may be a contraindication for IUD use for some women; however, the addition of progesterone into the IUD (Progetasert-T) has decreased the problem of menorrhagia (Hatcher et al., 1990). Women who have just discontinued OCs after several years of use may have heavier periods than the withdrawal bleeding that they recently experienced.

A single episode of heavy bleeding may signal an early pregnancy loss such as a spontaneous abortion or ectopic pregnancy. This type of bleeding is often thought to be a period that is heavier than usual, perhaps delayed, and is associated with abdominal pain or pelvic discomfort. When early pregnancy loss is suspected, a hematocrit and pregnancy test should be done. Although pregnancy tests are often done, a negative result may reflect a nonfunctioning placenta and thus no production of HCG rather than a lack of conception. Hematocrit values may be normal because the bleeding is too recent in onset to be reflected in the hematocrit.

Infectious and inflammatory processes, such as acute or chronic endometritis and salpingitis, may cause heavy menstrual bleeding. With an endometrial infection, normal endometrial clotting properties may be disturbed, resulting in painful, heavy bleeding. This may be the reason a woman with chronic infection seeks care.

Although rare, systemic diseases of nonreproductive origin also can cause hypermenorrhea. Blood dyscrasia accounts for about 20% of adolescent women who seek care for menorrhagia (Long & Gast, 1990). Among the most common diseases are von Willebrand's disease, idiopathic thrombocytopenia purpura, and prothrombin deficiency. Women with these diseases report either extraordinarily heavy flow or extended duration of flow and often have ovulatory cycles. Liver disease, such as cirrhosis, reduces the liver's ability to metabolize estrogens as well as decreases the production of fibrinogen and other coagulation factors and may cause menorrhagia. Renal disease interferes with normal excretion of estrogen and progesterone, thus disrupting normal endocrine control of menstruation.

In obese women, anovulation caused by increased peripheral conversion of androstenedione to estrogen may develop and manifest itself as menorrhagia. Medications also may cause abnormal bleeding. Chemotherapy, anticoagulants, neuroleptics, major tranquilizers, and steroid hormone therapy all have been associated with excessive flow.

Uterine leiomyomata (fibroids or myomas) are a common cause of menorrhagia. Fibroids are benign tumors of the smooth muscle of the uterus whose etiology is unknown. Although all myomas begin in the central area of the myometrium of the uterus, their location may change. Commonly, they are found in the uterine wall (intramural), protruding from the uterine cavity (submucosal), and bulging through the uterine wall (subserosal) (Jackson, 1990). Fibroids occur in 10% of white and 30% of black women by age 30; by age 50, this prevalence increases to 30% and 50%, respectively (Wallach, Hammond, Goldfarb, & Kempers, 1983). Submucosal and intramural fibroids are usually associated with heavy menses. Some women also may report pressure symptoms resulting from large myomas or ones located on the cervix or near the bladder or rectosigmoid colon. Myomas are usually found on bimanual pelvic examination. Uterine enlargement and/or irregularity with unusually firm, mobile, nontender, smooth nodules is characteristic. Sonogram may be used to obtain a baseline measurement and remeasurement in 3 to 4 months. Because bimanual examination may miss masses smaller than 5 cm, sonograms are useful when a woman's symptoms suggest myomas and none is found on a bimanual exam. A hemoglobin and hematocrit should always be done to assess the presence and extent of anemia.

Adenomyosis is another common cause of heavy menses, as well as intermenstrual or premenstrual spotting and often dysmenorrhea. Adenomyosis, or the presence of functional endometrial tissue deep in the uterine myometrium not connected with the endometrium, usually occurs in multiparous women in their 40s or 50s. This condition is often confused with fibroids or tumors of the uterus, which frequently are also present. With adenomyosis, the uterus is enlarged and may be irregular in contour and somewhat tender. However, it is rarely enlarged as much as is seen with fibroids. This condition is diagnosed only by histopathology following hysterectomy.

Other uterine growths ranging from endometrial polyps to adenocarcinoma and endometrial cancer are frequent causes of heavy menstrual bleeding as well as intermenstrual bleeding. Diagnosis is by endometrial curettage.

Treatment for menorrhagia depends on the cause of the bleeding. If the bleeding is related to contraception, the nurse can acknowledge the distress this may cause the client, present factual information and reassurance, and discuss other contraceptive options. In some instances, the woman may decide to use another contraceptive method. The degree of disability and discomfort associated with fibroids and the woman's plans for childbearing will influence treatment decisions. Most fibroids can be followed by frequent examinations to judge growth, if any, and correction of anemia, if present. Women should be warned not to use aspirin for pain relief because of its tendency to increase bleeding. Hormonal therapy may be tried in an effort to reduce the size of the tumors. If the woman wishes to have children, a myomectomy may be done. Myomectomy or removal of the tumors only is particularly difficult if multiple myomas must be removed. Most physicians consider the uterine scarring from this procedure to be an indication for future cesarean delivery. If the woman does not want to preserve her childbearing function or if she has severe symptoms (severe anemia, severe pain, considerable disruption of lifestyle), hysterectomy is often done. The treatment for adenomyosis is also surgical. Hormonal treatment does not seem to be of benefit; however, minimal disease may be treated with prostaglandin inhibitor analgesics such as ibuprofen (Motrin). Malignant disease always requires a staging workup and extensive therapy.

Dysfunctional Uterine Bleeding

Dysfunctional uterine bleeding (DUB), or abnormal endometrial bleeding without demonstrable organic pathology, is associated with a wide variety of menstrual irregularities, most often excessive bleeding of some type: too frequent flow, too heavy flow, too prolonged flow, or irregularities. DUB is most frequently caused by anovulation. When there is no luteinizing hormonal surge or if there is not sufficient progesterone produced by the corpus luteum to support the endometrium, it will begin to involute and shed. This most often occurs at the extremes of a woman's reproductive years—when the menstrual cycle is just becoming established at menarche or when it draws to a close at menopause. (See Chapter 3 for further information on this topic.)

Although estrogen breakthrough bleeding, in which the endometrium is continually stimulated by estrogen in the absence of progesterone, is most commonly seen in perimenarcheal teenagers and perimenopausal women, it can be seen with any condition that gives rise to chronic anovulation associated with continuous estrogen production. Such conditions include obesity, hyper- and hypothyroidism, polycystic ovarian syndrome, and any of the endocrine conditions discussed in the sections on amenorrhea and oligomenorrhea.

DUB is a diagnosis of exclusion (Clark-Coller, 1991) and is diagnosed only when all other causes of abnormal bleeding have been ruled out. Once the diagnosis has been made, therapy is begun, following five principles: (a) control of bleeding, (b) prevention of recurrence, (c) preservation of fertility, (d) correction of any coexisting conditions, and (e) establishment of ovulation in women wishing to have children. If the bleeding is severe, a physician is notified immediately. If possible, the nurse should obtain a complete initial database and assessment as previously described in this chapter. Hormonal therapy is the preferred treatment for DUB (Speroff et al., 1989). If uterine bleeding has been extensive or the woman has been taking oral or intramuscular progestins, the endometrium is apt to be shallow and atrophic and thus unable to form decidual tissue. In this case, the treatment is Premarin, 25 mg intravenously every 4 hours until bleeding stops or slows significantly (Clark-Coller, 1991). This is also the appropriate treatment for a woman who may not return or be able to return for additional visits.

In most cases, unless the woman is taking OCs or has exceptionally heavy bleeding, she probably has sufficient endometrium to form a pseudodecidual layer. Treatment should then be intensive progestin-estrogen combination therapy, such as OCs four times a day for 7 days (Clark-Coller, 1991). Once the acute phase has passed, the woman is maintained on cyclic, low-dose OCs for at least 3 months. If she wishes contraception, she should remain on OCs. If she has no need for contraception, the treatment is progestin therapy, such as Provera, 10 mg each day, for 10 days prior to the expected date of her menstrual period. Women on this therapy should be treated on a long-term basis so that they do not have persistent anovulation (Clark-Coller, 1991); this will prevent chronic unopposed endogenous estrogen hyperstimulation of the endometrium, which can result in eventual atypical tissue changes. Such long-term treatment also will help prevent recurrence of the pattern of dysfunctional uterine bleeding and hemorrhage.

D & C may be done to control severe bleeding and hemorrhage. An endometrial biopsy may be collected at the same time to evaluate endometrial tissue or rule out endometrial cancer. If the recurrent, heavy bleeding is not controlled by hormonal therapy or D & C, ablation of the endometrium through laser treatment may be performed. Nursing roles are informing clients of their options, counseling and educating as indicated, and referring clients to the appropriate specialists and health care services.

Menopausal/Postmenopausal Bleeding

Abnormal vaginal bleeding in the perimenopausal woman can be caused by complications of pregnancy, organic lesions, systemic diseases, side effects of drugs, and hormonal disorders. Although pregnancy is less common in women over the age of 40, the incidence of spontaneous abortion and other complications of pregnancy is increased and should be considered when a woman over 40 presents with abnormal bleeding. In addition, neoplasms, infections, systemic diseases, and hormonal disorders may also cause bleeding in the perimenopausal woman.

Any bleeding 6 months or more after menopause should be considered a serious symptom and pathological until proved otherwise because of the association of such bleeding with endometrial, ovarian, or cervical cancer. Malignancies always must be suspected in this age group and ruled out (see Chapter 27). Other etiologies include vaginitis, polyps, cervical pathology, and vulvitis. Often, postmenopausal bleeding is secondary to an atrophic endometrium from low estrogen levels (see Chapter 3). Another cause of postmenopausal bleeding is injudicious use of menopausal hormonal therapy (see Chapter 5 for a discussion of this issue).

Diagnosis of bleeding in menopausal and postmenopausal women incorporates a complete physical exam, with particular attention to indicators of chronic disease. Pap smears, cone biopsy, hysteroscopy, or hysterosalpingography are frequently used diagnostic tools (Connell, 1989). If histological studies show atypical endometrial hyperplasia, the D & C and Pap smear should be repeated in 3 months.

Pain

Among the most common gynecologic symptoms that women have is pain in the pelvic area and is one for which women frequently seek care. It can be transitory and benign in nature, or it can signal a serious, possibly life-threatening pathology. Gynecologic pain can be acute, chronic, or cyclic in nature.

For many women, pain associated with the reproductive organs may be particularly frightening because of its double significance: reproductive and sexual. Women may fear that they will be unable to fulfill reproductive or sexual functions and this fear influences pain perception. For example, the early cramps of a spontaneous abortion may be felt as excruciating pain because of their additional significance—loss of a pregnancy.

Cultural norms are significant influences on an individual's reactions to and expectations of pain, as are moral and religious teaching. The traditional view that women must suffer in childbirth has both a religious foundation and a moralistic message that a woman's lot is to suffer. Thus anticipation of pain as unavoidable in childbirth is a learned response.

Common Causes

Acute pelvic pain is sudden and new in onset. Chronic pain is well established and burning or aching in nature. Cyclic pain is intermittent and occurs repetitively and predictably in a certain phase of the menstrual cycle.

It is often difficult to determine the origin or cause of pelvic pain; women may have difficulty describing or localizing it; the site identified by women may not be the source of the pain but its referred site; and the meaning pain has for an individual influences her ability to describe pain. Pain can originate from two primary sources: One source is cutaneous and muscle innervations involving nerve fibers, responsible for acute pain and often described as stinging, pinprick, or knifelike. Often the woman can locate this pain with some accuracy. Pain of this type may originate in the labia, vagina, or abdominal wall. Another source of pain is visceral innervations involving C fibers, responsible for the burning and aching that are usually characteristic of chronic pain. Often, pain originating in C fibers is referred pain; thus pain originating in the ovaries, fallopian tubes, uterus, or bladder may be experienced directly or referred to other sites, such as the back, abdomen, or thighs. Furthermore, although the parenchyma of internal organs is not supplied with pain receptors, the arterial wall and peritoneum contain a rich network of nerve fibers. Pain from the fundus of the uterus is most commonly referred to the hypogastrium and is experienced as midline abdominal pain. Pain from the cervix is felt as pain in the lower back and sacral area and may also be transmitted to the hypogastrium or radiate down the leg. Pain originating in the ovarian area is very difficult to interpret because of the intercommunication of the ovarian and pelvic nerve plexuses and the variability of ovarian location. Usually, the ovarian parenchyma is insensitive to pain, and ovarian pain is a late manifestation caused by stretching of the surrounding peritoneum or vascular structures (Litcher & Warfield, 1985). Painful stimuli from the bladder is experienced in the lower abdomen from the umbilicus to groin or lower sacral area or buttocks. The client may also experience pain in these sites from causes other than gynecologic ones, which underscores the need for a meticulous assessment.

Although much of the gynecologic pain experienced by women is associated with menstruation and reproduction (e.g., dysmenorrhea, mittelschmerz, and ectopic pregnancy), other common causes of gynecologic pain include endometriosis and infectious processes. Among the most common infections are sexually transmitted diseases (STDs) (discussed in Chapter 24), toxic shock syndrome, and urinary tract infections. Premenstrual syndrome (PMS) also involves considerable gynecologic discomfort and disruption for many women. In addition, pain may be associated with some of the conditions explored previously in the discussion of bleeding (e.g., spontaneous abortion, adenomyosis, and myomas).

General Assessment

At times, the source of gynecologic pain is obvious, as in the client who presents with severe perineal pain associated with the ulcerations and excoriation of genital herpes; more frequently, however, the source is less obvious. A meticulous assessment that includes a careful history, thorough physical examination, and indicated laboratory studies is essential.

History

Careful history taking is perhaps the most critical component of assessing gynecologic pain. A number of questions should be asked each time a client reports gynecologic pain (Table 23.5).

The onset or way the pain begins often suggests its cause. Pain that begins suddenly and reaches intensity rapidly suggests perforation, rupture, or ischemia (for example, rupture of an ectopic pregnancy or abruptio placentae). Pain that begins gradually and develops over several days and weeks or pain for which an exact time of onset cannot be determined is more apt to be the result of obstruction, infection, inflammation, or congestion. Examples of this type of pain are chronic pelvic inflammatory disease, endometriosis, and dysmenorrhea.

The location of the pain can indicate the location of the pathological process. Unilateral lower quadrant pain may indicate an ectopic pregnancy, ovarian cyst, or mittelschmerz. Cystitis is experienced often as suprapubic pain. Pelvic tumors may cause midabdominal or lower back pain. Infectious processes cause pain that is often bilateral and involves the entire abdomen.

Clients are asked to describe their pain in their own words. Adjectives commonly used to describe gynecologic pain are shown in Table 23.6.

The duration and cyclical nature of some gynecologic pain can also suggest its cause. Pelvic pain that has an acute onset and rapid progression may result from a sudden event, such as rupture of a tubo-ovarian abscess, ectopic pregnancy, or ovarian cyst. On the other

Table 23.5 Gynecologic Pain Assessment

Characteristic	*Questions to Be Asked*
Onset	When did the pain first occur? How did the pain begin—suddenly or gradually? Did it wake you up from sleep? What were you doing when it first began? When it first began, was it related to exercise, activity, eating or not eating, specific food, medication, injury, trauma, coitus, menses, urination, or bowel movements? Does its recurrence relate to any of these? What was relation of onset to your menstrual cycle?
Location	Exactly where is the pain? Is it localized or does it radiate? If it radiates, to where? Is it internal or external? Deep or on the surface?
Character	What type of pain is it?
Frequency	Is the pain constant or intermittent? If intermittent, how often does the pain come?
Duration	How long does the pain last?
Intensity	Is the pain mild, moderate, or severe? Is it incapacitating? Can you carry out your normal daily activities when you have this pain? Do you have to stay in bed?
History of pain	Have you ever had this type of pain before, and, if so, how often? Has it been getting better or worse, or has it changed in any way since you first had it or since the last time you had the pain?
Relief measures	What do you do for the pain when you have it? Does this help? To what extent? Have you ever seen a health care provider for the pain? What was the previous diagnosis? What was the previous treatment, if any? Was this helpful? effective?
Associated symptoms	Are there any symptoms that occur before, during, or after the pain, such as nausea, vomiting, diarrhea, constipation, vaginal discharge or bleeding, or urinary frequency, urgency, or burning?

Table 23.6 Character of Gynecologic Pain

Cramping	This is intermittent, short-term, poorly localized pain indicating congestion, obstruction, irritation, or inflammation.
Sharp	This is intense, stabbing wavelike pain that may be characterized by cycles of intense pain followed by pain-free or dull, aching intervals. Location can often be pinpointed. Pain is often associated with neoplasms, thrombosis, and urethral stones.
Burning	This pain may be associated with a feeling of heat; it is often acute and may be caused by mucosal irritation (e.g., of the bladder or urethra). Pain may be present with many vaginal infections.
Aching	This is dull, continuous, steady pain that may be generalized and fluctuate in severity. Congestion, muscle spasm, and swelling may cause this type of pain.
Throbbing	This is a pulsing sensation, a regular waxing and waning of painful feeling. It is seen with infections, inflammation, and arterial spasms.
Fullness	This is a feeling of bloating or distention that may be experienced with conditions such as premenstrual tension syndrome.

NOTE: Women should be asked to describe their pain in their own words, as specifically as possible. Their choice of words will reflect their vocabulary and educational level, what they think is the cause of the pain, level of medical knowledge and understanding, and prior experience with pain.

hand, pain that is more chronic and is present for 3 months or more may represent pelvic inflammatory disease, adenomyosis, or endometriosis. Pain that occurs only at time of menses may be attributable to dysmenorrhea.

Intensity or severity of pain is not an accurate indication of the seriousness of a condition, because individuals differ greatly in their perception and communication of pain. It is important to ask how much interference with normal activities the pain causes. Interference with sleep patterns also can give clues to the severity of the pain as can the type of pain relief measures being used and their level of success.

It is important to explore with the client what precipitates pain, what makes it worse, and what relieves or diminishes it. These factors may assist in determining the etiology of the pain. For example, if a client reports that constipation makes her pain worse, she may have endometriosis that has seeded on the bowel. It is also important to ask about urinary and bowel habits. For example, pain that occurs during or after urination and is accompanied by frequency or hematuria is usually the result of urinary tract infection; pelvic pain associated with a history of diarrhea, constipation, nausea, vomiting, or mucus in the stools tends to suggest the gastrointestinal tract as the source of the pain.

The woman's age may provide pertinent clues to the nature of her problem. Although congenital anomalies of the reproductive tract associated with an outflow obstruction, such as imperforate hymen or blind uterine horn, manifest themselves with pain at menarche or soon after, the majority of problems causing pelvic pain occur during childbearing years. These problems are commonly related to sexual activity, contraceptive practices, and maturation of endometrial and ovarian function. Gynecologic malignancies usually occur later in life, during the perimenopausal and postmenopausal years.

Attention should be paid to the client's reproductive and menstrual history. Her obstetric history may suggest the etiology of her pain. A history of chronic pelvic pain with regularly occurring menses and intercourse without contraception, but with no pregnancies having occurred in 1 to 2 years, suggests conditions such as chronic pelvic inflammatory disease or endometriosis. Acute abdominal pain following one or two missed periods should be evaluated immediately for a potential ectopic pregnancy. Determination of the date of the client's last normal menstrual period is important in formulating a possible diagnosis. For example, a woman with a history of regular menstrual periods and amenorrhea for 1 or 2 months and with pelvic pain may be pregnant. The client should be asked when the pain occurs in relation to menstrual flow. Pain occurring about midcycle suggests mittelschmerz, whereas pain occurring after menstrual flow may be related to salpingitis. Menstruation may exacerbate chronic pelvic inflammatory disease: Pain associated with endometriosis often begins in the second half of the cycle.

A sexual history may suggest an origin of the gynecologic pain. Pain that occurs with vaginal penetration may be related to infection or inflammation of the vulva or vagina. Endometriosis, tumors, and pelvic inflammatory disease can cause deep pelvic pain associated with deep penetration during intercourse.

The client's past medical and surgical history is explored to ascertain whether prior illness or surgery is responsible for current pain. For example, abdominal or pelvic surgery or pain after acute appendicitis with rupture might suggest pelvic adhesions, whereas a history of gonorrhea or chlamydia might suggest pelvic inflammatory disease. Often, women do not know the specific names of previous problems but can remember their symptoms or how they were treated. Asking them to describe how they felt and what the health care provider did may yield valuable information. Ask when they had their last Pap smear, if they have had any abnormal Pap smears, and if so, what, if any, follow-up or treatment they received.

Finally, the woman's current lifestyle and recent changes and stressors should be noted. The nurse should assess the client's current level of stress and professional and personal circumstances, because stressful situations can be translated into somatic distress.

Physical Examination

Vital signs are always taken: Temperature elevations indicate infection or inflammation, and rapid pulse and respiration are associated with fever as well as with extreme anxiety or severe pain. Hypotension and tachycardia are clues to acute blood loss; when associated with fever, they may indicate a ruptured tubo-ovarian abscess. Blood pressure and pulse should be taken with postural changes: Although they may be stable in the supine position, they may be altered precipitously when the patient is upright. Alterations in blood pressure may signal shock associated with hemorrhage, as when an ectopic pregnancy ruptures. Color of palpebral conjunctiva, nail beds, and palmar surfaces can provide a rough assessment of red cell volume and possible hemorrhage.

An abdominal examination is always done. The contour is noted because distension may occur as abnormal fluid in the peritoneal cavity causes elevation and dilation of loops of the bowel. Careful observation of the abdomen may also reveal the outline of a distinct mass. Auscultation is performed, and the presence or absence of bowel sounds as well as their quality, if present, is noted. Percussion will give valuable information about the presence of an abdominal mass or fluid.

During the abdominal assessment, any areas of tenderness, rigidity, or guarding are noted, and a pelvic and rectal examination is done. Gentleness is essential when doing the pelvic exam. It must be remembered that the client is already uncomfortable, and the necessary examinations may add to discomfort. The external genitalia are inspected for concurrent disease and the presence of blood or purulent discharge in the introitus. Using an unlubricated, warm speculum, the vagina is inspected for mucosal abnormalities, fistulae, bleeding, or discharge. The cervix is inspected for presence of tissue in the os, purulent discharge, blood, or IUD strings. During the bimanual examination, any areas of tenderness, masses, thickening, and fullness are noted. Cervical tenderness on gentle movement (Chandelier's sign) associated with adnexal fullness or masses suggests an infectious process, twisted adnexa, or ectopic pregnancy. During the bimanual exam, palpation of the uterus is done to determine the size, shape, contour, consistency, and position in the pelvis and whether pain is elicited during the examination. Uterine tenderness is often associated with endometriosis.

The adnexa are assessed for pain and masses. If a mass is located, is it fixed, mobile, firm, tender, defined, or diffuse? Examination of the adnexa is done gently and carefully to avoid rupturing any cystic masses present. At times, a distinct mass cannot be felt, but rather the adnexal areas feel thickened, as when they are chronically inflamed. A rectal examination may reveal masses not detected vaginally. The displacement of the uterus and status of the uterosacral ligaments can be assessed during the rectal examination, during which time the presence of tumors and stool blood also may be checked.

Laboratory Studies

When indicated, various laboratory tests may be performed to provide additional data. Complete blood counts are often ordered. An elevated white count may indicate infections such as pelvic inflammatory disease, whereas a lowered hematocrit and hemoglobin may suggest a ruptured ectopic pregnancy. An elevated erythrocyte sedimentation rate may suggest pelvic inflammatory disease. A clean-catch urine is always collected when there is any suggestion of urinary tract infection; indeed, the nurse may want to incorporate such collection as part of the routine assessment of all clients who present with gynecologic pain.

Dysmenorrhea

Dysmenorrhea is one of the most common gynecologic problems of women, yet considerable confusion exists as to what exactly it is (Brown & Woods, 1984). Although the literal translation of the Greek term is "difficult menstruation," it is more commonly defined as painful menses or uterine cramping. Beyond this, definitions differ as to when dysmenorrhea pain occurs, how it should be classified, and how encompassing it is.

Almost all women have some indication or awareness that their period is about to start (e.g., a sense of pelvic fullness or slight discomfort); this awareness is not necessarily perceived as pain and is not considered to be dysmenorrhea. Symptoms of dysmenorrhea generally begin with menstruation, although some women will experience symptoms for several hours before the onset of flow. The symptoms may persist for several hours or several days. The range and severity of symptoms vary widely from woman to woman, and from month to month in the same woman. The pain is located in the suprapubic or lower abdomen and is described either as sharp, gripping, and cramping or as a steady dull ache. It may be accompanied by feelings of pelvic fullness and radiate to the lower back or upper thighs. Many women also experience systemic symptoms, including nausea and vomiting, bloating or fluid retention, headache, diarrhea, fatigue, dizziness or fainting, and nervousness.

Usually, dysmenorrhea is differentiated as primary or secondary. Primary dysmenorrhea, also labeled idiopathic, intrinsic, essential, or functional, traditionally has been defined as dysmenorrhea that occurs in the absence of anatomical abnormalities of pelvic pathology. This definition is no longer accurate, however, in view of recent research that has demonstrated that primary dysmenorrhea has a biochemical basis and the current understanding that the majority of primary dysmenorrhea is caused by abnormal uterine activity resulting from an excessive production of uterine prostaglandin stimulation. With full maturation of the ova, estrogen and progesterone are secreted, and this uterine hormonal environment promotes prostaglandin synthesis. In dysmenorrheic women, the prostaglandins stimulate increased activity of the myometrium, with consequent increased baseline tone and greater frequency and intensity of uterine contractions. The increase in uterine contractions with resulting vasospasm of the uterine arterioles leads to tissue ischemia and thus the cramping pain of primary dysmenorrhea (Avant, 1988; Sullivan, 1990; Treybig, 1989). Systemic effects of prostaglandins produce many of the symptoms commonly associated with primary dysmenorrhea—gastrointestinal disturbances, headache, flushing, and syncope. It is not clear whether dysmenorrheic women are more sensitive to normal levels of prostaglandins or synthesize more prostaglandins.

Thus although primary dysmenorrhea is not a normal condition, it does not have a pathological etiology; rather, a physiological alteration occurs. Primary dysmenorrhea usually develops within 6 to 12 months of menarche when ovulatory function is established. For the most part, anovualtory bleeding, common in the first few months or years after menarche, is painless. Both estrogen and progesterone are necessary for primary dysmenorrhea and thus it is found only with ovulatory cycles. Typically, women report painless irregular cycles initially followed in 6 to 12 months by ovulation and then regular menses and dysmenorrhea.

Secondary dysmenorrhea is acquired menstrually related pain that develops later in life, often after age 25. It is caused by pathology such as pelvic inflammatory disease, endometrial polyps, submucous or interstitial myomas, endometriosis, use of an intrauterine device, or adenomyosis (see Table 23.7). The pain associated with secondary dysmenorrhea can be differentiated from that of primary dysmenorrhea. The pain often starts a few days before menses begins, may be present at ovulation and continue through the first days of menses, or may begin after menstrual flow has begun. It may be present throughout most of the menstrual cycle, and the woman may experience a similar pain with intercourse. It is often characterized by dull, lower abdominal aching radiating to back or lower thighs and may be associated with feelings of bloating or pelvic fullness.

Although more than 50% of women report discomfort associated with menses, and 10% to 17% report severe dysmenorrhea (Avant, 1988; Busch, Costa, Whitehead, & Heller, 1988), the extent to which dysmenorrhea disrupts women's lives is difficult to assess; however, it has been estimated that 10% of women who experience dysmenorrhea will be incapacitated for 1 to 3 days each month (Avant, 1988) and that 600 million work hours are lost annually in the United States because of absenteeism from dysmenorrhea (Dawood, 1986). There is no doubt that dysmenorrhea is a serious health problem for some women; however, the incidence and implication of dysmenorrhea must be documented by accurate research. In addition, the social and economic effect of dysmenorrhea on productivity (compared with the common cold or lower back pain) need further study.

Assessment

A careful menstrual history and detailed description of the woman's pain as described earlier in the chapter are essential in obtaining an accurate diagnosis. For example, women who describe an onset of dysmenorrhea within 2 years after menarche are more apt to have primary dysmenorrhea, whereas women who describe menstrual pain that started later in life and increased in intensity are more likely to have an organic cause for their dysmenorrhea.

It is important for the nurse to note what form of contraceptive the client is using, because this may affect cramping. For example, the IUD is often associated with sudden, severe cramps. The client's reproductive history also is significant; cervical lacerations, infections, and gynecologic procedures all can predispose one to secondary dysmenorrhea. Often, primary dysmenorrhea diminishes or resolves completely following pregnancy, whereas painful menstrual periods associated with infertility suggest endometriosis or pelvic inflammatory disease.

The client should be asked about the extent to which dysmenorrhea causes disruption of her life: Can she continue with her usual daily activities or must she be in bed? How long the pain lasts and what seems to relieve it (and for how long) should be determined. The nurse should inquire about any other symptoms the woman experiences.

A complete physical examination is necessary to rule out pathological causes of dysmenorrhea. Pelvic exam findings in women with

Table 23.7 Causes of Dysmenorrhea

Cause	*Symptoms*	*History*	*Physical Examination*	*Laboratory Finding*
Physiological (prostaglandin)	Cramping pain, radiates to thighs and lower back Nausea and vomiting Headache/dizziness	Onset within 2 years of menarche Pain decreases with age Relief after pregnancy	Normal findings	None significant
Endometriosis	Aching, constant pain Pain before menses and persists after flow Abnormal vaginal bleeding	Dyspareunia Infertility Years of pain-free menses	Fixed, retroverted tender, nodular uterus Nodular, tender uterosacral ligaments	None significant
Pelvic inflammatory disease	Pelvic pain, fever, vaginal discharge Pain begins after flow begins May be sudden or insidious onset	History of pelvic pain, discharge Painless menses in past	Uterus fixed Uterosacral ligaments nontender	Elevated white blood cell count Adnexal mass
Leiomyoma of uterus	Menorrhagia Passage of clots Cramping pain with menses Bladder pressure, fullness	Dysmenorrhea usually develops after adolescence	Enlarged uterus Palpable spherical abnormalities	Anemia associated with menorrhagia
Adenomyosis	Menorrhagia with pain	Usually begins during 40s or 50s Pain pattern similar to endometriosis	Uterus boggy, tender	Possible anemia

NOTE: Dysmenorrhea has a number of etiologies, both physiological and pathological. An understanding of the causes of dysmenorrhea assists the nurse in assessment of the woman with this problem.

primary dysmenorrhea are normal. In contrast, women with secondary dysmenorrhea will have significant pelvic findings characteristic of their specific pathology. For example, the woman with fibroids will have an enlarged, possibly irregularly shaped uterus, whereas the woman who has endometriosis may have nodular thickening of the uterosacral ligaments or a fixed, retroflexed uterus.

Laboratory studies provide relatively little information in assessing dysmenorrhea because no specific laboratory test exists for dysmenorrhea. If secondary dysmenorrhea is suspected, however, appropriate laboratory tests may provide additional information.

Nursing Management

The management of dysmenorrhea is multifaceted and depends on the severity of the problem and the individual woman's response. The extent to which her activities must be curtailed because of dysmenorrhea and the presence of organic pathology will guide the types of interventions needed. Important aspects of care for the client with dysmenorrhea are information and support. An integral component of the alleviation of menstrual distress is education to facilitate positive attitudes. Nurses can do much to correct misinformation, provide facts about what is normal, and support their clients' feelings of positive sexuality and self-worth. Several alternatives for alleviating menstrual discomfort and dysmenorrhea may be suggested. The client thus can explore alternatives and decide which ones work best for her.

Nonpharmacological Treatments. Women with mild symptoms who wish to avoid medication may choose to try nonpharmacological remedies. Other women may elect to use such remedies in conjunction with medication to decrease the dosage needed to relieve the pain. These remedies are often very effective in minimizing menstrual distress; the individual client will need to find out which ones work best for her. Heat minimizes cramping, although it may not totally eliminate it, by increasing vasodilation and muscle relaxation, thus minimizing uterine ischemia. Many women find a heating pad, hot water bottle, or hot bath to be effective.

The beneficial effects of exercise in relieving the discomforts of dysmenorrhea are attributed to increased vasodilation and consequent decreased ischemia; release of endogenous opiates, specifically beta endorphins, during exercise, which can decrease pain perception; suppression of prostaglandins; and/or the shunting of blood flow away from the viscera, resulting in less pelvic congestion (Gannon, 1988; Israel, Sutton, & O'Brien, 1985; Treybig, 1989). Specific exercises suggested include those for the lower back, including the pelvic rock and plough supine yoga position ("heels over head"). In the plough position, the woman lies on her back, raises her straightened legs over her head as far as possible without discomfort, holds for 5 seconds, relaxes, and repeats.

Massaging of the lower back may reduce pain by relaxing the paravertebral muscles and increasing pelvic blood supply. Effleurage, a soft rhythmic rubbing of the abdomen in a circular motion, is often effective; it provides a distraction and alternate focal point. For some women, strong manual pressure on the abdomen is more successful. Biofeedback techniques, progressive relaxation, meditation, and Hatha Yoga also have been used successfully to decrease menstrual discomfort (Sullivan, 1990). To massage the lumbar spine, the woman brings her knees to her chest, chin to chest, wraps her arms around her knees, and gently rocks forward and backward on her spine.

Although maintenance of good nutrition at all times is essential for menstruating women, dietary changes may be helpful in decreasing some of the symptoms associated with dsymenorrhea. Decreasing sodium and refined sugar intake in the week or 10 days prior to menses may help reduce fluid retention. Natural diuretics such as asparagus, cranberry juice, watercress, parsley, peaches, and watermelon may also help decrease water retention, and avoiding excessive intake of red meats as a protein source may minimize dysmenorrhea symptoms. A diet high in fiber may help to prevent constipation, which may make menstrual symptoms worse. Dietary fat has been linked to prostaglandin levels and plasma estrogen levels. In a study of women with primary dysmenorrhea, symptoms decreased when they switched from a high-fat to a low-fat diet (Jones, 1987).

Pharmacological Agents. The current therapy for primary dysmenorrhea is focused on medications that are prostaglandin synthesis inhibitors, primarily nonsteroidal anti-inflammatory drugs (NSAIDs) (see Table 23.8). All NSAIDs have potential side effects; gastrointestinal side effects, including nausea, vomiting, and indigestion, are common. All women taking NSAIDs are instructed to report dark colored stools, as this may be an indication of gastrointestinal bleeding. Women with a history of aspirin sensitivity or allergy should avoid all NSAIDs. If the first NSAID prescribed does not relieve dysmenorrhea, a second one is prescribed. If the second drug is unsuccessful after a 4-month trial, OC therapy is often considered.

OCs inhibit ovulation and can decrease the amount of menstrual flow, which can decrease the amount of prostaglandin and thus decrease dysmenorrhea. OCs are often used in place of NSAIDs if the woman wishes oral contraception and has primary dysmenorrhea. Combination OCs with low estrogen-to-progestin ratio are reported to be more effective in relieving dysmenorrhea (Treybig, 1989). It should be remembered that OCs have side effects and that women not needing them or wanting them may not wish to use them for dysmenorrhea. OCs also may be contraindicated for some women (see Chapter 14).

Prior to the development of NSAIDs, numerous drugs were used to treat dysmenorrhea, including narcotics, antispasmodics, tranquilizers, and diuretics. Due to their potential harmful effects or undocumented effectiveness, these should no longer be used for the treatment of dysmenorrhea.

Over-the-counter preparations specifically for dysmenorrhea are generally less effective than

Table 23.8 Medications Used to Treat Dysmenorrhea

Drug	*Dosage*[a]	*Side effects*[b]	*Comments*
Aspirin	600-1200 mg 4 times a day (qid) to 5 gm	Gastrointestinal irritation Tinnitus with excess dosage	Does not reduce prostaglandin synthesis very much; usefulness limited
Fenoprofen (Nalfon)	300-600 mg qid to 2,400 mg	Nausea and vomiting, dyspepsia, constipation	
Ibuprofen (Motrin, Advil)	400-600 mg qid to 2,400 mg	Nausea, dyspepsia	Most commonly used Effective with minimal side effects. Take with meals.
Indomethacin (Indocin)	25-50 mg 3 times a day (tid) to 200 mg	Nausea dyspepsia, gastric irritation	Not as effective, side effects more likely. Take with meals.
Mefenamic acid (Ponstel)	500 mg initially, then 250 mg qid	Few reported	Very effective; potent prostaglandin synthesis inhibitor and antagonizes already formed prostaglandin
Naproxen (Anaprox, Naprosyn)	250-500 mg 2 times a day (bid) to 1 gm	Nausea, constipation, abdominal distress, dyspepsia	

NOTES: a. Dosages are current recommendations and should be verified before use.
b. Risk with all NSAIDs is gastrointestinal ulceration and possible bleeding.

prescription NSAIDs in doses above 200 mg. Some of the preparations have weak amounts of the same ingredients, especially aspirin. For example, Midol has an analgesic and NSAID (aspirin), caffeine, and another ingredient (cinnamedrine). In general, these medications are probably less effective than plain aspirin (Sullivan, 1990). Preparations containing acetaminophen rather than aspirin are even less effective, because acetaminophen does not have the antiprostaglandin properties of aspirin.

Mittelschmerz

Many women experience cyclic lower abdominal pain or discomfort associated with ovulation or mittelschmerz. The source of the pain is thought to be increased intrafollicular pressure prior to rupture or leakage of small amounts of follicular fluid or blood into the peritoneal cavity during ovulation itself. Although the pain may be sharp initially, ordinarily it is dull and aching in character and transient in nature, lasting less than 24 hours. Many women experience it every month to a mild degree, some only when they ovulate from one ovary more than the other and some never. When present, the pain is a reasonably reliable indicator of ovulation. Some women report an associated pinkish discharge (mittelstaining) occurring at the same time. The discomfort is rarely incapacitating and resolves spontaneously.

Endometriosis

Endometriosis is a common disease in women that can seriously interfere with well-being and enjoyment of life. It can cause severe discomfort and may be extremely debilitating. Women with endometriosis may have dysmenorrhea, dyspareunia, chronic noncyclic pelvic pain, and abnormal vaginal bleeding, including premenstrual spotting and DUB. Many women also report bowel symptoms, including diarrhea, pain with defecation, and constipation secondary to avoiding defecation because of the pain. Endometriosis has received much attention in recent years, primarily because of its relationship with infertility and spontaneous abortion. Chapter 25 discusses this gynecologic condition.

Ectopic Pregnancy

Ectopic pregnancy can be an extremely serious pregnancy complication, primarily because of hemorrhage. It is the leading cause of maternal death in the first trimester and accounts for 6% to 11% of all pregnancy-related deaths (Wardell, 1989). The risks associated with ectopic pregnancy include future problems delivering a live infant, increased probability of subsequent ectopic pregnancies, and infertility (Wardell, 1989). When implantation of the blastocyst occurs outside the endometrial cavity (ectopic pregnancy), pain often occurs. Trophoblastic invasion of the tubal wall results in lower abdominal or pelvic pain, which is first experienced as a dull ache and changes to a sharp localized pain as the pregnancy progresses. Tubal rupture is then imminent. Following tubal rupture, the pain is temporarily relieved; however, generalized abdominal and pelvic pain of increasing severity develops as blood flows into the peritoneum.

Ectopic pregnancy occurs when normal implantation of the fertilized ovum is interfered with. Although implantation may occur in a variety of abnormal sites, 97% occur in the fallopian tube. Among tubal implantations, the majority occur in the ampulla, the usual site of fertilization. Factors such as salpingitis or pelvic inflammatory disease, previous abdominal or tubal surgery, or congenital anomalies and benign tubal tumors that narrow the lumen of the fallopian tube, allowing upward migration of sperm but blocking transportation of the larger fertilized ovum, are common causes of ectopic pregnancies. Occasionally, an ectopic pregnancy may be a complication of tubal ligation, particularly if the procedure involved extensive destruction. More than 50% of ectopic pregnancies occur in fallopian tubes that are apparently anatomically and histologically normal (Clarke-Pearson & Dawood, 1990) and result from a disturbance in tubal physiology on a hormonal or neurological basis.

The incidence of ectopic pregnancies increased threefold between 1970 and 1987 (Ellerbrock, Atrash, Hogue, & Hughes, 1987; Nederlof, Laswon, Saftlos, Altrush, & Finch, 1989) related in part to a concurrent rise in pelvic inflammatory disease and an increase in the number of chlamydial infections. Risk for ectopic pregnancy is greater in nonwhite women and increases with age for women of all races; the highest rates occur in women aged 35 to 44 years (Horton, 1992). Other risk factors, such as past IUD use, lower genital tract infections, pelvic surgery, and post-abortion infection, are all probably associated with ectopic pregnancy through their relationship to pelvic infection (Horton, 1992).

Assessment

Women with an ectopic pregnancy most often seek care before the 12th week of gestation, and their symptoms differ depending on whether the tube is intact or ruptured. Usually, the woman with an unruptured ectopic pregnancy describes lower abdominal pain (often unilateral) and spotting or slight bleeding. The pain can be intermittent over several days, vague, and cramping or can progress rapidly with increasing severity. She may have a history of recent amenorrhea and suspected pregnancy or she may interpret the initial bleeding as a delayed menstrual period. About one fourth of women with diagnosed ectopic pregnancy have no history of amenorrhea (Jackson, 1990). The woman may have signs and symptoms of early pregnancy. If the ectopic pregnancy has ruptured, the client presents with severe, generalized abdominal pain, referred shoulder pain secondary to intra-abdominal bleeding, vertigo, fainting, and shock.

Although diagnosis of an ectopic pregnancy is sometimes clinically obvious, more often considerable ambiguity exists in the presenting picture. Many other conditions may present with similar physical findings (Table 23.9). The diagnosis of ectopic pregnancy should be considered in every woman of childbearing years who presents with lower abdominal pain and/or unusual vaginal bleeding. Ask the client about possible risk factors, such as smoking, and any predisposing history (e.g., previous pelvic inflammatory disease or chlamydial infection), and ask her to describe her symptoms in detail. Presence of referred pain, such as shoulder pain; symptoms associated with bleeding, such as fatigue and dizziness; and increase in pain should be noted because these suggest progression of the condition. A menstrual history is necessary, including what is normal for the woman and any recent variations she has noticed.

Traditional findings during physical examination include a normal or slightly softened or enlarged uterus with unilateral adnexal tenderness. However, abdominal tenderness is not always present, although rebound tenderness may be found. At times, physical exam findings may resemble more closely those of an early intrauterine pregnancy or a normal nonpregnant examination.

Pregnancy tests and sonograms are the most useful laboratory tests to obtain when an ectopic pregnancy is suspected. Radioimmunoassay (RIA) for B-HCG should be used to avoid the false-negative results obtained with less sensitive tests.

Table 23.9 Differential Diagnosis for Ectopic Pregnancy

Assessment Data	*Ectopic Pregnancy*	*Spontaneous Abortion*	*Acute Pelvic Inflammatory Disease*
Vaginal Bleeding	History of missed period, irregular spotting or bleeding Usually brownish red to scanty last menstrual period	Amenorrhea followed by dark red spotting Bleeding heavier than normal period, bright red	No amenorrhea May have metrorrhagia or hypermenorrhagia or both
Pain	Before rupture: unilateral, colicky abdominal/pelvic pain After rupture: sudden sharp abdominal/ pelvic pain Shoulder pain	Suprapubic cramps, backache Midline pain less severe	Bilateral pelvic pain
Abdominal examination	Abdominal tenderness and rebound Distention common after rupture	Usually normal No abdominal tenderness	Lower abdominal tenderness and usually rebound
Pelvic examination	Cervical motion pain/tenderness Tender adnexal mass Crepitant mass on one side or in cul-de-sac	Uterine enlargement Cervix softening, may be dilating Tissue may be seen in os	Cervical motion tenderness Masses only when pyosalpinx present
Other signs/symptoms	Signs of shock Uterine enlargement Nausea and vomiting Fainting	Temperature elevated if infected	Temperature elevation 100° to 103° F
Laboratory	RIA pregnancy test often positive Routine immunologic urine pregnancy test negative in 50% of cases Hemoglobin, hematocrit, red blood cell count low and falling after rupture White blood cell (WBC) count increased to 15,000/mm^3 Erythrocyte sedimentation rate (ESR) slightly elevated	Pregnancy test usually positive No anemia WBC count elevated to 30,000 mm^3 if infected	Pregnancy test normal Usually no anemia ESR markedly elevated

(continued)

Serum concentration of HCG doubles every 2 to 3 days through the first 6 weeks of pregnancy and then levels off. At 6.5 weeks after last menstrual period, the mean HCG level is 10,000 mlU per ml (Jackson, 1990). If this level is not reached by the appropriate gestational age or if HCG does not double in 48 hours, this suggests ectopic pregnancy.

Transabdominal ultrasonography can be used to diagnose an intrauterine pregnancy when HCG levels exceed 1,800 mlU per ml, and an intravaginal sonogram can be used when the HCG levels are 500 to 1,000 mlU per ml. Early intrauterine pregnancies can be demonstrated by the presence of the gestational sac at approximately 30 days after ovulation or 6 weeks after the last menstrual

Table 23.9 Continued

Assessment Data	*Corpus Luteum Cyst*	*Acute Appendicitis*	*Acute Pyelonephritis*
Vaginal bleeding	Amenorrhea followed by bleeding	None	None
Pain	Unilateral pelvic pain becomes generalized with progressive bleeding	Right lower quadrant Epigastric, periumbilical Rebound tenderness	Backache, dysuria, costovertebral angle tenderness
Abdominal examination	Lower abdominal tenderness and rebound	Localized tenderness in right side of abdomen Rebound present	Normal
Pelvic examination	No masses Tenderness over affected ovary	Normal	Normal
Other signs/symptoms	Hemoglobin, hematocrit , and red blood cell count low and falls with rupture No temperature elevation Rapid pulse with rupture	Nausea and vomiting Rapid pulse	Nausea and vomiting Urgency, frequency Temperature 101° to 105° F Rapid pulse
Laboratory	Pregnancy test negative WBC count normal	Pregnancy test negative No anemia WBC count elevated	Pregnancy test negative No anemia Elevated WBC count Pus in urine

NOTE: Although sometimes a woman's symptoms make a diagnosis of ectopic pregnancy obvious, more often, considerable ambiguity exists. Many other conditions have similar symptoms. It is important that nurses caring for women in their childbearing years know what these are and how they can be differentiated.

period. By 42 days after ovulation (8 weeks after last menstrual period), fetal heart motion can be detected by ultrasound.

Nursing Management

Once a diagnosis is confirmed or strongly suspected, medical management is necessary for prompt treatment. A ruptured ectopic pregnancy is an obstetric emergency, and surgery must be performed as soon as possible. When possible, the woman's desires for future pregnancies should be discussed prior to surgery. Conservative surgery aimed at preserving future childbearing ability is recommended when feasible.

The woman who has an ectopic pregnancy requires much physiological and emotional support. Initial care must be focused on prevention of life-threatening hemorrhage and infection. Throughout all procedures, tests, and examinations, the client should be told the working diagnosis, given information about the tests and what they reveal, and informed of the management plan. If Rh negative, she should receive RhoGam after surgery to prevent possible Rh sensitization. Often, the woman's physical condition is so serious that emergency surgery is done without the possibility of adequate preparation prior to surgery. She is in pain before and after the operation and may need blood and fluid replacement therapy. She may or may not have known that she was pregnant and the pregnancy may have been desired, unplanned, or unwanted. She may be afraid that she will not be able to conceive again or carry a subsequent pregnancy to term. Many women experience intense feelings of loss after an ectopic pregnancy and may go through a grieving process. Guilt may be present. Compassionate, supportive counseling should be provided and referrals made to social services, grief teams, and psychological counseling services as indicated.

Education regarding risk factors is indicated for all women who desire additional pregnancies. The risk of IUD usage to reproductive capability should be discussed. Women should be encouraged to seek care promptly for all sexually transmitted diseases and to have regular screening for these infections if they are at risk for them (see Chapter 24). The client should be fully informed in writing of the extent of her surgery in terms she can understand. Education regarding the symptoms of another ectopic pregnancy and salpingitis and the importance of early prenatal care should be emphasized. Early pregnancy testing is recommended. Women desiring to become pregnant again should be counseled to wait until postoperative healing has occurred (6 to 8 weeks) and normal menstrual cycles have resumed. Such a delay also will allow time for resolution of the grieving process.

Other Pregnancy-Related Pain

Pain is associated with other conditions of pregnancy, including spontaneous abortion, abruptio placentae, tension of broad and round ligaments of the uterus, and uterine contractions. (Bleeding is a more universal symptom of spontaneous abortion and therefore is discussed in the section on bleeding in this chapter.) Acute, severe abdominal pain that occurs late in pregnancy may be caused by abruptio placentae, a condition in which premature separation of the placenta occurs with retroplacental hematoma formation and infiltration of the myometrium with blood. The degree of pain is correlated with the degree of separation. The cardinal signs of abruptio placentae are vaginal bleeding after the 20th week of pregnancy and constant abdominal pain. Depending on the severity of the abruption, maternal and fetal well-being may be severely compromised. Management usually consists of immediate cesarean or vaginal delivery to preserve the life of a live fetus or prevent further bleeding with a dead fetus.

It is important to distinguish broad or round ligament pain, a common normal discomfort of pregnancy, from serious complications of pregnancy. Ligament pain originates from spasms that occur as the uterus enlarges and the fundus stretches the ligaments. This type of pain usually lasts less than 20 minutes, does not require medication, and may be relieved by change in position or flexing of the knees.

Pregnant women may also experience uterine contractions that vary in intensity from painless to uncomfortable. Commonly called *Braxton Hicks contractions,* these are intermittent, mild cramps or painless pressure in the abdomen and reflect twinges of the uterus or sensations of the "baby balling up" that may be noticed in early pregnancy and become more frequent after 28 weeks gestation. It was suggested that the contractions, traditionally thought to be harmless, play a role in preparing for labor by causing cervical changes late in pregnancy. However, Braxton Hicks contractions may not be as harmless as once was thought. Current thinking suggests that nurses do their clients an injustice when they consider increased uterine activity during the second and third trimester of pregnancy, painful or not, as normal and tell them not to worry about the cramping or contractions that they feel (Hill & Lambertz, 1990). Only when a cervical examination is done and a lack of cervical changes is documented can health care providers safely reassure their clients that all is well and the uterine activity they are feeling is normal.

Toxic Shock Syndrome

Toxic shock syndrome (TSS) is an acute, multisystem, potentially fatal illness that primarily affects menstruating women. It is thought to be caused by a toxin, toxic shock syndrome toxin 1 (TSST-1), produced by *staphylococcus aureus*. The precise pathogenic mechanisms of TSST-1 are uncertain. After it was first described in children in 1978 (Todd, Fishaut, Kapral, & Welch, 1978), the disorder was found to be associated with menstruation. A relatively rare condition today, affecting 3 to 14 women in 100,000 (Hatcher et al., 1994), TSS affected many more women in the early 1980s. It continues to be of concern to women's health care practitioners because it is potentially lethal and is related to menstruation and tampon usage. Although 1% to 5% of women have TSS-producing strains of staphylococcus aureus (Hoeprich & Jordan, 1989), certain factors seem to increase the risk of TSS by providing the toxin an entry to the systemic circulation:

- Use of high-absorbency tampons during menstruation
- Postoperative or postpartal infection
- Leaving barrier methods of contraception, such as the vaginal contraceptive sponge and diaphragm, in the vagina more than 24 hours (rare risk) (Hatcher et al., 1994)

TSS typically begins with high fever, vomiting, and profuse watery discharge, perhaps accompanied by sore throat, headache, and myalgia between days 2 and 4 of the menstrual period. Within 48 hours, it progresses to hypotensive shock and the patient develops a diffuse, macular, erythematous rash. The patient may be disoriented and combative, with marked hemoconcentration, elevated blood urea nitrogen levels, and enzyme abnormalities. Level of consciousness decreases, followed by renal failure, disseminated intravascular coagulation, and circulatory collapse.

No definitive treatment exists for TSS. Intensive care is warranted, and treatment should be aggressive, involving integrated support of all organ systems, antistaphlococcal antibiotic therapy, and steroid administration (McGregor & Todd, 1987).

Teaching and counseling are critical to the prevention and early detection of TSS. All menstruating women who use tampons and those who use (and possibly misuse) barrier methods of contraception should be particularly targeted for education. If a woman uses tampons, she should be taught the signs and symptoms of TSS and the following suggested recommendations (Lichtman & Smith, 1990):

- Not using tampons can greatly reduce your chances of contracting TSS.
- You can decrease your risk of TSS by not using superabsorbent tampons.
- Frequent changes of tampons may reduce your risk.
- Using pads during part of your menstrual period or at night may reduce your risk of TSS.
- Always read the tampon package inserts and be sure you understand them.
- Ask for help if you are not sure about proper use of tampons.
- Always wash your hands before inserting tampons.
- If you have had TSS, just delivered a baby, or had an abortion do not use tampons.
- If you develop any symptoms of TSS discontinue use of tampons immediately.
- Contraceptive sponges and diaphragms should not be left in place more than 24 hours. Neither should be used in the first 6 to 8 weeks after childbirth.

It also has been recommended that adolescents should not use high-absorbency tampons and that women under the age of 25 should be advised that the risk of TSS is greater for women 24 years or younger.

Urinary Tract Infections

Most women experience dysuria, or painful urination, at some point in their lives. A common cause of dysuria is urinary tract infections (UTIs). The most common UTIs, their symptoms, and diagnostic points are summarized in Table 23.10. These infections are among the most frequent infectious problems of women and are often seen in pregnant women. Several factors are involved in the high frequency of female UTIs: Infectious organisms are introduced to the urinary tract through the urethra; sexual intercourse, sexual stimulation, insertion of tampons, close-fitting clothing, and perineal pads all have the potential for bringing pathogenic organisms into contact with the meatus; and there can be urethral contamination by fecal soiling. Use of the vaginal diaphragm has been associated with occurrence of bacteriuria and/or UTIs (Peddie, Gorrie, & Bailey, 1986).

The anatomy of the female urinary system helps explain its predisposition to infection. The short female urethra and its close proximity to the anus make introduction of pathogens to the bladder more likely in women than in men. Changes in the vaginal epithelial cells and vaginal pH associated with menopause increase the chances of a symptomatic UTI. Other predisposing factors include overdistention and inadequate emptying creating a medium for bacterial growth. Overdistention commonly occurs because of the infrequent voiding pattern of many adult women. In addition, many women do not empty their bladder completely when voiding, leaving a reservoir of urine. There are also a number of factors that are protective and contribute to a favorable prognosis: Most clients are healthy and have normal urinary tracts; the majority of infecting organisms are relatively sensitive to available antibiotics; and most antibiotics are concentrated and excreted via the kidneys so that high levels of antibiotics are present at the infection site.

A woman who has a lower UTI has dysuria and, usually, urinary frequency and urgency. Few women can tolerate acute dysuria for any length of time. The pain is commonly felt at the end of urination and experienced suprapubically. Frequency makes a woman void more often, and urgency makes her feel she will lose control of her urine at any minute. Although she feels this way, the actual amount of urine flow may be diminished in volume. These symptoms make it impossible to concentrate, focus on

Table 23.10 Common Urinary Tract Infections

Disease	*Symptoms*	*Physical Examination*	*Laboratory Data*
Urethritis	Persistent dysuria; frequency and urgency; hematuria with initial voiding; no fever, malaise, nausea, or vomiting	No costovertebral angle (CVA) tenderness or abdominal discomfort	Urinalysis of first voiding shows significant white blood cells (WBCs) and bacteria; midstream voiding is negative; urine culture positive
Trigonitis	Persistent dysuria; frequency and urgency; often sexual intercourse 36 hours to 72 hours prior to onset of symptoms; no systemic symptoms or hematuria; postvoiding pain	No abdominal discomfort or CVA tenderness	Urine culture negative
Lower urinary tract infection	Constant dysuria; urgency and frequency; hematuria at end of voiding; systemic symptoms rare	Suprapubic tenderness; no CVA tenderness	Midstream voiding has WBCs and bacteria; urine culture positive
Interstitial cystitis	Frequency, urgency, often nocturnal; infra- and suprapubic pain; hematuria and hesitancy; perhaps generalized abdominal, back, and rectal pain; pain with bladder filling and relief with emptying	Usually negative; possible urethral/vaginal tenderness	Sterile urine, cytologically negative
Pyelonephritis	Fever (102°-105°F), malaise, nausea, and vomiting; back and flank pain; dysuria, urgency, frequency, and hematoma may or may not be present	Severe CVA tenderness, usually unilateral	Midstream voiding shows high concentration of WBCs and bacteria; pyuria may or may not be present; urine culture positive

NOTE: Women may experience infection at a number of different points in the urinary tract. Different sites manifest different symptoms. A knowledge of how infection at these different points present will assist the nurse in assessing her woman client accurately.

usual activities, or become comfortable. Relief is usually sought quickly.

Some women experience dysuria following sexual intercourse. The syndrome known as trigonitis or "honeymoon cystitis" often occurs when the pattern of sexual activity alters from little or no activity to vigorous and frequent activity. Symptoms of dysuria, urgency, frequency, and bladder irritation not associated with infection are characteristic of this noninfectious inflammatory process. It is caused by trauma to the urethra during prolonged or very active intercourse. It is more common in nulliparous women, whose perineum is high with a tight introitus and whose pelvic sling muscles have not been cut or damaged during childbirth. The penile shaft comes in close contact with the anterior vaginal wall; with frequent, vigorous thrusts under the urethra and against the base of the bladder, trauma, capillary rupture, edema, and inflammation can occur.

Changes in sexual patterns or sexual partners can introduce new pathogens and thereby cause an infection. Women may associate urinary problems with their sexuality. For the woman susceptible to trigonitis, sexual intercourse becomes closely associated with dysuria. The resultant pain and discomfort may make her less eager for sexual activity. Many women first experience urinary tract problems when they are pregnant. Many women have difficulty voiding postpartally, and urinary retention and infection are common problems. Inability to control urine flow completely may occur first during pregnancy or following a traumatic delivery.

Assessment

UTIs are diagnosed on the basis of the client's history, specific laboratory tests, and physical examination. It is important that clients describe their symptoms, including onset and duration of frequency and urgency, when and where the dysuria is experienced, and if suprapubic or back pain is present. Because vaginitis can cause urethritis, increased vaginal discharge, external or perineal discomfort, and pruritis can signal urethritis. Any history of UTIs and their treatment is noted. Ask clients about their usual sexual activity patterns, any recent changes in pattern or in partners, and contraceptive practices. Inquire about types of soaps and perineal products she uses and her tampon and pad practices. Recent childbirth, gynecologic procedures, and/or catheterization should be noted.

The client's vital signs are obtained to document the presence of fever. Percussion of the costovertebral angle (CVA) is essential; exquisite tenderness or sharp pain may indicate pyelonephritis. Suprapubic tenderness is assessed on abdominal examination. External genital examination will reveal the presence of a urethral discharge and any redness or irritation around the urethra. A vaginal examination with cultures and wet prep should be done if the client has reported symptoms suggestive of a vaginal infection (see section on vaginal discharge in this chapter).

Microscopic urinalysis and urine culture are standard diagnostic studies for UTIs. If pyelonephritis is suspected, a complete blood count may be useful. An accurate culture requires a midstream, clean-catch urine (CCU) specimen; catheterization is to be avoided because of the potential for introducing infection into the bladder. Never assume that clients know how to collect a CCU specimen; rather, review the procedures with them every time a specimen is collected.

Pyuria, the presence of white blood cells (WBCs) or pus in the urine, is the most important diagnostic parameter in a urinalysis. More than 8 to 10 WBCs per high power field is the standard for diagnosis of UTIs. Often, red blood cells and bacteria are seen as well. A culture identifies the pathogenic organism present in the urine. In specimens obtained by clean catch, colony counts greater than 100,000 bacteria are considered diagnostic of infection. Sensitivity studies should be done to determine which antibiotic will be effective against the infecting organism.

At times, a quick screening test that indirectly detects leukocytes or bacteria may be used. Correlations of rapid measurements of leukocytes in the urine with urine cultures have demonstrated that the tests are highly sensitive; thus a negative test has a high predictive value (97%) and reduces the need for urine culture. Because the test is relatively nonspecific, a positive test does not necessarily indicate a need for treatment. A rapid screen for bacteria (Bact-T-Screen) detects bacteria or WBCs quickly, with a sensitivity of 92% but a low specificity. Thus this test can also be used to exclude UTI with a high probability of accuracy (Lichtman & Duran, 1990).

Management

UTIs in women with symptoms and a positive urinalysis are treated with antibiotics. Whenever possible, the antibiotic should be one that the causative organism is sensitive to; however, in practice, treatment is often instituted before culture and sensitivity results are available. Many of the infections are caused by gram-negative bacteria (e.g., *Escherichia coli*), and drugs that are effective against these organisms are generally used. Table 23.11 summarizes the most common drugs and appropriate dosages. It is not necessary to treat asymptomatic bacteriuria, except in pregnant women or women with diabetes or sickle-cell anemia, because asymptomatic bacteriuria has not been shown to lead to UTI (Lichtman & Duran, 1990). Nonpregnant

Table 23.11 Medications Commonly Used for Urinary Tract Infections

Medication	*Dosage*[a]	*Side Effects*	*Comments*
Nitrofurantoin (Macrodantin)	50-100 mg by mouth (po) 4 times a day (qid) for 7-10 days *or* 3 gm po for 1 day	Allergic reaction Liver damage Acute and chronic pulmonary reaction, blood dyscrasias Neuropathy	Contraindicated in pregnancy at term Risk of side effects higher in women, increases with age Lower doses for small and older women Take with food to avoid nausea; works best when urine is acidic
Trimethoprim and sulfamethoxazole (Bactrim, Septra)	1 tablet po twice a day (bid) for 10-14 days *or* 2-3 tablets po for 1 day	Gastrointestinal (GI) disturbance Hypersensitivity: skin, GI, central nervous system reactions, drug fever, chills, and toxic nephrosis Hemolysis in G6PD deficiency patients; other blood dyscrasias	Less side effects with single dose therapy Not recommended in pregnancy Adequate fluid intake Take each dose with water
Amoxicillin	250-500 mg po 3 times a day (tid) for 10 days *or* 3 gm po for 1 day	Hypersensitivity: nausea, vomiting, epigastric distress, diarrhea Black "hairy tongue," fungal overgrowth	Contraindicated in women with previous hypersensitivity
Ampicillin	250 mg po qid for 10 days	Low toxicity, may result in hypersensitivity	Contraindicated in women with hypersensitivity to any penicillin
Sulfisoxazole (Gantrisin)	500 mg po qid for 10 days	See trimethoprim and sulfamethoxazole	Contraindicated in 3rd trimester of pregnancy Maintain adequate fluid intake Take on empty stomach
Tetracycline	250-500 mg tid po for 7-10 days	Allergic reactions: GI upset, rash	Contraindicated in pregnancy, breast-feeding, early childhood Take 30-60 minutes before or 1-2 hours after meals Dairy products and some antacids interfere with absorption Avoid direct sunlight

a. Dosages are current recommendations and should be verified before use.

patients with definite symptoms and a negative culture should be treated with tetracycline, doxycycline, or erythromycin; this recommendation is based on the assumption that there may be a bacterial cause for the symptoms, frequently chlamydia (Lichtman & Duran, 1990).

Length of treatment is somewhat controversial. Some researchers have found 1-day therapy with amoxicillin, sulfisoxazole (Gantrisin), or trimethoprim-sulfamethoxazole (Septra) to be approximately as effective as a 5- to 10-day regimen. Single-dose therapy has the advantages of fewer and less severe side effects, increased patient compliance, and lower cost. Risks associated with single-dose approach are lower cure rates in patients with pyelonephritis and resistance to longer term therapy after treatment failure (Hooton, Running, & Stamm, 1985). Single-dose therapy should not be used with any woman who has signs or symptoms of pyelonephritis.

In many instances, treatment will be 7 to 10 days in length. A test-of-cure culture 1 week after completion of the medication should always be done; a follow-up culture is done sooner if the patient remains symptomatic. A woman should be instructed to take the full course of medication even if her symptoms disappear within 48 to 72 hours. She should drink large amounts of fluids and void often. If the medication should not be taken with food, dairy products, or antacids, the client should be informed of this. Phenazopyridine hydrochloride (Pyridium) may be used for pain relief.

Because most women will experience at least one UTI in their lifetime, preventive measures are extremely important for all women, especially for those who experience recurrent infections. Proper technique in wiping (front to back) after voiding or defecation is essential to prevent bacterial contamination of the urethra from the anal area. Use of plain, white, unscented toilet tissue is recommended. The woman who has experienced repeated UTIs may wish to shower rather than take tub baths and to wash with soap and water after a bowel movement. Many women tend to void infrequently; they should be encouraged to urinate soon after they feel the urge so that urine does not stagnate. Increased fluid intake (up to 10 to 14 glasses per day) will flush urine out of the bladder regularly.

Emptying the bladder before and after intercourse will help to wash bacteria away from the urinary meatus. Women should be warned against sexual practices that bring fecal organisms to the vagina. Penile or digital vaginal contact after anal contact without washing should be avoided. Cleansing the perineal area prior to intercourse will also reduce the number of bacteria available to be introduced into the meatus. Women with recurrent UTIs who use a diaphragm as their contraceptive method may wish to choose an alternative method of birth control or try using a smaller diaphragm with a more flexible rim.

Measures primarily used to prevent vaginal infections, such as the avoidance of tight-fitting clothes, always wearing underpants and panty hose with cotton crotches, and not sitting around in a wet bathing suit may help prevent UTIs. Vaginal sprays, perfumes, and bubble baths should be avoided because they may provoke allergic responses.

Pain Related to Sexual Activity

Some women experience pain associated with sexual activity, most commonly dyspareunia, or pain with intercourse. Often, dyspareunia is a symptom indicative of another problem such as endometriosis (see Chapter 25), vaginal infections (discussed later in this chapter), or pelvic inflammatory disease (see Chapter 24).

Pelvic Masses

Pelvis masses can cause pain or abdominal discomfort experienced as a vague ache and a sense of fullness or heaviness in the pelvis. At times the pain is associated with intercourse, menstruation, or defecation. Acute pain is experienced when the mass twists on its pedicle, when bleeding into a cyst occurs, or when a cyst ruptures.

Women with an ovarian cyst often experience unilateral adnexal pain and dyspareunia. Bimanual examination may suggest the diagnosis, which is confirmed by ultrasound. Many ovarian cysts are functional and develop from the graafian follicle or corpus luteum. Follicular cysts, which can develop at any time during the reproductive years, are not neoplastic but variations of normal physiological events and are the most common cause of detectable ovarian enlargement. Although they usually do not cause symptoms, some women notice menstrual irregularities, mild pelvic discomfort, lower back pain, or deep dyspareunia. Most follicular cysts resolve with time, and management consists of reassurance and repeat evaluation after a menstrual cycle, when the cyst may have resolved. Corpus luteum cysts are found in ovulating women only and are apt to be symptomatic. Menstruation may be delayed and then prolonged and irregular. Unilateral pelvic discomfort is common. Acute abdominal pain occurs with ovarian cysts when hemorrhage into the cyst or rupture with intraperitoneal spillage occurs. Initial treatment of corpus luteum cysts includes observation because the majority of these cysts disappear spontaneously. When a hemorrhagic cyst is larger than 8 cm or does not resolve spontaneously or when evidence of active intraperitoneal bleeding exists on ultrasound, surgical excision is necessary. It is important that the possibility of very early gestation be considered, because the symptoms and associated adnexal mass are similar to those associated with threatened abortion or ectopic pregnancy.

Fibroids, or leiomyomas, are very common benign tumors in women. The discomfort associated with uterine fibroids is likely to be an aching or dragging fullness in the pelvis. Discomfort is often caused by encroachment on the adjacent bladder or rectum. Menorrhagia is also common with fibroid tumors. The reader is referred to the section on menorrhagia in this chapter for a fuller discussion of this condition.

Pelvic pain may also be caused by malignant neoplasms. Usually, this does not happen until increased size and/or metastasis have occurred. Gynecologic cancer is discussed in Chapter 27. Many of the surgical interventions used when women have gynecologic cancer are discussed in Chapter 26.

Premenstrual Syndrome (PMS)

PMS is a constellation of physical and psychological symptoms occurring in the luteal phase of the menstrual cycle. Almost all women experience some minor physical and emotional changes preceding menstruation—so much so that "they must be considered normal events in the lives of most women of reproductive age" (Reid, 1991, p. 1208). A much smaller percentage (thought to be about 5%) of women experience physical or psychological symptoms that reach severe or temporarily disabling proportions during the premenstrual period. Originally termed "premenstrual tension" or "premenstrual tension syndrome," this condition is now known as premenstrual syndrome, which takes into account the different clinical presentations that may occur.

The literature on PMS is full of unproved assumptions; on the one hand, many question whether PMS is a biological entity, whereas others blame PMS for antisocial behavior and female incompetence and offer it as the reason women should not hold positions of power and authority. The existence and diagnosis of PMS is hotly and widely debated. Parlee (1973) stated that there is no scientific proof that PMS exists, pointing to studies that fail to include control groups and questionnaires that bias responses by focusing on negative symptoms, retrospective accounts, and experiences just before and during menses. In a contrasting view, Katharina Dalton, who pioneered research on PMS from the 1950s through the 1970s, is convinced that the condition exists and that it drastically affects the lives of women who suffer from it. She cites examples of behavioral changes, including increased numbers of home, factory, and road accidents; poor school performance; and criminal activity (Dalton, 1960a, 1960b, 1980a). During the 1980s, PMS has been used successfully as a legal defense in criminal cases in Great Britain. Many feminists are concerned with this approach, however, fearing that such attention will lead to a revival of myths about raging hormones and female mental instability.

Because many women with severe premenstrual psychological changes are treated by psychiatrists, debate has surfaced about whether PMS should have its own diagnostic category in psychiatric nomenclature. In 1987, the American Psychiatric Association (APA) included a description of "late luteal-phase dysphoric disorder" in the appendix to the *Diagnostic and Statistical Manual of Mental Disorders* (3rd edition, revised; *DSM-III-R*). In 1994, the APA qualified that the transient mood changes that many women experience around the onset of menses should not be considered a mental disorder (APA, 1994). The introduction of a sex-specific diagnosis has the risk of stigmatization and unwarranted generalizations about all women. Clinically, the diagnosis could become a catchall and prevent appropriate investigation of a woman's individual symptoms and concerns.

Defining PMS has presented many difficulties because of the subjectivity and variety of its symptoms. However, certain basic facts have been agreed on (Peck, 1990): PMS is a clinical entity that is somatic rather than psychic in origin. Furthermore, PMS is a complex mechanism. Although its origin may be in disturbances of the ovarian cycle and hormonal balances, it also involves other endocrine glandular functions as well as the autonomic and central nervous system. In the broadest context, PMS may be defined as "the cyclic recurrence in the luteal phase of the menstrual cycle of a combination of distressing physical, psychological, and/or behavioral changes of sufficient severity to result in deterioration of interpersonal relationships and/or interference with normal activities" (Reid, 1991, p. 1208). This definition thus excludes women who experience mild premenstrual changes, such as acne, bloating, breast tenderness, or craving for sweets or salty foods, which rarely disrupt one's life or relationships. It includes severe luteal-phase symptoms, such as depression, anxiety, mood swings, fatigue, insomnia, and headaches, when these result in social withdrawal, deterioration of relationships, suicidal thoughts or actions, or impaired performance or cognition.

Minimal criteria for a diagnosis of PMS include the following (Peck, 1990; Walton & Youngkin, 1987):

- Symptoms occur in the luteal phase and resolve within a few days of the onset of menses.
- A symptom-free period occurs in the follicular phase.
- Symptoms are recurrent.

PMS may be diagnosed if the intensity of symptoms increases at least 30% in the 6 days prior to onset of menses compared with days 5 through 10 of the cycle; symptoms must occur in two consecutive months (Osofsky, Keppel, & Kuczmierczyk, 1988). Although these criteria clarify some ambiguities associated with diagnosing PMS by specifying temporal relationships, many PMS symptoms, such as depression, bloating, and anxiety, are not readily quantifiable (Hsia & Long, 1990). Most clinicians would find it difficult to detect a 30% increase in symptom intensity in a clinical setting.

Researchers have attempted to categorize PMS into several subtypes based on clusters of symptoms in an effort to understand etiology and guide treatment more effectively. Four categories of PMS or premenstrual tension syndrome (PMT) have been suggested (Abraham & Rumley, 1987): PMT-A—anxiety, irritability, and nervous tension; PMT-H—fluid retention, abdominal bloating, mastalgia, and weight gain; PMT-C—premenstrual cravings for sweets, increased appetite, and food binges; and PMT-D—depression, withdrawal, insomnia, forgetfulness, and confusion. However, it is difficult if not impossible to fit women into a single category because many often have symptoms from several classifications at the same time. Because of the overlap of symptoms in an individual woman, it is not clear how practical this method of subtyping is for clinicians, although the categories may be useful for research studies on the etiology and treatment of PMS.

Epidemiology

Reported estimates of the incidence of perimenstrual symptoms vary widely, from 20% to 95% of all women. However, estimates of the percentage of women who experience incapacitating symptoms are much smaller. Up to 20% to 40% report some degree of incapacitation (Peck, 1990) and between 3% and 5% report symptoms that reach severe or temporarily disabling proportions (Reid, 1991). PMS has been reported in all age groups; traditionally, however, reported rates have been higher among women in their 30s and 40s. Recent studies (Fisher, Trieller, & Napolitano, 1989; Wilson & Keye, 1989) found that adolescents also report experiencing premenstrual symptoms. PMS severity is associated with higher parity; however, age may be a confounding factor because it also correlates positively with parity (Hsia & Long, 1990).

Etiology

Numerous theories have been advanced to explain PMS; however, to date no one cause of PMS has been identified. Proposed hypotheses include hormones (estrogen, progesterone, thyroid, insulin), neurotransmitters, circadian rhythms, prostaglandins, vitamin B_6, nutritional factors, allergic reactions, stress, and psychological factors. Prolactin excess; endorphin deficiency; aldosterone excess; and prostaglandins, either in excessive or deficient amounts, have been implicated as further possible causes, but to date research has not supported any of these hypotheses consistently.

Progesterone deficiency is a popular theory in that PMS symptoms occur only in the luteal phase, the only time that progesterone is produced. Dalton (1980b) contends that it is not the progesterone or estrogen that is significant but, rather, the ratio between the two and that PMS results from an imbalance in this ratio. Neither of these theories has been supported consistently by research findings, however. Severino and Moline (1990) suggest that how cyclic ovarian hormonal changes influence the pattern of neurotransmitter release may ultimately explain the diversity of symptoms and their timing that are associated with PMS.

Symptoms

A wide variety of symptoms are associated with PMS, and individual experiences of a given symptom may range from mild to severe. Reported manifestations include the following:

- Gastrointestinal: abdominal bloating, nausea, vomiting, constipation, increased thirst
- Respiratory: colds, hoarseness, rhinitis, asthma, sinusitis, sore throats
- Urologic: oliguria, urethritis, cystitis
- Ophthalmologic: conjunctivitis, visual changes, glaucoma, sties
- Mammologic: breast tenderness, swelling, heaviness
- Dermatologic: acne, boils, urticaria, spot bruising, recurrence of herpes
- Neurological: headaches/migraines, aggravation of epilepsy, vertigo, syncope, fainting, parenthesis of hands or feet
- Behavioral: tension and irritability, depression, insomnia, fatigue, lethargy, lack of concentration, indecision, confusion, mood swings, crying episodes
- Miscellaneous: backache, joint pain, edema of extremities, weight gain, palpitations, pelvic/lower abdominal pain, cold sweats, hot flashes, food cravings, and compulsive eating

In a study of 256 women who sought treatment for premenstrual symptoms and were diagnosed with PMS, the most common physical symptoms were fatigue, headache, abdominal bloating, breast tenderness, and acne. The most common emotional complaints included anxiety, hostility or anger, and depression (Keye, 1987). Many of Keye's respondents complained of isolation from others, oversensitivity to rejection, paranoia, panic attacks, decreased or increased sexual drive, and disrupted interpersonal relationships. The most controversial symptoms attributed to PMS are those affecting cognitive and motor function (Coyne, Woods, & Mitchell, 1985).

Not all the symptoms reported in the PMS literature are negative, however. Stewart (1989) found that 66% of subjects reported at least one positive symptom, such as increased libido, more energy, more creative ideas, and increased ability to accomplish tasks.

Assessment

The client's age and parity are important as is a full description of her concern and symptoms. The nurse should inquire about age at onset of PMS, duration and precipitating factors, and circumstances surrounding the onset or exacerbation of PMS. Ask the client to list all of her symptoms and their timing and interval. If she has kept a record or diary, this should be reviewed. If the client has not kept a diary, she should be asked to for 3 months. The menstrual diary or calendar documents the occurrence of her symptoms in relation to timing of menses. To be considered diagnostic, the same symptoms should be present in three consecutive cycles; in addition, there should be a symptom-free stage in the cycle. The nurse should inquire as to what, if anything, makes symptoms better or worse. Have self-help measures been tried, and were they helpful? If the woman has seen other health care providers for her symptoms, what therapies were prescribed and to what effect? What effect have her symptoms had on her relationships with family, friends, and colleagues? Finally, the nurse asks the client what are her expectations concerning evaluation and therapy (Hsia & Long, 1990).

Assessment of PMS also includes obtaining menstrual, sexual, reproductive, family, medical, surgical, and psychiatric histories. This information is useful in ruling out other causes of symptoms. Clients are asked about dietary habits, medications, drug and alcohol use, and social and occupational history. Any health maintenance practices such as exercise and stress reduction efforts, for example, meditation that the client employs, are noted.

A screening physical, including a pelvic examination, is done to determine the client's general health status, confirm any subjective data from the history, and identify or rule out any gynecologic, neurological, endocrine, metabolic, or latent organic diseases. Weight and blood pressure should be noted.

No single laboratory test is diagnostic for PMS. Thus laboratory tests should be individualized, based on the woman's neurological, endocrine, emotional, or physical symptoms (Maxton, 1988). Osofsky and associates (1988) recommend that baseline data be obtained, including a complete blood count, urinalysis, blood sugar level, and thyroid status. Hormonal levels that might be obtained include FSH/LH, serum estradiol, serum progesterone, and serum prolactin.

These levels should be drawn 1 to 7 days prior to menstruation or at the time of the woman's most severe symptoms (Peck, 1990).

Nursing Management

The goal in the management of mild to moderate PMS is promotion and maintenance of a healthy lifestyle and the alleviation or amelioration of symptoms when possible. Nurses must recognize and accept the client's distress. The limited understanding of etiology, the multitude of symptoms of varying severity, and lack of agreement as to what are the best therapies to use mean that there is no one clear-cut treatment for the syndrome. Most of the treatments are based on hypotheses about etiology, attempts to provide symptom relief, or the desire to encourage healthy lifestyle behaviors.

Teaching and counseling are essential components of the management of PMS. The nurse and client should discuss the results and implications of the assessment process and diagnosis. It is important to be specific about the presence of normal findings as well as the absence of abnormal findings; these individual clarifications give the client realistic information about her situation and either remove or validate her concerns. Using a menstrual calendar, a woman can learn to identify her own symptoms and how they are primarily manifested. She can learn which events trigger or exacerbate her symptoms and, with the use of the calendar, will learn to anticipate more difficult times and plan accordingly.

Three important components of a self-help program for PMS are stress reduction, increasing the body's natural defenses as much as possible, and alleviation of symptoms (Peck, 1990). Self-care measures, including dietary changes, exercise, and a support network, may be helpful. For example, clients may wish to plan stressful activities so that, insofar as possible, these occur in the symptom-free part of their cycle, avoiding potential problems in their premenstruum. They may wish to put off important decisions or prepare for such decisions ahead of time. This is done not because women are incapable of making these decisions but, rather, because it may reduce the stress that is associated with PMS (Coyne et al., 1985). Because fatigue tends to decrease the body's natural defenses and exaggerate PMS symptoms, sleep should be a priority during the premenstruum. The woman can be encouraged to nap and use relaxation techniques to combat fatigue.

The client with PMS can be encouraged to discuss her problem. Because partners, children, parents, friends, and coworkers often experience the difficult times with the woman herself (Lindow, 1991), it is important that she be as honest as possible within her support system. Nurses may choose to invite family members and support persons to health care visits to discuss PMS. Support groups, counseling, or education sessions also may be of help to women with PMS and their families (Walton & Youngkin, 1987). Woman-run self-help groups are a forum for information sharing, discussing feelings, and providing mutual assistance, especially in the premenstruum.

Exercise has been recommended widely for relief of PMS symptoms (Gannon, 1988). It is thought that consistent aerobic exercise, which increases beta endorphin levels, may offset depressive symptoms and provide mood elevation. In a prospective study, 6 months of exercise training was associated with decreased premenstrual symptoms for 15 women compared with 6 women who did not alter their activities during the study period (Prior, Vigna, Sciaretta, Alajado, & Schulzer, 1987). Exercise programs for PMS should consist of at least 20 to 30 minutes of aerobic workout at least four times a week. Because symptoms such as headache or severe breast tenderness may make it difficult for women to do some exercises, a monthly exercise program that varies in intensity and type of exercise according to PMS symptoms is best. For example, a woman may choose to jog or do aerobic dance when she is symptom free and to swim when she has severe headaches or severe breast tenderness.

Although few studies have looked at the relationship of PMS to diet, and there is little research evidence to indicate that nutrition plays a role in the etiology of PMS, many women find that dietary changes improve their symptoms. Many adult women have poor eating habits and thus instruction regarding a balanced, nutritious diet is important for the prevention or relief of PMS throughout the menstrual cycle. Specific instructions regarding dietary revisions include the following (Peck, 1990):

- Limit consumption of refined sugar (< 5 tbsp/day), salt (< 3gms/day), red meat (up to 3 oz/day), alcohol (1 oz or less/day), and caffeinated beverages.

- Use fish, poultry, whole grains, and legumes rather than red meat and dairy products as sources of protein.
- Limit dairy products to 2 servings per day; use low-fat or no-fat products. (The practitioner may want to consider suggesting the use of calcium supplements if necessary.)
- Limit fat intake to less than 20% of total calories.
- Increase intake of complex carbohydrates to 60% to 70% of total calories.
- Increase intake of green, leafy vegetables, legumes, whole grains, and cereals (good source of B vitamins and magnesium).
- Have small, frequent meals to maintain steady blood sugar levels.
- Use natural diuretics such as water, cucumber, asparagus, and certain types of herbal teas to reduce fluid retention.

Nutritional supplements may be of use in reducing symptoms. Calcium, magnesium, vitamins A, B_6, and E, and evening primrose oil all have been suggested. Magnesium may be beneficial because many women with PMS symptoms have been shown to have low serum magnesium levels. Vitamin B_6 has been widely prescribed because of its role as a coenzyme in the synthesis of amino acids; controlled studies have had conflicting results, and an excess intake of this vitamin can lead to peripheral neuropathy. An acceptable dosage of vitamin B_6 is 100 mg by mouth daily throughout the menstrual cycle (Hsia & Long, 1990). Evening primrose oil has been used to treat prostaglandin E1 deficiency, although study findings of its efficacy are conflicting (Horrobin, 1990).

Multiple medications have been used in the treatment of PMS. At present no one medication has been found to alleviate all the symptoms of PMS. Many of the studies on the efficacy of various drug therapies have not been well controlled, and their results are inconclusive. Furthermore, there is a strong placebo effect in treating PMS. Medications often used include diuretics, prostaglandin inhibitors (NSAIDS), progesterone, OCs, bromocriptine, and psychotropic drugs.

Because edema during the luteal phase is one of the most common symptoms of women with PMS, diuretics frequently have been prescribed. Despite conflicting study results, Wicks (1988) suggests that a probable role for diuretics exists in the treatment of PMS. The drug of choice is the aldosterone antagonist spironolactone 25 mg four times a day, used during the luteal phase from 3 days prior to expected symptoms until onset of menses. Prostaglandin inhibitors have been shown to relieve symptoms in some studies. Because these are generally safe medications with few side effects, it is reasonable to prescribe them for symptom relief. Generally, naproxen sodium 500 mg twice a day begun 10 days prior to onset of menses and stopped 1 to 2 days after menses may alleviate symptoms.

Natural progesterone is widely used for treatment of PMS, although its use is highly controversial and its efficacy has not been established. Several double-blind studies have not shown any therapeutic benefit of progesterone over placebo (Maddocks, Hohn, Moller, & Reid, 1986; Maxton, 1988). Natural progesterone is administered either intramuscularly or by vaginal or rectal suppository. When given intramuscularly, the dose is 100 mg per day; given as a vaginal or rectal suppository, the usual dosage is 200 to 400 mg per day. It is given during the luteal phase of each cycle from ovulation to menses. The long-term side effects of progesterone therapy are unproven, and its effect on the breast, uterus, and cervical and vaginal epithelium are unknown. Despite this, clinicians consider it safe because the levels prescribed are lower than those found in pregnancy (Hsia & Long, 1990). Possible side effects may include vaginal irritation and discharge, yeast infections, pruritis, occasional delayed onset of menses, and dysmenorrhea; women using rectal suppositories often report diarrhea. Because of the lack of controlled studies consistently showing a positive effect of progesterone and in light of its inconvenience, discomfort, and expense, it should be used only when a more conservative approach has failed. Close supervision and follow-up are essential.

Birth control pills may provide some relief for some women with PMS and may be a reasonable option for women under 40 who also desire birth control. However, some women experience an exacerbation of symptoms while on birth control pills (Chihal, 1987). Danazol has been used by some physicians to suppress the menstrual cycle and thus improve PMS symptoms, particularly breast tenderness; but the unpleasant side effects (see Chapter 25) and cost make many women reluctant to use this medication. Bromocriptine has been used with varying success to treat PMS. Tranquilizers and sedatives are often prescribed for women who have severe behavioral manifestations of PMS such as anxiety, depression, and insomnia; these drugs, however, are habit forming with long-term use and are of little proven benefit. They should be used with great caution, if at all, in the treatment of PMS.

Because no single treatment is universally accepted as effective, the client has an important role in determining which therapies provide the best relief for her. Client input, coupled with educational and supportive measures to facilitate self-care and medication, will assist the clinician and woman in devising a therapeutic regimen that will provide maximum symptom relief.

Discharge and Pruritus

Although not life threatening, discharge and pruritis unquestionably diminish the quality of life for women who suffer from them. Vaginal discharge and itching of the vulva and vagina are among the most frequent reasons a woman seeks help from a health care provider. Indeed, more women complain of leukorrhea, or vaginal discharge, than any other gynecologic symptom. Different women perceive discharge and itching in unique ways; one woman may be extremely uncomfortable, another may feel only minor distress, a third may be very anxious, and a fourth may be mildly concerned. Women's reactions depend on many factors, including their previous experiences; knowledge; societal, religious, and cultural beliefs; and the number and severity of symptoms.

Normal Characteristics

Vaginal secretions are a normal, regularly occurring experience for women during their childbearing years. The numerous variations in the amount and characteristics of vaginal secretions are determined by physiology, emotions, and pathology. Women who have adequate endogenous or exogenous estrogen will have vaginal secretions.

The major source of vaginal secretion is the cervical mucosa. Small amounts are secreted by the Bartholin's, sebaceous, sweat, and apocrine glands of the vulva. The vaginal mucosa, which contains no glands, is not truly secretory; however, copious vaginal lubrication known as sweating does occur during sexual excitement. Normal vaginal secretions are clear to cloudy in appearance and may turn yellow after drying; the discharge is slightly slimy, nonirritating, and has a mild unoffensive odor. The alkaline, shiny mucoid substance secreted by the cervix, on the other hand, is more abundant than vaginal secretions and is less viscous at ovulation. Normal vaginal secretions are acidic, with a pH range of 3.8 to 4.2. Döderlein's bacillus are customarily seen in the vaginal secretions of women in their reproductive years. The amount of vaginal discharge a woman experiences is not, in itself, an indication of infection.

Life Cycle Changes

The female newborn may have a mucous discharge for 1 to 10 days following delivery as a result of in utero stimulation of the uterus and vagina by maternal estrogen. A similar mucoid discharge may be seen a few years before and after menarche as a result of increased estrogen production by the maturing ovary. Pregnancy often substantially increases mucus production, with a resulting profuse discharge. A similar discharge may occur in the woman taking OCs (Hatcher et al., 1994).

Before menarche and following menopause, when estrogen levels are low, vaginal secretions are minimal. The vaginal epithelium is inactive and thin, the cells contain very little glycogen, Döderlein's bacilli are absent, and the vaginal pH is between 6 and 7. Such inactive mucosa is particularly susceptible to infection, whereas the estrogen-stimulated vaginal mucosa during the reproductive years is less so.

Vaginal secretions normally vary throughout the menstrual cycle. During the immediate postmenstrual phase, when the estrogen level is low, the mucosa is thin and relatively inactive, with little cervical cell secretion present. Vaginal cells proliferate and exfoliate rapidly as estrogen production increases; at the same time, the cervical cells secrete more and more mucus. Maximal estrogen production occurs at ovulation and causes a profuse watery discharge, primarily from the cervix. Secretions then decrease until just prior to menstruation.

Common Causes

Common causes of vaginal discharge are summarized in Table 23.12. Among the most common causes of vaginal discharge are (a) infectious processes, such as bacterial vaginosis (BV), trichomoniasis, and candidiasis; (b) chemical and contact allergens; and (c) lower estrogen levels (atrophic vaginitis). Many sexually transmitted diseases also cause vaginal discharge. These will be discussed in Chapter 24. Chronic cervicitis accounts for most discharges not associated with itching, pain, or sensitivity. OCs and IUDs also have been found to cause vaginal discharge; each of these causes is associated with a fairly typical history and characteristic physical findings.

Discharge may also be a characteristic symptom of malignant neoplasms of the lower genital tract. Any growth in the genital area may cause a continuous serous, mucoid, sanguineous, or purulent discharge. Bloody discharge should be a clue to the possibility of malignancy. If the neoplasm becomes infected or necrotic, the discharge will be purulent and malodorous. Copious amounts of thin watery discharge, which drains from the cervix and collects in the vagina, may indicate fallopian tube carcinoma in the postmenopausal woman.

Parasites, particularly pinworms, can cause vaginitis in children. Diagnosis is usually made by microscopic examination of a piece of clear tape placed on the perineum of the child while asleep. The tape will show the typical ova of the pinworm, which are deposited outside the rectum at night.

In the sections that follow, general information appropriate when any pathological cause of vaginal discharge is suspected is presented and strategies to prevent discharge are outlined. In addition, the most common vaginal infections that cause discharge are described in detail, including etiology, prevention, risk factors, clinical presentation, and management.

General Assessment

There are three components of an accurate diagnosis: history, physical examination, and laboratory tests. This section outlines data collection steps to be used when any vaginal infection is suspected.

History

Table 23.13 outlines the essential information to be collected by the nurse. It is important to know when discharge began. Recent onset indicates an acute condition, whereas a chronic condition such as cervicitis is typified by symptoms of long duration. The color and consistency of the discharge can suggest specific causes. Discharge that is thick and purulent suggests bacterial infection; a white, curdlike discharge, however, is suggestive of Candida infection. The amount of discharge can be significant in suggesting a diagnosis (e.g., a woman who has trichomoniasis vaginal infection may report that her discharge is very heavy, saturating her panties). When asking about amount, it is important to have the woman quantify her answer, because amounts and the perception of amount can vary greatly. Discharge is considered copious if it soaks through the woman's underpants onto her outer clothing or stains her underpants sufficiently for her to require wearing a tampon or pad.

Itching is often associated with vaginal discharge. Trichomoniasis characteristically is associated with intense itching of the vulva, although any infection that causes labial and vulvar irritation and erythema can result in itching. Other symptoms often associated with vaginal discharge are dysuria resulting from local irritation of the urinary meatus, pelvic or groin pain, abdominal cramping, or a sense of pelvic fullness. Presence of fever, abnormal vaginal bleeding or spotting, and/or lesions should be noted as well. Ask about lifestyle behaviors, including personal hygiene. Douching may irritate vaginal tissue and alter the vaginal environment, thus predisposing the woman to infection. Sprays, deodorants, powders, perfumes, and antiseptic soaps or ointments used in the perineal area can cause irritation or allergic reactions. Nylon panties or tight fitting pants that do not allow free air flow and absorption of moisture can cause chafing and irritation. Thus any recent change in personal habits, including use of new detergents, vaginal deodorants, or perfume, and type of underwear should be noted. Any changes in type of douching solution or frequency are noted.

A complete sexual history is obtained because discharge can be a symptom of some STDs (trichomoniasis, gonorrhea). Chapter 24 provides information on risk screening for STDs. Because some infectious processes causing discharge are associated with menses, a menstrual history is gathered in order to detect such an association. A medical history will reveal the presence of system illnesses that are associated with vaginal infections (such as diabetes) and recent or ongoing treatment with antibiotics, which can predispose women to yeast infections.

Table 23.12 Vaginal Discharge

Condition	*History*	*Symptoms*	*Physical Examination Findings*	*Laboratory Data*
Normal	Associated with ovulation, pregnancy, relation to LMP Cyclical in occurrence	Normal body odor Discharge: white/clear, thin/mucoid	Absence of abnormality Spinnbarkheit	Vaginal pH 3.8-4.2 Wet smear: normal flora
Candidiasis (Monilia or yeast)	Recent antibiotic use Pregnancy/oral contraceptive, hormone use History of yeast infections Diabetes mellitus Obesity Symptoms occur or increase prior to menses, relief with menses Dyspareunia	Mild to severe pruritus Thick or thin, white adherent, "cottage-cheese" like discharge None/yeasty, musty odor External dysuria	Inflamed, friable cervix or vagina Inflamed labia or perineum Thick plaques adherent to vaginal walls Excoriations due to scratching Presence of characteristic discharge	Wet prep with potassium hydroxide (KOH); pseudo-hyphae with yeast buds White blood cell Nickerson culture vaginal pH6 = 4.5
Bacterial vaginosis	May be asymptomatic May report odor or partner may complain May report suprapubic discomfort May report increase in odor after intercourse	Discharge (if present) grayish-white, thin scanty Mild pruritus Fishy odor	None/occasional evidence of inflammation Pooling of discharge	Wet prep with saline solution (NaCl): positive cells Add KOH to discharge, fishy odor (whiff test) Increased bacteria
Trichomoniasis	Symptoms of urinary tract infection History of previous trichomoniasis Symptoms may increase during/after menses Use of hot tubs, whirlpool, shared towels History of exposure, multiple partners	Grayish-yellowish-green discharge, copious, frothy, odorous Vaginal burning, pruritus Dyspareunia Lower abdominal cramps, pain	Presence of characteristic discharge "Strawberry spots" on cervix Inflamed friable cervix, vagina Possible abdominal tenderness Possible lymphadenopathy	Wet prep with NaCl: motile trichomonas May be reported on Pap smear

Past episodes of similar symptoms; their diagnoses, course, and treatment; and the result of treatment are documented. Because yeast infections are thought by some to be associated with

Table 23.12 Continued

Condition	*History*	*Symptoms*	*Physical Examination Findings*	*Laboratory Data*
Allergic or chemical vaginitis	No abnormal discharge, odor Dyspareunia History of use of vaginal deodorant sprays, contraceptive cream or foam, soaps, detergents, bubble bath or oils, colored/ perfumed toilet paper Recent change in these	Pruritus External dysuria Vulvular rash Tenderness, pain	Possibly edema, erythema, blisters, ulcerations, rash, thickened patches	No pathogens found

Table 23.13 Historical Data Collected When the Client Complains of Vaginal Discharge

Chronology: onset, duration, course

Quantity and quality of discharge

History of risk factors: oral contraceptives, broad-spectrum antibiotics, sexual activity, pregnancy, use of vaginal sprays, douches

Presence of associated symptoms: itching, burning, dysuria, pelvic pain, fever, irregular vaginal bleeding

Self-treatment measures used

Medications: prescription, over-the-counter, how used

General health: last menstrual period, pattern of contraception, past medical history, previously diagnosed conditions, data and results of last Pap smear

Sexual history: recent contacts, symptoms of contacts, sexual practices, previous history of sexually transmitted diseases

excessive ingestions of dairy products, refined sugars, or artificial sweeteners, taking a diet history may be useful (Shesser, 1990).

Physical Examination and Laboratory Tests

After the history is taken, a pelvic examination, including speculum and bimanual examination, and collection of specimens are indicated. It is important that the examination be done when symptoms are present and the client has not douched or used any medication, so that adequate laboratory specimens can be obtained. The following points should be included in the pelvic examination: Abdominal palpation and palpation for CVA tenderness is done to rule out gastrointestinal or urinary tract problems. The vulva, perineum, and labia are examined for parasites, lesions, irritation, excoriation, discharge, signs of atrophy, and edema. These symptoms may be mild to severe and involve all or only a portion of the area. For example, bright red, inflamed labia are indicative of Candida infection. Any lesion that cannot be identified or that appears suspicious should be biopsied to rule out carcinoma. The vulva and entire vagina are palpated to determine the presence or absence of masses and tenderness. Examination with a warm, dry speculum is always done. No lubricating material should be used because it may alter the results of specimens taken. During the examination, inspect the vaginal walls and cervix for redness, petechial hemorrhages, lesions, discharge and its characteristics, and signs of atrophy. Appropriate laboratory tests may include wet smears with normal saline (NaCl) and potassium hydroxide (KOH), whiff test with KOH, Pap smears, cultures, serological tests, urinalysis, and/or urine culture and sensitivity.

Data gathered from the client's history, a description of symptoms, physical examination findings, and laboratory test results are combined to make a nursing diagnosis.

Preventive Measures

The nurse can do much to alleviate a client's discomfort by teaching preventive measures, instructing her in recognition of symptoms, and assisting her with self-care activities to prevent and treat vaginitis. Lichtman and Papera (1990b) recommend starting with an explanation of the normalcy of vaginal secretions and providing each woman with the opportunity to see her genitalia and normal secretions. The client also should be given time to ask questions, discuss cultural beliefs, and explore her feelings and concerns.

Preventive measures are important for all types of vaginal infection, particularly for women with recurrent vaginitis. Good general health may be a key to preventing frequent infections: Adequate rest, reduction of life stressors, and a healthy diet low in refined sugars may help to decrease the likelihood of infection. Good personal hygiene is essential for preventing vaginal infections. The perineal area needs to be washed frequently to remove perspiration and smegma accumulations. The client should be instructed to pat the area dry rather than rub it. Towels, washcloths, douche bags, contraceptive diaphragms or cervical caps, and underwear should be clean and never shared. Bathtubs should be washed after use. The proper technique of wiping after voiding and defecation should be taught: One should always wipe from front to back (never the reverse) to avoid introducing bacteria into the vagina or urethra. Sprays, soaps, powders, and deodorants that are perfumed or irritating in any way should not be used. Any chemicals that irritate the skin or vaginal mucosa or that alter the vaginal environment should be avoided. Clothing that is too tight, does not allow free airflow to the perineum, or traps moisture should be avoided. Underpants and panty hose should always have a cotton crotch. Douching should be avoided or kept to a minimum because it can strip the vagina of its normal flora, introduce bacteria, or aggravate inflammation.

Measures to prevent STDs, discussed in Chapter 24, are also helpful in preventing vaginal infections.

Frequent changes of tampons and sanitary pads should be recommended. The woman should be counseled to not wear tampons to bed and not to use them when flow is scanty, because they may become adherent to the vagina or cervix and cause trauma when removed.

Bacterial Vaginosis

Bacterial vaginosis (BV), formerly called nonspecific vaginitis, *hemophilus vaginalis*, vaginitis, or *Gardnerella vaginalis,* is the most common type of vaginitis today. Estimates of the prevalence of BV range from 10% in average gynecologic practice to 15% in childbearing women, 25% among university students, and 45% in populations at high risk for STDs (Paavonen et al., 1986; Steinmetz, 1986; Symposium, 1986). BV is extremely common in female jail and prison inmates.

The exact etiology of BV is unknown. The organisms thought to be possible etiologic agents, Gardnerella and *Mobiluncus,* are normal vaginal flora. Although it has been documented that BV occurs in conjunction with an increase in anaerobes in the vagina, the reason why this occurs is not known. What is known is that a decrease in the normal lactobacilli of the vagina occurs, which allows the growth of the normally repressed Gardnerella. This then allows a proliferation of anaerobes, raises the level of vaginal amines, and alters the normal acidic pH of the vagina. Epithelial cells slough and numerous bacteria attach to their surfaces (clue cells) (see Figure 23.1). When the amines are volatilized, the characteristic odor of BV is produced.

Most women with BV complain of a characteristic fishy odor; however, not all note it. The odor may be noticed by the woman or her partner after heterosexual intercourse as semen releases the vaginal amines. When present, the BV discharge is usually profuse, thin, and white or gray, or milky in appearance. Some women also

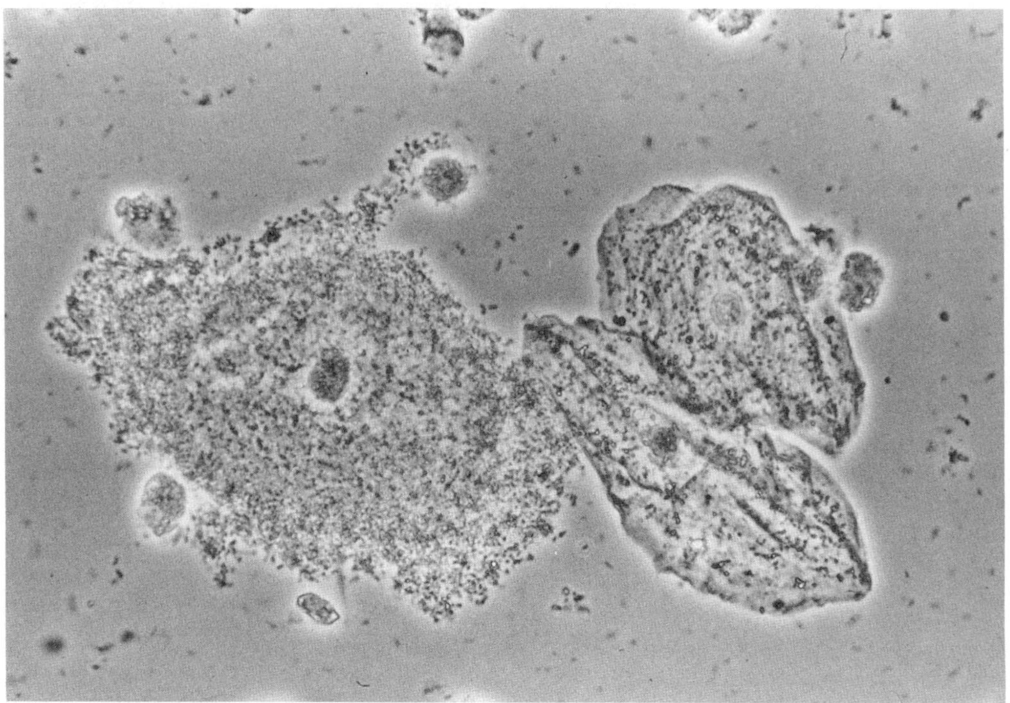

Figure 23.1. Bacterial Vaginosis

may experience mild irritation or pruritis. Women who develop discharge are often very uncomfortable, losing work time and making frequent visits to health care providers (Thomason, Gelbart, & Broekhuizen, 1989).

Assessment

A careful history may help distinguish BV from other vaginal infections if the woman is symptomatic. Reports of fishy odor and increased thin vaginal discharge are most significant, and report of increased odor after intercourse is also suggestive of BV. Previous occurrence of similar symptoms, diagnosis, and treatment should be asked about, because women with BV often have been treated incorrectly. However, because more than 50% of women with BV have no symptoms, the Centers for Disease Control (CDC, 1993) recommends that diagnosis be based on the presence of three of the four following criteria: (a) presence of clue cells on a wet smear, (b) homogeneous noninflammatory discharge that adheres to the vaginal walls, (c) vaginal fluids with a pH of higher than 4.7, and (d) a fishy odor of vaginal discharge before or after addition of 10% KOH (whiff test).

Microscopic examination of vaginal secretions is always done. Both normal NaCl and 10% KOH smears should be made. (The reader is referred to Chapter 9 for information on collection of wet smears.) If the woman has BV, the saline smear should show characteristic signs: decreased number of lactobacilli, characteristic curved rods and corkscrew motility of Mobiluncus, and few WBCs. The presence of clue cells (vaginal epithelial cells coated with bacteria) by wet smear is highly diagnostic, because the phenomenon is specific to BV. Vaginal secretions should be tested for pH and amine odor. Nitrazine paper is sensitive enough to detect a pH of 4.5 or greater. The fishy odor of BV will be released when KOH is added to vaginal secretions on the lip of the withdrawn speculum.

Management

The CDC (1993) recommends metronidazole (Flagyl) 500 mg orally, twice a day for 7 days or a single 2-gm oral dose of metronidazole, which is less expensive and easier to use. Alternative regimens recommended by the CDC are metronidazole gel, 0.75%, one applicator (5 gm) intravaginally, twice a day for 5 days; clindamycin (Cleocin) 300 mg, twice a day for 7 days; or clindamycin cream, 2%, one applicator (5 gm) intravaginally, at bedtime for 7 days.

Metronidazole is an antiprotozoal and antibacterial agent. It is contraindicated in women with hypersensitivity and those in the first trimester of pregnancy. Before metronidazole is prescribed, the nurse must rule out the possibility of early pregnancy. The drug is also contraindicated when the patient is breast-feeding, because high concentrations have been found in infants. If it is necessary to prescribe metronidazole for the lactating woman, she can suspend breast-feeding temporarily and resume it 48 to 72 hours after taking the last dose. Metronidazole is contraindicated in clients with blood dyscrasia or central nervous system disease, because in rare cases it may affect the hematopoietic or central nervous system.

Side effects of metronidazole are numerous, including sharp, unpleasant metallic taste in the mouth, furry tongue, central nervous system reactions, and urinary tract disturbances. When oral metronidazole is taken, the client is advised not to drink alcoholic beverages, or she will experience the severe side effects of abdominal distress, nausea, vomiting, and headache. Gastrointestinal symptoms are common whether alcohol is consumed or not.

Metronidazole has become the object of concern in light of studies reporting carcinogenesis and tumorigenesis in mice and rats given high doses of the medication. Although the carcinogenic potential in humans of the drug is not known, some drug manufacturers and authorities recommend avoiding unecessary use of metronidazole (Lichtman & Duran, 1990).

BV may be a factor in premature rupture of membranes and preterm labor in pregnant women (Gravett, Hummel, Eschenbach, & Holmes, 1986); thus close follow-up of pregnant women is essential. However, at this time, no data suggest that routine treatment is necessary, and until such studies have been done, the CDC states that routine treatment of pregnant women with BV should be at the option of the health care provider. Because metronidazole is contraindicated in the first trimester of pregnancy and its safety in the rest of pregnancy has not been established, treatment with clindamycin, 300 mg, twice a day for 7 days is recommended.

Response to metronidazole is variable, and recurrence of BV is a problem in up to 30% of cases. Currently the CDC does not recommend treatment of sexual partners, stating that sexual transmission of BV has not been proved (CDC, 1989). However, recent data have demonstrated males with the same organism isolated from urethral discharge as women with BV, suggesting that the disease may be sexually transmitted (Symposium, 1991). Therefore, treatment of partners should be considered in women with recurrent disease. Treatment is not recommended for women who are asymptomatic.

It is essential that the woman with BV understand the possible treatments available for her condition and be involved in the choice of treatment, particularly when a drug such as metronidazole is used. When metronidazole is prescribed, the nurse should thoroughly explain the medication regimen, including the need to take all the medication even if her symptoms disappear. Special instructions, such as avoiding alcohol 24 hours before, during, and 24 hours after finishing the medication and the necessity of taking the drug with food, must be given. Women planning a pregnancy should be informed of the risks of BV and advised to have the infection thoroughly treated prior to conception. It is important that the infection be irradicated to prevent the serious sequelae associated with BV: In addition to those associated with pregnancy, sequelae include increased postoperative infection following abdominal or vaginal surgery, pelvic inflammatory disease, postpartum endometritis, and recurrent UTIs.

Some women may wish to try a more natural treatment regimen than metronidazole. Acidification of the vagina may be helpful for women who experience recurrences. Vinegar and water douches, Aci-Jel, or lactobacillus tablets may also be used. Garlic suppositories have been used successfully by some women. Other suggestions are found in Table 23.14.

It is important that women understand the nature of BV. Because an unpleasant odor results from the condition and odor is associated with uncleanliness, a woman may believe that BV is caused by poor personal hygiene. She

Table 23.14 Alternative Therapy for Vaginitis

Intervention	*Dosage*	*Administration*	*Use*
Gentian violet	Few drops in water, 0.25% to 2%	Douche or local application	Yeast infection
Vinegar (white)	1 tbsp/pint water	Douche every 5-7 days; or twice a day (bid) for 2 days	Yeast infection or trichomoniasis
	1-2 tbsp/qt water	Douche 1-2 times a week	Bacterial vaginosis
Acidophilus culture	2 tbsp/pt water	Douche bid	Bacterial vaginosis, yeast infection
Yogurt	1 application to labia or vagina	Hourly, as needed	Yeast infection
Chaparral	Steep 1 handful in 1 qt water for 20 minutes	Douche 2-3 times a week	Trichomoniasis
Chickweed	Steep 3 tbsp in 1 qt water for 10 minutes, strain	Douche daily	Trichomoniasis
Goldenseal	1 tsp in 3 cups water, strain and cool	Douche	Bacterial vaginosis
Garlic clove	1 peeled clove wrapped in cloth dipped in olive oil	Overnight in vagina, change daily	Bacterial vaginosis
Boric acid powder	600 mg in gelatin capsule	Every day in vagina for 14 days	Bacterial vaginosis, yeast infection
Sassafras bark	Steep in warm water	Wash affected area	Itch
Cold milk, cottage cheese, yogurt	Compress	Apply to affected area	Itch

should be reassured that this is not so. Nor does sexual intercourse cause the infection, even though the odor may become stronger at such times.

Candidiasis

The incidence and prevalence of vulvovaginal candidiasis or yeast infection has increased throughout the world in greater proportions than the world population (Symposium, 1991). It is the second most common type of vaginal infection in the United States (Shesser, 1990), accounting for approximately 13 million cases of vulvovaginitis annually (Symposium, 1991). Three quarters of women in the United States will experience at least one yeast infection in their lifetime, often during pregnancy.

The most common organism is *Candida albicans*; it is estimated that 80% to 95% of the yeast infections in women are caused by this organism. However, in the past 10 years, the incidence of nonalbicans infections has risen steadily, from 10% to as much as 25% in some areas (Symposium, 1991). The nonalbicans organisms largely responsible for this increase are *Candida glabrata* and *Candida tropicalis.* Women with chronic or recurrent infections often are infected with a higher percentage of nonalbicans species than are women who are experiencing their first infection or who have few recurrences.

Numerous factors have been identified as predisposing a woman to yeast infections, including antibiotic therapy, particularly broad-spectrum antibiotics such as ampicillin, tetracycline, cephalosporins, and metronidazole; diabetes, especially when uncontrolled; pregnancy; obesity; diets high in refined sugars or artificial sweeteners; use of corticosteroids and exogenous hormones; and immunosupressed states. Clinical observations and research have suggested that tight-fitting clothing and underwear or panty hose made of nonabsorbent materials creates an environment in which the vaginal fungus can grow.

The most common symptom of yeast infections is vulvular and possibly vaginal pruritis. The itching may be mild or intense, interfere with rest and activities, and occur during or after intercourse. Some women report a feeling of dryness. Others may experience painful urination as the urine flows over the vulva; this usually occurs in women who have excoriations resulting from scratching. Vaginal discharge is variable in yeast infections. Some women complain of a discharge and others do not. Most often the discharge is white, lumpy, and cottage-cheese-like; however, it may be thin and watery. Often the discharge is found in patches on the vaginal walls, cervix, and labia. Commonly the vulva is red and swollen, as are the labial folds, vagina, and cervix. Although there is not a characteristic odor with yeast infections, sometimes a yeasty or musty odor is produced.

Assessment

In addition to listing the woman's symptoms, their onset, and their course, the history is a valuable screening tool for identifying predisposing risk factors. A nutritional history may help to identify dietary factors, whereas a review of personal hygiene habits may identify regular use of tight-fitting clothes or athletic clothing, douches, and feminine sprays. If the woman is of childbearing age and sexually active, a pregnancy test should be done for nonpregnant women.

Physical examination should include a thorough inspection of the vulva and vagina. A speculum examination is always done. Any discharge present should be inspected and smelled.

Although often overlooked, a complete laboratory workup is necessary even when the classic symptoms of yeast are present. Laboratory tests include NaCl and KOH wet smear, vaginal pH, and, less often, gram staining and latex agglutination tests. Vaginal pH is normal with a yeast infection; if the pH is higher than 4.5, one should suspect trichomoniasis or bacterial vaginosis. The characteristic pseudohyphae may be seen on a wet smear done with normal saline; however, they may be confused with other cells and artifacts. The KOH slide is diagnostic of Candida, because it lyses other vaginal cells and leaves the Candida intact. (The characteristic spores or hyphae of Candida can be seen in Figure 23.2.) The latex agglutination test is useful in identifying nonalbican strains.

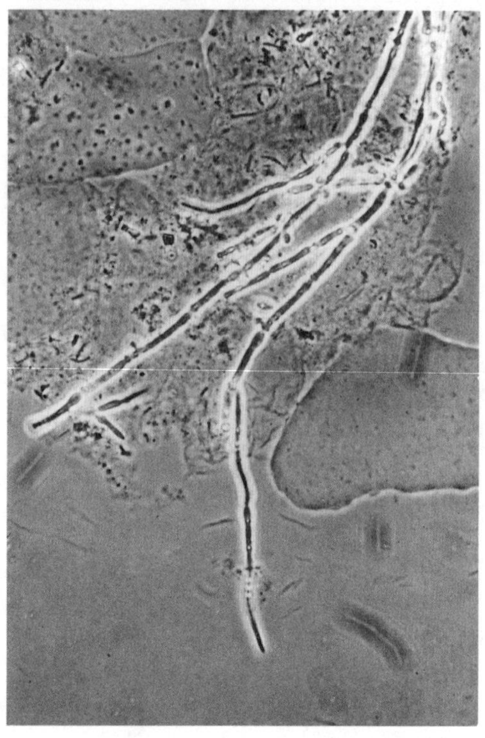

Figure 23.2. Candida

Nursing Management

A number of antifungal preparations are available for the treatment of infections by *Candida albicans.* CDC (1993) recommendations are as follows:

- Miconazole nitrate (Monistat) 200-mg vaginal suppository, intravaginally at bedtime for 3 days
- Miconazole nitrate cream, 2%, 5 gm for 7 days
- Miconazole nitrate 100-mg vaginal suppositories, 1 suppository intravaginally for 7 days
- Clotrimazole (Gyne-Lotrimin) 100-mg vaginal tablets, 1 tablet intravaginally at bedtime for 7 days
- Clotrimazole 100-mg vaginal tablets, 2 tablets intravaginally for 3 days
- Clotrimazole 500-mg vaginal tablets, 1 tablet intravaginally, single application
- Butaconazole (Femstat) cream, 2%, 5 gm, intravaginally at bedtime for 3 days
- Teraconazole (Terazol) 80-mg suppository, 1 suppository for 3 days
- Teraconazole cream, 0.4%, 5 gm intravaginally at bedtime for 7 days
- Teraconazole cream, 0.8%, 5 gm intravaginally at bedtime for 3 days
- Teraconazole ointment, 6.5%, 5-gm single application

In 1990, many of these medications (Monostat and Gyne-Lotrimin) were made available over the counter. The first time a woman suspects that she may have a yeast infection, she should see a health care provider for confirmation of the diagnosis and treatment recommendation. If she experiences another infection, she may wish to purchase an over-the-counter preparation and self-treat; if she elects to do this, she should always be counseled regarding seeking care for numerous recurrent or chronic yeast infections. Amankwaa and Frank (1991) tested another intervention for increasing the comfort of women with vulvovaginal candidiasis. In an experimental study using a sample of 20 women, the comfort of a control group who received routine care was compared to the comfort of the experimental group who received routine care plus vaginal debridement with a cotton swab followed by application of vaginal medication. Study results suggest that the experimental intervention was effective in decreasing the discomfort of women with yeast infections. Clinicians should be aware that recurrent, difficult-to-treat Candida infections may be an initial indication of HIV infection or AIDS. This topic is discussed in Chapter 24.

Women who have extensive irritation, swelling, and discomfort of the labia and vulva may find sitz baths helpful in decreasing inflammation and increasing comfort. Adding Aveeno powder to her bath may also increase the woman's comfort. Preventive, comfort measures discussed earlier are taught. Not wearing underpants to bed may help decrease symptoms and prevent recurrences. Completing the full course of treatment prescribed is essential in removing the pathogen, and women are instructed to continue medication even during menstruation. They should be counseled not to use tampons during menses because the medication will be absorbed by the tampon. If possible, intercourse is avoided during treatment; if this is not feasible, the woman's partner should use a condom to prevent introduction of more organisms.

Many women may wish to use self-help measures to prevent a fungal infection, relieve the discomfort of infection, or prevent recurrence of infection. (Table 23.14 lists many that are useful with yeast infections.) Some practitioners believe that certain women have a particular sensitivity to yeast and recommend a diet low in foods that grow yeast (Crook, 1986). Such foods include breads and pastries, cheeses, alcohol, malt products, condiments, sauces, vinegar, processed and smoked meats, teas and coffees, fruits such as melons, dried fruits, and leftovers. As another possible preventive measure, women should be taught to disinfect diaphragms and bathtubs after they have had an infection.

Trichomoniasis

Trichomonas vaginalis is almost always a STD. It is also a very common cause of vaginal infection and discharge and thus is discussed in this chapter rather than in Chapter 24.

Trichomoniasis is caused by *Trichomonas vaginalis*, an anaerobic one-celled protozoan with characteristic flagellae (see Figure 23.3). An estimated 180 million women worldwide have trichomoniasis each year; 2.5 million cases are reported annually in the United States (Shesser, 1990). Women attending STD clinics; teenagers; and single, pregnant women have increased numbers of infections (Hill, Luther, Young, Pereira, & Embil, 1988). Although the incidence peaks at ages 16 to 35, the disease is also common in women aged 30 to 50 (Lichtman & Duran, 1990).

In acute trichomoniasis, the discharge is characteristically yellowish to greenish, frothy, mucopurulent, copious, and malodorous. In some women, the discharge is more gray than green. Inflammation of the vulva, vagina, or both may be present, and the woman may complain of irritation and pruritis. Dysuria and dyspareunia are often present. Typically, the discharge worsens during and after menstruation. Symptoms often begin during or shortly after menses when the blood-buffering activity enhances multiplication of the Trichomonas organism (Stresser, 1990). Often, the cervix and vaginal walls will demonstrate the characteristic "strawberry spots" or tiny petechiae, and the cervix may bleed on contact. In severe infections, the vaginal walls, cervix, and, occasionally, the vulva may be acutely inflamed.

Trichomoniasis may be asymptomatic or chronic. A woman with an asymptomatic infection, however, may have a history of symptoms and may become symptomatic in the future. In an asymptomatic infection, the vaginal pH is 3.8 to 4.2 and organisms are present. Women with chronic infections will have abnormal vaginal discharge although the vulva and vagina are not affected and irritation may or may not be present.

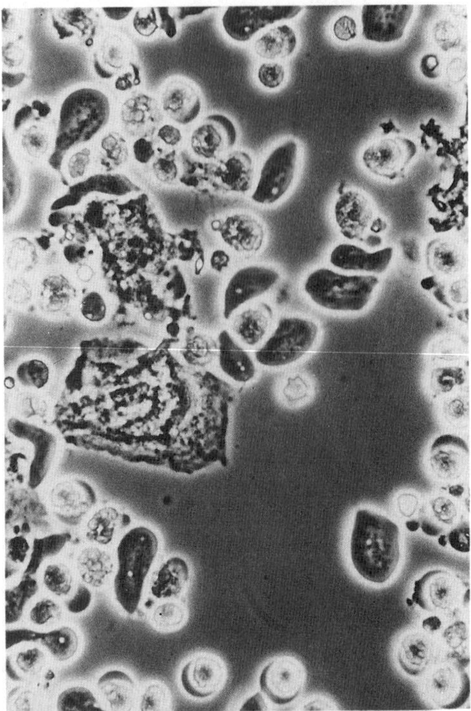

Figure 23.3. Trichomoniasis

Assessment

In addition to obtaining a history of current symptoms, a careful sexual history should be obtained because trichomoniasis is a sexually transmitted infection. Any history of similar symptoms in the past and treatment regimens used should be noted. The nurse should determine whether her client's partner was treated and if she has had subsequent relations with a new partner.

The vulva, vagina, and cervix are inspected, and the urethra should be milked for discharge. A speculum examination is always done, even though it may be very uncomfortable for the woman; relaxation techniques and breathing exercises may help the woman with the procedure. Any of the classic signs may or may not be present on physical examination.

Definitive diagnosis is made through demonstration of the organism, most easily done with a normal saline wet smear. (See Chapter 9 for instructions on obtaining a wet smear.) If there is any question of diagnosis, a KOH smear can be done to rule out Candida. The typical one-celled flagellate Trichomonas organisms are easily distinguished (see Figure 23.3). Trichomoniasis may also be identified on Pap smears; however, diagnosis should be confirmed by direct visualization or culture.

Because trichomoniasis is an STD, once diagnosis is confirmed, appropriate laboratory studies for other STDs should be carried out.

Nursing Management

Asymptomatic and symptomatic clients are treated. The recommended treatment is 2 grams of metronidazole orally in a single dose (CDC, 1993). Alternative therapy is metronidazole, 500 mg, twice a day for 7 days. If either regimen does not cure the disease, the woman should be retreated with metronidazole, 500 mg, twice a day for 7 days. If repeated failure occurs, the woman is treated with a single 2-gm dose of metronidazole daily for 3 to 5 days. Metronidazole is contraindicated in the first trimester of pregnancy, and its safety has not been established in the remainder of pregnancy. No other adequate therapy exists, however; therefore, after the first trimester of pregnancy treatment with 2 grams of metronidazole in a single dose may be considered for pregnant women with severe symptoms (CDC, 1989). Self-help measures for the treatment of trichomoniasis are found in Table 23.14.

Although the male partner is usually asymptomatic, it is recommended that he receive treatment also, because he often harbors the Trichomonas organism in the urethra or prostate. It is important that nurses discuss the importance of partner treatment with their clients. If partners are not treated, it is likely that the infection will reoccur.

Women with trichomoniasis need to understand the sexual transmission of this disease. It is important that the client know that the organism may be present without symptoms, perhaps for several months, and that it is not possible to determine when she became infected. Women should be informed of the necessity for treating all sexual partners and helped with ways to raise the issue with their partners. (See Chapter 24 for a detailed discussion.)

Clients should be given ample opportunity to ask any questions they may have and be provided with written information for themselves and their partners. Clients can be reassured that trichomoniasis is not a systemic infection and is not known to cause infertility.

Contact Vaginitis

Vaginitis can result from reactions to allergens, foreign bodies, or chemicals such as perfumes. No one specific discharge is characteristic of such vaginitis. The woman may experience an increase in the usual type and amount of secretions, as well as itching and burning. Rashes in the vulvar area are often present, although usually little upper vaginal or cervical irritation occurs. The diagnosis is often made by exclusion and confirmed by the alleviation of symptoms once the irritant or allergen is removed.

Foreign bodies in the vagina result in a foul-smelling, blood-tinged, serosanguineous or purulent discharge, which may be either thick or thin. With speculum examination, the foreign body should be visible; frequently, it is lodged in the posterior fornix of the vagina. Foreign bodies commonly found include tampons, diaphragms, and condoms. If there is a secondary infection with inflammation and purulent discharge, it should be cultured.

Removal of the allergen or irritant is the treatment for allergic or irritative vaginitis. The nurse should explore any possible areas of irritation; preventive health measures can be very effective with this type of vaginitis. When the client is experiencing considerable discomfort, local relief measures may help. Sitz baths several times a day can reduce inflammation, and hydrocortisone cream can be used to reduce the local inflammatory reaction. If vaginitis is caused by a foreign body, removal of the body will alleviate symptoms in a few days. If infection is present, specific antibiotic therapy should be started once the pathogen is identified.

Atrophic Vaginitis

Anything that decreases a woman's estrogen levels after menarche can result in vaginal thinning, loss of rugae, and decreased elasticity of vaginal tissues. As vaginal pH increases, lactobacilli growth is depressed and other bacteria tend to multiply; this combination of factors can lead to vaginitis. Most commonly, this is seen in breast-feeding women and women who have experienced menopause. It is called atrophic vaginitis, a misnomer for what is a normal process.

A woman with atrophic vaginitis may report a thin watery discharge that is variable in amount. Vaginal discharge may be watery, purulent, serosanguineous, or sticky. She may have a small amount of bleeding after intercourse, dysuria, dyspareunia, pruritis, or tenderness. Bladder symptoms such as dysuria may be present. In menopausal women, vulvular inflammation may be noted. Excoriation may be present.

Assessment

An important piece of historical data is the woman's age and menstrual status. Whether she has stopped menstruating or had a surgical menopause is noted. Ask about any other symptoms of menopause, such as hot flashes. If she is premenopausal, her lactation status is ascertained.

A complete pelvic examination is done and signs of atrophy watched for. Wet smears are done and will usually reveal decreased presence of lactobacilli and increased blood cells and bacteria. A Pap smear is always done if there is spotting or blood-tinged discharge. A maturation index from the upper lateral third of the vaginal wall can indicate decreased estrogenization of the vagina.

Management

When a diagnosis of atrophic vaginitis is made, water-soluble lubricants may be recommended for intercourse. A number are available over the counter. Masturbation without penetration, which decreases trauma to the vagina, may be an acceptable alternative for couples in the initial lactation period. Woman-on-top position during vaginal intercourse will allow her to control the depth of penile thrusting and may prove to be a more comfortable position. Women should always be counseled to discuss the problem with their partner and explain its physical basis. Vaginal or systemic estrogen replacement may be warranted for postmenopausal women (see Chapter 5). Treatment for any secondary infections is mandatory. Women need information about this condition and reassurance that it does not mean that their organs are atrophying or shriveling up. Any misconceptions about menopause should be explored and corrected.

Recurrent Vaginitis

Recurrent vaginitis can be extremely discouraging and frustrating for both the client and clinicians. It is important to identify the reason for the recurrence. Is it due to reinfection? Inadequate following of treatment regimen? Incorrect treatment? If the client does not complete an entire course of treatment, the organisms have probably not been eradicated, and another complete course of treatment is needed. Sometimes, medications are absorbed inadequately because heavy vaginal discharge has interfered or the woman has used tampons or douched shortly after inserting the medication. Douching should precede insertion of medication to clear away a heavy discharge. Tampons, which can absorb much of the medication, should be avoided.

Possible pockets of organisms in sheltered sites should be explored. Skene's glands, Bartholin's glands, the urethra, bladder, or rectum can all act as sources of reinfection. Sexual partner(s) should also be considered as a possible source of reinfection.

Summary

The symptoms of bleeding, pain, and discharge are common to women and cause discomfort, interference with lifestyle, and distress, both physical and emotional. The nurse can alleviate these adverse effects through intervention. Client education to facilitate self-care activities and interventions that support specific diagnosis and treatment measures are essential nursing roles. Permeating all nursing endeavors should be a relationship of mutual trust that enhances an honest communication with and support of the client.

References

Abraham, G., & Rumley, R. (1987). Role of nutrition in managing the premenstrual syndromes. *Journal of Reproductive Medicine, 32,* 405-422.

Amankwaa, L. C., & Frank, D. F. (1991). Vulvovaginal candidiasis: A study of immediate vs. delayed treatment on patient comfort. *Nurse Practitioner, 16*(6), 24, 26-27.

American Psychiatric Association. (1994). *Diagnostic and statistical manual of mental disorders* (4th ed.). Washington, DC: Author.

Avant, R. F. (1988). Dysmenorrhea. *Primary Care, 15,* 549-559.

Aycock, D. G. (1991). Ibuprofen: A monograph. *American Pharmacy, NS31*(3), 46-49.

Beischer, N. A., & MacKay, E. V. (1986). *Obstetrics and the newborn* (2nd ed.). Philadelphia: W. B. Saunders.

Brown, M. A., & Woods, N. F. (1984). Correlates of dysmenorrhea. *JOGNN, 13,* 259-265.

Busch, C. M., Costa, P. T., Whitehead, W. E., & Heller, B. R. (1988). Severe perimenstrual symptoms: Prevalence and effects on absenteeism and health care seeking in a non-clinical sample. *Women & Health, 14*(1), 59-74.

Centers for Disease Control. (1989). 1989 Sexually transmitted diseases treatment guidelines. *Morbidity and Mortality Weekly Report, 39*(Suppl. 8), 1-43.

Centers for Disease Control. (1993, September 24). Sexually transmitted disease—Treatment guidelines. *Morbidity and Mortality Weekly Report,* pp. 1-102.

Chihal, J. H. (1987). Indications for drug therapy in premenstrual syndrome patients. *Journal of Reproductive Medicine, 32,* 449-452.

Clark-Coller, T. (1991). Dysfunctional uterine bleeding and amenorrhea. *Journal of Nurse-Midwifery, 36*(1), 49-62.

Clarke-Pearson, D. L., & Dawood, M. Y. (1990). *Green's gynecology: Essentials of clinical practice* (4th ed.). Boston: Little, Brown.

Connell, A. (1989). Abnormal uterine bleeding. *Nurse Practitioner, 14*(1), 40, 43-44, 47, 50, 53, 56-57.

Coyne, C. M., Woods, N. F., & Mitchell, E. S. (1985). Premenstrual tension syndrome. *JOGNN, 14,* 446-453.

Crook, W. G. (1986). *The yeast connection* (3rd ed.). Jackson, TN: Professional Books.

Dalton, K. (1960a). Menstruations and accidents. *British Medical Journal, 2,* 1425-1426.

Dalton, K. (1960b). Schoolgirls' behavior and menstruation. *British Medical Journal, 2,* 1647-1659.

Dalton, K. (1980a). Cyclic criminal acts in premenstrual syndrome. *Lancet, 2,* 1070-1071.

Dalton, K. (1980b). Progesterone, fluid and electrolytes in premenstrual syndrome. *British Medical Journal, 281,* 61.

Dawood, M. Y. (1986). Current concepts in the etiology and treatment of primary dysmenorrhea. *Acta Obstetrica Gynecoligica Scandinavica* (Suppl. 138), 7-10.

DeBrovner, C. H. (1985, March 21). Initial work-up of dysmenorrhea. *Hospital Medicine,* pp. 63-65, 69-71, 75-77, 80.

Doody, K. M., & Carr, B. R. (1990). Amenorrhea. *Obstetrics and Gynecology Clinics of North America, 17,* 361-384.

Ellerbrock, T., Atrash, H., Hogue, C., & Hughes, J. (1987). Ectopic pregnancy mortality in the United States, 1979-1982. *MMWR CDC Surveillance Summaries, 36*(SS-2), 13-18.

Federation of Feminist Women's Health Centers. (1981). *A new view of a woman's body.* New York: Simon & Schuster, Touchstone.

Fisher, M., Trieller, K., & Napolitano, B. (1989). Premenstrual syndrome in adolescents. *Journal of Adolescent Health Care, 10,* 369-375.

Fogel, C. I. (1981). The gynecologic triad: Discharge, pain and bleeding. In C. I. Fogel & N. F. Woods

(Eds.), *Health care of women: A nursing perspective* (pp. 220-256). St. Louis, MO: C. V. Mosby.

Gaines, F. (1981). Secondary amenorrhea: Part II. Assessment and plans. *Nurse Practitioner, 6*(4), 14-23.

Gannon, L. (1988). The potential role of exercise in the alleviation of menstrual disorders and menopausal symptoms: A theoretical synthesis of recent research. *Women & Health, 14*(2), 105-127.

Gilbert, E. S., & Harmon, J. S. (1986). *High risk pregnancy and delivery: Nursing perspectives.* St. Louis, MO: C. B. Mosby.

Gravett, M. G., Hummel, D., Eschenbach, D. A., & Holmes, K. K. (1986). Preterm labor associated with subclinical amniotic fluid infection and with bacterial vaginosis. *Obstetrics and Gynecology, 67,* 229-237.

Hatcher, R. A., Trussell, J., Stewart, F., Stewart, G. K., Kowal, D., Guest, F., Cates, W., & Policar, M. S. (1994). *Contraceptive technology 1994-1996* (16th rev. ed.). New York: Irvington.

Hawkins, J. W., Roberto, D., & Stanley-Haney, J. L. (1994). *Protocols for nurse practitioners* (4th ed.). New York: Tiresias.

Hayashi, R. H., & Castillo, M. S. (1986). Bleeding in pregnancy. In R. A. Knuppel & J. E. Drukker (Eds.), *High-risk pregnancy: A team approach* (pp. 539-560). Philadelphia: W. B. Saunders.

Hill, L. V., Luther, E. R., Young, D., Pereira, L., & Embil, J. A. (1988). Prevalence of lower genital tract infections in pregnancy. *Sexually Transmitted Diseases, 15*(1), 5-10.

Hill, W. C., & Lambertz, E. L. (1990). Let's get rid of the term "Braxton Hicks contraction." *Obstetrics and Gynecology, 75,* 709-710.

Hooton, T. M., Running, K., & Stamm, W. E. (1985). Single-dose therapy for cystitis in women: A comparison of trimethoprim-sulfamethoxazole, amoxicillin and cyclacillin. *JAMA, 253,* 387-390.

Horrobin, D. F. (1990). Evening primrose oil and premenstrual syndrome. *Medical Journal of Australia, 153,* 630-631.

Horton, J. A. (1992). *The women's health data book.* Washington, DC: Jacobs Institute of Women's Health.

Hsia, L. S., & Long, M. H. (1990). Premenstrual syndrome. *Journal of Nurse-Midwifery, 35,* 351-357.

Israel, R. G., Sutton, M., & O'Brien, K. (1985). Effects of aerobic training on primary dysmenorrhea symptomatology in college females. *Journal of American College Health, 33,* 241-244.

Jackson, V. (1990). The uterus. In R. Lichtman & S. Papera (Eds.), *Gynecology well-woman care* (pp. 261-272). Norwalk, CT: Appleton & Lange.

Jones, D. Y. (1987). Physiology and behavior, influence of dietary fat on self-reported menstrual symptoms. *Physiology and Behavior, 40,* 483-487.

Keye, W. R. (1987). General evaluation of premenstrual symptoms. *Clinics in Obstetrics and Gynecology, 30,* 396-405.

Lichtman, R., & Duran, P. (1990a). The well-woman gynecologic interview. In R. Lichtman & S. Papera (Eds.), *Gynecology well-woman care* (pp. 19-28). Norwalk, CT: Appleton & Lange.

Lichtman, R., & Duran, P. (1990b). The urinary tract. In R. Lichtman & S. Papera (Eds.), *Gynecology well-woman care* (pp. 300-301). Norwalk, CT: Appleton & Lange.

Lichtman, R., & Papera, S. (Eds.). (1990a). *Gynecology well-woman care.* Norwalk, CT: Appleton & Lange.

Lichtman, R., & Papera, S. (1990b). The vulva and vagina. In R. Lichtman & S. Papera (Eds.), *Gynecology well-woman care* (pp. 173-201). Norwalk, CT: Appleton & Lange.

Lichtman, R., & Smith, S. M. (1990). Multiorganic disorders. In R. Lichtman & S. Papera (Eds.), *Gynecology well-woman care* (pp. 309-313). Norwalk, CT: Appleton & Lange.

Lindow, K. B. (1991). Premenstrual syndrome: Family impact and nursing implications. *JOGNN, 20*(2), 135-138.

Litcher, E. D., & Warfield, C. A. (1985, March 15). Pelvic pain syndrome. *Hospital Practice,* 32E, 32H, 32K.

Long, C. A., & Gast, M. J. (1990). Menorrhagia. *Obstetrics and Gynecology, 17,* 343-359.

Maddocks, S., Hohn, P., Moller, F., & Reid, R. L. (1986). A double-blind, placebo-controlled trial of progesterone vaginal suppositories in the treatment of premenstrual syndrome. *American Journal of Obstetrics and Gynecology, 15,* 573-581.

Maxton, W. S. (1988). Physiology of the normal menstrual cycle: A physiological basis for premenstrual symptoms. In W. R. Keye (Ed.), *The premenstrual syndrome.* Philadelphia: W. B. Saunders.

McGregor, J. A., & Todd, J. K. (1987, October). Toxic shock syndrome a decade later. *Physician's Assistant,* pp. 34, 37-38, 40, 43-44, 53-54.

Miller, L. G., & Prichard, J. G. (1990). Current issues in NSAID therapy. *Primary Care, 17*(4), 589-601.

Murata, J. M. (1990). Abnormal genital bleeding and secondary amenorrhea. *JOGNN, 19*(1), 26-36.

Nederlof, K. P., Laswon, H. W., Saftlos, A. F., Atrash, H. K., & Finch, E. L. (1989). Ectopic pregnancy. *Morbidity and Mortality Weekly Report, 39*(Suppl. 4), 9-17.

Olin, B. R. (1991). *Drug facts and comparisons.* Philadelphia: J. B. Lippincott.

Osofsky, H. J., Keppel, W., & Kuczmierczyk, A. (1988). Evaluation and management of premenstrual syndrome in clinical psychiatric practice. *Journal of Clinical Psychiatry, 49,* 494-497.

Ouellette, M. D., MacVicar, M. G., & Harlan, J. (1986). Relationship between percent body fat and menstrual patterns in athletes and nonathletes. *Nursing Research, 35,* 330-333.

Paavonen, J., Heinonen, P. K., Aine, R., Laine, S. & Grönroos, P. (1986). Prevalence of nonspecific vaginitis and other cervicovaginal infections in the third trimester. *Sexually Transmitted Diseases, 13*(1), 5-8.

Parlee, M. B. (1973). The premenstrual syndrome. *Psychological Bulletin, 80,* 454-465.

Peck, D. (1990). Premenstrual syndrome. In R. Lichtman & S. Papera (Eds.), *Gynecology well-woman care* (pp. 333-343). Norwalk, CT: Appleton & Lange.

Peddie, B. A., Gorrie, S. I., & Bailey, R. R. (1986). Diaphragm use and urinary tract infection. *JAMA, 255*(13), 1787.

Prior, J. C., Vigna, Y., Sciaretta, D., Alajada, N., & Schulzer, M. (1987). Conditioning exercise decreases premenstrual symptoms: A prospective, controlled 6-month trial. *Fertility and Sterility, 47,* 402-408.

Reid, R. L. (1991). Premenstrual syndrome. *New England Journal of Medicine, 324,* 1208-1210.

Scott, J. R. (1986). Spontaneous abortion. In D. N. Danforth & J. R. Scott (Eds.), *Obstetrics and gynecology* (5th ed., pp. 378-356). St. Louis: C. V. Mosby.

Scott, J. R., Disaia, P., Hammond, C., & Spellacy, W. N. (1994). *Danforth obstetrics and gynecology* (7th ed.). Philadelphia: J. B. Lippincott.

Severino, S. K., & Moline, M. L. (1990). Premenstrual syndrome. *Obstetrics and Gynecology Clinics of North America, 17,* 889-903.

Shesser, R. (1990, August). Diagnosis of common vaginal infection. *Physician's Assistant,* pp. 23-33.

Shulman, J. F. (1990). Bleeding disorders. In R. Lichtman & S. Papera (Eds.), *Gynecology well-woman care* (pp. 355-365). Norwalk, CT: Appleton & Lange.

Simmons, P. S. (1988). Common gynecologic problems in adolescents. *Primary Care, 15,* 629-642.

Speroff, L., Glass, R. H., & Kase, N. G. (1989). *Clinical gynecologic endocrinology and infertility* (4th ed.). Baltimore: Williams & Wilkins.

Steinmetz, K. S. (1986). Gardnerella vaginalis vaginitis. *Journal of Nurse-Midwifery, 31*(2), 87-92.

Stewart, D. E. (1989). Positive changes in the premenstrual period. *Acta Psychiatrica Scandinavica, 79,* 400-405.

Sullivan, N. (1990). Dysmenorrhea. In R. Lichtman & S. Papera (Eds.), *Gynecology well-woman care* (pp. 345-353). Norwalk, CT: Appleton & Lange.

Symposium: Establishing bacterial vaginosis. (1986). *Contemporary Ob/Gyn, 27,* 186-203.

Symposium: Vulvovaginitis—causes and therapies. (1991). *Clinical Courier, 9*(2), 1-12.

Thomason, J. L., Gelbart, S. M., & Broekhuizen, F. F. (1989). Advances in the understanding of bacterial vaginosis. *Journal of Reproductive Medicine, 34*(Suppl.), 581-586.

Todd, J., Fishaut, M., Kapral, F., & Welch, T. (1978). Toxic-shock syndrome associated with phage-group-1 staphylococci. *Lancet, 2,* 116-118.

Treybig, M. (1989). Primary dysmenorrhea or endometriosis? *Nurse Practitioner, 14*(5), 8, 15-17.

Wallach, E. E., Hammond, C., Goldfarb, A., & Kempers, R. (1983). Problems linked to uterine myomas. *Contemporary Ob/Gyn, 22,* 265-279.

Walton, J., & Youngkin, E. (1987). The effect of a support group on self-esteem of women with premenstrual syndrome. *JOGNN, 16*(3), 174-178.

Wardell, D. W. (1989). Ectopic pregnancy: A growing concern. *Journal of the American Academy of Nurse Practitioners, 1*(4), 119-125.

Wicks, S. L. (1988). Premenstrual syndrome. *Primary Care, 15*(3), 473-487.

Wilcox, A. J., Weinberg, C. R., O'Connor, J. F., Baird, D. D., Schlatterer, J. P, Canfield, R. E., Armstrong, E. G., & Nisula, B. C. (1988). Incidence of early loss of pregnancy. *New England Journal of Medicine, 319,* 189-194.

Wilson, C. A., & Keye, W. R. (1989). A survey of adolescent dysmenorrhea and premenstrual symptom frequency. *Journal of Adolescent Health Care, 10,* 317-322.

Wolner-Hanssen, P., Krieger, J. N., Stevens, C. E., Kaviat, N. B., Kowtsky, L., Critchlow, C., DeRouon, T., Hillier, S., & Holmes, K. K. (1989). Clinical manifestations of vaginal trichomoniasis. *JAMA, 261,* 571-576.

24

Sexually Transmitted Diseases

CATHERINE INGRAM FOGEL

Sexually transmitted diseases (STDs) are infections or infectious disease syndromes primarily transmitted by sexual contact. Caused by a wide spectrum of bacteria, viruses, protozoa, and ectoparasities (organisms that live on the outside of the body, such as a louse), STDs are a direct cause of tremendous human suffering, place heavy demands on health care services, and cost hundreds of millions of dollars to treat (Hatcher et al., 1994). Despite the U.S. Surgeon General's targeting STDs as a priority for prevention and control efforts (Public Health Service, 1979), STDs are among the most common health problems in the United States today (Cates, 1988).

Currently, more than 50 diseases and syndromes are recognized as being transmitted sexually (Cates, 1988). In the past, public health efforts were aimed at the control of the traditional venereal diseases of gonorrhea and syphilis; more recently, however, when it appeared that these diseases were controlled, concern focused on other diseases such as chlamydia, herpes simplex virus (HSV), human papillomavirus (HPV), and the human immunodeficiency virus (HIV). Unfortunately, such a shifting focus does not mean that gonorrhea and syphilis are no longer of concern. In recent years, drug-resistant strains of gonorrhea and upswings in the number of cases of syphilis reported have become common (Centers for Disease Control [CDC], 1989). The CDC estimates that there are 12 million cases of STDs every year (Division of STD/HIV Prevention, 1991). The most common STDs in women are chlamydia, condyloma acuminatum, gonorrhea, herpes simplex virus (HSV) type-2, syphilis, and HIV infection.

Although, historically, STDs were considered to be symptomatic illnesses usually afflicting men, it is actually women and their children who suffer the most severe symptoms and sequelae of these diseases (Fogel, 1990). The total cost for care of patients with STDs is high. If all STDs are considered, the costs are estimated at 5.5 billion dollars a year. The human costs are equally overwhelming (Fogel & Lauver, 1990). The lives of women with cervical cancer and chronic pelvic pain or who experience stillbirth or preterm delivery are full of suffering. Couples faced with a diagnosis of infertility may require invasive procedures, such as in vitro fertilization. The emotional costs are immeasurable.

Nurses have the responsibility for providing accurate, safe, sensitive, and supportive care for women with an STD. To meet a client's needs, a nurse must have up-to-date information about specific diseases and conditions, diagnostic measures, and treatment options. In this chapter, risk factors for STDs are considered and prevention strategies examined. Assessment and management strategies appropriate for all STDs are presented and specific entities discussed in terms of etiology and transmission, epidemiology, clinical presentation, complications and sequelae, assessment, and management.

Risk Factors

The chance of contracting, transmitting, or suffering complications from sexually transmitted diseases depends on a number of factors. Risk factors for STDs in women include (a) young age, (b) being black or Hispanic, (c) urban residence, and (d) certain sexual behaviors.

In women, STDs are primarily diseases of those aged 15 to 29 (Division of STD/HIV Prevention, 1991). The highest incidence is seen in women aged 20 to 24, with the next highest age group being 25- to 29-year-olds. Recent studies in urban areas have shown that the transmission of gonorrhea, syphilis, chancroid, and HIV infection has been closely associated with exchange of drugs for sex (Aral & Holmes, 1991; Rolfs, Goldberg, & Sharrar, 1990). To support their addiction, women, especially adolescent women, may have very large numbers of sexual partners.

STDs are concentrated more heavily in some racial and ethnic groups, affecting blacks and Hispanics more than whites or individuals of Asian ethnicity (Handsfield, 1991; Lichtman & Duran, 1990). Some of the differences seen may be attributable to reporting bias; blacks and Hispanics more often seek care at public clinics, where case reporting is more complete than in private offices.

STDs are the only illnesses whose spread is directly caused by the human urge to share sexual intimacy and reproduce (McGregor, French, & Spencer, 1989). Because intimate human contact is the common vehicle of transmission, sexual behavior is a critical risk factor for STDs. Risk factors for contracting an STD linked to sexual behavior include having multiple partners, early age at onset of sexual activity, increased frequency of intercourse, and choice of a high-risk partner.

Risk of contracting an STD is determined not only by the woman's actions but by her partner's as well. In addition to identifying the partner who is at high risk because of drugs and medical factors, it is important that the woman ascertain the sexual practices of her partner. However, this may be difficult to do because partners may lie about their risk history. A recent study of 18- to 25-year-old college students found that a sizable percentage of men reported having lied in order to have sex and that 68% of the sexually active men were involved with more than one partner simultaneously and their partners were unaware of this (Cochran & Mays, 1990). Women who engage in sexual activities with other women only may or may not be at risk for infection. Many women who identify themselves as lesbian have had intercourse with a man at one time by choice, by force, or by necessity. Their female partners may have had intercourse with a man. In addition, lesbians may use drugs and share needles, may receive blood transfusions, or may be artificially inseminated.

Sexual practices such as intercourse without latex condoms, anal intercourse, or oral-genital contact increase risk. Alcohol and drug use associated with sexual activity may also increase a woman's risk of contracting STDs because their use may result in lapses in clear thinking or judgment that could lead to high-risk behaviors.

Prevention of STDs

Preventing infection (primary prevention) is the most effective way of reducing the adverse consequences of STDs for individuals and for society. With the advent of serious and potentially lethal STDs that are not readily cured or are incurable, primary prevention becomes critical. Prompt diagnosis and treatment of current infections (secondary prevention) can also prevent personal complications and transmission to others.

Primary Prevention

Primary preventive measures are individual activities aimed at deterring infection. Risk-free options include complete abstinence from sexual activities that transmit semen, blood, or other body fluids or that allow for skin-to-skin contact

(Hatcher et al., 1994). Alternatively, involvement in a mutually monogamous relationship with an uninfected partner also eliminates risk of contracting an STD. When neither of these options is realistic for a woman, however, the nurse must focus on other, more feasible measures.

To be motivated to take preventive actions, individuals must perceive a disease as having serious consequences; one tends to underestimate the personal risk of infection present in a given situation, however. Thus many women may not perceive themselves as at risk for contracting an STD, and telling them that they need to carry condoms may not be well received. In addition, denial of personal risk may override the taking of self-protective measures (Mantell, Schinke, & Akabas, 1988). Although, generally, levels of awareness of STDs are high, widespread misconceptions or specific gaps in knowledge also exist (DiClemente, Zoan, & Temoshok, 1986; Price, Desmond, & Kukulka, 1985).

Safer Sex Practices. An essential component of primary prevention is counseling women regarding safer sex practices, including knowledge of her partner, reduction of number of partners, low-risk sex, and avoiding the exchange of body fluids.

No aspect of prevention is more important than knowing one's partner. Reducing the number of partners and avoiding partners who have had many previous sexual partners deceases a woman's chance of contracting an STD. Because many STDs are asymptomatic, infectious persons may be impossible to identify and avoid. Thus, logically, reducing the number of one's partners should reduce one's likelihood of exposure. Deciding not to have sexual contact with a casual acquaintance may also be helpful. Discussing each new partner's previous sexual history and exposure to STDs will augment other efforts to reduce risk. Unfortunately, recent research (Cochran & Mays, 1990) has shown that sizable percentages of men (39%) and women (10%) report lying in order to have sex. Thus women must be cautioned that safer sex measures are always advisable, even when partners insist otherwise. Critically important is whether or not male partners resist wearing condoms. This is crucial when women are not sure about their partner's history. Sexually active persons may also benefit from carefully examining a partner for lesions, sores, ulcerations, rashes, redness, discharge, swelling, and odor before initiating sexual activity. Although the efficacy of such modifications in sexual behavior is theoretical rather than empirically demonstrated (Stone, Grimes, & Magder, 1986), the potential benefits are obvious.

Women should be taught low-risk sexual practices and which sexual practices to avoid. Mutual masturbation is low risk as long as bodily fluids come in contact only with intact skin. Caressing, hugging, body rubbing, massage, and hand-to-genital touching are low-risk behaviors. Possible safer sex practices include deep kissing and oral sex with a woman who does not have her period or a vaginal infection (Hatcher et al., 1994). Rubber (dental) dams have been suggested to provide additional safety (Andrist, 1988; Hatcher et al., 1994); however, no studies have been done to confirm this as an adequate method of protection. Certain sexual practices should be avoided to reduce one's risk of infection. Abstinence from any sexual activities that could result in exchange of infective body fluids will help decrease risk. Anal-genital intercourse, anal-oral contact, and anal-digital activity are high-risk sexual behaviors and should be avoided (Stone et al., 1986). Sexual transmission occurs through direct skin or mucous membrane contact with infectious lesions or body fluids. Because mucosal linings are delicate and subject to considerable mechanical trauma during intercourse, often small abrasions occur, which facilitate the entry of infectious agents into the bloodstream. The rectal epithelium is especially easy to traumatize with penetration. Sexual practices that increase the likelihood of tissue damage or bleeding such as fisting (inserting a fist into the rectum) should be avoided. Deep kissing when lips, gums, or other tissues are raw or broken should also be avoided (Hatcher et al., 1994). Because enteric infections are transmitted by oral-fecal contact, avoiding oral-anal "rimming" (licking the anal area) and digital-anal activities should reduce the likelihood of infection. Vaginal intercourse should never follow anal contact unless a condom has been used and then removed and replaced with a new condom.

Currently, the sole physical barrier promoted for the prevention of sexual transmission of HIV and other STD infection is the condom (Stein, 1990). Because most of the condoms are now available to American women, active male cooperation is essential. Barriers to use of condoms have been well documented, including the opinion that condoms interfere with the pleasure of intercourse, the view that condoms are primarily a contraceptive device rather than a disease prevention strategy, and the conviction that condom use is unnatural (Siegel & Gibson, 1988; Valdiserri, Arena, Proctor, & Bonati, 1989; Worth, 1989). A key issue in condom usage as a preventive strategy is that in sexual encounters men must comply with a woman's suggestion or request that they use a condom. Such compliance is based in part on the power relationships among the sexes; in most instances, this is an unequal balance, with the woman having less power. Thus nurses must suggest strategies to enhance a woman's negotiating and communication skills (Smeltzer & Whipple, 1991). Suggesting that she talk with her partner about condom use at a time removed from sexual activity may make it easier to bring up the subject. Role-playing possible partner reactions with a woman and her alternative responses may also be useful. Women may fear that their partner would be offended if a condom were introduced. Gender role expectations regarding female dependency may prevent women from initiating sexual behavior changes to protect themselves (Fullilove, Fullilove, Haynes, & Gross, 1989); for instance, some women may fear rejection and abandonment, conflict, potential violence, or loss of economic support if they suggest the use of condoms to prevent STD transmission (Worth, 1989). For many individuals, condoms are symbols of extra-relationship activity. Introduction of a condom into a long-term relationship where they have not been used previously threatens the trust assumed in most long-term relationships. Many women do not anticipate or prepare for sexual activity in advance; embarrassment or discomfort in purchasing condoms may prevent some women from using them.

Cultural barriers may also impede the use of condoms. Latino gender roles make it difficult for Latina women to suggest using condoms to a partner (Worth & Rodriguez, 1987). If condoms are viewed only as contraceptive devices, their usage will be in conflict with cultural ideals of virility and womanhood. In many communities, asking a partner to use a condom would violate traditional normative behavior dictating that women assume a passive sexual role (Worth, 1989). Suggesting condom use implies that a woman is sexually active, that she is "available" for sex, and that she is "seeking" sex; these are messages that many women are uncomfortable conveying given the prevailing mores of our country. In a society that commonly views a woman who carries a condom as overprepared, possibly oversexed, and willing to have sex with any man (Hankins, 1990), expecting her to insist on the use of condoms in a sexual encounter is unrealistic. Moreover, condom usage must be renegotiated with every sexual contact, thus women must address the issue of control of sexual decision making every time they request a male partner to use a condom.

Condom Counseling. Using a condom helps prevent exchange of body fluids, and condom counseling is an essential component of safer sex counseling. Nurses can help to motivate clients to use condoms by first discussing the subject with them. This gives women permission to discuss any concerns, misconceptions, or hesitations they may have about using condoms. The nurse may initiate a discussion of how to purchase and use a condom. Information to be discussed includes importance of using latex rather than natural skin condoms and using only condoms with a reservoir and that are lubricated with nonoxynol-9. The nurse should remind women to use only condoms with a current expiration date and to store them away from high heat. Contrary to popular myth, a recent study found no increase in breakage after carrying condoms in a wallet for a lengthy period of time. Although not ideal, women may choose to carry condoms safely in wallets and shoes or inside a bra (Wheeler, 1992). Women can be taught the differences between condoms, price ranges, sizes, and where they can be purchased. Women should be reminded to use a condom only one time and to use condoms with every sexual encounter.

Often, women may require help in developing the social skills necessary for negotiating condom use with a partner. Specific scenarios can be role-played with the client. Asking a woman who appears particularly uncomfortable to rehearse how she might approach the topic can be helpful, particularly when a woman fears her partner may be resistant. The nurse might suggest that her client begin by saying "I need to talk with you about something that is important to both of us. It's hard for me and I feel embarrassed, but I think we need to talk about safe sex." If women are able to sort out their feelings and fears before talking with their partners, they may feel more comfortable and in control of the situation. Women can be reassured that it is natural to be uncomfortable and that the hardest part is getting started. Because it is easier for women to discuss safe sex if they are clear about their own feelings, nurses should help their clients clarify what they will and will not do sexually. Women can be reminded that their partner may need time to think about what they have said and that they must pay attention to their partner's response. If the partner seems to be having difficulty with the discussion, a woman may slow down and wait a while. She can be reminded that if her partner resists safer sex, she may wish to reconsider the relationship. Finally, women should be counseled to watch out for situations that make it hard to talk about and practice safer sex: These include romantic times when condoms are not available and when alcohol or drugs make it impossible to make wise decisions about safer sex.

Selection of a contraceptive has a direct impact on STD risk (Hatcher et al., 1994). Latex condoms and spermicidal agents containing nonoxynol-9 have been shown to be effective against many bacterial and viral STDs, including gonorrhea, genital herpes, condyloma acuminatum, and HIV infections (Hatcher et al., 1994). Condoms should protect women from transmission of organisms found in semen, infectious urethral discharge, infectious penile lesions, and possibly from asymptomatic shedding of HSV or HPV from penile skin. A properly placed diaphragm provides a mechanical barrier over the cervix, and concurrent use of spermicides should provide an additional mechanism of chemical protection. The contraceptive sponge is protective against gonorrhea and, possibly, other STDs (Hatcher et al., 1994). None of these provides complete protection against all STDs, however, and are most effective when used with other risk-reducing practices.

Secondary Prevention

Prompt diagnosis and treatment is predicated on the assumption that any person who believes he or she may have contracted an STD, has symptoms of an STD, has had sexual relations with someone who has symptoms of an STD, or has a partner who has been diagnosed with an STD will seek care. To obtain prompt diagnosis and treatment, clients must know how to recognize the major signs and symptoms of all STDs and obtain health care if they experience symptoms or have sexual contact with someone who had an STD. Nurses have the responsibility of educating their clients regarding the signs and symptoms of STDs: This may be done when a woman comes in for a well-woman examination, seeks contraception, obtains preconceptual care, or comes to her health care provider for prenatal care. Written information should be given to women to reinforce verbal instructions. Nurses also must ensure that clients know where and how to obtain care if they suspect they might have contracted an STD. Many local health departments have clinics specifically designed to treat STDs, and often, free treatment can be obtained at local emergency rooms.

It has been suggested that all women who are sexually active are at risk and should be screened regularly through history, physical examination, and laboratory studies. To identify those at risk, specific questions should be asked during the collection of a health history (see Figure 24.1 and Tables 24.1 and 24.2). A proposed schedule for screening follows:

- Women with unsafe sex practices (use no protection, use alcohol or drugs frequently, have multiple sex partners) should be screened every 1 to 3 months.
- Women with familiar partners, who use safe-sex practices sporadically and occasionally use alcohol or drugs should be screened every 3 to 6 months.
- Women who are primarily monogamous with partners at low risk and who always use safer sex practices should be screened every 6 to 12 months.

Any woman who has been diagnosed with an STD should be screened for other STDs, because many of these infections (e.g., chlamydia, gonorrhea, syphilis) can be asymptomatic in women.

Infected individuals should be asked to identify and notify all partners who might have been exposed. In addition, all persons infected with an STD must be thoroughly and appropriately treated. General procedures for reporting and treating STDs are discussed in the section in this chapter entitled "Caring for the Woman With an STD"; information specific to individual STDs is presented in the sections devoted to individual STDs.

Caring for the Woman With an STD

Women may delay seeking care for STDs because they fear social stigma, have little accessibility to health care services, or may be

Review of Systems	*No*	*Past*	*Now*	*Staff Comments*
Do you experience now or have you ever experienced				
Frequent or severe headaches/migraines				
Seizures/fainting spells				
Emotional problems/depression				
Abuse				
Vision problems				
Chest pain/difficulty breathing				
Numbness or tingling in arms, hands, legs, or feet				
Heart problems/murmurs				
High blood fat levels (i.e., cholesterol)				
High blood pressure				
Blood clots in veins/varicose veins				
Skin problems				
Anemia				
Breast lumps/surgery/nipple discharge				
Stomach/intestinal problems				
Gallbladder or liver disease/problems				
Kidney/bladder problems/infections				
Pain or burning with urination				

Menstrual/Gynecologic History	*No*	*Past*	*Now*	*Staff Comments*
Do you experience now or have you ever experienced				
*Frequent vaginal infections				
*Unusual vaginal discharge/odor				
*Vaginal itching/burning/sores/warts				
*Venereal disease: gonorrhea/syphilis/other				
*Abdominal pain				
*Pelvic inflammatory disease/infection of uterus, tubes, ovaries				
*Rape				
Uterine growths/fibroids/abnormality				
Abnormal Pap smear				
*Pain/bleeding with intercourse				
Unusual or missed periods in the past year				
Severe menstrual cramps				
Premenstrual discomforts				

Sexual History

The following practices put you at risk for AIDS: bisexual partners, intravenous (IV) drug use, intercourse with an IV drug user, anal intercourse, intercourse with a male hemophiliac.

*Do you consider yourself at risk?	☐ Yes	☐ No	☐ Unsure
Are you currently sexually active?	☐ Yes	☐ No	
Are you having any problems with sexual relations?	☐ Yes	☐ No	
Do you think you may be pregnant now?	☐ Yes	☐ No	☐ Unsure
Have you had sex without using birth control since your last period?	☐ Yes	☐ No	☐ Unsure
*Having sex with more than one partner increases the chance of sexual disease. Have you had a new sex partner in the past 2 months?	☐ Yes	☐ No	
*Have you had more than one sex partner in the past 6 months?	☐ Yes	☐ No	
*Does your sex partner have any other partners?	☐ Yes	☐ No	☐ Unsure

Figure 24.1. Sample Questions to Assess Risk of STDs in a Well-Woman Examination
* Questions that may indicate risk

Table 24.1 HIV Risk Assessment Questions

Sexual
Since 1977,[a] have you ever had sex with
A homosexual man
A bisexual man
A prostitute (male or female)
A person born in central, eastern, or southern Africa or some Caribbean countries
A person you thought or knew was infected with the AIDS virus[b]
Have you ever had an STD, such as gonorrhea, syphilis, herpes, or genital warts?
Have you had more than five sex partners in any one year since 1977?[c]
Have you ever had sex without latex condoms (except for long-term, mutually monogamous relationships)?

Drugs
Have you ever used injectable drugs and shared injection equipment (from 1977 to the present)?
Have you ever had sex with a person who uses or used needle drugs and shared injection equipment (from 1977 to the present)?
Have you ever blacked out from alcohol or drugs, especially during sex?[d]

Medical
Have you ever had a transfusion of blood or blood components (1977-1985)?
Have you ever had sex with a person who had a transfusion in 1977-1985 (1977 to the present)?
Have you ever received donor semen or eggs or transplanted organ or tissue (1977 to the present)?
Have you ever been exposed to blood in your work setting?[e]

SOURCE: Centers for Disease Control (1993).
NOTE: Assessment of risk for contracting HIV infection is an essential component of prevention. These questions should be included in every well-woman assessment and whenever a women seeks care for a gynecologic problem or treatment of an STD.
a. 1977 is chosen to mark the beginning of the HIV epidemic in the United States. The Red Cross uses 1977 in blood donor screening questions.
b. Some providers ask an additional question about sex with a person who has been in jail or prison, looking for partner risk factors such as voluntary or coerced sex, drug use with shared needles, or tattooing with shared needles.
c. There is no consensus about how many partners would constitute "multiple" partners. Some people ask about a total of more than five partners since 1977. Others use three in a lifetime. Our question is designed to pick up the more extreme end of the multiple continuum. Use of crack cocaine, epidemic in the United States, is often associated with very high numbers of sexual partners, because users exchange sex for money and sex for drugs.
d. This question helps flag lapses in clear thinking or judgment that could lead to high-risk sexual activity.
e. A yes answer need not indicate risk, but alerts the care provider to probe further.

asymptomatic or unaware that they have an infection. In this age of widespread and often sensational media publicity about STDs, being told she has any STD may be terrifying for a woman. She may not understand the difference between one infecting organism and another. Instead, she may hear a diagnosis of illness, possibly incurable. Symptoms such as increased vaginal discharge, malodor, and itching associated with some STDs may be perceived as "dirty," and the woman may be embarrassed and concerned that she will offend those caring for her. When a woman is diagnosed with an STD, her reactions may range from acceptance to hurt, disbelief, anger, or concern. These reactions may vary with the expectations in the woman's subculture and personal experience.

Assessment

The diagnosis of an STD is based on an integration of relevant historical, physical, and laboratory data (see Table 24.2). A history that is accurate, comprehensive, and specific is crucial to sound diagnosis. Because many women are embarrassed or anxious, the history should be taken first, with the woman dressed. Information should be collected in a nonjudgmental manner, using open-ended questions and avoiding assumptions of sexual preference. All partners should be referred to as partners and not by gender. Specific areas to address include the reason why the woman has sought care and any symptoms she has noticed; a sexual history, including a description of the date and type of sexual activity; number of contacts;

Table 24.2 Assessment of the Client With an STD

History	*Physical Examination*	*Laboratory Tests*
Current symptoms	Inguinal nodes	Wet smear with potassium hydroxide (KOH), normal saline (NaCl)
Vaginal discharge	External genitalia	Urinalysis
Lesions	sores	Gonorrhea culture of cervix, anus, urethra, and mouth as indicated
Itching, burning, swelling, rash	Whiff test with KOH	Chlamydia culture
Dysuria	Edema	Serology for syphilis, HIV, hepatitis B virus
Menstrual history	Erythema	Complete blood count
Last menstrual period	Tenderness	Pap smear
Sexual history	Parasites	Cultures of suspicious lesions
Type, time of sexual activity	Urethral meatus	Colposcopy
Partners: numbers, symptoms	Erythema	
Frequency	Edema	
Areas of contact	Discharge when stripped	
Sexual preference	Bartholin's glands	
General health history	Tender	
Allergies	Enlarged	
Adult health problems	Drainage	
Contraceptive method(s)	Vagina	
History of similar symptoms	Lesions, masses	
	Discharge: color, odor, amount, consistency	
	Cervix	
	Color	
	Lesions, masses	
	Discharge	
	Tenderness with movement	
	Bimanual examination	
	Tenderness in adnexa, uterus	
	Lesions, masses	

whether or not she has had contact with someone who recently had an STD; and potential sites of infection (mouth, cervix, urethra, rectum). Pertinent medical history includes anything that will influence the management plan: history of drug allergies, previously diagnosed chronic illnesses, and general health status. A menstrual history, including the date of the client's last menstrual period, must always be obtained so that pregnancy may be ruled out because certain medications used to treat STDs are contraindicated in pregnancy. When indicated, an HIV-oriented systems review should be conducted and should include the following (Hollander, 1988):

- General observation: weight loss, anorexia, fever, sweats
- Skin: rashes or pigmented lesions, generalized drying, pruritus
- Lymphatics: localized or generalized lymph node involvement, increase or decrease in size of any previously enlarged lymph nodes
- Head, eyes, ears, nose, and throat: headaches, nasal discharge, sinus congestion, changes in visual acuity, sore throat, whitish or painful lesions of the oral mucosa
- Cardiopulmonary: cough or shortness of breath
- Gastrointestinal: abdominal pain, change in bowel habits, diarrhea
- Musculoskeletal: myalgias, arthralgias
- Neurological: symptoms of depression, personality change, cognitive difficulties, bowel or bladder dysfunction, peripheral weakness or parenthesis

Any positive answers regarding symptoms should be followed up to elicit information about onset, duration, and specific characteristics, such as color, amount, and consistency of discharge.

Before the actual physical examination is performed, the nurse should discuss the exam with her client so that she is prepared for it. Careful visualization of the external genitalia, vagina, and cervix, including a speculum examination; thorough palpation of inguinal area and pelvic organs; milking of the urethra for discharge; and assessment of vaginal secretion odors is essential. Lesions should be evaluated and cultures obtained when appropriate. Because the speculum is usually not lubricated prior to insertion into the vagina because cultures of vaginal secretions may have to be obtained, insertion may be more uncomfortable than usual. Clients should be informed of this and reassured that every effort will be made to make the speculum exam as comfortable as possible. Appropriate laboratory studies will be suggested, in part, by the history and physical examination results. Because women are often infected with more than one STD simultaneously and many are asymptomatic, additional laboratory studies may be done, including Pap smear, wet mounts, gonococcal culture, and Venereal Disease Research Laboratory (VDRL) or rapid plasma reagent (RPR) for syphilis. Cultures for HSV are obtained when indicated by history or physical examination. The woman should be offered the HIV-antibody test. When indicated, a complete blood count, sedimentation rate, urinalysis, or urine culture and sensitivity should be obtained.

Nursing Management

The woman with an STD will need support in seeking care at the earliest stage of symptoms. Counseling women about STDs is essential for (a) preventing new infections or reinfection, (b) increasing compliance with treatment and follow-up, (c) providing support during treatment, and (d) assisting patients in discussions with their partner(s). Clients must be made aware of the serious potential consequences of STDs and the behaviors that increase the likelihood of infection.

Table 24.3 outlines necessary client education for all STDs. The nurse must make sure that her client understands what disease she has, how it is transmitted, and why it must be treated. Clients should be given a brief description of the disease in language that they can understand. This description should include modes of transmission, incubation period, symptoms, infectious period, and potential complications. Effective treatment of STDs necessitates careful, thorough explanation of treatment regimen and follow-up procedures. Thorough, careful instructions about medications must be provided, both verbally and in writing. Side effects, benefits, and risks of the medication should be discussed. Unpleasant side effects or early relief of symptoms may discourage women from completing their medication course. Clients should be strongly urged to continue their medication until it is used up regardless of whether their symptoms diminish or disappear in a few days. Comfort measures that decrease symptoms such as pain, itching, or nausea should be suggested. Providing written information is a useful strategy because this is a time of high anxiety for many clients and they may not be able to hear or remember what they were told. A number of booklets on STDs are already available, or the nurse may wish to develop literature that is specific to her practice setting and clients.

In general, women will be advised to refrain from intercourse until all treatment is finished and a reculture, if appropriate, is done. After the infection is cured, women should be urged to continue using condoms to prevent recurring infections, especially if they have had one episode of pelvic inflammatory disease (PID) or continue to have intercourse with new partners. Women may wish to avoid having sex with partners who have many other sexual partners. All women who have contracted an STD should be taught safer sex practices if this has not been done already. Follow-up appointments should be made as needed.

Addressing the psychosocial component of STDs is essential. Remember that a woman may be afraid or embarrassed to tell her partner, ask her partner to seek treatment, and admit her sexual practices, or she may be concerned about confidentiality. The nurse may need to help her client deal with the effect of a diagnosis of an STD on a committed relationship for the woman who is now faced with the necessity of dealing with "uncertain monogamy."

In many instances, sexual partners should be treated; thus the infected woman is asked to identify and notify all partners who might have been exposed. Often, she will find this difficult to do. Empathizing with the client's feelings and suggesting specific ways of talking with partners will help decrease anxiety and assist in efforts to control infection. For example, the nurse might suggest that the woman say, "I care about you and I'm concerned about you. That's why I'm calling to tell you that I have a sexually transmitted disease. My clinician is ______, and she will be happy to talk with you if you would like" (Fogel, 1988). Offering literature and role-playing situations with the client may also be of assistance. It is often helpful to remind the client that although this is an embarrassing situation, most persons would rather know than not know that they have been exposed. Health profession-

Table 24.3 Client Education for All Sexually Transmitted Diseases[a]

Take medication
- How
- When
- Things to avoid

Obtain repeat cultures after treatment for test-of-cure
- When
- Why
- What happens at the clinic

Recheck
- When
- Why
- What happens at the clinic

Sex partner(s)
- Need for medical care
- Need for a period of abstinence from sexual intercourse
- Health plan should include (a) how client is going to tell partner(s), (b) where client is going to refer partner(s), (c) when partner(s) will go, (d) where client can reach counselor for additional help, and (e) where counselor can reach client if needed

Future health
- Respond immediately to any unusual bumps, sores, rashes, discharges
- Return to the clinic occasionally—even if things appear normal

SOURCE: Fogel, C. I., & Lauver, D. (1990). *Sexual health promotion.* Philadelphia: W. B. Saunders. Reprinted with permission.
NOTE: Education for all women who have an STD is essential so that they can promptly identify symptoms, obtain treatment, follow medical instructions, refer partners for care, and protect themselves from contracting future STD infection.
a. Be sure the client leaves the clinic with *no* unanswered questions.

als who take time to counsel their clients on how to talk with their partner(s) can improve compliance and case finding.

Many STDs are reportable; all states require that the five traditional venereal diseases—gonorrhea, syphilis, chancroid, lymphogranuloma venereum, and granuloma inguinale—be reported to public health officials. Many other states require other STDs such as chlamydial infections, genital herpes, and genital warts to be reported. In addition, all states require that AIDS cases be reported; 35 states require that HIV infection be reported. The nurse is legally responsible for reporting all cases of those diseases identified as reportable and should make sure she knows what the requirements are in the state in which she practices. The client must be informed when a case will be reported and told why. Failure to inform the client that the case will be reported is a serious breech of professional ethics. Confidentiality is a crucial issue for many clients. When an STD is reportable, women need to be told that they may be contacted by a health department epidemiologist. They should be assured that the information reported to and collected by health authorities is not available to anyone without their permission. Every effort, within the limits of one's public health responsibilities, should be made to reassure clients.

The following sections outline the treatments for specific STDs following CDC guidelines. When possible, they also delineate self-help measures and preventive strategies. Instructions specific to individual diseases are given in the appropriate sections.

Chlamydia Infection

In the United States, genital infections caused by *Chlamydia trachomatis* (C. trachomatis) are the most common STDs in women. Although chlamydia is not a reportable disease, it is estimated that 3 to 4 million Americans are newly infected each year (Division of STD/HIV Prevention, 1991). These infections are often silent and very destructive; their sequelae and complications can be very serious. In women, chlamydial infections are difficult to diagnose; the symptoms, if present, are nonspecific and the organism is expensive to culture.

The major mode of transmission of chlamydia is sexual and, like many other STDs, chlamydial infections are epidemic in the United States today. Although in utero transmission has not been shown, the organism is transmitted during birth and has been transmitted in donor semen through artificial insemination (Mascola & Guinan, 1987).

Although the asymptomatic state is most common, some women may experience spotting or postcoital bleeding, mucoid or purulent cervical discharge, or dysuria.

Several risk factors for chlamydia have been documented: age 24 years or less; intercourse with a new partner in past 3 months; purulent or mucopurulent cervical discharge; cervical bleeding induced by swabbing the endocervical mucosa; and use of nonbarrier contraceptive method (Handsfield, Jasman, & Roberts, 1986). A study by Oh, Feinstein, Soileau, Cloud, and Pass (1989) suggests that oral contraceptive use may promote chlamydial infection of the cervix or enhance the detection of C. trachomatis in the cervix; in contrast Wolner-Hanssen et al. (1990b) found a decreased risk of chlamydial infections in women using oral contraceptives.

Acute salpingitis or PID is the most serious complication of chlamydial infections, and past chlamydial infections are associated with an increased risk of ectopic pregnancy (Chow et al., 1990) and tubal factor infertility (see Chapter 25, "Infertility," for a discussion of this problem). Furthermore, chlamydial infection of the cervix causes inflammation, resulting in microscopic cervical ulcerations, and thus may increase risk of acquiring HIV infection. Untreated chlamydia during pregnancy is associated with increases in premature rupture of the membranes, low birth weight, and decreased survival of infants (Ryan, Abdella, McNeeley, Baselski, & Drummond, 1990). Chlamydial infections can be passed to the newborn at time of delivery with a 60% to 70% chance that infants born through the infected birth canal will contract chlamydia; 25% to 50% of these infants will develop conjunctivitis in the first 2 weeks of life and 10% to 20% will develop pneumonia (Star, 1990a).

Assessment

In addition to obtaining information regarding the presence of risk factors, the nurse should inquire about the presence of any symptoms.

A thorough abdominal and pelvic examination should be done. The patient may have abdominal tenderness or rebound tenderness, palpable masses, or inguinal adenopathy. The Bartholin's glands should be examined for abnormal discharge and swelling and the cervix carefully inspected. The most important physical finding in chlamydial infection is a purulent or mucopurulent cervical discharge. The cervix often looks edematous, congested, and friable; cervical motion tenderness may be present. The physical findings associated with salpingitis and PID are discussed in a later section.

Diagnosis of chlamydia is by culture. Endocervical (columnar) cells are required; cell scrapings provide better specimens, so the cervix should be swabbed with cotton or rayon swabs prior to collecting the specimen to remove mucus and discharge from the cervical os. Special culture media and proper handling of specimens are important, so the nurse should always know what is required in her individual practice site. Chlamydial culture testing is not always available, primarily because of its expense, and may take several days to yield results.

Nursing Management

An important component of management of chlamydial infections is screening. The CDC (1989) strongly urges screening of asymptomatic, high-risk women in whom infection would otherwise go undetected. Whenever possible, all women with two or more of the risk factors for chlamydia should be cultured. In addition, all pregnant women should have cervical cultures for chlamydia at the first prenatal visit. Reculturing late in the third trimester (36 weeks) should be carried out if the woman was positive previously or if she is at high risk for STDs.

CDC (1993) recommendations for treatment of chlamydial infections are given in Table 24.4. Because chlamydia is often asymptomatic, the patient should be cautioned to take all medication prescribed. All exposed sexual partners should be treated. Test of cure evaluation is not necessary because antimicrobial resistance of C. trachomatis has not been observed (CDC, 1989).

Table 24.4 Recommended Primary Treatment Regimens

Chlamydial infection
- Nonpregnant woman
  - Doxycycline 100 mg orally 2 times a day for 7 days
  - *or*
  - Azithromycin 1 gm orally once
- Pregnant woman
  - Erythromycin base 500 mg orally 4 times a day for 7 days
  - *or*
  - Erythromycin base 250 mg orally 4 times a day for 14 days

Human papillomavirus (HPV)
- Cryotherapy with liquid nitrogen or cryoprobe
- Podophyllin, 10%-25% in compound tincture of benzoin applied to lesions for 1-4 hours once a week (*contraindicated in pregnancy*). Apply weekly for up to a total of 6 applications.
- Trichloroacetic acid (TCA), 80%-90% concentration, applied to warts. Repeat weekly, if necessary, up to a total of 6 applications

Gonococcal infection
- Ceftriaxone 125 mg intramuscularly (IM) once
- *or*
- Ciprofloxacin 500 mg by mouth (po) once
- *or*
- Cefixime 400 mg po once
- *or*
- Ofloxacin 400 mg po once
- *plus*
- Doxcycline 100 mg orally 2 times a day for 7 days

Herpes genitalis
- Initial infection
  - Acyclovir 200 mg orally 5 times a day for 7-10 days or until clinical resolution occurs
- Severe recurrent infection
  - Acyclovir 800 mg orally 2 times a day for 5 days

Syphilis
- Primary and secondary syphilis and early latent syphilis less than 1 year duration
  - Benzathine penicillin G 2.4 million units IM one dose
- Early latent syphilis
  - Benzathine penicillin G 7.2 million units, administer one dose
- Late latent or latent of unknown duration syphilis
  - Benzathine penicillin G 2.4 million units, administer in 3 doses of 2.4 million units IM 1 week apart for 3 consecutive weeks

SOURCE: Centers for Disease Control (1993).

Human Papillomavirus

Genital or venereal warts, an STD that was first described in 25 A.D. and is now one of the most common STDs seen in ambulatory health care settings are caused by HPV, part of the papovavirus family. This double-stranded DNA virus has over 40 known serotypes, 6 of which are known to cause genital wart formation and 8 of which are currently thought to have oncogenic potential (Enterline & Leonardo, 1989). HPV types 6 and 11 are responsible for most benign anogenital diseases.

Because health care providers are not required to report HPV infections, the true incidence of these infections is not known. However, genital warts appeared to be the most rapidly spreading STD from the mid-1960s until the onset of the AIDS epidemic (Aral & Holmes, 1991), with up to 1 million individuals infected yearly (Division of STD/HIV Prevention, 1991). HPV is considered to be highly infectious; it is thought that up to 85% of exposed sexual partners will develop lesions (Lynch, 1985).

In addition to the general risk factors for STDs noted earlier, cigarette smoking and use of oral contraceptives for more than 5 years have been found to be risk factors for HPV. A recent study (Deitch & Smith, 1990) suggests that women who have chronic yeastlike symptoms have a significant incidence of microscopic vulvular condyloma.

Genital warts in women are most frequently seen in the posterior part of the introitus; however, lesions are also found on the buttocks, vulva, vagina, anus, and cervix. Typically, the lesions present as small (2 to 3 mm in diameter and 10 to 15 mm in height), soft, papillary swellings occurring singularly or in clusters on the genital and anal-rectal region. Infections of long duration may appear as a cauliflower-like mass. In moist areas, such as the vaginal introitus, the lesions may appear to have multiple, fine, finger-like projections. Vaginal lesions are often multiple. Flat-topped papules, 1 to 4 mm in diameter, are seen most often on the cervix. Often, these lesions are visualized only under magnification. Cervical or vaginal lesions may be present in up to 70% of women with vulvular lesions (Lichtman & Duran, 1990). Warts are usually flesh-colored or slightly darker on Caucasian women, black on black women, and brownish on Oriental women (Enterline & Leonardo, 1989).

Genital warts are often painless but may also be uncomfortable, particularly when very large. They can become inflamed and ulcerated.

Previously thought to be a relatively benign condition, the HPV recently has been linked to genital squamous cell carcinoma in women (Enterline & Leonardo, 1989; Richart, 1987). HPV serotypes 16, 18, 31, 33, 35, and 39 are potentially oncogenic; more than 90% of cervical neoplasms have been associated with these serotypes. Not all women infected with these HPV serotypes develop cancer, however; current evidence suggests that infection with the virus alone is an insufficient condition for the development of precancerous lesions or cancer of the cervix and that cofactors (young age at first exposure, repeated infections, weak immunity, smoking) may be necessary for the development of cancer (Koss, 1987).

HPV infections seem to be more frequent in pregnant than nonpregnant women, probably due to increasing levels of progesterone (Ferenczy, 1989), with an increase in incidence from the first trimester to the third. Furthermore, a significant proportion of preexisting HPV lesions enlarge greatly during pregnancy, a proliferation presumably resulting from the relative state of immunosuppression present during pregnancy. Warts may become large enough during pregnancy to cause severe discomfort; secondary infection of the lesions from vaginal and rectal bacteria can develop and may be a source for intrapartum fetal infections, premature rupture of membranes, and chorioamnionitis (Ferenczy, 1989). Lesions may become large enough to impede delivery. Because the growths are vascular and could tear or be cut during an episiotomy, cesarean section is often done when extensive growths are present. However, initial observation of large growths can be misleading, suggesting that the entire vagina is involved. All of the growth may derive from one stalk, however, and, in such cases, it may be possible to push the large mass to the side, allowing the baby to pass through. HPV infection may be acquired by the neonate during delivery; the frequency of such transmission is unknown (Watts & Eschenbach, 1987). Juvenile laryngeal papilloma (JLP) can occur in children exposed to HPV during delivery. JLP can cause mortality or significant morbidity requiring multiple surgical or laser treatments in affected children. The exact incidence of JLP is not known, but it is thought to be rare.

Assessment

Viral screening and typing for HPV is not standard practice yet. History, evaluation of signs and symptoms, Pap smear, and physical examination are used in making a diagnosis. The only definitive diagnostic test for presence of HPV is by histological evaluation of a biopsy specimen.

A woman with genital warts may complain of symptoms such as a profuse, irritating vaginal discharge, itching, dyspareunia (painful intercourse), or postcoital bleeding. She also may report "bumps" on her vulva or labia. History of a known exposure is important; however, because of the potentially long latency period and the possibility of subclinical infections in men, the lack of a history of known exposure cannot be used to exclude a diagnosis of genital warts.

Physical inspection of the vulva, perineum, anus, vagina, and cervix is essential whenever HPV lesions are suspected or seen in one area. Because speculum examination of the vagina may block some lesions, it is important to rotate the speculum blades until all areas are visualized. When lesions are visible, the characteristic appearance previously described is considered diagnostic. However, in many instances, cervical lesions are not visible and some vaginal or vulvular lesions may also be unobservable to the naked eye. Because of the potential spread of vulvular or vaginal lesions to the anus, gloves should be changed between vaginal and rectal examinations (Lichtman & Duran, 1990).

Several laboratory tests are indicated when genital warts are suspected. Examination of genital tissues is facilitated by applying 5% acetic acid (ordinary white vinegar) liberally to the indicated areas with large cotton swabs. Acetic acid makes the large nuclei of the proliferating epithelium appear opaque (acetowhiting) because it causes the cytoplasm of the cells to shrink. After 1 to 5 minutes of exposure, flat lesions not ordinarily seen and papillary lesions will be enhanced. Sites are examined under magnification for blanching. Acetowhiting is not diagnostic for HPV; rather, it increases the index of suspicion in an otherwise unsuspicious area. False-positive whitening may occur after recent intercourse, yeast infections, genital irritation, and previously treated lesions.

Pap smears of the cervical transformation zone are used as a screening technique; however, because of false-negatives, a negative Pap smear does not indicate absence of disease. The general recommendation is that women with genital warts should have routine Pap smears and colposcopic examinations as indicated and that all atypical or persistent lesions should be biopsied (Enterline & Leonardo, 1989). Colposcopy and directed biopsy can confirm HPV infection in acetowhite or suspicious lesions.

Genital warts must be differentiated from condyloma latum and molluscum contagiosum. Molluscum contagiosum lesions are half-domed, smooth, flesh-colored to pearly white papules with depressed centers. Condyloma latum is a form of secondary syphilis and, generally, has lesions that are flatter and wider than genital warts. A serological test for syphilis would confirm the diagnosis of secondary syphilis.

Nursing Management

Treatment of genital warts is often very difficult. No therapy has been shown to eradicate HPV. The goal of treatment therefore is removal of warts and relief of signs and symptoms, not the eradication of HPV (CDC, 1989). Often, the client must make multiple office visits; frequently, many different treatment modalities will be used. Eradication of the virus is not considered conclusive even after there is no visible evidence of wart tissue because of the high incidence of recurrence (Enterline & Leonardo, 1989).

In most instances, cryotherapy with liquid nitrogen or cryoprobe is the indicated treatment for external genital and perianal warts (CDC, 1993). Cryotherapy is nontoxic, does not require anesthesia, and, when used properly, does not cause scarring (CDC, 1989). Podofilox, .05% solution, may be used for self-treatment of genital warts only. It is applied to the warts with a cotton swab daily for 3 days, followed by 4 days of no therapy. This cycle may be repeated as needed up to a total of 4 cycles (CDC, 1993). Podofilox is contraindicated in pregnancy (see Table 24.4 for information regarding other medications and dosages). Laser therapy and conventional surgery are used when genital warts are extensive or lesions are resistive. Because viable HPV particles have been found in the smoke plume associated with CO_2 laser therapy, it is extremely important to use vacuum suction (Allen & Marte, 1992).

In the past, genital warts have been treated with interferon. Current CDC guidelines (CDC, 1993), however, state that treatment with interferon is not recommended because of its relatively low efficacy, high frequency of adverse side effects, and expense. Interferon should not be used during pregnancy because it may interfere with normal liver, bone marrow, and immune functions (Ferenczy, 1989).

Women who have cervical warts must be evaluated for dysplasia before treatment is started and should be referred to an expert in the field of gynecologic dysplasia. Any concurrent vaginal infections or STDs should be treated. Women who are experiencing discomfort associated with genital warts may find that bathing with an oatmeal solution and drying the area with a cool hair dryer will provide some relief. Keeping the area clean and dry will also decrease growth of the warts. Cotton underwear and loose fitting clothes that decrease friction and irritation also may decrease discomfort. Women should be advised to maintain a healthy lifestyle to aid the immune system; women can be counseled regarding diet, rest, stress reduction, and exercise.

Patient counseling is essential. Women must understand the virus, how it is transmitted, that no immunity is conferred with infection, and that reacquisition of the infection is likely with repeated contact. Women need to know that their partners should be checked even if they are asymptomatic. Because HPV is highly contagious, the majority of women's partners will be infected and should be treated. All sexually active women with multiple partners or a history of HPV should be encouraged to use male or female latex condoms and a vaginal spermicide for intercourse to decrease acquisition or transmission of HPV. Spermicidal condoms should be used until both partners are lesion free and up to 9 months after appearance of lesions because subclinical lesions may be infectious (Lichtman & Duran, 1990).

Instructions for all medications and treatments must be detailed. Women should be informed prior to treatment of the possibility of posttreatment pain associated with specific therapies. The importance of proper thorough treatment of concurrent vaginitis of STD should be emphasized. The link between cervical cancer and the need for close follow-up should be discussed. Semiannual or annual health examinations are recommended to assess disease recurrence and screening for cervical cancer. At least annual Pap smears should be done on women who have been treated for HPV infections. When the cervix is treated, a Pap test should be done in 4 to 6 months; after two negative Pap smears at 6-month intervals, an annual Pap smear can be performed (CDC, 1989). Women should understand the advisability of treatment before becoming pregnant.

Women with HPV infection may radically alter their sexual practices both from fear of transmission to and from a partner and from genital discomfort associated with treatment, which may have a negative impact on their sexual relationships. Unless the partner accepts and understands the necessary precautions, it may be difficult for the woman to follow the treatment regimen.

The nurse can offer to discuss feelings that the woman may have and, when indicated, joint counseling can be suggested.

Gonorrhea

Gonorrhea is probably the oldest communicable disease in the United States and is the most commonly reported today. Although approximately 1 million new cases are reported annually, the CDC (1989) estimates that about 3 million cases a year occur in the United States. Often, cases are not reported by health care providers; moreover, the disease may go unrecognized because many cases of gonorrhea are asymptomatic. The incidence of drug-resistant cases of gonorrhea, in particular penicillinase-producing *Neisseria gonorrhoeae* (PPNG), is dramatically rising in the United States, from less than 5,000 antibiotic-resistant cases in 1980 to approximately 60,000 in 1990 (Division of STD/HIV Prevention, 1991).

Gonorrhea is caused by the aerobic, gram-negative diplococci *Neisseria gonorrhoeae.* In recent years antibiotic-resistant strains of gonorrhea have developed: PPNG, chromosomally mediated resistant *Neisseria gonorrhoeae* (CMRNG), and tetracycline-resistant Neisseria gonorrhoeae (TRNG). PPNG infections are associated with inappropriate and ineffective use of antibiotics in the treatment of gonorrhea and the indiscriminate use of penicillin in high-reservoir groups, such as prostitutes and individuals with multiple sexual partners. PPNG patients are predominantly inner-city residents, members of ethnic minority groups, and heterosexuals.

Gonorrhea is almost exclusively transmitted by the skin-to-skin contact of sexual activity. The principle means of communication is genital-to-genital contact; however, it is also spread by oral-to-genital and anal-to-genital contact. There is also evidence that infection may spread in females from vagina to rectum. Gonococcal infection has been transmitted by donor semen during artificial insemination (Mascola & Guinan, 1987). Gonorrhea can also be transmitted to the newborn in the form of ophthalmia neonatorum during delivery by direct contact with gonococcal organisms in the cervix.

Age is probably the most important risk factor associated with gonorrhea. The majority of those contracting gonorrhea are from 15 to 24 years old. Of particular concern is the high incidence (99.4 per 100,000 women) in very young women aged 10 to 14. Traditionally, the reported incidence of gonococcal disease has been higher in nonwhites, and this racial difference has been widening since 1984 (Aral & Holmes, 1991). Many of the apparent differences in infection rates can be explained by the disproportionate representation of blacks among the nation's poor and among inner-city dwellers. Rates of gonorrhea are higher in urban than rural areas, with even higher rates in the inner city. A direct correlation between prevalence of the disease and the number of sexual partners has been noted (Aral & Holmes, 1991).

Women are often asymptomatic; when symptoms are present, they are often less specific than the symptoms in men. Because concurrent infections with chlamydia and syphilis are common, it is difficult to describe the "typical" presentation of gonorrhea in women. They may have a purulent endocervical discharge, but discharge is usually minimal or absent. Menstrual irregularities may be the presenting symptom, or women may complain of pain—chronic or acute severe pelvic or lower abdominal pain or longer, more painful menses. Infrequently, dysuria, vague abdominal pain, or lower backache is what prompts the woman to seek care. Gonococcal rectal infection may occur in women following anal intercourse. Individuals with rectal gonorrhea may be completely asymptomatic or, conversely, experience severe symptoms with profuse purulent anal discharge, rectal pain, and blood in the stool. Rectal itching, fullness, pressure, and pain also are common symptoms, as is diarrhea.

A diffuse vaginitis with vulvitis is the most common form of gonococcal infection in prepubertal girls. There may be few signs of infection, or vaginal discharge, dysuria, and swollen, reddened labia may be present.

Gonococcal infections in pregnancy potentially affect both mother and infant. Women with cervical gonorrhea may develop salpingitis in the first trimester. Perinatal complications of gonococcal infection include premature rupture of membranes, preterm delivery, chorioamnionitis, neonatal sepsis, intrauterine growth retardation, and maternal postpartum sepsis. Amniotic infection syndrome manifested by placental, fetal, and umbilical cord inflammation following premature rupture of the membranes may result from gonorrheal infections during pregnancy. Opthalmia neonatorum, the most common manifestation of neonatal gonococcal infections, is very contagious and, if untreated, may lead to blindness of the infant (Brunham, Holmes, & Embree, 1990; Watts & Eschenbach, 1987).

Assessment

Although information about symptomatology is always important, it may not provide information specific enough to suggest a diagnosis of gonorrhea, particularly because many women are asymptomatic. Any positive answers should be followed up to elicit information about onset, duration, and specific characteristics, such as color, amount, and consistency of discharge. Each client should be asked about vaginal discharge, swelling or burning of the perineum, dysuria, urinary frequency, lower abdominal pain, cramping or pain localized in the perineum, rectal symptoms, and sore throat. Women should be asked about general indicators of infection such as fever, chills, nausea, or vomiting (Star, 1990b). A detailed menstrual history, such as is described in Chapter 9, "Well-Woman Assessment," should be gathered. A sexual history will provide information on the date of last sexual contact and the number of contacts the client has had in the past 2 months. It is important to know what types of sexual contacts the client has had—genital-genital, oral-genital, genital-rectal, oral-anal—in determining which type of physical examination to perform and what cultures to obtain. A history of exposure or symptoms in a woman's male partner(s) is significant, and a diagnosis of gonorrhea in a sexual partner is sufficient for treatment.

Vital signs should be taken during the physical examination. When indicated by history of oral-genital contact, a throat exam should be done. The nurse should examine the woman for local signs of infection and salpingitis. The lower abdomen, inguinal area, hands, palms, and forearms should be inspected for vesicles or pustules with a hemorrhagic base. The external genitalia, including perineum and anus, should also be inspected. Palpation for inguinal and femoral lymphadenopathy and abdominal tenderness and pain should be done. Skene's glands and urethra should be milked for discharge and Bartholin's glands palpated for swelling, tenderness, and exudate. Every woman should have a speculum and bimanual pelvic examination. Cervical friability, redness, or purulent or mucopurulent discharge should be noted. During the bimanual examination, presence of cervical motion tenderness, uterine tenderness or fixation, or adnexal tenderness or masses are evaluated.

Gonococcal infection cannot be diagnosed reliably by clinical signs and symptoms alone. Individuals may present with "classic" symptoms, with vague symptoms that may be attributed to a number of conditions, or with no symptoms at all. Cultures are considered the "gold standard" for diagnosis of gonorrhea. Cultures should be obtained from the endocervix, rectum, and, when indicated, the pharynx. Thayer-Martin cultures are recommended to diagnose gonorrhea in women. Any woman suspected of having gonorrhea should have a chlamydial culture and serological test for syphilis if one has not been done in the past 2 months. A Pap smear may be obtained; however, if the woman has cervicitis at the time of the examination, the Pap smear may be deferred unless it is unlikely that the patient will return for future care.

Nursing Management

Management of gonorrhea is straightforward, and the cure is usually rapid with appropriate antibiotic therapy. Single-dose efficacy is a major consideration in selecting an antibiotic regimen for women with gonorrhea. Another important consideration is the high percentage (45%) of women with coexisting chlamydial infections in some populations. Generally, women should be treated with an antibiotic that is effective against both organisms because simultaneous treatment may lessen the possibility of treatment failure due to antibiotic resistance (CDC, 1989). Current CDC (1989) recommendations for treatment of uncomplicated endocervical or rectal infections are found in Table 24.4.

All women with gonorrhea and syphilis should be treated for syphilis according to CDC guidelines (see discussion of syphilis in this chapter). All patients with gonorrhea should be offered confidential counseling and testing for HIV infection.

Gonorrhea is a highly communicable disease. Sexual partners should be examined, cultured, and treated with appropriate regimens. Most treatment failures result from reinfection: The client needs to be informed of this, as well as of the consequences of reinfection in terms of chronicity, complications, and potential infertility.

Gonorrhea is a reportable communicable disease. Health care providers are legally responsible for reporting all cases to the health authorities, usually the local health department in the client's county of residence. Women should be informed that the case will be reported, told why, and informed of the possibility of being contacted by a health department epidemiologist.

Treatment failure following combined ceftriazone/doxycycline therapy is rare; therefore, follow-up culture (test of cure) is not essential (CDC, 1989). A more cost-effective approach is reexamination with culture 1 to 2 months after treatment. This approach will detect both treatment failures and reinfections. Patients should also be counseled to return if symptoms persist after treatment. Patients treated with regimens other than ceftriaxone/doxycycline should be recultured 4 to 7 days after treatment.

Pelvic Inflammatory Disease (PID)

PID is an infectious process that most commonly involves the fallopian tubes (salpingitis), uterus (endometritis), and, more rarely, the ovaries and peritoneal surfaces. Multiple organisms have been found to cause PID, and most cases are associated with more than one organism. In the past the most common causative agent was thought to be *Neisseria gonorrhoeae*; however, *C. trachomatis* is now estimated to cause between one quarter and one half of all cases of PID (Clarke-Pearson & Dawood, 1990). In addition to gonorrhea and chlamydia, a wide variety of anaerobic and aerobic bacteria are recognized to cause PID. Because PID may be caused by a wide variety of infectious agents and encompasses a wide variety of pathological processes, the infection can be acute, subacute, or chronic and has a wide range of symptoms.

Most PID results from ascending spread of microorganisms from the vagina and endocervix to the upper genital tract. This spread most frequently happens at the end of or just after menses following reception of an infectious agent. During the menstrual period, several factors facilitate the development of an infection: The cervical os is slightly open; the cervical mucus barrier is absent; and menstrual blood is an excellent medium for growth. PID may also develop following an abortion, pelvic surgery, or delivery.

Each year, approximately 1 million women in the United States will have an episode of symptomatic PID (CDC, 1991b). Risk factors for acquiring PID are those associated with the risk of contracting an STD. In addition, recent research suggests that cigarette smoking is associated with PID (Marchbanks, Lee, & Peterson, 1990) and that douching may increase a woman's risk for acute PID (Wolner-Hanssen et al., 1990a). Until very recently it was believed that intrauterine device (IUD) use increased a woman's risk for acquiring PID. However, a reanalysis of data suggests that the risk was overestimated and that "IUDs do not increase the risk of PID" (Kronmal, Whitney, & Mumford, 1991, p. 110). The CDC (1991b) states that women who use IUDs are probably at increased risk for PID that may not be STD related and that most of this risk occurs in the first months after IUD insertion.

Women who have had PID are at increased risk for ectopic pregnancy, infertility, and chronic pelvic pain. After a single episode of PID, a woman's risk for ectopic pregnancy increases sevenfold compared with the risk for women who have never had PID. Other problems associated with PID include dyspareunia, pyosalpinx (pus in the fallopian tubes), tubo-ovarian abscess, and pelvic adhesions.

The symptoms of PID vary, depending on whether the infection is acute, subacute, or chronic; however, pain is common to all clinical presentations. It may be dull, cramping, and intermittent (subacute) or severe, persistent, and incapacitating (acute). The woman with acute PID also may complain of intermenstrual bleeding. Physical examination reveals adnexal tenderness, with or without rebound, and exquisite tenderness with cervical movement (Chandelier's sign). Pelvic tenderness is usually bilateral. There may or may not be a palpable adnexal swelling or thickening. A urethral or cervical discharge, often purulent in nature, may be present. A fever of 102° F or above is characteristic. Significant laboratory data include an elevated white blood cell count and markedly elevated erythryocyte sedimentation rate (ESR). Fever and peritonitis are more characteristic of gonococcal PID than of PID caused by other organisms, which are more likely to be "silent." Because PID caused by chlamydia is more commonly asymptomatic, it more often results in tubal obstruction from delayed diagnosis or inadequate treatment.

Subacute PID is far less dramatic, with a great variety in the severity and extent of symptoms. At times they are so mild and vague that the woman ignores them. Symptoms that suggest subacute PID are chronic lower abdominal pain, dyspareunia, menstrual irregularities, urinary discomfort, low-grade fever, lower backache, and constipation. Abdominal examination usually reveals no rebound tenderness; there is slight adnexal tenderness with cervical movement, and cervical or urethral discharge may be present.

Assessment

A careful history is necessary to distinguish between PID and other conditions that cause abdominal pain, such as an ectopic pregnancy or appendicitis. A pain history (see Chapter 23, "Common Symptoms") is critical in establishing a diagnosis of PID. Pain associated with appendicitis is generally unilateral and accompanied by nausea and anorexia. Unilateral pain without nausea or other gastrointestinal symptoms suggests ectopic pregnancy or ovarian cyst, whereas suprapubic pain is characteristic of a bladder infection. A menstrual history is useful in establishing the relationship of onset of pain to menses and in identifying any variations from normal in the cycle. Other relevant history includes recent pelvic surgery, delivery, abortion, or dilatation of the cervix; purulent vaginal discharge; irregular bleeding; and a longer, heavier menstrual period. A sexual history will assist in identifying possible increased risk for STD exposure. Symptoms of an STD in a woman's partner(s) should also be noted.

Vital signs should be taken and a complete physical examination performed. A careful abdominal examination and thorough pelvic examination will help identify the presence of lower abdominal tenderness, bilateral adnexal tenderness, and cervical motion tenderness. These findings are the minimal criteria for making a clinical diagnosis of PID (CDC, 1991b). Costovertebral angle (CVA) tenderness should be assessed to rule out pyelonephritis. Rebound tenderness, generally characteristic of appendicitis, may or may not be present. Whether the nurse should perform a pelvic examination on a woman she strongly suspects has PID is a serious question (Jackson, 1990). It is essential that as few pelvic examinations as possible be carried out because such exams have the potential for introducing additional infectious organisms and facilitating the spread of infectious organisms. In addition, a pelvic exam can be very painful for a woman with PID. Jackson (1990) recommends that if the diagnosis seems rather clear from history and abdominal examination, and the referring or consulting physician is available, it may be prudent to defer the pelvic examination. Essential laboratory data are a complete blood count (CBC) with differential and cervical cultures for gonorrhea and chlamydia.

Nursing Management

Perhaps the most important nursing intervention is prevention. Primary prevention would be education in avoiding acquisition of STDs, whereas secondary prevention involves preventing a lower genital tract infection from ascending to the upper genital tract. Instructing women in self-protective behaviors, such as practicing safer sex and using barrier methods, is critical. Also important is the detection of asymptomatic gonorrheal and chlamydial infections through routine screening of high-risk groups and in high-risk settings. Partner notification when an STD is diagnosed is essential to prevent reinfection.

The majority of women with PID are hospitalized, although occasionally outpatient management is carried out. The CDC (1993, p. 78) recommends hospitalization in the following situations:

- The diagnosis is uncertain
- Surgical emergencies such as appendicitis or ectopic pregnancy cannot be excluded
- A pelvic abscess is suspected
- The patient is pregnant
- The patient is an adolescent
- The patient has HIV infection
- Severe illness precludes outpatient management
- The patient is unable to follow or tolerate an outpatient regimen
- The patient has failed to respond to outpatient therapy
- Clinical follow-up within 72 hours of starting antibiotic treatment cannot be arranged

Many experts recommend that all women with PID be hospitalized so that parenteral antibiotic treatment can be done. It may be particularly important to hospitalize the adolescent patients because their compliance with therapy may be unpredictable and the long-term sequelae of PID can be particularly devastating for this group.

Although treatment regimens vary with the infecting organism, generally a broad-spectrum antibiotic is used. Several antimicrobial regimens have proved to be effective, and no single therapeutic regimen of choice exists (see Table 24.5). The woman with acute PID should be resting in bed in a semi-Fowler's position. Comfort measures include analgesics for pain and all other nursing measures applicable to a patient confined to bed. Few pelvic examinations should be done during the acute phase of the disease. During the recovery phase, the woman should restrict her activity and make every effort to get adequate rest and a nutritionally sound diet. Follow-up laboratory work after treatment should include endocervical cultures for a test of cure.

Health education is central to effective management of PID. Nurses should explain to women the nature of their disease and should encourage them to comply with all therapy and prevention recommendations emphasizing the necessity of taking all medication, even if symptoms disappear. Any potential problems, such as lack of money for prescriptions or lack of transportation to return to clinic for follow-up appointments, that would prevent a woman from completing a course of treatment should be identified and the importance of follow-up visits stressed. Women should be counseled to refrain from sexual intercourse until their treatment is completed. Contraceptive counseling should be provided. The nurse can suggest that the client select barrier methods, such as condoms, a contraceptive sponge, or a diaphragm. A woman with a history of PID should not choose an IUD as her contraceptive method.

The woman who suffers from PID may be acutely ill or experience long-term discomfort. Either or both take an emotional toll. Pain in itself is debilitating and is compounded by the infectious process. The potential or actual loss of reproductive capabilities can be devastating and can affect her self-concept adversely. Part of the nurse's role is to help her client adjust her self-concept to fit reality and to accept alterations in a way that promotes health. Because PID is so closely tied to sexuality, body image, and self-concept, the woman diagnosed with it will need supportive care. Her feelings need to be discussed and her partner(s) included when appropriate.

Herpes Genitalis

Unknown until the middle of the 20th century, genital herpes is now one of the most common STDs in the United States today, especially in women, who contract it far more often than do men. Herpes genitalis is a painful vesicular eruption of the skin and mucosa of the genitals caused by two different antigen subtypes of herpes simplex virus: herpes simplex virus 1 (HSV-1) and herpes simplex virus 2 (HSV-2). HSV-2 is usually transmitted sexually and HSV-1 nonsexually (Breslin, 1988). Although HSV-1 is more commonly associated with gingivostomatitis and oral labial ulcers (fever blisters) and HSV-2 with genital lesions, both types are not exclusively associated with the respective sites.

Although HSV infection is not a reportable disease, it is estimated that approximately 30 million Americans are infected with genital herpes (Johnson, Nahmias, Magder, Lee, Brooks, & Snowden, 1989) and that 200,000 persons contract an initial (or primary) infection each year; recurrent HSV infections are much more com-

Table 24.5 Treatment Regimens for Pelvic Inflammatory Disease

Inpatient Management

Regimen A

- Cefoxitin 2.0 gms intravenously (IV) every 6 hours or Cefotetan 2 gms IV every 12 hours
  plus
- Doxycycline 100 mg orally or IV every 12 hours
- Continue regimen for at least 48 hours after the patient shows substantial clinical improvement.
- Continue doxycycline 100 mg twice a day (bid) for 14 days of total therapy.

Regimen B

- Clindamycin 900 mg IV every 8 hours
  plus
- Gentamicin: loading dose IV or intramuscularly (IM) (2.0 mg/kg of body weight) followed by maintenance dose IV or IM (1.5 mg/kg) every 8 hours
- Continue for at least 48 hours after the patient shows improvement.
- Follow with doxycycline 100 mg orally bid or clindamycin 450 mg orally four times a day (qid) to complete 14 days of total therapy.

Outpatient Management

Regimen A

- Cefoxitin 2 gms IM *plus* probenecid 1 gm orally, concurrently, or ceftriaxone 250 mg IM or other third-generation cephalosporin (e.g., ceftizoxime or cefotaxime)
  plus
- Doxycycline 100 mg orally bid for 14 days

Regimen B

- Ofloxacin 400 mg orally bid, *plus either* clindamycin 450 mg orally qid *or* metronidazole 500 mg bid for 14 days

SOURCE: Centers for Disease Control (1993).

mon (Hatcher et al., 1994). HSV-2 antibodies are more commonly found in blacks than whites and, among blacks, women are more likely than men to have HSV-2 antibodies. Antibodies to HSV-2 are more prevalent in individuals living in inner cities and among persons of lower socioeconomic status (Aral & Holmes, 1991). Prevalence is higher in women with multiple sex partners. The greatest number of new cases occur in individuals between the ages of 15 and 34.

An initial herpetic infection characteristically has both systemic and local symptoms and lasts about 3 weeks. Generally, women have a more severe clinical course than do men. Often, the first symptoms following incubation (between 1 and 26 days, median time 6-8 days) are genital discomfort and neuralgic pain. Systemic symptoms appear early, peak about 3 to 4 days after lesions appear, and then subside over 3 to 4 days. Ulcerative lesions last 4 to 15 days before crusting over. New lesions may develop up to the 10th day of the course of the infection. Viral shedding, and thus infection, may last 6 to 8 weeks (Nettina & Kauffman, 1990).

Common systemic symptoms with the primary infection include fever, malaise, headache, and photophobia. Women with primary genital herpes have many lesions that progress from macules to papules, then form vesicles, pustules, and ulcers that crust and heal without scarring. These ulcers are extremely tender, and primary infections may be bilateral. Women may also have itching, inguinal tenderness, and lymphadenopathy. Severe vulvular edema may develop and women may have difficulty sitting. HSV cervicitis is also common with initial HSV-2 infections: The cervix may appear normal or be friable, reddened, ulcerated, or necrotic. A heavy, watery to purulent vaginal discharge is common. Extragenital lesions may be present because of autoinnoculation. Urinary retention and dysuria may occur secondary to autonomic involvement of the sacral nerve root.

Women experiencing recurrent episodes of HSV infections will commonly have only local symptoms, which are usually less severe than those associated with the initial infection. Systemic symptoms are usually absent, although the characteristic prodromal genital tingling is common. Recurrent lesions are unilateral, less severe, and usually last 7 to 10 days without prolonged viral shedding. Lesions begin as vesicles and progress rapidly to ulcers. Very few women with recurrent disease have cervicitis.

During pregnancy, maternal infection with HSV-2 can have adverse effects on mother and fetus. Viremia occurs during the primary infection, and congenital infection is possible although rare. Primary infections during the first trimester have been associated with increased spontaneous abortion rates. Primary infection in the second and third trimesters has been associated with increased incidence of preterm labor and delivery (Watts & Eschenbach, 1987). The most severe complication of HSV infection is neonatal herpes, a potentially fatal or severely disabling disease. Risk of neonatal infection is highest among women with primary herpes infection who are near term and is low among women with recurrent herpes (CDC, 1989). Neonates who develop HSV infection usually have severe disseminated or central nervous system infection resulting in mental retardation or death. Neonatal HSV infections usually occur in neonates born to asymptomatic mothers with primary infections at time of delivery.

An association between cervical cancer and HSV-2 has been observed. During the 1970s, many women infected with HSV-2 were counseled that they might be at serious risk for cervical cancer. Currently, it is thought that genital herpes is a marker for high-risk sexual behaviors that could transmit other STDs—including one that is the true cause of cervical cancer—and many researchers are examining HPV infections more closely (Aral & Holmes, 1991).

Assessment

A careful history provides much information when making a diagnosis of herpes. A history of exposure to an infected person is important, although infection from an asymptomatic individual is possible. A history of having viral symptoms, such as malaise, headache, fever, or myalgia, is suggestive. Local symptoms such as vulval pain, dysuria, itching, or burning at the site of infection and painful genital lesions that heal spontaneously are also very suggestive of HSV infections. The nurse should ask about prior history of a primary infection, prodromal symptoms, vaginal discharge, and dyspareunia (Nettina & Kauffman, 1990).

During the physical examination, the nurse should assess for inguinal and generalized lymphadenopathy and elevated temperature. The entire vulvular, perineal, vaginal, and cervical areas should be carefully inspected for vesicles or ulcerated or crusted areas. A speculum examination may be very difficult for the patient because of the extreme tenderness often associated with herpes infections.

Although a diagnosis of herpes infection may be suspected from the history and physical, it is confirmed by laboratory studies. Tests commonly used are Pap smear, Tzanck smear, and viral culture. A viral culture is obtained by swabbing exudate from an early-stage lesion and placing it in a viral medium. Results are available in 48 hours (Nettina & Kauffman, 1990). The Pap smear detects characteristic cell changes of the herpes virus. It is two thirds as sensitive as viral isolation techniques. The Tzanck smear is an air-dried scraping of the vesicular lesion stained with Wright or Giemsa preparation and observed for presence of multinucleated giant cells. It is one half as sensitive as the Pap smear (Breslin, 1988).

Nursing Management

Genital herpes is a chronic and recurring disease for which there is no known cure. Management is directed toward specific treatment during primary and recurrent infections, prevention, self-help measures, and psychological support.

The only FDA-approved medication is acyclovir, an antiviral agent that provides partial control of the signs and symptoms of herpes episodes and accelerates healing (CDC, 1989). It does not eradicate the infection or alter subsequent risk, frequency, or recurrences when the patient stops taking the drug. Treatment recommendations are given in Table 24.4. Safety and efficacy have been shown clearly in persons taking acyclovir daily for up to 3 years. After 1 year of continuous daily suppressive therapy, acyclovir should be stopped so that the patient's recurrence rate can be reassessed. Oral acyclovir therapy may be used during specific periods of high stress or when a woman wishes a period of certainty and control over outbreaks of the virus (Davies, 1990). In these instances, suppressive therapy is used in the same way as with severe recurrences. The safety of acyclovir therapy during pregnancy has not been established, and acyclovir should not be used with pregnant women unless life-threatening disease is present.

Cleaning lesions twice a day with saline will help prevent secondary infection. Bacterial infection must be treated with appropriate antibiotics. Measures that may increase comfort for women when lesions are active include warm sitz baths with baking soda; keeping lesions warm and dry by blowing area with a hair dryer set on cool or patting it dry with a soft towel; wearing cotton underwear and loose clothing; using drying aids such as hydrogen peroxide, Burrow's solution, and oatmeal baths; applying cool, wet black tea bags to lesions; and applying compresses with an infusion of cloves or peppermint oil and clove oil to lesions.

Oral analgesics such as aspirin or ibuprofen may be used to relieve pain and systemic symptoms associated with initial infections. Because the mucous membranes affected by herpes are very sensitive, any topical agents should be used with caution. Nonantiviral ointments, especially those containing cortisone, should be avoided (Davies, 1990). Zovirax (acyclovir) ointment is recommended by some authorities if the oral preparation is not used (Hawkins, Roberto, & Stanley-Haney, 1991). A thin layer of lidocaine ointment or an antiseptic spray may be applied to decrease discomfort, especially if walking is difficult (Lichtman & Duran, 1990). Women should be informed that occlusive ointments may prolong the course of infections (Nettina & Kauffman, 1990).

A diet rich in vitamins C, B-complex, and B6; zinc; and calcium is thought to help prevent recurrences. Daily use of kelp powder (2 capsules) and sunflower seed oil (1 tbsp) also has been recommended to decrease recurrences (Ammer, 1989). The amino acid L-lysine has been used in doses of 750 to 1,000 mg daily while lesions are active and 500 mg during asymptomatic periods. It is thought that L-lysine has an inhibitory effect on the multiplication of the herpes simplex virus.

Counseling and education are critical components of the nursing care of women with herpes infections. Information regarding the etiology, signs and symptoms, transmission, and treatment should be provided. The nurse should explain that each woman is unique in her response to herpes and emphasize the variability of symptoms. Women should be helped to understand when viral shedding and thus transmission to a partner is most likely and that they should refrain from sexual contact from the onset of prodromes until complete healing of lesions. Some authorities recommend consistent use of condoms for all persons with genital herpes (CDC, 1985). Condoms may not prevent transmission, particularly male-to-female transmission: This does not mean, however, that the partners should avoid all intimacy. Women can be encouraged to maintain close contact with their partners while avoiding contact with lesions. Women should be taught how to look for herpetic lesions using a mirror and good light source, and a wet cloth or finger covered with a finger cot to rub lightly over the labia. The nurse should ensure that patients understand that when lesions are active, sharing intimate articles (e.g., washcloths, wet towel) that come into contact with the lesions should be avoided. Plain soap and water is all that is needed to clean hands that have come in contact with herpetic lesions; isolation is not necessary or appropriate.

The nurse should explain the role of precipitating factors in the reactivation of the latent virus and recurrent episodes. Stress, menstruation, trauma, febrile illnesses, chronic illness, and ultraviolet light have all been found to trigger genital herpes (Davies, 1990). Women may wish to keep a diary to identify which stressors seem to be associated with recurrent herpes attacks for them so that they can then avoid them when possible. Referral for stress reduction therapy, yoga, or meditation classes may be done when indicated. The role of exercise in reducing stress can be discussed. Avoiding excessive heat and sun and hot baths and using a lubricant during sexual intercourse to reduce friction may also be helpful.

Women in their childbearing years should be counseled regarding the risk of herpes infection during pregnancy. They should be instructed to use condoms if there is any risk of contracting any STD from a sexual partner. If they are using acyclovir therapy, they should be counseled to use contraception due to the potential teratogenicity of acyclovir. Women currently breastfeeding should not use acyclovir.

Because neonatal HSV infection is such a devastating disease, prevention is critical. Current recommendations (CDC, 1993; Davies, 1990) include careful examination and questioning all women about symptoms at onset of labor. Diagnosis of genital herpes in any pregnant woman with active, visible lesions should be confirmed with culture. If visible lesions are not present at onset of labor, vaginal delivery is acceptable. Cesarean delivery within 4 hours after labor begins or membranes rupture is recommended if visible lesions are present. Infants who are delivered through an infected vagina should be carefully observed and cultured. Some experts recommend presumptive treatment of infants who were exposed to HSV at delivery. Weekly surveillance cultures from pregnant women with a history of HSV but who do not have visible lesions are not necessary or recommended (Binkin & Koplan, 1989).

Because HSV infection may be associated with cervical dysplasia, women must be encouraged to have yearly Pap smears and gynecologic examinations.

The emotional impact of contracting herpes is considerable. Media publicity regarding this disease has made receiving a diagnosis of genital herpes a devastating experience. No cure is available and most women will experience recurrences. At diagnosis, many emotions may surface—helplessness, anger, denial, guilt, anxiety, shame, or inadequacy. Women need the opportunity to discuss their feelings and help in learning to live with the disease. A woman can be encouraged to think of herself as a person who is not diseased but rather healthy and inconvenienced from time to time. Herpes can affect a woman's sexuality, her sexual practices, and her current and future relationships. She may need help in raising the issue with her partner or with future partners.

Syphilis

Syphilis, one of the earliest described STDs, is caused by *Treponema pallidum* (*T. pallidum*), a motile spirochete. Transmission is thought to be by entry in the subcutaneous tissue through microscopic abrasions that can occur during sexual intercourse. The disease can also be transmitted through kissing, biting, or oral-genital sex (Lichtman & Duran, 1990). Transplacental transmission may occur at any time during pregnancy; the degree of risk is related to the quantity of spirochetes in the maternal bloodstream. According to the CDC, syphilis reached its highest incidence, since the end of World War II, in 1990, when more than 50,000 new cases were reported (Division of STD/HIV Prevention, 1991). Much of the recent increase has been attributed to the use of crack cocaine and exchange of sex for drugs (Aral & Holmes, 1991). Other factors that seem to have contributed to the current syphilis epidemic are (a) an increase in syphilis transmission among medically hard-to-reach groups and (b) that persons in groups at increased risk for syphilis may not have access to health care.

Primary syphilis is characterized by a primary lesion, the chancre, that appears 5 to 90 days after infection; this lesion often begins as a painless papule at the site of inoculation and then erodes to form a nontender, shallow, indurated, clean ulcer several millimeters to centimeters in size. Although usually not painful, lesions that become secondarily infected, especially in the perianal region, may be painful. Associated regional lymphadenopathy usually appears 7 to 10 days later. Chancres may be multiple and extragenital (Nettina & Kauffman, 1990); if located in nongenital areas, they may not be clinically apparent. The primary chancre generally disappears in 2 to 6 weeks.

Secondary syphilis occurs 6 weeks to 6 months after the appearance of the chancre; however, primary and secondary syphilis may overlap in approximately 30% of cases (Star, 1990c). Secondary syphilis is characterized by a widespread, symmetrical maculopapular rash and generalized lymphadenopathy. The infected individual also may experience fever, headache, and malaise. Characteristically, the rash is seen on the palms and soles. Condyloma lata (wartlike infectious lesions) may develop on the vulva, perineum, or anus. If the patient is untreated, she enters a latent phase that is asymptomatic for the majority of individuals.

The early latent phase—1 year's duration—is symptomatic in about 25% of patients (Star, 1990c). Patients are potentially infectious through the early latency phase. The late latency period—greater than 1 year's duration—may last indefinitely. Some patients may no longer have a positive serology and most are healthy. If left untreated, however, about one third of patients will develop tertiary syphilis. Neuro/cardiovascular, musculoskeletal, or multiorgan system complications can develop in this third stage.

Pregnant women with primary or secondary syphilis when blood levels of *T. pallidum* are the highest are more likely to transmit the infection to their fetuses than those in the latent or late phases of the disease. During the primary and secondary phase, high rates of spontaneous abortion, stillbirth, premature delivery, and neonatal death occur. Congenital syphilis is a multisystem disease with manifestations similar to secondary syphilis; often, there is skeletal involvement with osteochondritis and periostitis. The mortality rate of infants with congenital syphilis symptomatic at birth is greater than 50%. However, most infants with early congenital syphilis are asymptomatic at birth, and active disease is not apparent until 10 days to 2 weeks of life. If untreated or inadequately treated, classic manifestations of late congenital syphilis will develop.

Assessment

Aspects of the history to be obtained include those discussed previously in the general assessment section. In addition, women should be asked about the presence of lesions, particularly nontender ones, on her or her partner's genitalia that followed sexual relations by 5 to 90 days and healed within 2 to 6 weeks. Any history of undiagnosed rashes or lesions, especially on the mucous membranes or soles and palms should be discussed. Patchy hair loss also may be significant.

The physical examination should include a thorough exam of cervical and inguinal lymph nodes, mouth, skin, hair, soles and palms, extremities, spleen, liver, external genitalia, vagina, cervix, and anus. Notation is made of the presence of lymphadenopathy; alopecia (hair loss); diffuse maculopapular rash on soles or palms; presence of chancres in mouth, vagina, vulva, or cervical or anal areas; mucous patches on lips, tongue, buccal mucosa, pharynx, tonsils, vaginal introitus; and condyloma lata. If indicated, a neurological exam should be done.

Definitive diagnosis of early syphilis is based on dark field examination and direct fluorescent antibody tests on lesions or tissue (CDC, 1989). These procedures are not done routinely and require an experienced microscopist. Presumptive diagnosis is based on serological testing and clinical presentation (Nettina & Kauffman, 1990). Two types of serological tests are used: nontreponemal and treponemal. Nontreponemal antibody tests, such as the VDRL or RPR, are used as screening tests, and false/positive results are not unusual, particularly when conditions such as acute infection, autoimmune disorders, malignancy, pregnancy, and drug addiction exist and after immunization or vaccination. The treponemal tests, fluorescent treponemal antibody absorbed (FTA-ABS) and microhemagglutination assays for antibody to *T. pallidum* (MHA-TP), are used to confirm positive results. Test results in patients with early primary or incubating syphilis may be negative. Seroconversion usually takes place 6 to 8 weeks after exposure, so testing should be repeated in 1 to 2 months when a suspicious genital lesion exists. Positive treponemal antibody tests stay positive for life regardless of treatment or disease activity (CDC, 1989).

Tests for concomitant STDs should be done, the HIV-antibody test offered, and, if indicated, wet preps carried out. All pregnant women should be screened for syphilis at the first prenatal visit and again in the late third trimester.

Nursing Management

Penicillin is the preferred drug for treating patients with syphilis. It is the only proven therapy that has been widely used for patients with neurosyphilis, congenital syphilis, or syphilis during pregnancy. Recommendations for treatment are given in Table 24.4. Although doxycycline, tetracycline, and erythromycin are alternative treatments for penicillin-allergic patients, both tetracycline and doxycycline are contraindicated in pregnancy, and erythromycin is unlikely to cure a fetal infection. Therefore, pregnant women with a history of penicillin allergy should be treated with penicillin after desensitization (CDC, 1993).

Patients treated for syphilis may experience a Jarisch-Herxheimer reaction. This is an acute febrile reaction often accompanied by headache, myalgias, and arthralgias that develop within hours of treatment (Star, 1990c). Women treated in the second half of pregnancy are at risk for preterm labor and delivery if treatment precipitates this reaction (Star, 1990c). They should be advised to contact their health care provider if they notice any change in fetal movement or have any contractions.

Monthly follow-up is mandatory so that retreatment may be given if needed. The nurse should emphasize the necessity of long-term serological testing even in the absence of symptoms. The patient should be advised to practice sexual abstinence until treatment is completed, all evidence of primary and secondary syphilis is gone and serological evidence of a cure is demonstrated. Women should be told to notify all partners who may have been exposed. They should be informed that the disease is reportable. Preventive measures presented earlier in this chapter should be discussed.

Viral Hepatitis

Hepatitis B (HB) infection is an STD caused by the HB virus (HBV), the virus most threatening to the fetus and neonate. It is caused by a large DNA virus and is associated with three antigens and their antibodies: HB surface antigen (HBsAg), HBV antigen (HBeAg), HBV core antigen (HBcAg), antibody to HBsAg (anti-HBs), antibody to HBeAg (anti-HBe), and antibody to HBcAg (anti-HBc) (Lichtman & Duran, 1990; Lommel, 1990). Screening for active or chronic disease or disease immunity is based on testing for these antigens and their antibodies.

The following factors are considered to place a woman at risk for HB infection (CDC, 1991a):

- Asian, Pacific Islander (Polynesian, Micronesian, Melanesian) or Alaskan Eskimo descent
- Haitian or sub-Saharan Africa birth
- History of acute or chronic liver disease
- Work or treatment in a dialysis unit
- Household or sexual contact with a hemodialysis patient
- Work or residence in institutions for the mentally retarded
- Previous rejection as a blood donor
- History of multiple blood transfusions
- Health care workers
- Public safety workers exposed to blood in the workplace
- Household contact with an HBV carrier
- History of multiple sexual partners
- History of multiple STDs
- History of intravenous (IV) drug use

HB infection is transmitted parentally and through intimate contact. It is 50- to 100-fold more contagious than HIV and is regarded as the most common STD in the world (Cefalo & Moos, 1990). HBV surface antigen has been found in blood, saliva, sweat, tears, vaginal secretions, and semen. Perinatal transmission most often occurs in mothers who have acute hepatitis infection with HBeAg late in the third trimester or during the intrapartum or postpartum periods from exposure to HBsAg-positive vaginal secretions, blood, amniotic fluid, saliva, and breast milk (Cefalo & Moos, 1990). Infants born to mothers who are highly infectious (positive for both HBsAg and HBeAg) have a 70% to 90% chance of acquiring perinatal HBV infection. Approximately 85% to 90% of infected infants will become chronic carriers. HBV has also been transmitted by artificial insemination. Although HBV can be transmitted via blood transfusion, the incidence of such infections has decreased significantly since testing of blood for HBsAg became routine. Drug abusers who share needles are at risk, as are health care workers who are exposed to blood and needlesticks.

HB is a disease of the liver and is often a silent infection. In the adult, the course of the infection can be fulminating and the outcome fatal. Early symptoms include skin eruptions, urticaria, arthralgias, arthritis, lassitude, anorexia, nausea, vomiting, headache, fever, and mild abdominal pain (Lichtman & Duran, 1990). Later, the patient may have clay-colored stools, dark urine, increased abdominal pain, and jaundice. Between 5% and 10% of individuals with HB have persistence of HBsAg and become chronic HBV carriers. Of chronic carriers, 25% will die from primary hepatocellular carcinoma or cirrhosis of the liver.

Assessment

All women at high risk for contracting HB infection should be screened on a regular basis. Screening only high-risk individuals may not identify up to 50% of HBsAg-positive women (Butterfield, Shockley, Miguel, & Rosa, 1990); therefore current CDC (1989) guidelines recommend screening for the presence of HBsAg in all women at the first prenatal visit. However, at least one study has found that universal prenatal HB testing is not cost-effective (Koretz, 1989).

Testing for HB infection is complex. Patients with acute HB generally have detectable serum HBsAg levels in the late incubation phase of the disease, 2 to 5 weeks before symptoms appear. Anti-HBs with a negative HBsAg test signals immunity. Anti-HBs with a positive antigen denotes a chronic carrier state; during this time, the disease can be transmitted. During the recovery phase, the patient may continue to be infectious even though HBsAg cannot be detected. This is called the "window phase" and is identified by anti-HBc in the absence of anti-HBs.

Components of the history to be obtained when HB is suspected include the inquiry about the symptoms of the disease and risk factors outlined earlier. Physical examination includes inspection of the skin for rashes, inspection of the skin and conjunctiva for jaundice, and palpation of the liver for enlargement and tenderness. Weight loss, fever, and general debilitation should be noted. If the HBsAg is positive, further laboratory studies may be ordered: anti-HBe, anti-HBc, SGOT (serum glutamic oxaloasetic transaminase), alkaline phosphatase, and liver panel. If the HBsAG is negative in early pregnancy and the woman could be in the window phase, or if high-risk behaviors continue during pregnancy, a repeat HBsAg should be ordered in the third trimester.

Nursing Management

There is no specific treatment for HB infection. Recovery is usually spontaneous in 3 to 16 weeks. Usually, pregnancies complicated by acute viral hepatitis are managed on an outpatient basis. Women should be advised to increase bed rest, eat a high-protein, low-fat diet, and increase their fluid intake. They should avoid medications metabolized in the liver, drugs, and alcohol. Women with a definite exposure to HBV should be given HB immunoglobulin (HBIG), 0.06 ml/kg, intramuscularly (IM) in a single dose as soon as possible within a 7-day period after exposure (CDC, 1989). Infants born to HBsAg-positive women should be given HBIG, 0.5 ml, IM within 12 hours after birth and subsequently should be immunized with HB vaccine. The first vaccination should be given at the same time and repeated at 1 and 6 months. The child should be tested for immunity at 12 to 15 months (Wilson, 1988).

All nonimmune women at high or moderate risk of hepatitis should be informed of the existence of HB vaccine. Vaccination is recommended for all individuals who have had multiple sex partners within the past 6 months or who were diagnosed as recently having contracted another STD (CDC, 1993). In addition, IV-drug users (IVDUs), residents of correctional or long-term care facilities, persons seeking care for STD, prostitutes, women whose partners are IVDUs or bisexual, and women whose occupation exposed them to high risk should be vaccinated. Vaccination is not associated with serious side effects and does not carry a risk for contracting HIV. The vaccine is given a series of three (some authorities recommend four) doses over a 6-month period with the first two doses given within 1 month of each other. The vaccine should be given in the deltoid muscle, never in the gluteal or quadriceps muscles (CDC, 1989).

Patient education includes explaining the meaning of HB infection, including transmission, state of infectivity, and sequelae. The nurse should also explain the need for immunoprophylaxis for household members and sexual contacts. To decrease transmission of the virus, women with HB infection or who test positive for HBV should be advised to maintain a high level of personal hygiene—wash hands after using the toilet; carefully dispose of tampons, pads, and Band-Aids in plastic bags; do not share razor blades, toothbrushes, needles, and manicure implements; have male partner use a condom if unvaccinated and without hepatitis; avoid sharing saliva through kissing or sharing of silverware or dishes; wipe up blood spills immediately with soap and water. They should inform all health care providers of their carrier state. Newly delivered women should be reassured that breast-feeding is not contraindicated if their infants have been immunized.

Human Immunodeficiency Virus (HIV) Infection

Although the first cases of AIDS in women were reported in 1981, only recently have health care providers recognized that HIV infection in women is a serious problem that continues to worsen (CDC, 1992).

Basic information about HIV, its effect on the immune system, the natural history of HIV infection, and modes of transmission is provided in Table 24.6. HIV is not highly contagious. Transmission is only through direct contact with body fluids rich in T-4 lymphocytes. Although HIV has been detected in many body fluids (blood, semen, vaginal secretions, cerebrospinal fluids, urine, tears, and saliva), only blood, semen, and vaginal secretions have been implicated in horizontal transmission (person-to-person) of HIV (Holman, 1989). The major routes of horizontal transmission are sexual contact and inoculation of blood. At least 75% of HIV infections in women worldwide were acquired through sexual intercourse (CDC, 1991d). Available data suggest that female-to-male transmission is less efficient than male-to-female transmission (O'Brien,

Shaffer, & Jaffe, 1992). HIV infection resulting from artificial insemination with HIV-infected semen has also been documented (Stewart, Cunningham, Driscoll, Gold, & Lamot, 1985). HIV is transmitted vertically (from mother to infant), and infection may occur during pregnancy, at delivery, or through breast milk (Seltzer & Benjamin, 1990). Precisely when and how HIV is transmitted from an infected mother to her infant is not yet known (Holman, 1989). Furthermore, because HIV has been found in breast milk, there is the additive risk of HIV infection from breast-feeding for infants born to women who are HIV-seropositive.

In the United States, the proportion of women with AIDS has increased steadily (CDC, 1990a) and women are now the fastest growing population of individuals with HIV infection and AIDS (CDC, 1992; Shayne & Kaplan, 1991). In the United States, the majority of women with HIV infection are women of color who live in large urban areas on the East Coast and are of reproductive age (Ellerbrock, Bush, Chamberland, & Oxtoby, 1991). However, the proportion of women with AIDS reported by smaller cities and rural areas is rising steadily. Although the reported incidence of AIDS in women of every race and ethnic group continues to increase, women of color are at significantly higher risk for acquiring HIV infection (CDC, 1991d). Slightly more than half the women with AIDS have a history of IV-drug use; in addition, more than one third are sexual partners of high-risk men. Lesbians represent a very small proportion of women with AIDS in the United States and most cases are related to IV-drug use (Chu, Buehler, Flemming, & Berkelman, 1990).

Among all cases of AIDS in women, 85% occur among women of childbearing age. HIV/AIDS is expected to become one of the five leading causes of death in women of reproductive age by the mid-1990s (Chu, Buehler, & Berkelman, 1990). The risk of perinatal transmission of HIV infection is estimated to be 15% to 39% (Peckham, 1994). Transmission rates vary by region of the world: In Europe, the rate is 15% to 20%; in Africa, 25% to 39%; and in the United States, 16% to 30% (Newell & Peckham, 1993). Increased vertical transmission has been associated with extreme prematurity (European Collaborative Study, 1992) and breast-feeding (Dunn, Newell, Ades, & Peckham, 1992). Furthermore, a meta-analysis of several studies of rates of vertical transmission from mother to child suggest that cesarean delivery has a protective effect (Peckham, 1994).

HIV Testing and Counseling

Screening, teaching, and counseling regarding HIV risk factors, indications for being tested, and testing are major roles for nurses caring for women today. A number of factors and behaviors have been identified that place women at risk for contracting HIV infection, including IV-drug use, high-risk sexual partners, multiple sex partners, and a previous history of multiple STDs. The CDC (1993) guidelines recommend offering HIV testing to all women who are at risk for HIV infection. It may be useful to allow women to self-select for HIV testing. After entry to the health care system, a woman can be handed written information about the risk factors for the AIDS virus and asked to inform the nurse if she believes she is at risk. She should be told that she does not have to say why she may be at risk, only that she thinks she might be.

When a woman requests HIV testing, it is the nurse's responsibility to assess her understanding of the information such a test would provide and to be sure her client thoroughly understands the emotional, legal, and medical implications of a positive or negative test before she is ready to take an HIV test. One's life is profoundly altered by knowledge that he or she is HIV seropositive. A unique stigma is associated with HIV infection that can have a profound impact on the quality of life of those infected. This stigma extends to those who are asymptomatic but seropositive. Given the current limitations of HIV testing, Kurth and Hutchinson (1989) suggest that the social implications of HIV seropositivity dictate that HIV testing be done only after careful consideration by clients and providers.

HIV testing and screening in pregnancy is a very sensitive issue. Minkoff and Landesman (1988) believe that informing infected women of their serological status is critically important and that routine testing (with consent, confidentiality, and counseling) is the only practical way to accomplish this goal. The CDC (1993) recommends that all pregnant women with a history of STDs be offered HIV counseling and testing, because recognition of HIV infection in pregnancy permits health care providers to inform women about the risks of transmission and continuing pregnancy.

Table 24.6 Human Immunodeficiency Virus (HIV) Infection

Organism

- It is a retrovirus isolated in 1983.
- It was first referred to as lymphodenopathy-associated virus (LAV) by its French discoverers and human T-cell lymphatropic virus, variant III (HTLV-III) by American discoverers.
- It was renamed human immunodeficiency virus (HIV) in 1986.
- As a retrovirus, it has a unique enzyme that allows the virus, a piece of RNA, to convert to DNA and become inserted into the nucleus of a host cell.

HIV's effect on the immune system

- HIV causes a defect in the immune system by invading and multiplying within T-4 lymphocytes.
- HIV depletes T-4 cells, limits proper function of remaining T-4 cells, and interferes with the ratio between T-4 (CD4+, helper) and T-8 (CD8+, suppressor) cells.
- This inhibits the ability of T-4 cells to recognize and defend against certain parasitic, viral, and fungal organisms.
- HIV also infects monocytes and macrophages; limited viral repletion occurs, and the host cell is not completely destroyed.
- When these cells circulate in the body, the virus infects other cells, including lung and bone marrow.

Natural history of HIV infection

- HIV infection is a continuum ranging from asymptomatic carrier state to extreme immunodeficiency.
  - Acute infection
    - Approximately 2 to 8 weeks after infection, a mononucleosis-like syndrome may develop with high fever, lymphadenopathy, rash, and headache. This may persist for 10 to 14 days. No more than 50% of infected individuals report a history of such an illness. Infected individuals would test negative for HIV antibody for a "window period" of 6 to 12 weeks. Generally, antibodies develop 2 to 12 weeks after exposure to the virus; in some limited instances, antibodies are not detectable for up to 6 months after exposure. CD4+ cell count is normal (400-1,200) to high (over 1,200).
  - Symptom free
    - No signs or symptoms of HIV infection are present.
    - The individual is seropositive and can transmit the virus to others.
    - This period of being free of symptoms may last from a few months to several years.
    - CD4+ cell counts are > than 500.
  - Early symptoms
    - Symptoms: generalized lymphadenopathy, fever, night sweats, diarrhea, severe fatigue, weight loss, reactivation of chronic viral infections, opportunistic infections such as oral or vaginal candidiasis, papillomavirus, and herpes
    - This phase is also known as AIDS-related complex (ARC), which is misleading because there are no separate syndromes but, instead, an ongoing, overlapping response to HIV.
    - CD4+ cell count is typically < 500.
  - Discrete illness to end stage
    - This is usually referred to as AIDS; the average interval from infection to AIDS is 11 years.
    - It is characterized by severe depletion of T-helper lymphocytes and disruption of almost every process of a normal immune system.
    - Opportunistic infections are seen, including *Pneumocystis carinii* pneumonia, disseminated Myco bacterium tuberculosis, cytomegalovirus, toxoplasmosis, and candidiasis.
    - Malignancies related to states of immune deficiency, such as Kaposi's sarcoma, occur.
    - Organ dysfunction, particularly in the nervous system, results in dementia and polyneuropathy.

SOURCES: Adapted from Sinclair (1990), Hatcher et al. (1994), and Levy (1992).

Given the strong social stigma attached to HIV infection, nurses must consider the issue of confidentiality and documentation before providing counseling and offering HIV testing to clients. If test results are placed in the patient's chart—the appropriate place for all health information—they are available to all who have access to the chart: The client must be informed of this before testing. The process of consent for HIV testing is also critically important. In some states, written consent is mandated; in others, it is not. Women's consent for HIV testing should be obtained in a manner analogous to consent for alpha-fetoprotein testing or amniocentesis (Moroso & Holman, 1990).

Pretest counseling should be provided for all clients regardless of their decision to be tested. During a counseling session, the nurse can provide women with knowledge about at-risk behaviors and ways to reduce risk. Information conveyed during pretest counseling should include (a) the spectrum of HIV disease and relationship to AIDS, (b) modes of HIV transmission, (c) which tests are used, (d) the meaning of negative and positive results, and (e) risk reduction behaviors (Moroso & Holman, 1990).

Adequate counseling also includes a discussion of perinatal transmission and why it is important to know one's HIV status. The importance of a woman knowing her HIV status should be stressed, but the client should never be coerced into being tested. Sexual partners should also be encouraged to consider testing. Nurses should assess the coping mechanisms and support systems of their clients during precounseling. Specific questions that might be asked include the following (Moroso & Holman, 1990): "Who are the supportive persons in your life? If you are HIV positive, who could you tell who would be supportive and keep this confidential? How do you usually react in stressful situations? How do you think you might deal with a positive HIV result?" It also may be necessary to assess suicide risk and previous psychiatric problems.

Generally, there is a 1- to 3-week waiting period following testing for HIV, which can be a very anxious time for the client; it is helpful if the nurse informs her that this time period between blood drawing and test results is routine. Test results, whatever they are, must always be communicated in person and women informed in advance that such is the procedure. Whenever possible, the person who provided the pretest counseling should also tell the client her test results. Occasionally, a test result will be reported as equivocal or indeterminate: When this happens, the test must be repeated with a new blood sample. Women should be told beforehand that this sometimes occurs and does not necessarily mean that the results will be positive. All pretest counseling should be documented.

When providing posttest counseling for the HIV-negative women, the nurse should make sure she reviews what a negative test means. Some women when informed of negative results may escalate their risk behaviors because of an equating of negativity with immunity. Others may believe that negative means "bad" and positive means "good." Women's reactions to a negative test should be explored, asking, "How do you feel?" HIV-negative-result counseling sessions are another opportunity to provide education. Emphasis can be placed on ways in which a woman can remain HIV-free and encouraged to stay negative. She should be reminded that if she has been exposed to HIV in the past 6 months she should be retested and that if she continues high-risk behaviors she should have ongoing testing.

When providing posttest counseling to an HIV-seropositive woman, privacy with no interruptions is essential. Adequate time for the counseling sessions should also be provided. Women's reactions to learning they are HIV-seropositive may vary from shame, to fear and sadness, to crying and shouting, to lack of comprehension and denial. The nurse should acknowledge the reasonableness of fear of suffering, of dying, and of repeated losses (physical strength, mental acuity, sexual freedom, self-sufficiency). HIV-seropositive women face telling others, some of whom will be deeply saddened and perhaps others who will be furious at being placed at risk. Rejection by partner, lover, family, or friends may occur. A woman may lose her job or be asked to leave housing, even though such discrimination is usually illegal. She will find it impossible to obtain new health or life insurance. Women must be allowed sufficient time to work through some of their emotions. The nurse should not attempt to minimize the gravity of a woman's situation nor should she attempt to assess a time frame for the development of AIDS. More than one counselor may be helpful, one to be the bearer of bad news and the other to function as a support person. The session should be initiated after a review of information about the client's support system and an anticipation of her referral needs.

The nurse should make sure that her client understands what a positive test means and review the reliability of the test results. Safer sex guidelines need to be discussed in the initial counseling session. Women may not wish to tell their sexual partners about their serostatus immediately but, rather, may wish to wait until they feel the timing is right. Women should be offered the opportunity to bring their partner(s) in to discuss the implications of HIV infection.

Before a woman leaves the initial counseling session, the nurse should ask her to identify a supportive person and discuss how she might tell that person and what his or her reactions might be. This may help decrease the negative consequences that could occur from poorly planned disclosure of a positive test result. The nurse should plan with her client how she will tell others and notify sexual contacts and rehearse ways to tell them. Referral for appropriate medical evaluation and follow-up should be made at the initial counseling session, and the need or desire for psychosocial or psychiatric referrals should be assessed. It is important that clients be reassured as to the continued availability of the nurse to discuss HIV infection. The nurse should obtain a phone number for the woman so that she can follow-up with her in 1 to 2 days. If the woman does not have a phone or is reluctant to give it to the nurse, she can be asked to call the nurse at a given time. An early follow-up appointment is recommended to reassess the client's emotional status and review material covered earlier that may not have been absorbed or retained.

Women in their childbearing years and not using birth control and/or desirous of pregnancy should be encouraged to postpone pregnancy until a knowledgeable decision can be made.

The importance of early medical evaluation so that a baseline assessment can be made and prophylactic medication begun should be stressed. If possible, the nurse should make a referral or appointment for the woman at the first posttest counseling session.

As the number of HIV-infected women escalates, prevention, education, and counseling activities must be directed toward all women. As nurses, it is very difficult to keep abreast of the ever changing picture of AIDS. Important sources of information are the National AIDS Hotline (1-800-342-2437, 1-800-344-7432 [Spanish] or 1-800-243-7889 [deaf]) and National AIDS Information Clearing House, P.O. Box 6003, Rockville, MD 20850 (1-800-458-5231).

Nursing Management

During the initial contact with an HIV-infected woman, the nurse should establish what the client knows about HIV infection. The nurse should ensure that her client is being cared for by a medical practitioner or facility with expertise in caring for persons with HIV infections, including AIDS. Psychological referral may also be indicated. Resources such as counseling for death and dying, suicide prevention, financial assistance, and legal advocacy may be appropriate. All women who are drug users should be referred to a substance abuse program. A major focus of counseling is prevention of transmission of HIV to partners.

Nurses counseling seropositive women wishing contraceptive information may recommend oral contraceptives and latex condoms, Norplant implants and latex condoms, or tubal sterilization/vasectomy and latex condoms (Hatcher et al., 1994). Spermicides, female condoms, or abstinence can be offered to women whose partners refuse to use condoms. Oral contraceptives were associated with increased risk for HIV infection in one Kenyan study (Holmes & Kreiss, 1988); however, a 1988 study of American women working in the sex industry (prostitution) found no relationship between HIV and oral contraceptives (Hatcher et al., 1994).

There is no cure available for HIV infections at this time. Rare and unusual diseases are characteristic of HIV-infections. Opportunistic infections and concurrent diseases should be managed vigorously with treatment specific to the infection or disease. When a woman's CD4+ count falls below 200, she is at increased risk for opportunistic infections, and prophylaxis with trimethoprim, sulfamethoxozole, or pentamidine may be initiated.

A number of experimental drugs such as zidovudine (ZDV, brand name Retrovir) and didanosine (DDI, brand name Videx) are used and appear to retard the progression of the disease. Very little is known about the effectiveness of these drugs in treating women with HIV infections, however, because until recently, many of the studies have made little or no effort to include women in the drug trials. Treatment guidelines for nonpregnant women and men with HIV infection are similar. As of September 1993, CDC (1993) treatment guidelines recommend treatment for symptomatic persons with fewer than 500 CD4+ T-4 cells or asymptomatic persons with fewer than 300 CD4+ T-cells. The recommended therapeutic regimen for ZDV is 500 mg (100 mg orally every 4 hours while awake). DDI is recommended for persons who are intolerant of ZDV or who have increased symptoms even with ZDV. The recommended therapeutic regimen for DDI is two 100 mg tablets every 12 hours for persons weighing more than 60 kg (132 lbs.); the recommended dose for adults weighing less than 60 kg is one 100 mg tablet and one 25 mg tablet every 12 hours. ZDV therapy given during pregnancy and/or labor and delivery has been shown to be associated with a significant reduction in vertical transmission (Boyer et al., 1994).

Alternative therapies, such as visualization, chiropractic, and holistic remedies, may be useful for individuals with AIDS. Nurses can also make available information regarding the variety of resources and services available to individuals with HIV infections/AIDS. Women with HIV infection should be encouraged and helped to make lifestyle changes that make them as healthy as possible. Specific strategies include eating a balanced diet, getting enough rest, and avoiding stress when possible; preventing infection by washing hands frequently; and avoiding places with unsanitary conditions or where people are sick. HIV-seropositive women should be counseled to avoid alcohol and drugs that may damage the immune system. Women who are seropositive should seek medical advice before getting a vaccination or having their children vaccinated with a live virus. Specific CDC (1993) guidelines regarding recommended immunizations for adult and adolescent women infected with HIV are: pneumonococcal vaccination and an annual influenza vaccination, hepatitis B vaccine for women who are at increased risk for acquired HBV or who lack immunity already.

Over half of the women with HIV infection are IVDUs or partners of IVDUs. The problems associated with HIV infection are compounded by their drug use. Most are disenfranchised, poor, and isolated. They may find it even more difficult than other women to practice safer sex. Alcohol and other drugs may disinhibit behavior that can result in unsafe sharing of needles and sexual practices and thus increase exposure to HIV. In addition, sex is often traded for drugs. Women IVDUs have poor self-esteem and higher levels of anxiety and depression, are generally nonassertive, have little sense of control, and hold very traditional beliefs about sex role behaviors (Williams, 1989); all these characteristics can prevent them from practicing self-protective behaviors to prevent the transmission of HIV.

Group involvement with others who also have AIDS has been identified by AIDS patients as of key emotional value (Lichtman & Duran, 1990). Women who discover that they have AIDS or HIV infection feel extremely isolated. They may not talk to family or friends for fear of becoming ostracized (Williams, 1989). Often, they must depend on health care professionals for support, but cultural differences and attitudes of mistrust limit the usefulness of this resource for them. Nurses working with women with HIV infections must be sensitive to the importance of social contacts for these women and help to decrease their social isolation in whatever way possible. Referral to community resources or peer support groups should always be offered.

Female-Specific Problems

Vaginal candidiasis has been described as one of the earliest manifestations of immunosuppression in women. Although vaginal candidiasis infections are common in healthy women, those seen in women with HIV infection are often more severe and persistent. Genital candidiasis lesions may be painful, coalescing ulcerations necessitating continuous, prophylactic therapy. Temporary symptomatic relief may be achieved with treatment, and symptoms reappear as soon as medication is discontinued (Carpenter, Mayer, Fisher, Desai, & Durand, 1989). In women with HIV disease, unexplained oral and vaginal candidiasis appears to be an indicator of a severely compromised immune system and advanced disease (Allen & Marte, 1992). Women with recurrent candidiasis should have antifungal vaginal creams or suppositories, such as clotrimazole or nystatin, available for self-administration. If the condition recurs or is resistant to topical therapy, oral imidazoles, such as ketoconazole, may be prescribed. When a woman has been asymptomatic for 2 weeks, maintenance therapy may be started: ketoconazole, 100 to 200 mg, by mouth, daily for 5 days each month at onset of menses (Allen & Marte, 1992). If a woman has ulcerative candidiasi, she may need higher initial doses of ketoconazole, up to 800 mg per day. Liver function tests should be monitored when a patient is taking ketoconazole.

Genital herpes infections occur more often in women with HIV infection than in women without HIV infection (Holmberg et al., 1988). The clinical picture in asymptomatic seropositive women with genital herpes is different from that in seronegative women; as immune system function deteriorates, lesions are more painful, widespread, and persistent. Patients are treated with oral acyclovir, 400 mg, four or five times a day initially and maintained with 200 mg one or two times a day indefinitely. Renal function should be monitored closely. This treatment may be supplemented with acyclovir 5% ointment applied at 3-hour intervals. If resistant strains of herpes develop following long-term acyclovir therapy, intravenous foscarnet (0.60 mg/kg every 8 hours) may be prescribed (Allen & Marte, 1992).

The clinical course of HPV infection in women with HIV infection is accelerated, and recurrence is more frequent. A greater incidence of abnormal cervical smears and cervical intraepithelial neoplasia (CIN) has been reported in women with HIV infection compared with noninfected women (CDC, 1990b). Trichloroacetic acid (95%) is used for vulvular and perianal lesions smaller than 2 cm; topical 5-fluorouracil (once weekly for 10 weeks or daily for 5 days) may also be used for vaginal lesions. Persistent or recurrent lesions should be treated with cryosurgery, surgical excision, or CO_2 (Allen & Marte, 1992).

HIV infection is associated with serious PID partly because of similar risk factors and alterations in the immune system. More lengthy hospitalizations are necessary and more frequent surgery for tubo-ovarian abscesses are required (Marte & Allen, 1991). Because symptoms that persist after usual treatment of PID may suggest a failing immune system, HIV should be considered in all women who seek care for symptoms suggestive of PID.

Routine gynecologic care for HIV-seropositive women should include a pelvic examination every 6 months. Careful Pap screening is essential because of the greatly increased incidence of abnormal findings on examination (Provencher et al., 1988). In addition, HIV-seropositive women should be screened for syphilis, gonorrhea, and chlamydia and other vaginal infections.

Coinfection with syphilis is common in HIV-infected women, and treatment failures with benzathine penicillin are frequent (Allen & Marte, 1992). Furthermore, HIV infection increases susceptibility to neurosyphilis, which is hard to differentiate clinically from HIV dementia.

HIV Infection and Childbearing

Of women with HIV infection, 85% are in their childbearing years, and questions related to childbearing are of critical importance. Alterations in the immune system occur normally during pregnancy to allow the fetus to survive. For instance, T-4 cells are present in decreased numbers in the blood of healthy pregnant women. The question of the effect of pregnancy on HIV infection has been raised: Does pregnancy accelerate the course of the disease? Early reports suggested that pregnancy accelerates HIV disease and shortens life (Biggar et al., 1989; CDC, 1985; Koonan et al., 1989). More recent research suggests that AIDS probably is not altered by pregnancy (Minkoff, 1989; Selwyn et al., 1989). The increased severity of illness at time of conception, failure to seek health care during pregnancy, and attribution of nonspecific symptoms, such as nausea, fatigue, loss of appetite, and malaise, to pregnancy often result in delayed diagnosis and may add to the impression that pregnancy accelerates HIV disease progression (Smeltzer & Whipple, 1991).

Early studies examining the effects of HIV infection on pregnancy outcomes suggested that there are adverse outcomes, whereas more recent studies suggest that HIV infection is not associated with early or late poor pregnancy outcomes. A registry of pregnancy-associated mortality with 20 women who died within a year of a pregnancy showed that all 16 children with follow-up had adverse birth outcomes, including prematurity and stillbirth (Koonan et al., 1989). In contrast, preliminary data from a study by Landesman (1989) suggest that HIV infection does not have an adverse impact on pregnancy outcomes. Rates of prematurity and low birth weight were comparable in HIV-seropositive women and their matched seronegative controls. Minkoff and colleagues (1990) found that HIV-seropositive women with low CD4+ cell counts were at markedly increased risk for serious infections during pregnancy. Maternal HIV infection does not appear to affect newborn health characteristics (Butz, Hutton, & Larson, 1991).

Although most infants born to HIV-seropositive women are not infected with HIV, all are seropositive at birth and in the first months of life because of transmission of maternal antibodies across the placenta. Loss of antibody and consistent seronegativity at 15 months of age indicate that an infant is not infected.

Careful, sensitive counseling must be provided to seropositive women regarding reproductive options. Nurses should raise the option of abortion for seropositive women who are in the first trimester or early second trimester of pregnancy. HIV-infected women considering pregnancy termination should be provided with factual, appropriate data regarding options in their community and state. Although many public health officials, physicians, policy makers, and the general public consider the birth of HIV-infected infants inexplicable, unjustifiable, or immoral (Levine & Dubler, 1990) and many states have suggested or are considering legislation that would require all pregnant women to be tested for HIV infection (Kurth & Hutchinson, 1989), the decision belongs to the individual woman. Nursing responsibilities include presenting information in a nondiscriminatory, noncoercive manner and maintaining clients' rights to full disclosure, complete confidentiality, and unbiased health care.

The nurse must consider that women infected with HIV may not choose to prevent or terminate pregnancy. Pronatalist sentiments are strong in the American culture, and reproduction may be viewed as an affirmation of life and a hope for survival. Childbearing may have a special symbolism for poor women of color. Latino and black cultures place great value on a woman's fertility (Mitchell, 1988), and childlessness is a very serious concern in communities of color (Nsiah-Jefferson, 1989). A baby may be viewed as something concrete to love or to be loved by and a visible sign of having been loved or touched by another person (Levine & Dubler, 1990). Disenfranchised and disadvantaged women may consider the 2 to 5 in 10 chance of having a child better than the risks routinely faced in other parts of their lives (Marte & Anastos, 1990). Knowledge of HIV positivity is not associated with choice of pregnancy termination or prevention of subsequent pregnancies (Efantis & Sinclair, 1990; Selwyn et al., 1989).

Nursing management of the pregnant HIV-seropositive woman includes all of the strategies previously discussed. In addition, assessing the woman's adaptation to the pregnancy throughout the perinatal period is critical. Pregnant women with HIV disease may experience conflict associated with guilt, and attachment may be affected (Acosta et al., 1992). Routine prenatal assessment should be supplemented with careful assessment for potential complications at each visit. Weight loss greater than 10% in the second or third trimester may indicate HIV wasting syndrome, and an elevated temperature an underlying infection or neoplasm (Hecht & Soloway, 1991). Fundoscopic and visual exam should be done every 3 months or if symptoms arise because cytomegalovirus, toxoplasmosis retinitis, and syphilitic optic neuritis are common complications of AIDS and can result in vision loss. The mouth should be inspected for oral candidiasis, hairy leukoplakia, and discolorations associated with Kaposi's sarcoma. Lymph node palpation at every visit is essential because lymphadenopathy may signal infection or malignancy (Acosta et al., 1992). Auscultation of the lungs to detect pulmonary compromise and liver and spleen palpation to detect enlargement associated with tuberculosis, lymphoma, or histoplasmosis should also be done at every prenatal visit (Hecht & Soloway, 1991).

In addition to routine prenatal laboratory studies, women with HIV disease should be closely monitored for cellular and serological markers of disease progression (Fekety, 1989; Nanda, 1990). Fetal surveillance (see Chapter 19, "High-Risk Childbearing," for a discussion of specific tests) is critical. Prenatal visits will be scheduled more often, and weekly fetal surveillance tests, such as nonstress testing, may be begun at 32 weeks gestation. Serial ultrasonography may help detect early intrauterine growth retardation, and biophysical profiles may provide data regarding fetal health status. Invasive fetal testing techniques, such as amniocentesis or chorionic villus sampling, should be done only for genetic or obstetric indications because there is a risk that invasive procedures may contaminate a noninfected fetus (Efantis & Sinclair, 1990).

Care of the pregnant women with asymptomatic HIV infection in labor does not differ significantly from routine intrapartal care. Intrapartum care of the woman with symptomatic HIV disease requires high-risk management techniques, a discussion of which is beyond the scope of this chapter.

Summary

STDs are among the most common health problems in the United States, and women experience a disproportionate amount of the burden associated with these illnesses, including complications of sterility, perinatal infections, genital tract neoplasm, and possibly death. Nurses can help to ameliorate the misery, morbidity, and mortality associated with STDs through accurate, safe, sensitive, and supportive care. In this chapter, information regarding the epidemiology of STDs and risk factors associated with STDs was presented. An important theme throughout the chapter was prevention of infection and diminution of complications. Specific STDs were discussed in terms of clinical presentation, complications, assessment, and nursing management.

The reader should be aware that knowledge of STDs in general and HIV infection specifically is increasing at an extraordinary rate, with new and improved diagnostic and treatment modalities continually being developed and reported. All nurses have a responsibility to stay current with these developments by reviewing current journal articles, attending conferences, and being knowledgeable about recommendations and bulletins from the CDC. Furthermore, it is important that nurses be aware of policies, recommendations, and guidelines of the state in which they practice, which also may change frequently.

References

Acosta, Y. M., Goodwin, C., Amaya, M. A., Tinkle, M. B., Acosta, E., & Jacquez, I. (1992). HIV disease and pregnancy: Part 2. Antepartum and intrapartum care. *JOGNN, 21*(2), 97-103.

Allen, M. H., & Marte, C. (1992, March 15). HIV infection in women: Presentations and protocols. *Hospital Practice,* pp. 155-162.

Ammer, C. (1989). *The new A-to-Z of women's health: A concise encyclopedia.* New York: Facts on File, Inc.

Andrist, L. C. (1988). Taking a sexual history and educating a client about safe sex. *Nursing Clinics of North America, 23,* 955-965.

Aral, S. O., & Holmes, K. K. (1991). Sexually transmitted diseases in the AIDS era. *Scientific American, 264,* 62-69.

Biggar, R. J., Pahwa, S., Minkoff, H., Mendes, H., Willoughby, A., Landesman, S., & Goedert, J. J. (1989). Immunosupression in pregnant women infected with human immunodeficiency virus. *American Journal of Obstetrics and Gynecology, 161,* 1239-1244.

Binkin, N. J., & Koplan, J. P. (1989). The high cost and low efficacy of weekly viral cultures for pregnant women with recurrent genital herpes: A reappraisal. *Medical Decision Making, 9,* 225-230.

Boyer, P. J., Dillon, M., Navaie, M., Deveikis, A., Keller, M., O'Rourke, S., & Bryson, Y. J. (1994). Factors predictive of maternal-fetal transmission of HIV-1. *JAMA, 271*(24), 1925-1930.

Breslin, E. (1988). Genital herpes simplex. *Nursing Clinics of North America, 23,* 907-915.

Brunham, R. C., Holmes, K. K., & Embree, J. E. (1990). Sexually transmitted diseases in pregnancy. In K. K. Holmes, P-A. Mardh, P. F. Sparling, & P. J. Wiesner (Eds.), *Sexually transmitted diseases* (2nd ed., pp. 771-783). New York: McGraw-Hill.

Butterfield, C. R., Shockley, M., Miguel, G. S., & Rosa, C. (1990). Routine screening for hepatitis B in an obstetric population. *Obstetrics and Gynecology, 76*(1), 25-27.

Butz, A., Hutton, N., & Larson, E. (1991). Immunoglobins and growth parameters at birth of infants born to HIV seropositive and seronegative women. *American Journal of Public Health, 81*(10), 1323-1325.

Carpenter, C. J., Mayer, K. H., Fisher, A., Desai, M. B., & Durand, L. (1989). Natural history of acquired immunodeficiency syndrome in women in Rhode Island. *American Journal of Medicine, 86,* 771-775.

Cates, W. (1988). The other STDs: Do they really matter? *JAMA, 259,* 3606-3608.

Cefalo, R., & Moos, M-K. (1990). Prenatal screening for hepatitis B virus. *Current Practices, 10*(1), 1-2.

Centers for Disease Control. (1985). 1985 sexually transmitted diseases treatment guidelines. *Morbidity and Mortality Weekly Report, 34*(Suppl. 4), 75S-108S.

Centers for Disease Control. (1989). 1989 sexually transmitted diseases treatment guidelines. *Morbidity and Mortality Weekly Report, 38*(Suppl. 8), 1-38.

Centers for Disease Control. (1990a). AIDS in women—United States. *Morbidity and Mortality Weekly Report, 39,* 845-846.

Centers for Disease Control. (1990b). Risk for cervical disease in HIV-infected women—New York City. *Morbidity and Mortality Weekly Report, 39,* 846-849.

Centers for Disease Control. (1991a, November 22). Hepatitis B virus: A comprehensive strategy for eliminating transmission in the United States through universal childhood vaccination: Recommendations of the Immunization Practices Advisory Committee. *Morbidity and Mortality Weekly Report,* 1-16.

Centers for Disease Control. (1991b, April). Pelvic inflammatory disease: Guidelines for prevention and management. *Morbidity and Mortality Weekly Report, 40,* 1-24.

Centers for Disease Control. (1991c). Women and HIV infection. *Clinical Courier, 9*(1), 1-8.

Centers for Disease Control. (1992). The second 100,000 cases of acquired immunodeficiency syndrome—United States. *Morbidity and Mortality Weekly Report, 41*(2), 28-29.

Centers for Disease Control. (1993, September 24). Sexually transmitted disease—Treatment guidelines. *Morbidity and Mortality Weekly Report,* 1-102.

Chow, J. M., Yonekura, M. L., Richwald, G. A., Greenland, S., Sweet, R. L., & Schachter, J. (1990). The association between *Chlamydia trachomatis* and ectopic pregnancy. *JAMA, 263,* 3164-3167.

Chu, S. Y., Buehler, J. W., & Berkelman, R. L. (1990). Impact of the human immunodeficiency virus epidemic on mortality in women of reproductive age, United States. *JAMA, 264,* 225-229.

Chu, S. Y., Buehler, J. W., Flemming, P. L., & Berkelman, R. L. (1990). Epidemiology of reported cases of AIDS in lesbians, United States 1980-89. *American Journal of Public Health, 80,* 1380-1381.

Clarke-Pearson, D. L., & Dawood, M. (1990). *Green's gynecology: Essentials of clinical practice* (4th ed.). Boston: Little, Brown.

Cochran, S. D., & Mays, V. M. (1990). Sex, lies, and HIV. *New England Journal of Medicine, 322*(11), 774-775.

Davies, K. (1990). Genital herpes: An overview. *JOGNN, 19,* 401-406.

Deitch, K. V., & Smith, J. E. (1990). Symptoms of chronic vaginal infection and microscopic condyloma in women. *JOGNN, 19*(2), 133-138.

DiClemente, R. J., Zoan, J., & Temoshok, L. (1986). Adolescents and AIDS: A survey of knowledge, attitudes, and beliefs about AIDS in San Francisco. *American Journal of Public Health, 76,* 1443.

Division of STD/HIV Prevention. (1991). *Sexually transmitted disease surveillance, 1990* (U.S. Department of Health and Human Services, Public Health Services). Atlanta: Centers for Disease Control.

Dunn, D., Newell, M. L., Ades, A., & Peckham, C. S. (1992). Risk of human immunodeficiency virus Type 1 transmission through breast feeding. *Lancet, 340,* 585-588.

Efantis, J., & Sinclair, P. B. (1990). Antepartum management of pregnant women with HIV infection. *NAACOG's Clinical Issues in Perinatal and Women's Health Nursing, 1*(1), 41-46.

Ellerbrock, T. V., Bush, T. J., Chamberland, M. E., & Oxtoby, M. J. (1991). Epidemiology of women with AIDS in the United States, 1981 through 1990. *JAMA, 265,* 2971-2975.

Enterline, J. A., & Leonardo, J. P. (1989). Comdylomata acuminata (general warts). *Nurse Practitioner, 14*(4), 8-16.

European Collaborative Study. (1992). Risk factors for mother-to-child transmission of HIV-1. *Lancet, 339,* 1007-1012.

Fekety, S. E. (1989). Managing the HIV-positive patient and her newborn in a CNM service. *Journal of Nurse-Midwifery, 34,* 253-258.

Ferenczy, A. (1989). HPV-associated lesions in pregnancy and their clinical implications. *Clinical Obstetrics and Gynecology, 32*(1), 191-199.

Fogel, C. I. (1988). Gonorrhea: Not a new problem but a serious one. *Nursing Clinics of North America, 23,* 885-897.

Fogel, C. I. (1990). Sexually transmitted diseases. *Women's Health Perspectives, 3,* 122-139.

Fogel, C. I., & Lauver, D. (1990). *Sexual health promotion.* Philadelphia: W. B. Saunders.

Fullilove, M., Fullilove, R., Haynes, K., & Gross, S. A. (1989, June). *Gender roles as barriers to risk reduction in black women.* Paper presented at Fifth International Conference on AIDS, Montreal.

Handsfield, H. H. (1991, July 15). Recent developments in STDs: I. Bacterial diseases. *Hospital Practice,* pp. 47-56.

Handsfield, H. H., Jasman, L. L., & Roberts, P. L. (1986). Criteria for selective screening for *Chlamydia trachomatis* infection in women attending family planning clinics. *JAMA, 255*(13), 1730-1734.

Hankins, C. A. (1990). Issues involving women, children, and AIDS primarily in the developed world. *Journal of Acquired Immune Deficiency Syndrome, 3,* 443-448.

Hatcher, R. A., Trussell, J., Stewart, F., Stewart, G. K., Kowal, D., Guest, F., Cates, W., & Policar, M. S. (1994). *Contraceptive technology 1994-1996* (16th rev. ed.). New York: Irvington.

Hawkins, J. W., Roberto, D., & Stanley-Haney, J. (1991). *Protocols for nurse practitioners in gynecologic settings* (3rd ed.). New York: Tiresias.

Hecht, F. M., & Soloway, B. (1991). The physical exam in HIV infection. *AIDS Clinical Care, 3*(1), 4-5.

Hollander, H. (1988). Work-up of the HIV-infected patient: Practical approach. In M. A. Sande & P. A. Volberding (Eds.), *The medical management of AIDS* (p. 108). Philadelphia: W. B. Saunders.

Holman, S. (1989). Epidemiology and transmission of HIV infection in women. *Journal of Nurse-Midwifery, 34,* 233-241.

Holmberg, S. D., Stewart, J. A., Gerber, A. R., Byers, R. H., Lee, F. K., O'Malley, P. M., & Nahmias, A. J. (1988). Prior herpes simplex virus type 2 infection as a risk factor for HIV infection. *JAMA, 259,* 1048-1050.

Holmes, K. K., & Kreiss, J. (1988). Heterosexual transmission of human immunodeficiency virus: Overview of a neglected aspect of the AIDS epidemic. *Journal of Acquired Immunodeficiency Syndrome, 1,* 602-610.

Jackson, V. (1990). The fallopian tubes. In R. Lichtman & S. Papera (Eds.), *Gynecology well-woman care* (pp. 273-286). Norwalk, CT: Appleton-Lange.

Johnson, R. E., Nahmias, A. J., Magder, L. S., Lee, F. K., Brooks, C. A., & Snowden, C. B. (1989). A seropositive screening of the prevalence of herpes simplex virus type-2 in the United States. *New England Journal of Medicine, 326,* 7-12.

Koonan, L. M., Ellerbrock, T. V., Atresh, H. K., Rogers, M. F., Smith, J. C., Hogue, C. J. R., Harris, M. A., Charkin, W., Parker, A. L., & Halpin, G. J. (1989). Pregnancy associated deaths due to AIDS in the United States. *JAMA, 261*(9), 1306-1309.

Koretz, R. (1989). Universal prenatal hepatitis B testing: Is it cost-effective? *Obstetrics and Gynecology, 74,* 808-814.

Koss, L. G. (1987). Cytologic and histologic manifestations of human papillomavirus infection of the female genital tract and their clinical significance. *Cancer, 60,* 1942-1950.

Kronmal, R. A., Whitney, C. W., & Mumford, S. D. (1991). The intrauterine device and pelvic inflammatory disease: The women's health study reanalyzed. *Journal of Clinical Epidemiology, 44*(2), 109-112.

Kurth, A., & Hutchinson, M. (1989). A context for HIV testing in pregnancy. *Journal of Nurse-Midwifery, 34*(5), 259-266.

Landesman, S. H. (1989). Human immunodeficiency virus infection in women: An overview. *Seminars in Perinatology, 13*(1), 2-6.

Levine, C., & Dubler, N. N. (1990). HIV and childbearing: 1. Uncertain risks and bitter realities: The reproductive choices of HIV-infected women. *Milbank Quarterly, 68*(3), 321-351.

Levy, J. A. (1992). Viral immunologic factors in HIV infection. In M. A. Sande & P. A. Volberding (Eds.), *The medical management of AIDS* (3rd ed., pp. 18-33). Philadelphia: W. B. Saunders.

Lichtman, R., & Duran, P. (1990). Sexually transmitted diseases. In R. Lichtman & S. Papera (Eds.), *Gynecology well-woman care* (pp. 203-248). Norwalk, CT: Appleton-Lange.

Lommel, L. L. (1990). Hepatitis B. In W. L. Star, M. T. Shannon, L. N. Sammons, L. L. Lommel, & Y. Gutierrez (Eds.), *Ambulatory obstetrics: Protocols for nurse practitioners/nurse midwives* (2nd ed., pp. 309-313). San Francisco: University of California Press.

Lynch, P. J. (1985). Condylomata acuminata (anogenital warts). *Clinical Obstetrics and Gynecology, 28,* 142-151.

Mantell, J. E., Schinke, S. P., & Akabas, S. H. (1988). Women and AIDS prevention. *Journal of Primary Prevention, 9*(1/2), 18-39.

Marchbanks, P. A., Lee, C., & Peterson, H. B. (1990). Cigarette smoking as a risk factor in pelvic inflammatory disease. *American Journal of Obstetrics and Gynecology, 162,* 639-644.

Marte, C., & Allen, M. (1991). HIV-related gynecologic conditions: Overlooked complications. *Focus, 7*(1), 1-4.

Marte, C., & Anastos, K. (1990). Women: The missing person in the AIDS epidemic. Part II. *Medical Care Review, 20*(1), 11-18.

Mascola, L., & Guinan, M. E. (1987). Semen donors as the source of sexually transmitted diseases in artificially inseminated women. *JAMA, 257,* 1093-1094.

McGregor, J. A., French, J. L., & Spencer, N. E. (1989). Prevention of sexually transmitted diseases in women. *Obstetrics and Gynecology Clinics of North America, 16,* 679-702.

Minkoff, H. L. (1989). AIDS in pregnancy. *Current Problems in Obstetrics, Gynecology, and Fertility, 12,* 205-228.

Minkoff, H. L., & Landesman, S. H. (1988). The case for routinely offering prenatal testing for human immunodeficiency virus. *American Journal of Obstetrics and Gynecology, 158,* 793-796.

Minkoff, H. L., McCalla, S., Delke, I., Stevens, R., Salwen, M., & Feldman, J. (1990). The relationship of cocaine use to syphilis and human immunodeficiency virus infections among inner city populations. *American Journal of Obstetrics and Gynecology, 163,* 521-526.

Minkoff, H. L., Willoughby, A., Mendez, H., Moroso, G., Holman, S., Goedect, J. J., & Landesman, S. H. (1990). Serious infections during pregnancy among women with advanced human immunodeficiency virus infection. *American Journal of Obstetrics and Gynecology, 162,* 30-34.

Mitchell, J. L. (1988). Women, AIDS, and public policy. *AIDS & Public Policy Journal, 3*(2), 50-52.

Moroso, G., & Holman, S. (1990). Counseling and testing for HIV. *NAACOG's Clinical Issues in Perinatal and Women's Health Nursing, 1*(1), 10-19.

Nanda, D. (1990). Human immunodeficiency virus infection in women in the United States. *Obstetrics and Gynecological Clinics of North America, 17,* 617-625.

Nettina, S. L., & Kauffman, F. H. (1990). Diagnosis and management of sexually transmitted genital lesions. *Nurse Practitioner, 15*(1), 20-39.

Newell, M. L., & Peckham, C. S. (1993). Risk factors for vertical transmission of HIV-1 and early markers of HIV-1 infection in children. *AIDS, 7*(Suppl. 1), 591-597.

Nsiah-Jefferson, L. (1989). Reproductive laws, women of color, and low-income women. In S. Cohen & N. Taub (Eds.), *Reproductive laws for the 1990s: A briefing handbook.* Clifton, NJ: Humana.

O'Brien, T. R., Shaffer, N., & Jaffe, N. W. (1992). Acquisition and transmission of HIV. In M. A. Sande & P. A. Volberding (Eds.), *The medical management of AIDS* (3rd ed., pp. 3-17). Philadelphia: W. B. Saunders.

Oh, M. K., Feinstein, R. A., Soileau, E. J., Cloud, G. A., & Pass, R. F. (1989). *Chlamydia trachomatis* cervical infection and oral contraceptive use among adolescent girls. *Journal of Adolescent Health Care, 10,* 376-381.

Peckham, C. S. (1994). Human immunodeficiency virus infection and pregnancy. *Sexually Transmitted Disease, 21*(Suppl. 2), 528-531.

Price, J. H., Desmond, S., & Kukulka, G. (1985). High school students' perceptions and misperceptions about AIDS. *Journal of School Health, 55*(3), 107-109.

Provencher, D., Valne, B., Averette, H. E., Ganjel, P., Donato, D., Penalver, M., & Selvin, B. U. (1988). HIV status and positive Papanicolaou screening: Identification of a high-risk population. *Gynecologic Oncology, 31*(1), 184-188.

Public Health Service. (1979). *Healthy people: The surgeon general's report on health promotion and disease prevention.* Washington, DC: Government Printing Office.

Richart, R. M. (1987). Causes and management of cervical intraepithelial neoplasia. *Cancer, 60,* 1951-1959.

Rolfs, R. T., Goldberg, M., & Sharrar, R. G. (1990). Risk factors for syphilis: Cocaine use and prostitution. *American Journal of Public Health, 80,* 853-857.

Ryan, G. M., Abdella, T. N., McNeeley, S. G., Baselski, V. S., & Drummond, D. E. (1990). *Chlamydia trachomatis* infection in pregnancy and effect of treatment on outcome. *American Journal of Obstetrics and Gynecology, 162*(1), 34-39.

Saag, M. S. (1992). AIDS Testing: Now and in the future. In M. A. Sande & P. A. Volberding (Eds.), *The medical management of AIDS* (3rd ed., pp. 33-53). Philadelphia: W. B. Saunders.

Seltzer, V., & Benjamin, F. (1990). Breast-feeding and the potential for human immunodeficiency virus transmission. *Obstetrics and Gynecology, 75,* 713-715.

Selwyn, P. A., Schoenbaum, E. E., Davenny, K., Robertson, V. J., Feingold, A. R., Shulman, J. F., Mayers, M.

M., Klein, R. S., Friedland, G. H. & Rogers, M. F. (1989). Prospective study of human immunodeficiency virus infection and pregnancy outcomes in intravenous drug users. *JAMA, 261,* 1289-1294.

Shayne, V. T., & Kaplan, B. J. (1991). Double victims: Poor women and AIDS. *Women & Health, 17*(1), 21-37.

Siegel, K., & Gibson, W. (1988, February). Barriers to the modification of sexual behavior among heterosexuals at risk for acquired immunodeficiency syndrome. *New York State Journal of Medicine,* pp. 66-70.

Sinclair, B. P. (1990). Epidemiology and transmission of infection by human immunodeficiency virus. *NAACOG's Clinical Issues in Perinatal and Women's Health Nursing, 1,* 1-9.

Smeltzer, S. C., & Whipple, B. (1991). Women and HIV infection. *Image, 23,* 249-256.

Star, W. L. (1990a). Chlamydia. In W. L. Star, M. T. Shannon, L. N. Sammons, L. L. Lommel, & Y. Gutierrez (Eds.), *Ambulatory obstetrics: Protocols for nurse practitioners/nurse midwives* (2nd ed., pp. 283-287). San Francisco: University of California Press.

Star, W. L. (1990b). Gonorrhea. In W. L. Star, M. T. Shannon, L. N. Sammons, L. L. Lommel, & Y. Gutierrez (Eds.). *Ambulatory obstetrics: Protocols for nurse practitioners/nurse midwives* (2nd ed., pp. 300-305). San Francisco: University of California Press.

Star, W. L. (1990c). Syphilis. In W. L. Star, M. T. Shannon, L. N. Sammons, L. L. Lommel, & Y. Gutierrez (Eds.), *Ambulatory obstetrics: Protocols for nurse practitioners/nurse midwives* (2nd ed., pp. 338-345). San Francisco: University of California Press.

Stein, Z. A. (1990). HIV prevention: The need for methods women can use. *American Journal of Public Health, 80,* 460-462.

Stewart, G. J., Cunningham, A. L., Driscoll, G. L., Gold, J., & Lamot, B. J. (1985). Transmission of human T-cell lymphotrophic virus type III (HTLV-III) by artificial insemination by donor. *Lancet, 2,* 581-584.

Stone, K. M., Grimes, D. A., & Magder, L. S. (1986). Primary prevention of sexually transmitted diseases. *JAMA, 255,* 1763-1766.

Valdiserri, R. O., Arena, V. C., Proctor, D., & Bonati, F. A. (1989). The relationship between women's attitudes about condoms and their use: Implications for condom promotion programs. *American Journal of Public Health, 79*(4), 499-501.

Watts, D. H., & Eschenbach, D. A. (1987). Sexually transmitted diseases in pregnancy. *Infectious Disease Clinics of North America, 1,* 253-275.

Wheeler, L. (1992). *Condom counseling.* Unpublished manuscript, University of Oregon, Eugene.

Williams, A. (1989). Counseling women with HIV infection. In J. B. Meisenhelder & C. L. LaCharite (Eds.), *Comfort in caring: The client with AIDS* (pp. 75-86). Boston: Little, Brown.

Wilson, D. (1988). An overview of sexually transmissible disease in the perinatal period. *Journal of Nurse-Midwifery, 33*(3), 115-128.

Wolner-Hanssen, P., Eschenbach, D. A., Paavonen, J., Stevens, C. E., Kiviat, N. B., Critchlow, C., DeRouen, T., Koutsky, L., & Holmes, K. K. (1990a). Association between vaginal douching and acute pelvic inflammatory disease. *JAMA, 263,* 1936-1941.

Wolner-Hanssen, P., Eschenbach, D. A., Paavonen, J., Kiviat, N. B., Stevens, C. E., Critchlow, C., DeRouen, T., & Holmes, K. K. (1990b). Decreased risk of symptomatic chlamydial pelvic inflammatory disease associated with oral contraceptive use. *JAMA, 263,* 54-59.

Worth, D. (1989). Sexual decision-making and AIDS: Why condom promotion among vulnerable women is likely to fail. *Studies in Family Planning, 20,* 297-307.

Worth, D., & Rodriguez, R. (1987). Latina women and AIDS. *SIECUS Report, 15*(3), 5-7.

Supplemental Readings

Abel, E., & von Unwerth, L. (1988). Asymptomatic chlamydia during pregnancy. *Research in Nursing and Health, 11,* 359-365.

Bureau of Hygiene and Tropical Diseases. (1988). *AIDS Newsletter, 3,* 2.

Alter, M. J., & Margolis, H. S. (1990). The emergence of hepatitis B as a sexually transmitted disease. *Medical Clinics of North America, 74,* 1529-1541.

Anderson, J. R. (1989). Gynecologic manifestations of AIDS and HIV disease. *Female Patient, 14,* 57, 61-62, 65-66, 68.

Aral, S. O., & Cates, W. (1989). The multiple dimensions of sexual behavior as risk factor for sexually transmitted diseases: The sexually experienced are not necessarily sexually active. *Sexually Transmitted Diseases, 16*(4), 173-177.

Bergeron, C., Ferenczy, A., & Richart, R. (1990). Underwear: Contamination by human papillomaviruses. *American Journal of Obstetrics and Gynecology, 162*(1), 25-29.

Bourcier, K. M., & Seidler, A. J. (1987). Chlamydia and condylomata acuminata: An update for the nurse practitioner. *JOGNN, 16*(1), 17-22.

Campbell, C. A. (1990). Women and AIDS. *Social Science Medicine, 30,* 407-415.

Cates, W. (1987). Epidemiology and control of sexually transmitted diseases: Strategic evolution. *Infectious Disease Clinics of North America, 1*(1), 1-23.

Centers for Disease Control. (1988). Relationship of syphilis to drug use and prostitution. *Morbidity and Mortality Weekly Report, 37,* 755-759.

Cohen, I., Veille, J-C., & Calkins, B. M. (1990). Improved pregnancy outcome following successful treatment of chlamydial infection. *JAMA, 263,* 3160-3163.

Cohen, J. A. (1989). Virology, immunology, and natural history of HIV infection. *Journal of Nurse-Midwifery, 34*(5), 242-252.

Darrow, W. W., & Seigel, K. (1990). Preventive holistic behavior and STD. In K. K. Holmes, P-A. Mardh, P. F. Sparling, & P. J. Wiesner (Eds.), *Sexually transmitted diseases* (2nd ed., pp. 52-89). New York: McGraw-Hill.

Debuono, B. A., Zinner, S. N., Daamen, M., & McCormack, W. M. (1990). Sexual behavior of college women in 1975, 1986, and 1989. *New England Journal of Medicine, 322,* 821-825.

Donegan, E. A. (1985). Epidemiology of gonococcal infection. *STD Statistics, 135,* 1-39.

Eagar, R. M., Beach, R. K., Davidson, A. J., & Judson, F. A. (1985). Epidemic and clinical factors of *Chlamydia trachomatis* in black, Hispanic and white female adolescents. *Western Journal of Medicine, 143,* 37-41.

Feldblum, P. J., & Fortney, J. A. (1988). Condoms, spermicides, and the transmission of human immunodeficiency virus: A review of the literature. *American Journal of Public Health, 78,* 52-54.

Flaskerud, J. H., & Cavillo, E. R. (1991). Beliefs about AIDS, health, and illness among low-income Latina women. *Research in Nursing and Health, 14,* 431-438.

Flaskerud, J. H., & Nyamanthi, A. M. (1989). Black and Latina women's AIDS-related knowledge, attitudes, and practices. *Research in Nursing and Health, 12,* 339-346.

Flaskerud, J. H., & Rush, C. E. (1989). AIDS and traditional health beliefs and practices of black women. *Nursing Research, 38,* 210-215.

Flaskerud, J. H., & Thompson, J. (1991). Beliefs about AIDS, health, and illness in low-income white women. *Nursing Research, 40*(5), 266-271.

Fullilove, M. T., Fullilove, R. E., Haynes, K., & Gross, S. (1990). Black women and AIDS prevention: A view towards understanding the gender rules. *Journal of Sex Research, 27*(1), 47-64.

Gollub, E. L., & Stein, Z. (1992). Nonoxynol-9 and the reduction of HIV transmission in women. *AIDS, 6,* 599-601.

Guinan, M. E., & Hardy, A. (1987). The epidemiology of AIDS in women in the United States, 1981-1986. *JAMA, 257,* 2039-2042.

Hayes, C. E., Sharp, E. S., & Miner, K. R. (1989). Knowledge, attitudes and beliefs of HIV seronegative women about AIDS. *Journal of Nurse-Midwifery, 34*(5), 291-294.

Holmes, K. K., Karon, J. M., & Kreiss, J. (1990). The increasing frequency of heterosexually acquired AIDS in the United States, 1983-1988. *American Journal of Public Health, 80*(7), 858-862.

Holmes, K. K., Mardh, P-A., Sparling, P. F., & Wiesner, P. J. (1990). *Sexually transmitted diseases* (2nd ed.). New York: McGraw-Hill.

Jemmott, L. S., & Jemmott, J. B. (1991). Applying the theory of reasoned action to AIDS risk behavior: Condom use among black women. *Nursing Research, 40,* 228-234.

Jones, D. A. (1991). HIV-seropositive childbearing women: Nursing management. *JOGNN, 20*(6), 446-452.

Karan, L. D. (1989). AIDS prevention and chemical dependence treatment needs of women and their children. *Journal of Psychoactive Drugs, 21*(4), 395-399.

Kerr, D. L. (1991). Women with AIDS and HIV infection. *Journal of School Health, 61*(3), 139-140.

Krebs, H. B. (1989). Management strategies-HPV. *Clinical Obstetrics and Gynecology, 32,* 200-213.

Landesman, S. H., Minkoff, H. L., & Willoughby, A. (1989). HIV disease in reproductive age women: A problem of the present. *JAMA, 261,* 1326-1327.

Lindner, L. E., Geerling, S., Nettum, J. A., Miller, S. L., & Altman, K. H. (1988). Clinical characteristics of women with chlamydial cervicitis. *Journal of Reproductive Medicine, 33,* 684-690.

Marks, G., Richardson, J. L., & Maldonado, N. (1991). Self-disclosure of HIV infection to sexual partners. *American Journal of Public Health, 81*(10), 1321-1322.

Matorras, R., Ariceta, J. M., Rementera, A., Corral, J., Gutierrez-deJerin, G., Diez, J., Montoya, F., & Rodiquez-Escubero, F. J. (1991). Human immunodeficiency virus-induced immunosuppression: A risk factor for human papillomavirus infection. *American Journal of Obstetrics and Gynecology, 164,* 42-44.

McBarnette, L. (1987). Women and poverty: The effects on reproductive status. *Women and Health, 12*(3-4), 55-81.

McDonald, M. G, Ginzburg, H. M., & Bolan, J. C. (1991). HIV infection in pregnancy: Epidemiology and clinical management. *Journal of Acquired Immune Deficiency Syndrome, 4,* 100-108.

McGregor, J. A., French, J. I., & Spencer, N. E. (1988). Prevention of sexually transmitted diseases in women. *Journal of Reproductive Medicine, 33,* 109-118.

McQuiston, C. M. (1989). The relationship of risk factors for cervical cancer and HPV in college women. *Nurse Practitioner, 14*(4), 18-26.

Mitchell, J. L., Tucker, J., Loftman, P. O., & Williams, S. B. (1992). HIV and women: Current controversies and clinical relevance. *Journal of Women's Health, 1*(1), 35-39.

Moran, J. S., Aral, S. O., Jenkins, W. C., Peterman, T. A., & Alexander, E. R. (1989). The impact of sexually transmitted diseases on minority populations. *Public Health Reports, 104*(6), 560-565.

Nyamathi, A., & Shin, D. M. (1990). Designing a culturally sensitive AIDS educational program for black and Hispanic women of childbearing age. *NAACOG's Clinical Issues in Perinatal and Women's Health Nursing, 1*(1), 86-98.

Pepin, J., Plummer, F. A., Brunham, R. C., Piot, P., Cameron, D. W., & Ronald, A. R. (1989). The interaction of HIV infection and other sexually transmitted disease: An opportunity for intervention. *AIDS, 3,* 3-9.

Powers, M. (1990). Ethical considerations in HIV screening programs for infected women and children. *AIDS Patient Care, 4*(5), 40-41.

Rapkin, A. J., & Erickson, P. I. (1990). Differences in knowledge of and risk factor for AIDS among Hispanic and non-Hispanic women attending an urban family planning clinic. *AIDS, 4,* 889-899.

Rhodes, J. L., Wright, C. D., Redfield, R. R., & Burke, D. S. (1987). Chronic vaginal candidiasis in women with human immunodeficiency virus infection. *JAMA, 257,* 3105-3107.

Rosenberg, M. J., Rojanapithayakorn, W., Feldblum, P. J., & Higgins, J. E. (1987). Effect of the contraceptive sponge on chlamydial infection, gonorrhea, and candidiasis: A comparative clinical trial. *JAMA, 257,* 2308-2312.

Schilling, R. F., Ei-Bassel, N., Schinke, S. P., Gordon, K., & Nichols, S. (1991). Building skills of recovering women drug users to reduce heterosexual AIDS transmission. *Public Health Reports, 108*(3), 297-304.

Shanis, B. S., Check, J. H., & Baker, A. F. (1989). Transmission of sexually transmitted diseases by donor semen. *Archives of Andrology, 23,* 249-257.

Smith, P. F., Mikl, J., Teuman, B. I., Lessner, L., Stevens, R. W., Lord, E. A., Broeddies, R. K., & Morse, D. L. (1991). HIV infections among women entering the New York state correctional system. *American Journal of Public Health, 81*(Suppl.), 35-40.

Sutton-DeBarros, C. (1989). How to clinically evaluate the pregnant substance abuser for HIV infection. *AIDS Patient Care, 3,* 29-32.

Wasser, S. C., Aral, S. O., Reed, D. S., & Bowen, G. S. (1989). Assessing behavioral risk for HIV infection in family-planning and STD clinics: Similarities and differences. *Sexually Transmitted Diseases, 16*(4), 178-183.

Westrom, L., & March, P. A. (1990). Acute pelvic inflammatory disease (PID). In K. K. Holmes, P. A. March, P. F. Sparling, & P. J. Weisner (Eds.), *Sexually transmitted diseases* (2nd ed., pp. 593-613). New York: McGraw-Hill.

Whelan, M. (1988). Nursing management of the patient with *Chlamydia trachomatis* infection. *Nursing Clinics of North America, 23,* 877-883.

Wilfert, C. (1991, May 15). HIV infection in maternal and pediatric patients. *Hospital Practice,* pp. 55-67.

Williams, A. B. (1990). Reproductive concerns of women at risk for HIV infection. *Journal of Nurse-Midwifery, 35*(5), 292-298.

Williams, A. B. (1991). Women at risk: An AIDS educational needs assessment. *Image, 23*(4), 208-213.

25

Infertility

CATHERINE GARNER

Care of the infertile couple has become an integral part of women's health care in the last decade, in that infertility is a condition affecting approximately one in five couples in their childbearing years (Congress, 1988). There has been a tremendous explosion of the knowledge base regarding human reproduction in the last decade, with concomitant developments in medical therapies. Although diagnosis can be made in 90% to 95% of cases and many high-tech therapies are available, only 50% to 60% of these couples can expect to achieve a pregnancy. This presents a tremendous challenge to the nurse who cares for couples who are infertile and for those who experience family building through birth or adoption. As many as 20% of couples seeking obstetric care may have had infertility problems and have unique needs for nursing care during the maternity cycle.

Demographics

Infertility is defined as the inability to conceive a child after a year or more of regular unprotected intercourse or the inability to carry a pregnancy to live birth (recurrent miscarriages). Primary infertility occurs when there has been no history of pregnancy. Secondary infertility is a condition in which previous pregnancy has occurred regardless of the outcome. Recurrent pregnancy loss is defined as two or more miscarriages in the first trimester. The traditional advice that a workup be initiated after three spontaneous abortions has been discarded and more recent thinking encourages an earlier workup.

Infertility affects an estimated 2.4 million married couples and an unknown number of unmarried couples and singles. Although the overall incidence of infertility remained relatively unchanged between 1965 and 1983, one age group, married couples with wives aged 20 to 24 years, exhibited an increase in infertility, from 3.6% to 10% infertile in 1982. This increase may be linked to the rate of gonorrhea in this age group—a rate that tripled between 1960 and 1977 (Congress, 1988). Women are at higher risk for sexually transmitted disease (STD) when they become sexually active at a younger age, have more than one sex partner, and change partners frequently. Pelvic inflammatory disease (PID) is common and is caused by a number of microorganisms producing irreparable damage to fallopian tubes, causing infertility and ectopic pregnancies. (See Chapter 24, "Sexually Transmitted Diseases," for additional information on this topic.)

It is noteworthy that not all infertile couples seek treatment. Only an estimated 51% of couples with primary infertility and 22% with secondary infertility seek treatment. Even with these statistics, the number of office visits to physicians for infertility services rose from about 600,000 in 1968 to about 1.6 million in 1984 (Congress, 1988).

Older women are experiencing infertility at high rates due to delayed childbearing. Although fertility rates in the United States are at historically low levels, one age group is having more babies—those women 30 to 34 years of age. This is occurring as women delay childbearing to pursue advanced education and careers and is significant because the maximum fertility in both men and women is the age of 24. Women over 30 have a higher incidence of ovulation problems, endometriosis, and have a greater length of time to be exposed to STDs and their consequences. Although the term *biological clock* may be unappealing, it is nonetheless accurate. The delay in childbearing past age 35 carries with it a higher probability of infertility. The percentage of women infertile at ages 20 to 24 is 10.6%; approximately 24% of women ages 35 to 39 are infertile (Mosher, 1987). Race is also significant when analyzing the statistical data on infertility. Black couples are more likely than white couples to be infertile. In 1982, the risk of infertility for black couples was 1.5 times that of white couples (Pratt et al., 1985).

Male infertility has also been recognized to be increasing, although much of this documented increase may be due to more sophisticated testing. Male fertility declines much more slowly than does female fertility, with no real significant change in sperm count until after the age of 55. Even then, men can father children throughout their life span.

The number of babies available for adoption has declined steadily since the early 1970s due to increased availability of effective methods of birth control, legalized abortion, and a sociological trend for single women to keep their babies. This narrowing of the adoption pool has fueled a consumer demand for medical care. Counseling couples about adoption requires that the nurse be knowledgeable about many alternative avenues (Hahn, 1991).

There is no evidence that the use of birth control pills or abortion has contributed to the rise in infertility. Although previous research findings have suggested that women who use an intrauterine device (IUD) as a method of contraception are at increased risk for tubal infection, recent reanalysis of data suggests that the risk was overestimated and that "IUDs do not increase the risk of PID" (Kronmal, Whitney, & Mumford, 1991, p. 110). Women who are at high risk for PID because of sexual behaviors do have a higher incidence of tubal infertility. (See Chapter 24 for additional information.)

Common Responses to Infertility

The couple experiencing infertility faces many uncertainties and multiple losses. Malhlstedt (1985) describes infertility as a loss of self-esteem, a dream, balance in a relationship, security, and fantasy. Grief follows much the same pattern for infertility as with all losses. Surprise is often experienced first, because few persons ever expect to be infertile. Guilt, anger, and blame are often a part of the emotional reaction. Multiple losses can cripple an individual emotionally, and support groups such as Resolve, the national support network for infertile couples, and individual counseling can be beneficial to the individuals involved and to a couple's relationship. Appropriate support is critical.

The nursing diagnosis will depend on the educational level of the couple, clinical diagnosis, and treatment decision as well as on the overall goal of the woman and her partner. Many myths still need to be addressed (see Table 25.1). It is simplistic to assume that the only goal is achievement of pregnancy. For some, the goal is the answer to the question of why the problem is occurring. For others it will be the achievement of a pregnancy that results from the biological union. For others still, it will be the process of becoming a parent, be it through pregnancy or adoption. The nurse can provide education, facilitate the diagnosis and treatment phases of infertility, assist with the decision-making process, and help with resolution of infertility, either by assisting the grief process or by facilitating parenting.

Resolution of grief associated with either unsuccessful individual treatment or the inability

Table 25.1 Myths About Infertility

Myth: A woman ovulates from the left ovary one month and the right ovary the next month.
Fact: Only one ovary actually ovulates each month. There is no set pattern.

Myth: The egg is fertilized inside the uterus.
Fact: The egg is fertilized in the outer third of the fallopian tube and gradually makes its way to implant in the uterus 3 to 4 days later.

Myth: Pillows under the hips during and after intercourse enhance infertility.
Fact: Sperm are already swimming in cervical mucus as sexual intercourse is completed and will continue to travel from the cervix up the fallopian tubes for the next 48 to 72 hours. The position of the hips really doesn't matter.

Myth: If you just relax, you'll get pregnant.
Fact: If pregnancy has not occurred after a year, chances are there is a medical condition causing infertility. There is no evidence that stress causes infertility.

Myth: I've never had symptoms of a pelvic infection, so I can't have blocked tubes.
Fact: Many pelvic infections have no symptoms at all but can cause damage, sometimes irreversible, to tubes.

Myth: A man's sperm count will be the same each time it is examined.
Fact: A man's sperm count will vary. Sperm number and motility can be affected by time between ejaculations, illness, and medication.

Myth: We should be having intercourse every day to achieve pregnancy.
Fact: Sperm remain alive and active in a woman's cervical mucus for 48 to 72 hours following sexual intercourse; therefore, it isn't necessary to plan your lovemaking on a rigid schedule.

SOURCE: Serono Laboratories (1990). Reprinted with permission from *Pathways to Parenthood*. Copyright CRC Press, Boca Raton, Florida.
NOTE: Education of the couple often begins with ascertaining and then dispelling their myths about infertility. Some of these common myths and their refutations are given here.

to achieve pregnancy requires time and energy. Feelings must be acknowledged to be dealt with openly and honestly. Resolution of infertility takes time. Depression is not uncommon, and significant clinical problems should be referred for appropriate mental health care. Resolution of infertility is not a finite phenomenon. The identity of oneself as an infertile person does not change even when pregnancy occurs. Even after adoption, many couples still describe themselves as infertile. A part of the resolution process is accepting this as a part of the whole identity rather than the whole identity. Couples must redefine their relationship and fantasies about the future and must learn to be comfortable living out their lives in a fertile world (Menning, 1988). Some couples cope by becoming proactive. Joining forces through Resolve for community education and legislative efforts are healthy ways to channel feelings and energies. Positive results that affect others experiencing the same difficulty can be tremendously rewarding.

Many couples assume that the achievement of pregnancy will solve all of the emotional problems associated with infertility. Pregnancy does not necessarily dissolve all of the anxiety and concerns that affected the couple before. Many times, the attainment of pregnancy does not bring all of the satisfaction the couple envisions. Couples are at risk for distress if they have unresolved marital issues, conflicts with the medical profession, self-image problems, general or specific anxiety, or unrealistic expectations about pregnancy. Nursing care should include discussion of the significance of the infertility diagnosis and treatment to both the individuals and the couple. Education about normal adaptations of pregnancy can alleviate some of the anxieties if pregnancy occurs. Reading materials, book lists, and emergency telephone numbers can help reassure couples. Frequent appointments early in pregnancy can have a positive influence. Crisis intervention should a spontaneous abortion or ectopic pregnancy occur is also essential.

Nursing research is urgently needed to study the response of the infertile couple to pregnancy and parenting. Anecdotal references outline a difference in attachment behaviors during pregnancy, sexual relationships after delivery, and early parenting behaviors. To effect appropriate nursing intervention, these must be scientifically documented using well-done research. Individual and couple skills that can help couples move through this process include open communication, positive self-esteem, and mutual support. Nursing support as educator, counselor, and facilitator can support this process. Couples should be told that the feelings about infertility will reoccur at various points. The birth of a baby into the extended family or to a friend or the anniversaries of a pregnancy loss may trigger feelings of sadness, envy, or decreased self-worth.

Open communication can decrease stress and circumvent resentment in the relationship. At the initiation of any therapy, the possibility should be raised that the medical therapy will not result in pregnancy. Steps to strengthen the relationship should be developed by the couple because infertility therapy may result in a pregnancy and leave the marriage in ruins. Sharing experiences unrelated to childbearing is important. A couple may schedule a dinner "date" once in a while to allow time to talk. Others deliberately seek out couples without children. Couples need to explore the possibilities of childlessness and adoption. This process cannot be rushed and must occur as the couple is ready. The nurse, however, must raise this possibility. The treatment phase is described as a roller coaster of emotions, as hopes rise early in the cycle, only to be dashed with the onset of menses. Patients should be encouraged to discuss their feelings and referred for counseling as appropriate.

Investigation of Infertility

Evaluation of the infertile couple must focus on both partners: 40% of infertility cases can be expected to be due to a male factor, 40% to a female factor, and 20% to both. To evaluate only one partner, even when the problem seems apparent, is inappropriate due to the high incidence of multiple problems. The most common female problems are ovulation disorders, tubal disease, and endometriosis.

It is usually recommended that the couple seek help after 1 year of attempting pregnancy. The reason for this is that the chance of conception in a "normal" couple is expected to be 60% at 6 months, 90% at 12 months, and 95% at 24 months (Tietze, Guttmacher, & Rubin, 1950). Simple problems such as coital frequency can have a significant effect on fertility rates. If a couple has intercourse once a week over 6 months, there is only about a 16% chance of pregnancy. If a couple increases this to four times per week around the time of ovulation, this rate increases to 83% over 6 months (Tietze et al., 1950). Often, simple counseling about expected time of ovulation and coital frequency can alleviate the problem.

Assessment of Infertility

The infertility evaluation can be divided into phases, looking at six areas: ovulation, male factor, sperm-mucus interaction, tubal and uterine anatomy, endometrial sufficiency, and pelvic factors (see Table 25.2). For pregnancy to occur, the following physiological conditions must function appropriately. Ovulation must, of course, occur for pregnancy to happen. Sufficient motile sperm must be present in the ejaculate, usually at least 20 million motile sperm per cc. At the time of ejaculation, sperm are deposited at the cervix. An initial vanguard of sperm is in the fallopian tubes within seconds. Numerous sperm remain within cervical mucus crypts, nourished by estrogenic cervical mucus, and are released intermittently, until mucus becomes hostile under the influence of progesterone. Fallopian tubes must be patent and normal in anatomy. The endometrium must be sufficiently developed to allow implantation to occur, and the uterus should be free of anatomic defects. Finally, the pelvis should be free of conditions that would preclude conception.

Testing can be organized to evaluate these factors according to the menstrual cycle in the woman who is ovulating. A history of regular menstrual cycles is presumptive of ovulation. A semen analysis can be obtained at any time that can be coordinated with the laboratory. A postcoital test (PCT) is done to evaluate sperm-mucus interaction at midcycle around the time of ovulation. A hysterosalpingogram (HSG), or X ray of the tubes, is performed after menstruation but before ovulation. A biopsy of the uterine lining to assess endometrial development is accomplished 1 to 2 days prior to expected menses. Thus five sixths of the infertility evaluation can be accomplished in one menstrual cycle in the ovulatory women. It is therefore inappropriate to drag the investigation out over several cycles, particularly in the older

Table 25.2 The Infertility Evaluation

Test	*Purpose*	*Timing*
Basal body temperature	Document ovulation	Chart entire cycle
Postcoital test	Evaluate sperm survival	1 to 2 days prior to ovulation
Hysterosalpingogram	X-ray study of the uterus and tubes	After menses, prior to ovulation
Endometrial biopsy	Evaluation of maturity of the uterine lining	1 to 2 days prior to expected menses
Laparoscopy	Visualize the pelvis	Prior to ovulation
Semen analysis	Evaluate sperm count, motility, morphology, volume, liquification, and PH	After 2 days, but no longer than 1 week, of abstinence
Antisperm antibodies	Document presence of antibodies in male semen and serum, female serum, and cervical mucus	Variable
Sperm penetration assay	Evaluate ability of sperm to penetrate egg	After 2 days, but no longer than 1 week, of abstinence

NOTE: The infertility evaluation must be accomplished according to specific time schedules.

female. Couples should be given an explanation of the evaluation process and allowed to choose testing intervals. This testing should be done in an efficient and logical sequence to minimize the stress and cost to the couple. The workup of an oligo- or anovulatory female will require induction of ovulation before the PCT or endometrial biopsy can be performed. However, the semen analysis and HSG should be performed prior to starting ovulation induction medications, such as clomiphene citrate.

Once these factors have been evaluated, a diagnostic laparoscopy is performed to assess whether pelvic adhesions or endometriosis are present in the pelvis. The laparoscopy should not be performed before the other testing is completed unless the woman is in severe pelvic pain or prior to ovulation induction with expensive agents such as Pergonal or Metrodin. A surgical procedure for infertility should always have a current semen analysis on the chart ruling out male factor. It is inappropriate to subject a woman to a surgery for infertility if her partner has no sperm.

At the start of the infertility evaluation, the nurse should explain the components of the infertility investigation, their purpose, and the reasons for exact timing. The rigid scheduling is often difficult for the couple, particularly if they have to travel some distance and arrange time away from the workplace. Where slight variations in time or date of appointment are reasonable, allowing a couple to choose the day and time of the appointment gives back some measure of control. The assessment process can be reviewed in phases, starting with ovulation disorders that occur in 20% to 30% of infertile women.

Ovulation Disorders

The only true way to document adequate ovulation is to document pregnancy. Other methods are considered presumptive of ovulation. Regular (every 26-36 days) menstrual cycles with premenstrual symptoms can be considered presumptive of ovulation. Another method to document ovulation is the use of a temperature chart. A woman takes her temperature every morning prior to any activity and records this on the chart. During the first half of the cycle, under the influence of estrogen, the basal body temperature is below 98° F. Within 24 hours after ovulation, under the influence of progesterone, the temperature rises approximately 1° F. This is called a *biphasic temperature chart.* Ovulation can be documented only in retrospect. Urinary luteinizing hormone (LH) kits are also used to document the presence of LH in the urine at midcycle and are also presumptive of ovulation.

Extensive evaluation is necessary if the woman has had episodes of irregular bleeding, a time lapse of greater than 40 days between periods, amenorrhea, significant weight loss or gain, excessive facial or body hair, or a history of discharge from the breast.

Disorders may originate in the hypothalamus, ovary, or pituitary or may be due to congenital anomalies of the reproductive tract. In rare cases, a chromosomal anomaly may first manifest as absence of menses. An evaluation of pituitary function should include follicle-stimulating hormone (FSH), LH, prolactin, and thyroid function tests. Physical examination is necessary to ascertain normal sexual development, which implies a normally functioning ovary and a normal reproductive tract.

An elevated prolactin level is commonly found when evaluating the reproductive-age female for amenorrhea. An elevated prolactin level, with or without galactorrhea, requires further evaluation with computerized axial tomography (CAT scanning) or magnetic resonance imaging (MRI) of the pituitary. The only exception is a woman who has been lactating within the last 6 months. In a majority of cases, the diagnosis will be a benign microadenoma of the pituitary. Less commonly, thyroid dysfunction, macroadenoma, and craniopharyngioma can cause hyperprolactinemia. Treatment for microadenoma is bromocryptine (parlodel) in doses titrated to achieve normal prolactin levels. Prolactin levels should be taken annually and CAT scans should be taken every 1 to 2 years. Bromocryptine should be started at low doses and gradually increased to therapeutic levels to avoid hypotensive side effects.

Once on bromocryptine, the woman may attempt pregnancy if she begins to ovulate spontaneously, but bromocryptine should be discontinued as soon as pregnancy is confirmed. In cases in which prolactin levels are normal and ovulation does not resume spontaneously, clomiphene citrate is needed to induce ovulation. Baseline visual fields should be documented prior to pregnancy, because monitoring prolactin levels during pregnancy will give no true indication of the growth of the prolactinoma. Excessive enlargement of the prolactinoma during pregnancy may result in visual field changes due to compression of the optic nerve and may be the first indication of complications.

Müllerian anomalies and conditions that obstruct the outflow tract should be ruled out during physical examination. An HSG may be necessary for accurate diagnosis. On rare occasion genetic disorders may cause amenorrhea. (See Chapter 23, "Common Symptoms: Bleeding, Pain, and Discharge," for additional discussion of amenorrhea.)

Elevated FSH and LH levels are indicative of ovarian failure. Ovarian failure prior to the age of 40 is considered premature, and a thorough reproductive endocrine workup is indicated, because the incidence of autoimmune disorders is significantly higher in these women. An evaluation is also indicated if menses occurs prior to the age of 8 (precocious puberty) or has not occurred by the age of 16.

An elevated LH to FSH ratio, with hirsutism and obesity is indicative of polycystic ovarian disease (PCOD). Further evaluation of testosterone and dehydroepiandrosterone sulfate (DHEAS) is indicated to rule out ovarian and adrenal tumors. These women are often readily susceptible to clomiphine citrate and may require 25-mg dosages rather than 50 mg.

Ovulation Induction

Proper treatment can be started once a diagnosis is established. If there is an imbalance in the hypothalamic-pituitary-ovarian response or a low FSH and LH, induction of ovulation is usually initiated. Only rarely is ovulation induction successful in a woman with an elevated FSH. Müllerian anomalies and uterine defects may be treated surgically.

Ovulation induction medications are often mistakenly referred to as "fertility drugs." These medications simply induce ovulation; they do not enhance fertility. In some cases in which a woman is already ovulating, these drugs can actually decrease fertility due to the antiestrogenic effects (see Table 25.3).

Clomiphene citrate (Clomid, Serophene) is the drug of choice for initiating ovulation induction. In a normally ovulating woman, a lack of circulating estrogen signals the hypothalamus to release gonadotropin-releasing hormone (GnRH) and initiate the menstrual cycle. It is thought that clomiphene citrate binds to estrogen receptors in the pituitary, blocking them from detecting circulating estrogen. The hypothalamus then releases more GnRH, stimulating pituitary release of FSH and LH, thus initiating a menstrual cycle.

Clomiphene citrate is administered on cycle days 5 through 9 in daily dosages of 50 mg. Women can be expected to ovulate approximately 14 days from the start of the clomiphene citrate, or cycle days 17 to 19, with menses occurring days 32 to 34. If the woman fails to ovulate at the 50 mg dose, dosage can be in-

Table 25.3 Drugs Used in the Treatment of Infertility

Drug	*Indication*	*Mechanism of Action*	*Dose*	*Side Effects*
Clomiphene citrate (Clomid, Serophene)	Ovulation induction: treatment of luteal phase inadequacy	Thought to bind to estrogen receptors in the pituitary, blocking them from detecting estrogen	Causes hypothalamus to release more gonadotropin-releasing hormone (GnRH), stimulating the release of follicle-stimulating hormone (FSH) and luteinizing hormone (LH)	Tablets, starting with 50 mg/day for 5 days; may increase to 200 mg/day
Human menopausal gonadotropins (HMG) (Pergonal)	Ovulation induction	Pergonal LH and FSH in 1:1 ratio Direct stimulation of ovarian follicle	IM injections, dosage regimen variable	Ovarian enlargement, ovarian hyperstimulation, local irritation at injection site, multiple births
Purified FSH (Metrodin)	Treatment of polycystic ovarian disease	IM injections, dosage regimen variable	Purified FSH, direct action on ovarian follicle	Ovarian enlargement, ovarian hyperstimulation, local irritation at injection site, multiple births
Human chorionic gonadotropin (HCG) (Profasi)	Ovulation induction	Acts directly on ovarian follicle to stimulate meiosis and rupture of the follicle	2,000-10,000 units IM	Local irritation at injection site
Danocrine (danazol)	Treatment of endometriosis	Combination of estrogen/progestin/androgen suppresses ovarian activity, eliminating stimulation to endometrial glands and stroma, with resultant shrinkage and disappearance	100-800 mg/day for 6 months	Mild hirsutism, acne, edema and weight gain, elevation of liver enzymes

(continued)

creased to 100 mg in the next cycle. Most of the pregnancies that occur as a result of clomiphene citrate occur at dosages of 50 to 100 mg. Clomiphene citrate can be given in amounts up to 250 mg per day before considering other therapies. Once ovulation has occurred at a specific dose, there is no advantage in increasing the dose (more does not make better). Once ovulation is established, the PCT and endometrial biopsy should be performed on all women, because the anti-estrogenic properties of clomiphene citrate can have an adverse effect on cervical mucus and endometrial development.

Side effects of clomiphene citrate include hot flashes, headaches, ovarian enlargement, and multiple gestation. Other infrequent symptoms include nausea and visual disturbances. These disappear after stopping the medication. Approximately 90% of clomiphene citrate pregnancies result in singleton deliveries. Nearly 10% result in delivery of twins with less than 1% being triplets or more. If pregnancy has not

Table 25.3 Continued

Drug	*Indication*	*Mechanism of Action*	*Dose*	*Side Effects*
GnRH agonists (Synarel, Lupron)	Treatment of endometriosis	Desensitization and down regulation of GnRH receptors of the pituitary, resulting in suppression of LH/FSH and ovarian function	Synarel: 200 μg intranasally twice a day for 6 months Lupron depot 375 mg every 28 days for 6 months Lupron subcutaneously 0.1 mg daily for 6 months	Synarel: nasal irritation, nosebleeds Synarel and Lupron: hot flashes, vaginal dryness, myalgia and arthralgia, headaches, mild bone loss (usually reversible within 12-18 months posttreatment)
Progesterone (progesterone in oil, Progestoral)	Treatment of luteal phase inadequacy	Direct stimulation of the endometrium	Vaginal suppositories 25-50 mg twice a day or 50 mg every night Rectal suppositories 12.25 mg every 12 hours Progesterone capsules 100 mg by mouth three times a day	Breast tenderness; local irritation, headaches

resulted in 6 to 12 months of therapy, laparoscopy, to rule out pelvic factors, and the use of other medications should be considered.

Pergonal (human menopausal gonadotropins) is a preparation of FSH and LH in a 1:1 ratio. This therapy is indicated with women who fail to ovulate with clomiphene citrate. Pergonal directly stimulates ovarian follicular development. Dosage is carefully monitored by daily serum estradiol levels and ovarian ultrasound. Once follicular maturation has occurred, ovulation is triggered by administration of human chorionic gonadotropin (HCG). Because Pergonal administration can result in the development of multiple follicles, HCG may be withheld when there are more than three mature follicles, to limit the chance of multiple gestation. Although 80% of Pergonal births will be singletons, the multiple gestation rate is 20%, with less than 5% of that being three or more. If the woman becomes pregnant with more than twins, the issue of selective reduction of one or more fetus must be discussed with the couple. The other serious side effect of Pergonal therapy is ovarian hyperstimulation. This syndrome presents with pelvic distension and weight gain. Early diagnosis and treatment is essential, because death can result if the condition progresses. Metrodin is purified human menopausal gonadotropins, with a resultant mixture of almost pure FSH. Metrodin is also used when amenorrhea is caused by an elevated LH:FSH ratio or by PCOD. Metrodin requires the same intensive monitoring as does Pergonal and has the same potential side effects.

Nursing care of the woman undergoing ovulation induction requires adequate patient education regarding mechanism of action, expected results, and potential side effects. Patient compliance with specified regimens is essential. Ovulation induction with Pergonal or Metrodin can be quite expensive and requires a time commitment due to the necessity of daily monitoring. Couples must be carefully counseled about the prospect of multiple births, and this counseling must be documented in the chart. The drugs used in ovulation induction often have significant side effects. The nurse should educate women and their partners about what to expect and should provide reassurance and support during the cycles. The cost of ovulation induction with Pergonal/Metrodin can run between $1,500 and $3,000 a year.

Male Factor

Very little is usually available to the women's health nurse on male infertility, and yet 40% to 60% of fertility is related to a male factor. Careful explanation of the normal physiology of the male and the evaluation components of the evaluation of the male and partner should be provided at the initial exam.

A systematic history of physical development, general health, and sexual habits is necessary to identify potential problems. Because spermatogenesis is an ongoing process, the male is much more susceptible to environmental factors, such as drug use and high scrotal temperatures. Questions about drug use, illnesses, past episodes of STD, and adequacy of ejaculation are essential to the male history.

Alcohol intake and cigarette smoking have been implicated in decreased sperm counts. Medications such as cimetidine (Tagamet) and aldomet can decrease sperm counts. The use of anabolic steroids causes a decline in testosterone and subsequently in sperm production.

Causes of male infertility include pituitary and hypothalamic dysfunction, which can be diagnosed by serum FSH and LH levels. Low FSH and LH may indicate hypothalamic or pituitary dysfunction, whereas elevated gonadotropins (FSH, LH) indicate testicular failure. Hormonal problems at the level of the testes can be detected by serum testosterone levels.

Undescended testes after the age of 2 may result in permanent damage due to high temperature of the testes. Hypospadias, a congenital anomaly in which the urethral outlet is on the shaft of the penis rather than at the end, may result in semen being deposited in the vagina rather than at the cervix. Hyposadias is being reported with increasing frequency in infants born to cocaine-addicted women. Mumps, particularly after adolescence, can result in permanent damage to the testes. Recurrent STD may cause scarring and blockage of the reproductive tract. A low-grade prostate infection can also affect sperm count. Any injury, such as testicular torsion, can result in ischemia to the testes and a decreased sperm count.

Antisperm antibodies may develop and cause fertility problems. Normally the male reproductive tract does not come into direct contact with the circulatory system. When there is a breakdown of the reproductive tract that allows sperm into the general circulation, the immune system forms antibodies to sperm. Conditions that can cause antibody formation include recurrent STD and vasectomy. The titer of antibodies, which can either immobilize or agglutinate sperm, is significant in projecting overall chances of pregnancy. Men should be counseled about obtaining a serum antisperm antibody titer prior to attempting a vasectomy reversal. Men with high antibody titers should be counseled regarding the poor prognosis of pregnancy and the other options available, including adoption and artificial insemination.

Laboratory Evaluation

Laboratory evaluation of the male starts with semen analysis. Traditionally done with a hemocytometer, the introduction of computerized technology is changing the procedure for semen analysis. Normal semen parameters are as follows:

- Volume 3 to 5 cc
- Count 20 million/cc
- Morphology (number of normally shaped sperm) greater than 60%
- Motility (number of sperm swimming progressively forward) greater than 60%

No semen analysis will have 100% motility or normal forms. The problem with low motility or abnormally developed sperm is that they are not able to navigate the cervix so that fertilization can occur in the fallopian tubes. Degrees of oligospermia (reduced count) or reduced motility and abnormal morphology will have bearing on the types of therapy available to the couple.

Ideally, the semen sample is collected by masturbation into a sterile container with no less than 2 days but no more than 7 days of abstinence. The sample should be examined within 2 hours of collection. Sterile, unlubricated condoms can be used for collection when there are religious or cultural objections to masturbation. Two or more abnormal samples must be obtained before a definitive diagnosis is made. Obtaining serum levels of FSH, LH, and testosterone and a physical examination are then appropriate for further diagnosis.

Additional testing for sperm-mucus interaction, antisperm antibodies, and sperm penetration may be necessary before a prognosis can be given and treatment recommended. The sperm penetration assay (SPA) is an evaluation of the functional ability of sperm to penetrate hamster eggs. Human eggs are not readily available to test for penetration, but there appears to be a correlation between the ability of sperm to penetrate human eggs and hamster eggs. This test may be ordered when there is a question about the ability of sperm to fertilize. Although the only true test of sperm is with human eggs, the SPA is the best test available at the present time.

A varicocele is a varicose vein in the scrotum and is commonly found on physical exam in males. It is theorized that this causes an elevation in scrotal temperature and thus affects spermatogenesis. The number of fertile males with varicoceles is unknown, but this condition is thought to be associated with male infertility.

Treatment

Treatment will be tailored to the individual problem. Medical therapies for low FSH and LH include clomiphene citrate and tamoxifen citrate, both anti-estrogens that stimulate FSH and LH production. Antibiotics are indicated when infection is present. Lifestyle changes may be necessary to correct self-induced fertility factors. Surgical therapy to correct blockages or ligate varicose veins may also be appropriate. There are data that say that 50% of men will see an improvement in semen parameters after variocelectomy, but there are no conclusive data that say that fertility rates are enhanced (Vermeulen & Vandewghe, 1984). Other therapies, such as artificial insemination and intrauterine insemination of the partner's semen, are directed at manipulation of the semen. Although 20 million motile sperm are required for natural conception, as few as 50,000 to 500,000 sperm are necessary for in vitro fertilization (IVF) or gamete intrafallopian transfer (GIFT). The availability of these procedures has led to an increase in couples choosing this because of male factor. These technologies are detailed later in the chapter.

Artificial Insemination

Artificial insemination of partner's sperm involves collection of the semen sample by masturbation and placing it into the cervix or directly into the uterus. This procedure minimizes semen loss and maximizes motility. Intrauterine insemination allows for direct placement of sperm into the uterus, thus bypassing the cervix when there is a problem with cervical mucus production. The semen sample is processed to remove the seminal plasma and concentrate the motile sperm prior to placement. This procedure is also performed when there is a low motility and low sperm count, although overall pregnancy rates for male factors are poor.

Both of these procedures require precise timing with menstrual cycles and may be quite taxing to the couple emotionally. Artificial insemination can provoke feelings of inadequacy and abnormality and often interferes with the satisfying sexual relationship of the couple. Nursing sensitivity to these issues is important. Insemination with the partner's sperm can be taught to couples so that this can occur at home. Use of milex clinicap is common.

Therapeutic Donor Insemination (TDI)

Insemination with donor semen is indicated in cases with severely low count or no sperm (azoospermia), sex-linked genetic diseases, and severe male antisperm antibodies. Couples require extensive counseling regarding this option, because there are a number of psychological issues involved. The couple may need to grieve over the inability to achieve a biological union as well as discuss any religious objections. Most donor insemination programs in the United States are coordinated by nurses, who counsel couples about the procedures, assist them in selecting a donor from a written description of the donor profile, and then perform the inseminations. The nurse must be able to detect problems with the couple's acceptance of the procedure and, ultimately, of the child produced. Nurses must be knowledgeable about the ethical, religious, legal, and medical aspects of the procedure (Hahn, 1991).

More single women who are approaching the end of their reproductive years are considering donor insemination. Frank discussions about the pros and cons of single parenting are an important part of the initial counseling. Single women, more than married couples, will have to address issues related to the societal acceptance of donor insemination and telling a child about donor parentage.

Sperm are usually obtained from a commercial bank that screens donors for STDs, health risk factors, and congenital defects. Sperm must be quarantined for 6 months and the donor retested for the human immunodeficiency virus (HIV) prior to release for use, because semen is a route of transmission for HIV. The sample is frozen in liquid nitrogen in the interim. Insemination is accomplished using thawed donor semen by intracervical or intrauterine insemination. An estimated 75,000 babies are born each year through donor insemination.

Cervical Factor

The precise role and relative importance of cervical mucus in human fertilization continues to be controversial. The secretions of the cervical canal serve as a filter for the millions of spermatozoa that are deposited into the vagina. Perhaps as few as 100 sperm pass through the cervical canal into the uterine cavity. Although there is no absolute proof that cervical mucus is necessary for fertilization, poor quantity and quality have been associated with infertility. Although the true incidence of abnormal cervical mucus-sperm interaction is unknown, it is estimated to be a causal factor in between 5% and 15% of infertility cases. Cervical factor infertility is on the rise due to more aggressive treatment of cervical dysplasia associated with the human papilloma virus. Destruction of the cervical mucus glands by cautery or laser vaporization causes permanent destruction of mucus glands.

Initial evaluation of the cervical mucus-sperm interaction is the PCT. The menstrual cycle is monitored by the woman at home using a urinary LH kit. When the test indicates evidence of the midcycle LH surge, couples are asked to have sexual intercourse and come to their health care provider within 24 hours. Cervical mucus is aspirated with a small catheter from the internal os and examined under a microscope for the presence of motile sperm. The results are reported as the number of sperm per high power field (HPF). Greater than five sperm per HPF is considered to be consistent with proven fertility. Sperm that are immotile or observed to "shake" may be related to antisperm antibodies.

The most common reason for a poor PCT result is poor timing. There is a window of only 48 to 72 hours when cervical mucus is receptive to sperm. At any other time, cervical mucus serves as a protective barrier. Thus a careful evaluation of timing in relation to ovulation is important. The urinary LH kits available today to consumers can be used to time this test more accurately and eliminate this factor.

Other reasons for a poor PCT result include coital difficulties, such as premature ejaculation and obesity, which causes the sperm to be deposited in the outer two thirds of the vagina. Other couples are simply unable to complete the act of intercourse "on demand." If repeated cancellations occur, the nurse should be alert to this possibility. Furthermore, poor cervical mucus can be caused by cervical stenosis, cervical infection, or cervical trauma due to removal of portions of the cervical canal through biopsy, cauterization, or resection. Coital lubricants, such as petroleum jelly, act as spermicides and should be avoided when attempting pregnancy.

Poor PCTs with normal cervical mucus may be due to cervical mucus antisperm antibodies (ASAB). Antibodies can be found in both the serum and cervical mucus of females. Antibodies in the female have several proposed mechanisms of action: prevention of mucus penetration, interference with acrosome reaction, activation of macrophages, and impaired sperm-egg interaction.

The type of therapy available to the couple with repeated poor postcoital testing will depend on the etiology. Highly cellular mucus is indicative of infection, which is treated with doxycycline, 100 mg twice a day for 10 days for both partners, starting on day 1 of menses. The PCT is then repeated in the next cycle. When problems are persistent, sperm are placed directly into the uterus using intrauterine insemination. It is generally recommended that three to four cycles of intrauterine insemination be performed. If the woman has not become pregnant, the couple should consider other therapies, such as IVF or GIFT, or consider discontinuing therapy. Repeated inseminations offer no additional advantage for fertility, and repeated failure with inseminations can be very damaging to a couple's self-esteem.

Tubal Factor

Damage or blockage of the fallopian tubes is one of the most common causes of female infertility and has been on the increase due to a rise in pelvic infections from chlamydia and gonorrhea. Evaluation of the uterine cavity and fallopian tubes is accomplished with an HSG. X rays are taken from several different angles after the uterus and tube are filled with a contrast media introduced into the uterus through a cannula. If tubal obstruction is present, the patient may experience moderate to severe discomfort.

Women report varying degrees of pain and cramping with the procedure, and prophylactic analgesia may be indicated. Because serious pelvic infections occur in between 0.3% and 1.3% of patients undergoing HSG, prophylactic antibiotics should be used when there is a history of PID or blocked tubes. Side effects of HSG include uterine cramping, bleeding, nausea, and dizziness. Vagal stimulation may occur with cervical manipulation, resulting in mild bradycardia, hypertension, and diaphoresis. There is a risk of uterine perforation and allergic reaction to the contrast media. Most women report some cervical bleeding after the procedure.

Tubal damage places the woman at much higher risk for ectopic pregnancy should conception occur. Women should be counseled to report for medical observation as soon as they suspect pregnancy. Early monitoring can result in more conservative treatment.

If the HSG shows extensive damage, it is the degree of tubal damage that dictates those therapeutic options available to the woman. Extensive internal damage is rarely able to be treated effectively. If there is limited damage to only a portion of the tube, the damaged portion of the tube may be removed and the healthy part is reanastamosed.

Microsurgery requires extensive training and experience. The fallopian tubes are delicate organs that, once damaged, never heal. Skill of the surgeon is critical in being able to offer a surgical solution to tubal problems. The goals of microsurgery are to correct the anatomic defect and to prevent pelvic adhesions. Any insult to the pelvis may result in further adhesion formation, so tissue handling must be delicate.

IVF was first developed as therapy for women with absent or irreparable damaged tubes and remains one of the primary options to be considered. Women should be counseled about the actual success rates of tubal surgery and risks of subsequent ectopic pregnancy versus the current success rates for IVF.

Disease processes outside the tube that can lead to tubal problems include appendicitis, endometriosis, ruptured ovarian cyst, or peritubular adhesions from abdominal or pelvic surgery. It is suspected that diethylstilbestrol (DES) exposure contributes to ectopic pregnancy because of tubal abnormalities now being documented in DES daughters. Ectopic pregnancy is discussed in Chapter 23.

Endometrial Development

Adequate development of the endometrium is necessary for normal implantation of the embryo. The endometrial glands and stroma respond to the progesterone secreted by the corpus luteum in the second half of the menstrual cycle or the luteal phase. Inadequate development during the luteal phase may be due to either inadequate progesterone stimulation from the ovarian follicle or an inappropriate response of the endometrium.

An endometrial biopsy using a pipelle aspirator or Novak curette is obtained 1 to 2 days prior to expected menses and is used to evaluate the endometrial response. The procedure causes one to two menstrual-like cramps. Discomfort will depend on the individual woman's pain threshold. Women should expect mild cramping and spotting after the procedure but should call with increase in temperature or severe cramping. The woman should be instructed to call with the date of her menstrual period, because this is essential to the proper interpretation of the biopsy. Occasionally, the endometrial biopsy is done during the cycle of conception, so patients may wish to use barrier contraception during the month of biopsy. If a sensitive urine pregnancy test is available, this should be performed immediately prior to the biopsy.

The biopsy specimen is examined microscopically and an approximate cycle date assigned to the endometrial pattern. A biopsy that is out of phase with where it is expected to be must be confirmed by a second biopsy in a subsequent cycle for a diagnosis of luteal-phase inadequacy, because all women occasionally experience an out-of-phase cycle.

Although serum progesterone sampling has been used to document luteal-phase inadequacy, there may be little or no correlation between the serum progesterone and the endometrial response due to the pulsating nature of progesterone secretion. Therefore, it is recommended that endometrial biopsy be obtained to establish a luteal-phase deficiency.

Treatment of a luteal-phase defect depends on the etiology. If the defect is present with other conditions, such as elevated serum prolactin or endometriosis, treatment of the underlying disorder may result in correction of the defect.

There is some debate about the treatment of luteal-phase deficiency. Some argue that because the etiology may involve faulty development of the ovarian follicle, the approach should be to enhance the follicular phase with ovulation induction agents. Others argue that a progesterone deficiency is best treated with luteal-phase progesterone. Both approaches have been successful.

Progesterone supplementation is usually accomplished with progesterone rectal or vaginal suppositories, 12.5 to 25 mg every 12 hours. The suppositories are begun 3 days after the midcycle rise of basal body temperature and are continued until menstruation, which is rarely delayed beyond 2 days by the progesterone. The dosage is modulated to achieve an adequate endometrial response. The progesterone is absorbed through the vaginal mucosa as the suppository melts, and the use of a sanitary pad may help protect undergarments. Side effects can include local irritation of the vagina and external genitalia. Some patients prefer to self-inject 12.5 mg of progesterone in oil intramuscularly on a daily basis. Oral progesterone has also been used. Should pregnancy occur, the progesterone is continued until an ultrasound scan at 6 to 8 weeks documents a viable pregnancy. At this time, the fetal-placental unit should be able to sustain itself through its own placental progesterone production. The corpus luteum declines at this time.

One third of recurrent spontaneous abortions are caused by a luteal-phase defect. If this is the indication for the biopsy, the couple should be cautioned to use a barrier method of contraception until the defect has been corrected.

Pelvic Factor

Once the initial phases of the infertility evaluation have been accomplished, factors that have been identified should be treated prior to laparoscopy. Ovulation induction should be established and the couple given an opportunity to achieve pregnancy. If pregnancy has not occurred after 6 to 9 months of ovulation, laparoscopy is indicated because direct intra-abdominal visualization may be necessary to establish a diagnosis. Laparoscopy allows direct visualization of the internal organs through a small incision in the umbilicus. A second, and occasionally a third, incision is necessary to manipulate the pelvic organs for complete evaluation. Six characteristics—the size; shape; surface; color; consistency; and mobility of the uterus, tubes, and ovaries—are noted during diagnostic laparoscopy.

Much operative work can be accomplished through the laparoscope, including lysis of adhesions, vaporization of endometriosis, and surgical excision of ectopic pregnancy. Postoperatively, many patients report some shoulder discomfort, due to the insufflation of carbon dioxide. This usually resolves within 24 hours and discomfort can be relieved by assuming the knee-chest position. A sore throat from the endotracheal intubation is not uncommon. The degree of abdominal discomfort will depend on the amount of surgical manipulation and the individual's threshold of pain. Nausea and vomiting may occur as a consequence of anesthesia or manipulation of the bowel during surgery.

Hysteroscopy is a similar procedure that examines the inside of the uterine cavity. This may be done at the time of laparoscopy or as a separate procedure. Evaluation and removal of a uterine septum, polyps, or intrauterine adhesions may be accomplished through the hysteroscope. It is particularly valuable for the lysis of adhesions with Ascherman's syndrome, a condition in which there is internal scarring of the uterus.

Endometriosis

Endometriosis is commonly observed at laparoscopy. This disease is defined as the presence of endometrial glands and stroma outside the uterine cavity. Endometrial tissue has been found on the ovary, uterine ligaments, pelvic peritoneum, cervix, inguinal area, cul-de-sac, and the rectovaginal septum. Endometrial lesions have been found in the vagina, vulva, perineum, bladder, and surgical scars. Some women have lesions of the gastrointestinal tract, usually in the sigmoid. Endometrial implants have also been found in sites far from the pelvic area, such as the thoracic cavity, limbs, gallbladder, and heart. Endometrial lesions contain glands and stroma and respond to cyclic hormones at times similar to the uterine endometrium but often out of phase with it. Blood may flow into endometrial lesions or into their surrounding tissue.

Symptoms result from the pathophysiological changes that occur, including the bleeding from the lesions, formation of endometriomas (cysts), adhesions, and/or anatomical distortions or obstructions. Pain results from inflammation, irritation, encroachment, and obstruction.

Although its exact incidence is difficult to determine, because it can exist without causing symptoms, a rough estimate is that 10% of all women in the reproductive age group and 25% to 35% of all infertile women have endometriosis (Cramer, 1987). Approximately one third to one half of all women having major gynecologic procedures are found to have endometriosis (Clarke-Pearson & Dawood, 1990). At one time it was thought that endometriosis was more prevalent in white middle- and upper-class women; however, more recently racial differences have been found to be nonexistent (Clarke-Pearson & Dawood, 1990). It was also once believed that problems attributed to lower socioeconomic groups, such as tubal blockage caused by gonorrhea, prevented the disease. It is more likely, however, that the symptoms once attributed to PID were actually symptoms of unrecognized endometriosis and that prejudicial attitudes may account for the belief that pelvic pain or other symptoms in black women were related to PID rather than to endometriosis (Clarke-Pearson & Dawood, 1990). The common belief that endometriosis occurs only in goal-oriented career women who have delayed their childbearing also has been discredited. Traditionally, endometriosis was considered a disease of women in their 30s and 40s; however, endometriosis is more common in adolescents than previously believed. In two series of laparoscopies of teenagers with disabling pain or abnormal vaginal bleeding, a significant percentage were found to have endometriosis. It also had been assumed that nulliparity was a risk factor for endometriosis; however, 30% to 40% of women with the disease are parous (Luciano & Pitkin, 1984). There appears to be a familial tendency to develop endometriosis; research has demonstrated that the incidence of severe endometriosis is higher (61.1%) in the family group than in the nonfamily group (23.8%) (Clarke-Pearson & Dawood, 1990).

Although endometriosis has been recognized as a clinical entity since the mid-1800s and many theories concerning it have been advanced, the etiology and pathology are still poorly understood. One of the most widely accepted, long-debated etiologies is that of retrograde flow of menstrual fluid through the fallopian tubes and subsequent implantation of viable fragments of endometrial tissue within the pelvic cavity. However, this explanation does not account for extrapelvic sites of endometriosis such as the lungs or limbs. Retrograde menstruation alone is unlikely to produce endometriosis; more probably, a genetic factor or susceptibility and a favorable hormonal milieu are needed for implantation and growth of transplanted endometrial tissue (Clarke-Pearson & Dawood, 1990). Other explanations for the development of endometriosis include genetic and immunologic factors, elevated prostaglandin levels, and the luteinized unruptured follicle syndrome in which a functioning corpus luteum exists but the egg does not leave the follicle.

Careful pain, menstruation, and reproductive histories should provide additional data to support the suspicion. In addition, the nurse should obtain a sexual history to document the presence of dyspareunia. The woman should be asked if any family members have experienced similar symptoms.

A complete pelvic examination is essential to confirm the diagnosis of endometriosis. In the pelvic exam, the most common indicator of endometriosis is nodularity of the uterosacral ligament. These nodules may be tender. The dyspareunia described by the woman often may be recreated with cervical manipulation that occurs during a pelvic or rectovaginal examination. A rectal examination should be done, because the uterus is often fixed in a retroverted position due to endometriosis, and the endometrial nodules present on the posterior uterine wall, cul-de-sac, and uterosacral ligament may be distinguished better rectally. No specific laboratory tests assess specifically for endometriosis. Definite diagnosis is done by laparoscopy.

Once the diagnosis is made, management is approached from the standpoint of both prevention and treatment. Although absolute prevention of endometriosis is not possible for most women, prophylaxis against some of the more disabling aspects of the disease and decreased fertility may be possible. Clarke-Pearson and Dawood (1990) recommend that the woman who has a family history of endometriosis and who wishes to have children should avoid undue delay in childbearing.

Treatment goals for endometriosis include prevention of disease progression, alleviation of pain, and establishment or restoration of fertility. Treatment options include observation alone, medical therapy, surgical therapy, or a combination of medical and surgical options. The woman's age, desire for children, presence or absence of significant adhesions, and severity of symptoms are major considerations in developing a treatment plan.

A young woman with mild endometriosis who wants children and does not have a fixed, retroverted uterus will have as good a chance of becoming pregnant without treatment as with either medical or surgical therapy (Garner & Webster, 1985). Moderate to severe disease with infertility but without significant tubo-ovarian adhesions or endometriosis may be treated medically if the woman is young enough to have time for medical suppression. Women with extensive disease, large endometriomas, or significant distortion of tubo-ovarian anatomy with adhesions will require surgical intervention in most cases.

The aim of medical therapy is to stop the growth of the ectopic tissue and allow regression of the disease. A variety of therapies have been used, including estrogen therapy with DES and progestins. Such therapies are rarely used today, however, because of the significant risk of endometrial hyperplasia and thrombophlebitis associated with estrogen therapy and the numerous side effects associated with progestins. Combination oral contraceptives have been used to produce a state of pseudopregnancy that should induce regression of the disease. When this therapy is stopped, patients experience high rates of recurrence of pain and other symptoms.

Hormonal antagonists such as Danazol and other GnRH antagonists (e.g., buserelinm nafarelin) have been used to suppress ovulation. Danazol acts to produce anovulation and hypogonadotropinism with resultant decreased ovarian secretion of estrogen and progesterone, thus allowing regression of the endometrium. Amenorrhea is seen in most users after 6 to 8 weeks of treatment, and some women experience other symptoms of menopause. The most commonly recommended daily dosage for effective treatment is 800 mg Danazol in four divided doses because of its short plasma half-life (Clarke-Pearson & Dawood, 1990). Symptoms improve in 70% to 93% of women with these regimen. With this regimen, fertility rates are between 40% and 76% depending on the stage of the disease (Clarke-Pearson & Dawood, 1990), with a recurrence rate of 5% to 15% 1 year after therapy (Garner & Webster, 1985). Side effects usually result from the androgenic and anti-estrogenic properties of the Danazol and include weight gain, acne and oily skin, edema, hirsutism, hot flushes, menstrual spotting, and a decrease in breast size. Danazol is contraindicated in women with hepatic dysfunction, severe hypertension, congestive heart failure, or borderline renal function. Usually, Danazol treatment is begun during menses, and women are counseled to wait one normal menstrual cycle after stopping the drug before attempting pregnancy. Danazol is expensive, which may be a problem for many women.

GnRH agonist therapy (Leuprolide, Synarel) is also often used to treat endometriosis. GnRH agonists act by inducing down regulation and desensitization of the pituitary. FSH/LH stimulation to the ovary declines markedly and ovarian function diminishes significantly. The hypoestrogenism leads to hot flashes in almost all women. There can be minor bone loss, most of which is reversible within 12 to 18 months after therapy.

Surgery is often necessary for severe, acute, or incapacitating symptoms. Decisions regarding the extent of the surgery depend on age, desire for children, and extent and location of the disease. In women who do not wish to conserve their reproductive capacity, hysterectomy and bilateral salpingo-oophorectomy are the only definitive cures. When the woman is in her childbearing years and wants children, and the disease does not preclude it, reproductive function should be retained through careful removal of all endometrial tissue with retention of ovarian function.

Counseling and education are important components of nursing management of the client with endometriosis. A frank discussion of the treatment options and potential risks and benefits is mandatory. Because pelvic pain is a subjective, personal experience that is often frightening, psychological support is important for women with endometriosis. Sexual dysfunction resulting from dyspareunia is common, and referral for psychological counseling may be indicated. Support groups for women with endometriosis are available in some locations, and Resolve, the organization for infertile couples, may also be of help to these women. Continuation or recurrence of pelvic pain may necessitate assisting the woman to manage her chronic pelvic pain and dysmenorrhea. The nursing strategies discussed in the section on dysmenorrhea in Chapter 23 are applicable here as well.

Unfortunately, no matter what the form of treatment, endometriosis returns in approximately 40% of cases. Thus, for many, endometriosis represents a chronic disease and will require nursing management of the manifestation of this condition, be it chronic pelvic pain or infertility. Peak fertility after treatment of endometriosis is in the first 12 to 18 months after therapy. This is one of the reasons for correcting other fertility factors prior to laparoscopy.

Unexplained Infertility

There is still much to be learned about human reproduction. In the early 1950s perhaps 40% to 50% of infertility cases were "unexplained." As the knowledge base has expanded, this diagnosis is now applied in less than 5% of cases. With further advances in diagnostic testing this number will continue to decline.

This is certainly the most difficult "diagnosis" for couples to accept. This diagnosis allows for the possibility of subsequent pregnancy but does not pose any specific factor that can be treated. Although many couples with this diagnosis do ultimately become pregnant, there are an equal number who do not. Psychological support is important for these couples.

Assisted Reproductive Technologies

IVF evolved as a procedure to assist women with blocked or absent fallopian tubes achieve pregnancy. It has since been used to treat couples with male factor, antisperm antibodies, cervical infertility, and unexplained infertility. Very simply, the ovaries are hyperstimulated using a combination of ovulation-induction agents to obtain a large number of oocytes. Once the ovary has been sufficiently stimulated, oocytes are removed via laparoscopy or vaginal ultrasound-guided aspiration and placed into an incubator with sperm. After 48 hours, if fertilization and division of oocytes has occurred, four to eight cell embryos are transferred into the uterus using a small catheter.

GIFT is a variation of IVF, in which oocytes are laparoscopically removed, identified, and then placed back into the ends of the fallopian tubes with the sperm (see Figure 25.1). The woman then recovers and fertilization occurs naturally. GIFT is an option for women with one normal fallopian tube, unexplained infertility, or recurrent endometriosis. Both IVF and GIFT are performed for men with compromised semen analysis, because as few as 50,000 to 100,000 are necessary for IVF/GIFT.

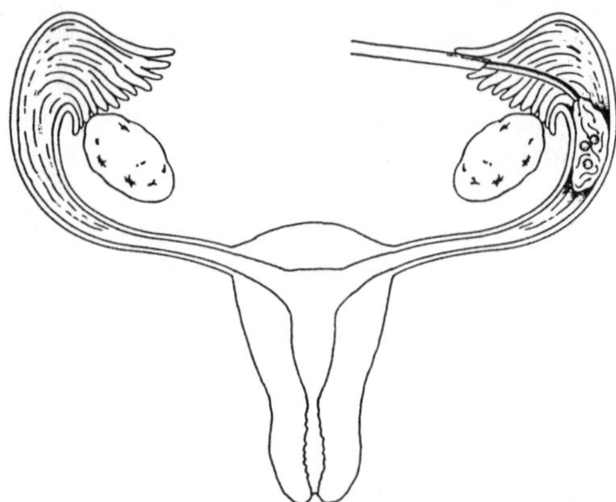

Figure 25.1. Gamete Intrafallopian Transfer (GIFT)
SOURCE: Serono Laboratories (1990). Reprinted with permission from *Pathways to Parenthood.* Copyright CRC Press, Boca Raton, Florida.

When transfer of embryos or oocytes is accomplished, one of the major concerns is the possibility of multiple births. Many fertility centers are limiting the number of eggs/embryos transferred to three to significantly decrease the likelihood of multiple gestation. Excess embryos can be frozen (cryopreserved) for indefinite periods of time, then thawed and transferred into the uterus, and progress through normal pregnancy and birth. Couples who do not become pregnant in the initial stimulation cycle can thus return in a subsequent menstrual cycle for a transfer of thawed embryos. When multiple embryos are transferred, the couple must be extensively counseled about the risk of multiple births, and this must be well documented.

The issue of cryopreservation of human embryos presents numerous ethical and religious dilemmas. Couples must be comfortable with their decisions and the lifelong consequences. What happens, for instance, if the couple dies prior to the transfer? Nursing roles must focus on education and working through alternatives with couples. The consent form must encompass possibilities such as death, divorce, or simply that the couple does not want the embryo at a later date.

Cost is a significant factor when couples are deciding about assisted reproductive technologies. The average cycle costs between $5,000 and $7,000, and very few insurance companies cover this procedure. With success rates averag-

the religious acceptance of procedures, feelings about cryopreserving human embryos, and family acceptance of their decision and their child's origins.

The reproductive technologies are expanding rapidly and currently allow for donor eggs, donated embryos, and transfer of an embryo into the uterus of a gestational surrogate mother. The ethical and legal implications have not been well researched.

Counseling About Options

The crux of counseling the infertile couple is the recognition that all aspects of diagnosis and treatment involve choices with emotional, ethical, and religious responses. What is acceptable to one individual may not be acceptable to another. The infertility evaluation may be personally invasive, and people have the option not to continue testing. Once the diagnosis has been made, options may be severely limited or may involve therapies that are religiously unacceptable. Many infertility therapies are simply unaffordable.

Nurses who are involved with infertile couples must be knowledgeable about adoption resources in the community so that they can do initial counseling and appropriate referral. Adoption workshops can be organized for couples, as can consumer seminars on infertility. The number of babies available for adoption has declined steadily, so the option of foster parenting or parenting older children should be discussed. Adoption involves a great deal of emotional investment in the decision-making process.

Implications for the Future

Infertility is a new area for the nurse specialist. Reproductive endocrine/infertility nursing was first considered a subspecialty area in the early 1980s. The first certification examination for reproductive endocrinology and infertility was offered by the NAACOG Certification Corporation in 1989. Although there is a paucity of nursing and psychological research in the area, this evolving specialty offers numerous opportunities for research and innovative clinical programs.

Research regarding the pregnancy and parenting experiences of previously infertile women is beginning to be done. Dunnington and Glazer (1991) compared the differences in maternal identity and early mothering behaviors in previously infertile women and never-infertile women. No significant differences between the two groups were found for quantitatively measured early mothering behaviors. Previously infertile mothers did demonstrate lower postpartum maternal identity scores, a delay in preparation of the home environment, and less self-confidence. Harris, Sandelowski, and Holditch-Davis (1991) studied the emotional impact of spontaneous abortion as well as the transition to parenthood in infertile couples. Couples defined miscarriage as both a loss and a gain. Some of the gains included knowing that a pregnancy was possible for them and having a sense of normalcy.

Further evaluation and understanding of the pregnancy and parenting experiences of infertile couples as well as the coping skills of infertile couples and what can be done to enhance a healthy outcome, from both a medical and psychosocial standpoint, is needed. Assisted reproductive technologies are expanding rapidly, although little has been done to study the effects in the families that are created. Maternal/child and women's health nurses have the essential background to initiate and maintain research in this area.

As advances such as pre-implantation genetic screening of embryos and gene therapy take off in the next few years, nurses must be at the forefront of education and research. Too little is known about parenting and pregnancy after infertility. Does the infertile couple need earlier prenatal education? What can be done to enhance attachment? Are there interventions needed during pregnancy to repair the damage of infertility to marital communication and sexuality? These and other questions are the future of nursing.

References

Clarke-Pearson, D. L., & Dawood, M. Y. (1990). *Green's gynecology: Essentials of clinical practice* (4th ed.). Boston: Little, Brown.

Congress of the United States. Office of Technology Assessment. (1988). *Infertility: Medical and social choices.* Washington, DC: Government Printing Office.

Cramer, D. W. (1987). Epidemiology of endometriosis. In E. A. Wilson (Ed.), *Endometriosis* (pp. 5-22). New York: A. R. Liss.

Dunnington, R. M., & Glazer, R. (1991). Maternal identity in previously infertile and never infertile women. *JOGNN, 20*(4), 309-318.

Garner, C. H., & Webster, B. W. (1985). Endometriosis. *JOGNN, 14*(Suppl.), 10s-20s.

Hahn, S. (1991). Caring for couples considering alternatives in family building. In C. H. Garner (Ed.), *Principles of infertility nursing* (pp. 179-206). Boca Raton, FL: CRC Press.

Harris, B. G., Sandelowski, M., & Holditch-Davis, D. (1991). Infertility and new interpretations of pregnancy loss. *MCN, 16*(4), 217-220.

Kronmal, R. A., Whitney, C. W., & Mumford, S. D. (1991). The intrauterine device and pelvic inflammatory disease: The women's health study reanalyzed. *Journal of Clinical Epidemiology, 44*(2), 109-112.

Luciano, A. A., & Pitkin, R. M. (1984). Endometriosis: Approaches to diagnosis and treatment. *Surgery Annals, 16,* 297-312.

Malhlstedt, P. (1985). The psychological component of infertility. *Fertility and Sterility, 43,* 335-346.

Menning, B. E. (1988). *Infertility: A guide for the childless couple* (2nd ed.). New York: Prentice Hall.

Mosher, W. D. (1987). Infertility: Why business is booming. *American Demographics, 9*(1), 42-43.

Pratt, W. F., Mosher, W. D., Bachrach, C. A., & Horn, M. C. (1985). Infertility—United States, 1982. *Morbidity and Mortality Weekly Report, 34,* 197-199.

Serono Laboratories. (1990). *Pathways to parenthood.* Nowell, MA: Author.

Tietze, C., Guttmacher, A. F., & Rubin, S. (1950). Time required for conception in 1727 pregnant patients. *Fertility and Sterility, 1,* 338-441.

Vermeulen, A., & Vandewghe, M. (1984). Improved fertility after varicocele correction: Fact or fiction? *Fertility and Sterility, 42,* 249-256.

26

Reproductive Surgery

DEITRA LEONARD LOWDERMILK

Since the 1970s, when the women's health movement aroused public awareness of issues regarding women's health, interest in providing consumers as well as practitioners with information about reproductive surgery has continued to increase. Prior to the movement, women were often subjects for new surgical procedures without their full knowledge, which would have allowed them to give informed consent. Surgical procedures were often excessive or unnecessary, and alternatives were not always offered (Sloane, 1985). Today, there is still a concern that a number of surgical interventions, especially hysterectomies, are not necessary. Technological advances have introduced new diagnostic and surgical procedures that may provide alternatives to major surgery, such as laser surgery and microsurgery, but they may also increase the potential for unnecessary intervention (Littlefield, 1986). Women undergoing reproductive surgery expect to be involved with health care professionals in decision making about care, and practitioners need to be able to provide information to them about these procedures so that they can truly be informed consumers.

Assessment

The nurse must recognize women who are at risk for reproductive surgery and the factors that influence this at-risk state so as to inform clients of the potential risk and to counsel them about ways in which the health care system can meet their needs.

The most common signs and symptoms of reproductive problems that may require surgical intervention are vaginal bleeding, pelvic pain, and pelvic or abdominal masses. The significance of these symptoms varies with the woman's age and race (Herbst, Mishell, Stenchever, & Droegemueller, 1992). During the adolescent years (age at onset of menses to age 19), bleeding problems related to menstruation can lead to diagnostic surgery such as dilatation and curettage (D & C). The reproductive years (20-44) may involve a number of surgical procedures in addition to operative procedures associated with pregnancy (cesarean delivery, forceps delivery). A high number of sterilizations are performed on women 25 to 35 years of age; surgery for infertility problems is also prevalent in this age group. Furthermore, women of all ages are at risk not only for problems related to menstruation but also for benign tumors and cervical cancer. These latter conditions might lead to hysterectomy. For example, black women are three times as likely as white women to be at risk for uterine fibroids and subsequent surgery (Herbst et al., 1992). All women in their 40s are at risk for gynecologic malignancies that may require surgery (Adams, 1986). During the perimenopausal and postmenopausal years, surgery may be done for dysfunctional bleeding related to changing ovarian function and for malignancies, especially endometrial cancer (Greenwood, 1988). Finally, there is a high incidence of pelvic surgery in the older female (60-69 years of age). This fact is correlated with the increased longevity of women and the concomitant increased risk of cancer and pelvic relaxations (Nichols, 1990).

Regular health screening to identify any existent health problems is an essential part of the care of women. A record of obstetric and gynecologic problems can facilitate data collection. (See Chapter 9, "Well-Woman Assessment," for information regarding obtaining a gynecologic history.)

Diagnosis

Prior to the 1980s, the gynecologist relied on bimanual examination, exploratory laparotomy, or laparoscopy to obtain the information needed to make a diagnosis. Today, accurate assessment of problems can be made without the disadvantages of surgery. Thus diagnostic radiology plays an important role in diagnosis of pelvic problems. These and other diagnostic procedures that may be used prior to surgery will need to be explained to the client to facilitate her decision making and to encourage her to be an active participant in treatment. For all diagnostic procedures, the client needs to be informed about what to expect during the procedure, why it is being done, what preparations she can expect (i.e., dietary restrictions, enemas), where the procedure will be performed (clinic, physician's office, or hospital), the cost, and whether or not third-party payers will pay for the procedure.

These procedures include intravenous pyelograms, barium studies, ultrasonography, culposcopy, hysteroscopy, computer tomography, magnetic resonance imaging, laboratory tests (e.g., Pap smear, pregnancy tests, complete blood count), and X rays.

Consultations and Informed Decision Making

Once a diagnosis has been made, it is important that the health care team thoroughly inform the woman about the disease or condition requiring surgery. This dialogue should include family members if possible and should be explained at the client's level of understanding. The physician should discuss the indications for surgery, the potential risks involved, advantages and disadvantages, and any available alternatives to the surgery. The reasons why the physician has chosen a particular treatment, the predicted outcome of the surgery, and possible complications must also be discussed during the consultation (Boston Women's Health Collective [BWHC], 1992; Disaia & Walker, 1990). There should also be time set aside for the woman to ask any questions she has concerning the surgery. The role of the nurse is to complement the physician's explanations—to make sure that the woman understands what has been said to her by reemphasizing important points and making further explanations when necessary. At all times, the nurse should emphasize the woman's right to control her body and her right to make informed decisions.

Some women have general concerns about surgical procedures that may influence their decision to have surgery. These include fears of death or disability, fear of postoperative pain, and concerns about anesthesia—loss of control with general anesthesia or feeling pain if awake under regional anesthesia; length of hospitalization and the recovery period; welfare of the family during hospitalization; and financial concerns (especially if surgery means loss of income or paying for all surgical costs not covered by third-party payers). The nurse listens to the concerns, answers questions, and refers the client to other resources when necessary to address unanswered concerns.

Women may also have concerns about gynecologic surgery that may need to be discussed. Reproductive surgery can affect a woman's self-concept and may be seen as a threat to her femininity, particularly if a woman's self-esteem is related to her ability to bear children (Chapin,

1988). The client should be informed whether the surgery will affect her childbearing ability or alter her sexual performance. Often clients have misconceptions about these topics that can be cleared up prior to surgery.

Health care providers should inform the woman of her right to consult other health care providers prior to consenting to surgery. Many third-party plans require second opinions for major gynecologic surgery or costs may not be covered, and a gynecologist is preferred to a general surgeon for most second opinions (Holt & Weber, 1982).

Prior to surgery, a woman is asked by the physician to sign a written consent that legally authorizes the surgery and acknowledges the information explained to her.

Management Strategies

After the decision for surgery has been made, the nurse must plan the pre- and postoperative care of the client on the basis of identified needs. In the following discussion of surgical procedures, attention is given not only to the usual techniques but to alternative procedures as well. The goals of nursing care are to meet the physiological and emotional needs of women undergoing the procedures.

Dilatation and Curretage

Indications

Dilatation of the cervix and curettage of the endometrium is one of the most frequently performed uterine operative procedures. Indications for this procedure include diagnosis of uterine malignancy, evaluation and control of dysfunctional uterine bleeding, incomplete abortion, therapeutic abortion, evaluation of causes of infertility, and relief of dysmenorrhea. The diagnostic purpose of endometrial curettage is to differentiate abnormal bleeding related to hormonal function from bleeding related to malignancy. The therapeutic value of curettage is to control abnormal bleeding by removing the endometrium (Herbst et al., 1992).

Technique

D & C is frequently done as an outpatient procedure, but it can also be performed in the hospital. Preoperatively, the woman may be given analgesics or a local anesthetic; however, brief general anesthesia or regional anesthesia may be used if a thorough internal examination is needed (Nichols & Randall, 1989). For the D & C, the woman is placed in a lithotomy position. A bimanual examination is done to determine the position of the uterus. A speculum is inserted into the vagina to expose the cervix. A sound (elongated instrument) is introduced into the uterus to measure the uterine cavity, and the cervix is gradually dilated with metal dilators. A curette is then introduced into the uterine cavity and the endometrium is scraped away. Suction curettage may be used instead of a curette. The specimen is sent to a pathology laboratory for analysis and confirmation of the preoperative diagnosis.

Complications

Secondary hemorrhage, lacerations of the cervix perforation of the uterus, and infection are risks after a D & C (Nichols & Randall, 1989).

Nursing Care

Usually, there is no preoperative preparation except that the client consumes nothing by mouth past midnight the day of the surgery.

Postoperatively, the nurse should check vital signs every 15 minutes until they are stable. The amount of vaginal bleeding and/or pad count should also be assessed. Mild analgesics may be given for pain, and diet is usually dictated by the client's wishes.

Prior to discharge, the nurse informs her client about the following facts and procedures:

- Slight bleeding is normal. If bleeding is as heavy as your normal period or if bleeding lasts more than 2 weeks, call your physician.
- Abdominal cramping is not unusual during the first few days following discharge. For relief, you can take mild analgesics, such as acetominophen (Tylenol), or place a heating pad or hot water bottle on the abdomen.

- Temperature should be taken once a day for 2 days. If your temperature is more than 100° F (38° C), call your health care provider.
- Sexual intercourse, tub bathing, and the use of tampons should be avoided for 2 weeks to allow healing and to prevent infection (Lowdermilk, 1986).

Cryosurgery

Indications

Cryosurgery is used in the treatment of chronic cervicitis, endocervicitis, erosions, and nabothian cysts. It is also used as a preventive measure to treat dysplasia (intraepithelial neoplasia) (Herbst et al., 1992).

Technique

Treatment is usually performed in the clinic or physician's office and without anesthesia. During the procedure, a large speculum is inserted into the vagina. Nitrous oxide is circulated through a special cryoprobe that is placed on the area to be treated. Nitrous oxide causes local freezing, allowing necrosis of the affected or diseased tissues to occur. The tissues slough off and the remaining healthy tissue heals cleanly (Herbst et al., 1992). Cryosurgery is best performed 1 week after the end of a menstrual period. Performing the surgery at this time avoids freezing a uterus with an early pregnancy and permits the most active phase of cervical regeneration to take place prior to the onset of the next menstrual period.

Complications

Occasional spotting and cervical stenosis (hardening) with resultant infertility may occur. Injuries to normal tissue can occur if touched by the probe.

Nursing Care

The client will need to know that she must remain in a lithotomy position until the tissues are frozen because movement can cause damage to normal tissues. After the treatment, the client can expect to have a profuse watery vaginal discharge for 2 to 3 weeks. Perineal pads may be necessary. If the discharge has a strong odor, cornstarch applications to the opening of the vagina may help (Ammer, 1989). Avoidance of sexual intercourse, douching, use of tampons, tub bathing, or swimming for up to 2 weeks may also be recommended to allow for healing.

Biopsy of the Cervix and Endometrium

Indications

A cervical biopsy is recommended whenever there is a need to investigate suspicious cervical tissue as seen with colposcopy to diagnose or rule out cervical cancer in its earliest stages. Conization is indicated if atypical squamous cells are found in cytology smears and colposcopy examinations. An *endometrial biopsy* is widely used to diagnose infertility problems and to detect uterine malignancies.

Techniques

Cervical tissues may be obtained by several methods. A *punch biopsy* is a technique in which a needle is inserted into tissue to remove a column of tissue when a lesion is clearly visible. This procedure is almost painless and is usually performed as an office procedure without anesthesia. If bleeding occurs after the biopsy, cauterization of the biopsy site with a silver nitrate stick will usually control bleeding. Cervical tissues can also be obtained by conization (see Figure 26.1). This procedure can be performed under local, regional, or general anesthesia in office or hospital settings. A colposcopy is used to visualize the lesion for the procedure. The size of the cone of tissue to be removed by a scalpel is determined by the extent of the lesion.

Endometrial biopsy is usually performed in an office or clinic setting and may or may not require anesthesia. The procedure is used to obtain a cytological specimen of endometrium with a curette or a suction device. If performed for infertility studies, the biopsy is scheduled for the last half of the menstrual cycle. It is done in the immediate premenstrual phase to evaluate menstrual disturbances and at any time for postmenopausal evaluations (Ignatavicius & Bayne, 1991).

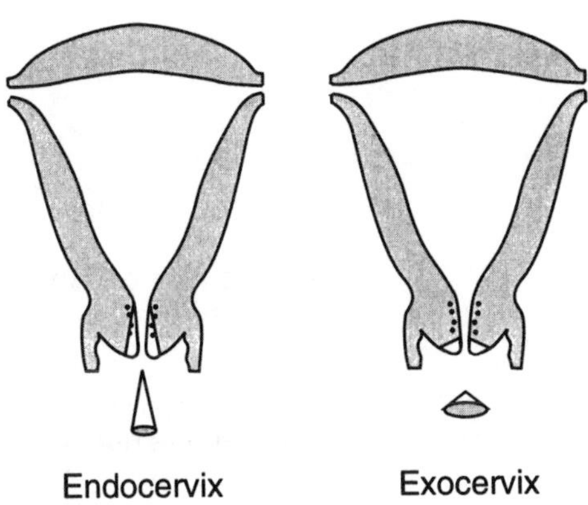

Figure 26.1. Conization Biopsy of the Endocervix and Exocervix

Complications

Secondary hemorrhage, cervical stenosis, and cervical infection can occur after cervical and endometrial procedures.

Nursing Care

The client should be informed about what to expect during the procedure and postoperatively. Women may be anxious before the procedure, especially if it is being done to evaluate a potential malignancy, and they may need time to express their feelings. During the procedure, use of relaxation and breathing techniques may relieve discomfort caused by uterine cramping.

Follow-up care instructions will vary with each procedure. After a conization, the client may have profuse or prolonged menstrual periods for several cycles. Bleeding that is more than a normal period for the client as well as signs of infection (fever, severe abdominal pain, foul-smelling vaginal discharge) should be reported. Douching, use of tampons, and sexual intercourse should be avoided until the biopsy site has healed (at least 1 week). After endometrial biopsy, the client should report any signs of infection or excessive bleeding to the physician and avoid sexual intercourse until bleeding has stopped.

Laparoscopy

Indications

Laparoscopy is a procedure by which the pelvic organs are visualized and examined by insertion of a laparoscope through the abdominal wall (Figure 26.2). Laparoscopy can be used instead of an exploratory laparotomy to diagnose endometriosis, malignancy, and ectopic pregnancy. It is invaluable for infertility evaluations in which tubal patency and ovulation need to be determined.

Technique

Although laparoscopy can be performed as an inpatient procedure, it is most often performed as an outpatient procedure. Short-acting general anesthesia or local or regional anesthetic agents may be used. Usually, clients can go home within 2 hours after surgery.

During the laparoscopic procedure, the client is placed in a modified Trendelenburg position. A small (2-3 cm) incision is made in the skin of the lower rim of the umbilicus. A needle attached to an insufflation apparatus is inserted. Carbon dioxide or nitrous oxide is used to distend the abdomen and separate the organs; the endoscope is then inserted into the incision for visualization. Often, a second instrument is inserted into an incision made in the area above the symphysis pubis to allow the surgeon to visualize the whole pelvic cavity and to perform operative procedures. After the surgery is completed, as much gas as possible is expelled from the peritoneal cavity. Clips or sutures are used to close the puncture sites.

Complications

Insufflation can cause pulmonary embolism or cardiac or respiratory problems. In addition, hemorrhage and infection are always risks. If electrocautery is used, burns to the abdominal and bowel tissue can occur, leading to necrosis and peritonitis (Herbst et al., 1992).

Nursing Care

Preoperatively, the client usually consumes nothing by mouth past midnight on the day of

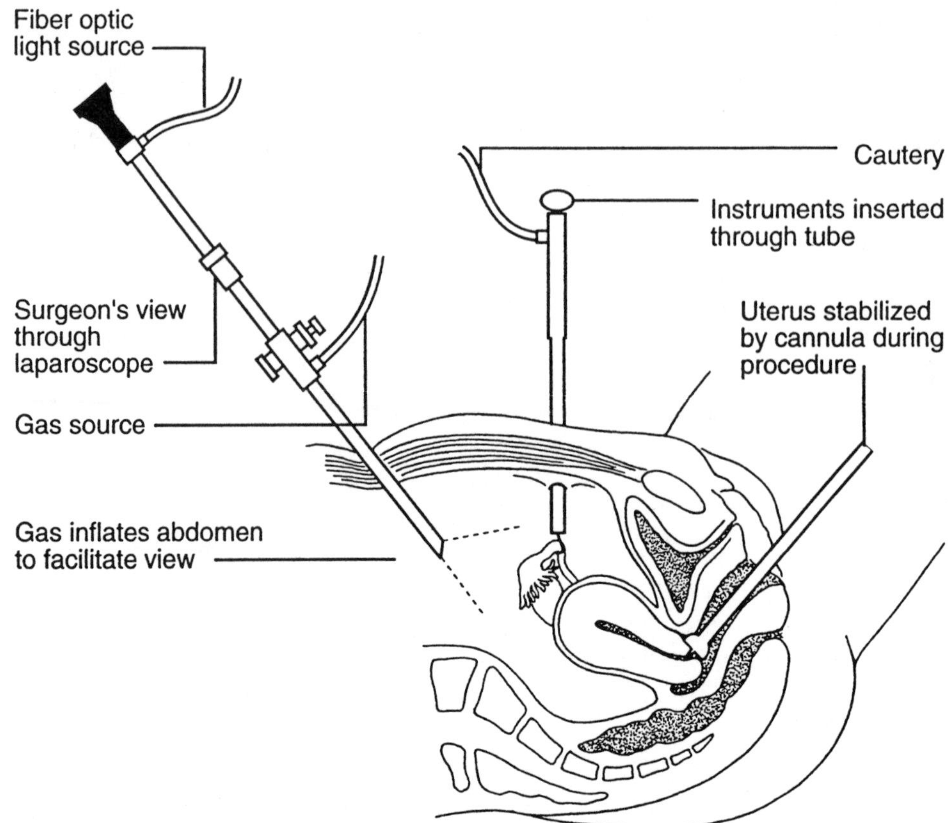

Figure 26.2. Laparoscopy

surgery. Postoperatively, the client's vital signs are usually taken frequently during the first hour or until they are stable. Prior to discharge, instructions should be given regarding convalescence. The client may have a sore throat from intubation and discomfort at the incision site; mild analgesics may alleviate the pain. The greatest discomfort will likely be from transient shoulder pain caused by residual gas in the peritoneal cavity. This will usually disappear within 48 hours. The client should observe the incision for signs of infection or bleeding, and the bandage over the incision should be changed as needed. If the client is concerned about body image, she should be informed that the incision scar will barely be noticeable. Showers are recommended over tub baths until the incision has healed. No heavy lifting or strenuous exercise should be done for at least 1 week after the surgery. Sexual intercourse is usually not restricted.

Tubal Surgery

Sterilization and infertility procedures are the primary reasons for tubal surgery, but surgery may also be performed for malignancy, infection, and tubal pregnancy.

Tubal Sterilization

Female sterilization is the most popular method of birth control for couples over the age of 35 in the United States and is reportedly the most widely used contraceptive method in the world (Hatcher et al., 1994). (See Chapter 14, "Fertility Control," for additional information on this topic.)

Methods and Selection of Procedures. Several techniques for tubal sterilization have been developed to interrupt ovum transport through

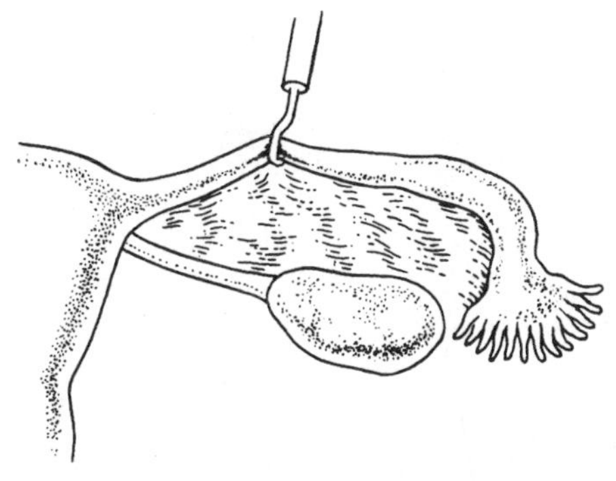

Figure 26.3a. Electrocauterization
Electrocauterization is used after the tube is located to seal it by "melting" the tissue. This procedure is almost 100% effective but also has a low potential for reversibility because of tissue destruction.

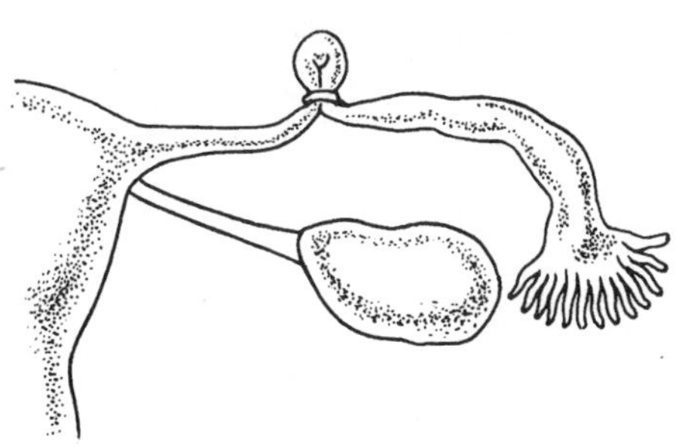

Figure 26.3b. Ring Technique
Plastic rings are placed around a loop of the tube to occlude it. Failure rates range from 2.9% to 11.2% but have approximately 90% success rate for reversibility (Rioux & Soderstrom, 1988; Saidi & Zainie, 1980).

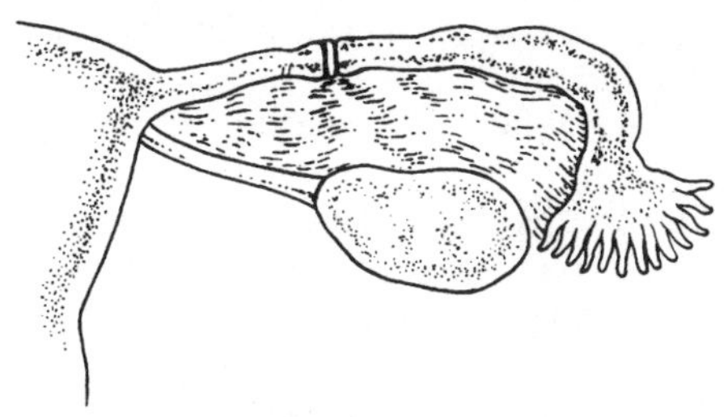

Figure 26.3c. Clip Technique
Clips are placed around the tube to occlude it. Failure rates and potential for reversibility are similar to those of the ring technique.

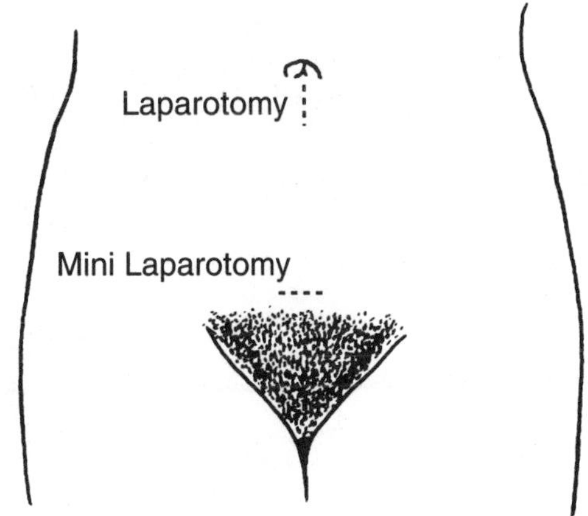

Figure 26.4. Laparotomy/Mini Laparotomy

the fallopian tube. The choice of technique depends on the woman's life situation and specific needs. For example, sterilization can be performed within 24 to 48 hours after a vaginal delivery or at the time of a cesarean delivery, after abortion, and as an interval procedure—that is, 6 weeks after a delivery, anytime between pregnancies, or anytime for women who have never been pregnant.

Sterilization can be performed abdominally or vaginally using traditional surgical techniques or endoscopic approaches. The most popular abdominal approach in the United States is the laparoscopic approach (see Figure 26.2) by electrocauterization (see Figure 26.3a), the most frequently used technique. Laparoscopic procedures are commonly performed as interval procedures and can be compared to vasectomy in terms of safety and efficacy (Rioux & Soderstrom, 1988). The failure rates (pregnancy) are low (0.1-0.2%), but because of tissue destruction, potential for reversibility is also low (Saidi & Zainie, 1980). Mechanical devices that obstruct the fallopian tubes, such as plastic clips or rings (see Figures 26.3b and 26.3c), can also be used with laparoscopy. Although these devices have a higher potential for reversibility (90%), failure rates are reportedly higher (2.9-11.2%) (Rioux & Soderstrom, 1988). Other abdominal approaches, such as the laparotomy (a subumbilical incision) or minilaparotomy (suprapubic incision), are more commonly performed after vaginal delivery (see Figure 26.4). Methods of tubal occlusion with these approaches usually involve ligation and/or resection of the fallopian tubes.

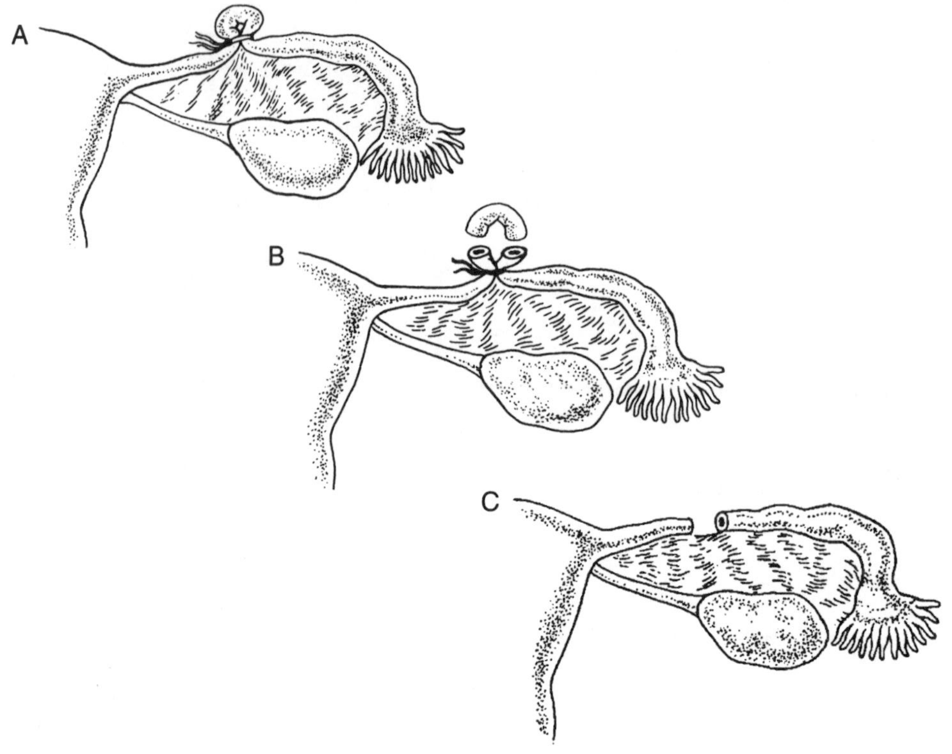

Figure 26.5a. Pomeroy Technique

The most popular postpartum method of tubal occlusion is the Pomeroy technique (see Figure 26.5a). With this method, a loop is formed in the midportion of the tube, which is ligated and resected. Infection and bleeding are the principal complications; however, the reported failure rate is less than 1% (Rioux & Soderstrom, 1988). Another abdominal occlusion method is the Irving technique (see Figure 26.5b), commonly used after a cesarean delivery. The fallopian tubes are cut in the isthmic portion and ligated (Frame A). The ends nearest the uterus are embedded in the uterine musculature and the distal ends are buried in the broad ligament (Frame B). This procedure is almost 100% effective (Rioux & Soderstrom, 1988). Fimbriectomy, removal of the fibriated end and ligation of the end of the tube (see Figure 26.5c), is another occlusion method, and it is almost totally irreversible.

Hysteroscopic techniques are also currently being used for sterilization. A hysteroscope (a viewing instrument similar to a laparoscope) is inserted vaginally through a dilated cervix into the uterus under local or regional anesthesia, and an occlusion technique such as electrocauterization is performed. Complications such as uterine perforation, bleeding, and cervical lacerations can occur. Nonsurgical methods of tubal sterilization via the hysteroscopic approach continue to be under investigation. Although not yet approved by the Food and Drug Administration (FDA), chemical blocking agents that cause necrosis and fibrosis of the tubes and silicone plugs that "block" the tubes are being used in investigational studies. The former are usually not reversible, but the latter have potential for reversibility because, theoretically, the plugs can be removed (Papera, 1990; Shuber, 1989).

Nursing Care. Recovery from sterilization procedures is usually fast. If local anesthesia is used and if the sterilization is performed in an outpatient setting, the client can usually go home within 1 to 2 hours, although she should not drive herself home. Postpartum hospitalization

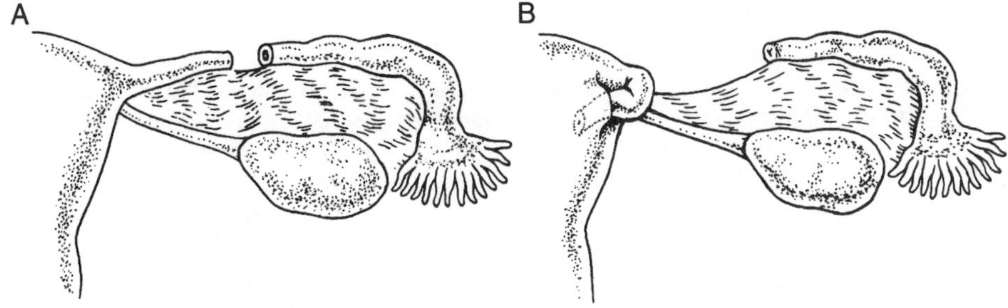

Figure 26.5b. Irving Technique

usually is prolonged by only a day. Most women can resume normal activities within 24 to 48 hours after surgery. Women should be taught to monitor for signs of infection at the incision site and to report abnormal signs, such as vaginal or incisional bleeding or severe abdominal pain. Signs of ectopic pregnancy (abdominal pain or vaginal bleeding) should also be taught, because this can also be a complication after tubal sterilization (Kjer & Knudsen, 1989). Mild analgesics are usually suggested to relieve postoperative pain.

Discharge instructions should include an explanation of the physical and emotional changes that may occur following sterilization. The woman should be informed that she will continue to menstruate and that the menstrual period may vary in length of cycle, duration of flow, or amount of flow. These changes will probably be mild, if present at all, and will seldom require treatment. Women continue to ovulate, and the ovum will be reabsorbed. There should be no physiological effect on hormones, weight, or sexual response.

Women should also be assessed postoperatively for psychological responses. Studies of women's responses after sterilization report that most women have no regrets after surgery. Many report increased sexual satisfaction because they are no longer worried about getting pregnant. Women who were awake and aware during the procedure have reported a positive psychological response and have attributed this feeling to being able to participate fully with the health care team and to being in control of themselves (Penfield, 1986). Those who expressed regrets were usually women who felt pressured to have surgery; who did not feel fully informed, especially about irreversibility; and those whose marital status changed or whose partners reacted negatively to the sterilization (Gonzales, 1983; Rioux & Soderstrom, 1987).

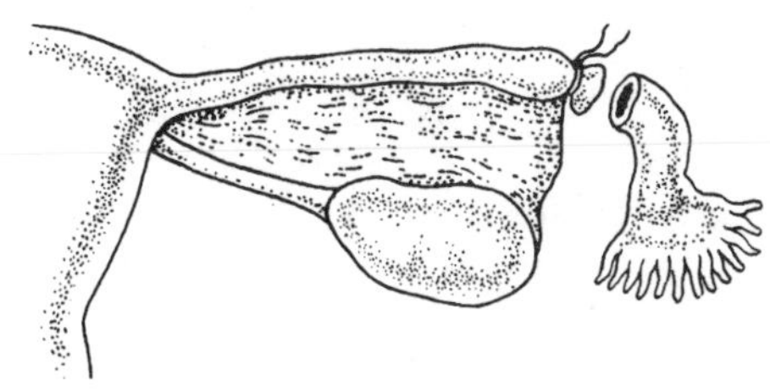

Figure 26.5c. Fimbriectomy

Salpingectomy

Salpingectomy is the removal of one or both fallopian tubes through laparoscopic or abdominal surgery. Reasons for this removal may include malignancy, pelvic inflammatory disease, and sepsis. Salpingectomy may be used as treatment for ruptured ectopic pregnancy, but salpingostomy (incision into the tube to remove its contents) is more likely to be performed because this will allow for the preservation of future fertility (Sloane, 1985). Salpingectomy is not recommended for sterilization because of its irreversibility (Saidi & Zainie, 1980).

Nursing care for clients having a salpingectomy is similar to care for those undergoing tubal sterilization.

Tuboplasty

Currently, there is an increased number of requests for tuboplasty or tubal reconstruction after sterilization. Most of these requests come from women who have been divorced and remarried and who desire to have a baby by their new spouse.

Death of a child, a change in lifestyle, and a change in economic status that allows for a larger family are other factors that motivate requests for reversal of sterilization (Rioux & Soderstrom, 1988). Additional information on this topic is found in Chapter 25, "Infertility."

The clip and ring techniques have a greater potential for successful reversibility (up to 90%) because these methods cause less interference with tubal blood supply than cauterization or ligation (Rioux & Soderstrom, 1988). Fibriectomy usually cannot be reversed. In general, the shorter the tube after reanastomosis, the smaller the chance of pregnancy. Reversal surgery may not be covered by insurance or federally funded medical care.

Another major reason for tuboplasty is for correction of infertility problems related to tubal occlusions. Microsurgery is a recent technique for both reversal of sterilization and tubal occlusions. During this procedure, the surgeon uses magnification and microsurgical techniques that allow exact alignment and approximation of the remaining portion of tubes to be reconstructed. Microsurgery appeared to offer the best opportunity for restoring tubal patency with reported rates of success of 60% to 80% (Penfield, 1983); however, more recent reports range from 10% to 90% (Papera, 1990). Microsurgery is reportedly less successful if the interval since sterilization is greater than 5 years (Dahl, Kjaer, Bagger, & Staheman, 1988). Reformation of adhesions after surgery also interferes with the success of surgery, and ectopic pregnancy may occur (Kjer & Knudsen, 1989).

Nursing care after tuboplasty is similar to care after sterilization.

Ovarian Surgery

Oophorectomy

Oophorectomy is the removal of one or both ovaries through an abdominal incision. Reasons for surgery may include ectopic pregnancy, ovarian cysts, pelvic inflammatory disease, and malignancy. Although the ovaries may be removed electively when a menopausal woman has a hysterectomy, removal of the ovaries as a routine procedure should be questioned for women of any age. One reason given for removal of ovaries in menopausal women is to prevent ovarian cancer, which affects about 1% of American women over the age of 50. Removal of ovaries in premenopausal women can contribute to increased incidence of osteoporosis and coronary heart disease (Sloane, 1985). Removal of healthy ovaries in premenopausal women is not recommended because hormone replacement therapy is inferior to natural hormone production (Herbst et al., 1992).

Surgical menopause occurs when both ovaries are removed in premenopausal women. Symptoms of surgical menopause may include hot flashes, vaginal atrophy, decreased libido, and decreased vaginal lubrication. These symptoms are often treated with estrogen replacement therapy. (See Chapter 5, "Midlife Women's Health," for discussion of hormonal replacement therapy.) Complications of oophorectomy include infection and hemorrhage. Clients should be informed of the risks and benefits of this therapy, as well as available alternatives, so that they can make informed decisions about accepting therapy.

Nursing care for the woman having an oophorectomy is similar to care of the client having tubal sterilization.

Uterine Surgery

Myomectomy and hysterectomy are the most common surgical procedures performed on the uterus.

Myomectomy

Leiomyomas, or uterine fibroids, are the most common benign tumors of women. They are more common in nulliparas. For women in their 40s and 50s, vaginal bleeding is usually the first sign of a fibroid. Symptoms vary with the size of the fibroid but usually include pain and discomfort, increased menstrual flow, or irregular bleeding. For women with small fibroids causing discomfort or infertility who want to maintain their childbearing potential, periodic evaluation of the fibroids or myomectomy (an incision into uterine muscle to remove myomas with preservation of the uterus) may be the treatment of choice. Often, fibroids will decrease in size after menopause, and surgical treatment may not be necessary if they are asymptomatic and do not increase in size (Myers, 1986). If surgery is needed, and the uterine size is no larger than that at 12 to 14 weeks gestation, myomectomy is usually recommended. However, early myomectomy may mean subsequent surgery because there is a 30% risk of recurrence of fibroids (Sanz & Hoyne, 1988; Smith & Uhlir, 1990). About 25% of all women having a myomectomy will subsequently have a hysterectomy (Herbst et al., 1992).

Myomectomy is usually a major surgical procedure with all the risks of such surgery. Preoperative preparations are similar to those of abdominal hysterectomy, if the abdominal approach is used, or to vaginal hysterectomy, if the vaginal approach is used. Surgery is usually performed in the proliferative phase (days 5-14) of the menstrual cycle to avoid the possibility of unsuspected pregnancy and to minimize blood loss. The procedure includes a skin incision (if abdominal), an incision into the uterus where the fibroids are located, removal of all fibroids, and reconstruction of the uterus without injury to the fallopian tubes and ovaries. Incision into the uterine cavity is avoided except if needed for removal of fibroids. If the uterine cavity is entered, cesarean delivery may be recommended in subsequent pregnancies to avoid the risk of uterine rupture. The pregnancy rate after myomectomy is approximately 50% (Sanz & Hoyne, 1988).

Laser surgery can also be used to destroy small fibroids using a laparoscopic or hysteroscopic approach. See "Laser Surgery for Gynecologic Problems" on page 640.

Postoperative nursing care after myomectomy is similar to care after hysterectomy. Postoperative hemorrhage is a significant problem because the incised uterus can bleed into the peritoneal cavity. A gonadotropin-releasing hormone agonist may be given to the client 6 to 8 weeks before surgery to decrease blood supply to the uterus, cause the fibroid(s) to atrophy, lessen blood loss, and shorten surgical time. The laser can also be used with surgery to improve hemostasis and decrease the occurrence of postoperative adhesions (Sanz & Hoyne, 1988; Smith & Uhlir, 1990).

Clients need counseling regarding the risks and benefits of myomectomy. As previously discussed, it is not a procedure that will benefit all women with fibroids, but it may be an alternative for those who want to maintain their fertility.

Hysterectomy

Health care professionals, consumer groups, government agencies, and third-party payers all have concerns about the number of hysterectomies performed in the United States. With the exception of procedures related to childbirth, it is the most frequently performed major surgery for all women (Horton, 1992). Of all hysterectomies performed, 65% are for women who are between 30 and 49 years old, with the average age being 43 years (Greenwood, 1988; National Center for Health Statistics, 1988).

As many as 30% to 40% of all hysterectomies performed may be unnecessary; for certain problems, alternative procedures may be better (Ammer, 1989; BWHC, 1992). However, there is a lack of agreement about what is necessary. The quality of the woman's life before and after surgery and the risks and benefits of having or not having the procedure need to be considered before judging whether a hysterectomy is necessary (Easterday, Grimes, & Riggs, 1983). Women need to know that there may be alternatives to hysterectomy, and they should consider getting a second opinion before making a decision to have surgery.

In spite of the adverse publicity and controversy, women are still having hysterectomies. Because the number of hysterectomies being performed is large, the nurse needs knowledge about the physiological and psychological changes that occur after the surgery so that comprehensive care can be given.

Indications

Although there is some disagreement among physicians about the absolute indications for hysterectomy, certain conditions are usually treated with this procedure. Usually, cancer of the uterine endometrium or ovary is treated with hysterectomy. Cancer of the cervix may be treated with hysterectomy; however, radiation therapy may be as effective (Herbst et al., 1992). If there is persistent bleeding or if no further childbearing is desired, abdominal hysterectomy may be performed for fibroid tumors that are larger than a 12- to 14-week gestation size (Smith & Uhlir, 1990).

Other conditions that may be treated by abdominal hysterectomy are chronic pelvic infections, life-threatening hemorrhage, and rupture of the uterus if suturing is not possible. Abdominal procedures are usually performed if the ovaries and fallopian tubes are to be removed or if the woman has had previous abdominal surgery.

Laser Surgery for Gynecologic Problems

Laser treatment for gynecologic problems has been used for over 10 years and is increasingly being used as an alternative to certain surgical procedures, including D & C, conization, cryosurgery, hysterectomy, and vulvectomy. It can be used to vaporize small fibroids, ovarian cysts, condylomas, and some ectopic pregnancies and treat pre-invasive cancer of the cervix and vulva (Lomano, 1988; Wilson, 1988).

Laser surgery converts energized light into heat to vaporize tissues and cause necrosis. The invisible, highly concentrated laser beam can be precisely focused through a laparoscope (abdominal) or hysteroscope (vaginal) for internal procedures or without these viewing devices for external procedures and is used as a "thermal" scalpel (Baggish, 1988).

Laser surgery can be performed on an inpatient or outpatient basis under local or general anesthesia. Cervical application may require no anesthesia, although clients may feel transient shoulder pain due to heat transfer during the procedure. Therefore, premedications such as nonsteroidal inflammatory drugs may be suggested.

Women who are interested in laser surgery as an alternative treatment need to be counseled regarding its risks and benefits. For example, fertility is conserved with vulvar procedures, but endometrial vaporization (ablation) for dysfunctional bleeding or endometriosis will cause uterine scarring and, likely, sterility. Therefore, if a woman wants to keep her childbearing function, laser surgery for these latter conditions may not be an option in place of D & C or other traditional procedures (Goldrath, 1990). Also, if laser therapy is used to treat dysfunctional bleeding, it may not be 100% effective, and additional treatment may be needed (Ball, 1988). Normal tissues can be destroyed during the procedure and hemorrhage can occur (Martin, 1990).

Nursing care after laser surgery will depend on the type of procedure done. If external genitalia were treated, the woman should be taught to keep the treated areas clean and dry and to wear loose underclothing. For all procedures, she should report signs of infection, such as fever higher than 100° F (38° C). If the cervix or vagina was treated, the woman should not douche, wear tampons, or have intercourse until healing has taken place (3 to 6 weeks) (Yandell, Dinh, & Hannigan, 1990). Most clients are discharged the day of surgery and can resume normal activities in 1 to 2 days. Analgesics or nonsteroidal inflammatory drugs may be prescribed for postoperative pain. Serosanguineous vaginal discharge may be present for 4 to 6 weeks after uterine ablation. Sitz baths or warm compresses may be suggested for vulvar surgery (Ball, 1988; Wright, 1990).

Indications for vaginal hysterectomy generally include uterine prolapse (which usually occurs in the older woman) and pelvic relaxation due to impaired bladder or rectal supports (common in multiparous women). It can also be used to remove fibroids, if only small fibroids are present, or to treat severe dysfunctional bleeding, although alternatives should be tried first (Ammer, 1989). Hysterectomy is usually not considered justifiable as a method of sterilization in women without pelvic pathology (Ammer, 1989; Herbst et al., 1992).

The woman must understand all options for treatment. Preoperative counseling should include information about whether the alternative procedures will be as beneficial as hysterectomy; information about hospital admission, the procedure, anesthesia, postoperative care, convalescence, and resumption of activities must also be provided. If the ovaries are to be removed, an explanation of surgical menopause and information about estrogen replacement therapy is warranted. Making sure the woman is fully informed about risks, benefits, and alternatives is a step toward eliminating unnecessary hysterectomies.

Techniques

When hysterectomy is indicated, it can be performed abdominally or vaginally; abdominal procedures account for 70% of all hysterecto-

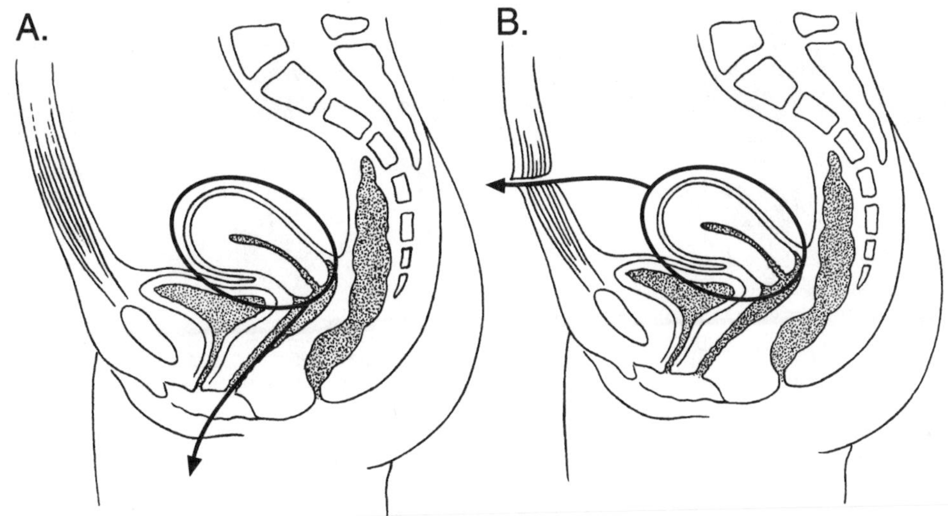

Figure 26.6a. Vaginal Hysterectomy
A. The uterus is removed through the vaginal opening, and the incision is internal.

Figure 26.6b. Abdominal Hysterectomy
B. The uterus is removed through an abdominal incision. If the tubes and ovaries are to be removed at the same time, usually this procedure is used.

mies. In both the vaginal hysterectomy (see Figure 26.6a) and the abdominal hysterectomy (see Figure 26.6b) the procedure consists of removing the uterus from its supporting ligaments. These ligaments (broad, round, and uterosacral) are attached to the vaginal cuff so that normal depth of the vagina is maintained.

Total hysterectomies (removal of the entire uterus) (Figure 26.7a) account for more than 95% of all procedures. Subtotal hysterectomy, in which the cervix is not removed, is rarely performed because of the high risk of cervical cancer. In a radical hysterectomy, the lymph nodes are dissected and may be removed along with the upper third of the vagina and the parametrium. This procedure may be done if malignancy is present (Ignatavicius & Bayne, 1991). Panhysterectomy (Figure 26.7b), or total abdominal hysterectomy with bilateral salpingo-oophorectomy, refers to the removal of the uterus, fallopian tubes, and ovaries and is often seen abbreviated as "TAH-BSO" in client charts. The ovaries are not usually removed in premenopausal women because oophorectomy causes surgical castration and menopause (Clarke-Pearson & Dawood, 1990).

Anterior and Posterior Repairs

As noted earlier, uterine prolapse and pelvic relaxation are two major indications for vaginal hysterectomy. Repair of the anterior and posterior vaginal walls is included when there is displacement of one or more of the pelvic organs, including urethra, bladder, uterus, and rectum. Displacement of these organs usually results from weakening of the pelvic supporting structures by repeated childbearing, obstetric injury, or age. At least 40% of all pelvic relaxation problems are seen in women over the age of 60 (Nichols, 1990). Complaints include a heaviness in the pelvis and a bearing-down sensation. There is a strong familial history of these disorders, and they are seen more frequently in whites than blacks. Obesity increases the symptoms (Ignatavicius & Bayne, 1991).

A specific complaint related to weakening of bladder support is loss of urine whenever there is increased intra-abdominal pressure, such as that produced by laughing or coughing (stress urinary incontinence). Weakening of the rectal wall causes constipation and difficult defecation. These symptoms are distressing and women are often embarrassed to describe them to their physician. An alert nurse can assess these problems during history taking and physical examination.

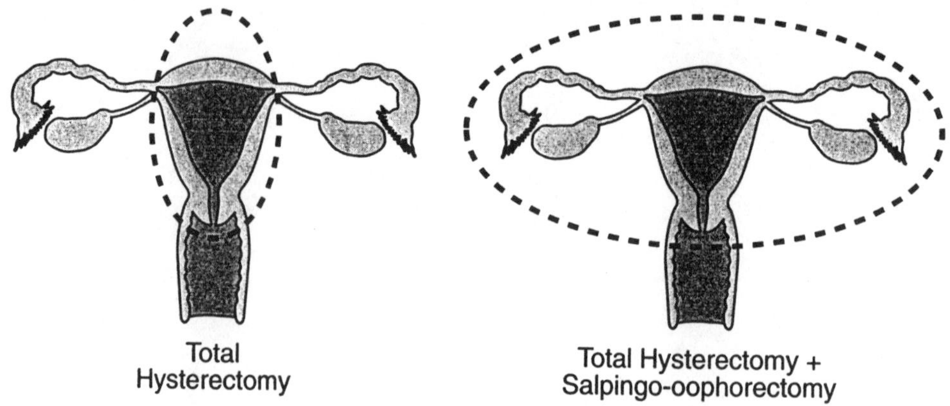

Figure 26.7 Total Hysterectomy Versus Total Hysterectomy Plus Salpingo-Oophorectomy
In the total hysterectomy, the total uterus and nothing else is removed. In the total hysterectomy plus bilateral salpingo-oophorectomy (TAH-BSO), the uterus, both tubes, and ovaries are removed.

An anterior colporrhaphy or anterior repair can tighten up the pelvic muscles for better bladder support. Alternatives to surgery for mild cases of stress urinary incontinence include use of Kegel exercises to increase pelvic tone, use of vaginal tampons or pessaries to support the bladder neck, and weight reduction in obese women.

A posterior colporrhaphy or posterior repair can correct rectal displacement, strengthen pelvic supports, and reduce bulging. Alternatives to surgery for these conditions focus on promoting bowel elimination through high-fiber diets, stool softeners, or laxatives. Fecal incontinence is relieved only by surgical repair (Nichols & Randall, 1989; Richardson & Ostergard, 1988).

Nursing Care

Preoperative Assessment. The nurse is often responsible for physiological and psychological preparation of the preoperative hysterectomy patient. Women may have concerns about surgery in general as well as hysterectomy in particular. Concerns specifically related to hysterectomy depend on the significance of the uterus for the woman. Hysterectomy can be a threat to self-image in several ways. Body image is affected whenever there is a loss of a body part—even though there is no outward change in appearance with hysterectomy, the loss may be felt strongly by the woman.

Many women have misconceptions about the effects of hysterectomy—for example, that it is associated with masculinization, weight gain, and accelerated aging. Hysterectomy can also be a threat to femininity, especially in cultures in which women's roles are primarily childbearing and motherhood. Since the 1970s, the importance of these roles in the United States has decreased as women have developed other rewarding roles, such as careers (Drummond & Field, 1984; Kaltrieder, Wallace, & Horowitz, 1979; Kruger et al., 1979; Roeske, 1978).

Physical assessment in the preoperative period includes finding out a woman's knowledge of pre- and postoperative procedures. A general guide for preoperative preparation for hysterectomy includes the following (Faro, 1989; Disaia & Walker, 1990; Nichols & Randall, 1989):

- Signed consent: The nurse should make sure that this is informed consent.
- Laboratory work: complete blood count, hematocrit, type and cross match of blood, urinalysis, chest X ray, electrocardiogram
- Vaginal examination or complete physical examination
- Surgical preparation: abdominal mons or perineal shave if ordered
- NPO (nothing by mouth or *nil per os*) past midnight
- Empty bladder immediately prior to surgery
- Preoperative medication and intravenous fluids
- No makeup or nail polish
- Removal of glasses, dentures, and so on
- Identification band in place
- Prophylactic antibiotics that may be given for patients at high risk for complications

- Teaching postoperative care such as turning, coughing, and deep breathing

Preoperative care should also include a psychological assessment: The nurse may particularly be alert for a grief reaction. The woman's initial response may be shock and disbelief or denial, especially if the hysterectomy is to be performed as an emergency procedure. The woman may react angrily to having an intrusive procedure that will result in physical loss of child-bearing potential or a conceptual loss, such as loss of femininity. Depression can occur preoperatively if the woman is reminded of her impending loss through an encounter with a pregnant woman or if she is worried about losing her attractiveness (Stanfill, 1982).

Psychological assessment also includes an assessment of the significance of the loss to the individual woman. Some women will be relieved by loss of menses, especially if bleeding is a problem; others will be sad if menses is seen as a sign of youth or as a cleansing process. In addition, impaired sexual function can occur in women who feel that their sexuality is dependent on the presence of the uterus (Lalinec-Michaud & Engelsmann, 1984). Assessment of the woman's support system is also needed because some women fear rejection by their husbands or significant others.

Postoperative Assessment. Postoperative assessment begins in the operating room immediately after surgery and continues until convalescence is complete. Physiological care after abdominal hysterectomy is similar to other abdominal surgery postoperative care. Usual interventions for both vaginal and abdominal hysterectomy clients include monitoring vital signs every 15 minutes until stable and then every 4 hours for at least 48 hours. Maintaining an unobstructed airway is critical. Turning, coughing, and deep breathing should be performed at frequent intervals (every 2 hours) for the first 24 hours. After abdominal hysterectomy, assisting the woman to splint her abdomen with her hands or a pillow as she coughs may be helpful. Incentive spirometry may also be ordered.

Stimulating circulation with leg exercises (passive or active) is also done. Administration of heparin or antiembolism stockings may be ordered until the woman is ambulating satisfactorily. These measures will help prevent thrombophlebitis. All patients should be observed for signs of bleeding that can lead to hemorrhage. This is accomplished by assessing the amount of drainage on the abdominal dressing and/or perineal pads. Vaginal bleeding is usually minimal, but a saturated pad in 1 hour should be reported to the physician. A drop in blood pressure, signs of shock, or a decrease in hematocrit or hemoglobin may also indicate bleeding.

When assessing for pain relief, the type of surgery and individual tolerance for pain need to be considered. Analgesics (narcotics) are usually ordered every 3 to 4 hours for the first 24 hours. Patient-controlled analgesia (PCA) or epidural narcotics are also used (Disaia & Walker, 1990). As discomfort lessens, the amount and strength of medication is reduced. Nursing measures for pain relief should be used with, or as alternatives to, medications. These may include use of breathing and relaxation techniques, position changes, guided imagery, and back rubs. Ambulation or application of heat to the abdomen may relieve discomfort produced by intestinal gas. Warm sitz baths, ice packs, or heat lamps may relieve pain after vaginal hysterectomy.

Fluid intake should be carefully monitored. Intravenous fluids and ice chips or clear liquids are given after surgery. Maintenance needs as well as replacement of lost fluids are important. Urinary output should be monitored accurately to assess achievement of fluid balance. Foley catheters are usually discontinued after 24 hours or sooner. After surgery for prolapse with repairs, retention of urine is a problem and, often, a catheter (foley or suprapubic) must be left in place for 7 days. These clients are at risk for urinary infections and may be given prophylactic antibacterial or antibiotic medications (Nichols & Randall, 1989). Bowel sounds and function are also monitored. Stool softeners or mild laxatives are usually not needed unless posterior repair has been done. Enemas are usually not given unless laxative treatment is ineffective.

Early ambulation is encouraged because it improves circulation, muscle tone, lung expansion, and bowel function. Clients are usually encouraged to get out of bed by at least the first postoperative day. Ambulation may be delayed if the woman has had extensive surgery or if her condition warrants bed rest. The woman may need to be assisted to get out of bed without straining. To do this, the woman is told to roll on her side, bring her knees up so that her thighs are at right angles to the abdomen, put her feet over the side of the bed, push up on her elbow, and sit up.

Diet usually progresses from clear liquids to solid foods as tolerated. Sugar in foods, milk products, and carbonated beverages tends to cause gas production and may need to be kept at a minimum if the client is experiencing problems with intestinal gas.

Assessing abdominal and vaginal incisions is another important nursing function following hysterectomy. When dressings are removed, the incision is assessed for intactness and signs of infection. Clips or sutures are usually removed by the fourth postoperative day. Superficial drains (Hemovacs) may be present the first 24 to 48 hours. With vaginal hysterectomy, sutures are usually absorbable. Vaginal packing may be used to control bleeding and hematoma formation in the first 24 to 48 hours. The vagina is assessed for signs of infection or hemorrhage.

The nurse should be aware of the woman who is at risk for postoperative complications. Women over 65 are at risk for all complications. Obese women are at risk especially for thrombophlebitis. Women who have a history of medical problems such as diabetes or cardiac or pulmonary problems are at a higher risk for complications (Disaia & Walker, 1990; Graber & Feldman, 1988; Nichols & Randall, 1989). Complications associated with hysterectomy include the following (Clarke-Pearson & Dawood, 1990):

- Hemorrhage: Hemorrhage may be early (within 24 hours) or late (10 to 30 days postoperatively) and internal or external. Hemorrhage is more frequently seen with vaginal hysterectomy.
- Urinary tract complications: Urinary tract infections, such as cystitis or pyelitis, or urinary retention occur more frequently with vaginal hysterectomies and may not appear for up to 6 months after surgery.
- Infection: Wound infection is more frequent after vaginal hysterectomy. An elevated temperature (100° F or 38° C) is often the first sign, with redness and swelling of the wound area also noted.
- Intestinal obstruction or paralytic ileus: Intestinal complications are more common after abdominal hysterectomy. The chief symptoms are constipation and vomiting, followed by abdominal distention. Bowel sounds are absent with paralytic ileus.
- Thromboembolism: Thromboembolism is a late complication involving the deep veins of the lower extremities and is more common after abdominal hysterectomy. Preventive measures as previously described are the best treatment. Bed rest with the leg(s) elevated is also implemented.
- Pulmonary complications: Pulmonary complications occur more often after abdominal hysterectomy, and atelectasis is the most common problem.
- Evisceration: Wound dehiscence occurs more often after abdominal hysterectomy. Secondary closure of the wound may be required.

Psychosexual Assessments. The nurse should continue psychosexual assessments during the postoperative period to identify problems and intervene appropriately. An association between loss of the uterus and psychological problems has been posed for hundreds of years. Although there is controversy about whether hysterectomy is the cause of these reactions, nurses working with women who undergo hysterectomy need to know what responses research studies have attributed to the surgery and the factors affecting these responses.

Early studies found depression to be the most frequently reported symptom after hysterectomy, with 4% to 23% of all clients reporting this complaint; occurrences of these reactions range from 3 months to 5 years after surgery has taken place (Barker, 1968; Chynoweth, 1973; Lindemann, 1941; Melody, 1962; Richards, 1973). In the 1970s, the term *posthysterectomy syndrome* was coined by Richards (1974) after he observed that more women complained of depression after hysterectomy than after any other type of abdominal surgery. He also noted that many women who have had hysterectomies also had symptoms of hot flashes, headaches, insomnia, fatigue, or urinary symptoms and that estrogen replacement often alleviated these symptoms in women who also had bilateral oophorectomy. Because many of the studies reporting depression after hysterectomy have not considered ovarian status postoperatively, it is difficult to attribute adverse psychological reactions solely to hysterectomy (Bachmann, 1990).

Women who have been reported to experience psychosexual problems following hysterectomy are (a) those who have a preoperative history of depression, other psychological disturbances, or sexual dysfunction; (b) those under 35 to 40 years of age with limited educational attainment who are uncertain about future childbearing; (c) those who have misunderstandings or misconceptions about the surgery and its outcome; (d) those who believe the uterus has unique significance to their self-concept and/or sexual functioning; and (e) those who do not have pelvic malignancy (Barker, 1968; Drummond & Field, 1984; Green, 1973; Humphries, 1980; Lalinec-Michaud & Engelsmann, 1985; Roeske, 1978; Salter, 1985; Sloan, 1978).

There are studies that do not demonstrate an increase in psychological problems after hysterectomy. Furthermore, these studies indicate that women feel better postoperatively if the surgery has eliminated a preoperative condition (bleeding, pain, cancer, etc.); others report relief at ending the need to use contraceptives (Coppen & Bishop, 1981; Salter, 1985).

There is no consensus as to whether hysterectomy causes sexual dysfunction. The incidence of sexual problems after hysterectomy ranges from 10% to 40%, but most studies report either no change or an improvement in sexual function (Bachmann, 1990). Factors proposed to explain the increase in sexual desire include absence of fear of pregnancy and absence of the pain related to the condition requiring hysterectomy; decrease in desire has been related to fear of postoperative pain related to vaginal shrinkage and decreased lubrication and lack of desire for recreational sex (rather than for procreation), particularly among women who associate sex with reproductive function (Drummond & Field, 1984).

Sexual dysfunction seems to be more prevalent in women who have declining ovarian hormone function postoperatively, possibly related to decreased vaginal lubrication. Although effects of hysterectomy can contribute to dyspareunia, decreased libido and absent or decreased orgasm are not agreed-upon effects (Coppen & Bishop, 1981; Zussman, Zussman, Sunley, & Bjornson, 1981). Emotional distress can also cause sexual dysfunction (Anderson, 1987).

The nurse must take time to inform the woman privately about the possible psychological reactions. The client should be encouraged to express her feelings about the surgery. Partners may be included in these discussions if both the woman and partner agree. Use of support groups as previously discussed can also provide women with opportunities to share their surgical experiences and express their feelings and concerns. Incidence of psychological reactions often decrease after counseling and teaching sessions (Drummond & Field, 1984).

Specific information about sexual functioning after hysterectomy and repair surgery may need to be provided to assist women and their partners in resuming sexual activity but there is no one best approach to this counseling. Male sexual partners may have concerns or misconceptions about sexual functioning with a woman who has had a hysterectomy. Often, it is important to include the husband or sexual partner in discussions about sexual functioning, but in other instances, classes for men only or provision of information in written format suffice (Drummond & Field, 1984; Dulaney, Crawford, & Turner, 1990).

In general, nursing interventions after hysterectomy include providing or reinforcing information about the reproductive system and what it means to have part of it removed surgically. Humphries (1980) suggests a preoperative assessment of a woman's sexual behavior to determine postoperative needs. Specific information that may assist the woman in sexual adjustment after hysterectomy includes the following:

- Sexual intercourse is usually restricted after abdominal hysterectomy for 4 to 6 weeks; however, it may be several months before the woman is comfortable due to abdominal soreness and a temporary shrinkage of the vagina, which makes it feel narrow and short. Reassuring the couple that coitus will help stretch the vagina is a necessary support measure.
- Decreased sexual response may be caused by both hormonal (if ovaries are removed) and anatomical changes (Zussman et al., 1981). As many as one third of women having hysterectomies report decreased orgasm and excitement related to absence of cervical stimulation and decreased pelvic congestion (Greenwood, 1988).
- Use of foreplay to arouse the woman before penile penetration may be helpful. Also, use of water-soluble lubricants may be helpful for a dry vagina (Shell, 1990).
- If the abdomen is tender, positions other than those with the male on top may be more comfortable.
- Intercourse after vaginal hysterectomy may be painful at first, especially if anterior or posterior repair surgery was performed. Sexual functioning is poorly preserved after repair surgery because of narrowing and shortening of the vagina, resulting in stenosis. Resumption of intercourse within 6 weeks will help keep stenosis to a minimum. Use of dilators and lubricants may also relieve some vaginal tightness.

Discharge Teaching and Follow-Up. Preparation for home care should begin in the early postoperative period. The woman may be discharged as early as the day of surgery if she has had a vaginal hysterectomy in an ambulatory care facility, or in 3 days if she has had abdominal surgery and has not developed complications.

The nurse should be aware of the information needs of the woman postoperatively. The physician is responsible for providing the client with information relevant to recovery, both physically and emotionally, and the nurse should be available to answer or clarify questions as needed.

Clients should be reminded that following hysterectomy, weakness and fatigue are normal and that they will no longer menstruate and can no longer become pregnant. They should be reassured that masculinization, weight gain, and so on are merely old wives' tales. The possibility that they may have phantom pains (uterine cramping) should be mentioned. Numbness around the incision site will be present after an abdominal hysterectomy, and some women will experience a temporary loss of vaginal sensation after vaginal hysterectomy.

Women are cautioned to increase physical activities and exercise. No active sports (e.g., tennis, jogging, aerobics) should be undertaken for 1 month. Heavy housework (vacuuming, hanging out clothes, picking up objects weighing more than 10-25 pounds) should be deferred at least 1 month. Driving may be resumed about 2 weeks after discharge (some sources allow driving earlier, but many suggest delaying the activity for longer than 2 weeks). Women are cautioned to avoid sitting for long periods because this can cause pelvic congestion. They can resume their usual diet when they feel ready to do so; however, foods high in protein, iron, and vitamin C are encouraged because they promote healing and repair of tissues. Increasing intake of fluids and foods that are high in fiber may be helpful if constipation is a problem. Although showers and washing the hair are not restricted, tub baths may be restricted after abdominal hysterectomy because the difficulty of getting into the tub can cause strain on the sutures.

Sexual intercourse may be resumed in 4 to 6 weeks, depending on degree of comfort, healing, and desire. Suggestions such as those previously described can be given to assist in sexual adjustment after surgery. A postoperative checkup may be suggested as early as 1 week, with a follow-up checkup scheduled 1 month to 6 weeks after discharge (Nichols & Randall, 1989).

If ovaries are removed in premenopausal women, they will experience surgical menopause; estrogen therapy may be prescribed in these cases. (See Chapter 5 for information on hormonal replacement therapy.)

Signs of physical complications should also be reviewed because these can occur after discharge, especially infection, hemorrhage, and bladder problems.

Review of emotional reactions, especially depression, that can occur need to be included in discharge teaching because reactions can occur 3 months to 3 years after surgery. Women who are identified at high risk for psychological problems may need long-term follow-up or referral to a community agency or support group.

Extensive Gynecologic Surgery

Extensive gynecologic surgical procedures, such as vulvectomy and pelvic exenteration, are usually reserved for treatment of reproductive malignancies.

Vulvectomy

Carcinoma in situ (CIS) or pre-invasive cancer of the vulva can be treated with one of the following surgical procedures, although laser surgery may be used for premalignant lesions. A local wide excision may be used to remove abnormal tissue, or a simple vulvectomy may be used to remove the vulva, labia majora and minora, and possibly the clitoris; the latter procedure is not often performed for CIS because it is disfiguring (scarring, loss of pubic hair, etc.). Instead, a "skinning" vulvectomy may be performed; this includes removal of the superficial vulvar skin without clitoral removal following skin graft replacement. This procedure is less disfiguring and causes fewer effects on sexual functioning (Ignatavicius & Bayne, 1991). More radical procedures are performed for invasive cancer of the vulva. A radical vulvectomy is the removal of the entire vulva, including skin, labia, clitoris, subcutaneous tissues, and possibly inguinal and femoral nodes.

Preoperatively, a woman needs extensive explanation of the procedure she is undergoing, information about whether alternatives are possible, encouragement to talk about her fears and concerns about adjustment to physical changes and sexual functioning, and information about pre- and postoperative procedures. Specific preoperative procedures may include a mons or perineal skin shave, enema, and douche.

Postoperative interventions may include care of suction drains to the wound for 7 to 10 days, use of an indwelling bladder catheter for urinary drainage to prevent urethral stenosis and wound contamination, and frequent, meticulous wound care. Wound care is usually done with a solution of one-half strength hydrogen peroxide followed by a rinse with normal saline. Both solutions may be applied with a large bulb syringe or an automatic irrigating device such as a water pic. The wound is dried with either application of a heat lamp or use of a hair dryer on cool setting. Analgesics are usually ordered for postoperative pain and as premedication for wound care. Wound infection and breakdown occur in almost 50% of clients after radical vulvectomy; subsequently, healing may take as long as 6 months (Ignatavicius & Bayne, 1991; Rostad, 1988).

If radical surgery is performed, women may experience discomfort in everyday situations. Sitting for long periods will be uncomfortable due to the loss of perineal fatty tissue. Chronic edema of lower extremities after lymph node dissection can continue for years and may cause problems with mobility. Many women have problems controlling urine flow after surgery if the urethra has been removed or reconstructed. Using a funnel or standing up while voiding are techniques women have used with varying degrees of success for this problem (Shell, 1990).

If a radical vulvectomy is performed, clitoral removal may mean loss of orgasm; dyspareunia can occur due to loss of part of the vagina and introital stenosis (Jenkins, 1988; Wabrek & Gunn, 1984). The woman and her partner can be counseled to include alternative measures of giving and receiving sexual pleasure, such as breast stimulation. Vaginal dilators can be used to stretch the remaining vaginal tissues, and water-soluble lubricants and using a side-lying or woman on top position can decrease discomforts of intercourse. Use of Kegel exercises can increase perineal muscle tone (Shell, 1990). The woman may need to be encouraged to express her feelings about loss of normal sexual function.

A vulvectomy may affect the woman's self-image. The sudden disfigurement may cause a negative body image or low self-esteem. She may fear rejection by her sexual partner or other significant persons and may withdraw from intimate relationships (Dozier, 1986). Women and their significant others may need counseling and encouragement to express their fears and concerns. The nurse can use knowledge of the client's beliefs about feminine roles and sexual practices to identify appropriate interventions.

Pelvic Exenteration

Pelvic exenteration is one of the most radical surgical procedures performed. It is performed for recurrent cancer of the cervix and some vaginal and vulvar lesions (but only when the tumor is confined to the pelvis and there is no lymph node involvement) (Lawhead, Clark, Smith, Pierce, & Lewis, 1989). Exenteration procedures can include the anterior, posterior, or whole pelvis. Anterior exenteration includes the removal of the uterus, ovaries, fallopian tubes, vagina, bladder, urethra, and pelvic lymph nodes; an ileal conduit is created for urinary diversion. Posterior exenteration includes the removal of the uterus, ovaries, fallopian tubes, descending colon, rectum, and anal canal; a colostomy is created for passage of feces. A total exenteration includes removal of all pelvic organs with creation of both ileal conduit and colostomy.

Preoperative nursing measures include providing the woman with information about physical preparation, postoperative care, and recovery. Specific attention is given to assessing psychological readiness for surgery, including exploration of fears and concerns about surgery, death, and changes in body image and evaluation of support systems. Sexual assessment is critical because of the potential impact of surgery on sexual functioning related to alterations in excretory function and removal of the vagina. Vaginal reconstruction may be possible, and discussion is needed about this option. Significant others need to be involved in discussions when possible, because their reactions are critical for postoperative adjustment (Dozier, 1986; Shell, 1990).

Preoperative physical preparation begins with extensive tests to rule out spread of cancer outside the pelvis. Extensive bowel preparation (enemas) is performed, and stoma sites are selected. Information is given to the woman regarding immediate postoperative recovery care because this recovery takes place in an intensive care setting. She is also told what to expect with regard to pain management and invasive procedures (for example, nasogastric suctioning, intravenous lines, arterial catheters) (Ignatavicius & Bayne, 1991).

Postoperative nursing care immediately following surgery focuses on stabilizing the client and assessing for complications. Because of the extent of surgery, the woman is at risk for cardiovascular complications such as shock and hemorrhage; pulmonary complications, such as atelectasis and pneumonia, and fluid and electrolyte imbalance; and urinary complications (Ignatavicius & Bayne, 1991). After the client is stabilized, she returns to the gynecologic/surgical unit for continued postoperative care. Assessments are made for pain, infection, deep vein thrombosis, pulmonary embolus, paralytic ileus or other gastrointestional complications, and wound dehiscence (Ignatavicius & Bayne, 1991). Care of the ileal conduit and colostomy is initiated, as is wound care. The wound is usually cleaned with a solution of one half hydrogen peroxide and one half normal saline applied with a large bulb syringe. After cleaning, the wound is dried with a heat lamp or hair dryer on cool setting. Sitz baths may also be used.

After a hospital stay of several weeks, the client may be discharged to home or to an extended-care facility, depending on her rate of recovery and need for nursing care. The woman will need assistance at home, because she will not be able to do any strenuous activities for up to 6 months. She will need to be taught colostomy and ureterostomy care or have family members who are willing to assist with care. She will also require information regarding (a) diet, including foods that promote healing as well as foods that can be tolerated; (b) perineal care; (c) range of motion exercises and physical activities that are permitted by the physician; (d) signs of complications, such as infection or bowel obstruction; and (e) the importance of follow-up care.

Psychosocial adjustment is an integral part of postoperative recovery and adaptation to an altered body image. Usually, the woman expresses grief about her mutilated body. Initially, she may refuse to look at the wound or stoma sites as a form of denial. She may then become angry, hostile, or depressed and withdrawn. As she accepts the changes in her body, she will become active in self-care.

Pelvic exenteration patients will experience sexual disruption. If vaginal reconstruction is not done after anterior or total exenteration, the woman will not be able to have vaginal intercourse. Even with reconstruction surgery, women report decreased vaginal sensation of penile enclosure, increased chronic discharge, or say the neovagina is too large or too short. Often a waiting period of 12 to 18 months before resumption of sexual intercourse is advised to allow for healing. Another concern is that the presence of a colostomy or ureterostomy may cause odor or leakage during sexual activities. The bags can be emptied prior to engaging in sexual activity to decrease the chance of an accident. The client may also be worried about her altered physical appearance. Information about alternative techniques and options for sexual expression may need to be offered. These include touching and fondling other sensitive areas such as breasts and buttocks and bringing their partner to orgasm with hand or mouth stimulation (Dozier, 1986; Shell, 1990). Open communication between partners is essential in resolving problems related to sexual expression, and couples may need further sexual counseling to help promote this communication.

Summary and Implications for Research

This chapter has attempted to provide the nurse with a broad knowledge base to use with gynecologic clients, focusing specifically on the areas of preventive teaching and counseling, technical nursing skills, and restorative physiological and psychological care. More research is needed in the area of gynecologic nursing; the focus of this research should be on identifying nursing interventions that are effective and on ways to promote preventive health practices. Specific research needs include (a) identification of interventions that are effective in preventing problems related to pelvic supports, such as pelvic exercises; (b) identification of interventions that prevent psychological complications after hysterectomy; and (c) identification of effective nonpharmacologic or nutritional interventions for menopausal symptoms.

References

Adams, B. N. (1986). The middle years woman: Education for health and promotion. In V. M. Littlefield (Ed.), *Health education for women: A guide for nurses and other health professionals* (pp. 323-344). Norwalk, CT: Appleton-Century-Crofts.

Ammer, C. (1989). *The new A-to-Z of women's health.* New York: Facts on File.

Anderson, B. (1987). Sexual functioning complications in women with gynecologic cancer: Outcomes and directions for prevention. *Cancer, 60,* 2123-2128.

Bachmann, G. A. (1990). Psychosexual aspects of hysterectomy. *Women's Health Issues, 1*(1), 41-49.

Baggish, M. S. (1988). Intra-abdominal laser applications. In L. E. Sanz (Ed.), *Gynecologic surgery* (pp. 343-351). Oradell, NJ: Medical Economics Books.

Ball, K. A. (1988). Laser endometrial ablation treatment of dysfunctional uterine bleeding. *AORN Journal, 48*(6), 1153-1164.

Barker, M. G. (1968, April). Psychiatric illness after hysterectomy. *British Medical Journal,* pp. 91-95.

Boston Women's Health Collective. (1992). *The new our bodies, ourselves.* New York: Simon & Schuster.

Chapin, D. S. (1988). Preoperative counseling. In E. A. Friedman, M. Borton, & D. S. Chapin (Eds.), *Gynecological decision-making* (2nd ed., pp. 228-229). Toronto: B. D. Decker.

Chynoweth, R. (1973, June). Psychological complications of hysterectomy. *Australian and New Zealand Journal of Psychiatry,* pp. 102-104.

Clarke-Pearson, D., & Dawood, M. J. (1990). *Greene's gynecology: Essentials of clinical practice* (4th ed.). Boston: Little, Brown.

Coppen, A., & Bishop, M. (1981). Hysterectomy, hormones and behaviour: A prospective study. *Lancet, 1,* 126-128.

Dahl, C., Kjaer, S., Bagger, P., & Staheman, G. (1988). Microsurgical reversal of female sterilization. *Acta Obstetricia et Gynecologia Scandinavica, 67,* 223-224.

Disaia, P. J., & Walker, J. L. (1990). Perioperative care. In J. R. Scott, P. J. Disaia, C. B. Hammond, & W. N. Spellacy (Eds.), *Danforth's obstetrics and gynecology* (6th ed., pp. 875-885). Philadelphia: W. B. Saunders.

Dozier, A. M. (1986). Extensive gynecologic surgery. In V. M. Littlefield (Ed.), *Health education for women: A guide for nurses and other health professionals* (pp. 503-546). Norwalk, CT: Appleton-Century-Crofts.

Drummond, J., & Field, P. (1984). Emotional and sexual sequelae following hysterectomy. *Health Care for Women International, 5,* 261-271.

Dulaney, P. E., Crawford, V. C., & Turner, G. (1990). A comprehensive education and support program for women experiencing hysterectomies. *JOGNN, 19,* 319-329.

Easterday, C. L., Grimes, D. A., & Riggs, J. A. (1983). Hysterectomy in the United States. *Obstetrics and Gynecology, 62*(2), 203-212.

Faro, S. (1989). Antibiotic prophylaxis. *Obstetrics and Gynecology Clinics of North America, 16*(2), 279-289.

Goldrath, M. H. (1990). Intrauterine laser surgery. In W. R. Keye, Jr. (Ed.), *Laser surgery in gynecology and obstetrics* (2nd ed., pp. 151-157). Chicago: Yearbook Medical Publishers.

Gonzales, B. L. (1983). Psychosexual responses to female sterilization. In D. A. van Lith, L. G. Keith, & E. V. Van Hall (Eds.), *New trends in female sterilization* (pp. 195-201). Chicago: Yearbook Medical Publishers.

Graber, E. A., & Feldman, G. B. (1988). Geriatric gynecologic surgery. In L. E. Sanz (Ed.), *Gynecologic surgery* (pp. 432-439). Oradell, NJ: Medical Economics Books.

Green, R. L., Jr. (1973). The emotional aspects of hysterectomy. *Southern Medical Journal, 66*(4), 442-444.

Greenwood, S. (1988). Hysterectomy and ovarian removal: A major health issue in the perimenopausal years. *Western Journal of Medicine, 149*(6), 771-772.

Hatcher, R. A., Trussell, J., Stewart, F., Stewart, G. K., Kowal, D., Guest, F., Cates, W., & Policar, M. S. (1994). *Contraceptive technology 1994-1996* (16th rev. ed.). New York: Irvington.

Herbst, A. L., Mishell, D. R., Stenchever, M. A., & Droegemueller, W. (1992). *Comprehensive gynecology* (2nd ed.). St. Louis, MO: C. V. Mosby.

Holt, L. H., & Weber, M. (1982). *The American Medical Association book of woman care.* New York: Random House.

Horton, J. A. (1992). *The women's health data book.* Washington, DC: Jacobs Institute of Women's Health.

Humphries, P. T. (1980). Sexual adjustment after hysterectomy. *Health Care of Women, 2*(2), 1-14.

Ignatavicius, D., & Bayne, M. (1991). *Medical surgical nursing.* Philadelphia: W. B. Saunders.

Jenkins, B. (1988). Patients' reports of sexual changes after treatment for gynecologic cancer. *Oncology Nursing Forum, 15,* 349-354.

Kaltrieder, N. B., Wallace, A., & Horowitz, M. D. (1979). A field study of the stress response syndrome: Young women after hysterectomy. *JAMA, 242,* 1499-1503.

Kjer, J., & Knudsen, L. (1989). Ectopic pregnancy subsequent to laparoscopic sterilization. *American Journal of Obstetrics and Gynecology, 160,* 1202-1204.

Kruger, J. C., Hassell, J., Goggins, D. B., Ishimatsu, T., Pablico, M. R., & Tuttle, E. J. (1979). Relationship between nurse counseling and sexual adjustment after hysterectomy. *Nursing Research, 28*(3), 145-150.

Lalinec-Michaud, M., & Engelsmann, F. (1984). Depression and hysterectomy: A prospective study. *Psychosomatics, 25,* 550-558.

Lalinec-Michaud, M., & Engelsmann, F. (1985). Anxiety, fear and depression related to hysterectomy. *Canadian Journal of Psychiatry, 30*(1), 44-47.

Lawhead, R. A., Clark, G. C., Smith, D. H., Pierce, V. K., & Lewis, J. L., Jr. (1989). Pelvic exenteration for recurrent or persistent gynecologic malignancies: A 10-year review of the Memorial Sloan-Kettering Cancer Center experience (1972-1981). *Gynecologic Oncology, 33,* 279-282.

Lindemann, E. (1941). Observations on psychiatric sequelae to surgical operations in women. *American Journal of Psychiatry, 98*(1), 132-139.

Littlefield, V. M. (1986). Health education for women: Why? In V. M. Littlefield (Ed.), *Health education for women: A guide for nurses and other health professionals* (pp. 33-43). Norwalk, CT: Appleton-Century-Crofts.

Lomano, J. (1988). Endometrial ablation with the Nd: YAG laser. In L. E. Sanz (Ed.), *Gynecologic surgery* (pp. 370-374). Oradell, NJ: Medical Economics Books.

Lowdermilk, D. L. (1986). Reproductive surgery. In J. Griffith-Kenney (Ed.), *Contemporary women's health* (pp. 604-621). Menlo Park, CA: Addison-Wesley.

Martin, D. C. (1990). Laser safety. In W. R. Keye, Jr. (Ed.), *Laser surgery in gynecology and obstetrics* (2nd ed., pp. 35-45). Chicago: Yearbook Medical Publishers.

Melody, G. F. (1962). Depressive reactions following hysterectomy. *American Journal of Obstetrics and Gynecology, 83,* 410-413.

Myers, M. (1986). The enlarged uterus. In C. Havens, N. Sullivan, & P. Tilton (Eds.), *Manual of outpatient gynecology* (pp. 51-56). Boston: Little, Brown.

National Center for Health Statistics. (1988). *Hysterectomy in the United States, 1965-1984* (DHHS Publication No. PHS 88-1753). Washington, DC: Government Printing Office.

Nichols, D. H. (1990). Relaxation of pelvic supports. In J. R. Scott, P. J. Disaia, C. B. Hammond, & W. N. Spellacy (Eds.), *Danforth's obstetrics and gynecology* (6th ed., pp. 887-903). Philadelphia: W. B. Saunders.

Nichols, D. H., & Randall, C. L. (1989). *Vaginal surgery* (3rd ed.). Baltimore: Williams & Wilkins.

Papera, S. (1990). Sterilization. In R. Lichtman & S. Papera (Eds.), *Well-woman care* (pp. 465-472). Norwalk, CT: Appleton & Lange.

Penfield, A. J. (1983). Trends in sterilization: The American experience. In D. A. van Lith, L. G. Keith, & E. V. Van Hall (Ed.), *New trends in female sterilization* (pp. 27-42). Chicago: Yearbook Medical Publishers.

Penfield, A. J. (1986). *Gynecologic surgery under local anesthesia.* Baltimore/Munich: Urban & Swarzenberg.

Richards, D. H. (1973). Depression after hysterectomy. *Lancet, 2,* 430-433.

Richards, D. H. (1974). A post-hysterectomy syndrome. *Lancet, 2,* 983-985.

Richardson, D. A., & Ostergard, D. O. (1988). Evolution of surgery for stress urinary incontinence. In L. E. Sanz (Ed.), *Gynecologic surgery* (pp. 191-193). Oradell, NJ: Medical Economics Books.

Rioux, D., & Soderstrom, P. M. (1987). Sterilization revisited. *Contemporary Obstetrics and Gynecology, 30*(2), 80-104.

Rioux, J. E., & Soderstrom, R. (1988). Review of techniques for tubal sterilization. In L. E. Sanz (Ed.), *Gynecologic surgery* (pp. 304-318). Oradell, NJ: Medical Economics Books.

Roeske, N. C. (1978). Hysterectomy and other gynecologic surgeries: A psychological view. In M. T. Notman & C. C. Nadelson (Eds.), *The woman patient: Medical and psychosocial interfaces: Vol. I. Sexual and reproductive aspects of women's health care* (pp. 217-231). New York: Plenum.

Rostad, M. E. (1988). The radical vulvectomy patient: Preventing complications. *Dimensions of Critical Care, 7,* 289-294.

Saidi, M. H., & Zainie, C. M. (1980). *Female sterilization: A handbook for women.* New York: Garland.

Salter, J. R. (1985). Gynecological symptoms and psychological distress in potential hysterectomy patients. *Journal of Psychosomatic Research, 29,* 155-159.

Sanz, L. E., & Hoyne, P. M. (1988). Myomectomy. In L. E. Sanz (Ed.), *Gynecologic surgery* (pp. 331-339). Oradell, NJ: Medical Economics Books.

Shell, J. A. (1990). Sexuality for patients with gynecologic cancer. *NAACOG'S Clinical Issues in Perinatal and Women's Health, 1*(4), 479-494.

Shuber, J. (1989). Transcervical sterilization with use of methyl-2-cyanoacrylate and a newer delivery system (the femcept device). *American Journal of Obstetrics and Gynecology, 160,* 887-889.

Sloan, D. (1978). The emotional and psychosexual aspects of hysterectomy. *American Journal of Obstetrics and Gynecology, 131,* 598-605.

Sloane, E. (1985). *Biology of women* (2nd ed.). New York: John Wiley.

Smith, D. C., & Uhlir, J. K. (1990). Myomectomy as a reproductive procedure. *American Journal of Obstetrics and Gynecology, 162*(6), 1476-1482.

Stanfill, P. H. (1982). The psychosocial implications of hysterectomy. *JOGNN, 11*(5), 318-320.

Wabrek, A. J., & Gunn, J. L. (1984). Sexual and psychological implications of gynecologic malignancy. *JOGNN, 13,* 371-376.

Wilson, E. A. (1988). Surgical therapy for endometriosis. *Clinical Obstetrics and Gynecology, 31*(4), 857-865.

Wright, V. C. (1990). Laser therapy of the vulva and vagina. In W. R. Keye, Jr. (Ed.), *Laser surgery in gynecology and obstetrics* (2nd ed.) (pp. 100-120). Chicago: Yearbook Medical Publishers.

Yandell, R. B., Dinh, T. V., & Hannigan, E. V. (1990). Laser surgery of the cervix. In W. R. Keye (Ed.), *Laser surgery in gynecology and obstetrics* (2nd ed., pp. 130-137). Chicago: Yearbook Medical Publishers.

Zussman, L., Zussman, S., Sunley, R., & Bjornson, E. (1981). Sexual response after hysterectomy-oophorectomy: Recent studies and reconsiderations of psychogenesis. *American Journal of Obstetrics and Gynecology, 140,* 725-729.

27

Chronic Illnesses and Women

JANET PRIMOMO

Diabetes stays with you for the duration. It's not something you can take a vacation from. It's there every day of the year, constantly, and never goes away. Sometimes, it would be nice just to turn it over to someone to take care of, but you know you can't do that. You get tired of it all. Just like anything else, you need break from the routine, but you can't get one.

Woman with diabetes

Chronic illness is permanent and progressive and requires ongoing adaptation and management. Chronic illness is the most prevalent form of illness in the United States today and poses one of the country's most pressing and challenging health care problems (Rothenberg & Koplan, 1990). In spite of the pervasiveness of chronic illness, the U.S. health care system has revolved around the treatment of acute illness and injury. Scientific knowledge about living with chronic illness is relatively new (Burish & Bradley, 1983). In this chapter, chronic illness is described, and the epidemiology, prevention, and treatment of selected chronic diseases in women are reviewed.

Defining Chronic Illness

Chronic illness is differentiated from acute illness on a number of dimensions (Burish & Bradley, 1983). An acute illness is brief in duration or course. It has a sudden onset and produces signs and symptoms soon after exposure to the disease. Acute illness responds to treatment or is self-limiting and usually does not have long-term consequences. Recovery usually occurs after a short time, and people with acute illness are expected to return to their full level of pre-illness functioning.

In contrast, chronic illness persists over a long period of time and involves the permanent loss of functioning of an organ system (Feldman, 1974). The Commission on Chronic Illness defined chronic illness as "all impairments or deviations from normal that have one or more of the following characteristics: are permanent, leave residual disability, are caused by non-reversible pathological alterations, require special training of the patient for rehabilitation, and/or may be expected to require a long period of supervision, observation, or care" (Mayo, 1956).

Other characteristics of chronic illness include the long period of latency when the disease process has begun, but symptoms have not appeared (Rothenberg & Koplan, 1990). For example, with many types of cancers, it is thought that precursors such as cellular differentiation, hormones, or genetic factors may be present for many years even though there is no manifestation of the disease process. The cause or etiology of chronic illness is often uncertain. For example, the causes of multiple sclerosis and breast cancer are not known. With proper treatment and management, the symptoms of chronic disease may be controlled and complications may be minimized, but there is not a definite cure (Strauss et al., 1984). Often, chronic illness requires attention by the individual, family, and health care providers over the person's lifetime.

The words *disease* and *illness* are often used interchangeably. However, a distinction can be made between the terms. *Disease* refers to the observed or objective indicators that reflect a disorder of bodily functions, systems, or organs (Dimond & Jones, 1983). Each disease has a set of signs and symptoms associated with it, specific physical alterations, and a recognized causative agent or agents. In contrast, *illness* refers to how the person experiences and describes the signs and symptoms of biological dysfunction or disease. For most individuals, the illness (fatigue, nausea, pain) they experience is the result of a disease process. Because some chronic diseases are not easy to diagnose, a person may experience symptoms without having a "disease." Conversely, the disease process may be present, but symptoms of the disease may not be. Clinicians and researchers are increasingly aware of the influence that the person's experience with disease has on the course of disease. Therefore, in this chapter, the term *chronic illness,* which encompasses both the objective disease focus and how the person experiences the disease, is used predominantly.

Disability is a concept sometimes associated with chronic illness. "Disability refers to the state of being limited, due to a chronic health condition or set of conditions, in the type or amount of activities that a person would otherwise be expected to perform" (LaPlante, 1988, p. 4). Chronic illness may or may not result in disability. Human beings are tremendously resilient creatures and learn to accommodate their daily lives to challenging situations (Benoliel, 1970; Corbin & Strauss, 1988; Williams & Wood, 1988). Illness-related factors such as the types of symptoms, the severity of the illness, and the treatment regimen play a role in whether disability results from an illness (Burish & Bradley, 1983; Craig & Edwards, 1983; Dimond & Jones, 1983). Personal factors such as individual coping ability might influence whether disability results from chronic illness, too. Finally, the amount of social dependency may influence whether or not disability is associated with chronic illness (Eisenberg, Sutkin, & Jansen, 1984).

In summary, chronic illness is long-term, progressive, and requires ongoing care. The onset of chronic illness is often gradual, and symptoms are sometimes insidious. For each specific chronic illness, there are known pathological manifestations. Chronic illness may have a profound influence on the individual and family. Fortunately, there is a growing body of knowledge about the psychosocial, family, and economic implications of chronic illness.

The Trajectory of Chronic Illness

The term *chronic illness trajectory* refers to the overall course or voyage a person experiences as a result of an illness. Trajectory covers not only the physiological changes but also the nonmedical aspects, including social or role performance changes, self-identity alterations, and the evolving sequence of work to manage the disease (Corbin & Strauss, 1988). In general, the trajectory for all chronic illnesses is a downward progression; however, the rate of progression varies. The trajectory depends on the type and severity of disease as well as on individual coping efforts and family and social factors.

Phases of the chronic illness trajectory have been described (see Figure 27.1) (Corbin & Strauss, 1988; Rolland, 1984). The illness phases involve a period of crisis, a chronic phase, and a terminal phase. The course of illness begins with the onset and diagnosis of a chronic illness. A person who has been healthy may begin to

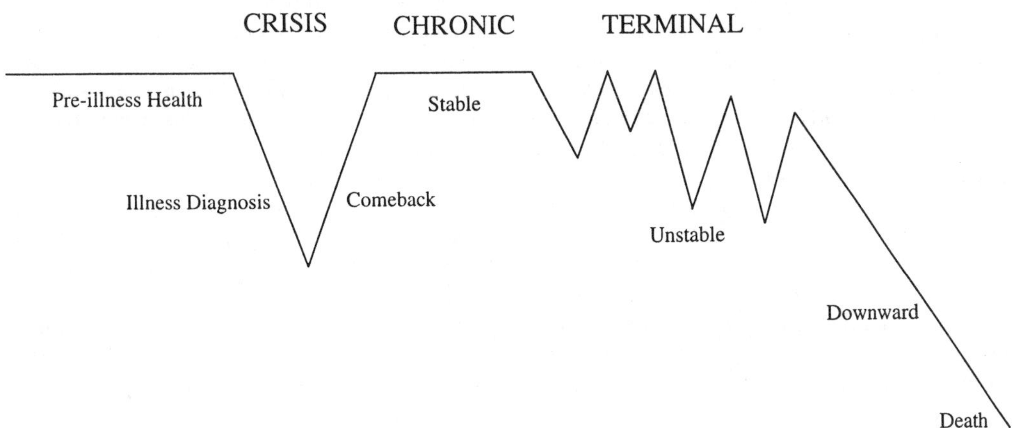

Figure 27.1. Phases of the Chronic Illness Trajectory
SOURCE: Adapted from Corbin and Strauss (1988) and Rolland (1984).

experience signs and symptoms of illness and seek medical attention, including diagnostic tests. Observable signs, such as elevated blood pressure, lumps, or a productive cough, are used in the diagnosis of disease. Symptoms, a person's report of some abnormal function or sensation, may include nausea, pain, or headache. A number of models have been described that elaborate on the processes people use for seeking help about their signs and symptoms of illness (Dimond & Jones, 1983). Why people seek help seems to be dependent on the visibility, perceived severity, frequency, and persistence of the symptoms; the degree to which their usual activities are disrupted; competing demands; cultural values; threshold tolerance; alternative explanations about the symptoms; and accessibility to treatment (Mechanic, 1978).

The illness diagnosis phase is a highly stressful period full of uncertainty for the person and family (Lewis, 1986; Strauss et al., 1984). At the time of the initial diagnosis, a period of crisis may be experienced as the person and family begin to face the realities of a chronic and possibly life-threatening illness. Alterations in roles and lifestyles occur as the individual and family assimilate routines to manage a "disordered body" (Williams & Wood, 1988). This adjustment may be sudden, as in a heart attack, or gradual, as in multiple sclerosis. Initial medical or surgical treatment is started once the diagnosis has been made. In some diseases, such as advanced cancer, palliative or supportive care may be started if treatment is not considered to be beneficial or if it is not desired by the individual and family. During this phase, the person may become increasingly ill if side effects of the treatment are experienced, as with some chemotherapy and radiation therapies used in cancer treatment. Once the treatment is completed, the person may enter the comeback phase when strength gradually returns and pre-illness activities of daily living are resumed. For many persons, a stable phase follows. The term *remission* is used to describe this stable period when symptoms have subsided.

Later in the course of the illness when symptoms reappear and the disease process is active again, the terms *exacerbation* or *flare-up* are used (Lewis, 1986). This unstable phase is highly stressful for the individual and family (Worden, 1989). During the unstable phase, acute medical crises may occur, requiring hospitalization or intensified contact with health care providers. For people with cancer, this may occur when the disease has spread or metastasized to other parts of the body. Treatment decisions must be made once again; the individual may experience not only the symptoms of the disease but the side effects of treatment as well. As in many types of advanced cancer, chemotherapy and radiation become highly toxic and are no longer effective in battling the disease progression. The downward trend begins and supportive or palliative care replaces attempts to cure the disease. At this final phase of the trajectory, people may be referred to specialized services such as Hospice.

To better understand the psychological and social similarities and differences of various chronic illnesses over their course, a classification or typology of chronic illnesses was developed (Rolland, 1984). The broad dimensions used in the chronic illness classification scheme include the (a) onset, (b) course, (c) outcome, and (d) degree of incapacitation caused by the illness.

The onset of chronic illness may be sudden or acute, as in a stroke or myocardial infarction. In contrast, multiple sclerosis, arthritis, and chronic obstructive pulmonary disease have a gradual onset. Whether or not an illness has a rapid or slow onset may have implications for how the individual and family respond (Adams & Lindemann, 1974). When a chronic illness suddenly presents itself, a crisis may occur and the person and family may be required to mobilize their resources rapidly to cope with the changes. In the gradual onset of illness, the family has time to adjust to the slow progression of symptoms. Rolland (1984) categorized the course of chronic illness to be progressive, constant, or relapsing/episodic. In progressive illnesses, such as cancer, emphysema, and Type I (insulin-dependent) diabetes, symptoms are generally always present and the severity increases. The person and family must continually adapt to changing health status and increasing care needs. A progressive illness can be contrasted and compared with one that has a constant or stable course. When a person has a stroke, the illness course tends to be one of a constant nature. Once the initial adjustments are made to manage the residual physical, cognitive, or emotional limitations, the course of day-to-day events is generally predictable.

A relapsing or episodic course of illness occurs in illnesses such as asthma, ulcerative colitis, and the early stages of cancer. Periods of relatively good health are interrupted by episodes of high symptomatology. The fatal, life span shortening or nonfatal nature of various chronic illnesses is another important dimension in Rolland's (1984) typology. Illnesses such as Type I diabetes and cardiovascular disease may possibly be fatal, can shorten the person's life span, and may lead to an early death. These illnesses may be unpredictable and create a high level of uncertainty. An individual and family may respond very differently to nonfatal arthritis than they would to illnesses that are fatal, such as AIDS or metastatic cancer.

The degree and type of incapacitation caused by an illness is a final dimension in the typology. Some illnesses such as multiple sclerosis and arthritis may physically impair a person. Depending on the stage of Alzheimer's disease, incapacitation may be cognitive or physical. AIDS, a highly stigmatized and fatal illness, carries with it a fear of contagion and social incapacitation due to the visibility of symptoms as well as the stigma attached to the disease itself.

In summary, although each chronic illness has a unique trajectory or course, in general, people with chronic illness experience an onset or crisis phase, a chronic phase, and a terminal phase of illness. The actual illness course experienced by the individual may be dependent on the specific illness; characteristics of the individual, including age and gender; and psychological, family, and social factors. The concept of illness trajectory helps to delineate the specific needs of individuals and families as they move through the ups and downs of life with chronic illness.

The Work of Managing Chronic Illness

The work involved in managing chronic illness has four dimensions: (a) managing the illness itself, (b) care of the ill person, (c) biographical work, and (d) everyday life work (Strauss, Fagerhaugh, Suczek, & Weiner, 1985). This work and the associated tasks are related more to the management of the symptoms of illness and the person's integration with others than to the disease process itself. The first dimension of work is the major task of managing the physical manifestations of illness (Corbin & Strauss, 1988). The types of work involved in managing the illness itself include the process of the diagnostic workup, work with machinery (such as respirators, glucometers, or oxygen tanks), measures to enhance the ill person's comfort, work to ensure the ill person's safety and well-being when involved with the health care system, and "sentimental work" or efforts on the part of the family to help the ill person endure the illness situation (Strauss et al., 1985). Tasks in managing chronic illness have been identified and include preventing and managing medical crises through the administration of medications and home diagnostic tests; managing regimens that may require changing patterns and habits, such as diets; controlling and managing symptoms; adhering to treatment regimens, such as exercise routines; and managing limitations of activity (Strauss et al., 1985).

Caring for the ill person is a special dimension of work (Corbin & Strauss, 1988). The tasks include assisting the person in the performance of activities of daily living, such as bathing, dressing, and toileting; participating in the person's rehabilitation; and preventing and living with the social isolation that may be imposed by the illness. The need for independence must be balanced with the need for assistance from others. Energy conservation, planning and pacing activities, nutritional support, and the use of adaptive equipment become critical factors in managing chronic illness.

Biographical work involves coming to terms with the illness and reconstructing a personal biography to include the illness and limitations imposed by the illness (Corbin & Strauss, 1988). Self-concept changes occur due to bodily changes, and the person may take on a new identity as someone with an illness (Benoliel, 1970).

Finally, the individual and family must attend to the normal routines of daily living in addition to managing the illness, caring for the ill person, and biographical work (Corbin & Strauss, 1988). This "everyday life work" includes occupational work, maintaining a household, raising children, nurturing a marriage, maintaining social and community ties, and articulating work or coordinating all the work necessary to integrate daily routines.

In summary, the heterogeneous nature of chronic illness cannot be understood without attention to the family and social context. Disease-related factors; individual characteristics, including age and duration of illness; and the family and social environment all play a role in how the illness trajectory unfolds (Craig & Edwards, 1983). Health care workers are challenged to develop an understanding of the complex nature of the chronic illness experience to help individuals and families cope. It is imperative to give the chronically ill individual and family choices, support, and autonomy in managing the work of chronic illness (Williams & Wood, 1988).

Women Managing Chronic Illness

Despite the pervasiveness of chronic illness, knowledge about women with chronic illness is minimal. The growing body of literature on women's roles, development, and cognitive processes is helpful in considering how chronic illness may affect women's lives. In general, women value their connections to others and their interdependence with others. Women live their lives around the themes of caring for others, responsibility, and empathy (Belenky, Clinchy, Goldberger, & Tarule, 1986; Gilligan, 1982). For women with chronic illness, then, the family and social context become crucial in understanding how women are affected by and manage chronic illness.

The impact of chronic illness on women's self-esteem, roles, and social support has been documented (Foxall, Ekberg, & Griffin, 1985). Chronic illness combined with life transitions may contribute to the loss of individual and family cohesion (Foxall et al., 1985). Some researchers have suggested that younger women ages 27 to 30 may have greater difficulty adjusting to chronic illness than older women due to the high number of transitions occurring in their lives (Foxall et al., 1985; Rankin & Weekes, 1989). Furthermore, there is ample evidence to suggest that social support systems are important factors in women's adjustment to chronic disease (Lambert, Lambert, Klipple, & Mewshaw, 1989; Primomo, Yates, & Woods, 1990; Sexton & Munro, 1986).

Recent studies examined the intrapersonal, interpersonal, and environmental demands or hardships imposed on women by chronic illness (Haberman, Woods, & Packard, 1990; Packard, Haberman, Woods, & Yates, 1991). Women with diabetes, cancer, and fibrocystic breast disease described domains of demands, including (a) direct disease effects, (b) personal disruption (integrity, normalcy), and (c) environmental transactions (social response, treatment processes, and patient-provider interaction) (Packard et al., 1991). Similarly, Haberman et al. (1990) reported a multidimensional construct of demands of illness that included physical symptoms, personal meaning, family functioning, social relationships, self-image, symptom monitoring, and treatment issue demands. It is important to point out that women also reported family functioning demands, such as child care difficulties, yet they did not attribute these demands to their chronic illness. Women with chronic illness must cope not only with their illness but with the day-to-day struggles of life as well.

In one study, the processes by which women managed diabetes and the factors that influenced adjustment to illness were examined (Primomo,

1989). An open-ended interview guide was used to generate data on the behaviors and strategies women used to manage their diabetes routines on a day-to-day basis. Six patterns or styles of diabetes management were developed. The patterns are described next, followed by women's descriptions of their management style.

The first pattern was called "revolving around the social milieu." This management pattern reflected women's priorities in life. Although women knew how to manage their diabetes well, their diabetes routines were secondary to the needs of their families, work responsibilities, or social lives. For example, one woman stated:

> I test before dinner and then take my shot . . . that's the one where I really have problems because I've got hungry kids and I'm trying to get dinner done and the baby wants to eat. And for a while there I wasn't always getting that evening shot because I hate to take a shot without testing. It's just something I never do so I skip the shot and end up with blood sugars of 180 or higher at bedtime. (Primomo, 1989, p. 142)

"Calculating adjusters" juggled the diabetes routines to achieve the flexibility and freedom that fit their own desired lifestyles. Careful planning helped these women to take control of their diabetes rather than allow diabetes to dominate their lives.

> You have to decide whether you really want to do something and then you can always find a way to do it. I discovered I could pack up my insulin and testing equipment and bring it with me. We can be on vacation and leave the hotel in the morning, wander around and never come back until after dinner. I don't have to go all the way back to our hotel just to take a shot and then go back to eat so it all works out. You can always figure out some way to do it. (Primomo, 1989, p. 143)

Diabetes routines dominated women's lives in subtle ways for the women who were being "driven by the clock." The day-to-day existence was characterized by a very regimented and scheduled life that was centered around diabetes treatments.

> My family watched a TV program about a month ago where they were talking about a mother who had diabetes and how the entire family vacation revolved around when the mother had to eat next. My 16-year-old son just looked at me and said, "sound familiar?" (Primomo, 1989, p. 144)

"Straight arrows" tried to maintain very tight control of their blood sugar. To do this, they were almost hypervigilant about their diabetes regimens. These women were comfortable juggling their diet, exercise, and insulin doses and were not afraid to experience low blood sugar reactions.

> What I'm giving you is my minimum testing times as far as 7, 10, 12, 3 and then at 5 again before dinner . . . and let's see at bedtime. I usually test between 10:30 and 11:00. And then I always test before I drive . . . it just makes me feel more comfortable. It's more like a habit. I don't think about it too much I just do it. (Primomo, 1989, pp. 145-146)

"Chancers" were inconsistent and haphazard in managing their diabetes routines. These women admitted to guessing or playing around with their routines and not really knowing what would happen.

> I don't know the routines yet or the formulas to use to make it all that precise. I know that there's a way you're supposed to measure, eat so much or shoot up with so many units of this in order to eat so much of that. Or shoot up so many of this if your blood sugar happens to be this much higher. I don't have those down yet. Up to this point, it's all been a lot of guess work. That's the word, a lot of guess work. (Primomo, 1989, p. 145)

A final pattern was that of "minimizing the routines." Minimizers demonstrated a sense of denial or avoidance in relation to their diabetes routines. They tried to compartmentalize their diabetes and do as little as possible. Concealing diabetes from others and limiting the intrusion of diabetes routines on social interaction were common.

> There's this part of me that always wants to pretend that it's not there or just push it away or turn away from it. And then I have this part of me that's kind of a perfectionist and would like to do well but the other part doesn't even admit diabetes is part of me. . . . I don't like to feel different from everybody else and that comes up at work and just different places where you're with people who don't know you . . . because you're different when you have diabetes and I hate that and so that's another

part of what makes this hard. (Primomo, 1989, pp. 146-147)

The management patterns just described ranged from highly flexible (almost chaotic) to highly rigid and provided insight into how women manage chronic illness. Women whose management style was most chaotic had few anchors in their lives, such as other family members; were not employed; and had the lowest incomes. These women were the most anxious and depressed. Furthermore, they had the lowest stage of psychosocial development. Women with higher stages of psychosocial development were more likely to take control of their diabetes regimens and adjust their regimens to accommodate the demands of family and work (Primomo, 1989). These results complement studies about the importance of a personality characteristic identified as hardiness or a sense of commitment, control, and challenge. Women with the ability to take charge of their lives may be better able to cope with chronic illness (Lambert et al., 1989).

Further research is indicated to determine if patterns or styles of management are found in other women with diabetes and different chronic illnesses. Although there may not be a body of knowledge to guide interventions with chronically ill women at this time, it is vital that health care professionals attend to the variations in women's personal, family, and social lives as they attempt to help women manage their chronic illness.

Families and Chronic Illness

Although a woman may be the diagnosed "patient" with a chronic illness, the family often assumes responsibility for her care (Stuifbergen, 1987). Chronic illness may require pervasive alterations in every aspect of the family's life together (Corbin & Strauss, 1988). Occupational, sociocultural, and family roles may be disrupted temporarily or permanently (Burish & Bradley, 1983; Entmacher, 1983). A chronic illness may impose changes in a couple's sexual activity, thereby affecting the marital relationship (Lewis, 1986). Physical changes may necessitate dependency on family members to provide for personal, social, financial, and health care needs. The potential for social isolation and loneliness is great when a family member has a chronic illness. The family, therefore, is an important caregiving resource and may provide assistance with all activities of daily living, including emotional and tangible support (Burish & Bradley, 1983; Corbin & Strauss, 1988; Stuifbergen, 1987).

Psychological adjustment to chronic illness may include changes in self-identity, self-concept, and self-image (Strauss et al., 1984). Often, the family is the context for self-identity and making meaning of the illness (Lewis, 1986). The family may function as a buffer zone in helping to derive a sense of purpose in life and feelings of self-worth.

Women with chronic illness may be concerned about their ability to maintain role expectations at home or at work. Indeed, family roles may be altered depending on the chronically ill person's needs (Holmes, 1988; Lewis, Woods, & Ellison, 1986; Strauss et al., 1984). For example, a male partner who has not previously been involved in running a household may have to assume new responsibilities for grocery shopping, meals, laundry, child care, and housekeeping when his spouse becomes unable to fulfill previous roles. Similarly, women with a weakened physical state may strive to redefine roles and make adjustments so that they can still participate in family life. A mother might make out a shopping list rather than shop herself and plan and oversee meal preparations, thereby maintaining an active role in daily living.

Women with chronic illness who have children may have a special set of concerns (Lewis et al., 1986; Packard et al., 1991; Stetz, Lewis, & Primomo, 1986; Thorne, 1990). Some women expressed concerns about their ability to perform mothering roles because of fatigue or activity limitations imposed by their physical condition (Thorne, 1990). They may be less available to their children for daily events or special occasions. Women may feel dependent on their children for emotional or tangible support, such as help with chores, shopping, meals, or child care. On a positive note, the constant presence of the mother's chronic illness may enhance children's compassion for others (Thorne, 1990).

The treatment regimens for some chronic illnesses may require major adjustments on the part of family members. With diabetes, family meals may revolve around the person with diabetes because of her need to eat "on schedule." Family members must live with the mood changes caused by fluctuations in glucose levels (Lewis et al., 1986; Packard et al., 1991).

Exactly how families are affected by chronic illness is not known. It is likely that many factors affect how families adapt to chronic illness (Lewis, 1986). The effects of chronic illness on families may depend on the illness itself, the individual family members, or the family life cycle stage (Rankin & Weekes, 1989). For example, a young woman diagnosed with diabetes, a chronic disease that may be hereditary and is associated with birth defects and complications as well as a shortened life span, may find her childbearing decisions influenced by her illness (Ahlfield, Soler, & Marcus, 1985; Primomo, 1989). In contrast, an elderly woman who has a grown family may be concerned about not becoming a burden to her family (Jenny, 1984).

Families may experience financial insecurity and limited access to health care as a result of chronic illness. Economic disruptions may occur if work or career opportunities are limited because of disability. Because work is often associated with health insurance coverage, if an individual is not able to work and health care insurance is not financially affordable, access to health care may be limited. Access to employment, economic opportunities, and health insurance are valid concerns for people with chronic conditions (Entmacher, 1983).

The types of problems that families with chronic illness experience may not be all that different from those of "normal families." Families are tremendously resilient and attempt to normalize as much as possible. In one study (Lewis et al., 1986), the challenges and strains identified by families with chronic illness fell into seven general categories:

1. Household management issues (changes in routines, time scheduling, and transportation)
2. Financial and business strains (unemployment, work demands, or decisions about the allocation of money)
3. Situational and development challenges (learning to drive a car, remodeling the home, or adding a family pet)
4. Family network transitions (the gain or loss of a family member through death, divorce, or remarriage)
5. Intrafamilial strains (behavioral problems at home, conflict, tension, or communication problems in the family)
6. School strains (problems with grades, behavior, or school events)
7. Family illness or injury (illness, injury, or symptoms of a family member)

Furthermore, most of the coping strategies that families used to manage their problems were similar to those reported by other families (Stetz et al., 1986) and included passive acceptance, reframing, seeking support and assistance from both within and outside the family, and participating in alternative activities. Unique patterns of coping for families with chronic illness included reducing their involvement in activities, discretionary nonaction, and altering the management of their household to cope with problems. The recognition that families with chronic illness have similar yet unique problems and solutions to their problems merits further attention.

Supporting families with chronic illness, then, becomes a critical issue for health care providers. The type, timing, nature, and source of support appropriate to families varies depending on the specific illness, the characteristics and needs of the family members, and the sources of support available (Woods, Yates, & Primomo, 1989). Dimensions of support for families include emotional, instrumental (for example, tangible help with meals, transportation, child care), and informational support. The type of support needed may be determined in part by the phase of the illness trajectory. Emotional support may be needed throughout all phases of the illness due to uncertainty about the consequences of the illness. In contrast, tangible assistance may be crucial at the initial phase of an illness diagnosis and at the terminal phases. Informational support may be most important during transitional phases (Woods et al., 1989). Furthermore, the best source of support may vary according to the expressed need. For example, emotional support from the partner may be most effective in preventing depression, maintaining marital quality, and enhancing family functioning (Primomo et al., 1990). Clearly, more research is needed to determine how to best support families with chronic illness. However, health care professionals should consider the various types, sources, and timing of support to facilitate women's coping with chronic illness.

Epidemiology of Chronic Disease in Women

Epidemiology is the study of the determinants and distribution of diseases in humans

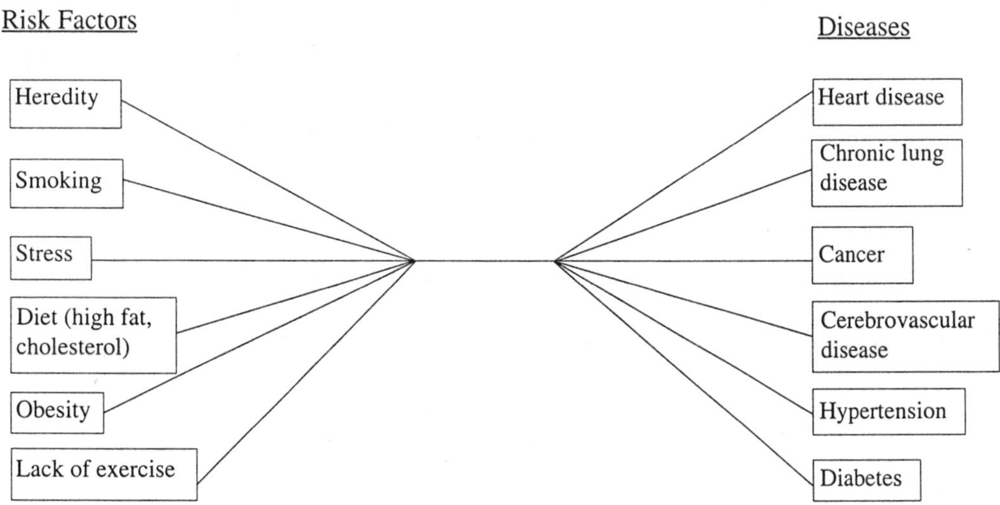

Figure 27.2. Interaction of Multiple Risk Factors and Diseases

(Mausner & Kramer, 1985). Information generated from epidemiological studies is useful in understanding the patterns and causes of disease (Dever, 1991). Epidemiology provides vital evaluative information on the effectiveness of illness prevention programs, screening techniques, and treatment modalities. The planning of health care services is heavily dependent on the data from epidemiological studies as well.

Determining the causes and patterns of chronic illness and disease is highly complex. For many diseases, including cancer and diabetes mellitus, the exact cause is not well understood. Therefore, diagnostic tests have not been developed for many chronic diseases. Because the onset of chronic disease is often gradual, it is difficult to track the exact number of cases at any one time. With some chronic diseases, there is a long period of time or latency between exposure to the causing agents and the development of the disease. For example, the development of colon cancer, considered to be related to diets high in refined food and low in fiber, may have a long latency period.

Multiple factors contribute to the development of multiple chronic diseases (see Figure 27.2). Causative factors may interact and combine in specific ways to place the individual at higher risk for developing disease than if a single causative factor were present alone. In other words, a multiple-cause/multiple-effect model is the appropriate model to guide epidemiological investigations rather than a model implicating one causative agent with one disease (Dever, 1991). For example, if a smoker has an occupational exposure to certain industrial chemicals or asbestos, the risk for lung cancer is much greater than for a smoker who does not have the work exposure. Although smoking is the leading contributing factor to lung cancer deaths, smoking is associated with heart disease, stroke, chronic obstructive pulmonary disease (COPD), other types of cancer, and complications of diabetes as well. Similarly, stress, a diet high in saturated fat and cholesterol, obesity, inactivity, and hereditary factors all contribute to cardiovascular and heart disease.

In spite of the difficulties in generating information on chronic illness, some data that describe the distribution and determinants of chronic disease are available. These data are useful in determining patterns of illness in the population, risk factors, and health care services needed.

Today, about 71% of deaths are attributable to chronic diseases, such as heart disease, cancer, stroke or cerebrovascular diseases, diabetes, COPD, and cirrhosis (U.S. Bureau of the Census, 1991). Although the death rates from heart disease, cerebrovascular disease, and diabetes have decreased between 1970 and 1987, the rates for malignant neoplasms (cancer), COPD, and AIDS have increased (see Table 27.1). The lower death rate from heart disease, stroke, and diabetes may be attributed to better treatment modes in recent years than in the previous two decades. One of the most striking features of

Table 27.1 Age-Adjusted[a] Death Rates in Women and Men, by Selected Causes, 1970 and 1987 (rates per 100,000 population)

	Women		*Men*	
Causes	*White*	*Black*	*White*	*Black*
Heart disease				
1970	167.8	251.7	347.6	375.9
1987	116.3	180.8	225.9	287.1
Malignant neoplasms				
1970	107.6	123.5	154.3	198.0
1987	109.7	132.0	158.4	227.9
Cerebrovascular disease				
1970	56.2	107.9	68.3	122.5
1987	26.3	46.7	30.3	57.1
Chronic obstructive lung disease				
1970	9.2	6.3	26.7	20.9
1987	13.7	9.5	27.4	24.0
Diabetes				
1970	12.8	30.9	12.7	21.2
1987	8.1	21.3	9.5	18.3
Human immunodeficiency virus (HIV)				
1987	0.6	4.7	8.3	25.4

SOURCE: U.S. Bureau of the Census (1991).
NOTE: By comparing death rates over time, it is possible to identify trends in disease prevention and treatment efforts. For example, the death rates for heart disease and cerebrovascular disease have dropped markedly over the past two decades. However, chronic lung problems are increasing.
a. Standardized for age distribution of population.

Table 27.1 is the racial gap; African Americans have significantly higher death rates from the major chronic illnesses than do whites. The disparity between whites and blacks is evident in average life expectancy, too. White women have a life expectancy of 78.9 years, followed by black women (73.6 years), white men (72.0 years), and finally, black men (65.6 years) (U.S. Bureau of the Census, 1991).

Although death rates are useful indicators, they provide very little information about the day-to-day lives of people with chronic illness. To generate data about morbidity or illness, the National Center for Health Statistics conducts an annual National Health Interview Survey. The survey is a national probability sample of the civilian noninstitutionalized U.S. population and includes about 40,000 households. A wide range of interview questions about health and health practices are used. The information compiled from the survey provides a rough picture of the chronic health care needs of the U.S. population. For the purposes of the survey, chronic conditions are defined as conditions that were noticed 3 months or more prior to the survey or conditions that are known to be chronic regardless of when they began (National Center for Health Statistics, 1988).

The most common conditions reported differ according to gender (see Table 27.2) as well as race, income, and geographic location. Arthritis, chronic sinusitis, high blood pressure, orthopedic deformities, heart conditions, chronic bronchitis, and diabetes are the most common conditions reported by women. Women report chronic conditions more often than men. Hypertension, heart conditions, chronic lung disease, and diabetes are not only the highest causes of death but the most frequently reported conditions as well.

In the National Health Interview Survey, activity limitations, such as the inability to take care of personal needs, work, attend school, maintain a household, or participate in leisure activities, are assessed. Chronic conditions causing the highest percentage of limitation in activity include mental retardation, multiple sclerosis, cancer, paralysis, lung diseases, stroke, and diabetes (see Table 27.3). Lung cancer, one of the highest causes of death and most common chronic conditions, is a disease that limits the activities of almost 70% of those with the disease. Similarly, stomach and colon cancers limit the activities of almost half of the people with the illness. About 40% of people with chronic lung diseases and cardiovascular disease report

Table 27.2 Prevalence of Self-Reported Selected Chronic Conditions in Women and Men[a]

Conditions	*Rate*	
	Women	*Men*
Arthritis	169.8	91.3
Chronic sinusitis	147.1	117.3
Hypertension	129.6	106.9
Deformities or orthopedic impairments	115.6	116.9
Heart conditions	87.3	77.2
Chronic bronchitis	60.7	41.5
Diabetes	27.9	27.8

SOURCE: U.S. Bureau of the Census (1991).
a. Conditions per 1,000 persons.

activity limitations due to the disease. Diabetes limits activities for about 35% of those with the illness.

In general, when all respondents with chronic conditions in the survey are considered, slightly more women (14.4%) than men (13.6%) were limited in day-to-day activities (see Table 27.4). Heart conditions were an exception, with more men than women reporting activity limitations. As might be expected, the percentage of the population with limitations in activity increased with age. For example, almost 40% of all persons over 65 years of age reported limitations in activity compared with only 7% under the age of 45 years. Furthermore, when people have chronic conditions, their activity limitations increase similarly with age. This trend has important implications for the health care needs of older adults.

The Management of Specific Chronic Illnesses

A thorough review of the causes, treatment, nursing implications, and prevention of chronic diseases is beyond the scope of this chapter, and the reader is referred to a general medical-surgical nursing text for a complete description of chronic conditions and their management (Phipps, Long, Woods, & Cassmeyer, 1991). A brief description of some of the most common chronic diseases in women is provided in order of their prevalence.

Arthritis

Arthritis is two to three times more common in women than in men (see Table 27.2). It is the most prevalent chronic condition reported by women overall, and its prevalence increases with age. Although only 37 of every 1,000 women under the age of 45 years report arthritis, over half (550) of every 1,000 women over 65 experience arthritis (Adams & Benson, 1990). About 25% of women with arthritis experience some limitations in activity because of their condition (see Table 27.4).

There are more than 100 arthritic diseases, and some cause more debilitation and pain than others. The most common form of arthritis is degenerative joint disease or osteoarthritis. This form of arthritis affects the cartilage and surrounding tissues, whereas rheumatoid arthritis is a systemic illness and may involve other organ systems of the body. The most common symptoms of arthritis include pain, fatigue, deformity, joint stiffness, and swelling. Although the causes of osteoarthritis tend to be related to trauma, infections, or wear and tear on the joints, the cause of rheumatoid arthritis is not known but thought to be related to the immune system, metabolic factors, or infection processes.

Women with arthritis must deal with an uncertain prognosis, a medical regimen, and multiple losses (Lambert et al., 1989). A loss in mobility, the inability to work, an altered self-identity due in part to a changed bodily appearance, and changes in leisure activities frequently accompany rheumatoid arthritis (Cornwell & Schmitt, 1990). In fact, a woman's perception of self-esteem may vary depending on whether she is in a stable period or experiencing a flare-up in the inflammatory process (Cornwell & Schmitt, 1990).

Prevention of osteoarthritis involves avoiding obesity and repeated trauma to the joints as well as the use of joint protection techniques, especially in the occupational setting. Treat-

Table 27.3 Selected Chronic Conditions Causing Highest Percentage of Limitation in Activity, in Rank Order, and Percentage of Persons With Condition Who Are Limited in Activity

Chronic Condition	*Rank*	*Percentage of Persons With Limitation of Activity*
Mental retardation	1	85.6
Multiple sclerosis	2	76.8
Malignant neoplasms (lungs and bronchus)	3	68.2
Paralysis of extremities (complete or partial)	4	59.8
Paralysis, other sites (complete or partial)	5	50.4
Intervertebral disc disorders	6	48.8
Malignant neoplasms (gastrointestinal)	7	48.6
Epilepsy	8	46.7
Emphysema	9	42.5
Occupational lung diseases	10	38.2
Cerebrovascular disease	11	37.6
Diabetes	12	35.5

SOURCE: Adapted from National Center for Health Statistics and Collins (1988).

Table 27.4 Percentage of Persons With Activity Limitations, by Selected Chronic Conditions, Sex, and Age

	Sex		*Age Group*		
Condition	*Women*	*Men*	*< 45 years*	*45-65 years*	*>65 yrs*
Heart conditions	16.7	18.2	4.7	21.5	27.1
Arthritis and rheumatism	24.6	12.4	5.4	22.8	29.7
Hypertension	12.8	7.9	2.9	15.2	14.2

SOURCE: U.S. Bureau of the Census (1991).
NOTE: Chronic conditions are often accompanied by limitations in the duration, type, and frequency of daily activities. Overall, about 14.4% of all Americans have some limitations in activity due to a chronic condition. As expected, the percentage of people with limitations increases with age.

ment involves prescribed medications, a balance of rest and activity, exercise and special equipment as prescribed by the physician or physical therapist, joint protection, good nutrition, avoiding weight gain, and pain management. Surgical intervention may be used to remove fragments of bones or joints, or to realign, fuse, or replace joints. In addition, recent studies have shown the importance of identifying and cultivating support systems for women with arthritis to promote and maintain well-being (Lambert et al., 1989). Nurses can help women identify supportive people in their networks and refer women to support groups or specific community services.

Hypertension

Hypertension is the third most common chronic condition (National Center for Health Statistics, 1988) and affects about 22 million or 30% of women 18 to 74 years of age (Makuc, Freid, & Kleinman, 1989). As with most chronic illnesses, the prevalence increases with age. About 36 of every 1,000 women under 45 years of age have hypertension. In comparison, over 430 of every 1,000 women over 65 years of age report hypertension (Adams & Benson, 1990). Almost 13% of women with hypertension report activity limitations due to their high blood pressure (see Table 27.4). Hypertension is more common in African Americans than in whites (Rothenberg & Koplan, 1990). Risk factors associated with hypertension include family history, obesity, smoking, atherosclerosis, high salt diet, alcohol use, and emotional stress. High blood pressure is a major contributing factor to heart, vascular, and kidney diseases (U.S. Department of Health and Human Services [DHHS], 1988).

Hypertension, or high blood pressure, is defined as elevated blood pressure on at least two occasions. Technically, readings of systolic blood pressure higher than 140 mm HG and/or diastolic blood pressure of higher than 90 mm HG are diagnosed as hypertension (U.S. DHHS,

1988). Because blood pressure can be affected by multiple external factors, its measurement should be taken carefully. To ensure accuracy, the appropriate size of blood pressure cuff must be used, the person should have been in a resting state for 5 minutes or more, the bared arm should be positioned at heart level, and smoking or caffeine ingestion should not have occurred within 30 minutes prior to measurement. Health care providers are encouraged to measure blood pressure at each patient visit.

The evaluation and treatment of hypertension depend on the severity of the blood pressure reading and a thorough physical examination and health history, including family history, medications, and other diseases, such as heart disease, kidney disease, diabetes, and vascular disease. Because oral contraceptive use is a risk associated with hypertension, contraception methods must be explored.

Blood pressure readings lower than 140/90 are the desirable treatment outcome. The treatment of hypertension includes nonpharmacological approaches, such as weight reduction, exercise, salt restriction, moderation of alcohol consumption, tobacco avoidance, biofeedback and relaxation, and reduced intake of saturated fats. These treatment modalities may lower blood pressure and, if drug treatment is used, improve the effectiveness of the drugs. Drug therapy is highly effective in reducing high blood pressure. Antihypertensive drugs fall into at least five categories. The most common category is diuretics or drugs that increase the excretion of urine. As with all drugs, undesirable side effects may occur and must be monitored. The reader is referred to the National Institutes of Health document on detection, evaluation, and treatment of high blood pressure (U.S. DHHS, 1988) for further information.

Lifestyle factors, including cultural background, are important considerations in the treatment of hypertension. Diet, cultural beliefs, education and literacy, language barriers, and environmental conditions, including access to care, require special attention on the part of health care providers when working with women of various backgrounds. Nurses caring for women with hypertension should teach them about the need to continue with blood pressure monitoring and medication regimens. Nurses can help women to adjust their activities to facilitate their therapeutic regime and avoid activities or events that may increase arterial pressure.

Heart Disease

Heart disease is the leading cause of death and is the fifth most common chronic disease in women (National Center for Health Statistics, 1988). These data suggest that women are less likely than men to have heart attacks, but if they do, more die as a result. In spite of the grave statistics, most research on heart disease has been completed on men, thus limiting knowledge about the usefulness of diagnostic tests on and interventions with women (Cochrane, 1992). Heart disease is reported as a chronic condition by about 34 of every 1,000 women under 45 years of age. In the group of women over the age of 65, about 265 of every 1,000 women report heart disease (Adams & Benson, 1990), a frequency similar to reports by men. Overall, about 17% of all women with heart disease are limited in their activities (see Table 27.4). Furthermore, heart disease in women is thought to be qualitatively different than in men in part because of physiological, family, and sociocultural factors that influence women's lives (Cochrane, 1992; Rankin, 1990). Women may present with different symptoms of heart disease, such as angina, whereas men have a myocardial infarction (Cochrane, 1992). Interestingly, there has been a decline in mortality from coronary heart disease since the mid-1960s for all population groups, with the greatest decline in white women and men. Once again, these statistics underscore the overrepresentation of the socially disadvantaged among groups who have chronic illness.

There are many classes or types of heart disease, including (a) congenital, inflammatory, valvular, and coronary artery diseases; (b) aortic aneurysms; and (c) congestive heart failure (Phipps et al., 1991). Diseases of the heart may result from hypertension and atherosclerosis, a slow, progressive narrowing of the arteries by fatty deposits commonly called plaques. Plaques build up on the inner layer of the heart's arterial walls and block the flow of blood to the heart. When circulation of blood to and from the heart is obstructed, the loss of nutrients and oxygen may cause tissue damage and a heart attack may occur. Other reasons for heart attacks include arteriosclerosis (narrowed arteries) leading to the heart muscle and aneurysms or bulges in the artery walls that may rupture.

The cardinal symptom of heart disease is angina or pain in the chest. The diagnosis of heart disease is made on the basis of a thorough physical and history, laboratory tests, electrocardiography, ultrasound, stress tests, radiography, and invasive monitoring techniques, such as cardiac catheterization and angiography. Risk factors for heart disease include elevated blood pressure, triglyceride and cholesterol levels, cigarette smoking, family history, obesity, changes on electrocardiograms, diabetes, lack of exercise, and Type A personality profile (aggressiveness, need to excel, and urgency) (Murdaugh, 1986). Women on oral contraceptives and who smoke are also at greater risk for heart disease.

As women increasingly occupy traditionally male roles in the workforce and take on habits similar to those of men (less exercise and leisure, stressful work environments), it is possible that heart disease may increase in women. At the present time, the relationship between occupational stress in women and heart disease is not clear. Although some studies show increased risk of heart disease for women in traditionally male-dominated work settings, other studies show that women in managerial positions are healthier than unemployed women. Although employment may increase stress for women who have dual or multiple roles (wife, mother, worker), employed women have higher economic independence, social support, and self-esteem (Murdaugh, 1986).

Prevention of heart disease includes a diet low in cholesterol, triglycerides, and saturated fats; regular exercise; avoiding cigarette smoking; and preventing and treating hypertension. Because younger women are thought to be somewhat protected from heart disease by female sex hormones present before menopause compared with older women, estrogen replacement in older women is considered by some a means of preventing heart disease (Murdaugh, 1986). Treatment of heart disease includes medications, prescribed exercise, diet, and surgical interventions (see Phipps et al., 1991). The coronary artery bypass graft (CABG) is one procedure used to treat coronary artery disease. Interestingly, women seem to have longer recovery periods, greater complications, and a higher death rate following CABG surgery than do men (Rankin, 1990). This may be due to the smaller size of women's arteries, more severe physical state, or late referral for surgery (Rankin, 1990).

During the acute phases of cardiac illness, nurses are involved in constant surveillance of the person's cardiac condition. Once women are stabilized, nurses can teach them about lifestyle modifications, such as diet, exercise, medication regimens, and sexual activity, to promote optimal physical and psychosocial adjustment to the illness.

Diabetes

Diabetes is the fifth highest cause of death for women (see Table 27.1). Life expectancy for people with diabetes is one third less than for persons without diabetes. Diabetes is reported as a chronic condition by about 9 of every 1,000 women younger than 45 years of age and more than 98 of every 1,000 women over 65 (Adams & Benson, 1990). Women, older adults, Hispanics, African Americans, and Native Americans have higher rates of diabetes than the general population.

In the United States, diabetes limits the activities of over 35% of people with the illness (National Center for Health Statistics, 1988). Diabetes is the leading cause of disability for people over 45 years of age; the leading cause of new legal blindness for individuals under 65 years of age; a major cause of neurological and vascular disorders, which may necessitate the loss of limbs; and a leading cause of kidney failure, which may require dialysis (Carter Center, 1985). People with diabetes are more prone to complications of stroke, peripheral vascular and coronary heart disease, adverse outcomes of pregnancy, ketoacidosis, blindness, kidney disease, and amputations than the general population.

Diabetes affects the way that food is metabolized by the body. Carbohydrate, fat, and protein metabolism are altered due to a deficiency in the quantity or efficiency of insulin, a hormone needed by the body to regulate glucose levels (Davidson, 1986). The altered metabolism is manifested in chronic high blood sugars that contribute to vascular diseases, including changes in vision, hypertension, and heart disease. Although the etiology of diabetes is not clear, scientists suggest a genetic, environmental, or infectious origin. Obesity and physiological or emotional stress also predispose women to diabetes.

There are three types of diabetes. Gestational diabetes affects some pregnant women due to high demands occurring during pregnancy. Type I or insulin-dependent diabetes accounts for 5% to 10% of diabetes. Because people with Type I diabetes do not produce insulin, treatment requires the injection of insulin at least once daily. Type II or non-insulin-dependent diabetes accounts for about 85% to 93% of people with diabetes. Treatment of Type II diabetes involves diet, weight loss, exercise, and oral medications or insulin to improve the efficiency of insulin produced by the body (Davidson, 1986).

Signs and symptoms of diabetes include fatigue, increased thirst and drinking, appetite changes, excessive urination, urination at night, weight changes, poor concentration, and menstrual changes. Women may have chronic yeast or other vaginal infections. Diagnosis is made on the basis of blood glucose and other laboratory values, symptoms, and physical exams. People with diabetes may experience visual changes; neurological and vascular changes, such as bowel and bladder dysfunction; and pain and weakness in the extremities.

To live with diabetes, the person and family become "health care practitioners 24 hours a day" (Benoliel, 1970). Dramatic lifestyle changes are required of people with diabetes to manage the illness and prevent or minimize complications. People with diabetes must engage in a complex self-care regimen, including (a) diet planning; (b) the timing and spacing of meals and snacks; (c) self-monitoring of blood and urine glucose; (d) administration of oral medications or insulin injections adjusted for the current blood glucose level; (e) exercise; (f) monitoring of hypoglycemia, hyperglycemia, and symptoms; and (g) close observation of the feet and skin for signs of infections (Carter Center, 1985). As described earlier, women with diabetes must integrate the complex diabetes regimen into their family, social, and work lives (Lundman, Asplund, & Norberg, 1990; Primomo, 1989). Extensive education and support about medications and tests, foot care, and the need for periodic screening of eyes and blood pressure are needed to provide the person with diabetes with as much information as possible to prevent complications from the disease. Psychosocial and peer support may help the person with diabetes and her family cope with the burdens of the disease.

The onset of non-insulin-dependent diabetes may be delayed or prevented through the maintenance of normal weight, weight reduction, exercise, and a balanced diet. Persons at high risk for developing diabetes, those who are obese or elderly, those with a family history of diabetes, or women who give birth to babies weighing more than 9 pounds, should be screened for diabetes.

Cancer

Cancer is the second leading cause of death for women in the United States and is responsible for over 22% of all deaths. The mention of cancer evokes fears and uncertainty for most people. However, progress in the early detection of some cancers and treatment advances have increased the length of survival for half of the people with a cancer diagnosis to 5 years or more.

As with many other chronic diseases, cancer is not a single disease but multiple diseases. The most common types of cancer in women are lung, breast (see Chapter 28, "Problems of the Breast"), colon/rectal, pancreatic, and ovarian. The signs and symptoms, diagnostic and screening tests, treatment, and prognosis vary according to the site, type, and extent of cancer in the individual. Cancer occurs when cells reproduce in an uncontrolled manner, invade normal cells, and subsequently change them to abnormal cells. The malignant or cancerous cells multiply, take over the blood supply from the normal tissue, and may spread to other parts of the body. In general, treatment for cancer relies on surgical procedures, chemotherapy, radiation therapy, or a combination of methods. A relatively new experimental treatment of cancer is the autologous bone marrow transplantation.

In general, there are few screening tools for cancer. Furthermore, the general population has limited knowledge about the value of early diagnosis and screening. This minimal knowledge about prevention and early diagnosis is more pronounced in people with lower educational levels and leads to a sense of fatalism about cancer.

Risk factors for cancer are largely related to lifestyle and include smoking, diet, age, family history, occupational hazards, radiation, sunlight, and environmental pollutants. Specific risk factors have been identified for different types of cancer as well. For example, a diet with low consumption of fiber and increased fat is associated with cancer of the colon. Overexposure to the sun is a risk factor for skin cancer. Early identification and treatment of cancer is the best way to increase the survival rate. The American Cancer Society recognizes seven danger signals for cancer that require further examination by a health care professional:

1. Change in bowel and bladder habits
2. A sore that does not heal
3. Unusual bleeding or discharge
4. Thickening or lump in the breast or elsewhere
5. Indigestion or difficulty swallowing
6. Obvious change in wart or mole
7. Nagging cough or hoarseness

Risk factors, signs and symptoms, and treatment of cancers increasingly common in women are discussed specifically in the following sections.

Lung Cancer

Lung cancer is now the leading cause of cancer deaths among women and has surpassed the death rate from cancer of the breast. About 41,100 women died from lung cancer in 1986. That same year, almost 50,000 women were diagnosed with lung cancer, and it is estimated that only 16% of women survive 5 years or more (Itri, 1987). Lung cancer is a highly debilitating illness, with almost 70% of all people limited in activity due to the condition (National Center for Health Statistics, 1988).

Cigarette smoking causes about 75% of all lung cancer in women. In fact, the 500% increase in lung cancer deaths between 1950 and 1985 is directly attributable to the number of women who began smoking during and after World War II (Itri, 1987). With tobacco advertising targeting teens, young women, and minorities, the grim statistics will show no improvement in the near future. Other causes of lung cancer include asbestos, radioactivity, industrial chemicals, air pollution, and secondary smoke.

Symptoms associated with lung cancer include a persistent cough, blood-streaked sputum, chest pains, or recurring pneumonia or bronchitis (Kirkpatrick, 1986). Unfortunately, lung cancer is very difficult to diagnose in its early stages, and signs and symptoms do not appear until the disease is advanced. A diagnosis of lung cancer is made on the basis of chest X ray, bronchoscopy, and sputum testing. Treatment (surgery, radiation, and/or chemotherapy) depends on the type of lung cancer and the stage of development (Kirkpatrick, 1986). Non-small-cell carcinoma accounts for about 80% of lung cancers and is treated with surgery if the tumor has not spread to other parts of the body (about 20% of cases). Fewer than half of those women whose cancer is surgically removed survive 5 years. Women who have inoperable lung cancer live on the average 6 months after diagnosis. Radiation and chemotherapy tend to be palliative in nature and may enhance the woman's comfort level but do not necessarily increase survival. Small-cell carcinoma occurs in about 20% of women with lung cancer. Small-cell carcinoma is treated with radiation and chemotherapy because the cancer has usually spread to distant sites by the time of diagnosis (Itri, 1987).

For the most part, lung cancer is a preventable disease. Widespread public education campaigns that educate young people about the risks of smoking are needed. Eliminating tobacco advertising, especially ads geared toward young women and underrepresented ethnic groups, may help reduce the number of young people who start to smoke. Smoking cessation is effective in lowering the risk of developing lung cancer, but it takes years to reduce the risk. Because smoking is a physical and psychological addiction, professional help may facilitate the process of quitting.

Uterine Cancers

Uterine cancers (cervical and endometrial) account for about one third of gynecologic malignancies (Cashavelly, 1987). In the United States, cervical cancer caused 4,508 female deaths or 5% of female cancer deaths in 1985 (Makuc et al., 1989). The number of deaths represents a 38% decline since 1973. One study documented shorter survival and greater tumor size among younger women than older women (Kaplan, 1989).

Viral agents such as herpes and papillomavirus may play a role in the development of cervical cancer. Cervical cancer seems to be associated with women who have had multiple sexual partners, those who became sexually active at a younger age, and those who use oral contraceptives (Kirkpatrick, 1986). Preventing sexually transmitted diseases may help reduce the incidence of cervical cancer.

Often, women with cervical cancer have no symptoms. If they do have symptoms, they include unusual bleeding or discharge that is sometimes associated with douching or intercourse. Treatment of cervical cancer includes surgery and radiation therapy. An annual Pap test, a screening test for early detection of cervical cancer, is recommended by the American College of Obstetricians and Gynecologists (Makuc et al., 1989). The American Cancer Society recommends less frequent screening. A reasonable recommendation based on expected benefits, risks, and cost is for screening at least every 2 to 3 years for women from the ages of 20 to 65 if two previous Pap smears are normal. Unfortunately, in a recent study of minority women, about 28% gave histories of inadequate recent screening (Rostad, 1990). Women who never had a Pap smear were older, had infrequent contact with the health care system, and did not recall ever having been advised to receive screening (Rostad, 1990). It is imperative that providers take the opportunity to screen women for cancer during their encounters with the health care system.

Endometrial cancer is most common during the sixth and seventh decades of women's lives. Women at high risk for endometrial cancer include women who have never had children and those who experienced late menopause and/or early menarche. Other factors associated with endometrial cancer include obesity, high socioeconomic status, and a family history of breast cancer. Hormonal activity, including an excess of estrogen, is recognized as having a role in the development of endometrial cancer (Kirkpatrick, 1986). Symptoms include abnormal bleeding, and an enlarged uterus may be detected on exam. Sampling vaginal secretions and endometrial biopsy of high-risk women may help detect this type of cancer early. Treatment includes hysterectomy and radiation therapy.

Fear, mutilation, insults to self-esteem and sexuality, changed body image, and uncertainty surround the diagnosis and treatment of cancer. Factors that reduced uncertainty for women with gynecologic cancers such as cervical cancer include social support, familiarity with the procedures involved in diagnosis and treatment, and perceiving the health care provider as a credible authority (Mishel & Braden, 1988). Cervical cancer has been associated with negative changes in sexual functioning. Women who had cervical cancer reported decreased frequency of intercourse, orgasm, feeling of desire, and enjoyment (Jenkins, 1988). Surprisingly, nearly 60% of women received no information about potential sexual changes. The need to provide support and information to women about the scope of potential changes they may experience is underscored by these studies.

Ovarian Cancer

Ovarian cancer causes more deaths than any other gynecologic cancer and accounts for 6% of all cancers in women. (See Chapter 26, "Reproductive Surgery.") Approximately 10,000 women die annually from ovarian cancer. Postmenopausal women up to the age of 70 have the highest incidence and mortality rates for ovarian cancers. Unfortunately, there are no symptoms associated with early ovarian cancer, and it is difficult to detect during its early stages, when cure rates are high. Some women may report vague symptoms such as intestinal upset or shoulder pain; these should be investigated if no other apparent cause is found.

About 60% to 70% of women with ovarian cancer are diagnosed with advanced disease; the 5-year survival rate is as low as 0% to 30% (Yoder, 1990). Diagnosis of ovarian cancer is based on findings on a pelvic exam followed by ultrasound and biopsy. The treatment of ovarian cancer depends on the stage of disease. As with other malignancies, treatment may include surgical removal of the tumor, hormonal therapy, chemotherapy, or radiation.

The major risk factors associated with ovarian cancer suggest endocrine dysfunction. Factors associated with higher risk for developing ovarian cancer include infertility, nulliparity, celibacy, high-fat diet, higher socioeconomic status, and occupational exposure to talc and asbestos (Yoder, 1990). Health care providers should pay special attention to women's family, socioeconomic, and occupational histories for clues about ovarian cancer risks. Currently, the periodic pelvic examination is the only screening method for ovarian cancer. Education for all women and health care providers about the importance of regular gynecologic exams is needed.

The nursing care associated with various types of cancers varies depending on many factors, such as the site and extensiveness of the cancer, the treatment modalities, and the woman's age. Psychosocial support and health teaching about the treatment and its side effects, the importance of follow-up care, and warning signs of recurrences are some of the important nursing interventions (see Chapter 26).

Prevention of Chronic Illness

Unless efforts are made to prevent chronic disease, the prevalence will continue to increase

Table 27.5 Selected Risk Factors, by Sex and Race

Risk Factor	*Women*		*Men*	
Prevalence (Percentage)	*White*	*Black*	*White*	*Black*
Cigarette smoking	27.0	27.9	30.7	40.3
Hypertension (age 35-44)	9.9	17.4	15.2	33.2
Overweight (age 35-44)	24.8	40.8	28.2	40.9
Elevated cholesterol (age 35-44)	13.3	14.3	20.1	24.5

SOURCE: Adapted from Rothenberg and Koplan (1990).
NOTE: Risk factors contribute to the development of many chronic diseases. In this table, the prevalence of smoking, high blood pressure, overweight, and cholesterol are shown to vary across both gender and race.

over time. Activities that prevent chronic disease occur on three levels (primary, secondary, and tertiary) of a continuum.

Primary Prevention

Primary prevention includes health promotion, health protection, and disease prevention activities that may inhibit the disease process from starting. Primary prevention of some communicable and chronic diseases (e.g., polio) is accomplished by vaccine. Primary prevention of most chronic diseases is difficult because the exact causes of many conditions are unknown and highly complex. Hereditary, occupational, environmental, and nutritional factors may contribute to the development of chronic disease. For hereditary conditions, genetic counseling may be used to detect those people who have a high probability of passing some chronic conditions on to their offspring.

Clearly, there are many opportunities starting early in life during which health-promoting activities may be established to reduce the risk of chronic illness. Educational efforts and associated behavioral changes in lifestyle, tobacco and alcohol intake, diet, exercise, and stress management during the school-age years and throughout the life span may help slow down the rate of chronic illness. Research on personal health practices and risks (see Table 27.5) shows that there is room for progress in reducing smoking and increasing personal health practices such as regular exercise.

Another aspect of primary prevention, specific protection against disease, merits discussion. Protection against carcinogens and occupational hazards that contribute to chronic disease is possible through the use of protective clothing, masks, and monitoring devices. Specific factors related to the onset of many chronic conditions, such as heart disease and hypertension, are known as well. Data from population studies show that low salt intake, weight reduction, and moderation of alcohol consumption may prevent blood pressure from rising. Groups at risk for developing high blood pressure (individuals who have family members with the disease, African Americans, obese persons) may benefit from these primary prevention strategies (see Table 27.5 for risk factors). Specific risk factors associated with cancer have been identified, too. Cancer prevention strategies such as education about the risks of smoking, alcohol, diet, radiation exposure, excessive sunlight exposure, occupational exposures, and environmental pollution may help to reduce or prevent malignant diseases.

Nurses can participate in primary prevention activities in all health care settings. In hospitals, nurses might teach the family of a patient with heart disease about prevention through diet, exercise, and lifestyle changes. In community settings, nurses can teach children about preventing sunburn and limiting exposure to the sun's harmful rays to reduce skin cancer in later life. Worksite education by occupational health nurses might include stress reduction techniques.

Secondary Prevention

Secondary prevention measures such as screening surveys, physical examinations, and diagnostic tests are used to diagnose the disease process in the early stages. Examples include the use of the Pap test to detect cervical cancer and health risk appraisals to identify risk factors for chronic illness.

Since 1973, increases in recent use of clinical breast examinations, Pap tests, and blood pressure screening, especially for older women and black women, have been documented (Makuc et al., 1989). However, despite the increased rates of screening, the rate still remains low among older women and the poor. Health care providers are in a position to expand secondary prevention by including screening measures during routine contact with patients. Nurses in occupational settings might teach women about breast self-examination and provide regular blood pressure screenings. Furthermore, it is critical for nurses to be advocates so that health insurance plans reimburse providers for primary and secondary prevention.

Tertiary Prevention

Rehabilitation and prevention of further complications constitutes tertiary prevention. The ultimate goal of tertiary prevention in chronic illness is to maximize the person's level of functioning within the limitations imposed by the chronic illness. Community facilities that provide rehabilitation, housing, vocational training, and supportive services to families with chronic illness fall within tertiary prevention. Community-based health services, such as home health care, including nursing, social work, physical, occupational, and speech therapy, are often required to maximize optimal functioning for persons with chronic illnesses.

Because of the pervasive changes caused by chronic illness, tertiary prevention of chronic illness for women must include a broad range of services in addition to traditional medical treatment. Health care providers may provide a variety of supportive services to women based on their needs. These may include information on the diagnosis and treatment of the illness, anticipatory guidance on the illness course, assistance with interpreting emotions and symptoms of the illness or treatment, and access to needed services, such as home care or child care (Lewis, 1986). Women may be referred to specific classes or support groups. As problems arise for the woman and her family, services specific to the problem may be useful (for example, transportation to doctor's appointments). Finally, it may be necessary to refer women and families experiencing extreme psychosocial distress to counseling services (Lewis, 1986).

Summary

Women with chronic illness live with symptoms and disabilities that must be managed for their entire lifetime. Living with chronic illness requires careful and thorough planning so that treatments are integrated into the ongoing activities of women's lives. Health care providers who work with women experiencing chronic illness must develop collaborative partnerships with them and their families. Partnerships are best developed by providing information on managing treatment regimens, available resources, and emotional and tangible assistance. It is vital to understand the perspective of the woman with chronic illness, her particular phase in the illness course, and her own and her family's needs. A holistic approach to care with attention to physiological, psychological, spiritual, cultural, social, environmental, and economic needs is vital in providing dignified care to women with chronic illness.

References

Adams, J., & Lindemann, E. (1974). Coping with long-term disability. In G. Coehlo, D. Hamburg, & J. Adams (Eds.), *Coping and adaptation* (pp. 127-138). New York: Basic Books.

Adams, P. F., & Benson, V. (1990). Current estimates from the National Health Interview Survey, 1989. *Vital and health statistics.* Washington, DC: Government Printing Office.

Ahlfield, J., Soler, N., & Marcus, S. (1985). The young adult with diabetes: Impact of the disease on marriage and having children. *Diabetes Care, 8*(1), 52-56.

Belenky, M., Clinchy, B., Goldberger, N., & Tarule, J. (1986). *Women's ways of knowing.* New York: Basic Books.

Benoliel, J. Q. (1970). The developing diabetic identity: A study of family influence. In M. Batey (Ed.), *Communicating nursing research* (Vol. 3, pp. 14-32). Boulder, CO: Western Interstate Commission for Higher Education.

Burish, T. G., & Bradley, L. A. (1983). *Coping with chronic disease: Research and applications.* New York: Academic Press.

Carter Center of Emory University. (1985). Closing the gap: The problem of diabetes mellitus in the United States. *Diabetes Care, 8*(4), 391-406.

Cashavelly, B. J. (1987). Cervical dysplasia: An overview of current concepts in epidemiology, diagnosis, and treatments. *Cancer Nursing, 10*(4), 199-206.

Cochrane, B. (1992). Acute myocardial infarction in women. *Critical Care Nursing Clinics of North America, 4*(2), 279-289.

Corbin, J., & Strauss, A. (1988). *Unending work and care: Managing chronic illness at home.* San Francisco: Jossey-Bass.

Cornwell, C., & Schmitt, M. (1990). Perceived health status, self-esteem and body image in women with rheumatoid arthritis or systemic lupus erythematosus. *Research in Nursing and Health, 13,* 99-107.

Craig, H. M., & Edwards, J. F. (1983). Adaptation in chronic illness: An eclectic model for nurses. *Journal of Advanced Nursing, 8,* 397-404.

Davidson, M. (1986). *Diabetes mellitus: Diagnosis and treatment* (2nd ed.). New York: John Wiley.

Dever, G. E. A. (1991). *Community health analysis* (2nd ed.). Gaithersburg, MD: Aspen.

Dimond, M., & Jones, S. L. (1983). *Chronic illness across the life span.* East Norwalk, CT: Appleton-Century-Crofts.

Eisenberg, M., Sutkin, L., & Jansen, M. (1984). *Chronic illness and disability through the life span.* New York: Springer.

Entmacher, P. (1983). Economic aspects: Employability and insurability. In M. Ellenberg & H. Rykin (Eds.), Diabetes mellitus: Theory and practice (3rd ed., pp. 1053-1061). New York: Medical Examining Publishing.

Feldman, D. (1974). Chronic disabling illness: A holistic view. *Journal of Chronic Diseases, 27,* 287-291.

Foxall, M., Ekberg, J., & Griffin, N. (1985). Adjustment patterns of chronically ill middle-aged persons and spouses. *Western Journal of Nursing Research, 7,* 425-444.

Gilligan, C. (1982). *In a different voice: Psychological theory and women's development.* Cambridge, MA: Harvard University Press.

Haberman, M. R., Woods, N. F., & Packard, N. J. (1990). Demands of chronic illness: Reliability and validity assessment of the demands of illness inventory. *Holistic Nursing Practice, 5*(1), 25-35.

Holmes, D. (1988). The person and diabetes in psychosocial context. *Diabetes Care, 9*(2), 201-211.

Itri, L. (1987, July-August). Women and lung cancer. *Public Health Reports Supplement,* pp. 92-96.

Jenkins, B. (1988). Patients' reports of sexual changes after treatment for gynecological cancer. *Oncology Nursing Forum, 15*(3), 349-354.

Jenny, J. (1984). A comparison of four age groups' adaptation to diabetes. *Canadian Journal of Public Health, 75*(3), 237-244.

Kaplan, M. (1989). Investigation of age as a prognostic factor in early stage invasive cancer of the cervix: Implications for nursing. *Cancer Nursing, 12*(3), 177-182.

Kirkpatrick, C. (1986). *Nurse's guide to cancer care.* Lanham, MD: Rowman & Littlefield.

Lambert, V., Lambert, C., Klipple, G., & Mewshaw, A. (1989). Social support, hardiness and well-being in women with arthritis. *Image, 21*(3), 128-131.

LaPlante, M. P. (1988). *Data on disability from the National Health Interview Survey, 1983-1985. An InfoUse report.* Washington, DC: U.S. National Institute on Disability and Rehabilitation Research.

Lewis, F. (1986). The impact of cancer on the family: A critical analysis of the research literature. *Patient Education and Counseling, 8,* 269-289.

Lewis, F. M., Woods, N. F., & Ellison, E. (1986). *The family impact study: The impact of cancer on the family* (Division of Nursing Grant R01-NU-01000). Seattle: University of Washington.

Lundman, B., Asplund, K., & Norberg, A. (1990). Living with diabetes: Perceptions of well-being. *Research in Nursing and Health, 13,* 255-262.

Makuc, D., Freid, V., & Kleinman, J. (1989). National trends in the use of preventive health care by women. *American Journal of Public Health, 79*(1), 21-26.

Mausner, J. S., & Kramer, S. (1985). *Mausner and Kramer epidemiology: An introductory text* (2nd ed.). Philadelphia: W. B. Saunders.

Mayo, L. (Ed.). (1956). *Guides to action on chronic illness. Commission on Chronic Illness.* New York: National Health Council.

Mechanic, D. (1978). *Medical sociology* (2nd ed.). New York: Free Press.

Mishel, M., & Braden, C. J. (1988). Finding meaning: Antecedents of uncertainty in illness. *Nursing Research, 37*(2), 98-103.

Murdaugh, C. (1986, October-December). Coronary heart disease in women. *Progress in Cardiovascular Nursing,* pp. 2-8.

National Center for Health Statistics, & Collins, J. G. (1988). Prevalence of selected chronic conditions, United States, 1983-1985. *Advance data from vital statistics* (No. 155, DHHS Pub. No. PHS 88-1250). Hyattsville, MD: Public Health Service.

Packard, N. J., Haberman, M. R., Woods, N. F., & Yates, B. C. (1991). Demands of illness among chronically ill women. *Western Journal of Nursing Research, 13*(4), 434-457.

Phipps, W., Long, B., Woods, N. F., & Cassmeyer, V. (1991). *Medical-surgical nursing* (4th ed.). St. Louis, MO: C. V. Mosby.

Primomo, J. (1989). *Patterns of chronic illness management, psychosocial development, family and social environment, and adaptation among women with diabetes.* Unpublished doctoral dissertation, University of Washington, Seattle.

Primomo, J., Yates, B., & Woods, N. (1990). Social support for women during chronic illness: The relationship among sources and types to adjustment. *Research in Nursing and Health, 13,* 153-161.

Rankin, S. (1990). Differences in recovery from cardiac surgery: A profile of male and female patients. *Heart & Lung, 19*(5), 481-485.

Rankin, S., & Weekes, D. (1989). Life-span development: A review of theory and practice for families with chronically ill members. *Scholarly Inquiry for Nursing Practice: An International Journal, 3*(1), 3-22.

Rolland, J. (1984). Toward a psychosocial typology of chronic and life-threatening illness. *Family Systems Medicine, 2,* 245-262.

Rostad, M. (1990). Advances in nursing management of patients with lung cancer. *Nursing Clinics of North America, 25*(2), 393-403.

Rothenberg, R., & Koplan, J. (1990). Chronic disease in the 1990's. *Annual Review of Public Health, 11,* 267-296.

Sexton, D., & Munro, D. (1986). Living with a chronic illness: The experience of women with chronic obstructive pulmonary disease. *Western Journal of Nursing Research, 10*(1), 26-44.

Stetz, K., Lewis, F., & Primomo, J. (1986). Family coping strategies and chronic illness in the mother. *Family Relations, 35,* 515-522.

Strauss, A., Corbin, J., Fagerhaugh, S., Glaser, B., Maines, D., Suczek, B., & Weiner, C. (1984). *Chronic illness and the quality of life* (2nd ed.). St. Louis, MO: C. V. Mosby.

Strauss, A., Fagerhaugh, D., Suczek, B., & Weiner, C. (1985). *The social organization of medical work.* Chicago: University of Chicago Press.

Stuifbergen, A. (1987). The impact of chronic illness on families. *Families and Community Health, 9*(4), 43-51.

Thorne, S. E. (1990). Mothers with chronic illness: A predicament of social construction. *Health Care for Women International, 11,* 209-221.

U.S. Bureau of the Census. (1991). *Statistical abstract of the United States: 1990* (110th ed.). Washington, DC: Government Printing Office.

U.S. Department of Health and Human Services. (1988). The 1988 report of the Joint National Committee on Detection, Evaluation, and Treatment of High Blood Pressure. *Archives of Internal Medicine, 148*(5), 1023-1038.

Williams, G., & Wood, P. (1988). Coming to terms with chronic illness: The negotiation of autonomy in rheumatoid arthritis. *International Disability Studies, 10*(3), 128-133.

Woods, N., Yates, B., & Primomo, J. (1989). Supporting families during chronic illness: What, who, when and why. *Image, 21*(1), 46-50.

Worden, J. W. (1989). The experience of recurrent cancer. *Ca—A Cancer Journal for Clinicians, 39*(5), 305-310.

Yoder, L. (1990). The epidemiology of ovarian cancer: A review. *Oncology Nursing Forum, 17*(3), 411-415.

28

Problems of the Breast

BARBARA NETTLES-CARLSON

Breast problems range from women's concerns about normal life cycle changes to infections, chronic pain, lumps, and cancer. In this chapter, evaluation and management of breast symptoms will be presented as well as ambulatory care of well women, including breast health in the life cycle, teaching breast self-examination, and performing breast clinical examination. Problems of atypical breast size or symmetry are described, followed by a discussion of various types of breast plastic surgery. Breast cancer epidemiology, prevention, early detection, diagnosis, and treatment are presented in the final section. Fear of cancer as well as the breast's association with sexuality contributes to the anxiety often evoked by breast symptoms. It is important for clinicians to understand that women react to breast problems within a sociocultural context of meanings and symbols, and that these meanings also influence clinical care.

Sociocultural Context of Breast Problems

Nurturance and Sexuality

Throughout the ages, the female breast has symbolized nurturance and sexuality. The physiological function of lactation, providing life-giving nourishment to the infant, connotes a strong association of the breast with survival of the species. In fact, the presence of mammary glands is a defining characteristic of Mammalia, the vertebrate class to which the human species belongs. A breast surgeon observed that "Women worry about their breasts in a different way than they worry about the rest of their bodies—and for good reason" (S. Love, 1990, p. xvii).

Unlike the hidden uterus, the breasts are external, incontrovertible signs of femaleness. In paintings and sculpture of primitive times, and even up to the present day, the breasts identify the female body as the penis does the male body. In contemporary times in the United States, the meanings of the breast, as reflected in the media, more often focus on explicit sexuality than on nurturance. Advertisements for products ranging from blue jeans to cars and perfume show women in frankly sexual poses with their breasts prominently displayed, and the breasts of film stars are often promoted as models of the "ideal" sexually attractive shape and size.

Illustrative of societal ambivalence about the breasts' sexual and nurturant symbolism are the inconsistent mores regarding exposure. Although it is socially acceptable for a woman to wear a minimal bikini on the beach, exposing the breast while nursing a baby in a public place is not. Similarly, in films barebreastedness is pictured often in sexual encounters but appears rarely in domestic scenes of a woman nursing a baby. In fact, a breast-feeding mother may experience pressure from her family or work associates to confine nursing to the home. Not surprisingly, clinicians have observed that many women seem to experience their breasts with a mixture of pride and shame (S. Love, 1990).

Clearly, the loss of a breast is potentially threatening to feminine identity. Rosemary, a 26-year-old with breast cancer, said after her mastectomy,

> My mom changed the bandages for me the first week because I couldn't—I just couldn't bear to look at myself. Finally one day in the shower, I thought, "I'm going to change the bandages myself." So finally I got up enough nerve to change them. It took me a week. I sat on the edge of the tub and cried again. I mourned for the loss of my breast. It's part of your femininity, so you mourn the loss. (Oktay & Walter, 1991, p. 46)

Medical Approaches

Past medical approaches to breast disease contribute to the care environment within which women experience breast problems. Traditionally, medicine has focused on aggressive surgical treatment of breast cancer with much less interest in treatment of or clinical research on noncancerous breast problems. In the past, after the possibility of cancer was ruled out, women with worrisome chronic breast symptoms often received cursory treatment and little follow-up. Chronic breast pain was frequently attributed to psychological causes, although some early empirical studies described its epidemiology and treatment (Patey, 1949; Preece, Mansel, & Hughes, 1978).

Until the 1970s, the standard treatment for breast cancer was radical mastectomy, in which all the breast tissue, the axillary lymph nodes, and the pectoral muscle were removed. Prior to a biopsy under anesthesia, the patient customarily consented to undergo mastectomy immediately if the biopsy confirmed cancer. At that time physicians believed the advantages of the "one-step" procedure, as it was called, were expeditious removal of the cancer before potential spread of the disease and avoidance of risks of a second anesthesia. The patient, however, lost decision-making control over the timing of this extensive and mutilating surgery. It is now known that the results of pathological examination of a frozen specimen are less accurate than when the specimen is prepared in a 24- to 48-hour process. Radical mastectomy is no longer the standard treatment for localized breast cancer, but medical attitudes and practices are slow to change. Some patients (Gross & Ito, 1991), clinicians (S. Love, 1990), and women's health activists (Soffa, 1991) assert that a surprising number of surgeons still advise mastectomy without sufficient consideration of equally effective breast-conserving treatments.

Controversial medical issues, which have an impact on clinical care, include the (a) multiplicity and unclear effectiveness of the treatment options for early breast cancer, (b) the safety and regulation of breast implants, (c) the high cost and underuse of mammography, (d) the value of breast self-examination, (e) whether or not to participate in clinical trials, and (f) the paucity of federal funding for basic research on breast cancer and other diseases affecting women (Knobf, 1990; Pearson, 1991; "Politics of Breast Cancer," 1990; Zones, 1991). Conflict regarding unresolved issues at times fosters an adversarial rather than a collaborative relationship between clinicians, patients, and women's advocacy groups.

Illness Paradigm

Traditionally, the delivery of health care services in the United States has been in actuality largely illness oriented. Although this is changing, a problem still exists with adequate resources and incentives that ensure the delivery of clinical preventive services, such as breast cancer screening. For example mammography services are not accessible to all women in the population, and the costs, which may be as much as $100, are usually not reimbursed by insurers. Although the use of mammography was increased according to a recent regional survey (Zapka, Hosnmer, Costanza, Harris, & Stoddard, 1992), in a nationwide survey, fewer than half of American women reported adequate breast cancer screening (Dawson & Thompson, 1989). Moreover, clinicians have little incentive to perform breast physical examinations and teach breast self-examination, both of which are labor-intensive tasks that generate less practice revenue than do procedures for diagnosis and management of illness. Furthermore, physicians and nurses, having been educated largely in tertiary care, often lack expertise in the delivery of clinical preventive services. Even with well women, who comprise two thirds to three quarters of all asymptomatic patients in ambulatory settings, the traditional clinician is more comfortable with the focus on problem evaluation and management than on prevention.

Breast Health

The concept of breast health is an appropriate framework for providing clinical services to well women in ambulatory care settings. Education for self-care, rather than problem management, is the central intervention. Parts of the framework are (a) active listening; (b) collection and evaluation of relevant historical and physical data, including clinical breast examination; (c) information sharing that results in mutual planning; (d) anticipatory guidance regarding breast changes expected during the life cycle; (e) appropriate consultation and referral patterns; and (f) availability for follow-up and continuing care offered to the patient. This framework affirms the woman as a self-care agent, able to make health decisions in her best interest, with the clinician as a knowledgeable, supportive health guide. Availability over time, and the extent and expertise of consultation and referral networks, will enhance the clinician's effectiveness, as will the clinician's knowledge of current information about breast changes, variations in development, plastic surgery options available for women with atypical breast size, teaching breast self-examination, and performing clinical breast examination.

The Breast in the Life Cycle

Fetal Development, Infancy, Childhood. Breast development begins at about the 5th week of fetal life with the formation of a "milk streak." In humans, primitive breast tissue, called the mammary ridge, continues to develop only in the thorax and regresses elsewhere. Incomplete regression of the mammary ridge accounts for the fact that extra breasts (polymastia) or nipples (polythelia) occur in about 1% of females; this inherited condition can also occur in males (Romrell & Bland, 1991). Found on the milk line from the axilla to the groin, these rarely cause any problems. Accessory nipples can be mistaken for a pigmented mole, and accessory breasts may become engorged and produce milk (Osborne, 1991).

From about the 20th week of fetal life, mammary ducts and lobes develop under the influence of estrogen and progesterone; from about the 32nd week, the fetal mammary tissue increases fourfold, and the nipple and areola become pigmented. The newborn's breasts may be enlarged due to hormonal stimulation during fetal life, and in 80% to 90% of neonates, colostrum (a secretion of the mammary glands) can be expressed for 4 to 7 days after birth. Called "witches' milk," this fluid subsides after 3 to 4 weeks as the influence of placental hormones disappears. Rarely, congenital absence of a breast and nipple (amastia) is seen in a newborn (Osborne, 1991).

Little happens developmentally in the breast between infancy and puberty. During this period, estrogen levels are low and the breast bud remains quiescent beneath the nipple. However, if the breast bud is removed or injured during childhood it will not grow back; no further breast tissue will develop at puberty.

Puberty and the Menstrual Cycle. Breast development is one of the earliest visible signs of puberty. Shortly after pubic hair appears and about a year or so before menarche, breast tissue begins to grow, beginning with a swelling subareolar bud that may be itchy. At puberty, marked increases in tactile sensitivity of the breast have been found in females compared to males (Robinson & Short, 1977). Phases of breast development during puberty are described further in Chapter 3, "Women's Bodies."

Women remember experiencing their pubertal breast development intensely and in varying ways. One survey showed that about half of the women remembered being pleased, 33% felt "shy," 24% were embarrassed, and 10% were worried or unhappy (S. Love, 1990, p. 14). During preventive care visits, the clinician can offer the adolescent female anticipatory guidance about breast development and perhaps suggest that she discuss her feelings and reactions with her mother. Most women can recollect vividly their adolescent feelings about their breasts; sharing these with their daughters can be affirming to both.

The hormonal influences of the menstrual cycle are responsible for waxing and waning breast size and tactile sensitivity, although the exact mechanism by which this occurs remains unclear. Premenstrually, the average increase is 15 cm to 30 cm; this is thought to be due to duct proliferation under the influence of estrogen and to lobular edema mainly caused by progesterone (Osborne, 1991; Romrell & Bland, 1991). Postmenstrually, edema subsides and minimum breast size is observed from 5 to 7 days after menses (Osborne, 1991). Similarly, breast sensitivity is least during menses and 2 weeks afterward; it is greatest at ovulation (Robinson & Short, 1977).

The Mature Breast. By about 20 years of age, a woman's breasts have reached their full development. The anatomy of the mature breast and breast changes in the sexual response cycle are described in Chapter 3.

Pregnancy and Lactation. Early in the first trimester, marked growth begins in the ducts, lobes, and alveoli; a sensation of breast fullness and heaviness may be experienced as the first bodily change signaling pregnancy. Dramatic sprouting and branching of the ducts occurs under the influence of estrogen as early as the 3rd to 4th week of gestation. By the 5th to 8th week, noticeable breast changes include enlargement, enlargement of the superficial veins, and increased pigmentation of the nipple and areola.

In the second trimester, proliferation of ducts and lobules, stimulated by the hormone progesterone, results in increased breast size; stretch marks, called striae, may appear on the skin. From the second half of pregnancy on, the increasing size of the breast is due less to proliferation of the ducts and lobules than to accumulating secretion of colostrum in the alveoli and hypertrophy of the mammary epithelial cells, connective tissue, and fat (Osborne, 1991; Romrell & Bland, 1991). During pregnancy, the hormone prolactin is released progressively; this is thought to stimulate both epithelial growth and milk secretory activity in the mammary gland (Neville, Allen, & Watters, 1983).

After birth, cessation of placental hormones triggers the release of prolactin through a feedback mechanism, beginning the transition of the breast from a nonsecretory to a lactating state. For 4 to 5 days postpartum, breast enlargement continues due to accumulation of colostrum in the alveoli and ducts. During this transition, the release of prolactin is also stimulated and maintained when the newborn is brought to the breast and suckles the colostrum.

As the transition continues, the infant's suckling stimulates nerve endings in the nipple; sensory impulses are then relayed to the hypothalamus, triggering release of the hormone oxytocin into the general circulation. Oxytocin then acts to contract the nipple's myoepithelial cells, and milk is ejected through the lactiferous ducts. Often called the "let-down reflex," this process can be activated by sounds, sights, smells, and thoughts of the infant and inhibited by emotions such as fear and embarrassment. During the milk ejection process, increases of intramammary ductal pressures of 20 mm Hg to 30 mm have been observed; this is thought to be related to mammary blood flow (Osborne, 1991). In all species in which it has been measured, mammary blood flow rises markedly during lactation; in animal studies, some correlations between mammary blood flow, stress, and milk production have been found. No relationship has been observed between breast size, milk production, and mammary blood flow (Neville et al., 1983).

Enhanced tactile sensitivity of the breast after parturition has been demonstrated (Robinson & Short, 1977), supporting the clinical observation that many nursing mothers find breast-feeding a sensually pleasurable experience, some noting vaginal lubrication. The breasts of the lactating woman are larger, heavier, and more pendulous than those in the nonlactating state. After weaning, the mammary gland becomes inactive, followed by atrophy of the lobular structures and degeneration of alveolar secretory cells (Osborne, 1991).

Mature breast milk is produced by about 30 days postpartum. Rich in protein, fat, and lactose, it also contains immunoglobulins, vitamins, minerals, and trace elements. Breast milk is thin and bluish in color, whereas colostrum is thick and yellowish. Dietary changes during lactation are more likely to affect the fat than the protein content of breast milk. Adding protein supplement to an inadequate diet tends to increase the total yield (Casey & Hambridge, 1983).

Menopause and Aging. The breasts age along with the rest of the body. After menopause, involution of ducts and lobes occurs due to cessation of cyclic hormones; fat and connective tissue largely replace these glandular structures. In old age, the breast shrinks and becomes pendulous. Hormone replacement retards sagging somewhat, but will not restore a youthful contour.

Atypical Size

Most women's breasts are within normal size limits. To judge what is "within normal limits," a few reference points may be helpful. According to one author (Osborne, 1991) the "average" breast measures 10 cm to 12 cm in diameter and 5 cm to 7 cm in thickness centrally. A "typical" nonlactating breast has been reported to weigh between 150 gm and 225 gm (Romrell & Bland, 1991). Among 55 women studied, researchers found that mean volume of the right breast was 276.46 ml (range 94.6 ml to 889.3 ml), and the left breast was 291.69 ml (range 106.9 ml to 893.1 ml) (Smith, Palin, Katch, & Bennett, 1986).

"Ideal" breast size is culturally determined. For a variety of reasons, a woman may express concern that her breasts are too small, too large, or asymmetrical. Many women's breasts are slightly asymmetrical in size; this is a normal variation that the clinician may not even notice unless the patient points it out. The variety of shapes and sizes is equaled by the variety of perceptions women have about what is large or small breastedness. The breasts can enlarge rapidly concurrently with pregnancy or overall weight gain; this is not considered an abnormality, but the increased size may be undesired. Huge breasts can be an embarrassment, and their weight is physically uncomfortable; on physical examination bra strap marks on the shoulders may be seen as well as Candida skin infections that thrive in the warm airless environment of the inframammary fold.

A woman's concerns about atypical size or asymmetry should receive careful initial evaluation. By exploring the meaning of her concern, obtaining a history, and performing a physical examination before discussing options such as breast enlargement or reduction, the clinician can do much to help a woman clarify feelings and expectations and inform her about available options. Too often, however, women receive from the clinician premature reassurance of normality or a referral to a plastic surgeon without any initial discussion and evaluation.

The clinician should be aware of the following specific abnormal conditions of atypically large or asymmetrical breasts. A history should be obtained of the chronology of this problem, whether any other women in the family have similar breasts, and what, if any, medications the woman is taking.

Early in puberty, very large breasts can develop and keep on growing out of proportion to the rest of the body. This abnormality is called *virginal (juvenile, adolescent) hypertrophy.* It may be familial. Usually bilateral, it occasionally occurs in only one breast. A drug-induced condition called *breast gigantism* has also been described (Bland & Romrell, 1991).

Rarely, absence of the breast is observed on physical examination; this condition may be congenital or acquired. *Amastia* is the congenital absence of nipples and breasts. *Amazia* is the presence of nipples with no breast tissue. Amazia may be acquired iatrogenically during childhood through biopsy of a precociously developing breast, by radiation treatment to the chest, or through trauma such as a burn. *Hypoplasia* is congenital underdevelopment; it may be bilateral or unilateral. In 90% of women with amastia or severe hypoplasia, the pectoral muscle is also underdeveloped, resulting in an abnormal sunken appearance of the anterior chest. Unilateral hypoplasia of the breast, thorax, and pectoral muscle is a congenital condition called *Poland's syndrome* (Bland & Romrell, 1991).

Breast Plastic Surgery. The principal types of mammoplasty are procedures that decrease breast size (reduction) and increase breast size (augmentation) (see Figures 28.1 and 28.2). The clinician should discuss these surgical options with the patient, considering the benefits and risks in the context of data previously obtained in the history and physical examination. Breast plastic surgery is a highly specialized field; the clinician should be knowledgeable about local and regional referral sources. The clinician should help clarify expectations and goals with any woman considering mammoplasty before referring her to a specialist. What results would she

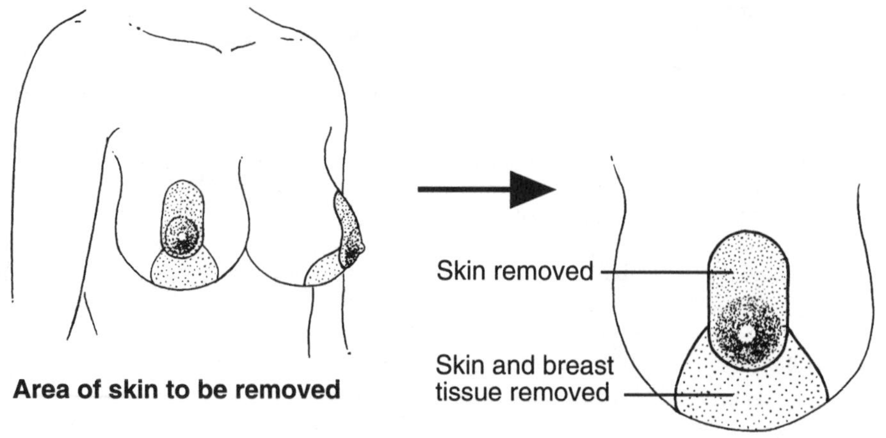

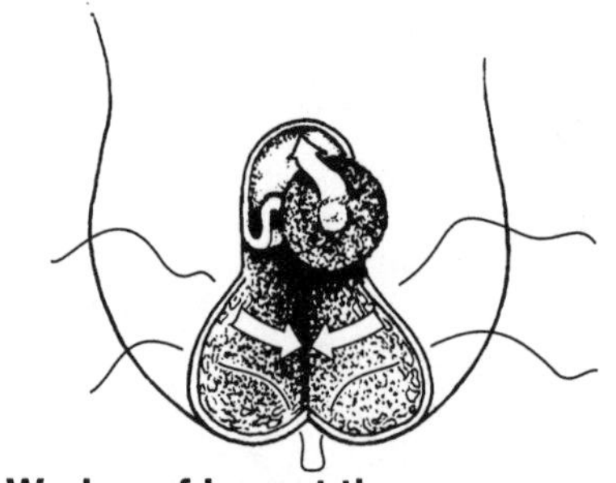

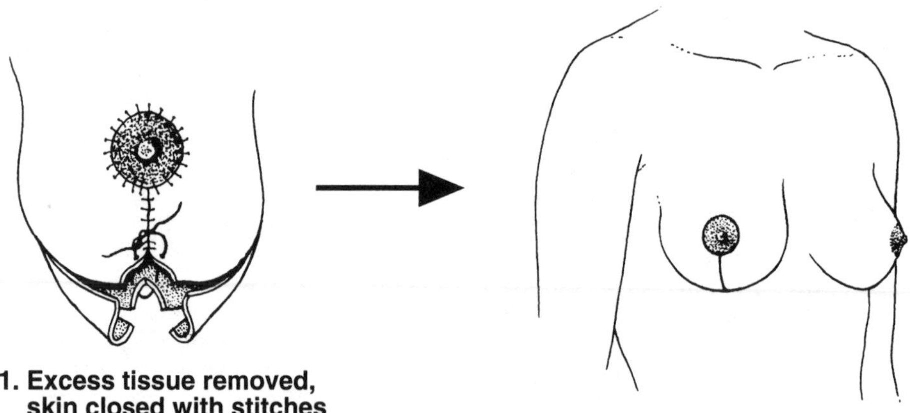

Figure 28.1. Breast Reduction
SOURCE: Adapted from Love, S. M. *Dr. Susan Love's Breast Book.* Reading, MA: Addison-Wesley Publishing Company, Inc. (1990), p. 64. Used with permission.

like to achieve? What does she want the procedure to accomplish and for whom? Women who want to please themselves are more likely to be satisfied with the results than are those motivated by others' wishes.

Breast reduction is the oldest type of mammoplasty. The procedure, which may require 3 to 4 hours to complete, is performed under general anesthesia. Tissue is removed from around the nipple, which is usually left intact on a pedicle. Scars from this procedure run horizontally along the inframammary fold, vertically up the breast, and circumferential to the nipple.

Reduction is considered quite safe in terms of general surgical risks, but there are some side effects and complications. Reduction surgery decreases lactation capability (about half can breast-feed) as well as tactile sensitivity on the breast, nipple, and areolar skin. In addition, postoperative necrosis and subsequent loss of the nipple and areola can occur (< 5% of cases); this can be corrected only by artificial reconstruction. Necrosis of these structures is due to compromised blood supply when tissue is removed from around them. Postoperative weight gain, although not a complication of surgery, may result in reversal of the desired results, as the breasts will get larger again, just as they would have before reduction surgery (Goldwyn, 1976; S. Love, 1990). Breast cancer risk is unaffected by reduction surgery.

Breast augmentation techniques were developed in the 1960s. An estimated 2 to 3 million women in the United States have had augmentation mammoplasty. Before access to breast implants was restricted in 1992, about 150,000 procedures were done annually, of which 20% were postmastectomy reconstructions and the remainder were considered cosmetic (Silverstein et al., 1988; Zones, 1991). The procedure takes about 2 hours to complete and may be done on an outpatient basis. Placement of implants is through an incision in the axilla (the inframammary fold) or circumferential to the areola (see Figure 28.2, Locations of incisions). The patient returns for follow-up care and suture removal in about 10 days.

Breast implants may be made of silicone, saline solution, or autologous tissue grafted from the woman's abdomen or thigh. Formerly, liquid silicone was injected directly into the breast, but this is no longer done. Silicone-gel-filled implants have been most often used, followed by those filled with saline solution. Silicone produces more natural looking and feeling results than do saline implants although the latter have fewer medical complications. Autologous implants, although safe, are less commonly used than other types; the procedure is costly, requiring more extensive surgery than do other implants.

Implants may be positioned between the breast tissue and the pectoral muscle, or underneath the pectoral muscle (see Figure 28.2, Locations of implants). Advantages of the latter positioning are less risk that the implant will conceal a future breast cancer or lead to a postoperative complication known as contractures—that is, thick scar tissue that forms around the implant. Contractures, which detract greatly from the desired aesthetic results of the surgery, are accompanied by hardening of the implant, with an unpleasantly firm, almost wooden feeling to the breast, and an unattractive spherical shape. Massage may help to reduce the firmness caused by contractures; further surgical procedures that correct this complication can be attempted but are not always successful. Contractures occur more often (18% to 50% of cases) when the implant is positioned between breast tissue and pectoral muscle than when it is placed beneath the pectoral muscle (1% to 18% of cases); the latter technique, however, takes longer to perform surgically, making it a more expensive choice for the patient (S. Love, 1990).

Rupture of the implant, which can occur years after its implantation, is an uncommon but serious complication of augmentation mammoplasty. The reported incidence of rupture varies from 0.2% to 6%; its true incidence is unknown (Kessler, 1992). After rupture, which may occur either spontaneously or after a blow to the breast, immediate surgery is indicated to remove the implant and all the silicone that can be found. Other complications of augmentation mammoplasty are postoperative infection or bleeding (1%) and permanent loss of sensation in the nipple or areola (2%) (S. Love, 1990).

The safety of silicone implants is unclear; remarkably little longitudinal research has been done on these devices. In two cohort studies, augmentation was not associated with the risk of breast cancer (Berkel, Birdsell, & Jenkins, 1992; Deapen, Pike, Casagrande, & Brody, 1986). However, the clinical concern that implants may delay diagnosis of breast cancer was supported in one case control study comparing stage of disease in nonaugmented and augmented women with breast cancer. The researchers found that augmented women had presented with more advanced disease, a higher percentage of invasive

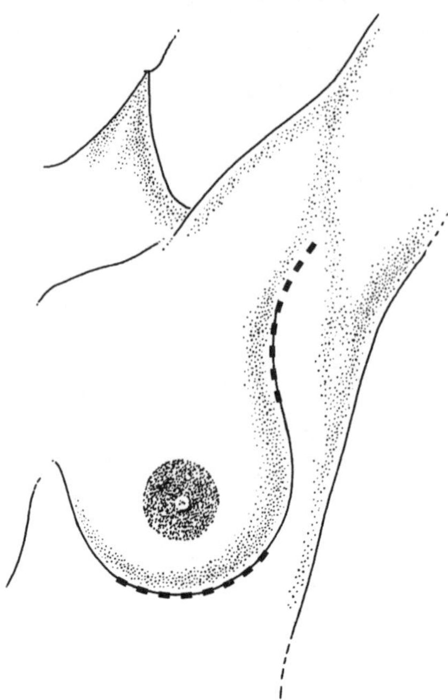

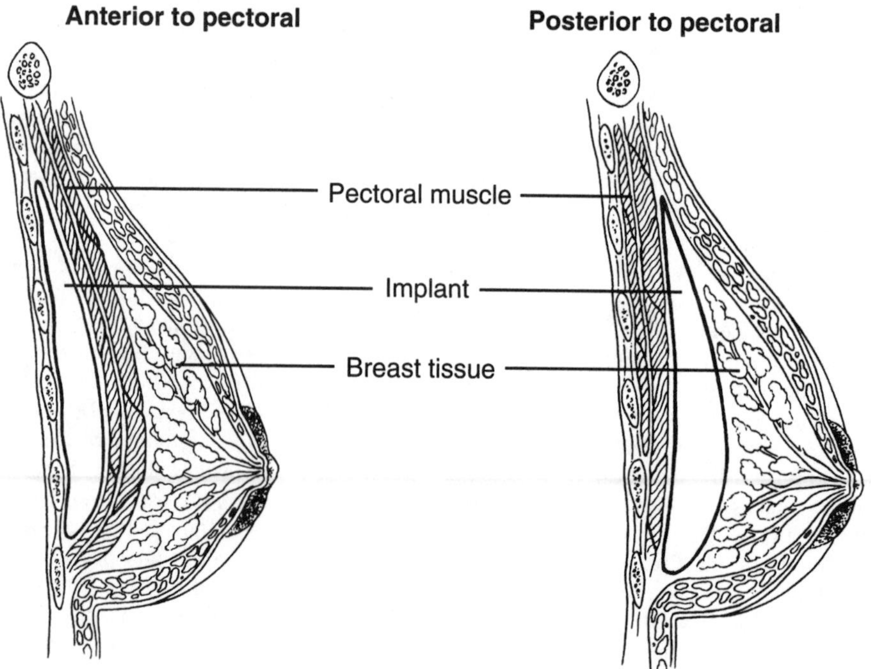

Figure 28.2. Breast Augmentation
SOURCE: Adapted from Love, S. M. *Dr. Susan Love's Breast Book.* Reading, MA: Addison-Wesley Publishing Company, Inc. (1990), p. 68. Used with permission.

lesions, and more positive axillary nodes than did nonaugmented women (Silverstein et al., 1988).

Association between silicone implants and the development of scleroderma (Spiera, 1988) and other autoimmune diseases has also been suggested but has not been shown conclusively. A concern is that silicone migrates to other body organs or systems and causes nonspecific symptoms. In breast implant litigation, women have alleged that their symptoms, which suggested autoimmune disorders, were not diagnosed or related to their history of breast implants (Henry, 1992).

After investigating the numerous concerns about silicone implants, an advisory panel of the Food and Drug Administration (FDA) recommended that access to these devices be limited until their safety and effectiveness were demonstrated. Subsequently, in April 1992, the FDA announced that silicone gel breast implants would be available only through controlled clinical studies and that women who needed implants for reconstruction would be assured of access to these studies. This decision has been very controversial (Fisher, 1992; Kessler, 1992).

Women's health clinicians should stay informed regarding rapidly changing developments on the regulation of breast implants and regarding research on their safety and effectiveness. Although there is general agreement that long-term safety of silicone implants has yet to be demonstrated, major controversy exists regarding what research is needed and the degree to which the use of implants should be regulated now (Zones, 1991). Litigation involving breast implants has become much more frequent (Henry, 1992). The National Women's Health Network and the Boston Women's Health Collective have prepared packets of information about silicone gel implants, one for women who are considering cosmetic augmentation and another for women considering breast reconstruction following mastectomy; these may be obtained from the Network offices (1325 G Street, NW, Washington, DC, 20005) for $10. In addition, free information is available from the FDA (1134 Parklawn Building, 5600 Fishers Lane [HFV-40], Rockville, MD 28057).

Other Breast Surgeries

There are also procedures that firm and uplift sagging breasts (mastopexy) and evert inverted nipples.

In *mastopexy,* excess skin and fat are removed and the nipple is elevated. The effects, like those of a face-lift, are not permanent. *Inverted nipples* can be everted by a simple procedure done under local anesthetic, with stitches removed in about 2 weeks. A drawback is that inversion may recur; but the procedure can be repeated. For women with *assymetry,* one breast can be augmented or the other reduced or a combination of these. Women with Poland's syndrome can have an artificial breast reconstructed similar to that for women postmastectomy, using flaps of skin, muscle, and fat from the back or abdomen (Bland & Romrell, 1991; Goldwyn, 1987).

Breast Self-Examination

Women could enhance their body awareness and become much more accurate self-observers through performing breast self-examination (BSE). A woman who examines her breasts regularly and proficiently is a more informative historian from the clinician's point of view. Clinical services that nurses should be providing include instruction on how to examine the breasts, periodic reinforcement of this skill during office visits or in other settings, clinical follow-up, and telephone availability regarding worrisome changes found on BSE.

According to a national survey of ambulatory care in the United States, 47% of women patients over 40 reported BSE monthly or more often, 32% reported performing BSE "infrequently"; 11% said they did not know how, and 10% said they never performed BSE despite knowing how to do so. In the same survey, the proportion of women who did not perform BSE increased with age, and education and income were strongly associated with BSE, even when age and race were taken into account (Dawson & Thompson, 1989). In other studies, a variety of health beliefs and perceptions, such as confidence in technique, feeling susceptible to breast cancer, and perceiving few barriers, have been associated with regular self-examination (Champion, 1988; Lashley, 1987; Meyerowitz & Chaiken, 1987; Nettles-Carlson & Smith, 1988; Rutledge, 1987; Wyper, 1990).

Having received personal instruction from a nurse or doctor increases frequency, but not necessarily accuracy, of BSE performance (Baines, Wall, Risch, Kuin, & Fan, 1986; Mamon &

Zapka, 1985). Brief instruction on technique may be as effective as more intensive counseling-oriented interventions (Lauver, 1989; Nettles-Carlson, Field, Friedman, & Smith, 1988). Detailed instructional information may increase thoroughness among women already performing BSE (Lauver, 1989), and BSE technique improves with periodic instruction over time (Baines, To, & Wall, 1990). Women who perform BSE much more often than recommended (overadherence) may do so because of inadequate BSE technique and low confidence in what they are doing (Lauver & Angerame, 1990).

Although few women in the population report regularly examining their breasts, the majority of breast cancers are still discovered by women themselves, often accidentally. Most self-discovered lumps are greater than 1 centimeter. In experimental studies, however, researchers have shown that after instruction, women can correctly detect small lumps (< 1 cm) in breast models (Saunders, Pilgrim, & Pennypacker, 1986), and improved skill also remains over time (Fletcher et al., 1990). However, BSE as it is currently practiced by most women appears to be less accurate in detecting early breast cancer than is a combination of mammography and clinical examination by a professional. Although some retrospective studies indicate that BSE is associated with earlier detection of breast cancer or longer survival, no prospective studies have yet linked BSE with reduced mortality (U.S. Preventive Services Task Force, 1987). Although the efficacy of BSE remains unknown, its potential sensitivity in early cancer detection may be far greater than is currently thought. The clinician, then, is faced with hard choices in terms of how best to incorporate BSE teaching into the care process.

When teaching women how to perform BSE (see Figure 28.3) the clinician should begin with inspection but should place special emphasis on palpation technique, which has been shown to be a predictor of accurate lump detection (Fletcher et al., 1990). Demonstrate palpation using the pads, not tips, of the fingers to examine all quadrants of the breast and the axillary tail. A circular or up-and-down search pattern is acceptable; researchers in one study found that women using the latter pattern performed a more thorough examination (Saunders et al., 1986). Emphasize that the purpose is not to make a diagnosis but, rather, to become familiar with one's breasts to recognize changes over time. Use nonmedical words to describe palpation findings, such as those women have used to describe the feel of normal breast tissue (see Table 28.1). An anatomical diagram of the breast is a helpful aid. Written information supplements but never substitutes for clear verbal explanations.

After instruction, ask the client to demonstrate the steps of the examination, give her feedback on technique, and reinforce continued efforts. A positive approach emphasizing body awareness and the development of self-observation skills is preferable to focusing exclusively on detection of breast cancer. The clinician's BSE instruction and availability for telephone follow-up can do much to dispel barriers that women frequently express, such as low confidence in ability to perform BSE and not knowing what to do if one "finds something" (Nettles-Carlson, 1989).

Clinical Breast Examination

Periodic physical examination of the breast, usually termed *clinical breast examination* (CBE), is an essential part of the clinician's evaluation of both asymptomatic and symptomatic patients. A woman's concerns about variations such as inverted nipples or assymetry, as well as more sensitive issues such as fear of breast cancer, often surface during a physical examination; this context of shared observation of her body may prompt comments or questions she would hesitate to utter in a less private setting. Effective responses will be nonjudgmental, empathetic, and factual. During CBE, the clinician has an ideal opportunity to offer anticipatory guidance regarding life cycle changes appropriate to the individual's age and stage.

The technique of inspection and palpation in this examination is essentially the same as that of BSE. When beginning CBE with the woman sitting, first inspect the breast contour and skin for rashes, prominent veins, dimpling, and retraction of the nipple. Asking her to assume various positions, such as arms raised above the head and then extended forward and placed on the examiner's shoulders, is useful when examining a symptomatic woman; in asymptomatic women these procedures are time-consuming with low yield of positive findings (Fletcher & O'Malley, 1986). Arm extension is indicated for the woman with large breasts; it may reveal dimpling or abnormal contour if a mass adherent to underlying muscle is preventing free movement of the breast tissue.

Here's what you should do to check for changes in your breasts.

1. Stand in front of a mirror that is large enough to let you see your breasts clearly. Check both breasts for anything unusual. Check the skin for puckering, dimpling, or scaliness. Look for any discharge from the nipples.

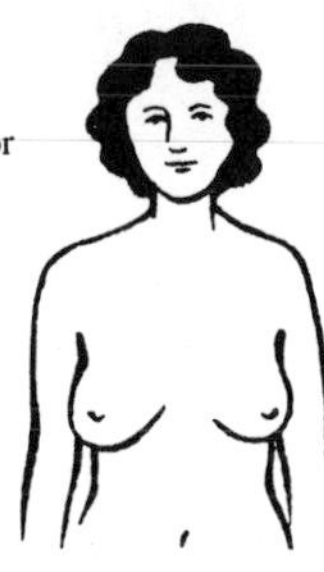

Do steps 2 and 3 to check for any change in the shape or contour of your breasts. As you do these steps, you should feel your chest muscles tighten.

2. Watching closely in the mirror, clasp your hands behind your head and press your hands forward.

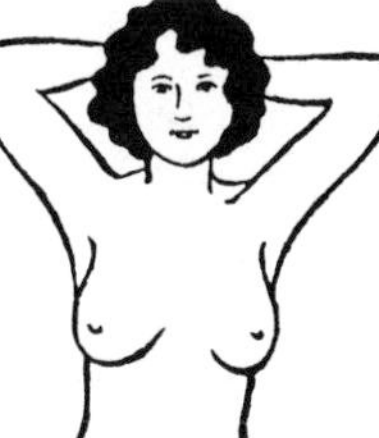

3. Next, press your hands firmly on your hips and bend slightly toward the mirror as you pull your shoulders and elbows forward.

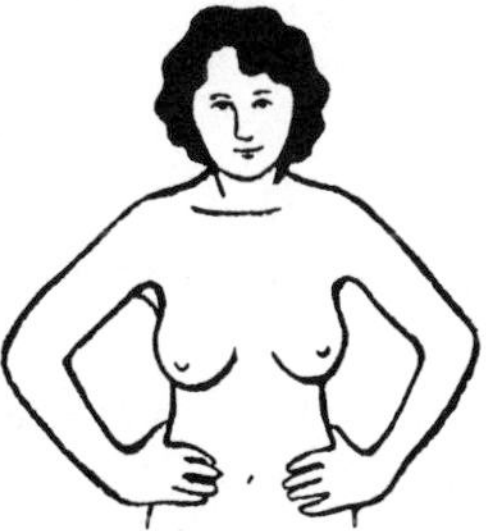

4. Gently squeeze each nipple and look for a discharge.

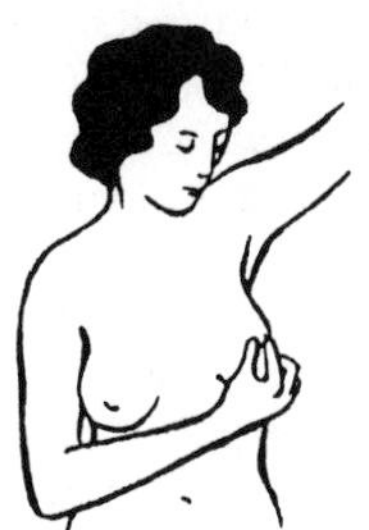

Some research suggests that many women do BSE more thoroughly when they use a pattern of up-and-down lines or strips. Other women feel more comfortable with another pattern. The important thing is to cover the whole breast and to pay special attention to the area between the breast and the underarm, and to the underarm itself. Check the area above the breast, up to the collarbone and all the way over to your shoulder.

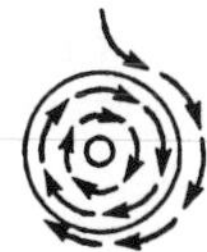

CIRCLES: Beginning at the outer edge of your breast, move your fingers slowly around the whole breast in a circle. Move around the breast in smaller and smaller circles, gradually working toward the nipple. Don't forget to check the underarm and upper chest areas, too.

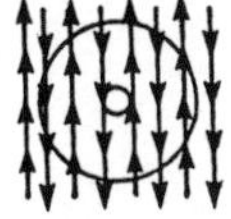

LINES: Start in the underarm area and move your fingers downward little by little until they are below the breast. Then move your fingers slightly toward the middle and slowly move back up. Go up and down until you cover the whole area.

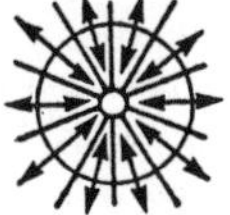

WEDGES: Starting at the outer edge of the breast, move your fingers toward the nipple and back to the edge. Check your whole breast, covering one small wedge-shaped section at a time. Be sure to check the underarm area and the upper chest.

5. Raise one arm. Use the flat part of the fingers of your other hand to check the breast and the surrounding area—firmly, carefully, and thoroughly. Some women like to use lotion or powder to help their fingers glide easily over the skin. Feel for any unusual lump or mass under the skin.

Feel the tissue by pressing your fingers in small, overlapping areas. To be sure you cover your whole breast, take your time and follow a definite pattern: lines, circles, or wedges.

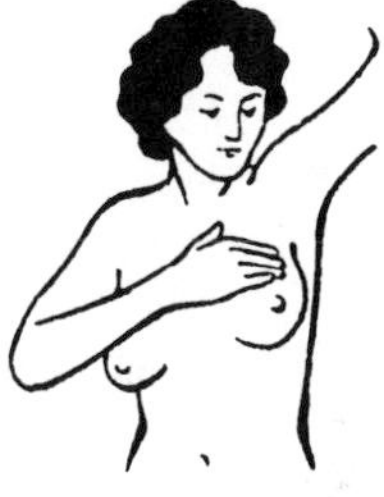

6. It's important to repeat Step 5 while you are lying down. Lie flat on your back, with one arm over your head and a pillow or folded towel under the opposite shoulder. This position flattens the breast and makes it easier to check. Check each breast and the area around it very carefully using one of the patterns described above.

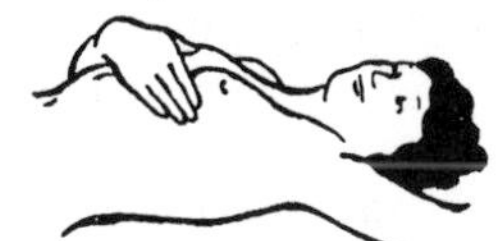

7. Some women repeat Step 5 in the shower. Your fingers will glide easily over soapy skin, so you can concentrate on feeling for changes underneath.

If you notice a lump, a discharge, or any other change during the month—whether or not it is during BSE—contact your doctor.

Figure 28.3. Breast Self-Examination (BSE)
SOURCE: From The National Cancer Society (1994).
NOTE: Do BSE once a month, about a week after your period. If you're not having periods, choose a regular time, such as the first day of each month. The important thing is to learn how your breasts feel. If you notice anything unusual or detect any changes, talk to your nurse or doctor.

Table 28.1 Descriptors of Normal Breast Tissue[a]

Descriptor	Endorsement	
	Number	*Percentage*
Soft	20	80
Movable	19	76
Fatty fullness	17	68
Pliable	16	64
Fleshy, lumpy; like fat beneath the skin	15	60
Mild lumpiness	14	56
Thick	13	52
More firm underneath	12	48
Teeny little balls that move around; like muscle; irregular	11	44
Bumpy; little knots; softer than bread dough	10	40
Marshmallow-like; little gel-like balls all in one place	8	32
Spongy; squishy; like a Nerf ball; like a pillow; regular	7	28
Like foam rubber; grainy	6	24
Like a grapefruit, with fibers and squishy; like tiny little peas	5	20
Like lumpy oatmeal; like ridges; like little bundles of grapes	4	16
Like farina; like flowerets on top of cauliflower	3	12
Smooth, like a steak	2	8
Like rice	1	4

SOURCE: From *Health Care for Women International, 12*(1), 78, Lauver, D., and Keenan, C. (1991). Taylor & Francis, Inc., Washington, DC. Reproduced with permission.
a. Generated by women scheduled for screening mammograms ($N = 26$) and ranked by their frequency of endorsement among women attending mammography appointments ($N = 25$).

Duration and thoroughness of clinical palpation have been positively correlated with accurate lump detection (Fletcher, O'Malley, & Bunce, 1985). When palpating the breast, the tissue should be as flat as possible. To accomplish this, ask the patient to lie on her hip opposite the breast being examined, rotate her shoulders to the supine position, and place the ipsilateral hand on her forehead; this position is not as uncomfortable as it may sound. If her breasts are large or pendulous, place a folded towel or pillow under the scapula to elevate and further flatten them. Thorough CBE can be completed in 5 to 10 minutes, depending on breast size.

Palpate the entire breast, including the axillary tail. Palpate with the pads of the three middle fingers held together. Powder or lotion will help the clinician's fingers to slip more easily over the skin, increasing their tactile sensitivity. The fingers should move in circles that are about the size of a dime; at each point a circular motion should be performed using variable pressures (light, medium, deep). A circular search pattern starting at the nipple and extending in concentric circles may be used; an up-and-down pattern (sometimes called stripping) is equally acceptable. Inspect and palpate the nipple, noting any skin irritation or discharge. "Milk" the nipples by pressing the areolar skin inward with both hands and lifting the nipple upward. This maneuver will express any nipple discharge more thoroughly than will squeezing. Finally, palpate the axilla and supraclavicular area, noting any enlarged lymph nodes.

Nonmalignant Breast Disorders

Nonmalignant breast problems are traditionally referred to in the medical literature as *benign breast disease.* In this discussion a classification system based on symptoms and physical findings will be used (Love, Schnitt, Connolly, & Shirley, 1987). The descriptive classifications are (a) physiological, cyclic swelling, and tenderness; (b) nodularity; (c) mastalgia or mastodynia, which is severe breast pain that may be cyclic or noncyclic; (d) infections and inflammations; (e) nipple discharge; and (f) dominant lumps.

Assessment of symptoms and physical findings will assist the clinician in initially classifying the problem, deciding whether to proceed with further diagnostic evaluation through a consultation or referral process, and instituting a plan of management. Although, often, the possibility of breast cancer needs to be considered in the evaluation, the evaluation process is often therapeutic in itself when the outcome relieves the woman's fear that her symptoms were due to breast cancer. It is helpful if the clinician can offer the patient continuing care, particularly being available to respond to telephone calls regarding any current breast concerns or changes found on BSE.

Physiological, Cyclic Swelling and Tenderness

Cyclic swelling and tenderness are normal variations in a woman's breasts due to hormonal influences during the menstrual cycle. Although usually mild, these variations cause considerable discomfort for some women. Their cyclic nature can be documented by asking the woman to monitor her breast changes while keeping a menstrual calendar for several months and by comparing the volume and tenderness of the breast in clinical examinations at different times in the menstrual cycle. The distinction between normal sensitivity and swelling and mastalgia is one of both degree and persistence of these changes (Love et al., 1987).

Nodularity

Nodularity refers to the breast tissue feeling lumpy or grainy on palpation, without the presence of a dominant lump. Although the degree of nodularity usually varies with the menstrual cycle, it may remain stable over time. Nodularity is usually bilateral but may be more marked in one breast than the other. Nodular breasts may be painless or painful; the relationship between nodularity and later cyst formation is unclear. The terms *fibrocystic disease* and *fibrocystic condition* have often been used inaccurately to describe nodularity (Schnitt & Connolly, 1991).

On palpation, the clinician may be uncertain whether nodularity or a dominant lump is felt; in this case, medical consultation or referral to a breast specialist for diagnostic evaluation is appropriate. Nodularity is not in itself abnormal; its principal significance is that distinguishing a dominant lump is more difficult in women with nodular breasts. The clinician may examine a woman with nodular breasts more often and may ask a colleague to examine the patient to validate findings.

Mastalgia

Cyclic mastalgia, the most frequent type of breast pain, is associated with the menstrual cycle. In this condition, women experience significantly more pain than the usual premenstrual swelling and tenderness. Although usually accompanied by nodularity, pain may exist in the absence of any specific physical finding (Souba, 1991). Pain is felt bilaterally in about half the cases and may extend to the axilla. One group of researchers found a significant correlation between the degree of breast pain, tenderness, and engorgement perceived by the patient and the degree of objective findings on physical examination (Goodson, Mallman, Jacobson, & Hunt, 1985). The onset of cyclic mastalgia is frequently in the mid-30s; it may persist until menopause, and the etiology is poorly understood.

Treatment of Cyclic Mastalgia. A complete history, physical examination, and mammography (in women over 35) are important in excluding pain arising from outside the breast and in excluding a dominant mass as the source of the pain (Morrow, 1991a). Discuss honestly with the patient that the cause of this condition is not well understood, that a number of treatments have been tried, some treatments have helped individuals, but none has proved generally effective. Thorough explanation and reassurance that the pain is not caused by cancer is essential. For some women, the simple measure of a sturdy supporting bra proves very helpful. Numerous pharmacological treatments have been tried with varying success.

Treatment with hormones and their inhibitors is based on theories that breast pain is due to hormonal imbalance, such as relative insufficiency of progesterone in the luteal phase of the cycle (Ayers & Gidwani, 1983; Sitruk-Ware, Sterkers, & Mauvais-Jarvais, 1979). Although many women report pain relief with oral progesterone (Provera), randomized trials of its efficacy have had mixed results (Love et al., 1987). Danocrine (danazol) relieves breast pain and tenderness in many women; it is expensive and has androgenic side effects, such as menstrual irregularities, weight gain, lowered voice, and growth of facial hair. Bromocriptine (Parlodel), a prolactin antagonist, has shown some efficacy in reducing pain and nodularity; its use is based on observed elevation of prolactin levels in women with cyclic mastalgia (Pye, Mansel, & Hughes, 1985). Thyroxine (Synthroid) and the estrogen antagonist tamoxifen citrate, are two other hormonal therapies that have shown some evidence of effectiveness (Love et al., 1987).

Failure to respond to one drug does not preclude good response to another. In one study, an excellent response (no residual pain) or a good response ("tolerable" residual pain) was obtained with evening primrose oil in 45% of women with cyclic mastalgia, with Danocrine in 70% of these women, and with bromocriptine in 47% (Pye et al., 1985). Dietary restriction of methylxanthine (coffee, tea, cola, chocolate) results in less breast swelling and tenderness for some individuals, although, again, research has not confirmed clear evidence of its benefit (Lubin et al., 1985; Morrow, 1991a). Diuretics have also been used with limited success. Some women report reduced tenderness and cyst size after taking vitamin E, but in a randomized trial no difference was found between the effects of vitamin E and placebo (London et al., 1985).

Noncyclic mastalgia remains constant throughout the cycle or is intermittent but unrelated to menses. This type of breast pain may originate outside the breast and is rarely helped by hormone therapy. Localized mastalgia can be due to trauma such as a blow to the breast or surgical procedure; mastalgia may persist for years and may be associated with fat necrosis or a hematoma. *Costochondritis,* which is an inflammation at the junction of the anterior ribs and the sternum, is a cause of musculoskeletal pain that women have described as aching breast pain. On palpation, localized tenderness can be elicited over the costochondral junction. Anti-inflammatory agents usually help to relieve pain in this condition, which often takes 6 to 8 weeks or longer to resolve. *Cervical radiculopathy,* that is, compression of nerve roots in the cervical spine (often C6 and C7), can cause pain felt as chronic unilateral breast pain. In one case series, pain extended into the neck and along the outer border of the arm, and some women had abnormal motor and sensory findings on neurological examination; all were successfully treated with physiotherapy, cervical collar, or traction. Although cancer or gross cysts can cause localized breast pain, pain is an unusual presentation for these conditions (Morrow, 1991a).

Infections and Inflammations

Breast infections are marked by varying degrees of localized pain, heat, redness, tenderness, and fever. Most infections occur during the puerperium, the most common being *lactational mastitis,* a condition that begins with simple milk stasis in a clogged duct. It usually responds to frequent breast-feeding, combined with 20-minute warm soaks and massage three or four times daily. If, however, the ducts remain obstructed, a medium for bacterial growth is set up in the back flow of milk, causing infectious mastitis to develop; this is followed clinically by the degree of heat, redness, and fever and by obtaining leukocyte counts and cultures. The causative organisms are usually normal skin inhabitants, such as staphylococci or streptococci; the infection is treated with broad-spectrum antibiotics. In less than 10% of cases, infectious mastitis does not respond to antibiotic therapy, a lactational breast abscess forms, and surgical incision and drainage are necessary. This procedure may require general anesthesia unless the abscess is very small, in which case it can be drained by needle aspiration under local anesthetic (S. Love, 1990).

Nonlactational mastitis and abscesses are most likely to occur in the presence of lowered resistance to infection, such as in diabetes, radiation treatment, or compromised immune status. Localized streptococcal mastitis can extend to acute systemic illness with cellulitis and bacteremia, requiring hospitalization for antibiotic therapy.

A condition that fails to respond to antibiotics is marked by repeated episodes of abscesses that form beneath the areola; these drain spontaneously, followed by periods of quiescence and the formation of fistulous tracts to the skin. The etiology of these chronic recurrent subareolar abscesses is not well understood; they are thought to be due to blockage and subsequent infection of the lactiferous ducts or the Montgomery's glands. Women with inverted nipples are more likely to get these abscesses, which can be extremely difficult to cure (Bland, 1991). Referral to a skilled breast surgeon is indicated when mastitis fails to respond promptly to antibiotics or the clinician suspects an abscess.

An inflammatory reaction most often occurs in the breast in response to internal rupture of a gross cyst, with symptoms of mastitis, such as marked local swelling, tenderness, and fever. Another type of inflammatory process occasionally seen on the breast is a tender, red, inflamed cord on the skin that may extend from the axilla, around the breast to the epigastric area of the abdomen. This is a phlebitis of the thoracoepigastric vein called *Mondor's disease,* after the physician who first identified it. The phlebitis is caused by irritation and trauma to the aforementioned vein, due to diagnostic procedures, surgery, or radiation. It resolves spontaneously over several weeks to months.

Rarely, breast cancer can present with inflammatory symptoms of pain, swelling, heat, and tenderness. Finally, because the skin of the breast forms part of the integument, infections extrinsic to the breast, notably tuberculosis and syphilis, can also present as breast lesions, although this is a rare occurrence (Bland, 1991).

Nipple Discharge

Nipple problems include discharge and itching. The breasts of most nonlactating women of all ages are capable of secreting fluid when the nipple is squeezed; such normal reactive secretions are nonspontaneous, usually bilateral, serous, and arise from multiple ducts. This type of discharge is physiological and requires no further evaluation or treatment.

Bilateral milky discharge occurring spontaneously in a nonlactating female is an abnormal condition called *galactorrhea.* Galactorrhea is usually due to elevated prolactin levels, some causes of which are pituitary tumor, thyroid disorders, and medications, such as oral contraceptives and neuroleptic drugs. Galactorrhea may be accompanied by amenorrhea. Appropriate initial evaluation of a woman with galactorrhea includes drug history, menstrual history, physical examination, thyroid function tests, and serum prolactin levels (Morrow, 1991b).

Other types of abnormal nipple discharge are grossly bloody, serous, or clear with a sticky consistency. Pathological discharge is usually unilateral, spontaneous, and can often be localized to a single duct. These women should be referred to a breast surgeon for further diagnostic evaluation, which will probably include cytological examination of the discharge and a biopsy, often preceded by a ductogram to identify the origin of the discharge.

The most frequent cause of bloody nipple discharge is *intraductal papillomas,* nonmalignant tumors of the lactiferous ducts that occur most often among women from 30 to 50 years of age. Papillomas may be solitary or multiple (intraductal papillomatosis); the latter are more subject to malignant transformation. Rarely, the presence of papillomas causes nipple retraction. Bloody nipple discharge may also be caused by intraductal carcinoma in situ or, rarely, invasive cancer (Morrow, 1991b).

A condition that causes pasty, sticky discharge is *duct ectasia,* also called *periductal mastitis.* It is most common around menopause, and its natural history is not entirely understood, although it is thought to be due to chronic inflammation and dilation of the lactiferous ducts. In either duct ectasia or intraductal papillomas, a subareolar mass may be palpable or seen on mammogram. The treatment is local excision of either the affected duct(s) or all the ducts if the woman does not plan to breast-feed in the future or if she is past reproductive age.

Itchy nipples are most often due to local skin dryness, chapping, or eczema; it is bilateral and responds to symptomatic therapy. If, however, these symptoms are unilateral, with scaling and itchiness of one nipple persisting several weeks or months without improvement, a surgical referral is indicated. Persistent itching and scaliness are symptoms of a type of breast cancer called *Paget's disease,* which is diagnosed with a punch biopsy of the areolar skin. Paget's disease almost never occurs bilaterally.

Dominant Lumps

On physical examination, a dominant lump is a palpable mass that stands out from the rest of the breast tissue and remains relatively unchanged after repeated examinations. The majority of dominant lumps are not caused by breast cancer. Noncancerous causes include gross cysts, fibroadenomas, and "pseudolumps."

Gross Cysts. Cysts, the most frequent cause of dominant breast lumps, are fluid-filled sacs that are usually tender on palpation. Less commonly, they may be painless. Although the natural history of cysts is incompletely understood, it is thought that they form in the glandular breast tissue in response to cyclic hormonal activity. After repeated menstrual cycle enlargement or lactation, some of the terminal lobules and ducts remain enlarged and eventually become encapsulated. As one might expect from their natural history, cysts are more likely to appear after a woman has been menstruating a number of years. A milk-filled cyst, called a *galactocele,* can form due to blockage of the lactiferous ducts. After menopause, breast cysts shrink unless a woman takes estrogen replacement therapy.

On examination, a cyst that is close to the surface feels smooth and regularly shaped and is ballottable. If, however, a cyst is located deep in the breast its consistency feels harder and less fluid filled. When a cyst is suspected, the lump may be aspirated. Cystic fluid can be a variety of colors but is seldom bloody; the amount ranges from 0.5 ml to 50 ml or more.

The character of a suspected cyst may also be evaluated by a mammogram followed by ultrasound examination; on a mammogram, a fluid-filled mass will appear as an area of density but will form no dense shadow on ultrasound. Masses thus demonstrated on ultrasound to be cysts do not have to be aspirated unless they are painful, in which case aspiration will provide immediate relief. Although it is more usual for only a few palpable cysts to occur in a lifetime, it is possible for a woman to have multiple recurrent cysts, and this patient should be followed by a specialist, who may examine her as frequently as every 3 months and regularly aspirate the cysts. One risk of having cysts is that the woman may not seek medical attention for new lumps because she believes they are "just cysts."

The incidence of malignancy within a cyst itself is very small (1%). This rare cancer, called *intracystic papillary carcinoma,* has little invasive potential. The relationship between the occurrence of breast cysts and the later development of cancer in another part of the breast is unclear. Although most researchers have found no relationship, in one study, an association was found between gross cysts and the later development of breast cancer (Haagensen, 1977); and in another, the researchers found an increased risk of breast cancer only among those women who had gross cysts and a first-degree relative (mother, sister) with breast cancer (Dupont & Page, 1987).

Fibroadenomas. Fibroadenomas are noncancerous, painless, solid tumors that develop mostly in younger women. When they are found in older women it is thought that they have been there for years and are discovered because the shrinking of glandular tissue with advancing age makes them easier to identify by mammography or palpation. Fibroadenomas occur more often in African Americans than in Caucasians and less often in contraceptive users. On palpation, fibroadenomas feel like firm rubber and are freely movable; their shape is rounded, lobed, or spherical. Ranging in size from less than a centimeter to 5 centimeters (giant fibroadenomas), they are easily distinguishable from the rest of the breast tissue. Some enlargement of fibroadenomas may be noted during the luteal phase of the menstrual cycle. Also, dramatic enlargement can occur in adolescence or during pregnancy. Fibroadenomas may become calcified, and in this case the lump may have a rock-hard consistency. The treatment of fibroadenomas is simple excision.

The presence of fibroadenomas does not increase the risk of later developing cancer elsewhere in the breast. Rarely, however, a cancer called *cystosarcoma phyllodes* develops within the fibroadenoma itself. The incidence of this type of cancer is about 1%; it usually occurs in giant fibroadenomas (Love et al., 1987).

Pseudolump. This term is used to describe a lumpy area of the breast that is worrisome to the clinician because it is prominent, but it does not have the clear characteristics of a cyst, fibroadenoma, or a cancerous lump. Some causes of these pseudolumps are prominent ribs pushing up the tissue and making it feel hard or a large lobular area that feels discrete but does not clearly stand out from the rest of the breast tissue. Hardened pieces of silicone in women who have had breast implants can feel like lumps, and fat necrosis from trauma can also form a hard lumpy area in the breast (S. Love, 1990). The decision of what to call a lump can be somewhat subjective. When such a worrisome lumpiness occurs, depending on the patient's age, history, and risk factors, the generalist clinician will obtain mammograms, examine the patient at different times of the menstrual cycle, and may subsequently refer the patient to a breast surgeon for a definitive diagnosis. When such lumpy areas are biopsied and found to be noncancerous, the pathologist may call this fibrocystic condition or fibrocytic changes, and the specific type of change should be described on the pathology report (Consensus Statement, 1986). One specific type of fibrocystic change called *atypical hyperplasia* is associated with an increased risk of future breast cancer (Dupont & Page, 1987).

Initial Evaluation of a Lump. Although definitive diagnosis of the cause of a dominant lump can be made only on the basis of pathological examination of the tissue, the initial evaluation begins with a chronological account of the complaint; a history of previous breast disease and treatment; major risk factors, such as older age and history of breast cancer in a first-degree relative; physical examination; and mammography for women over 35. Then a working hypothesis can be formulated.

An important part of the initial evaluation is sharing and interpreting the clinician's working hypotheses with the patient in a factual and empathetic manner. Offer her anticipatory guidance regarding what to expect in a further diagnostic evaluation, if that is being recommended. Usually, a needle aspiration will be done to determine whether the lump is solid or cystic. Biopsy is necessary when the results of aspiration are equivocal or when a cyst is recurrent even after aspiration. Continuity of care with regular follow-up is very important, especially for women with a history of nodularity and/or recurrent cysts.

Breast Biopsies. Today, the recommended approach is the two-step procedure, which is a biopsy under local or general anesthesia, followed by histological examination of the tissue and further discussion of treatment options. In this approach, the patient and family have time to participate in the decision-making process.

For patients who are being referred and will probably undergo a breast biopsy, the clinician should provide the patient anticipatory guidance on the types of biopsies that are commonly done and encourage her to clarify with the breast specialist what type will be done in her case and why.

There are four types of biopsies. Closed (needle) biopsies include those performed with a small needle that removes only a few cells and those using a larger needle that removes a small piece of the lump. Open (surgical) biopsies include the incisional type, which removes a wedge of tissue, and the excisional type, which removes the entire lump and a margin of surrounding tissue; the latter may require general anesthesia. Complications of breast biopsies include infection and hematomas (Kinne, 1991; S. Love, 1990).

Breast Cancer

Because of its high prevalence and seriousness, breast cancer is an important problem for women's health clinicians. In the United States, a woman's estimated lifetime risk of developing breast cancer is one in nine (American Cancer Society [ACS], 1992). Clinically speaking, about 1 of 12 lumps examined in premenopausal women and about half those detected in postmenopausal women are found to be breast cancer (S. Love, 1990). Scientific understanding of the natural history and pathogenesis of breast cancer is incomplete. A decade ago, breast cancer was thought to be a local disease of the breast tissue. The current view guiding treatment and research is that breast cancer, almost from its inception, is a systemic disease.

Epidemiology

In terms of prevalence, breast cancer is the second leading cause of cancer death among American women (ACS, 1992). Rising breast cancer incidence, increasing by about 3% each year since 1980, remains largely unexplained; earlier detection and better reporting systems may account for some, but not all, increased incidence of the disease (Newman, 1990). Overall mortality due to breast cancer has remained unchanged since the 1950s (ACS, 1992). Although the 5-year survival among women with localized breast cancer has improved from 78% in 1940 to 91% in 1990, 5-year survival for regionally invasive disease (69%) and metastatic disease (18%) has remained unchanged (ACS, 1992).

Risk Factors. The principal risk factors are not modifiable through behavioral change. The major at-risk condition is advancing age; 90% of breast cancer occurs in women over 40 years of age. Cancer in one breast increases the subsequent risk of the disease in the contralateral breast. Family history of breast cancer in a first-degree relative (mother, sister, or daughter) is termed a major risk factor, especially if the disease occurred premenopausally, in which case the relative risk is two- to threefold that of the general population. Previous exposure to ionizing radiation is also a known risk factor (Hildreth, Shore, & Dvoretsky, 1989; Miller, 1991).

Other factors associated with increases in breast cancer risk include early menarche (age 12 or younger) and late menopause (age 55 or older), nulliparity, first birth after age 30, having taken diethylstilbestrol during early pregnancy, prolonged use of oral contraceptives before first-term pregnancy, and prolonged postmenopausal estrogen replacement therapy. A specific type of pathological report on biopsy, indicating "proliferative atypical hyperplasia," appears to be associated with the later development of breast cancer (Bergkvist, Adami, Persson, Hoover, & Schairer, 1989; Dupont & Page, 1987; Henderson & Bernstein, 1991; Miller, 1991).

Dietary Factors. A link between dietary fat and subsequent breast cancer was first proposed in the 1940s. Low rates of breast cancer in human females were observed in Japan and other countries where dietary fat is only 12% to 15% of calories. In animal studies, increased incidence of breast cancer was found in rats fed a very high fat diet (Miller, 1991). The hypothesized link between dietary fat and breast cancer in women was not supported in a cohort study (Willet et al., 1987a); it has been argued, however, that the dietary fat consumption among women in that cohort was too high to show any effect on breast cancer incidence. The feasibility of an intensive intervention that helps women reduce dietary fat to less than 25% of daily calories has been successfully tested; a randomized trial showed that, in the women studied, a very low fat diet could be implemented and maintained over a 2-year period (Henderson et al., 1990). Whether maintenance of such a diet will result in reduced breast cancer incidence over time has not been shown; a planned prospective trial has not yet been implemented (Pearson, 1991).

Further dietary factors hypothesized to protect against breast cancer are vitamins A, C, and E combined with selenium, an essential trace element that functions as an antioxidant enzyme in human metabolism (Bakemeier, 1988). Decreased breast cancer incidence has been found in regions where the soil is high in selenium, and among animals given a diet high in selenium; a protective effect of dietary selenium however, has not yet been confirmed in humans (Meyer & Verreault, 1987; Willet et al., 1987b). It is hypothesized that low levels of vitamins A and E, combined with low selenium, may increase susceptibility to cancer more than lack of one of the elements alone.

Other Factors. Other than specific components of the diet, there is some evidence that obesity contributes to breast cancer risk, as does a history of moderate alcohol consumption beginning before age 30 (Willet et al., 1987b). It is important for the clinician to remember that because breast cancer is so prevalent, a history of risk factors in the context of a comprehensive health database should be obtained for all women patients. For high-risk women, the use of tamoxifen citrate, an antiestrogenic agent, has been proposed for prophylaxis (Jordan, 1990), and a clinical trial of its effectiveness is in progress. Subcutaneous mastectomy has also been used prophylactically for women at very high risk for breast cancer (S. Love, 1990). When counseling women with regard to reducing their modifiable breast cancer risks through behavioral change, the clinician should keep in mind that no causal link has been demonstrated between a behavioral risk factor and breast cancer, such as that found between smoking and lung cancer. However, it seems likely that, on the basis of the existing evidence, high fat and calorie intake play a role in susceptibility to breast cancer. Professional and consumer educational materials on diet and prevention are available (Bakemeier, 1988; National Cancer Institute, 1984).

Early Detection

Early detection through periodic screening is the principal determinant of survival. This is best accomplished with a combination of mammography, CBE, and BSE. The benefits of periodic screening with mammography and CBE in reducing breast cancer mortality, especially among women over 50 years of age, have been demonstrated in several large landmark studies (Baker, 1982; Shapiro, 1977; Tabar, Fagerberg, & Gad, 1985). The earliest and perhaps best known is a randomized clinical trial in which 62,000 women were assigned to either an experimental group that received annual CBE and mammography for 4 years or a control group that received usual medical care. When the women were followed over time, those over the age of 50 in the experimental group had a 30% decrease in breast cancer mortality compared with that of the control group.

Mammography remains underused despite its demonstrated benefits in the early detection of breast cancer. There is thus far no evidence of radiation-induced cancer from mammography. A two-view mammogram with today's techniques delivers one rad or less of radiation; moreover, the sensitivity of breast tissue to radiation decreases sharply after age 35 (Miller, 1991). In a survey of primary care physicians,

Table 28.2 Screening Recommendations for Early Detection of Breast Cancer in Asymptomatic Women

	Screening Maneuvers[a]		
Expert Group	*Mammography*	*Clinical Exam*	*Breast Self-Exam (BSE)*
American Cancer Society (1988)	Baseline at age 35-39; every 1-2 years from age 40-49; annually at age 50 and above	Every three years from age 20-40; annually from age 40	Monthly from age 20
U.S. Preventive Services Task Force (1987)	Annually from age 50	Annually from age 40	Teach BSE from age 40[b]
Canadian Task Force on Periodic Examination (1986)	Annually from age 50	Annually from age 40	Teach BSE from age 40[b]

SOURCE: In Nettles-Carlson, B. (1989). Early detection of breast cancer. *JOGNN, 18,* 373-381. Used with permission.
a. Clinicians may elect to recommend earlier or more frequent screening for the special category of women at high risk, especially those with a family history of premenopausally diagnosed breast cancer in a first-degree relative.
b. Clinicians may elect to teach BSE on grounds of clinical prudence, although there is insufficient evidence of the maneuver's efficacy to support a recommendation for inclusion in or exclusion from the periodic health examination.

reasons reported for not ordering screening mammograms were belief that they were unnecessary, disagreement with the recommended guidelines, concern about radiation risk, and concern about cost to the patient of mammograms compared to that for CBE (ACS, 1988). Women who have a regular provider and higher education and income are more likely to receive mammograms (Dawson & Thompson, 1989; Zapka et al., 1992). In one study, women with a family history of breast cancer were more likely to have had mammograms (Zapka et al., 1992), but another researcher found that high-risk women were no more likely to have had mammograms than women in the general population (Kaplan, Weinberg, Small, & Herndon, 1991).

Screening Recommendations. All women should receive age-appropriate periodic screening with a combination of mammography, CBE, and BSE teaching (see Table 28.2). Recommendations of expert groups vary in detail and emphasis (Fink, 1991; U.S. Preventive Services Task Force, 1987). The clinician should keep in mind that about 70% of women who develop breast cancer are not at high risk, and age is by far the most important factor in determining when to begin screening. Because of the high prevalence of breast cancer, selectively screening only very high-risk women on the basis of factors other than age would result in an estimated two thirds of all breast cancers being missed.

Diagnosis and Staging

The classic "warning signals" of breast cancer are a persistent lump, thickening, swelling, dimpling, skin irritation or scaliness, distortion of the breast contour, and skin or nipple retraction (ACS, 1992). Often the clinical presentation is a lump discovered by the patient. Cancerous lumps are more likely than benign lesions to be hard, not clearly localized, not freely movable, and irregularly shaped. A palpable lump, whether found by clinician or patient, should be biopsied even in the presence of negative mammograms; mammography has a 10% to 15% false-negative rate. More nonpalpable lesions are being discovered on mammography screening; in a recent study of such women who subsequently underwent mammography-assisted needle biopsies, the malignancy rate was 24% (Thompson, Bowen, & Dorman, 1991). Due to more early detection in the past decade, the clinician is less likely to see the "grave" signs of locally advanced breast cancer described by Haagensen (1986), which include (a) breast skin edema or *peau d'orange,* (b) breast skin ulceration, (c) tumor fixation to chest wall, (d) axillary lymph node fixation to skin or deep tissues, and (e) enlarged axillary lymph nodes (> 2.5 cm in diameter). Localized pain and tenderness is an unusual presentation except in advanced disease.

Definitive diagnosis is accomplished by microscopic examination of biopsied breast tissue, which identifies the histological type of the cancer and assigns a grade, from undifferentiated to well differentiated. The purpose of staging is then to determine the extent of disease and the prognosis for tumor progression, so that appropriate therapy can be instituted. Many staging classifications have been described (Yeatman & Bland, 1991); the method most widely used is the tumor-node-metastasis (TNM) system recommended by the American Joint Committee on Cancer Staging (1988). There are five stage groupings in the TNM system. Stage 0 tumors have the best prognosis and are almost 100% curable. Women with Stage I tumors have approximately an 80% chance of surviving 10 years without evidence of disease, compared with 60% with Stage II, 40% of women with Stage III, and less than 10% of women with Stage IV cancer (Yeatman & Bland, 1991). During the staging process, various studies may be done on the basis of the common sites of metastasis, which include lung, bone, liver, and adrenal glands.

Prognosis. There is general agreement that the most important known prognostic indicators are the degree of invasiveness of the tumor, tumor size, and axillary node status; the best single indicator being the number of involved metastatic axillary lymph nodes (Goodman & Harte, 1990; Yeatman & Bland, 1991). There is as yet no unified hypothesis regarding the biology of breast cancer, and various hypothesized biological prognostic factors are an important and complex area of current research, a discussion of which is beyond the scope of this chapter. Some factors being investigated are histological grade, tumor growth rate and cell kinetics, steroid hormone receptivity, the presence of certain biological markers, and monoclonal antibodies (Clark et al., 1989; Leis, 1991; Sigurdsson et al., 1990).

Psychological and social factors that have been associated with a favorable prognosis are positive adjustment to illness; emotional expressiveness with an attitude of fighting the disease rather than passive compliance or resignation; expressed "will to live"; and a high degree of social involvement, such as not living alone and the presence of supportive friends, family, or social organizations (Jamison, Burish, & Wallston, 1987; Leis, 1991; Marshall & Funch, 1983).

Treatment Alternatives

Many more diagnostic and treatment modalities are available to women now than a decade ago. A patient may face an array of choices, the benefits and disadvantages of which are seldom clear-cut, especially in the treatment of early disease (Knobf, 1990; Soffa, 1991). Taking into account the medical situation and the patient's preferences, surgery, radiation, and chemotherapy may be used singly or in combination. Breast reconstruction with good cosmetic results is now possible immediately after mastectomy, and this has become an important part of treatment and rehabilitation (Goldwyn, 1987; McCraw, Cramer, & Horton, 1991). Treatment, especially at the regional cancer centers, is prescribed collaboratively by medical subspecialists to whom the patient must relate at various times, such as the surgeon, the medical oncologist, and the radiologist. Regional breast cancer centers offer a woman the advantage of a formal multidisciplinary approach; these services may be used either for the definitive plan of therapy or to obtain a second opinion (Goodman & Harte, 1990).

The patient and her family are called on to make difficult decisions in a short period of time. Illustrative examples, which are by no means exhaustive, are deciding whether to have a one-step or two-step procedure, whether to have breast-conserving therapy or mastectomy, the type of mastectomy, whether to participate in clinical trial protocols if these are available, and the timing of the surgery. Some research suggests that patients with breast cancer who are offered a choice of treatment are better satisfied and less worried about recurrence than those to whom a specific treatment is recommended (Knobf, 1990). It appears that patients choose on the basis of an interplay of medical factors and personal characteristics (Fallowfield & Baum, 1991). The knowledge base on which treatment options are proposed to patients is complex and changing constantly with the results of current research; hence there will be differences of approach at various institutions. The clinical nursing specialist can be of great assistance as an advocate, coordinator, and guide as the patient goes through this process (Brown, Eyles, & Bland, 1991; Grossage, 1990).

Surgical Treatment. Generally, surgical interventions have become much more conservative. Various types of mastectomy involve removal of different amounts of tissue (see Figure 28.4). Most patients with operable breast cancer are candidates for *modified mastectomy,* which is also termed *total mastectomy,* with axillary lymph node dissection and preservation of the pectoralis major muscle. In this procedure, considerable variation exists in surgical technique and the number of axillary nodes removed (Kinne, 1991). In less extensive procedures, called *partial mastectomy* and *quadrantectomy,* less breast tissue is removed. The clinician should be aware that there may be local and regional variations of terminology, definitions of procedures, and surgical techniques that are termed *breast conserving.*

For women with potentially curable primary breast cancer, research has shown that lumpectomy is as effective as mastectomy (Fisher et al., 1985). The recommended technique for lumpectomy is excision of the tumor with at least 3 centimeters of normal tissue around it (Kinne, 1991). Clinical trials of breast cancer treatment have supported the effectiveness of lumpectomy in patients with Stage I or Stage II disease, staged according to criteria defined by the American Joint Committee on Cancer Staging (1988). Furthermore, in patients treated with lumpectomy, radiation reduced the probability of subsequent local recurrence (Fisher et al., 1989). In 1990, recommendations from the National Institutes of Health stated that for the majority of women with Stage I or II breast cancer, lumpectomy with axillary dissection, followed by radiation therapy, was preferable to mastectomy (NIH Consensus Conference, 1991).

Despite the research evidence and consensus recommendations on lumpectomy, there is no unanimity of practice. A regional population-based cancer registry showed underuse of breast-conserving therapy for Stage I and II disease, especially in older women; a majority of the 8,095 women studied received mastectomies (Lazovich, White, Thomas, & Moe, 1991).

Surgical treatment varies for Stage 0 disease, that is, ductal carcinoma in situ (DCIS) and lobular carcinoma in situ (LCIS). These conditions are sometimes referred to as "precancerous conditions" or "noninvasive cancer." DCIS is generally believed to be a more aggressive precursor of invasive carcinoma, but the recommendations for treatment are not generally agreed on for either LCIS or DCIS. The management of DCIS has been described as one of the most important and controversial areas in breast cancer treatment (Harris, Schnitt, & Kinne, 1991).

Many more pre-invasive lesions are now being detected on mammography, where the most common abnormality associated with them is clustered microcalcifications. The relationship between DCIS and the later development of invasive cancer is incompletely understood, and knowledge of the natural history of DCIS is limited because in the past most women with this condition had mastectomies. It appears likely, however, that not all DCIS has the potential to progress to invasive disease: Current evidence suggests that one subtype (comedo type) has the greatest malignant potential. Women with DCIS may elect a range of treatments, based on various prognostic factors. The rate of recurrence after breast-conserving surgery for DCIS is greater than following mastectomy, and how much irradiation decreases the rate of recurrence has not been established (Harris et al., 1991).

Women react to breast cancer surgery in different ways in accordance with their individual ways of coping. Before surgery, some themes uppermost in women's minds are whether the surgeon will be able to "get all" of the cancer, anticipatory grieving for loss of the breast, and feelings of impaired femininity. Other feelings are relief that an operation can be done to potentially cure the cancer or, conversely, anger—feeling that losing a breast is a very high price to pay for cure (Goodman & Harte, 1990).

In a study of newly diagnosed patients during their initial hospitalization for surgical treatment with mastectomy, women who minimized the seriousness of a cancer diagnosis had less mood disturbance. The authors concluded that distress during the initial hospitalization was decreased among those patients who reacted to the diagnosis with denial rather than an active confrontational coping response (Watson, Greer, Blake, & Shrapnell, 1984).

Both preoperatively and during the postoperative recovery period, the patient may benefit from participation in support groups or a visit from Reach to Recovery, a national program sponsored by the American Cancer Society in which women volunteers who have had breast surgery visit and provide practical information and support to patients in the hospital. Also at this time and during the postoperative recovery period, patients may receive support and feel assisted in working out their own personal issues by reading books written by and about women who have experienced breast cancer (Dackman, 1990; Gross & Ito, 1991; Oktay & Walter, 1991; Rollin, 1986).

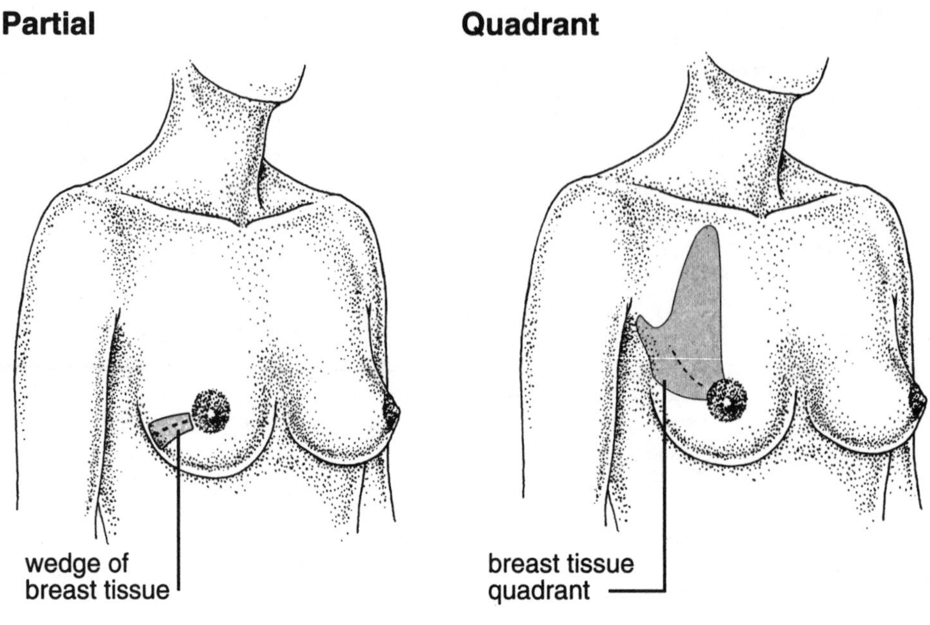

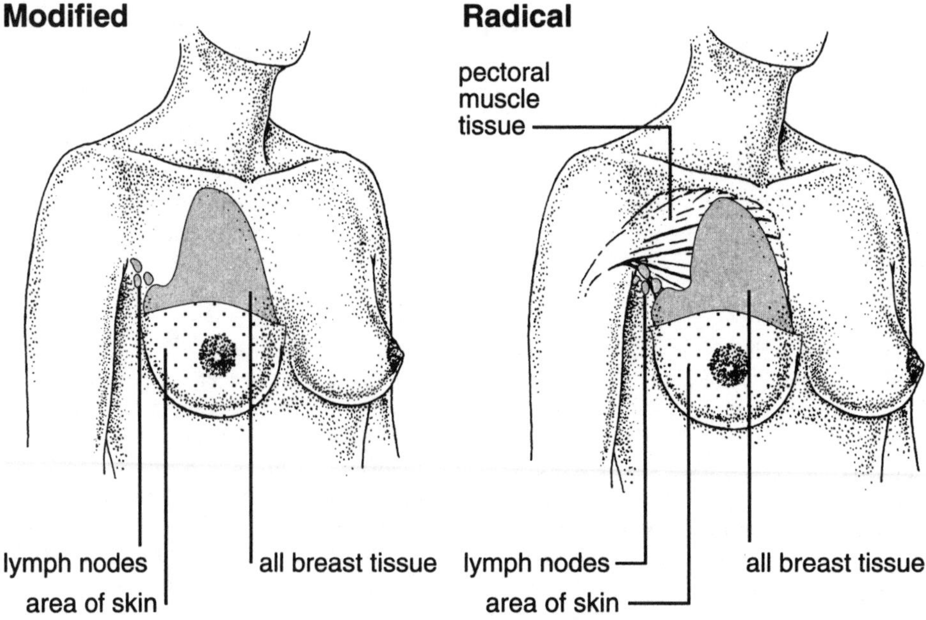

Figure 28.4. Tissue Removed in Various Mastectomy Procedures
SOURCE: Adapted from Love, S. M. *Dr. Susan Love's Breast Book.* Reading, MA: Addison-Wesley Publishing Company, Inc. (1990), p. 285. Used with permission.

The period of hospitalization for women undergoing mastectomy may be as brief as 3 to 5 days. Although a description of postoperative care of the mastectomy patient is beyond the scope of this discussion, the goals of immediate postoperative management include preserving the integrity of the skin flaps over the chest wound, minimizing edema and loss of function of the arm, preventing infection, pain management, and prevention of postsurgical complications. The risk of an infectious complication is increased with extensive axillary dissection and when the patient is undergoing adjuvant radiation (Goodman & Harte, 1990). After surgery, reconstruction may be undertaken immediately, particularly if the woman is not having adjuvant radiation; if she is, the more usual practice is to wait 3 months to a year after completion of adjuvant therapy before beginning reconstruction. There are some issues regarding the benefits and disadvantages of immediate versus delayed reconstruction, and informational resources are available to assist the clinician in discussing these with patients (Gaskin, Doss, Kelly, & Colburn, 1991; S. Love, 1990, p. 402; Snyder, 1989).

Radiation Treatment. Radiation, like surgery, is a form of local treatment for breast cancer. Used to treat both early and metastatic disease, radiation has proved effective in tumor control and preserving the breast. Radiotherapy may be an adjunctive treatment used postoperatively after mastectomy, or it may be the primary treatment. Preceded by an excisional biopsy and sampling of the axillary nodes, radiation has been used as the definitive therapy for Stage I or II disease; clinical trials have shown this to be an effective alternative to mastectomy (Fisher et al., 1989).

The timing of radiotherapy within an overall treatment plan is variable; radiation may be given before or after surgery or sequentially with chemotherapy.

The process of radiation treatment is often difficult for the patient. Side effects can be substantial, and the treatments are time-consuming and can be physically and emotionally exhausting. Before the treatments start, planning sessions are necessary. The patient lies on a table while the exact area to be irradiated is delineated and then outlined on the skin, customarily with a nonwashable tattoo that may feel disfiguring to the patient. A series of outpatient treatments lasts 4 to 6 weeks, usually 5 days a week. During treatment, anorexia and nausea are common. Skin dryness, desquamation, and/or hyperpigmentation usually occur. Skin changes, although often extensive, resolve in 1 to 3 weeks after completion of therapy. Possible adverse effects of breast irradiation are rib fractures, lymphedema, shortness of breath, pneumonitis, pleural effusions, and pericarditis (Goodman & Harte, 1990; S. Love, 1990).

Systemic Treatment. Chemotherapy and hormonal therapy are systemic treatments used in both early and metastatic breast cancer (Henderson, 1988; Kiang, Gay, Goldman, & Kennedy, 1985). In metastatic disease, systemic treatment is palliative, the goal being to relieve symptoms. In recent years, systemic agents have become increasingly important as adjuvant therapy for early disease. In early disease, the use of adjuvant chemotherapy and/or adjuvant tamoxifen citrate prolongs the time to recurrence; such treatment is given routinely in premenopausal and postmenopausal patients who have positive lymph nodes and/or estrogen receptor-positive tumors (Henderson, 1991). However, research and medical opinion on the appropriate use of adjuvant therapy in node-negative breast cancer is not unanimous (DeVita, 1989; McGuire, 1989).

In early and metastatic disease, the type, dose, and duration of drug therapy is individualized. Some chemotherapeutic drugs in use are cyclophosphamide (Cytoxan), methotrexate sodium, 5 fluorouracil (5-FU), doxorubicin hydrochloride (Adriamycin), chlorambucil (Leukeran), melphalan (L-PAM), thiotepa, vincristine sulfate, vinblastine sulfate (Velban), mitomycin, and mitoxantrone hydrochloride. Nausea, anorexia, stomatitis, fatigue, hair loss, and leukopenia are common adverse effects of most chemotherapeutic agents. Less toxic are the hormonal agents, which include tamoxifen citrate (Nolvadex), progestins (Megace), aminoglutethimide, diethylstilbestrol (DES), fluoxymesterone (Halotestin), and prednisone. Hormonal agents are generally well tolerated; side effects are infrequent; some of these are hot flashes, weight gain, breast tenderness, fatigue, nausea, Candida vaginitis, mood changes, and lowered voice (Brown et al., 1991; Brown-Daniels & Blasdell, 1990; Early Breast Cancer Trialists' Collaborative Group, 1988; Scanlon, 1991).

In women with advanced disease and hormone-receptor positive tumors, over half will respond to hormonal treatment, and remission lasts an average of a year (R. L. Love, 1989).

Use of a combination of chemotherapy and hormonal agents was shown to improve the response rates in a group of women with advanced disease, although overall survival was unaffected. In another study, quality of life was found to be improved with continuous rather than intermittent treatment (Coates et al., 1987).

Recurrence

Up to 70% of patients experience recurrence, which is strongly correlated with more advanced disease at diagnosis. Unfortunately, early detection of recurrence does not significantly affect survival time (Ellis & Bland, 1991). The majority of recurrences happen within 36 months of treatment but can occur years later, necessitating an indefinite period of follow-up. Usually women are followed in 3 months after initial treatment, then every 6 months for 5 years, then annually. Periodic clinical evaluation, with attention to a thorough history of symptomatology, and careful physical examination are the most effective modes of detecting recurrent disease. It is unwise to subject the patient to batteries of laboratory and radiologic testing, which at the present time have insufficient sensitivity or specificity to justify routine use.

Conclusions

Primary prevention of breast cancer is still a goal for the future. Nursing interventions that promote early detection of breast cancer include advocating for full implementation of mammography screening recommendations and an expanded role in performing clinical examinations and teaching self-examination during routine office visits of asymptomatic women.

Breast cancer treatment is in a state of flux, with new drugs and combinations of systemic and local treatments under intense investigation. Multicenter clinical trials of various treatments are currently being conducted; however, only about 3% of breast cancer patients are enrolled in these trials. Some of the issues concern whether or not insurance payers will cover the use of investigational therapies, the advantages and disadvantages of patients' participation in these trials, and the reasons why clinicians may be reluctant to enter eligible patients in clinical trials (Antman, Schnipper, & Frei, 1988; Tannock, 1987; Taylor, Margolese, & Soskolne, 1984). The women's health nurse should keep abreast of continuing research and debate on treatment choices and the controversies surrounding various aspects of breast cancer detection and treatment.

In view of the many treatment alternatives for breast cancer, the substantial recurrence rate, and in many cases the uncertain benefit to be gained from a specific course of treatment, it is especially important for the nurse to be well informed and to support informed choice of the patient. Choices for nontraditional cancer therapies, such as imagery techniques and special diets, may be reasonable alternatives and/or complements to medical treatment and should be supported. Quality-of-life issues as well as length of survival are of increasing concern to clinicians and researchers. The relationship of sociopsychological factors to survival and time to relapse is unclear. Psychosocial variables may play a much more crucial role in quality than in quantity of life experienced by women with breast cancer, and this is an important area for nursing research (Cassileth, Lusk, Miller, Brown, & Miller, 1985; Fallowfield & Baum, 1991).

There is hope for the future in the research efforts underway on the etiology and prevention of breast cancer, but meanwhile our best hope is in early detection, prompt treatment, and attention to quality-of-life issues. The women's health nurse can be influential through educating women, their families, and the public regarding the benefits of early detection, by being an advocate in behalf of the breast cancer patient and her family during treatment and rehabilitation, and through an ongoing caring relationship. Finally, the frequency and potential seriousness of breast problems as well as the complex sociocultural meanings associated with breast disease are reasons for the nursing clinician to seek a deeper understanding of this important aspect of women's health.

References

American Cancer Society. (1988). *Summary of current guidelines for the cancer-related checkup.* New York: Author.

American Cancer Society. (1992). *Cancer facts and figures: 1992.* Atlanta, GA: Author.

American Joint Committee on Cancer Staging. (1988). *Manual for staging of cancer* (3rd ed.). Philadelphia: J. B. Lippincott.

Antman, K., Schnipper, E., & Frei, E. III. (1988). The crisis in clinical cancer research: Third-party insurance and investigational therapy. *New England Journal of Medicine, 319,* 46-48.

Ayers, J. W. T., & Gidwani, G. P. (1983). The luteal breast: Hormonal and sonographic investigation of benign breast disease in patients with cyclic mastalgia. *Fertility and Sterility, 40,* 779-784.

Baines, C. J., To, T., & Wall, C. (1990). Changes in breast self-examination behavior achieved by 89,835 participants in the Canadian National Breast Screening Study. *Cancer, 66,* 570-576.

Baines, C. J., Wall, C., Risch, H. A., Kuin, J. K., & Fan, I. J. (1986). Changes in breast self-examination behavior in a cohort of 8214 women in the Canadian National Breast Screening Study. *Cancer, 57,* 1209-1216.

Bakemeier, A. H. (1988). The potential role of vitamins A, C, and E and selenium in cancer prevention. *Oncology Nursing Forum, 15*(6), 785-791.

Baker, L. (1982). Breast cancer detection demonstration project: Five-year summary report. *Cancer, 32,* 194-203.

Bergkvist, L., Adami, H. O., Persson, I., Hoover, R., & Schairer, C. (1989). The risk of breast cancer after estrogen and estrogen-progestin replacement. *New England Journal of Medicine, 321,* 293-297.

Berkel, H., Birdsell, D. C., & Jenkins, H. (1992). Breast augmentation: A risk factor for breast cancer? *New England Journal of Medicine, 326,* 1649-1653.

Bland, K. I. (1991). Inflammatory, infectious, and metabolic disorders of the mamma. In K. I. Bland & E. M. Copeland III (Eds.), *The breast: Comprehensive management of benign and malignant dosages* (pp. 87-112). Philadelphia: W. B. Saunders.

Bland, K. I., & Romrell, L. J. (1991). Congenital and acquired disturbances of breast development and growth. In K. I. Bland & E. M. Copeland III (Eds.), *The breast: Comprehensive management of benign and malignant diseases* (pp. 69-86). Philadelphia: W. B. Saunders.

Brown, M., Eyles, H., & Bland, K. (1991). Nursing care for the patient with breast cancer. In K. I. Bland & E. M. Copeland III (Eds.), *The breast: Comprehensive management of benign and malignant diseases* (pp. 1053-1066). Philadelphia: W. B. Saunders.

Brown-Daniels, C. J., & Blasdell, A. (1990). Early-stage breast cancer: Adjuvant drug therapy. *American Journal of Nursing, 90*(11), 32-33.

Canadian Task Force on the Periodic Examination. (1986). The periodic health examination. Canadian Medical Association Journal, 134, 721-729.

Casey, C. E., & Hambridge, K. M. (1983). Nutritional aspects of human lactation. In M. C. Neville & M. R. Neifert (Eds.), *Lactation: Physiology, nutrition and breast-feeding* (pp. 199-248). New York: Plenum.

Cassileth, B. R., Lusk, E. J., Miller, D. S., Brown, L. L., & Miller, C. (1985). Psychosocial correlates of survival in advanced malignant disease? *New England Journal of Medicine, 312,* 1551-1555.

Champion, V. L. (1988). Attitudinal variables related to intention, frequency and proficiency of breast self-examination in women 35 and over. *Research in Nursing and Health, 11,* 283-291.

Clark, G. M., Dressler, L. G., Owens, M. A., Pounds, G., Oldaker, T., & McGuire, W. L. (1989). Prediction of relapse or survival in patients with node-negative breast cancer by DNA flow cytometry. *New England Journal of Medicine, 320,* 627-633.

Coates, A., Gebski, V., Bishop, J. F., Jeal, P. N., Woods, R. L., & Snyder, R. (1987). Improving the quality of life during chemotherapy for advanced breast cancer: A comparison of intermittent and continuous treatment strategies. *New England Journal of Medicine, 317,* 1490-1495.

Consensus Statement. (1986). Is "fibrocystic" disease of the breast precancerous? *Archives of Pathology and Laboratory Medicine, 110,* 173.

Dackman, L. (1990). *Up front: Sex and the post-mastectomy woman.* New York: Penguin.

Dawson, D. A., & Thompson, G. B. (1989). Breast cancer risk factors and screening: United States, 1987. *Vital and health statistics* (Series 10, No. 172, DHHS Publication No. PHS 90-1500). Washington, DC: Government Printing Office.

Deapen, D. M., Pike, M. C., Casagrande, J. T., & Brody, G. S. (1986). The relationship between breast cancer and augmentation mammoplasty: An epidemiologic study. *Plastic and Reconstructive Surgery, 77,* 361-367.

DeVita, V. T. (1989). Breast cancer therapy: Exercising all our options. *New England Journal of Medicine, 320,* 527-529.

Dupont, W. D., & Page, D. L. (1987). Breast cancer risk associated with proliferative disease, age at first birth, and a family history of breast cancer. *American Journal of Epidemiology, 125,* 769-773.

Early Breast Cancer Trialists' Collaborative Group. (1988). Effects of adjuvant tamoxifen and of cytotoxic therapy on mortality in early breast cancer: An overview of 61 randomized trials among 28,896 women. *New England Journal of Medicine, 319,* 1681-1692.

Ellis, L. M., & Bland, K. I. (1991). General considerations for follow-up. In K. I. Bland & E. M. Copeland III (Eds.), *The breast: Comprehensive management of benign and malignant diseases* (pp. 1001-1011). Philadelphia: W. B. Saunders.

Fallowfield, L. J., & Baum, M. (1991). Psychosocial problems associated with the diagnosis and treatment of breast cancer. In K. I. Bland & E. M. Copeland III (Eds.), *The breast: Comprehensive management of benign and malignant diseases* (pp. 1081-1092). Philadelphia: W. B. Saunders.

Fink, D. J. (1991). Cancer detection: The cancer-related checkup guidelines. In A. I. Holleb, D. J. Fink, & G. P. Murphy (Eds.), *American Cancer Society textbook of clinical oncology* (pp. 153-176). Atlanta, GA: American Cancer Society.

Fisher, B. F., Redmond, C., Fisher, E. R., Bauer, M., Wolmark, N., Wickerham, D. L., Deutsch, M., Montague, E., Margolese, R., & Foster, R. (1985). Ten year results of a randomized clinical trial comparing radical mastectomy and total mastectomy with or without radiation. *New England Journal of Medicine, 312,* 674-681.

Fisher, B. F., Redmond, C., Poisson, R., Margolese, R., Wolmark, N., Wickerham, L., Fisher, E., Deutsch, M., Caplan, R., Pilch, Y., Glass, A., Shibata, H., Lerner, H., Terz, J., & Sidorovich, L. (1989). Eight-year results of a randomized clinical trial comparing total mastectomy and lumpectomy with or without irradiation in the treatment of breast cancer. *New England Journal of Medicine, 320,* 822-828.

Fisher, J. C. (1992). The silicone controversy—When will science prevail? *New England Journal of Medicine, 326,* 1696-1698.

Fletcher, S. W., & O'Malley, M. S. (1986). Clinical breast examination. *Hospital Practice, 21*(5), 80-89.

Fletcher, S. W., O'Malley, M. S., & Bunce, L. A. (1985). Physicians' abilities to detect lumps in silicone breast models. *Journal of the American Medical Association, 253,* 2224-2228.

Fletcher, S. W., O'Malley, M. S., Earp, J. L., Morgan, T. M., Lin, S., & Degnan, D. (1990). How best to teach women breast self-examination. *Annals of Internal Medicine, 112,* 772-779.

Gaskin, T. A., Doss, M. C., Kelly, P. A., & Colburn, J. M. (1991). Rehabilitation. In K. I. Bland & E. M. Copeland III (Eds.), *The breast: Comprehensive management of benign and malignant diseases* (pp. 1067-1075). Philadelphia: W. B. Saunders.

Goldwyn, R. M. (1976). *Plastic and reconstructive surgery of the breast.* Boston: Little, Brown.

Goldwyn, R. M. (1987). Breast reconstruction after mastectomy. *New England Journal of Medicine, 317,* 1711-1714.

Goodman, M., & Harte, N. (1990). Breast cancer. In S. L. Groenwald, M. H. Frogge, M. Goodman, & C. H. Yarbro (Eds.), *Cancer nursing: Principles and practice* (2nd ed., pp. 722-750). Boston: Jones & Bartlett.

Goodson, W. H., Mallman, R., Jacobson, M., & Hunt, T. K. (1985). What do breast symptoms mean? *American Journal of Surgery, 150*(8), 271-274.

Gross, A., & Ito, D. (1991). *Women talk about breast surgery: From diagnosis to recovery* (1st Harper Perennial ed.). New York: Harper Collins.

Grossage, J. (1990). Early-stage breast cancer: How nurses help. *American Journal of Nursing, 90*(11), 31.

Haagensen, C. D. (1977). The relationship of gross cystic disease of the breast and carcinoma. *Annals of Surgery, 185,* 375.

Haagensen, C. D. (1986). *Diseases of the breast* (3rd ed.). Philadelphia: W. B. Saunders.

Harris, J. R., Schnitt, S. J., & Kinne, D. W. (1991). In-situ carcinoma. In J. R. Harris, S. Hellman, I. C. Henderson, & D. W. Kinne (Eds.), *Breast diseases* (2nd ed., pp. 229-244). Philadelphia: J. B. Lippincott.

Henderson, B. E., & Bernstein, L. (1991). The role of endogenous and exogenous hormones in the etiology of breast cancer. In J. R. Harris, S. Hellman, I. C. Henderson, & D. W. Kinne (Eds.), *Breast diseases* (2nd ed., pp. 126-135). Philadelphia: J. B. Lippincott.

Henderson, I. C. (1988). Adjuvant therapy for breast cancer. *New England Journal of Medicine, 318,* 443-444.

Henderson, I. C. (1991). Adjuvant systemic therapy of early breast cancer. In J. R. Harris, S. Hellman, I. C. Henderson, & D. W. Kinne (Eds.), *Breast diseases* (2nd ed., pp. 427-486). Philadelphia: J. B. Lippincott.

Henderson, M. M., Kushi, L. H., Thompson, D. J., Gorbach, S. L., Clifford, C. K., Insull, W., Moskowitz, M., & Thompson, R. S. (1990). Feasibility of a randomized trial of a low-fat diet for the prevention of breast cancer: Dietary compliance in the Women's Health Trial Vanguard Study. *Preventive Medicine, 19,* 115-133.

Henry, P. E. (1992). Overview of breast implant litigation. *Nurse Practitioner Forum, 3*(4), 189-190.

Hildreth, N. G., Shore, R. E., & Dvoretsky, P. M. (1989). The risk of breast cancer after irradiation of the thymus in infancy. *New England Journal of Medicine, 321,* 1281-1284.

Jamison, R. N., Burish, T. G., & Wallston, K. A. (1987). Psychogenic factors in predicting survival of breast cancer patients. *Journal of Clinical Oncology, 5,* 768-772.

Jordan, V. C. (1990). Tamoxifen for the prevention of breast cancer. In V. T. DeVita, S. Hellman, & S. A. Rosenberg (Eds.), *Cancer prevention* (pp. 1-12). Bethesda, MD: National Cancer Institute.

Kaplan, K. M., Weinberg, G. B., Small, A., & Herndon, J. L. (1991). Breast cancer screening among relatives of women with breast cancer. *American Journal of Public Health, 81,* 1174-1175.

Kessler, D. A. (1992). The basis of the FDA's decision on breast implants. *New England Journal of Medicine, 326,* 1713-1715.

Kiang, D. T., Gay, J., Goldman, A., & Kennedy, B. J. (1985). A randomized trial of chemotherapy and hormonal therapy in advanced breast cancer. *New England Journal of Medicine, 313,* 1241-1246.

Kinne, D. W. (1991). Biopsy of a palpable lesion. In J. R. Harris, S. Hellman, I. C. Henderson, & D. W. Kinne (Eds.), *Breast diseases* (2nd ed., pp. 107-111). Philadelphia: J. B. Lippincott.

Knobf, M. T. (1990). Early-stage breast cancer: The options. *American Journal of Nursing, 92*(11), 28-30.

Lashley, M. E. (1987). Predictors of breast self-examination practice among elderly women. *Advances in Nursing Science, 9*(4), 25-34.

Lauver, D. (1989). Instructional information and breast self-examination practice. *Research in Nursing and Health, 12,* 11-19.

Lauver, D., & Angerame, M. (1990). Overadherence with breast self-examination recommendations. *Image: The Journal of Nursing Scholarship, 22,* 148-152.

Lauver, D., & Keenan, C. (1991). Identifying women's description of breast tissue for the promotion of breast self-examination. *Health Care of Women International, 12,* 73-81.

Lazovich, D., White, E., Thomas, D. B., & Moe, R. E. (1991). Underutilization of breast-conserving surgery and radiation therapy among women with stage I or II breast cancer. *Journal of the American Medical Association, 266,* 3433-3438.

Leis, H. P. (1991). Prognostic parameters of breast carcinoma. In K. I. Bland & E. M. Copeland III (Eds.), *The breast: Comprehensive management of benign and malignant diseases* (pp. 331-350). Philadelphia: W. B. Saunders.

London, R. S., Sundaram, G. S., Murphy, L., Manimekalai, S., Reynolds, M., & Goldstein, J. (1985). Effect of vitamin E on mammary dysplasia: A double-blind study. *Obstetrics and Gynecology, 65,* 104-106.

Love, R. L. (1989). Tamoxifen therapy in primary breast cancer: Biology, efficacy, and side effects. *Journal of Clinical Oncology, 7,* 803.

Love, S. L., with Lindsey, K. (1990). *Dr. Susan Love's breast book.* Reading, MA: Addison-Wesley.

Love, S. M., Schnitt, S. J., Connolly, J. L., & Shirley, R. L. (1987). Benign breast disorders. In J. R. Harris, S. Hellman, I. C. Henderson, & D. W. Kinne (Eds.), *Breast diseases* (1st ed., pp. 15-53). Philadelphia: J. B. Lippincott.

Lubin, R., Ron, E., Wax, Y., Black, M., Funaro, M., & Shitrit, A. (1985). A case-control study of caffeine and methylxanthines in benign breast disease. *Journal of the American Medical Association, 253,* 2388-2392.

Mamon, A., & Zapka, J. G. (1985). Improving frequency and proficiency of breast self-examination: Effectiveness of an educational program. *American Journal of Public Health, 75,* 618-624.

Marshall, J. R., & Funch, D. P. (1983). Social environment and breast cancer: A cohort analysis of patient survival. *Cancer, 52,* 1546-1550.

McCraw, J. B., Cramer, A. R., & Horton, C. E. (1991). Breast reconstruction after mastectomy. In K. I. Bland & E. M. Copeland III (Eds.), *The breast: Comprehensive management of benign and malignant diseases* (pp. 656-693). Philadelphia: W. B. Saunders.

McGuire, W. L. (1989). Adjuvant therapy of node-negative breast cancer. *New England Journal of Medicine, 320,* 525-527.

Meyer, F., & Verreault, R. (1987). Erythrocyte selenium and breast cancer risk. *American Journal of Epidemiology, 125,* 917-919.

Meyerowitz, B. E., & Chaiken, S. (1987). The effect of message framing on breast self-examination attitudes, intentions, and behavior. *Journal of Personality and Social Psychology, 52,* 500-510.

Miller, A. B. (1991). Causes of breast cancer and high-risk groups. In J. R. Harris, S. Hellman, I. C. Henderson, & D. W. Kinne (Eds.), *Breast diseases* (2nd ed., pp. 119-126). Philadelphia: J. B. Lippincott.

Morrow, M. (1991a). Breast pain. In J. R. Harris, S. Hellman, I. C. Henderson, & D. W. Kinne (Eds.), *Breast diseases* (2nd ed., pp. 63-73). Philadelphia: J. B. Lippincott.

Morrow, M. (1991b). Nipple discharge. In J. R. Harris, S. Hellman, I. C. Henderson, & D. W. Kinne (Eds.), *Breast diseases* (2nd ed., pp. 73-77). Philadelphia: J. B. Lippincott.

National Cancer Institute. (1984). *Diet, nutrition and cancer prevention: A guide to food choices* (NIH Publication No. 85-2711). Washington, DC: National Institutes of Health.

NIH Consensus Conference. (1991). Treatment of early-stage breast cancer. *Journal of the American Medical Association, 265,* 391-395.

Nettles-Carlson, B. (1989). Early detection of breast cancer. *JOGNN, 18,* 373-381.

Nettles-Carlson, B., Field, M. L., Friedman, B. J., & Smith, L. S. (1988). The effectiveness of teaching breast self-examination during office visits. *Research in Nursing and Health, 11,* 41-50.

Nettles-Carlson, B., & Smith, L. S. (1988). Self-examination in the early detection of breast cancer: Critical review of the literature. *Health Care for Women International, 9,* 337-352.

Neville, M. C., Allen, J. C., & Watters, C. (1983). The mechanisms of milk secretion. In M. C. Neville & M. R. Neifert (Eds.), *Lactation: Physiology, nutrition and breast-feeding* (pp. 49-102). New York: Plenum.

Newman, P. A. (1990). Breast cancer incidence is on the rise—but why? *Journal of the National Cancer Institute, 82,* 998-1000.

Oktay, J. S., & Walter, C. A. (1991). *Breast cancer in the life course: Women's experiences.* New York: Springer.

Osborne, M. P. (1991). Breast development and anatomy. In J. R. Harris, S. Hellman, I. C. Henderson, & D. W. Kinne (Eds.), *Breast diseases* (2nd ed., pp. 1-13). Philadelphia: J. B. Lippincott.

Patey, D. H. (1949). Two common non-malignant conditions of the breast. *British Medical Journal, 1,* 96-97.

Pearson, C. (1991). The trials of the Women's Health Trial. *The Network News: National Women's Health Network, 16*(1), 1, 3.

Politics of breast cancer. (1990, December 10), *Newsweek,* pp. 62-68.

Preece, P. E., Mansel, R. E., & Hughes, L. E. (1978). Mastalgia: Psychoneurosis or ordinary disease? *British Medical Journal, 1,* 29-30.

Pye, J. K., Mansel, R. E., & Hughes, L. E. (1985). Clinical experience of drug treatments for mastalgia. *Lancet, 2,* 373-376.

Robinson, J. E., & Short, R. V. (1977). Changes in breast sensitivity at puberty, during the menstrual cycle, and at parturition. *British Medical Journal, 1,* 1188-1191.

Rollin, B. (1986). *First, you cry.* New York: New American Library.

Romrell, L. J., & Bland, M. (1991). Anatomy of the breast, axilla, chest wall and related metastatic sites. In K. I. Bland & E. M. Copeland III (Eds.), *The breast: comprehensive management of benign and malignant diseases* (pp. 17-35). Philadelphia: W. B. Saunders.

Rutledge, D. (1987). Factors related to women's practice of breast self-examination. *Nursing Research, 36,* 117-121.

Saunders, K. J., Pilgrim, C. A., & Pennypacker, H. S. (1986). Increased proficiency of search in breast self-examination. *Cancer, 58,* 2531-2537.

Scanlon, E. F. (1991). Breast cancer. In A. I. Holleb, D. J. Fink, & G. P. Murphy (Eds.), *American Cancer Society textbook of clinical oncology* (pp. 177-193). Atlanta, GA: American Cancer Society.

Schnitt, S. J., & Connolly, J. L. (1991). Pathology of benign breast disorders. In J. R. Harris, S. Hellman, I. C. Henderson, & D. W. Kinne (Eds.), *Breast diseases* (2nd ed., pp. 15-30). Philadelphia: J. B. Lippincott.

Shapiro, S. (1977). Evidence on screening for breast cancer from a randomized trial. *Cancer, 399*(June Suppl.), 2772-2782.

Sigurdsson, H., Baldetorp, B., Borg, A., Dalberg, M., Ferno, M., Killander, D., & Olsson, H. (1990). Indicators of prognosis in node-negative breast cancer. *New England Journal of Medicine, 322,* 1045-1053.

Silverstein, M. J., Handel, N., Gamagami, P., Waisman, J. R., Gierson, E. D., Rosser, R. J., Steyskal, R., & Colburn, W. (1988). Breast cancer in women after augmentation mammoplasty. *Archives of Surgery, 123,* 681-687.

Sitruk-Ware, R., Sterkers, N., & Mauvais-Jarvais, P. (1979). Benign breast disease I: Hormonal investigation. *Obstetrics and Gynecology, 53,* 457-460.

Smith, D. J., Palin, W. E., Katch, W. L., & Bennett, J. E. (1986). Breast volume and anthropomorphic measurements: Normal values. *Plastic and Reconstructive Surgery, 78,* 331-335.

Snyder, M. (1989). *An informed decision: Understanding breast reconstruction.* New York: M. Evans.

Soffa, V. (1991, September). Breast cancer surgery: Taking time to choose. *The Network News: National Women's Health Network,* pp. 1-2, 11.

Souba, W. W. (1991). Evaluation and treatment of benign breast disorders. In K. I. Bland & E. M. Copeland III (Eds.), *The breast: Comprehensive management of benign and malignant diseases* (pp. 715-729). Philadelphia: W. B. Saunders.

Spiera, H. (1988). Scleroderma after silicone augmentation mammoplasty. *Journal of the American Medical Association, 260*(2), 236-238.

Tabar, L., Fagerberg, D., & Gad, A. (1985). Reduction in mortality from breast cancer after mass screening with mammography: Randomized trial from the Breast Cancer Screening Working Group of the Swedish National Board of Health and Welfare. *Lancet, 1,* 8299-8332.

Tannock, I. F. (1987). Treating the patient, not just the cancer. *New England Journal of Medicine, 317,* 1534-1535.

Taylor, K. M., Margolese, R. G., & Soskolne, C. L. (1984). Physicians' reasons for not entering eligible patients in a randomized clinical trial of surgery for breast cancer. *New England Journal of Medicine, 310,* 1363-1367.

Thompson, W. R., Bowen, R., & Dorman, B. A. (1991). Mammographic localization and biopsy of nonpalpable breast lesions. *Archives of Surgery, 126,* 730-734.

U.S. Preventive Services Task Force. (1987). Recommendations for breast cancer screening. *Journal of the American Medical Association, 257,* 2196.

Watson, M., Greer, S., Blake, S., & Shrapnell, K. (1984). Reaction to a diagnosis of breast cancer: Relationship between denial, delay and rates of psychological morbidity. *Cancer, 53,* 2008-2012.

Willet, W. C., Stampfer, M. J., Colditz, G. A., Rosner, B. A., Hennekens, C. H., & Speizer, F. E. (1987a). Dietary fat and the risk of breast cancer. *New England Journal of Medicine, 316,* 22-28.

Willet, W. C., Stampfer, M. J., Colditz, G. A., Rosner, B. A., Hennekens, C. H., & Speizer, F. E. (1987b). Moderate alcohol consumption and the risk of breast cancer. *New England Journal of Medicine, 316,* 1174-1180.

Wyper, M. A. (1990). Breast self-examination and the health belief model: Variations on a theme. *Research in Nursing & Health, 13,* 421-428.

Yeatman, T. J., & Bland, K. I. (1991). Staging of breast cancer. In K. I. Bland & E. M. Copeland III (Eds.), *The breast: Comprehensive management of benign and malignant diseases* (pp. 313-330). Philadelphia: W. B. Saunders.

Zapka, J. G., Hosnmer, D., Costanza, M. E., Harris, D. R., & Stoddard, A. (1992). Changes in mammography use: Economic need and service factors. *American Journal of Public Health, 82,* 1345-1351.

Zones, J. (1991, June/July/August). New developments in silicone breast implant regulations. *The Network News: National Women's Health Network,* pp. 1, 4.

29

Out of Eden

Philosophical Perspectives on Reproductive Technology

MARGARETE SANDELOWSKI

Few factors have influenced the health and lives of American women more than reproductive technology. Since the increasingly widespread use beginning in the 1970s of techniques such as intrauterine contraception, electronic fetal monitoring, cesarean delivery, amniocentesis, and in vitro fertilization (IVF), reproductive technology has become the focus of growing public debate and private concern. Adam and Eve were evicted from the Garden of Eden for eating the forbidden apple; Pandora unwittingly released evil into the world by opening the forbidden box; Prometheus dared to play with fire; and Icarus dared to fly. Reproductive technology evokes these biblical and mythological images of the promise and peril of having too much knowledge and of trying to master nature. Science fiction has become fact as fully planned "brave new babies" (Andrews, 1989) now increasingly inhabit our world. Perhaps, as Lilford (1989) remarked, women used to just have babies; but they now have the means to decide when and if they will have them, to choose which ones they will have, to reverse the reproductive decisions they once made, and to remove or bypass impediments that used to preclude conception and childbearing. These means, and their possibilities and dangers for women's health and nursing practice, are the subject of this chapter.

Definitions

Reproductive technology typically includes (a) contraceptive technology for preventing conception and terminating pregnancy or the ability to become pregnant, (b) conceptive technology for inducing conception or enhancing fertility, (c) prenatal technology for monitoring the fetus and intrauterine environment and for diagnosing and treating fetal impairments, and (d) childbirth technology for managing labor and birth. These technologies are emphasized in this chapter.

Other technologies that can be included in the category of reproductive technology are (a) menstrual technology, including such devices as sanitary napkins, tampons, and deodorants, for maintaining hygiene; (b) periconceptive technology, including the equipment and techniques for ovulation prediction and pregnancy testing; and (c) neonatal technology, including equipment and techniques for artificial infant feeding, expression of milk from the breast, and intensive medical and nursing care of the preterm infant.

Bush's (1983) definition of technology emphasizes the interaction of people and tools to achieve some human purpose and the distinctions between tool, technique, and technology. Using her definitions, reproductive technology is defined as the organized systems of interactions of people, tools, and techniques for the purposes of regulating fertility and controlling the process and product/outcome of childbearing. Examples of the tools of this technology are the intrauterine device, the laparoscope, the ultrasound machine, and forceps. Examples of the techniques of this technology are sterilization (which involves the use of a variety of surgical tools), amniocentesis (which involves the use of such tools as the ultrasound machine and needles), IVF (which involves the instruments and devices necessary for hormonal stimulation of ovaries, the retrieval of oocytes, the capacitation of sperm, the laboratory fertilization of eggs, and the transfer of the resulting embryos into a woman's body), and cesarean delivery (which involves the use of an array of surgical devices). Examples of the organized systems of interactions of this technology include the health care delivery systems required to use these tools and techniques, such as maternal/fetal and neonatal intensive care units, prenatal testing and genetic counseling programs, and the social exchanges and division of labor between nurses, patients, physicians, and other people in the application and use of reproductive techniques.

Although, typically, scholars in the field of technology do not conceive of pharmacological agents as tools or devices, the drugs used to regulate various reproductive processes (for example, the birth control pill and chemical agents used to induce conception and labor or to retard labor) frequently appear in discussions of reproductive technology. Accordingly, for the purposes of this chapter, pharmacological agents are considered as technological devices.

Perspectives on Technology

There are varying perspectives on the nature, meaning, and consequences of technology.

Technology as Knowledge

Technology may be viewed "as knowledge" (Layton, 1974) or as a distinctive way of knowing or engaging nature. The instruments, devices, and machines of a technology are themselves tangible "systems of concepts" that human beings work out in the metals, plastics, woods, or other materials of which their tools are made (Pirsig, 1974). Drawing from the work of philosopher Martin Heidegger, Klawiter (1990) proposed that modern Western technology is the "congealed form . . . of knowledge that approaches a problem with a readiness to challenge, order, and regulate" (p. 74). Western technology is a way of engaging nature that is characterized by an oppositional stance toward it: a countering or controlling of, rather than a working with, nature. This philosophical position is reflected in the long-standing Western exploitation of nature (currently being exposed and opposed by animal rights, environmental, and ecological activists in Western countries) and in increasing efforts to manage, conquer, and even eliminate natural phenomena (Merchant, 1980; White, 1968). Some feminist scholars have argued that modern Western technology constitutes a masculinist worldview in which nature, historically conceived of as female, has been subjugated to men's will (Merchant, 1980).

A critical historical development affirming Western men's wariness of natural phenomena and their efforts to master them is that reproductive functions have increasingly been brought under technological surveillance and management. There is now no part of the reproductive cycle for which technological intervention is not available or recommended. Proponents of reproductive technology seek to improve on, duplicate, control, or at the very least, keep a close eye on events in the reproductive cycle. For example, the superovulation techniques commonly used in infertility therapy were developed to improve on nature by hormonally inducing a greater number of mature ova per month than would normally occur in a natural menstrual cycle. Physicians employ cesarean delivery when they view labor contractions and vaginal delivery as causing the fetus too much stress. Techniques such as IVF and husband/donor insemination imitate or substitute for the biological milestones in natural reproduction. Uterine contractions are induced, augmented, or impeded to control the force, progression, and timing of labor. And techniques such as ultrasonography and amniocentesis reveal natural and potentially pathological processes once hidden from view.

In American culture, in particular, what is known as "natural is man's artifice" (Fletcher, 1988, p. 44). Women, couples, and caregivers often expand their concept of nature to include reproductive technology. For example, infertile couples undergoing IVF have expressed their view that IVF is natural because nature allowed it to succeed, because the child produced is biologically related to its parents, and because the pregnancy and birth following the procedure are themselves natural processes wholly comparable to the experiences of naturally conceiving couples (Sandelowski, 1991).

Technology as a Subsystem of Culture

Technology may also be viewed as a producing and using subsystem of culture, manifesting the preoccupations, choices, and values of particular groups of people at particular historical moments (Lechtman & Steinberg, 1979). A technology produces culture to the extent that it can act as a force for change, altering factors such as values, norms, practices, and social relations. A technology uses culture to the extent that it can act to maintain the status quo, reinforcing existing values, norms, practices, and social relations (Harding, 1978).

There are many ways in which reproductive technology has acted as a force for change. For example, reproductive technology has irrevocably altered the way sexuality, conception, pregnancy, childbirth, and motherhood are viewed and experienced. Reproductive technology has been instrumental in bringing these events into the domain of medical surveillance, diagnosis, and treatment. These life experiences are now increasingly viewed and experienced as either pathogenic, placing individuals at risk for disease, or as pathological, themselves constituting disease. Reproductive technology is both the means by which a medicalized view has been operationalized and, in its devices, instruments, and machines, a material expression of that view (Eakins, 1986).

Reproductive technology has also changed the experiences of time, space, and social relations in conception and gestation. Contraceptive and conceptive techniques have severed the link between sexual intercourse and procreation; engaging in sexual relations no longer necessarily entails conception nor does conception necessarily involve having engaged in sexual activity. Conceptive techniques have fragmented maternity, permitting different women to be the genetic (or ovarian), gestational (or uterine), or social mother of the same child. Conceptive and neonatal technologies have shortened the period of time an embryo/fetus may spend inside a woman's body, thus undermining the unique biological role the female has played in reproduction, confounding existing notions of fetal viability, and reframing debates about the personhood and moral claims to rights of the fetus vis-à-vis the pregnant woman (Callahan, 1986; Taub, 1989). Tocolytic agents, in turn, have prolonged pregnancies threatened by premature contractions.

With IVF, a new periconceptional period is added; the process of getting pregnant is experientially prolonged as women undergoing the procedure consciously experience each step leading to conception and each step immediately following it (Sandelowski, Harris, & Holditch-Davis, 1990). Techniques used for early pregnancy diagnosis also serve to make pregnancy experientially longer, with women now obtaining positive pregnancy tests within days of conception. Importantly, periconceptive, conceptive, and prenatal technology together have contributed to the earlier parental, medical, and social recognition of the fetus as a baby and as a patient (Blank, 1984). Women may, accordingly, become invested in their babies earlier in pregnancy, deriving more enjoyment from pregnancy but also becoming increasingly subject to grief responses should the pregnancy/baby be lost. Prior to the development of external fertilization and early pregnancy diagnosis techniques, early pregnancy losses were likely to remain unnoticed. Similarly, increasing medical, ethical, and legal attention is now directed to the fetal patient who can be seen, diagnosed, and, to a very limited extent, treated (Goodlin, 1979; Evans, Quigg, Kappitch, & Schulman, 1989; Kaufmann & Williams, 1985; Liley, 1972/1986; Pritchard, MacDonald, & Gant, 1985; Walters, 1986).

Reproductive technology has also created new patients, new orientations to existing patients, and new areas of professional practice. In addition to the creation of the fetal patient, reproductive technology has contributed to the discovery of other new populations of patients to monitor, diagnose, and treat. Women and couples who used to be advised against childbearing for medical or genetic reasons may now feel safer attempting to have children because of new and refined surveillance and management techniques, such as fetal stress testing and cesarean delivery, and because of new diagnostic techniques that provide them with information about a pregnancy that they may subsequently elect to maintain or terminate. Many women and couples who would not have been able to conceive because of a biological impairment now have the biotechnical means available to them to overcome or circumvent impediments to reproduction.

Moreover, reproductive technology has expanded the potential population of individuals eligible for or seeking medical services, in part, by redefining certain conditions. For example, as more women in their 40s seek infertility services, what used to be viewed as the physiological, or natural, infertility of midlife is increasingly being viewed medically as a treatable condition. In addition, couples who have delayed childbearing and have left themselves less time in which to conceive are increasingly seeking infertility services after only a few months of effort; consumers of conceptive technology now include couples who were once not considered infertile until they had been trying to conceive without success for at least one year. In addition, normally fertile women now undergo reproductive techniques such as superovulation, artificial insemination, and IVF when they volunteer to become egg donors and when they have male partners with fertility impairments. Congress (Congress of the United States, Office of Technology Assessment, 1988) has estimated that the increasing demand for services has probably surpassed any actual increase in the overall percentage of couples with fertility impairments. Reproductive technology has, accordingly, created a new market for professional services. Nurses and physicians can now be certified as experts in the use of reproductive technology, which has led to the establishment of such new advanced practice areas as maternal/fetal medicine, perinatal nursing, and infertility/reproductive endocrinology.

Reproductive technology has engendered many profound changes, but it has also reinforced existing cultural values and social practices and arrangements. In fact, many social critics have argued that reproductive technology has largely perpetuated the status quo, allowing prevailing social relations and gender, race, and class inequalities to remain unchallenged. For example, although regional block techniques for relieving childbirth pain have introduced new practices in the labor room, they have also reinforced in a material way the view of childbearing as a medical condition subject to medical intervention, and the division of mind from body characteristic in Western culture. Such techniques can be used only in a medical context, and they fragment women's personae, separating them from their bodies' functions. Moreover, the laboring woman under the influence of epidural anesthesia becomes a less reliable informant about the progress of her labor than her unanesthetized counterpart; clinicians must, accordingly, rely on other sources of information, such as the electronic fetal monitor (Sandelowski, 1984). Although new, techniques such as IVF reinforce rather than challenge the cultural emphasis on the importance of having a biological child and the tendency to treat women, even for male dysfunctions (Lorber, 1988, 1989; Modell, 1989). Contraceptive techniques, which have been developed for and used by women almost exclusively, reinforce the cultural expectation that women are responsible for the outcomes of sexual relations. Reproductive technology has also perpetuated race and class inequalities in health care; fertility-enhancing and prenatal techniques are much more available to the economically privileged, whereas fertility control techniques are more likely to be directed to the less economically privileged (Clarke, 1984; Nsiah-Jefferson & Hall, 1989). Significantly, it can be argued that in the case of reproductive technology, the more things have changed, the more they have stayed the same.

Technology as a Force for Liberation/Oppression

Reinforcing the view that technology acts as a force for cultural change is the prevalent Western belief that any technological innovation means progress and, therefore, constitutes a force for good. Menstrual hygiene products, for example, have permitted women a freedom in dress and a presence in society they probably did not have before the mass production and distribution of sanitary napkins and tampons (Schroeder, 1976). In a similar emancipatory vein, contraceptive techniques have given women the material means to control their lives, to pursue goals other than motherhood, and to protect themselves from the physical and psychic ravages of unwanted and untimely pregnancies. Contraceptive techniques have freed women to enter the mainstream of American life in equal partnership with men because they have allowed women to regulate a major biological function that has historically impeded equal partnership: maternity (Gordon, 1976).

In contrast, many critics of technology view it as a force for oppression and as a threat to health and humanity. Critics of contraceptive and conceptive techniques have described the iatrogenic harm caused by ineffective and/or unsafe devices and therapies, evident in the morbidity and mortality caused by the use of diethylstilbesterol (DES) in the treatment of threatened miscarriage, the Dalkon Shield for intrauterine contraception, and hormonal drugs that enhance fertility (Arditti, Klein, & Minden, 1984; Klein & Rowland, 1989). Far from liberating women, these devices, which are virtually all designed for use by women and not by men, reinforce in a material way the cultural idea that women are responsible for and, therefore, ought to shoulder the burdens (including injury and death) of preventing birth and inducing conception. Conceptive techniques are charged with fragmenting motherhood and thereby preserving patriarchy by permitting three different women to be (genetic or ovarian, gestational or surrogate, and nurturing) mothers of a child, none of whom has an exclusive claim to that child and all of whom have a connection to procreation as limited and tenuous as men's (Corea, 1985; Spallone & Steinberg, 1987; Stanworth, 1987; Taub, 1989). In an important literature critical of mainstream American childbirth practices, scholars and social critics have lamented the pervasive medicalization of the natural experiences of gestation, birth, and early parenting engendered by increasing technological surveillance and intervention. According to these critics, this technology has contributed to the disruption of intimate family bonds, the denigration and virtual effacement of childbearing women as persons, and the further subordination of women/patients to male/physician control (Eakins, 1986; Edwards & Waldorf, 1984; Haire, 1972; Michaelson, 1988; Oakley, 1986; Rothman, 1982).

Technology as Active/Passive

Related to the opportunity and threat associated with technology is the debate concerning whether technical things (machines, tools, instruments) are in and of themselves passive or neutral, deriving their influence solely from the way people use them (guns do not kill people, people do), or whether they have properties that actively dictate the way they are used (guns are for destroying, maiming, and killing people and animals and to choose to use a gun is to choose to destroy, maim, or kill). Bush (1983) proposed that tools, techniques, and technologies have "valences" or charges that tended to "pull or push" behavior in one direction or another (p. 155) in much the same way that atoms have positive, negative, or neutral charges. Conceiving a tool as being passive or neutrally charged can be a basis for the argument that the ultrasound machine, for example, is beneficial or harmful to the extent that professionals use it properly. In contrast, conceiving a tool as being active, or positively or negatively charged, provides a basis for the argument that the ultrasound machine is itself valenced toward fetal differentiation; by producing a visual and animated image of the fetus in utero, it causes the fetus to be recognized earlier in its development as a baby. This quality of the machine can, in turn, be used either to enhance women's enjoyment of pregnancy or to manipulate their behavior. The ultrasound machine has been described as useful in promoting maternal investment in pregnancy, inducing women to engage in more healthful behaviors on behalf of the fetus, and as an antiabortion propaganda device, serving to reduce the likelihood that women will terminate pregnancies (Cox et al., 1987; Hyde, 1986; Kohn, Nelson, & Weiner, 1980; Milne & Rich, 1981; Petchesky, 1987; Reading & Cox, 1982).

Also affirming the active quality of technology is the distinctive arrangement of power and authority (Winner, 1985) that a technology permits, creates, or reinforces by virtue of the context in which it is used and also by its very design. Critics of reproductive technology maintain that it tends to preserve the power and authority of the physician in matters of reproduction because it is used in, controlled by, and designed to achieve the purposes of a health care delivery system dominated by physicians and oriented to increasing technological intervention. Preventive health measures are typically "low-tech" and available without physician services and fees. For example, the conventional design of electronic fetal monitoring equipment confines women to and restricts their mobility in bed. Newer telemetry devices that allow women more mobility also permit them more freedom. Significantly, fetal monitoring equipment has the flexibility in design to allow different arrangements of power and authority; one design preserves the conventionally prone and subordinate patienthood of the childbearing woman, whereas the other design permits her a more active role vis-à-vis her caregivers. In other respects, however, this machine offers few alternative possibilities for power. Although the electronic fetal monitor can be designed to give women more comfort and freedom of mobility, women remain under the aegis of physicians who ultimately control the use of and access to this machine.

In contrast to surveillance technology, periconceptive and contraceptive technologies seem to allow truly different arrangements of power and authority. Over-the-counter birth control devices and pregnancy and ovulation testing kits allow women to manage their own reproductive lives. If more devices and techniques were redesigned to emphasize male methods or methods that do not require medical prescription or supervision, contraceptive technology could further alter the social relations between women and men by shifting the locus of power between them.

Technology as Expanding/ Contracting Human Capabilities

Technology extends human capabilities, but it also limits them, often eliminating or replacing human functions (Illich, 1973). Reproductive technology has been variously described as extending caregivers' senses, allowing them to see more and thereby to evaluate better the progress of reproductive functions. According to this view, fetal surveillance and diagnosis techniques, for example, reveal what used to be hidden in nature to the clinical gaze. As mentioned previously, this technology has also expanded caregivers' professional opportunities and skills.

Interestingly, although it expands human capabilities, technology also creates more work. Technology is labor creating, rather than laborsaving, in that it tends to create new and higher standards for human activity (Cowan, 1983). The replacement of the fetoscope with the electronic fetal monitor, for example, means that nurses have more to do in appraising fetal status. With machine technology, monitoring protocols are much more complex and demand more time and labor to learn and execute them. Although a popular image of machine monitoring implies that one nurse, seated at a bank of screens, can care for more laboring women and thus reduce the numbers of people needed to provide services, the proper use of this technology (given the complexity of monitoring protocols and the maintenance and repair that machines always require) demands more time and labor per patient on the part of nurses and maintenance personnel. A tool may make labor less physically taxing, as in the case of automated beds, but it typically does not reduce the time and energy human beings have to invest in achieving the purposes for which they use technology.

Reproductive technology is also popularly viewed as expanding women's and couples' choices and permitting them reproductive opportunities once unavailable to them. Couples can now choose when and if to have children; couples can overcome or circumvent impediments to conception, gestation, and birth; and, with the advent of fetal diagnosis techniques and safer pregnancy termination and surgical procedures, couples who would not have attempted (or who would have been advised against) having children for medical or genetic reasons now have this option increasingly available to them.

Yet the expansion of options with which this technology is associated is also illusory. Although individuals (especially the socioeconomically privileged) expect to be able to control the timing and nature of their reproductive experiences, complete birth control is ultimately an unattainable goal. Reproductive technology may now permit the exercise of more control over reproductive events than ever before, but many unplanned pregnancies still occur (Jones, Forrest, Henshaw, Silverman, & Torres, 1989), only 50% of infertile couples will achieve pregnancy in treatment (Congress, 1988), sterilizations and attempts to reverse sterilizations still fail (Hatcher et al., 1990), and impaired infants are still born. Americans' high expectations for regulating the processes and outcomes of reproduction often lead to frustration, anger, and regret (Gomel, 1978; Marcil-Gratton, 1988) concerning the real limits of both technology and nature.

Moreover, for every choice made available by reproductive technology, another choice is made increasingly unavailable. Reliance on cesarean delivery in complicated childbirth situations, for example, has "deskilled" (Sarah, 1987, p. 67) physicians in such techniques as forceps delivery and external version (Jordan, 1984). Reliance on electronic fetal monitoring has deskilled nurses in the use of the fetoscope and in behavioral observation and palpation (Sarah, 1987). With the advent of these techniques, nurses and physicians have less educational emphasis on, training in, and practice experience with the procedures or skills they replaced. Reliance on the pregnancy test has made women less confident in their abilities to validate the existence of pregnancy (Jordan, 1977; Patterson, Freese, & Goldenberg, 1986). The advent of bottle-feeding has deskilled women in breastfeeding. Significantly, by replacing human functions, technology simultaneously demands that human beings develop new capabilities and abandon others.

Moreover, the very existence of techniques such as amniocentesis to detect fetal impairment and IVF to treat infertility make the option not to choose to use these techniques less acceptable. Analyses of women's and couples' decision making in relation to techniques such as these indicate how difficult it has become to turn them down. Opportunities become mandates; the freedom to choose becomes the imperative to choose, with women and couples now bearing the burden of choosing from an array of technological options (Beck-Gernsheim, 1989; Rothman, 1984; Rowland, 1987). One uniquely contemporary and Western phenomenon associated with this burden is regret: (a) the regret that individuals anticipate if they decide against a technology offered to them (DeZoeten, Tymstra, & Alberda, 1987; Sandelowski, Harris, & Holditch-Davis, 1989; Tymstra, 1989) and (b) the regret following specific choices made in the past, such as "sterilization regret" (Gomel, 1978; Marcil-Gratton, 1988).

Innovations in medical technology also produce a chain of burden because one choice made in the past leads to other mandates to choose. For example, the couple choosing to have an amniocentesis that shows the presence of a genetically impaired fetus must then decide whether to terminate or maintain the pregnancy, a dilemma that did not exist before the advent of amniocentesis (Rapp, 1988b; Rothman, 1988). Significantly, reproductive technology certainly expands opportunities, but it also constrains them and coerces choice in frequently subtle ways. Moreover, the increasing reliance on this technology in the routine and customary care of women and couples calls into question the new meaning of choice and informed consent in a social system that, in effect, forces both patients and their caregivers to choose technology to substantiate their claims to responsible and lawful action and care. Increased reliance on technology often characterizes the practice of "defensive medicine," and it has become integral to what some physicians, lawyers, and others consider being a good mother. Physicians may feel forced to monitor patients electronically or to perform cesarean operations for fear of malpractice claims; women have been forced against their will to undergo cesarean delivery on behalf of the fetus (Taub & Cohen, 1988).

Technology Assessment: A Framework and Illustrations

Technology has made profound inroads into the American mind and experience, yet we remain "gadget-rich and assessment poor" (Bush, 1983, p. 168). Only recently have clinicians, social scientists, and a variety of policy makers given significant attention to evaluating technology in health care, as evident in the emergence of a literature on technology, an office of technology assessment, consensus development conferences on such techniques as the use of ultrasonography in pregnancy (Consensus Development Conference, 1984) and cesarean delivery (Consensus Development Conference, 1981), and efforts to set policy and research agendas.

Technology assessment is the systematic study of the effects of a technology on society, including its intended or first-order consequences and its side effects, including second- and third-order consequences that may be unintended or delayed (Coates, 1971). Although it is an attempt to base practice and policy on a rational, objective foundation, technology assessment remains a subjective enterprise because of the difficulty in predicting outcomes and because values enter the very process of assessment. Technology assessment inevitably involves issues of equity and values and, therefore, should include analyses of who benefits and who suffers from technological innovations and what values ought to prevail (Bush, 1983).

The remainder of this chapter is devoted to a description of a framework that may be particularly useful to nurses in assessing reproductive technology and to illustrations of how such an assessment might proceed. Elements of the framework are presented in a linear fashion; yet in actual practice, these elements are interrelated. Case examples of analyzing a tool, a technique, and a technology are given. Although these analyses are necessarily abbreviated and simplified, they nevertheless serve to illuminate issues typically obscured in medical and nursing discussions of technology. Exposing these issues alone can assist nurses in raising scientific and ethical questions about the technological basis for practice, including (a) how and even whether a particular technology should continue to be incorporated into practice, (b) how nurses can enhance the value and minimize the harm to women and their families associated with a particular technology, and (c) how and whether a technology advances or retards the caring mission of nursing.

Evaluating the Nature of Technology

What Is the Nature of the Tool/Technique/Technology?

1. What is its scientific/technical basis?
2. How does it work?
3. How effectively does it do its work?
4. How dependent/independent of the user context is it for its effectiveness?
5. What are its properties or valence?

This category of assessment focuses on the characteristics of "the things themselves" (E. Husserl, cited in Winner, 1985, p. 27) and the ways in which the tools we use by their very nature define and constrain our work and our behavior (Cowan, 1983). The case in point is the electronic fetal monitor.

Illustration 1: The Electronic Fetal Monitor. The electronic fetal monitor is a machine that permits continuous indirect or direct surveillance via Doppler ultrasound devices and electrocardiography of the frequency, duration, and intensity of uterine contractions and of the baseline of and fluctuations and variability in the fetal heart rate. It is used antepartally to determine the fetus's ability to withstand labor (fetal [non]stress testing) and intrapartally to monitor fetal status during labor. In indirect, or external, monitoring, a transducer emitting continuous sound waves is placed at the point on a woman's abdomen where the fetal heart is best heard. A water-soluble gel applied to the transducer facilitates the conduction of fetal heart sounds. The technique is based on the principle that any moving structure, such as the heart wall and valves, will send a signal via the transducer in the form of a reflected wave that changes in frequency. The results are recorded on a screen and on graph paper. Uterine contractions are monitored externally via a tocodynamometer, a device that transmits an electrical signal created by the uterine pressure exerted against it. In direct, or internal, monitoring, an electrode capable of providing a continuous recording of the fetal heart rate is attached to the fetal head or buttocks. An intrauterine catheter provides a record of uterine contractions via a pressure-responsive strain gauge connected to the monitor (Olds, London, & Ladewig, 1988).

The effectiveness of the electronic fetal monitor is very dependent on the way it is used and on the way the information it provides is interpreted. For example, if a tocodynamometer is too tightly attached to the maternal abdomen, a contraction may appear more intense than it really is. When a laboring woman moves, the information obtainable from external monitoring may be seriously compromised. Clinicians interpreting information obtained from direct and indirect surveillance frequently do not agree on the meaning of this information and on the clinical action required (Cohen, Klapholz, & Thompson, 1982; Dawes, Moulden, & Redman, 1990; Lotgering, Wallenberg, & Schouten, 1982). In addition, such factors as the speed of the paper (typically, 3 cm/minute in the United States) can alter beat-to-beat variability and make the detection of late and variable decelerations more difficult (Parer, 1986). Significantly, the operations of the electronic fetal monitor are directly influenced by the skill of clinicians in connecting a woman to the machine, recognizing and then controlling factors that can interfere with the accurate detection and recording of information, and reliably and accurately interpreting the contraction and fetal heart rate patterns the machine displays. Despite the fact that electronic fetal monitoring provides more information than auscultation with the fetoscope, the clinical interpretation of this information is more complicated and, therefore, more subject to error (Grant, 1989).

Studies of the effectiveness of electronic fetal monitoring in improving perinatal outcomes have demonstrated an equivocal scientific basis for the routine use of this machine, even in high-risk situations (Haverkamp, Thompson, McFee, &

Centrulo, 1976; Haverkamp et al., 1979; Kelso et al., 1978; Langendoerfer et al., 1980; Leveno et al., 1986; Luthy et al., 1987; MacDonald, Grant, Sheridan-Pereira, Boylan, & Chalmers, 1985; Wood et al., 1981). Importantly, the electronic fetal monitor has become part of standard obstetric management for virtually any woman laboring in a hospital that has the machine, despite the absence of clear scientific evidence that it reduces perinatal morbidity and mortality (Banta & Thacker, 1979; Haverkamp & Orleans, 1982). (The exigencies of conducting randomized clinical trials evaluating the effectiveness and safety of the fetal monitor make it difficult to draw scientifically valid conclusions.) Accordingly, both the American College of Obstetricians and Gynecologists and the American Academy of Pediatrics have stated that intermittent auscultation is equivalent to continuous electronic fetal monitoring, even in high-risk patients (Huddleston, 1990).

By virtue of its operations and the procedures its use mandates, the electronic fetal monitor can be viewed as a machine valenced toward (a) vigilance, (b) social isolation, and (c) intervention. In contrast to the fetoscope, the electronic fetal monitor is a machine that permits and demands more vigilance of fetal and uterine status because it provides a continuous (as opposed to intermittent) material record of many more discrete intrauterine events. This record has an existence apart from the events it represents, rhythm strips now constituting evidence in court cases. Moreover, the machine permits clinicians to detect factors that could not be detected when the fetoscope and the hand were the only instruments used to monitor contractions and fetal heart rate. Once known of, an event, such as late deceleration, can no longer be unknown; once seen, such an event becomes searched for in appraising the health of every fetus. Late deceleration is a good example of an event created by the machine that can detect it because it did not exist as a separate appraisal or diagnostic category—as an object for vigilance—until the advent of the electronic fetal monitor. The electronic fetal monitor allows more to be seen, but it also creates what is seen.

The electronic fetal monitor is also valenced toward social isolation in that the mere presence of the machine in the room draws people's attention to it and away from each other. The machine's pull is, in part, explained by its valence toward vigilance—the mandate that the information it produces be looked at and interpreted. Yet it also pulls human beings to it by such factors as its sounds, flashing lights, paper movement, and by the general fascination that Americans, in particular, seem to have with "gadgets." Starkman (1976) found that laboring women themselves personified the machine, variously thinking of it as a protector of their babies; an extension of themselves, their babies, or the physician; or as a "mechanical monster" that caused them discomfort and competed with them for attention.

In addition, the presence of the machine can impose social isolation on the woman monitored because the procedures it requires for use have a tendency to inhibit verbal and tactile contact between the woman and her caregiver. The information desired about contractions is obtained from the machine instead of from uterine palpation and from observing and asking the woman herself; and uterine palpation is itself made more difficult in external monitoring by the presence of the apparatus on the woman's abdomen connecting her to the machine. The use of the electronic fetal monitor tends to increase the likelihood that women will be left alone in labor (Grant, 1989). Moreover, machine-generated knowledge by itself tends to be viewed by both clinicians and patients as more objective (reliable and valid) than patients' subjective reports or behaviors (Oakley, 1986; Reiser, 1978).

Finally, and perhaps most important, the electronic fetal monitor is valenced toward intervention, in that the very presence of the machine raises the likelihood that cesarean section and other invasive procedures will be performed (Consensus Development Conference, 1981; Grant, 1989; Haverkamp & Orleans, 1982). Contributing to this valence is the need to improve the accuracy, or specificity and sensitivity, of machine monitoring by using other techniques (for example, fetal scalp blood sampling) to determine whether an ominous fetal heart rate pattern is accurately reflecting fetal distress. In addition, the procedures that the use of the machine requires, such as restricting a woman's activity in labor and rupturing the amniotic membranes for direct monitoring, may themselves cause the fetal distress that necessitates intervention. Moreover, because an increasing number of events can now be detected by the monitor, they become subject to interpretations or diagnoses, such as fetal distress or failure to progress, that warrant some action.

The electronic fetal monitor is a machine that tends to bend interactions toward it by its very design and presence. More important, the machine does not so much discover information as it produces information about the fetus and uterine contractions that makes it possible to (a) discuss such new entities as late and variable decelerations and (b) diagnose and treat such new problems as fetal distress and failure to progress. Most significant, the monitor produces information that human beings have to interpret; the putatively objective knowledge obtainable from the machine has no meaning without this subjective human element.

Evaluating the Context of Technology

What Is the Social/Political/Cultural Context of the Development and Use of the Tool/Technique/Technology?

1. What were the circumstances of its emergence?
2. What problem(s) is it supposed to solve?
3. What values/norms/prescriptions does it reinforce or create?
4. Who controls it?

This category of assessment focuses on the historical and sociocultural context in which technology is developed and deployed and illuminates the difficulty often encountered in identifying the problem(s) that a technology is intended to resolve and the role of technology in creating the new and/or reinforcing the old. What appears novel in the matter of technology may, on closer examination, be very familiar after all. The case in point is in vitro fertilization.

Illustration 2: In Vitro Fertilization. IVF, a technique for achieving fertilization of an ovum outside the woman's body, was first successfully performed in 1978 with the birth of Louise Brown. The birth of the first "test-tube" baby followed decades of research with human eggs and mammalian fertilization and the invention of a variety of techniques, including rapid and accurate measurement of hormone levels, ultrasound imaging of the pelvis, and laparoscopy (Corea, 1985; McShane, 1988). Accordingly, IVF is a technique that depended on the invention of other techniques for its development.

Contrasting views exist on the reasons for the emergence of this technique. For example, IVF is viewed as an inevitable culmination of human curiosity and the search for more knowledge about human reproduction; it is also viewed as the result of a long-standing male desire to create babies and to regulate the process and product of birth in the interests of male power and reproductive efficiency and quality. Importantly, IVF is a technique that was ostensibly invented to treat infertility, but it may also be construed as an example of a "socially camouflaged" (Maines, 1989) technique in that artificial conception has always been envisioned as contributing to other less visible, more controversial, and potentially destructive eugenic and patriarchal goals (Corea, 1985; Spallone & Steinberg, 1987; Stanworth, 1987), such as the creation of the "perfect" baby and the reduction of the distinctively female role in conception and childbearing.

In the American health care system, technology is generally viewed as solving problems. For example, with the refinement of the skills and techniques of anesthesia and surgery, cesarean section is now a technique that in the vast majority of cases successfully solves the mechanical problem of a fetus who is too large to be born vaginally. Cephalopelvic disproportion is a problem that typically escapes debate about whether it is a "real" or socially constructed problem dependent on such factors as history, class, and culture for its construction. No one would disagree that a fetus too large for its mother is a life-threatening problem necessitating medical intervention or that cephalopelvic disproportion constitutes the same problem whether it occurs in the United States or some other country or in white or black women. Moreover, no one would disagree that the best solution to the problem is to accomplish birth in a way that preserves the good health and life of both mother and infant. Although rising rates of cesarean section in the United States have engendered considerable controversy, resorting to the technique in cases of cephalopelvic disproportion has typically not been considered an abuse of this technique.

Unlike the problem of cephalopelvic disproportion, however, most problems for which reproductive technology is offered as solution are not as simply defined. In the case of IVF, what problem does it solve? Is it, for example, infertility—the inability to procreate—or is it childlessness—the lack of a desired child to parent? If the problem is identified as infertility, then conceptive technology becomes the only solution to the problem. If the problem is identified as childlessness, then conceptive technology becomes only one of a number of solutions that include adoption and fostering. Yet even when infertility is defined as the problem, IVF does not cure but, rather, circumvents the impairment causing infertility. IVF does not make obstructed oviducts patent, nor does it eliminate or ameliorate any other biological problem impeding conception. In addition, IVF is notoriously ineffective in producing babies; in 1989, the overall live delivery rate for IVF (based on 15,392 retrievals performed in 163 clinics in the United States) was only 14% (Medical Research International, 1991). Accordingly, if infertility is defined as the inability to reproduce, IVF still does not solve that problem. If, however, infertility is defined as the inability to produce a child who is in some way biologically related to either a woman or a man or both in a reproductive partnership, then IVF (and its variations, as well as other conceptive techniques) remains the only solution to the problem. Importantly, when IVF is offered as a solution to the problem of infertility, it is the inability to achieve some form of biological (genetic or gestational) parenthood that is emphasized, not the inability to procreate per se.

Infertility is also typically conceptualized as a problem affecting heterosexual married couples. This depiction of infertility reflects a cultural mandate for married couples to have children and a cultural proscription against having children outside of marriage or in gay partnerships; such a depiction of the problem serves to limit the access of these groups to conceptive techniques. Moreover, cultural emphases on having a biological child of one's own serve to make IVF appear as a necessary last chance and, paradoxically, a natural solution to the problem of infertility and to make other solutions, such as adoption and fostering, appear unnatural or second-best. In addition, because it operates in the treatment of individual couples rather than in the prevention of social and environmental factors contributing to infertility, IVF serves to reinforce an individualistic as opposed to social view of health problems and to perpetuate the American health care system orientation to intervention rather than prophylaxis and health promotion. Developed and used in such a cultural milieu, IVF has become a sensationalized and favored solution to infertility over efforts to prevent pelvic inflammatory disease, iatrogenically caused reproductive impairments, environmental hazards impeding procreation, and other factors contributing to infertility (Taub, 1989). The increasing use of techniques such as IVF also serves to obscure the fact that eliminating these hazards would also eliminate much of the need for conceptive technology (Scritchfield, 1989).

Although IVF and its variations (including gamete intrafallopian transfer, or GIFT, zygote intrafallopian transfer, or ZIFT, and the use of donor spermatozoa and ova) have created new types of parental relationships and opportunities for having a biologically related child not possible only 15 years ago, these techniques have also served to perpetuate the status quo. Conceptive techniques such as IVF preserve the usual power arrangement between physicians and patients and nurses. Women and couples consume the techniques, and nurses and laboratory technicians implement them; but physicians have the power to offer and withhold them. They create the medical and social criteria determining who can be a candidate for these procedures. In some IVF programs, criteria are intentionally broadened to expand the availability of the technique and, therefore, to expand the market for it and the profits to be made from it. In other programs, stricter criteria exist to allow in only those deemed most likely to conceive by IVF, because better success rates would result. Overall, physicians decide on the basis of criteria such as finances and fitness to parent, in addition to medical criteria, such as which couples are good candidates for the technique. In this way, physicians as members of their culture help to reinforce cultural prescriptions concerning who should be helped to have children. Judgments about fitness to parent and the ability to pay for infertility therapy determine, as much as any medical criteria, who will have access to conceptive techniques such as IVF (Damewood, 1990; Nsiah-Jefferson & Hall, 1989; Somerville, 1982).

Although IVF and its variations are increasingly promoted as both first-line and last-chance (Modell, 1989) solutions to the problem of infertility as it is variously conceptualized, these techniques do not cure any disease process contributing to infertility, nor are they especially successful in leading to viable pregnancies. Despite its ineffectiveness and the difficult nature of the problem it is supposed to solve, however, IVF continues to be viewed by couples and the medical community as worthy of continued use and refinement, in large part because it is a technique that reinforces a familiar cultural refrain—the importance of having a flesh-and-blood child of one's own (if not on one's own).

Evaluating the Consequences of Technology

What Are the Intended and Other Consequences of the Tool/Technique/Technology?

1. What new resources/procedures/skills/technology does it mandate?
2. What procedures/skills/technology does it replace?
3. What new orientations to people, events, or problems does it create?
4. What effect does it have on social interactions?
5. What are its health and other benefits/liabilities?
6. What are its costs?

This category of assessment emphasizes the intended and, frequently, unintended consequences of technological innovations. By inventing and using technology to achieve goals, human beings may not desire all of the outcomes that are produced. A technology, for example, may have the effect of diminishing women's autonomy, but this outcome may not have been intended by its inventors or deployers. The case in point is prenatal surveillance and diagnostic technology.

Illustration 3: Prenatal Surveillance and Diagnostic Technology. Prenatal surveillance and diagnostic technology includes techniques such as ultrasonography, chorionic villus sampling, alpha-fetoprotein testing, amniocentesis, and fetal stress testing, and the systems required to apply these techniques. This technology provides knowledge primarily about fetal but also about maternal status during pregnancy that assists childbearing couples and their caregivers to make decisions about the future course of pregnancy and to prepare emotionally and medically for medical complications and the birth of an impaired child. Prenatal technology is generally considered safe when used by experienced clinicians, although techniques such as chorionic villus sampling and amniocentesis may cause pregnancy complications and loss in small numbers of cases.

Prenatal technology has been a key factor in the development of the advanced practice areas of perinatal medicine and nursing and in the development of new disciplines, such as genetic counseling. (Nonphysicians and nonnurses may now obtain advanced academic degrees in this newly established field [Rothman & Detlefs, 1988].) This technology has also necessitated the proliferation of prenatal testing centers and facilities and the development of new diagnostic and surveillance skills. To a certain extent, techniques such as ultrasonography have reduced the need for physicians (but not necessarily for nurse-midwives) to be skilled in the assessment by hand of the growth and placement of the fetus; ultrasonography and amniocentesis have replaced the X ray as a means of intrauterine diagnosis.

Prenatal technology has had a critical impact on the way pregnancy is experienced and approached. First, this technology has had the effect of replacing conventional biological rhythms and milestones of pregnancy with technological ones (Beeson, 1984). For example, the ultrasound picture often replaces quickening as an initial validater of pregnancy and as a stimulus to the evolving maternal-fetal relationship (Reading & Cox, 1982). When performed early in pregnancy, it precedes quickening, a woman's first felt recognition of fetal movement. By providing an animated visual image of the fetus, this technique tends to induce fetal differentiation earlier—recognition of the fetus as a person separate from the mother—and it substitutes seeing for feeling as the critical sensory modality in achieving this awareness of the fetus. With ultrasonography, a woman's perception of the fetus is visual and publicly shared, as opposed to privately felt (Sandelowski, 1988; Stewart, 1986). In addition, a woman's recognition of the fetus is shaped by clinicians' or technicians' interpretations of the ultrasonic image projected. A "baby" often exists in the mind of a woman only after the image has been clinically interpreted as being a baby (Rapp, 1988a). Ultrasonography has transformed women's and couples' recognition of the fetus from a private event beginning somewhere in the middle of pregnancy into a medical/technical event occurring very early in pregnancy (Fletcher & Evans, 1983).

Amniocentesis has also been found to affect the "living" of pregnancy by altering the conventional periodization of pregnancy from three trimesters into two stages. With amniocentesis, pregnancy is often lived by women, or divided experientially into two periods: before prenatal testing and after the results of testing are known

(Beeson, 1984; Rothman, 1986). Several investigators have found that women increasingly do not invest in their pregnancies until after 4 to 5 months have passed, spending the first half of pregnancy waiting to undergo testing and then waiting for the test result that will provide them assurance of a healthy infant (Beeson, 1984; Beeson & Golbus, 1979; Sala, 1983; Silvestre & Fresco, 1980). Amniocentesis has, in a sense, created a new waiting period within the waiting period of pregnancy (Dixson et al., 1981).

Second, prenatal technology, which is directed almost exclusively to fetal (as opposed to maternal) surveillance and diagnosis, has emphasized and even created the fetal patient who has arguably achieved a higher medical priority than the pregnant woman (Goodlin, 1979; Liley, 1972/1986; Pritchard et al., 1985). This technology expresses the duality of the pregnant woman-fetal unit, it affirms a view of the pregnant woman as maternal vessel or vehicle for the fetal patient, and it has increasingly legitimated manipulating the behavior and treatment of the pregnant woman (sometimes against her will) on behalf of the fetus she carries (Hubbard, 1982; Irwin & Jordan, 1987). Prior to the development of this technology, the fetus was medically inaccessible, hidden from view, and generally treated as part of and one with the pregnant woman's body.

Third, prenatal technology has created a body of knowledge that both couples and caregivers cannot "unknow." Even couples who do not have ultrasonic images of their own fetus are increasingly exposed to them in print and other media. Some clinicians and researchers have suggested that the knowledge that can now be obtained about the fetus and intrauterine environment is beneficial in that it (a) promotes earlier parental attachment to the fetus and, therefore, more responsible parental, especially maternal, behavior; (b) provides reassurance in the vast majority of cases that pregnancy is proceeding normally; (c) produces an information base ensuring more rational clinical intervention; (d) permits couples who would otherwise not have attempted pregnancy (for medical/genetic reasons) a chance to have a child of their own; and (e) expands individuals', couples', and clinicians' choices in childbearing.

Yet the knowledge obtainable from this technology may also create or favor anxiety and other negative emotions in pregnancy (Astbury & Walters, 1979; Evers-Kieboom s, Swerts, & Van Den Berghe, 1988; Fava et al., 1982, 1983; Robinson, Hibbard, & Laurence, 1984; Robinson et al., 1988; Tabor & Jonsson, 1987; Tsoi, Hunter, Pearce, Chudleigh, & Campbell, 1987; Verjaal, Leschot, & Treffers, 1982) and make the burden of choice heavier (Sandelowski, Harris, & Holditch-Davis, 1991). For example, couples have to decide whether they want to know the sex of the fetus, information that is available as a by-product of fetal diagnosis. Alpha-fetoprotein testing is associated with a significant number of false-positive interpretations leading to further testing and increased maternal anxiety (Burton, Dillard, & Clark, 1985; Evans, Belsky, Greb, Dvorin, & Drugan, 1988; Fearn, Hibbard, Laurence, Roberts, & Robinson, 1982). Much of the foreknowledge that ultrasonography, chorionic villus sampling, and amniocentesis provide has "nondecisional value" (Berwick & Weinstein, 1985, p. 883) for those couples unwilling to abort any fetus; there is no action they or their physicians can take to reverse a disorder such as Down syndrome. Moreover, these techniques cannot provide knowledge about the degree of severity of conditions such as Down syndrome. Although having knowledge about an impaired fetus in advance of birth may be useful in preparing for the child, it also means living with this knowledge for a longer period of time and before the infant is born. For some couples, the prospect of this type of knowing is too disturbing and spoils the enjoyment of pregnancy; in addition, no one can fully prepare emotionally for such an event in advance of its occurrence (Sandelowski et al., 1991).

The very existence of prenatal technology offers couples options that did not exist prior to its development and widespread availability. Couples have to choose for or against a test and they must, then, bear the consequences of the decisions they have made. Importantly, this technology gives childbearing couples the option to choose, but it also imposes on them the burden of choosing. Women and couples may find it harder to resist a technology once it has become part of routine medical practice (Tymstra, 1989). Moreover, there is an expectation that certain women and couples will choose these techniques. Being 35 and pregnant is, for example, in itself considered an indication for prenatal testing because of the higher risk with increasing age of having a genetically impaired child. (Interestingly, however, more infants with Down syndrome are born to women under 35 because more babies are born to younger women [Evans et al., 1989].) Being a good and responsible mother now may imply that women will choose available technology on behalf of their fetuses, even if it is at the mothers' own expense (Henifin, Hubbard, & Norsigian, 1988; Poland, 1989). Some women have described the considerable peer and other pressures to undergo ultrasound examinations and amniocentesis (Sandelowski et al., 1991). In a similar vein, by emphasizing the production of the perfect child and the treatment or elimination of the imperfect child, prenatal technology has expanded the idea of social responsibility to include employing available means to prevent the birth of impaired infants. A by-product of the increasing use of prenatal technology is the perpetuation of cultural prejudices against disability; disability becomes even less acceptable when a means exists to prevent its occurrence (Asch, 1988).

Prenatal technology has economic, social, and psychological costs. Couples have to weigh the costs of having an impaired child against the cost of losing a healthy infant because of the procedure or the cost of selective pregnancy termination. Couples, caregivers, and society may mark different points at which prenatal technology is worth the risks associated with the procedure (Lippman, Perry, Mandel, & Cartier, 1985; McGovern, Goldberg, & Desnick, 1986; Pauker & Pauker, 1987). The financial costs of prenatal technology make it less accessible to any couple who might want to use it. For any one couple, the costs of prenatal technology have to be evaluated on an individual basis. Yet given the finite resources of American health care, balancing the costs of this technology against the costs of not employing it is also a societal burden.

Technology for monitoring and diagnosing the fetus has been both beneficial and detrimental to the well-being of women, their families, and society. Although its use provides reassurance (Roghmann & Doherty, 1983) and may reduce the anxieties and risks of childbearing, the technology often also increases them. Prenatal technology has elevated the fetus to primary patient status, emphasized the person of the fetus as separate from and even as opposed to its mother, and expanded the idea of good mothering to include compliance with technological surveillance in pregnancy. Prenatal technology has expanded clinicians' ability to see events once hidden from view and it has, to an important extent, replaced the hand, the X ray, and clinical intuition in determining the status of pregnancy. Most significant, prenatal technology has demystified pregnancy by exposing the fetus and the womb to the clinical gaze, and it has raised standards for infants and mothers, placing a higher premium on and creating new expectations for the "perfect" baby and the "good" mother (Richards, 1989; Taub & Cohen, 1988).

Reproductive Technology and the Nurse

A special domain of assessment for the nurse is the evaluation of the effect of reproductive technology on nursing practice itself. Very little work has been done in this area. The framework for technology assessment just described and illustrated is a useful starting point for such an investigation because it permits nurses to include themselves and their work in their evaluation of the nature, context, and consequences of reproductive technology. Some examples of the influence of this technology on practice have already been given. In this concluding section, the distinctive challenge that reproductive technology poses for nurses is discussed.

Nurses have played an important role in the dissemination and application of reproductive technology. Nurses have educated women and families about reproductive techniques, translating them into language that is meaningful to them. Nurses have informed patients of these techniques, assisting them to make decisions concerning whether they will use them. Nurses have humanized these techniques, enhancing patients' acceptance and even enjoyment of these techniques and preventing or ameliorating the anxiety, discomfort, and other causes of suffering they can engender. Nurses have incorporated reproductive techniques into their practice. In cases that fall into the infertility/reproductive technology domain, these techniques have even come to define nursing practice as nurses' function as coordinators of health care teams deploying a technology. In addition, it is largely nurses who apply techniques such as electronic fetal monitoring and compose systems such as the maternal/fetal and neonatal intensive care units. Importantly, nurses have sought to use reproductive technology in the interests of women's health and well-being.

As these technological developments have changed nursing practice, they have also posed a unique challenge to nurses: how to remain nurses oriented to the whole person on the frontier of a health care delivery system increasingly characterized by the fragmentation of technological surveillance, diagnosis, and treatment. Historically, medical technology has drawn nurses away from and distorted their caring mission. Although seeming to promise nurses opportunities for caring and for expanding their sphere of influence in the health care delivery system, technology has also been instrumental in limiting the evolution of their practice. "Seizing" the technology controlled by physicians and that is intended to achieve medical purposes and performing medical work delegated to them by physicians have consistently failed nurses as strategies to gain autonomy and respect. New technologies create new roles (for example, the perinatal specialist, the IVF nurse coordinator, the genetic counselor), but by themselves they cannot constitute a force for change within the prevailing social structure of the health care professions because their use has served to perpetuate that social structure (Krause, 1977). Medical technology has tended to reinforce the status quo for nursing.

Koenig's (1988) study of plasma exchange technology for purifying the blood illustrates the way that making medical technology the center of nursing practice can deceive nurses. The findings of this research suggest that when a technique is still new and experimental, nurses and physicians share an egalitarian relationship; physicians work alongside nurses in becoming familiar with the technique and frequently perform it themselves. As the technique becomes routinized, this egalitarian relationship reverts to the traditional hierarchical nurse-doctor relationship. The physician now "orders" the nurse to perform the technique and the nurse alone becomes responsible for "managing trouble" caused by the technique. The nurse assumes the role of the "ritual specialist," guarding the unit routines newly mandated by the technique and ensuring that it is properly used. As the nurse moves to the front line in the implementation of the technique, the physician moves to the background, as far as the work is concerned, yet ultimately maintains control over the technique *and* the nurse who applies it.

Other studies have also suggested the role of medical technology in preserving the dominant-subordinate relationship between physician and nurse (Gamarnikow, 1978; Rosengren & DeVault, 1963; Strauss, 1966). Significantly, technological innovations may temporarily improve the social position of the nurse, but the long-term effect on the nurse-physician relationship is to preserve its inequality. Moreover, in adding to nurses' (and subtracting from physicians') work, technology tends to free physicians to develop other medical therapies, whereas it inhibits nurses from developing nursing care. Technology tends to act as a force for liberation and power for physicians but as an oppressive force for nurses because it characteristically involves the exploitation of nursing labor. What is expanded when nurses incorporate such techniques into their practice is not nursing but, rather, medicine.

Nurses have been challenged to explore the nature of their collaboration with physicians in the medicalization of reproductive experiences (Sandelowski, 1983, 1988; Shearer, 1988; Williams, 1989). Although critics of reproductive technology in a variety of disciplines have exposed the hidden agendas and detrimental effects of reproductive technology on women's health, nurses have continued, for the most part, to embrace this technology uncritically, having incorporated the prevailing medical and cultural view that technology represents a force for good. In their literature and continuing education conferences, nurses tend to emphasize the technical and administrative tasks mandated by this technology rather than the human responses and alterations in life experiences and practice engendered by it. These responses are left to psychologists, social workers, and others to explore, appraise, and treat (Damewood, 1990; Smith, 1985). Nurses are, accordingly, left with little time or reason to engage in such activities as advocacy and counseling while, as in one depiction of nurses' infertility work, they give Pergonal injections, do sonograms, coordinate semen collection and egg donation services, and "walk carefully with eggs" (a reference to eggs retrieved for IVF) (Garner, 1988, p. 2). Nurses are in danger of becoming deskilled in the very acts of care defining nursing, as they become ever more skilled as technicians and physician extenders.

Reproductive technology makes it more difficult to nurse because it tends to impede certain caring functions of the nurse. A definition of *nurse care* is "supreme covenant . . . above even cure . . . into which nurse and patient can enter" (Gadow, 1988, p. 6). This "covenant of care" involves the nurse's "commitment to alleviating [the patient's] vulnerability" (pp. 6-7). Reproductive technology may be viewed as threatening this covenant of care because in achieving its effects through the exercise of power, it necessarily increases the vulnerability of the women monitored and treated by it. Although such techniques as amniocentesis, IVF, and electronic fetal monitoring may be intended for benevolent purposes, they cause a vulnerability that must itself be alleviated. Perhaps the distinctive role of the nurse vis-à-vis reproductive technology must be alleviating this iatrogenic vulnerability and the "technocogenic" (Oberst, 1986, p. 235) or "technologic syndromes" (Reiser, 1986, p. 11), or illnesses, generated by it.

For example, the increase in prenatal testing has generated iatrogenic test anxiety (Rothenberg & Sills, 1968). Although favorable test results can provide reassurance, the very process of testing raises the specter of tragedy and loss and brings into conscious awareness that something can be wrong (Sandelowski et al., 1991). In some couples, contraceptive techniques have engendered a contraceptive "habit," by which couples who express their desire for a child cannot decide to stop using contraception because they have been doing it for so long (Daniels & Weingarten, 1983, p. 45). Conceptive techniques may contribute to a "treatment addiction" (Greil & Porter, 1988) in infertile couples, causing them to make a "career" (Conrad, 1987) out of trying to conceive a child. The "never-enough quality" of these techniques can cause couples anguish as they repeatedly try and fail to set limits on when they will end treatment (Sandelowski, 1991).

These types of responses and "syndromes" ought to be at the center of nursing concerns and activities. Technology assessment for the nurse ought to include an exploration of the means by which the goal of ameliorating the iatrogenic vulnerability inherent in these responses may be accomplished and whether it can be achieved at all. Within a covenant of care framework, the character of nurses' current involvement with applying a technique such as IVF may be difficult to justify because IVF creates a vulnerability so extreme that current nursing activities are not able to alleviate it. One feminist critic of IVF techniques specifically appealed to nurses and other women caregivers to terminate their involvement with these procedures (Williams, 1989). But is this a solution that would favor women?

Another way in which reproductive technology impedes care is by interfering with the nurse's role as empathetic toucher. There is a caring touch and there is a touch that is antithetical to care, the only purpose of which is to palpate and manipulate (Gadow, 1990). In the caring touch, the nurse seeks to know and comfort the patient—to achieve a "tactile apprehension" or knowledge of the patient (Wyschogrod, 1981). In the anti- or noncaring touch, touch is simply a proxy for sight because it is used largely for its information yield—to get rather than to give. For example, the very design of machines such as the electronic fetal monitor, with its parts covering a woman's abdomen, and the very procedures mandated by ultrasound examinations, cesarean section, and artificial insemination force the nurse to touch more in the interest of applying the technology and for its information yield than in the interest of comfort and relationship building.

Importantly, nurses strive to oppose fragmentation in health care, yet they are everywhere confronted with a technology valenced to fragmentation that contributes to women being viewed as "other" and as "object" (Gadow, 1984), as manipulatable vessels for fetuses as opposed to autonomous persons in their own right, and that transforms body parts—eggs, sperm, reproductive organs—into interchangeable and marketable medical resources (Corea, 1985; Hubbard, 1982). Although this technology is also "employed out of concern" for the well-being of women and infants, its operations and the social context in which it is used often "mask" (Gadow, 1984, p. 68) and pervert that concern. With continued uncritical acceptance of this technology and without critical assessment of the dilemmas and challenges it creates, nurses will continue to believe they are in control of a technology that continues to manipulate and constrain their development as "existential advocates" (Gadow, 1983) for women and their families—as "entire" selves assisting women in the "authentic" exercise of their freedom of self-determination (pp. 45, 55). Without education and careful inquiry concerning the place of technology in culture, nurses will continue to miss opportunities to humanize the application of technology and to develop nursing alternatives to technological surveillance, diagnosis, and treatment. As Sarah (1987) suggested, although few patients and nurses would be willing to forego reproductive technology entirely, they do not have to accept its inappropriate use as the price of its significant but "rare" (p. 61) benefits.

Finally, without technology assessment of the type described here, nurses will be like the apprentices who do not learn the sorcerer's lesson. Cowan (1983) observed that tools do have a "life of their own" and they "define and constrain" behavior (p. 9). As she further admonished, "Our tools are not always at our beck and call. The less we know about them, the more likely it is that they will command us, rather than the other way around" (p. 10).

References

Andrews, L. (1989). *Between strangers: Surrogate mothers, expectant fathers, and brave new babies.* New York: Harper & Row.

Arditti, R., Klein, R. D., & Minden, S. (Eds.). (1984). *Test-tube women: What future for motherhood?* London: Pandora.

Asch, A. (1988). Reproductive technology and disability. In N. Taub & S. Cohen (Eds.), *Reproductive laws for the 1990s: A briefing handbook* (pp. 59-101). Newark, NJ: State University of New Jersey, Rutgers.

Astbury, J., & Walters, W. A. (1979). Amniocentesis in the early second trimester of pregnancy and maternal anxiety. *Australian Family Physician, 8,* 595-599.

Banta, H. D., & Thacker, S. B. (1979). Assessing the costs and benefits of electronic fetal monitoring. *Obstetrics/Gynecology Survey, 35,* 627-642.

Beck-Gernsheim, E. (1989). From the pill to test-tube babies: New options, new pressures in reproductive behavior. In K. S. Ratcliff (Ed.), *Healing technology: Feminist perspectives* (pp. 23-40). Ann Arbor: University of Michigan Press.

Beeson, D. (1984). Technological rhythms in pregnancy: The case of prenatal diagnosis by amniocentesis. In T. Duster & K. Garrett (Eds.), *Cultural perspectives on biological knowledge* (pp. 145-181). Norwood, NJ: Ablex.

Beeson, D., & Golbus, M. S. (1979). Anxiety engendered by amniocentesis. *Birth Defects: Original Article Series, 15,* 191-197.

Berwick, D. M., & Weinstein, M. C. (1985). What do patients value? Willingness to pay for ultrasound in normal pregnancy. *Medical Care, 23,* 881-893.

Blank, R. H. (1984). *Redefining human life: Reproductive technologies and social policy.* Boulder, CO: Westview.

Burton, B. K., Dillard, R. G., & Clark, E. N. (1985). The psychological impact of false positive elevations of maternal serum alpha-fetoprotein. *American Journal of Obstetrics and Gynecology, 151,* 77-82.

Bush, C. G. (1983). Women and the assessment of technology: To think, to be; to unthink, to free. In J. Rothschild (Ed.), *Machina Ex Dea: Feminist perspectives on technology* (pp. 151-170). New York: Pergamon.

Callahan, D. (1986). How technology is reframing the abortion debate. *Hastings Center Report, 16,* 33-42.

Clarke, A. (1984). Subtle forms of sterilization abuse: A reproductive rights analysis. In R. Arditti, R. D. Klein, & S. Minden (Eds.), *Test-tube women: What future for motherhood?* (pp. 188-212). London: Pandora.

Coates, J. F. (1971). Technology assessment: The benefits, the costs, the consequences. *Futurist, 5,* 225-231.

Cohen, A. B., Klapholz, H., & Thompson, M. S. (1982). Electronic fetal monitoring and clinical practice: A survey of obstetric opinion. *Medical Decision Making, 2*(1), 79-95.

Congress of the United States. Office of Technology Assessment. (1988). *Infertility: Medical and social choices* (OTA-BA-358). Washington, DC: Government Printing Office.

Conrad, P. (1987). The experience of illness: Recent and new directions. *Research in the Sociology of Health Care, 6,* 1-31.

Consensus Development Conference. National Institute of Child Health and Human Development and National Center for Health Care Technology. (1981). *Cesarean childbirth* (NIH Publication No. 82-2067). Bethesda, MD: U.S. Department of Health and Human Services.

Consensus Development Conference. National Institute of Child Health and Human Development, Office of Medical Applications of Research. (1984). *Diagnostic ultrasound imaging in pregnancy* (NIH Publication No. 84-667). Bethesda, MD: U.S. Department of Health and Human Services.

Corea, G. (1985). *The mother machine: Reproductive technologies from artificial insemination to artificial wombs.* New York: Harper & Row.

Cowan, R. S. (1983). *More work for mother: The ironies of household technology from the open hearth to the microwave.* New York: Basic Books.

Cox, D. N., Wittmann, B. K., Hess, M., Ross, A. G., Lind, J., & Lindahl, S. (1987). The psychological impact of diagnostic ultrasound. *Obstetrics and Gynecology, 70,* 673-676.

Damewood, M. D. (Ed.). (1990). *The Johns Hopkins handbook of in vitro fertilization and assisted reproductive technologies.* Boston: Little, Brown.

Daniels, P., & Weingarten, K. (1983). *Sooner or later: The timing of parenthood in adult lives.* New York: Norton.

Dawes, G. S., Moulden, M., & Redman, C. W. (1990). Limitations of antenatal fetal heart rate monitors. *American Journal of Obstetrics and Gynecology, 162,* 170-173.

DeZoeten, M., Tymstra, T., & Alberda, A. T. (1987). The waiting-list for IVF: The motivations and expectations of women waiting for IVF treatment. *Human Reproduction, 2,* 623-626.

Dixson, B., Richards, T. L., Reinsch, S., Edrich, V. B., Matson, M. R., & Jones, O. W. (1981). Midtrimester amniocentesis: Subjective maternal responses. *Journal of Reproductive Medicine, 26,* 10-16.

Eakins, P. S. (Ed.). (1986). *The American way of birth.* Philadelphia: Temple University Press.

Edwards, M., & Waldorf, M. (1984). *Reclaiming birth: History and heroines of American childbirth reform.* Trumansburg, NY: Crossing Press.

Evans, M. I., Belsky, R., Greb, A., Dvorin, E., & Drugan, A. (1988). Wide variation in maternal serum alpha-fetoprotein reports in one metropolitan area: Concerns for the quality of prenatal testing. *Obstetrics and Gynecology, 72,* 342-345.

Evans, M. I., Quigg, M. H., Kappitch, J. D., & Schulman, J. D. (1989). First trimester prenatal diagnosis. In M. I. Evans, A. O. Dixler, J. C. Fletcher, & J. D. Schulman (Eds.), *Fetal diagnosis and therapy: Science, ethics, and the law* (pp. 17-36). Philadelphia: J. B. Lippincott.

Evers-Kiebooms, G., Swerts, A., & Van Den Berghe, H. (1988). Psychological aspects of amniocentesis: Anxiety feelings in three different risk groups. *Clinical Genetics, 33,* 196-206.

Fava, G. A., Kellner, R., Michelacci, L., Trombini, G., Pathak, D., Orlandi, C., & Bovicelli, L. (1982). Psychological reactions to amniocentesis: A controlled study. *American Journal of Obstetrics and Gynecology, 143,* 509-513.

Fava, G. A., Trombini, G., Michelacci, L., Linder, J., Pathak, D., & Bovicelli, L. (1983). Hostility in women before and after amniocentesis. *Journal of Reproductive Medicine, 28*(1), 29-34.

Fearn, J., Hibbard, B. M., Laurence, K. M., Roberts, A., & Robinson, J. O. (1982). Screening for neural-tube defects and maternal anxiety. *British Journal of Obstetrics and Gynecology, 89,* 218-221.

Fletcher, J. C., & Evans, M. I. (1983). Maternal bonding in early ultrasound examinations. *New England Journal of Medicine, 308,* 392-393.

Fletcher, J. F. (1988). *The ethics of genetic control: Ending reproductive roulette.* Buffalo, NY: Prometheus.

Gadow, S. (1983). Existential advocacy: Philosophical foundation of nursing. In C. P. Murphy & H. Hunter (Eds.), *Ethical problems in the nurse-patient relationship* (pp. 41-58). Boston: Allyn & Bacon.

Gadow, S. (1984). Touch and technology: Two paradigms of patient care. *Journal of Religion and Health, 23,* 63-69.

Gadow, S. (1988). Covenant without cure: Letting go and holding on in chronic illness. In J. Watson & M. Ray (Eds.), *The ethics of care and the ethics of cure* (pp. 5-14). New York: National League for Nursing.

Gadow, S. (1990). The advocacy covenant: Care as clinical subjectivity. In J. Stevenson & T. Tripp-Reimer (Eds.), *Knowledge about care and caring* (pp. 5-17). Kansas City, MO: American Academy of Nursing.

Gamarnikow, E. (1978). Sexual division of labour: The case of nursing. In A. Kuhn & A. M. Wolpe (Eds.), *Feminism and materialism: Women and modes of production* (pp. 96-123). London: Routledge & Kegan Paul.

Garner, C. (1988, February). *IVF nurse coordinator: The past—the present—the future* [syllabus]. Paper presented at the Third Annual Conference for IVF Nurse Coordinators, Scottsdale, AZ.

Gomel, V. (1978). Profile of women requesting reversal of sterilization. *Fertility and Sterility, 30,* 39-41.

Goodlin, R. C. (1979). *Care of the fetus.* New York: Masson.

Gordon, L. (1976). *Woman's body, woman's right: A social history of birth control in America.* New York: Penguin.

Grant, A. (1989). Monitoring the fetus during labor. In I. Chalmers, M. Enkin, & M. J. Keirse (Eds.), *Effective care in pregnancy and childbirth: Vol. 2. Childbirth* (pp. 846-882). Oxford, UK: Oxford University Press.

Greil, A. L., & Porter, K. L. (1988, November). *Explaining "treatment addiction" in infertile couples.* Paper prepared for presentation at the annual meeting of the National Council of Family Relations, Philadelphia, PA.

Haire, D. (1972). *The cultural warping of childbirth* [pamphlet]. Milwaukee, WI: International Childbirth Education Association.

Harding, S. (1978). Knowledge, technology, and social relations [book review]. *Journal of Medicine and Philosophy, 3,* 346-358.

Hatcher, R. A., Stewart, F., Trussell, J., Kowal, D., Guest, F., Stewart, G. K., & Cates, W. (1990). *Contraceptive technology, 1990-1992* (15th ed., rev.). New York: Irvington.

Haverkamp, A. D., & Orleans, M. (1982). An assessment of electronic fetal monitoring. *Women and Health, 7*(3/4), 115-134.

Haverkamp, A. D., Orleans, M., Langendoerfer, S., McFee, J., Murphy, J., & Thompson, H. E. (1979). A controlled trial of the differential effects of intrapartum fetal monitoring. *American Journal of Obstetrics and Gynecology, 134,* 399-412.

Haverkamp, A. D., Thompson, H. E., McFee, J. G., & Centrulo, C. (1976). The evaluation of continuous fetal heart rate monitoring in high-risk pregnancy. *American Journal of Obstetrics and Gynecology, 125,* 310-320.

Henifin, M. S., Hubbard, R., & Norsigian, J. (1988). Prenatal screening. In N. Taub & S. Cohen (Eds.), *Reproductive laws for the 1990s: A briefing handbook* (pp. 127-154). Newark, NJ: State University of New Jersey, Rutgers.

Hubbard, R. (1982). Legal and policy implications of recent advances in prenatal diagnosis and fetal therapy. *Women's Rights Law Reporter, 7,* 201-218.

Huddleston, J. F. (1990). Electronic fetal monitoring. In R. D. Eden & F. H. Boehm (Eds.), *Assessment and care of the fetus: Physiological, clinical, and medicolegal principles* (pp. 449-457). Norwalk, CT: Appleton & Lange.

Hyde, B. (1986). An interview study of pregnant women's attitudes to ultrasound scanning. *Social Science and Medicine, 22,* 587-592.

Illich, I. (1973). *Tools for conviviality.* New York: Harper & Row.

Irwin, S., & Jordan, B. (1987). Knowledge, practice, and power: Court-ordered cesarean sections. *Medical Anthropology Quarterly, 1,* 319-334.

Jones, E. F., Forrest, J. D., Henshaw, S. K., Silverman, J., & Torres, A. (1989). *Pregnancy, contraception and family planning services in industrialized countries.* New Haven, CT: Yale University Press.

Jordan, B. (1977). The self-diagnosis of early pregnancy: An investigation of lay competence. *Medical Anthropology, 1*(2), 1-38.

Jordan, B. (1984). External cephalic version as an alternative to breech delivery and cesarean section. *Social Science and Medicine, 18,* 637-651.

Kaufmann, C. L., & Williams, C. L. (1985). Fetal surgery: The social implications of medical and surgical treatment of the unborn child. *Women and Health, 10*(1), 25-37.

Kelso, I. M., Parsons, R. J., Lawrence, G. F., Arora, S. S., Edmonds, D. K., & Cooke, I. D. (1978). An assessment of continuous fetal heart rate monitoring in labor: A randomized trial. *American Journal of Obstetrics and Gynecology, 131,* 526-532.

Klawiter, M. (1990). Using Arendt and Heidegger to consider feminist thinking on women reproductive/infertility technologies. *Hypatia, 5*(3), 65-89.

Klein, R., & Rowland, R. (1989). Hormone cocktails: Women as test-sites for fertility drugs. *Women's Studies International Forum, 12,* 333-348.

Koenig, B. A. (1988). The technological imperative in medical practice: The social creation of a "routine" treatment. In M. Lock & D. Gordon (Eds.), *Biomedicine examined* (pp. 465-496). Dordrecht, The Netherlands: Kluwer.

Kohn, C. L., Nelson, A., & Weiner, S. (1980). Gravidas' responses to realtime ultrasound fetal image. *JOGNN, 9*(2), 77-80.

Krause, E. A. (1977). *Power and illness: The political sociology of health and medical care.* New York: Elsevier North-Holland.

Langendoerfer, S., Haverkamp, A. D., Murphy, J., Nowick, K. D., Orleans, M., Pacosa, F., & Van Doorninck, W. (1980). Pediatric follow-up of a randomized controlled trial of intrapartum fetal monitoring techniques. *Journal of Pediatrics, 97*(1), 103-107.

Layton, E. (1974). Technology as knowledge. *Technology and Culture, 15*(1), 31-41.

Lechtman, H., & Steinberg, A. (1979). The history of technology: An anthropological point of view. In G. Bugliarello & D. B. Doner (Eds.), *The history and philosophy of technology* (pp. 135-160). Urbana: University of Illinois Press.

Leveno, K. J., Cunningham, G., Nelson, S., Roark, M., Williams, M. L., Guzick, D., Dowling, S., Rosenfeld, C. R., & Buckley, A. (1986). A prospective comparison of selective and universal electronic fetal monitoring in 34,995 pregnancies. *New England Journal of Medicine, 315,* 615-619.

Liley, A. W. (1986). The fetus as personality. *Fetal Therapy, 1*(1), 8-17. (Original work published 1972)

Lilford, R. J. (1989). "In my day we just had babies." *Journal of Reproductive and Infant Psychology, 7*(3), 187-191.

Lippman, A., Perry, T. B., Mandel, S., & Cartier, L. (1985). Chorionic villi sampling: Women's attitudes. *American Journal of Medical Genetics, 22,* 395-401.

Lorber, J. (1988). In vitro fertilization and gender politics. *Women and Health, 13*(1/2), 117-133.

Lorber, J. (1989). Choice, gift, or patriarchal bargain? Women's consent to in vitro fertilization in male infertility. *Hypatia, 4*(3), 23-36.

Lotgering, F. K., Wallenberg, H. C., & Schouten, H. J. (1982). Interobserver and intraobserver variation in the assessment of antepartum cardiotocograms. *American Journal of Obstetrics and Gynecology, 144,* 701-705.

Luthy, D. A., Shy, K. K., Van Belle, G., Larson, E. B., Hughes, J. P., Benedetti, T. J., Brown, Z. A., Effer, S., King, J. F., & Stenchever, M. A. (1987). A randomized trial of electronic fetal monitoring in preterm labor. *Obstetrics and Gynecology, 69,* 687-695.

MacDonald, D., Grant, A., Sheridan-Pereira, M., Boylan, P., & Chalmers, I. (1985). The Dublin randomized trial of intrapartum fetal heart monitoring. *American Journal of Obstetrics and Gynecology, 152,* 524-539.

Maines, R. (1989). Socially camouflaged technologies: The case of the electromechanical vibrator. *IEEE Technology and Society Magazine, 8*(2), 3-9.

Marcil-Gratton, N. (1988). Sterilization regret among women in metropolitan Montreal. *Family Planning Perspectives, 20,* 222-227.

McGovern, M. M., Goldberg, J. D., & Desnick, R. J. (1986). Acceptability of chorionic villi sampling for prenatal diagnosis. *American Journal of Obstetrics and Gynecology, 155,* 25-29.

McShane, P. M. (1988). In vitro fertilization, GIFT and related technologies: Hope in a test tube. *Women and Health, 13*(1/2), 31-46.

Medical Research International, Society for Assisted Reproductive Technology, & the American Fertility Society. (1991). *In vitro* fertilization-embryo transfer (IVF-ET) in the United States: 1989 results from the IVF-ET registry. *Fertility and Sterility, 55,* 14-23.

Merchant, C. (1980). *The death of nature: Women, ecology, and the scientific revolution.* San Francisco: Harper & Row.

Michaelson, K. L. (Ed.). (1988). *Childbirth in America: Anthropological perspectives.* South Hadley, MA: Bergin & Garvey.

Milne, L. S., & Rich, O. J. (1981). Cognitive and affective aspects of the responses of pregnant women to sonography. *Maternal-Child Nursing Journal, 10*(1), 15-39.

Modell, J. (1989). Last chance babies: Interpretations of parenthood in an in vitro fertilization program. *Medical Anthropology Quarterly, 3*(2), 124-138.

Nsiah-Jefferson, L., & Hall, E. J. (1989). Reproductive technology: Perspectives and implications for low-income women and women of color. In K. S. Ratcliff (Ed.), *Healing technology: Feminist perspectives* (pp. 93-117). Ann Arbor: University of Michigan Press.

Oakley, A. (1986). *The captured womb: A history of the medical care of pregnant women.* New York: Basil Blackwell.

Oberst, M. T. (1986). Nursing in the year 2000: Setting the agenda for knowledge generation and utilization. In G. E. Sorensen (Ed.), *Setting the agenda for the year 2000: Knowledge development in nursing* (pp. 229-237). Kansas City, MO: American Academy of Nursing.

Olds, S. B., London, M. L., & Ladewig, P. A. (1988). *Maternal-newborn nursing: A family-centered approach* (3rd ed.). Menlo Park, CA: Addison-Wesley.

Parer, J. T. (1986). The Dublin trial of fetal heart rate monitoring: The final word? *Birth, 13,* 119-121.

Patterson, E. T., Freese, M. P., & Goldenberg, R. L. (1986). Reducing uncertainty: Self-diagnosis of pregnancy. *Image: Journal of Nursing Scholarship, 18*(3), 105-109.

Pauker, S. P., & Pauker, S. G. (1987). The amniocentesis decision: Ten years of decision analytic experience. *Birth Defects: Original Article Series, 23,* 151-169.

Petchesky, R. P. (1987). Fetal images: The power of visual culture in the politics of reproduction. *Feminist Studies, 13,* 263-292.

Pirsig, R. M. (1974). *Zen and the art of motorcycle maintenance: An inquiry into values.* New York: Bantam.

Poland, M. (1989). An anthropological perspective. In M. I. Evans, A. O. Dixler, J. C. Fletcher, & J. D. Schulman (Eds.), *Fetal diagnosis and therapy: Science, ethics, and the law* (pp. 12-14). Philadelphia: J. B. Lippincott.

Pritchard, J. A., MacDonald, P. C., & Gant, N. F. (1985). *Williams' obstetrics* (17th ed.). Norwalk, CT: Appleton-Century-Crofts.

Rapp, R. (1988a). Chromosomes and communication: The discourse of genetic counseling. *Medical Anthropology Quarterly, 2*(2), 143-157.

Rapp, R. (1988b). The power of "positive" diagnosis: Medical and maternal discourses on amniocentesis. In K. L. Michaelson (Ed.), *Childbirth in America: Anthropological perspectives* (pp. 103-116). South Hadley, MA: Bergin & Garvey.

Reading, A. E., & Cox, D. N. (1982). The effects of ultrasound examination on maternal anxiety levels. *Journal of Behavioral Medicine, 5,* 237-247.

Reiser, S. J. (1978). *Medicine and the reign of technology.* Cambridge, UK: Cambridge University Press.

Reiser, S. J. (1986). Assessment and the technologic present. *International Journal of Technology Assessment in Health Care, 2,* 7-12.

Richards, M. P. (1989). Social and ethical problems of fetal diagnosis and screening. *Journal of Reproductive and Infant Psychology, 7*(3), 171-185.

Robinson, G. E., Garner, D. M., Olmsted, M. P., Shime, J., Hutton, E. M., & Crawford, B. M. (1988). Anxiety reduction after chorionic villus sampling and genetic amniocentesis. *American Journal of Obstetrics and Gynecology, 159,* 953-956.

Robinson, J. O., Hibbard, B. M., & Laurence, K. M. (1984). Anxiety during a crisis: Emotional effects of screening for neural tube defects. *Journal of Psychosomatic Research, 28*(2), 163-169.

Roghmann, K. J., & Doherty, R. A. (1983). Reassurance through prenatal diagnosis and willingness to bear children after age 35. *American Journal of Public Health, 73,* 760-762.

Rosengren, W., & DeVault, S. (1963). The sociology of time and space in an obstetrical hospital. In E. Friedson (Ed.), *The hospital in modern society* (pp. 266-292). New York: Free Press.

Rothenberg, M. B., & Sills, E. M. (1968). Iatrogenesis: The PKU anxiety syndrome. *Journal of the American Academy of Child Psychiatry, 7,* 689-692.

Rothman, B. K. (1982). *In labor: Women and power in the birthplace.* New York: Norton.

Rothman, B. K. (1984). The meanings of choice in reproductive technology. In R. Arditti, R. D. Klein, & S. Minden (Eds.), *Test-tube women: What future for motherhood?* (pp. 23-33). London: Pandora.

Rothman, B. K. (1986). *The tentative pregnancy: Prenatal diagnosis and the future of motherhood.* New York: Viking.

Rothman, B. K. (1988). The decision to have and not to have amniocentesis for prenatal diagnosis. In K. L. Michaelson (Ed.), *Childbirth in America: Anthropological perspectives* (pp. 90-102). South Hadley, MA: Bergin & Garvey.

Rothman, B. K., & Detlefs, M. (1988). Women talking to women: Abortion counselors and genetic counselors. In A. Statham, E. M. Miller, & H. O. Mauksch (Eds.), *The worth of women's work: A qualitative synthesis* (pp. 151-165). Albany: State University of New York Press.

Rowland, R. (1987). Technology and motherhood: Reproductive choice reconsidered. *Signs: Journal of Women in Culture and Society, 12,* 512-528.

Sala, I. (1983). Psychological aspects of prenatal diagnosis. In A. Albertini & P. G. Crosigani (Eds.), *Progress in perinatal medicine: Biochemical and biophysical diagnostic procedures* (pp. 245-256). Amsterdam: Excerpta Medica.

Sandelowski, M. (1983). Perinatal nursing: Whose specialty is it anyway? *MCN, 8,* 317-322.

Sandelowski, M. (1984). *Pain, pleasure, and American childbirth: From the twilight sleep to the Read method, 1914-1960.* Westport, CT: Greenwood.

Sandelowski, M. (1988). A case of conflicting paradigms: Nursing and reproductive technology. *Advances in Nursing Science, 10*(3), 35-45.

Sandelowski, M. (1991). Compelled to try: The never-enough quality of conceptive technology. *Medical Anthropology Quarterly, 5*(1), 29-47.

Sandelowski, M., Harris, B. G., & Holditch-Davis, D. (1989). Mazing: Infertile couples and the quest for a child. *Image: Journal of Nursing Scholarship, 21*(5), 220-226.

Sandelowski, M., Harris, B. G., & Holditch-Davis, D. (1990). Pregnant moments: The process of conception in infertile couples. *Research in Nursing and Health, 13,* 273-282.

Sandelowski, M., Harris, B. G., & Holditch-Davis, D. (1991). Amniocentesis in the context of infertility. *Health Care for Women International, 12,* 167-178.

Sarah, R. (1987). Power, certainty, and the fear of death. *Women and Health, 13*(1/2), 59-71.

Schroeder, F. E. (1976). Feminine hygiene, fashion, and the emancipation of American women. *American Studies, 17*(2), 101-110.

Shearer, M. (1988). Some effects of assisted reproduction on perinatal care [editorial]. *Birth, 15*(3), 131-133.

Silvestre, D., & Fresco, N. (1980). Reactions to prenatal diagnosis: An analysis of 87 interviews. *American Journal of Orthopsychiatry, 50,* 610-617.

Smith, P. (1985). The role of the office nurse in infertility care. In M. G. Hammond & L. M. Talbert (Eds.), *Infertility: A practical guide for the physician* (2nd ed., pp. 25-41). Oradell, NJ: Medical Economics Books.

Somerville, M. A. (1982). Birth technology, parenting, and "deviance." *International Journal of Law and Psychiatry, 5*(2), 123-153.

Spallone, P., & Steinberg, D. L. (Eds.). (1987). *Made to order: The myth of reproductive and genetic progress.* Oxford, UK: Pergamon.

Stanworth, M. (Ed.). (1987). *Reproductive technologies: Gender, motherhood, and medicine.* Minneapolis: University of Minnesota Press.

Starkman, M. N. (1976). Psychological responses to the use of the fetal monitor during labor. *Psychosomatic Medicine, 38,* 269-277.

Stewart, N. (1986). Women's views of ultrasonography in obstetrics. *Birth, 13*(Suppl.), 34-38.

Strauss, A. (1966). The structure and ideology of American nursing: An interpretation. In F. Davis (Ed.), *The nursing profession: Five sociological essays* (pp. 60-108). New York: John Wiley.

Tabor, A., & Jonsson, M. H. (1987). Psychological impact of amniocentesis on low-risk women. *Prenatal Diagnosis, 7,* 443-449.

Taub, N. (1989). Feminist tensions: Concepts of motherhood and reproductive choice. In J. Offerman-Zuckerberg (Ed.), *Gender in transition: A new frontier* (pp. 217-225). New York: Plenum.

Taub, N., & Cohen, S. (Eds.). (1988). *Reproductive laws for the 1990s: A briefing handbook.* Newark: State University of New Jersey, Rutgers.

Tsoi, M. M., Hunter, M., Pearce, M., Chudleigh, P., & Campbell, S. (1987). Ultrasound scanning in women with raised serum alpha fetoprotein: Short term psychological effect. *Journal of Psychosomatic Research, 31,* 35-39.

Tymstra, T. (1989). The imperative character of medical technology and the meaning of "anticipated decision regret." *International Journal of Technology Assessment in Health Care, 5,* 207-213.

Verjaal, M., Leschot, N. J., & Treffers, P. E. (1982). Women's experiences with second trimester prenatal diagnosis. *Prenatal Diagnosis, 2,* 195-209.

Walters, L. (1986). Ethical issues in intrauterine diagnosis and therapy. *Fetal Therapy, 1,* 32-37.

White, L. (1968). Historical roots of our ecologic crisis. In L. White, *Machina Ex Deo* (pp. 75-94). Cambridge: MIT Press.

Williams, L. S. (1989). The overlooked role of women professionals in the provision of in vitro fertilization. *Resources for Feminist Research, 18*(3), 80-82.

Winner, L. (1985). Do artifacts have politics? In D. MacKenzie & J. Wajcman (Eds.), *The social shaping of technology: How the refrigerator got its hum* (pp. 26-37). Philadelphia: Open University Press.

Wood, C., Renou, P., Oats, J., Farrell, E., Beischer, N., & Anderson, L. (1981). A controlled trial of fetal heart rate monitoring in a low-risk obstetric population. *American Journal of Obstetrics and Gynecology, 141,* 527-534.

Wyschogrod, E. (1981). Empathy and sympathy as tactile encounter. *Journal of Medicine and Philosophy, 6*(1), 25-43.

List of Acronyms

AA Alcoholics Anonymous

AAOHN American Association of Occupational Health Nurses Journal

ABC alternative birth centers

ACOG American College of Obstetricians and Gynecologists

ACTH adrenocorticotropic hormone

ADP adenosine diphosphate

AFDC Aid to Families with Dependent Children

AHCPER Agency for Health Care Policy and Research

AIDS acquired immunodeficiency syndrome

AJMCN American Journal of Maternal Child Nursing

ANA American Nurses Association

AOD alcohol and other drug

ARC AIDS-related complex

ASAB antisperm antibodies

AT anaerobic threshold

ATP adenosine triphosphate

BBT basal body temperature

B-HCG B subunit of human chorionic gonadotrophin

BMI body mass index

BPD biparietal diameter

bpm beats per minute

BPP biophysical profile

BRI brief risk intervention

BSI breast self-examination

BV bacterial vaginosis

CABG coronary artery bypass graft

CAT computerized axial tomography

CBC complete blood count

CBE childbirth education

CBE clinical breast examination

CBT cognitive behavioral therapy

CCU clean-catch urine

CDC Centers for Disease Control

CHD coronary heart disease

CIN cervical intraepithelial neoplasia

CIS carcinoma in situ

CMRNG chromosomally mediated resistant *Neisseria gonorrhoeae*

C.N.M. Certified Nurse Midwife

CPD cephalopelvic disproportion

CR consciousness raising
CRF corticotropin releasing factor
CRL crown-rump length
CRT cathode ray tube
CST contraction stress test
CVA cerberal vascular accident, costovertebral angle

D & C dilatation and curettage
D & E dilatation and evacuation
DCIS ductal carcinoma in situ
DDI didanosine
DES diethylstilbestrol
DHA dehydroisoandrosterone
DHAS dehydroisoandrosterone sulfate
DHHS Department of Health and Human Services
DID dissociative identity disorder
DIS Diagnostic Interview Schedule
DP diastolic pressure
DRG diagnostic related grouping
DUB dysfunctional uterine bleeding

ECA Epidemiological Catchment Area
EDD estimated date of delivery
EEG electroencephalogram
ERT estrogen replacement therapy
ESR erythryocyte sedimentation rate

FAE fetal alcohol effects
FAS fetal alcohol syndrome
FDA Food and Drug Administration
FHS follicle-stimulating hormone

GI gastrointestinal
GIFT gamete intrafallopian transfer
GnRH gonadotropin-releasing hormone

HB hepatitis B
HBcAb HBV core antigen
HBeAg HBV antigen
HBIG HB immunoglobulin
HBM health belief model
HBsAg hepatitis B virus surface antigen
HBV hepatitis B virus
HCG human chorionic gonadotropin
Hct hematocrit
HDL high-density lipoprotein
HDL-C high-density lipoprotein cholesterol
Hgb hemoglobin
HPF high power field
HPV human papillomavirus
HRT hormone replacement therapy
HSG hysterosalpingogram
HSV herpes simplex virus—HSV-1 and HSV-2
HTLV-III human T-cell lymphotropic virus, variant III

IDDM insulin-dependent diabetes mellitus
IHM integrated health model
IMB intermenstrual bleeding
IPT interpersonal therapy
IUD intrauterine device
IVDU intravenous drug use, intravenous drug user
IVF in vitro fertilization

JAMA Journal of the American Medical Association
JLP juvenile laryngeal papilloma
JOGNN Journal of Obstetric, Gynecologic and Neonatal Nursing

KOH potassium hydroxide

LAM lactational amenorrhea methods
LAV lymphadenopathy-associated virus
LCIS lobular carcinoma in situ
LDL low-density lipoprotein
LDL-C low-density lipoprotein cholesterol
LH luteinizing hormone
LMP last menstrual period
LNMP last normal menstrual period
LPN licensed practical nurse

MADD Mothers Against Drunk Driving
MAOI monoamine oxidase inhibitor
MAP mean arterial pressure
MRI magnetic resonance imaging
MSAFP maternal serum alpha-fetoprotein

NaCl saline solution
NCEP National Cholesterol Education Program
NCHS National Center for Health Statistics
NHANES National Health and Nutrition Examination Survey
NIA National Institute on Aging
NIDDM non-insulin-dependent diabetes mellitus
NIH National Institutes of Health
NSAID nonsteroidal anti-inflammatory drug
NSCST nipple stimulation contraction stress test
NSFG National Survey of Family Growth
NST nonstress test

OB/GYN obstetrics/gynecology, obstetrician/gynecologist
OC oral contraceptive
OCD obsessive-compulsive disorder
OCT oxytocin challenge test
OGTT oral glucose tolerance test

PCA patient-controlled analgesia
PCOD polycistic ovarian disease
PCP phencyclidine
PEL permissible exposure level
PEPI postmenopausal estrogen and progestin intervention
PGL phosphatidylglycerol
PHS Public Health Service
PID pelvic inflammatory disease
PIH pregnancy-induced hypertension
PMS premenstrual syndrome
PMT premenstrual syndrome tension
po by mouth
POMC propiomelanocorticotropin
PPNG penicillinase-producing *Neisseria gonorrhoeae*
PTH parathyroid hormone
PTSD posttraumatic stress disorder

RBC red blood cell
RDA recommended daily allowance
RIA radioimmunossay
RN registered nurse
RPE rate of perceived effort
RPM relapse prevention model
RPR rapid plasma reagin

SAB spontaneous abortion
SDAT senile dementia of the Alzheimer type
SES socioeconomic status
SGOT serum glutamic-oxaloacetic transaminase
SGPT serum glutamic-pyruvic transaminase
SIDs sudden infant death syndrome
SP systolic pressure
SPA sperm penetration assay
SRM self-regulation model
SSI supplemental security income

TC total cholesterol
TDI therapeutic donor insemination
TNM tumor-node-metastasis
TRNG tetracycline-resistant *Neisseria gonorrhoeae*
TSH thyroid-stimulating hormone
TSS toxic shock syndrome
TSST-1 toxic shock syndrome toxin 1
TWA time-weighted average

UI urinary incontinence

VBAC vaginal birth after cesarean
VDRL Veneral Disease Research Laboratory
VDT video display terminal

WBC white blood cell
WCTU Women's Christian Temperance Union
WHI Women's Health Initiative
WIC women, infants, and children

Index

About the Contributors

Kathryn Rhodes Alden is Clinical Assistant Professor in the School of Nursing at the University of North Carolina at Chapel Hill. Her primary focus is education of undergraduate students in the areas of maternal-newborn nursing and women's health. She has authored chapters for maternity texts on endocrine disorders in pregnancy and has developed curricula for childbirth preparation classes on vaginal birth after caesarean. Her research interests include infant-feeding decision making and migraine headaches related to the reproductive cycle.

Linda A. Bernhard is Associate Professor of Nursing and Women's Studies at the Ohio State University, Columbus. She is a product of the Chicago School of Thought in Women's Health, University of Illinois at Chicago (PhD, 1986) and she has been a women's health educator, researcher, and activist for more than 15 years. She teaches courses including Promotion of Health in Adults, Women's Health Issues, and Politics of Women's Sexuality. Her primary research interests are hysterectomy and menopause. Her publications appear in *Nursing Research, Advances in Nursing Science, Journal of Obstetric, Gynecologic and Neonatal Nursing,* and *Health Care for Women International.* She is a member of the Board of Directors, International Council on Women's Health Issues.

Cheryl A. Cahill, RN, PhD, is the Amelia Peabody Professor of Research at the Massachusetts General Institute of Health Professions. She received her diploma in nursing from the St. Joseph's Hospital School of Nursing in Syracuse, New York. She holds a BSN from Boston College; an MN from the University of Washington, Seattle; and a PhD in nursing from the University of Michigan, Ann Arbor. She is a member of the Society for Menstrual Cycle Research; the Society for Neuroscience; and the American Nurses' Association, Council of Nurse Researchers. She is also a member of Sigma Theta Tau and Sigma Chi, the Scientific Research Society. She held positions at the University of Maryland, Baltimore; the University of Arizona, Tucson; and the University of Kansas Medical Center, Kansas City, before assuming her current position. She has published in *Nursing Research,* and *Journal of Clinical Endocrinology and Metabolism,* among others. Her research study, Psychobiological Correlates of Perimenstrual Symptoms, was funded by a grant from the National Institutes of Health, Center for Nursing Research (#NR01399).

Jacquelyn C. Campbell received her baccalaureate nursing degree from Duke University; her master's degree in community health nursing from Wright State University in Dayton, Ohio; and her doctorate in nursing from the University of Rochester, New York. Her clinical experience includes a variety of community health nursing positions in inner-city Dayton, including school nursing, community mental health, and childbirth education. She was at Wayne State University College of Nursing from 1980 to 1993. She is currently the Anna D. Wolf Endowed Professor at the Johns Hopkins University School of Nursing. Her awards include Fellowship in the American Academy of Nursing and in the Kellogg National Leadership Program and being Principle Investigator on two research grants on battering funded by the National Institutes of Health. She has authored and coauthored more than 20 articles and chapters, mainly about battered women and family violence. She is coauthor with Janice Humphreys of the recently published text *Nursing Care of Survivors of Family Violence* and coeditor of the 1992 book *Sanctions and Sanctuary: Cultural Perspectives on the Beating of Wives.* She also has been working with wife abuse shelters for the last 10 years, including leading support groups and being on the Board of Directors at My Sister's Place, one of the shelters in Detroit.

Sharon Deevey is a doctoral candidate at the Ohio State University College of Nursing and works part-time at Hospice at Riverside in Columbus, Ohio. She obtained a BSN from Case Western Reserve University in 1981 and a master's degree at Ohio State University. Her major contribution has been increasing the visibility of lesbian health issues in nursing. As an openly admitted lesbian nurse, she has published articles on health-seeking behaviors in lesbian women over the age of 50. Her articles have appeared in *Journal of Psychosocial Nursing, Journal of Gerontological Nursing,* and *Health Care of Women International.* Her dissertation research focuses on bereavement experiences in lesbian kinship networks in Ohio.

Margaret Dimond, RN, PhD, FAAN, is Professor in the Department of Physiological Nursing, School of Nursing, at the University of Washington, Seattle. She was formally Project Director for a Robert Wood Johnson foundation teaching nursing home and directed the University of Utah Gerontology Center. Her research, teaching, and clinical interests center on older adults, with a more focused interest on bereavement, loss, chronic illness, and the delivery of health care to the older adult population in the community and in long-term care institutions. She has been a regular reviewer for research proposals to the National Institutes of Health and has served also as an ad hoc reviewer for the British Columbia Health Care Research Foundation and the Medical Research Council of Canada. She chaired the American Nurses Foundation Research Committee from 1991 to 1992 and chaired the NINR Priority Expert Panel on Long Term Care for Older Adults. She has published widely, most recently in *Clinical Nursing Research, Oxford Textbook of Geriatric Medicine,* and *Journal of Gerontological Nursing.* She has provided consultation to individual researchers, schools of nursing, and long-term care facilities and has presented her research at national and international meetings.

Anne Hopkins Fishel, PhD, RN, CS, is Associate Professor at the University of North Carolina at Chapel Hill. She has over 25 years of teaching experience. She has received a university teaching award and was recognized in the *Carrington Quarterly* for excellence in teaching. She is certified by ANCC as a clinical specialist in adult psychiatric-mental health nursing. She has served as chair of the Board on Certification in Psychiatric Mental Health Nursing for ANCC as well as a member of the test development committee. She has practiced as a crisis counselor, psychiatric nursing consultant, outpatient individual and family therapist, and clinical case manager for families with emotionally disturbed children and youth. Recent clinical interests include family violence and healing touch therapy. Research interests include women's health and family relations—especially parenting after divorce and family violence. Most recently, she has studied nurse administration of as-needed psychotropic medications. She has made numerous presentations and published in journals such as *Journal of Divorce, Journal of Psychosocial Nursing, Health Care for Women*

International, Journal of Family Violence, and *Journal of Child and Adolescent Psychiatric Mental Health Nursing.*

Catherine Ingram Fogel is Associate Professor of Nursing at the University of North Carolina at Chapel Hill, a certified OB/GYN nurse practitioner, and a fellow of the American Academy of Nursing. She is an advocate for women's health care, especially care of socioeconomically disadvantaged women, such as women prisoners. She is considered an expert on the physical and mental health of incarcerated women, pregnant prisoners, and incarcerated mothers. She has conducted nine (six funded) research studies with disadvantaged women and has received paper and presentation awards for her clinical research. She has given numerous national and regional presentations about disadvantaged women and has published databased articles on women prisoners in nursing, social science, and lay journals. Her publications on clinical aspects of women's health have had a major impact on nursing practice. *Health Care of Women* (with Nancy Fugate Woods, 1981) received AJN and NLN Book of the Year Awards, and *Sexual Health Promotion* (with Diane Lauver, 1990) also won an AJN Book of the Year Award. She developed and continues to be the primary care provider in the first nurse-run clinic for poor women at risk for preterm labor in North Carolina. She also implemented one of the first prenatal classes offered at a maximum-security prison. As a result of her research on risk appraisal for preterm labor, the risk appraisal tool used at all North Carolina Health Department prenatal clinics was changed to more accurately identify women at risk for preterm births. Her clinical contributions were recognized by the 1993 AWHONN National Excellence in Practice Award. In 1994, she was elected to the National Academy of Nursing.

Catherine Garner is President of Mature Strategies, a consulting firm specializing in strategic planning and development of women's health program. She is also Clinical Assistant Professor in the School of Nursing at the University of North Carolina at Chapel Hill. Her background includes positions with Vanderbilt University; the University of Kansas School of Medicine, Wichita; and the Tennessee Department of Public Health. She also served as the corporate consultant in women's health at Hospital Corporation of America. She has a master's degree in nursing from Vanderbilt University and a master's degree in public administration from the University of Tennessee. She is a doctoral candidate in public health policy at the University of North Carolina at Chapel Hill and is certified as an OB-GYN nurse practitioner. She is a widely published author. She served as president of NAACOG, the National Association of Obstetric, Gynecologic and Neonatal Nurses, in 1992 and is a fellow in the American Academy of Nursing.

Betty Glenn Harris, RN-C, PhD, is Clinical Associate Professor in the School of Nursing at the University of North Carolina at Chapel Hill. She has over 25 years of experience with nursing education for undergraduate and graduate students, as well as for practicing nurses through continuing education courses. Her primary teaching emphasis is maternal-infant care, with particular emphasis on high-risk pregnancy, preparation of couples for parenthood, and general women's health. She is certified in in-patient obstetrics by the National Certification Council. Past research projects include the impact of pregnancy loss and the transition to parenthood of infertile couples; current research is focused on nursing support of breast-feeding women. A current clinical focus involves identifying and applying information about different cultures to maternal-infant nursing. She has authored and coauthored a number of articles and book chapters reflecting these interests.

Joellen Hawkins is Professor in the School of Nursing at Boston College and a practicing OB-GYN Nurse Practitioner. Her research focuses on women as consumers and providers of health care and currently includes examination of the development of advanced practice roles for nurses; the portrayals of women and of nurses in advertisements in medical and nursing journals; outcomes of nurse-managed models of prenatal care delivery; women's self-care during pregnancy; abnormal Pap smears, STDs, and contraception; and women's use of contraception. Her historical research focuses on nurses and nursing in Massachusetts, the evolution of school nursing, and biographical work on Edna Foley and Jane Hitchcock. Her most recent publication is *Protocols for Nurses in Gynecologic Settings and Advanced Practitioner: Current Practice Issues,* coauthored with nurse practitioner colleagues.

Kären Landenburger is Assistant Professor of Nursing at the University of Washington, Tacoma Campus. She received her PhD in nursing from the University of Washington, Seattle, and she completed her postdoctoral work in women's health at the same institution. Her area of expertise is community health nursing with an emphasis on women as a population at risk. Her current research and practice focus on violence against women. She is actively involved on a community and state level in educating health professionals about domestic violence as a social issue and about the needs of women who seek care. She has written journal articles on the abuse of women as a cumulative and interactive process and on therapeutic approaches for working with women who are in abusive relationships. She is a member of the Nursing Network on Violence Against Women and the Nursing Research Consortium on Violence and Abuse.

Carol J. Leppa, RN, PhD, is Assistant Professor in Nursing, RN Baccalaureate Program, at the University of Washington in Bothell. Her research interests include women as health care providers, the nature of nursing work in varied environments and long-term care in particular, and the nursing work environment in relation to patient outcomes. Her most recent funded research is a pilot study on measuring nursing work in long-term care. Her pedagogical interests include the following topic areas: women's health explored through scientific and lay literature, cultural pluralism in the curriculum, ethics in health care, and gender autobiography in the exploration of self in society.

Dona J. Lethbridge, PhD, RN, is Associate Professor and Research Facilitator at the College of Nursing at the University of Alabama in Huntsville. Her past research has been mainly in areas of women's health—contraceptive use, breast-feeding, and the experience of midlife. Her current work and interests relate to health behaviors among very poor women.

Lynne Porter Lewallen is Assistant Professor in the School of Nursing at the North Carolina Agricultural and Technical State University in Greensboro. She is also a doctoral candidate in the School of Nursing at the University of North Carolina at Chapel Hill. Her research interests include prenatal care, health promotion in pregnancy, and women's health. She is a member of the American Nurses Association, AWHONN, Sigma Theta Tau, and the Southern Nursing Research Society.

Deitra Leonard Lowdermilk, RNC, PhD, is a Clinical Professor in the School of Nursing, Department of Health of Women and Children, at the University of North Carolina at Chapel Hill. She has been in nursing education for 24 years while maintaining a limited clinical practice in women's health nursing. She has taught continuing education programs and made presentations on women's health topics at local, state, national, and international levels. She has authored numerous chapters in nursing texts, has published articles in refereed journals, and developed and published computer-assisted instructional programs in maternity nursing. She has been an associate editor for two nursing textbooks and is currently coauthor of a maternity nursing text. Her research interests include identifying effective educational interventions for facilitating breast-feeding, identifying cultural influences on maternity nursing care, and identifying effective teaching strategies for fostering critical thinking skills in nursing students. She is active in the Association for Women's Health, Obstetric, and Neonatal Nurses, serving as the North Carolina Section Vice Chair.

Peggy S. Matteson, PhD, RNC, is Assistant Professor in the College of Nursing at Northeastern University, Boston, Massachusetts, teaching graduate students primary care and developing clinical sites for a community partnership program funded by the Kellogg Foundation. Her research interests are in women's health with current projects investigating "Clinical Assessment of a Woman's Ability to Implement a Contraceptive Method" and "Commonalities Among Women Who Do Not Return for Care After Abnormal Pap Smears." Recent publications include "What Women Use and Why They Change Family Planning Methods," in *Health Care for Women International, 14*, "Facilitating the Nurse Practitioner's Research Role: Using a Microcomputer for Data Entry in Clinical Settings," in the *Journal of the American Academy of Nurse Practitioners* (with Joellen Hawkins), and *Advocating for Self-Factors Influencing Women's Patterns of Fertility Regulation.*

Ellen Sullivan Mitchell is Associate Professor at the University of Washington School of Nursing and is an affiliate with the Center for Women's Health Research. She earned a PhD in Nursing

Science at the University of Washington, Seattle. She is acting coordinator of the Women's Primary Care Nurse Practitioner program in the School of Nursing. She has also had a private practice for the past 17 years as a nurse practitioner, with a focus on the primary care of women as well as on menstrual cycle problems. Her research interests include symptom experiences related to the menstrual cycle and menstrual cycle changes. She is interested in promoting the integration of health, illness, and wellness into primary care practice.

Barbara Nettles-Carlson, RN, MPH, SpClN, CS, is Associate Professor and Coordinator of the Primary Care Advanced Practice Area, Department of Community and Mental Health, University of North Carolina at Chapel Hill. A certified family nurse practitioner, she maintains a faculty practice and serves as a clinical preceptor for nurse practitioner students in a general adult medicine clinic at the University of North Carolina Hospitals. Her most recent articles have appeared in *Hospital Topics, Journal of Continuing Education in Nursing, Tar Heel Nurse,* and *Journal of the American Academy of Nurse Practitioners.* Her research interests focus on early detection of breast cancer through breast self-examination, and her publications range from cancer prevention to faculty practice and professional issues. She is a member of Sigma Theta Tau, ANA, AWHHON, and APHA.

Janet Primomo is Assistant Professor at the University of Washington, Tacoma and a member of the Graduate Faculty. She received her Bachelor of Science in Nursing from Russell Sage College, Troy, New York, after which she served 4 years in the United States Navy Nurses Corps. She received her Masters of Nursing in Community Health and her Doctorate of Philosophy from the University of Washington, School of Nursing. She has coauthored articles on women with chronic illness, which have been published in *Research in Nursing and Health* and *Image: The Journal of Nursing Scholarship.* Her current research focuses on health policy and population-based care.

Bonnie Rogers is Associate Professor of Nursing and Public Health and Director of the Occupational Health Nursing Program at the University of North Carolina, School of Public Health, at Chapel Hill. She received her diploma in nursing from the Washington Hospital Center School of Nursing in Washington, DC; her baccalaureate in nursing from George Mason University, Fairfax, Virginia; and her master's degree in public health and doctorate in public health with a major in occupational health nursing from The Johns Hopkins University, Baltimore, Maryland. She holds a postgraduate certificate as an adult health clinical specialist and is certified in occupational health nursing and community health nursing. She was invited to study ethics as a visiting scholar at the Hastings Center in New York and was granted a NIOSH career award to study ethical issues in occupational health. In addition to the managerial, consultant, and educator/researcher positions she has held, she also practiced for many years as a public health nurse, occupational health nurse, and occupational health nurse practitioner. She has published numerous articles and book chapters and is the senior author of the book *Occupational Health Nursing Guidelines for Primary Clinical Conditions.* She is a strong advocate of occupational health nursing research, and her research interests focus primarily on hazards to health care workers, particularly nurses, and ethical issues in occupational health nursing. She serves on numerous editorial panels and as an ethics consultant.

Margarete Sandelowski, PhD, RN, FAAN, is Professor in the School of Nursing, Department of Women's and Children's Health, at the University of North Carolina at Chapel Hill. She has conducted research on various aspects of reproductive technology, including cesarean birth, conceptive technology, and technology for fetal diagnosis. She is currently exploring how couples construct and manage positive prenatal diagnoses. Her most recent publication is *With Child in Mind: Studies of the Personal Encounter With Infertility.*

Eleanor Smith Tabeek, PhD, CNM, is Coordinator of the Parent Child Nursing Program, Evening/Weekend Division at Lawrence Memorial Hospital School of Nursing, Meford, Massachussets. She is also Director of Natural Family Planning, Archdiocese of Boston.

Christine Vourakis, BSN, MN, DNSc, is Associate Professor in the Department of Nursing at Samuel Merritt College, Oakland, California. She is also a consultant for the California Board of Registered Nursing's Substance Abuse and

Mental Illness Diversion Program. She is certified in addictions nursing and is a member of the American Nurses Association Task Force on Drug Abuse. She has clinical and managerial experience in critical care, psychiatric, and substance abuse settings. She has published many articles and book chapters and is coeditor of *Substance Abuse: Pharmacologic, Developmental, and Clinical Perspectives* (1st ed.) with G. Bennett and D. S. Woolf. She is editor of *Perspectives on Addictions Nursing,* the official publication of the National Nurses Society on Addictions (NNSA). Her research interests include the pain management needs of chemically dependent patients in general hospital and primary care settings. She was recently invited by the National Institute on Drug Abuse to join an interdisciplinary team of pain and addition specialists in Washington, DC, to identify the research priorities for treatment of pain in addicts. Currently, she is a postdoctoral fellow in the Department of Psychosocial Nursing at the University of Washington.

Debbie Ward is Associate Professor in the Department of Community Health Care Systems at the School of Nursing, University of Washington, Seattle. Her bachelor's degree in government is from Oberlin College, her master's in nursing from Yale, and her PhD in health policy from Boston University. She started her work life in health care as a home health aide. She teaches health policy and politics to graduate and undergraduate students and is coordinator of the Primary Care Nurse Practitioners programs in family, adult/geriatric, women's, and pediatric practice. Her research interests include public health policy and a variety of women's health issues, including low-paid and unpaid caregiving by women. Her most recent publications have appeared in *Second Opinion, Socialist Review, Holistic Nursing,* and *Western Journal of Nursing Research.*

Linda Wheeler is Associate Professor at Oregon Health Sciences University in Portland. She teaches in the school's Nurse-Midwifery Education Program and practices full-scope nurse-midwifery. She is fascinated by the uniqueness of individuals. This led to her interest in how teachers can adapt their teaching styles to facilitate student learning and how childbirth educators can adapt their classes to take advantage of the personality types and personal needs of expectant parents. Her article, "Teaching Strategies for Preceptors of Beginning Intrapartal Students," is upcoming in the *Journal of Nurse-Midwifery.*

Nancy Fugate Woods received a bachelor of science degree in nursing from the University of Wisconsin-Eau Claire in 1969, a master's degree in nursing from the University of Washington in 1969, and a PhD in epidemiology from the University of North Carolina at Chapel Hill in 1978. Since the mid-1970s, she has provided leadership in the development of women's health as a field of study in nursing science. Her early research focused on the relationship of women's social environments and their health, emphasizing the consequences of women's multiple roles and social structural supports for health. Since the late 1970s, she has led several large research projects focusing on women's perimenstrual symptom experiences. With her collaborators at Duke University and the University of Washington, she conducted the first prevalence study of perimenstrual symptoms in American women. Her subsequent research has focused on women's social environments, physiologic dimensions of stress response, and ovarian hormones in the etiology of menstrual cycle symptoms. In collaboration with colleagues at the University of Washington, she established the Center for Women's Health Research, focusing on women's health across the life span. Her current research focuses on midlife women, their health, and their health-seeking behavior patterns. She has been active in professional organizations, having served as president of the American Academy of Nursing and the Society for Menstrual Cycle Research and was a member of the National Advisory Council on Nursing Research for the National Center for Nursing Research, National Institutes of Health, and the Women's Health Task Force of the National Institutes of Health. She recently received the American Nursing Foundation Distinguished Contribution to Nursing Research Award and was elected to the Institute of Medicine, National Academy of Sciences.

Bonnie Worthington-Roberts is Professor of Nutritional Sciences/Epidemiology at the University of Washington, Seattle. Her area of interest is maternal and child nutrition; her textbook, *Nutrition in Pregnancy and Lactation,* is in its fifth edition. She has been extensively involved in lecturing throughout North America on issues related to diet and nutrition as they affect reproduction.